Psychiatric-Mental Health Nursing

Adaptation and Growth

Barbara Schoen Johnson
Ph.D., R.N., C.S.

Coordinator/Instructor
Nursing
El Centro College
Brookhaven College Satellite
Dallas, Texas

With 37 contributors

Psychiatric-Mental Health Nursing

Adaptation and Growth

2ND EDITION

J.B. Lippincott Company

Philadelphia   London   Mexico City   New York   St. Louis   São Paulo   Sydney

Sponsoring Editor: Nancy Mullins
Coordinating Editorial Assistant: Ellen Campbell
Art Director: Susan Blaker
Cover Designer: Miriam Recio
Interior Illustrations: Soheila V. Sanavi
Compositor: Circle Graphics
Printer/Binder: The Murray Printing Company

Second Edition

5   6   4

Library of Congress Cataloging-in-Publication Data

Psychiatric-mental health nursing : adaptation and growth.

  Includes bibliographies and index.
  1. Psychiatric nursing.   I. Johnson,
Barbara Schoen.
RC440.P737   1989   610.73′68   88-13903
ISBN 0-397-54688-2

Any procedure or practice described in this book should be applied
by the health-care practitioner under appropriate supervision in
accordance with professional standards of care used with regard to
the unique circumstances that apply in each practice situation. Care
has been taken to confirm the accuracy of information presented
and to describe generally accepted practices. However, the authors,
editors and publisher cannot accept any responsibility for errors or
omissions or for consequences from application of the information
in this book and make no warranty, express or implied, with respect
to the contents of the book.

Every effort has been made to ensure drug selections and dosages
are in accordance with current recommendations and practice. Because of ongoing research, changes in government regulations and
the constant flow of information on drug therapy, reactions and
interactions, the reader is cautioned to check the package insert for
each drug for indications, dosages, warnings and precautions, particularly if the drug is new or infrequently used.

to Barry

Contributors

Cheryl Lindamood Anderson, M.N., PH.D., R.N.
President
Educational Resources and Services, Inc.
Dallas, Texas
Lecturer
College of Nursing
Texas Woman's University
Dallas, Texas

Deborah Jackson Antai-Otong, M.S., R.N., C.S.
Psychiatric Clinical Nurse Specialist
Psychiatric Triage Unit
Dallas Veterans' Administration Medical Center
Dallas, Texas

Virginia Trotter Betts, M.S.N., J.D., R.N.
Associate Professor, Psychiatric-Mental Health Nursing
School of Nursing
Vanderbilt University
Nashville, Tennessee
Robert Wood Johnson Health Policy Fellow, 1987–1988

Patriciann Furnari Brady, M.A., M.S., R.N.
Assistant Professor, Department of Nursing
Mount Marty College
Yankton, South Dakota

Patricia Flatley Brennan, PH.D., R.N.
Assistant Professor of Nursing and Systems Engineering
Frances Payne Bolton School of Nursing
Case Western Reserve University
Cleveland, Ohio

Sharon Byers, M.S.N., R.N., C.S.
Nurse Coordinator, Adolescent Unit
Vanderbilt Child and Adolescent Psychiatric Hospital
Nashville, Tennessee

Sandra Carter Chandler, M.S., R.N.
Instructor, Nursing
El Centro College
Dallas, Texas

Barbara G. Tunley Crenshaw, M.S., R.N.
Professor, Department of Nursing
Front Range Community College
Westminster, Colorado

Joy Randolph Davidson, M.S.N., R.N.
Instructor, Nursing
El Centro College
Dallas, Texas

Susan D. Decker, PH.D., R.N.
Associate Professor of Nursing
University of Portland
Portland, Oregon

Cheryl Steudtner Detwiler, M.S.N., R.N.
Coordinator of Research and Evaluation/Instructor,
  Nursing
El Centro College
Brookhaven College Satellite
Dallas, Texas

M. Suzanne Doscher, M.S., R.N.
Associate Professor
College of Nursing
Medical University of South Carolina
Charleston, South Carolina

Peggy J. Drapo, PH.D., R.N.
Professor
College of Nursing
Texas Woman's University
Denton, Texas

Sally Francis, M.S., M.A.
Director, Child Life—Child Development Department
Children's Medical Center of Dallas
Assistant Professor of Clinical Pediatrics
Southwestern Medical Center
Dallas, Texas

Judith A. Greene, PH.D., R.N., C.S.
Nursing Coordinator
Westcott Center for Alcohol and Drug Abuse and
    Psychiatric Treatment
Hamilton Medical Center
Dalton, Georgia

Christina R. Hogarth, M.S., R.N., C.S.
Consultant
Mental Health Program Development
Dayton, Ohio

Mary Huggins, M.A., R.N.
Program Specialist, Division of Mental Health
Hennepin County
Minneapolis, Minnesota

Marilyn Jaffe-Ruiz, ED.D., R.N., C.S.
Dean and Professor
Lienhard School of Nursing
Pace University
New York, New York

Susan Kah, M.N., ED.D., R.N.
Professor and Chairperson
Special Programs in Nursing
Miami-Dade Community College
Miami, Florida

Nina A. Klebanoff, M.S.N., R.N., C.S.
Psychosocial Clinical Specialist
Dallas, Texas

Patricia Murphey Lucas, M.S., R.N.
Formerly Instructor, Nursing
El Centro College
Dallas, Texas

Maureen McCausland, D.N.SC., R.N.
Associate Vice President of Nursing
Beth Israel Hospital
Boston, Massachusetts

James McColgan, Jr., M.S., PH.D. CAND., R.N.
Major, U.S. Army Nurse Corps
Hanscom Air Force Base
Bedford, Massachusetts

Mary Snyder McElvain, M.S., R.N., C.S.
Nursing Coordinator/Education
West Valley Camelback Hospital
Glendale, Arizona

Patricia N. Mahon, PH.D., R.N.
Psychotherapist, Private Practice
Psychologist, Mental Health Clinic
Consultant, Nursing Home Care Unit
Bonham Veterans' Administration Medical Center
Bonham, Texas

Bruce Payne Mericle, M.S., R.N.
Assistant Professor of Nursing
Trenton State College
Trenton, New Jersey

Cynthia Ann Pastorino, M.S.N., R.N., O.N.C.
Clinical Nurse Specialist, Orthopaedics
Methodist Medical Center
Dallas, Texas
Specialist, School of Nursing
University of Texas at Arlington
Arlington, Texas

Katherine Pritchett, M.S., R.N.
Curriculum Coordinator/Instructor, Nursing
El Centro College
Dallas, Texas

Juliann Casey Reakes, ED.D., R.N., C.S., L.P.C.
Professor of Nursing
Chair, Baccalaureate Program
Abilene Intercollegiate School of Nursing
Abilene, Texas

S. Robin Shanks, M.S.N., J.D., R.N.
Adult Program Coordinator
Oak Valley Psychiatric Unit
Huntsville Hospital
Huntsville, Alabama

Margie N. Slaughter, M.S., R.N.
Dean, Health Occupations
Central Florida Community College
Ocala, Florida

Diane M. Snow, M.S.N., PH.D. CAND., R.N.
Specialist, School of Nursing
University of Texas at Arlington
Arlington, Texas

Mary Anne Sweeney, PH.D., R.N.
Dean for Research/Professor
School of Nursing
University of Texas Medical Branch at Galveston
Galveston, Texas

Barbara A. Thurston, M.S., R.N.
Associate Professor, Department of Nursing
New Hampshire Technical Institute
Concord, New Hampshire

Anne Warner Toothaker, B.S.N., R.N.
Staff Nurse
The Veterans' Administration Medical Center
Boise, Idaho

Sylvia M. Anderson Whiting, PH.D. CAND., R.N., C.S.
Director
The New Hope—D. Seth Mason Adolescent Residential
  Treatment Center
Charleston, South Carolina

Rhea P. Williams, PH.D., R.N.
Professor of Nursing
Azusa Pacific University
Azusa, California

Preface

As I was preparing this second edition of our textbook, *Psychiatric-Mental Health Nursing: Adaptation and Growth,* my son, then in fourth grade (he was barely out of toddlerhood when I first launched the idea of writing a book . . .), was studying adaptations in plants and animals in science. What a marvelous concept, I again thought, the idea of an organism becoming better fitted to survive and do well in its environment.

Isn't that what we are about, becoming increasingly skilled at surviving in, adjusting to, mastering, and even creating our internal and external environment? And isn't that what psychiatric-mental health nursing aims to provide for clients, communities, and populations? Aside from the wonderful understanding of adaptation which Selye has given us, we can gaze at the simple biological meaning of the term and find applications in the process of professional nursing.

This is also a book about growth. Growth is what happens when an individual recovers from a rape, a depression, an addiction. Perhaps the person has lowered his or her anxiety from a destructive, to a manageable and productive level. Perhaps the family has begun to change their former patterns of discounting, demeaning communication. Growth results in the understanding and empathy of a person and family who have resolved problems, faced crises, accepted challenges, and become, as Sally Francis reminds us in the words of Hemingway, "stronger in the broken places."

The text now has forty-eight chapters. Every chapter has been revised; six chapters are new. These new chapters cover the content of eating disorders, anxiety disorders, nursing theory, and the crisis of perinatal loss and depression. The community mental health chapter has been expanded into a community mental health section, with chapters on the foundational material, psychosocial home care, and community support and rehabilitation.

The preparation of the second edition of *Psychiatric-Mental Health Nursing: Adaptation and*

Growth has built on the goals and strengths of the first edition, namely its accuracy and up-to-dateness of information, clarity of writing, and attention to affective learning. And to attain these objectives, I turned to the thirty-seven nurse-writers, the experts in psychiatric-mental health nursing, and asked them to be comprehensive yet concise, factual yet inspiring, thorough yet exact.

Once again they delivered brilliantly. Judith Greene, for example, presents the newest material on anxiety disorders, including post-traumatic stress disorder and panic state, and personality disorders and reinforces with nursing care plans and case studies. Mary Huggins addresses the issues of caring for clients with long-term mental disorder and homelessness and appropriate program development for clients in the community in her chapter, Community Support and Rehabilitation. Susan Decker updates the reader on the latest information in diagnosing and treating clients with eating disorders. The newest information about the specialties within psychiatric nursing, child and adolescent, mental retardation, and geropsychiatry, are discussed by Mary McElvain, Peggy Drapo, and Pat Brady. Pattie Lucas and Kathy Pritchett bring to our awareness and emotions the experience of perinatal loss and depression.

The addition of the chapter, Nursing Theory and Psychiatric-Mental Health Nursing Practice, strengthens the theoretical underpinnings of this edition. Diane Snow has revised the Nursing Diagnosis chapter and demonstrated mental health nursing applications of the latest work of both NANDA and ANA's Task Force on the Phenomena of Concern to Psychiatric Nursing. The most current material in the field of psychiatric-mental health nursing has been added to every section of the book such as the inclusion of cognitive therapy in the chapter, Behavioral Approaches, the newest medications and their uses in Psychopharmacology, the ever-surfacing data on the neurobiological aspects of mental disorders, the topic of AIDS in the Sexuality and Sexual Concerns and Death and Dying chapters, latest research on addictions in Substance Abuse: the Drug Dependencies, and help for families with a member with Alzheimer's Disease in the chapter, Organic Mental Disorder.

The clarity and conciseness which marked the first edition are purposefully repeated in this edition. In fact, of the frequent praises which the first edition brought to the authors and editor, many of those focused on the book's clarity and directness, and its ability to lead readers to understand the difficult, complex material in a manner relatively free of confusing psychiatric jargon. The text's contributors carefully chose their words, descriptions, and examples to paint a precise, vivid picture for the reader. We know, for example, that although all of us know what it feels like to be depressed or "blue," we do not all know what it is like to be so intensely depressed that arising in the morning to face another day appears an insurmountable task. This was one of our tasks as authors—to make the subject matter come alive for the reader.

And, affectively, how can we make this experience come alive for the reader? First of all, we want the reader to become aware of and appreciate what is entailed in the day-to-day existence of a client with schizophrenia, an addiction to substances or food, a personality disorder, agoraphobia, a panic level of anxiety, etc., and how the client's disorder affects his or her family, neighborhood, and community. In addition, the reader must recognize that the affective realm of nursing—self-understanding, acceptance, trust, hope, and respect for human dignity—is a critical medium for healing and often the beginnings of change in the client and family's life.

Many experts add their own special knowledge in the form of an insert within chapters. Herbert Barr poignantly recounts his family's view of living with, and working toward better care of, a mentally ill member; he explains how the Alliance for the Mentally Ill is trying to improve the quality of mental health services for all families. Nancy Kupper describes the current public education campaign of the National Institute of Mental Health, D/ART (Depression/Awareness, Recognition, and Treatment), and its goals for all citizens. Karen Perkins provides an algorithm for the diagnosis and treatment of panic states. These and other fascinating inserts deepen the textual material and bring it to a new level of meaningfulness for the reader.

The Career Profiles, brief excerpts of actual psychiatric-mental health nurses telling about their daily work, are again featured. This was a popular part of the first edition; readers told me that they appreciated hearing, in first-person accounts, the various paths that psychiatric-mental health nursing and nurses had taken.

This book, like its predecessor, is a story of people, real people who also happen to be clients. They are neither "clinical cases" nor creatures from another world. They are more like us than not. They are people who, in the words of Dr. Suzanne Lego in the foreword to the first edition, "might be our mother, brother, friend, or lover. We are drawn," she continues, "into the existential world of the clients and their families and are helped to understand their feelings and actions. In turn, we learn about ourselves."

As psychiatric-mental health nurses, it is essential that we learn as much about ourselves as possible. Our self-awareness and understanding contribute powerfully to the degree of assistance we can offer to others. This, after all, is a book about nursing, that kind of aid, support, and intervention offered by educated and experienced individuals to others in need of those services to reach or regain health, wellness, and independence.

Some of the noteworthy features of the text include:

attention to the cultural aspects of health and disorder;

a humanistic approach to the care of any individual, family, community;

strong theoretical bases for discussions of mental health, disorder, and treatment;

a nursing process orientation, with nursing assessment and diagnosis guidelines, integrated throughout the text;

elaboration of the theoretical discussions of disorder with examples of nursing care plans, case studies, therapeutic dialogues, historical perspectives, and associated points of interest;

a focus on the value of the nurse's contribution as a collaborator with other members of the mental health team;

an emphasis on the affective, as well as the cognitive and behavioral, realms of psychiatric-mental health nursing practice;

the comprehensiveness of the content from crisis material and situations, to applications to the medical/surgical/pediatric/obstetric patient, to the developmental issues of aging and sexuality, to the organic mental disorders and psychophysiologic disorders, to the mild to severe emotional problems of clients at all ages; and,

an eclectic approach to the therapeutic possibilities for any client.

As this edition of *Psychiatric-Mental Health Nursing: Adaptation and Growth* goes to print, I am content that we have maintained and furthered the quality of writing, content, meaning, and usefulness begun in the first edition. I am proud of the result and hope that it will continue to interest and inspire readers to explore the challenges of psychiatric-mental health nursing.

Barbara Schoen Johnson, Ph.D., R.N., C.S.

Preface to the First Edition

When I undertook to write this textbook of psychiatric-mental health nursing, I had several goals in mind. First, I wanted to compile accurate, comprehensive, and up-to-date material that would stimulate the reader to seek out more information and experience in this area of nursing. Second, I wanted to produce good-quality writing that would not only communicate in a clear, concise, and interesting manner, but also touch the reader's emotions as well as his thinking processes. Third, I wanted to expose the reader to some exciting applications of psychiatric-mental health nursing concepts not ordinarily found within the realm of the traditional textbook.

As *Psychiatric-Mental Health Nursing: Adaptation and Growth* becomes a reality, I feel confident that I have achieved what I set out to do. The outcome of striving toward those three goals is contained within these pages.

To produce a textbook with current, comprehensive, and factual content, I turned to the 29 nurse practitioners, educators, and researchers who became the book's contributing authors. Each nurse-writer had specific tasks to accomplish—to research the topic of the chapter thoroughly, gather both the classic and the newest material, and put the chapter together in a comprehensive and logical manner.

The results, I believe, are significant. Patricia Brennan's chapter on suicide also addresses the needs of the survivor-victims; her chapter on trends in psychiatric-mental health care examines the issue of the impaired nurse and the approaches being considered to move beyond punishment to rehabilitation. Christina Hogarth's chapter on families and family therapy includes the topic of children of divorce. Virginia Betts' and Robin Shanks' discussion of least restrictive treatment environment provides clear guidelines to this legal implication of psychiatric nursing. Judith Greene's chapter on milieu therapy explains why and how the milieu benefits psychiatric clients.

These, of course, are just a few examples of the thought-provoking content that the contributing authors have brought to this new book.

My second goal focused on the affective domain. Nursing, after all, is more than an aggregate of cognitive and psychomotor learnings. Psychiatric-mental health nursing requires the integration into one's professional repertoire of certain affective behaviors such as self-awareness, objectivity, and acceptance of the other. The use of the self as a therapeutic instrument calls on a person's ability to employ honesty, openness, trustworthiness, and caring within a professional nursing role.

The writing in *Psychiatric-Mental Health Nursing* has been designed to impact the reader's emotions as well as his understanding and knowledge. Discussing individual therapy, Joy Davidson writes, "People hope for more happiness and less pain. They fear change in themselves and in the people they love." In her chapter on mood disorders, Susan Kah describes depression as a "lonely, loveless, and hopeless state." These and similar examples seek to speak to the reader directly, meaningfully, and without the interference of confusing jargon.

There are also personal accounts, the recounting of unique experiences generously shared by the authors. In the chapter on family violence, a member of Parents Anonymous describes the abuse of her own children and her present work, as a sponsor of other abusing parents, to prevent child abuse. In the chapter on death and dying, Fela Alfaro relates her personal experiences with death, from her earliest awareness that her mother died giving birth to her to her more recent encounters, as an adult, with the deaths of family members and friends. Explaining the need of the rape victim to be believed, Sally Francis uses the words of a victim to make the point: "A part of me was relieved when the police came—that I looked so bad, that there was blood, that the door had been broken open, the house was torn up, and there were fingerprints. 'There couldn't be any doubt that something awful had happened to me."

The third goal, that of including in this work a variety of topics not ordinarily found in psychiatric-mental health nursing textbooks, warrants the reader's attention. Besides the usual topics included in a psychiatric nursing book, *Psychiatric-Mental Health Nursing* has a section on the emotional aspects of medical care—trauma, surgery, and critical care, the physically ill or handicapped child, women's health issues of pregnancy, childbearing, mastectomy, and hysterectomy, and death and dying. There is also a section on crisis situations, with chapters on crisis theory and intervention, rape, suicide, and abuse. Other content that is not ordinarily found in psychiatric-mental health nursing textbooks includes the topics of mental retardation, organic mental disorder, sociocultural aspects of nursing care, mental health of the aging, trends in psychiatric-mental health care, nursing research, and career profiles of psychiatric-mental health nurses.

Selye's stress/adaptation theory forms the conceptual framework for this book. According to this theory, stress is an ever-present human state, and any biophysical or psychosocial factor causes stress to a human being. These stressors, or factors requiring a response or change in the individual, are perceived in various ways by different individuals. A person's perception of the stressor influences his manner of coping with it. Adaptation, says Selye, is the end-state of adjusting to the changes in a person's internal or external environment.

This book is also about growth—using one's problems or crises to grow to higher levels of mental health and toward self-awareness and empathy.

Nursing process is a strong emphasis that is integrated throughout *Psychiatric-Mental Health Nursing*. Rather than focusing on the client's mental disorder, its etiology, symptoms, and medical treatment, with nursing interventions tucked in, almost as an afterthought, at the end of each discussion, this book is a book about *nursing*, first and foremost. *Psychiatric-Mental Health Nursing* demonstrates the application of the nursing process in a wide variety of client situations.

Several noteworthy features of the book include

a clear, concise manner of presentation;

an emphasis on nursing process integrated throughout the text;

nursing assessment and nursing diagnosis guidelines;

attention to the guiding principles of psychiatric-mental health nursing and the specific nursing actions derived from those principles;

a theoretical framework built on stress and adaptation;

a humanistic approach that catches up the whole person;

adherence to the current DSM-III criteria of mental disorders;

attention to the affective realm—the development of empathic responses, insight, respect for human dignity, and growth through experiential exercises;

the exemplification of behavioral dysfunctions and their theoretical bases through clinical case studies, nurse-client dialogues and interactions, and a view of the nursing process at work through nursing care plans;

a focus on self-awareness in the nurse, that is, the nurse as a very human being, a person in touch with his or her own feelings;

an emphasis on cross-cultural aspects of psychiatric-mental health nursing;

reinforcement of the nurse's significance and role in the collaborative efforts of the entire mental health team; and

an eclectic approach to the therapeutic possibilities for any client.

It has been a joyful experience to put together *Psychiatric-Mental Health Nursing: Adaptation and Growth*. I believe that it will help open up for the reader the exciting world of psychiatric-mental health nursing. That was, and is, my most important goal.

Barbara Schoen Johnson, R.N., M.S.

Acknowledgments

There arrives in any big project (the writing of a book, the painting of a picture, the running of a race) that dreaded moment when you must stop and acknowledge the many people who helped you on your way. This is, for me, the most difficult part of writing a book. There are so many to thank . . . where do I start?

Perhaps I should first thank the dear, generous friends—the ones who "keep smiling, keeping shining"—who day in and day out encourage, support, and accept me. And so I thank you, Barbara Burke, Juanita Zapata Flint, Sondra George Flemming, Felicitas "Fela" Alfaro, Sandy Chandler, Dana Stahl, Marjorie Schuchat, Jane Weil, Sue McLelland, Cheryl Detwiler, Susan Wegman, Gayle Varnell, Dayna Davidson, Betty Nelson, Diana Reding, Beth Perdue, Carol Hardin, Debi Trammell, Margie Slaughter, Pattie Murphey Lucas, Kathy Pritchett, Elizabeth Winslow, Nancy Breed, Mandie Turner, Sharon Sonkin, and the others I may have forgotten here. My life would be very different, and not terribly enticing, without the gifts you constantly bring me.

I also express appreciation to my mentors whose intervention in my life has led me to a greater love and gratitude for my work. And so I thank you, Helen Czarnecki, Dolores Cleveland, Catherine Thayer, Marianne Mosley, Pat Mahon, and Helen Bush.

I am grateful that I work in growth-producing environments and for that I acknowledge the efforts of my Dean, Kay Kiefer Eggleston, and Associate Dean, Carol Lipin Speyerer, El Centro College, and Larry Darlage, Vice President of Instruction, Brookhaven College.

I have been fortunate to work with some of the best of Lippincott's Nursing Division. I thank Nancy Mullins, Senior Editor, for maintaining her faith in my ability, and Ellen Campbell, Editorial Assistant, for keeping up with every detail involved in these 900 pages and doing it all with the greatest of humor and grace. I also thank Annette Hall, Vice-President of Editing, Design, and Production, who has, with care and conscientiousness, brought this book from manuscript pages to its production.

I thank Ginny Kimsey, Director of Library Services of Texas Woman's University in Dallas, for designing and running endless numbers of computer searches so that every author could have access to the latest research and writings available to augment her or his chapter content.

And then there are my neighbors, Bethann and Darwin Scratchard, Jeannine and Doug Robinson, and Linda and Mark Prewitt, who think they should be mentioned. And I imagine they should be recognized if computer repair and assistance, emotional support, cheerful faces, and even temperaments count for anything.

What about my students who help me look at events and behaviors in new ways, through the eyes of the uninitiated? It is for you that I have tried to write in clear, precise words.

And what about the clients who teach me about the labyrinth of schizophrenic thought? the depths of inertia and depression? the fearful uncertainties of suicide attempts? the unwielding chain of dependencies? I hope that the authors and I have accurately represented the realities of disturbance and distress, and that these pages will lead other nurses to create new and better ways to provide psychiatric-mental health nursing to those in need.

Now, to the toughest part of all, acknowledging my family.

I thank my parents, Marie and Roy Schoen, for their undiminishing belief in me and their wholehearted support of anything I try.

I thank my sisters, brother, brothers- and sisters-in-law, Roberta and Fred Ravagnani, Mary Ellen and Don Makkos, Jeff Schoen, Bonnie and Denny Balcer, and Dee and Bryan Johnson, for their continuing kindnesses and encouragement over the years.

My children, Eric and Jessica Schoen Johnson, are the ones who give meaning to my life. They bring me their wonder, love, delight, and discoveries. I thank them for being the most wonderful children I could ever want to share my life.

And what do I say about my husband, Barry, the person who, for the past twenty years, has shared my best and worst moments—and the millions of moments in between. The man who first told me he thought I could return to college and take English 101? The man who does it all—children, work, home—and does it all so well and happily, so that I can reach my dreams? Your "slow and steady fire" has sustained me, enriched me, shaped me, and helped me to grow. I thank you and love you.

Contents

13 Individual Psychotherapy 183
Joy Randolph Davidson

14 Groups and Group Therapy 199
Barbara G. Tunley Crenshaw

15 Families and Family Therapy 222
Christina R. Hogarth

16 Behavioral Approaches 248
Juliann Casey Reakes

17 Psychopharmacology   268

Deborah Jackson Antai-Otong

IV DEVELOPMENTAL ISSUES IN PSYCHIATRIC-MENTAL HEALTH NURSING

18 Development of the Person   297

Sylvia M. Anderson Whiting
Deborah Jackson Antai-Otong

19 Sexuality and Sexual Concerns   311

Sharon Byers

24 Retreat from Reality: The Schizophrenic Disorders 415

Barbara Schoen Johnson

25 Suspicious, Hostile, and Aggressive Behavior: The Delusional and Acting-Out Disorders 440

Mary Snyder McElvain

26 Substance Abuse: The Drug Dependencies 464

Barbara A. Thurston

31   Organic Mental Disorders   603

Cheryl Steudtner Detwiler

32   Psychophysiologic Disorders   622

M. Suzanne Doscher

VII   CRISIS

33   Crisis Theory and Intervention   641

Sandra Carter Chandler

IX MENTAL HEALTH INTERVENTION WITH THE MEDICAL PATIENT

41 Trauma, Surgery, and Critical Care 777
Cynthia Ann Pastorino

42 The Child of Risk: Illness, Disability, and Hospitalization 794
Sally Francis

43 Issues in Women's Health Care 816
Rhea P. Williams

PART 1

Foundations of Psychiatric–Mental Health Nursing

1 Introduction to Psychiatric–Mental Health Nursing

Barbara Schoen Johnson

I do not know what causes insanity or what can cure it, and I don't really believe that anyone else knows either. I do not even think that it is a constant condition, much less an "illness," or that the crazy people live over there on that side of the line, and the rest of us over here. I think that madness is part of all of us, all the time, that it comes and goes, waxes and wanes....I myself don't think that madness can be fully understood, only experienced—in oneself or in one's friends or in the people one sees crumbling at the office or on the streets.

Otto Friedrich,
Going Crazy: An Inquiry
into Madness in Our Time,
1976

Chapter Preview

This chapter introduces the reader to the field of psychiatric–mental health nursing. Often mystifying or frightening to the novice, psychiatric–mental health nursing draws upon the knowledge bases of mental health and nursing to create an integrated and unique discipline. The principles of psychiatric–mental health nursing permeate all areas of nursing practice, such as helping new parents recognize and respond to the needs of their infant, calming the fears of a hospitalized child, talking with an adult facing surgery, or intervening in a disturbed family system.

This chapter examines mental health and mental disorder, the present and past roles of psychiatric–mental health nursing, and the application of the nursing process to client problems. It explores nurses' and clients' views of each other, their feelings, reactions, expectations, and attitudes and values regarding mental health. The individual's responses to stress and his use of coping mechanisms are also discussed.

The importance of nurses' taking care of themselves and attending to their own needs is emphasized throughout the chapter. Measures such as ventilation to understanding friends or colleagues, attention to one's physical health through diet and exercise, and involvement in absorbing hobbies or activities are explored as concrete ways to reduce stress and burnout and to promote optimal effectiveness in psychiatric–mental health nursing.

Learning Objectives

On completion of this chapter, you should be able to accomplish the following:

1. discuss the parameters of mental health and mental illness
2. identify the challenges facing mental health care, including prevention of mental disorder and care of the person with long-term mental illness
3. differentiate between stress and distress
4. explain the three stages of the General Adaptation Syndrome
5. give examples of coping mechanisms
   denial
   regression
   displacement
   projection
   reaction formation
   repression
   suppression
   identification
   rationalization
   fantasy
   intellectualization
6. describe the roles of psychiatric–mental health nurses
7. compare the views and perceptions of psychiatric nurses and clients
8. discuss nurses' reactions to clients exhibiting disturbed behavior
9. identify measures to prevent job stress and burnout in psychiatric–mental health nursing
10. describe the steps of the nursing process

Mental Health and Mental Illness

The states of health and illness are defined according to the values of a society. Generally, when a person's behavior is adaptive to his environment, we say that he is healthy, and when his behavior is maladaptive, we say that he is ill. Culture greatly influences these determinations about health and illness. Behavior that is acceptable in one cultural group may or may not be tolerated in another group. (For a fuller description of cultural influences on mental health and illness, see Chap. 6, "Sociocultural Aspects of Care.")

Mental Health

The World Health Organization defines health as "a state of complete physical, mental and social well-being, not merely the absence of disease or infirmity." The significance of this definition is that it emphasizes the positive—a state of well-being—and does not focus on the lack of illness, disease, or disorder.

In this aforementioned state of emotional well-being, or *mental health,* the person functions comfortably within his society and is satisfied with himself and his achievements.[15]

We say that someone is mentally healthy when we observe in the person a balance between the integrated body, mind, and spirit and the environment.[48] The fact is, though, that no generally accepted definition of mental health exists. Rather, we infer the presence or absence of mental health from an individual's behavior.

Mental health implies mastery in the areas of life involving love, work, and play. Some definitions of mental health also include the criterion of happiness as an important aspect.

Some of the components of mental health follow:

Self-governance. The person demonstrates autonomy, a sense of detachment, independence, and a tendency to look within for guiding values and rules to live by. He acts independently, dependently, or interdependently as the need arises, without permanently losing his independence.

Growth orientation. The person is willing to depart from the status quo, or equilibrium, to progress toward self-realization, androgyny, and maximization of his capacities.

Tolerance of uncertainty. The person faces the uncertainty of living and the certainty of death by means of faith and hope.

Self-esteem. The person's self-esteem is built on self-knowledge and awareness of his talents, abilities, and limitations.

Mastery of the environment. The person is effective, capable, competent, and creative in dealing with and influencing his environment.

Reality orientation. The person distinguishes fact from fantasy, the real world from a dream world, and acts accordingly.

Stress management. The person experiences appropriate depression, anxiety, and so forth in daily life and can tolerate high levels of stress, knowing that the feeling is not going to last forever. He is flexible and can experience failure without berating himself. Usually he copes with crises without needing help beyond the support of family and friends.

Evidence of mental health is usually seen in a person's meaningful work, enjoyment of life, humor, ability to benefit from rest and sleep, optimism, spontaneity, satisfying relationships with others, ability to work well alone and with others, sound judgments and decisions, acceptance of responsibility for actions, ability to give and receive, behavior that is generally accepted by the group, and direct expression of emotions, including strong feelings. Variables affecting mental health may be biological, sociocultural, or psychological. *Biological factors* are prenatal and perinatal influences, physical health, neuroanatomy, and physiology. *Sociocultural factors* are family stability, child-rearing patterns, economic level, housing, membership in a minority that may experience the effects of prejudice or inadequate health resources, religious influences, and values. *Psychological factors* are parent- and sibling-infant/child interactions, intelligence quotient (IQ), self-concept, skills, talents, creativity, and emotional developmental level.[7, 32, 37, 43, 48]

Freedoms of the Mentally Healthy

Five "freedoms" that mentally healthy people demonstrate, according to Satir and associates, are as follows:

1. The freedom to see and hear what is here instead of what should be, was, or will be
2. The freedom to say what one feels and thinks, instead of what one should say
3. The freedom to feel what one feels, instead of what one ought to feel
4. The freedom to ask for what one wants, instead of always waiting for permission
5. The freedom to take risks in one's own behalf, instead of choosing to be only "secure" and not rocking the boat[39]

Androgyny in Mentally Healthy Persons

Androgyny is the interaction and balance of "feminine" and "masculine" characteristics in an individual. Sex-role stereotypes, such as "Men should be strong and not express their feelings" or "It's OK for women to cry and ask for help," are often inflexible and limit a person's adaptive and interpersonal effectiveness. Androgyny, on the other hand, allows an individual to adapt his or her behavior according to different situations or needs.

As we begin to realize that roles assigned on the basis of gender only are restricting, many people are challenging these old roles and substituting new roles according to individual inherent abilities and traits. The androgynous person integrates "masculine" and "feminine" characteristics in an adaptive manner, leading to both a greater behavioral repertoire and a greater risk of role strain due to conflicting internal and societal expectations. A person who accumulates new roles without resolving the conflict between personal and societal demands, and who tries to meet all the demands of multiple roles, will experience increased stress, role strain, and risk of illness.[18] Instead of adding new behaviors to old ones, the person must relinquish or renegotiate roles not personally satisfying.

The result of androgyny may be a greater degree of mental health and personal fulfillment. One study, however, suggests that there may be a double standard of mental health for men and women among mental health professionals. Androgynous behavior, in this study, was seen as more acceptable in female than male clients.[25] Another study examined whether depressed individuals were experiencing sex-role strain and whether individuals with traditional masculine or feminine sex roles would have deeper depression than those with nontraditional androgynous roles. The findings of this study supported the hypothesis that there is a direct relationship between sex-role strain and depression.[18]

Mental Illness or Disorder

Historical Views of Mental Illness

Historically, mental illness was viewed as demonic possession, the influence of ancestral spirits, the result of violating a taboo or neglecting a cultural ritual, and spiritual condemnation.[15] The mentally ill have been ridiculed, neglected, banned, persecuted, and deprived of their freedoms.

The common belief that mental disturbance was related to supernatural phenomena meant that healing, if it were to take place at all, must involve supernatural intercession. Other beliefs have held that the "passions" that interfered with proper reasoning were responsible for mental illness. Melancholia, now called depression, at one time was thought to result from an imbalance of body systems, which caused an excess of bile in the body.[15]

In the 19th century, mental illness was viewed as incurable and little, if any, humane treatment existed. Until 1820, the mentally ill were exhibited, for a fee, as diversion and entertainment for the public. Until 1886, the mentally ill were restrained in iron manacles.[11]

Beginning in the 1950s, pharmacotherapy changed the picture of mental health care. The discovery of neuroleptic and, later, antidepressant drugs brought about a more hopeful attitude regarding the prognoses of the mentally ill, particularly those with psychotic disorders.[22] The psychoactive drugs gave the psychotic client some relief from his symptoms and allowed him greater benefits from other therapies.

Defining Mental Disorder

Precise definitions of mental illness or disorder are elusive and impractical. Some would define mental illness as "psychiatric disease."[15] A noted nurse–author describes mental distress as "the mind expressing its discomfort through thoughts, feelings, and behaviors."[7] General criteria for *mental disorder* include the following:

Dissatisfaction with one's characteristics, abilities, and accomplishments
Ineffective or unsatisfying interpersonal relationships
Dissatisfaction with one's place in the world
Ineffective coping or adaptation to the events in one's life as well as a lack of personal growth

Although it has often been said that 10% of the American population is affected by mental illness, it is now estimated that perhaps 15% of Americans suffer some form of emotional disorder during a year. It is further estimated that of these 32 million people, nearly 7 million receive no care at all.[4]

Attitudes Toward Mental Illness

When our attitudes toward understanding and accepting mental illness are examined over centuries, we find that they have not progressed dramatically.[14] Our approaches to the mentally ill are determined not only by medical and psychiatric theory, but also by the political and social climates of the time. In the mid-1800s, for example, a schoolteacher from New England, Dorothea Lynde Dix, investigated the deplorable conditions in mental institutions in the United States and appealed to state legislatures for better treatment of the mentally ill. Almost single-handedly she began a revolution in mental health care.[23] In more recent years, on February 5, 1963, President John F. Kennedy delivered his well-known "bold new approach" address to the United States Congress. The result of this address and subsequent legislation was the creation and growth of the community mental health movement in the United States. Unfortunately, after the 1970s, interest in community mental health waned, and currently there are vastly unserved and underserved populations in our country (see Chaps. 38 and 47).

The judicial system in the United States is influential in psychiatric–mental health treatment issues. In recent years court decisions have affirmed individuals' right to treatment, right to refuse treatment, and right to treatment in the least restrictive setting.[14] These rulings influence our attitudes about mentally disturbed persons and their rights and responsibilities (see Chap. 45, "Legal Implications of Psychiatric–Mental Health Nursing").

An individual's values and personal beliefs affect his attitudes about mental illness, people with mental disorders, and treatment of mental illness. If, for example, a person holds independence and being a "self-made man" as strong values, he may disdain the apparent dependence or weakness of a disturbed individual. If a person values his liberty and personal freedom highly, he may fail to appreciate the need for physical or chemical restraint of an aggressive client. If he values stoicism, he may find it difficult to understand the usefulness of the expression of feelings in regaining or maintaining one's mental health.

There still exists a stigma surrounding individuals who need or use psychiatric–mental health services. The need continues for public education to modify or alter misconceptions about mental illness and persons with mental disorders.

Mental Health Care Today

Many problems face mental health care today. Psychiatric–mental health treatment is costly, and until recently, most medical insurance plans did not cover treatment for mental disorders. If a client is hospitalized in a state institution for the mentally ill, he is removed from his support system and often receives little more than custodial care. The lack of governmental support for community mental health centers hastened the centers' narrowing of services and populations served.

Consumer Advocacy

There exists in the United States unequal access to health care. Consumer advocate groups have not demanded improved mental health care, although their voice is now becoming stronger (see Chap. 38).[47]

In all "mental patient" self-help groups, says one activist in the mental patients' liberation movement, there is some degree of advocacy base, that is, a dissatisfaction with the present mental health care system.[49] To achieve their aims, the self-help groups have created new, alternative programs of mutual support.

Care of the Aged

The 1971 White House Conference on Aging acknowledged the need for comprehensive health care (including mental health care) for the aged.[46] It called for the diagnosis, treatment or safe transfer to a more adequate site for care, and rehabilitation of aged persons with emotional disorders, as well as their return home to family and community. The Conference also recommended alternatives to institutional care: training of mental health care providers to work with the aged, an allotment of an increased amount of research monies to the treatment of the aged, and the development of innovative therapeutic services to currently institutionalized older persons.[46]

The Chronically Mentally Ill

Deinstitutionalization of state mental hospitals, which took place during the 1970s, created many problems related to the delivery of services to the long-term mentally ill in this country. Chronic mental patients typically encounter many barriers that limit their access to services and prevent continuity of care.[2]

Prevention

Prevention of mental or emotional disorders is a popular topic in mental health fields today. It is suggested that prevention must begin with institutions—the peer play institutions and the school—serving families and prospective families, the key integrative social systems of our society.[5] We usually expect that when these institutions fail, the mental health care system comes into action. Yet, before the treatment interventions of the mental health care system become necessary, preventive interventions could have occurred.

Studies of psychosocial resilience aim to discern why some people succumb to stress and adversity, while others escape its damage. The available results thus far show that "protective processes" reduce the impact of the risk situations (such as a threatening event), reduce the negative chain reactions stemming from the encounter with the risk situation, promote self-esteem and self-efficacy through secure and supportive relationships and successful task accomplishment, and open up opportunities for the individual. Protection resides in the ways in which individuals perceive and deal with life changes and what they do about their stressful life circumstances.[38] Another study of stress-resistant factors in children is ongoing; this research developed out of studies of adaptive and maladaptive schizophrenic adults and, later, studies of children vulnerable to psychopathology.[17] It is hoped that at some point the results of this kind of research will lend guidance and direction to our preventive activities.

Late in 1986, the National Institute of Mental Health began its first major educational campaign, which was entitled D/ART—Depression/Awareness, Recognition, Treatment. This education program about depressive disorders is aimed at both public and professional groups (see Chart 1-1).

Stress: Mechanisms and Responses

Hans Selye, a renowned biological scientist, defines *stress* as the "nonspecific response of the body to any demand made upon it."[41] Although *stressors*, or stress-producing factors, are different, such as the physical stressors of heat and cold and the psychological stressors of failure, success, and a new challenge, they elicit essentially the same biologic stress response. It is even immaterial, he claims, whether the situation or challenge we face is a pleasant one (success) or an unpleasant one (failure). Stress is not a synonym for distress; it is not anxiety or tension, nor is it something to be avoided at all costs. The absence of all stress, in fact, is death.

General Adaptation Syndrome

To cope with any type of increased demand made upon it, the body responds in a stereotyped manner, with identical biochemical changes.[41] These responses

CHART 1-1
The National Institute of Mental Health's D/ART Program

Nancy Kupper M.S.N., R.N.
Assistant Professor of Nursing
Tarrant County Junior College, Fort Worth, Texas

The National Institute of Mental Health (NIMH) launched the first major, national educational campaign in its 40-year history late in 1986. Known as D/ART (Depression/Awareness, Recognition, Treatment), the campaign is intended to be a systematic application of the knowledge gained from years of research. NIMH views D/ART as a return on the public's investment in mental health research, which over the past 20 years has included research on psychobiology, natural history, epidemiology, and the treatment of affective disorders.

Although NIMH initiated and organized D/ART, its purpose is to create national and local partnerships linking professional and lay mental health agencies and groups, business, government, professional organizations, and service providers in an effort to educate the public about the symptoms and treatment of depressive disorders. Local D/ART Community Partnerships are being organized to parallel the national D/ART group in an education campaign that combines media and community activities.

Project D/ART was developed to disseminate a consistent message:

—Depression is a disorder that, when recognized, can be treated.
—Effective medications and psychological treatments exist and often are used in combination.
—Even the most serious forms of depressive disorders respond rapidly to treatment.

Education and training programs will encompass both the professional and public sectors. The professional education program aims to provide health care providers with the most up-to-date information on the diagnosis and treatment of depressive disorders. Primary care providers will be helped to recognize, assess, treat, and when necessary refer patients with affective illnesses. Mental health professionals will be made aware of the latest treatment approaches and taught to incorporate them into their practices. Short-term clinical training grants will be awarded to medical schools, university psychiatry departments, and nursing, social work, and psychology graduate schools. In addition, brief education courses will be offered at professional meetings and at sites around the nation.

The public education program aims to create changes in the attitudes and behaviors of the general public. This is expected to help people to recognize depression in themselves or their friends and families, to understand that it is treatable, and to learn how to seek treatment. Enhanced public awareness of its symptoms and treatment will reduce the effects of depression in personal, family, and work life.

D/ART's Community Partnership Program has been established to help implement the education campaign. Lead organizations, chosen by the D/ART Program (typically mental health association state and local affiliates), will disseminate electronic and print materials and products developed by D/ART. The duplication and use of these materials will be encouraged to spread D/ART's message and to support the campaign's goals.

Media kits with electronic and print materials are being distributed nationally and to participating community partnership programs. Some bilingual pamphlets will be distributed. Guidelines are available to allow participating organizations to use the D/ART logo and theme on materials they duplicate. Local partnerships may also develop their own materials; these, after approval by D/ART, may bear the logo.

By coordinating national and local efforts, using multiple channels for communication, and coordinating community programs with media efforts, NIMH hopes to maximize D/ART's effectiveness. The project's name describes its goals of enhancing public awareness and encouraging help-seeking behavior. Public and professional participation and involvement will help meet these goals through the education of individuals, families, employers, school counselors and teachers, the media, and the public at large.

are termed the *General Adaptation Syndrome* (GAS). The General Adaptation Syndrome demonstrates the body's manifestations of stress as they develop over a period of time.

The General Adaptation Syndrome evolves in three stages.

1. *Alarm reaction* is the stage in which the body begins to respond and adjust to the stressor; the body's resistance is being diminished and death may occur if the stressor is sufficiently strong.
2. *Stage of resistance* is the stage in which the body continues to resist the stressor and no longer evidences signs of the initial reaction; the person's level of resistance is greater than normal.
3. *Stage of exhaustion* is the stage in which the body's ability to resist the stressor, or adaptation energy, becomes exhausted following lengthy exposure to the same stressor; the signs of the initial reaction return but are irreversible and the person dies.[41]

For a more in-depth look at the body's physiological response to stressors, see Figure 1-1.

Distress

Damaging or unpleasant stress is *distress*. The body's biologic responses to stressors cause psycho-physiological disorders. According to Selye, damaging stressors (*e.g.*, anxiety, frustration, insecurity, and aimlessness) may result in a variety of physical and emotional disorders, such as migraine headaches, peptic ulcers, myocardial infarctions ("heart attacks"), hypertension, suicide, mental illness, and "hopeless unhappiness."[41]

What is the ultimate aim of people? Is it, as Selye suggests, to express ourselves as fully as possible, according to our own talents and desires, and to achieve a sense of security? If so, then we must learn how to accomplish this. Selye's solution is to find our own optimal stress level and then to use our adaptive energy at a rate and in a direction adjusted to our own qualifications and preferences.[41]

Selye's own philosophy gives us a guideline for using our adaptive energy:

> "Fight for your highest attainable aim
> But never put up resistance in vain."[41]

Coping Mechanisms

Coping mechanisms are also referred to as ego-defense mechanisms, mental mechanisms, and defense mechanisms. Coping mechanisms function to protect the ego from overwhelming anxiety; for the most part, they operate on an unconscious level. See Chart 1-2,

"Coping Mechanisms," for many examples of these mechanisms in everyday life.

Denial

Denial is a commonly used coping mechanism wherein a person denies the existence of some external reality. The person using denial is unaware that he is using it. When a patient is informed of his medical diagnosis, for example, he usually denies its existence for some period of time.

> "Oh no, this is a mistake."
> "It's not true."
> "There's nothing wrong with me."
> "I can't have diabetes (multiple sclerosis, cancer, heart attack), I'm too young and healthy."

For a brief or lengthy periods of time, denial generally operates as a protective and often a healthy mechanism, protecting the individual from the shock of reality until he is better able to deal with it. In time, denial usually diminishes and the person gradually begins to face, accept, and deal with the harsh realities.

There are varying degrees of denial. A person who has been told that he has had a heart attack, which caused a great deal of damage to the heart muscle, may deny that he has had a heart attack at all. Another person facing the same diagnosis may acknowledge that he has suffered a heart attack and recognize the need for treatment and for modification of his lifestyle, but may not believe that the extent of heart damage is as serious as his doctors have described.

Denial may also have treatment implications. If a child exhibits overtly disturbed behavior but his parents deny that a problem exists, the parents will not seek treatment for their child and may, in fact, become indignant when a teacher or school nurse recommends psychological assessment of the child.

A person may deny selectively, that is, deny certain facts but accept, or seem to accept, others.

> A husband and wife in their early thirties were told by the pediatric neurologist that their son, 10 months of age, had static congenital encephalopathy, commonly called cerebral palsy, evidenced in right-sided hemiparesis. While dealing with their shock, anger, and the other facets of grief, they began to plan and implement various therapies needed by their son—passive exercising of his right arm and leg and an active swimming program.
> Eight months after the diagnosis of the child's condition, the couple sat in their living room watching the Summer Olympic Games on television. The woman turned to her husband and asked, "Do you think someday our son will be an olympic athlete?" "What?!" replied the man, looking at his wife in disbelief.
> *(Text continues on p. 13)*

Figure 1-1. *The body's response to stress.* (From Kozier B, Erb G: Fundamentals of Nursing: Concepts and Procedures, 3d ed, p 328. Menlo Park, CA, Addison-Wesley, 1987)

CHART 1-2
Coping Mechanisms

Joann W. Bohm, M.S., R.N.
Instructor/Coordinator
Associate Degree Nursing
Grayson County College
Denison, Texas

Nursing Perspective

Defense, or coping, mechanisms protect the ego in times of anxiety. Generally, they operate on an unconscious level. When they become conscious, they lose their effectiveness. Everyone uses coping mechanisms at one time or another. The formation begins in infancy; most coping mechanisms become well-embedded into the personality by adolescence. If coping mechanisms are over-used, they become ineffective, or ego-defeating.

Nursing students often become quite anxious when they are first assigned to psychiatric units. They normally use many defense mechanisms to cope with these anxieties. An understanding of your use of coping mechanisms will allow you to improve your adjustment to psychiatric nursing, as well as your skills in problem-solving.

MECHANISM	EXAMPLE	MECHANISM	EXAMPLE
Denial: A person denies the existence of some external reality.	A nursing student thinks that a psychiatric client should not be hospitalized because he acts so normal.	*Repression:* A person forces certain thoughts or feelings into his unconscious.	A nursing student's mother died at a state psychiatric hospital, but the student has no memory of visiting her.
Regression: A person returns to an earlier, more comfortable time in his life.	A nursing student begins to cry and cling to her friends when she enters her assigned, locked psychiatric unit.	*Suppression:* A person consciously excludes certain thoughts or feelings from his mind.	A nursing student's care plan is due tomorrow afternoon. She decides that she will go to a movie that evening and get up early in the morning to complete the plan.
Displacement: A person transfers an emotion from its original object to a substitute object.	A nursing student's assigned client does not keep his appointment. Her process recording of an interaction with this client is due that afternoon. When she returns to her room, she throws her books on the floor.	*Identification:* A person unconsciously adopts the personality characteristics, attitude, values, and behavior of another person.	A nursing student is very impressed with a psychiatric nurse's communication techniques. She incorporates these into her communication with clients.
Projection: A person displaces generally negative feelings onto another individual.	A female nursing student is sexually attracted to a nice-looking client and accuses him of flirting with her.	*Rationalization:* A person substitutes acceptable reasons for the real or actual reasons motivating behavior.	A nursing student who does not want to dance with clients during their evening activities says she does not know how to dance.
Reaction formation: A person acts in a way that is the opposite of how he feels.	A nursing student dislikes psychiatric nursing, yet asks repeatedly to be assigned to a psychiatric client.		

(Continues on p. 12)

MECHANISM	EXAMPLE	MECHANISM	EXAMPLE
Fantasy: A person uses non-rational mental activity to escape from daily pressures and responsibilities.	During relaxation therapy, a nursing student dreams that she has identified the cause of mental illness and that all clients will be cured.	*Intellectualization:* A person uses his intellectual powers of thinking, reasoning, and analyzing to blunt or avoid emotional stress.	Asked how she felt when a client became hostile toward her, a nursing student responded by identifying the precipitating factors of the incident and the therapeutic techniques which could have prevented it.

Client Perspective

MECHANISM	EGO-BUILDING (EFFECTIVE) EXAMPLE		EGO-DEFEATING (INEFFECTIVE) EXAMPLE
	Pre-Adult	*Adult*	
Denial: A person denies the existence of some external reality.	A 5-year-old child who is allergic to chocolate is told not to eat it. She sneaks a candy bar at every opportunity.	A 22-year-old male has been told he has diabetes and must follow a special diet with no sugar for the rest of his life. He says to his doctor and nurse, "Oh, no. You must be mistaken. I can't have diabetes."	A diabetic man does not follow his diet and goes into a coma.
Regression: A person returns to an earlier more comfortable time in his life.	A child is frightened on the first day of school and begins to suck his thumb.	A young woman who has difficulties with her husband returns to her parents' home.	A young woman goes to bed and assumes the fetal position when she and her husband have any disagreement.
Displacement: A person transfers an emotion from its original object to a substitute object.	A child is mad at his mother, so he goes to his room to break his favorite toy.	After an argument with his wife, the husband leaves and slams the door.	Each time a man is in a situation where others do not agree with him, he becomes physically abusive.
Projection: A person displaces generally negative feelings onto another individual.	A toddler who is afraid of the dark tells her parents her teddy bear is afraid.	A neighbor makes fun of a young wife who is afraid to stay alone at night when her husband is working.	A person says there are demons in the night and refuses to leave his home after the sun sets.
Reaction formation: A person acts in a way that is the opposite of how he feels.	An 8-year-old boy hates all girls. He says he wouldn't be caught dead talking to one.	A young male who is a well-established banker thinks that all women are after his money.	A young male refuses to talk to anyone with feminine characteristics.
Repression: A person forces certain feelings or thoughts into his unconscious.	A female child is not aware of her jealousy of her cousin, whom the relatives describe as "darling."	At a family reunion a young woman "forgets" her pretty cousin's name when she begins to introduce her husband to this cousin.	A woman has no memory of a large part of her formative childhood years.

Client Perspective (continued)

MECHANISM	EGO-BUILDING (EFFECTIVE) EXAMPLE		EGO-DEFEATING (INEFFECTIVE) EXAMPLE
	Pre-Adult	*Adult*	
Suppression: A person consciously excludes certain thoughts or feelings from his mind.	A school age child "forgets" to bring his books home to do his homework.	A man "forgets" to get all the information he needs to complete his income tax return.	A man files his income tax return late and has to pay a penalty.
Identification: A person unconsciously adopts the personality characteristics, attitudes, values, and behavior of another person.	An adolescent has her hair cut like her favorite recording star.	When buying clothes, a woman always checks to see what style is being worn by the President's wife.	A woman thinks she is the President's wife.
Rationalization: A person substitutes acceptable reasons for the real or actual reasons motivating behavior.	A child is not invited to a birthday party and says, "I didn't really want to go anyway."	An older woman was not invited to a big social event. She copes by thinking her invitation was lost in the mail.	A person denies that she may have some unacceptable qualities others do not like. She feels she is perfect.
Sublimation: A person transforms unacceptable sexual or aggressive drives into socially acceptable pursuits.	A 6-year-old boy who is aggressive plays cowboys and Indians.	A young man who is very competitive and aggressive uses this energy to become a pro football player.	A pro football player spends all of his time working out or at football practice, and he has no time left to spend with his family.
Fantasy: A person uses non-rational mental activity to escape from daily pressures and responsibilities.	A child pretends she is a fairytale princess.	A housewife faced with a sink full of dirty dishes dreams she has a live-in maid.	A lady lives in a fantasy world and makes no effort to tend to her basic needs. She stays in bed all day and commands "the slaves" to care for her.
Intellectualization: A person uses his intellectual powers of thinking, reasoning, and analyzing to blunt or avoid emotional stress.	When a teenager is asked about her first day of high school, she responds by giving the criteria for the positive adjustment of teenagers in striving for adulthood.	An older adult is asked to share her feelings on death. She reviews all the stages of death and dying as identified by Kubler-Ross.	A college professor talked at length about the fact that existence equaled doubt and he was on both sides of the metaphysical equation. He was trying to say he was suicidal.

Denial takes many forms and serves many functions. In this situation, it protected the woman from the full force of her grief over the loss of the ideal or "perfect" child.

Regression

Through the use of *regression,* a person avoids anxiety by returning to an earlier, more comfortable time in his life, a time when his needs were met more completely.

A 3-year-old child might regress in response to the birth of a sibling and begin again to soil her pants, suck her thumb, talk "baby talk," and ask for a bottle. An adult undergoing any physical or emotional stress might regress by becoming irritable, demanding, and whining; or the adult might take to his bed for a "sick day," thereby giving up his responsibilities for the day and allowing others to meet his needs.

Play is one important form of regression. It is our way of voluntarily relinquishing our adult concerns and duties and engaging in a childlike state of spontaneity and enjoyment. For children, of course, play serves many functions, including fantasy, learning, and opportunity for mastery of physical and emotional challenges.

Like the other coping mechanisms, regression may be a useful and healthy response to stressors, but may become maladaptive if used excessively or exclusively.

Displacement

Displacement is the transfer of an emotion from its original object to a substitute object. For example, if a person is angry with his superior at work or school, he may feel too threatened to confront that individual with his anger; instead, he may go home and vent his anger on a family member. The person has displaced his feeling (anger) from its original object (his superior) to a substitute object (a family member).

It is likely that the individual who displaces his feelings has no awareness that he is using displacement. Later, however, he may look back on the events and realize that, because he was angry with someone to whom he could not comfortably express his feeling, he "took it out" on a member of his family.

Projection

Projection is the displacement of feelings, usually feelings perceived as "negative," onto another individual. If, for example, a person feels guilty (or angry, dependent, aggressive, or hostile) and this feeling is unacceptable to him, he may project it onto another rather than owning it.

> "I'm not angry, but she's mad at me."
> "I don't have any bad feelings toward him, but he sure hates me."

Individuals with paranoid behavior frequently overuse the mechanism of projection. If the person is fearful of his environment, he may project those feelings onto the external world and develop the delusion that forces in the environment, such as the FBI, CIA, or Soviet spies, are "out to get him." He may believe that others are constantly watching him and plotting his demise.

Sometimes, projection of feelings functions as an adaptive mechanism, protecting us from feelings that we find unacceptable in ourselves until we can learn to own up to them and acknowledge that having both "positive" and "negative" feelings is part of our humanity.

Reaction Formation

When a person uses *reaction formation,* he acts in a way that is the opposite of how he feels. For example, if a person feels aggressive or hostile toward another, he

might, because these feelings are unacceptable to him, behave very kindly and politely toward the object of his feelings. The individual who uses reaction formation is not consciously aware of the great disparity between his feelings or ideas and his actions.

> A student seemed to be angry at one particular instructor. She was displeased with her grades on the instructor's exams and with the many criticisms and corrections she received from the instructor. When she interacted with the instructor, however, she wore a frozen, continuous smile on her face, was excessively polite, and talked in a high-pitched, "little girl" tone of voice. Frequently, she gave the instructor gifts.

If a person cannot acknowledge his own feelings of dependency, he may behave in ways that emphasize his independence. He may assert that he "needs no one" and verbally and nonverbally drive others away.

Repression

Through *repression,* an individual forces certain feelings or thoughts into his unconscious. The repressed material, such as painful memories or feelings, remains in the person's unconscious, although it may surface from time to time in his dreams or "slips of the tongue." Repression is a mechanism that occurs at the unconscious level.

The usefulness of repression, again, is to protect the individual from overwhelming anxiety. He involuntarily "forgets" certain events or feelings that evoke a great deal of anxiety.

Suppression

Suppression takes place when a person consciously excludes certain thoughts or feelings from his mind. The excluded thoughts or feelings are those that cause him anxiety. This coping mechanism operates at the conscious level. When a person decides to "put something out of his mind" or "not worry about it until tomorrow," he is using suppression.

> A student was assigned a major research paper to write. Every time he thought about the length and depth of the paper and the amount of hard work it would require, he felt extremely anxious.
> To overcome his anxiety and initiate work on the paper, he decided he would not think about it as a total, completed project, but would break it down into smaller, more manageable units. He listed each component of the assignment—choosing and delineating the topic, outlining the scope of the topic, researching each subtopic, and so on—and then proceeded to tackle each component systematically.
> When his anxiety surfaced from time to time, he forced himself to push aside fears about the total undertaking and concentrate on the smaller unit of work before him.

Identification

Identification is the unconscious adoption of the personality characteristics, attitudes, values, and behavior of another person. Children frequently identify with their parents, favorite aunts, uncles, or teachers, and even well-known public figures in sports or entertainment. Adults also use identification as a means of continued growth by adopting some of the attributes of their role models. When this process becomes conscious, however, it is called *imitation.*

The person using identification is unaware of doing so, although others may recognize that he is identifying with another. Overuse of identification may result in a person developing low self-esteem and little individuality because he has relied heavily on the advice and support of others.

Rationalization

Rationalization is the substitution of acceptable reasons for the real or actual reasons motivating behavior. Through rationalization, a person justifies his behavior or conceals his disappointments.[31] For example, if a person interviews for a job but is not hired, he may rationalize that the interviewer for the company did not spend enough time with him to get a fair impression of his strengths. He may also rationalize that he did not really want the job or that the job would have required more time than he was willing to devote to it. In each of these rationalizations, the person covers his real feelings of failure and disappointment with ones that will protect him from the anxiety associated with failure and disappointment.

Fantasy

Fantasy is nonrational mental activity that allows an individual to escape from his daily pressures and responsibilities.[48] Through fantasy, a person temporarily breaks through the boundaries of reality and enters a place where he can daydream about whatever is most pleasurable to him. For example, if a person is overwhelmed by the pressures of a task he has undertaken, he may imagine the completion of the task and the feelings of satisfaction and pride he will experience at its completion. These feelings may spur him on to work harder toward his goal.

The thinking of children, particularly young children, is characterized by fantasy. Often, adults become stifled by the realities of the world and abandon their use of fantasy. The ability to fantasize, however, provides an effective escape valve for people of all ages and promotes childlike creativity. The excessive use of fantasy, on the other hand, reduces an individual's contact with reality and may render him incapable of dealing with the demands of his life.

Intellectualization

Through *intellectualization,* a person uses his intellectual powers of thinking, reasoning, and analyzing to blunt or avoid emotional issues. Talking about or dealing directly with feelings is too threatening or painful for him.

Sometimes, an individual with significant emotional problems (*e.g.,* a severe lack of interpersonal skills) will intellectualize his problems. He may discuss Sullivan's interpersonal theory and the effect of childhood interpersonal experiences on adult functioning and he may weigh the value of one therapeutic intervention over another, but he will avoid the more difficult discussion of his feelings. Feelings are often the heart of the issue in psychiatric–mental health nursing, but they require a degree of courage and confidence to face.

The usefulness of these various coping mechanisms lies in their protection of the person from intolerable anxiety. We all use these mechanisms at one time or another, particularly in situations that elicit threatening or painful feelings; however, their value depends on their judicious use. The continuous, exclusive use of these mechanisms would inhibit or prevent the person from learning other, more effective, ways to cope with, adapt to, and grow in relation to his environment.

Psychiatric–Mental Health Nursing

One of the most significant figures in the history of psychiatric care in the United States was Dorothea Lynde Dix (1802–1887). During her time, the standard treatment of the mentally ill ranged from negligence to brutality. She found patients confined in cages and cellars, chained, and beaten.[11] She pioneered the crusade for reforms in the treatment of the mentally ill and gained the support of influential citizens by describing to them the abhorrent conditions in which mental patients lived.

By 1940, there were few more than 4000 graduate nurses working in state mental hospitals. In some states psychiatric nursing was not even taught, although those states operated psychiatric hospitals. Nurses may have learned how to care for the mentally ill in a general hospital school of nursing, a psychiatric hospital school of nursing, or through their experience in a psychiatric institution. Some leaders in nursing were beginning to recognize that the responsibilities and role of the psychiatric nurse might differ from those of a nurse caring for the physically ill. Some nurses began to see the importance of interaction, acceptance, respect for other human beings, and what today would be called the therapeutic use of self.[23]

In July 1946, the United States passed the National Mental Health Act, administered by the National Institute of Mental Health (NIMH), to finance mental health research, training programs, and community mental health services. The NIMH traineeship program, begun in 1948, was a significant support for graduate-level education of psychiatric nurses.[23]

Psychiatric–mental health nursing has evolved into a unique discipline. It now combines the knowledge, experience, and skills of nursing and mental health. In actuality, the name psychiatric–mental nursing implies two different areas of nursing that often interact and overlap. Psychiatric nursing focuses on the care and rehabilitation of those with identifiable emotional disorders. Mental health nursing focuses on well populations; it intervenes in crisis situations and with high-risk individuals or groups to prevent the development of mental illness or disorder.

Roles of Psychiatric–Mental Health Nurses

Some of the roles of the psychiatric–mental health nurse are skilled communicator, role model of adaptive behavior, director of the therapeutic milieu, advocate for the client and family, member of the mental health care team, primary nurse for specific clients, and therapist with individuals, groups, and families. This last role, nurse-therapist, requires advanced education, supervision, and experience. Many of these roles are approached in depth in other chapters of this book (see Chaps. 4, 5, 12, 13, 14, 15, 16, and 33). The reader is encouraged to explore these and other chapters for a greater understanding of the many roles of nursing.

One important nursing role or function, for example, is that of helping the client develop social skills. The challenge of this function lies in focusing interventions and individualizing them for clients. A novice nurse may observe psychiatric staff sitting and talking to clients, or playing cards or other games with them, and wonder why a certain activity was chosen for a particular client. By first identifying specific ego strengths and problems (frustration tolerance, impulse control, relatedness to others, thought processes, judgment, reality testing), the nurse begins to determine the therapeutic value of an activity for a client. Nursing observations should examine such issues as: Who initiated the activity or interaction? How much is the client participating? What is the degree of the client's mechanical ability to perform the activity? What is the client's emotional tone and anxiety level during the activity? What is his response to interruptions? The psychiatric staff member faces the challenge of remaining in the professional role rather than becoming absorbed in the activity.[33]

Nurses' Reactions to Disturbed Behavior

Like everyone else, nurses are affected by the behavior of the people around them. When nurses work with clients with psychiatric problems, they may encounter various forms of disturbed behavior—bizarre, aggressive, hostile, suspicious, dependent, and violent. Their reactions to these behaviors are likely to reflect the range of their experiences and values.

The nurse reacting to disturbed behavior may be offended, repulsed, threatened, annoyed, angered, surprised, or shocked. She may be confused and frightened by these feelings. She may view her feelings as "unprofessional" and be ashamed of them. If the goal of nursing is to provide the highest quality nursing care for patients, then nurses must first examine their own values, feelings, and reactions. Self-exploration and working through difficult issues, such as how to interpret and deal with manipulation or hostility, are critical developments in the nurse's professional growth.

There is no one "right way" to intervene therapeutically in disturbed behavior. Mental health care providers explore their thoughts and feelings, follow certain broad guidelines, and experiment with what works for them. Nurses and other care providers cannot impart wisdom to anyone, but they can give of themselves—their caring and hopes—to the other.[24]

Views of Novice Nurses

The impressions, perceptions, and fears of nurses new to psychiatric–mental health nursing are important to examine. If unexamined or ignored, they may hamper the nurse's effectiveness in intervention. A noted psychiatric–mental health nurse and author, Ann W. Burgess, has described the feelings common to nursing students facing their first psychiatric nursing experiences. They are listed below:

Feeling useless
Fear of appearing like a novice
Anxiety
Fear of being rejected by the client
Fear of hurting the client
Fear of being hurt by the client
Depression
Anger
Embarrassment
Concerns about their own mental health[7]

Chart 1-3 will help mental health nurses prepare for their experiences.

C H A R T   1-3
Preparing for Psychiatric–Mental Health Nursing Experiences

Johnnie Bonner, M.S.N., R.N.
Coordinator, Child and Adolescent Crisis Stabilization Unit
Dallas County Mental Health Mental Retardation
Dallas, Texas

Philosophies and theories about the nature of human behavior and what constitutes competent, ethical treatment of individuals with emotional disorders vary greatly. In addition to these philosophic and theoretical differences, treatment settings, researchers, educators, and the literature usually focus on limited aspects rather than the entire continuum of possible services and knowledge. You may be exposed to a variety of settings or you may realize that your textbook or instructor describes different kinds of treatment from what you observe. If you think of the inconsistencies as differences and refrain from making judgments about "right or wrong" or "good or bad," you may be more open to learning from what you see and hear.

Sometimes, the structure or the day-to-day tasks and functions are not as easy to identify on a psychiatric unit as they are in other services. This apparent lack of specific treatments and tasks may leave you wondering whether you can make any meaningful or helpful contribution to clients and the agency providing the learning experience for you. Most psychiatric–mental health professionals and agencies believe that contributing to your learning experience is an investment that is expected to pay off indirectly; it will also pay off in the long term by adding some of you to the ranks of clinicians or by providing you with a constructive awareness of psychiatric nursing, regardless of the field within nursing that you choose for a career. Psychiatric–mental health staff do not expect you to do anything but learn; however, they also know from experience that you will make significant contributions. Your energy and enthusiasm are refreshing. Your relatively unbiased exploration of what staff are doing and why will raise important questions and issues that need to be reviewed in the ongoing process of evaluating care.

You may wonder, particularly during your initial psychiatric nursing experience, "What will I discuss with the client?" The client may choose to keep the process of your interactions superficial, partially due to the dynamics of his problems and partially due to the reality that the time limits of a student's rotation will not allow the development of an in-depth therapeutic alliance. Focus initial questions or interview openings on what led to the client's or others' decision to seek treatment. This will help you become acquainted with the client and give him an opportunity to reflect again on the nature of his difficulties or treatment issues. Discussing the decision to seek treatment can be genuinely helpful, even when it is repeated many times, because it is an opportunity to examine the same set of circumstances from a different perspective. The simplicity of these natural and expected kinds of questions does not negate their therapeutic value.

There are also other areas that you may invite clients to explore with you. These include their expectations of the treatment facility and services and their responses to them. Thoughtful reflection on progress in the course of treatment can help build the client's self-esteem and hope for change.

The issue of confidentiality assumes an important and perhaps somewhat different perspective within the psychiatric–mental health team. The potential situation exists in which you are asked by the client not to share some information that he has revealed. I can think of *no* situation in which agreeing to this kind of request would be therapeutic. This may be a difficult dilemma, often preceded by the client's flattering comments about your attributes as a good listener or an understanding and trustworthy person. You may even be lured by the hope that the client will reveal something that will have great impact on his treatment. The client will need to be reminded, kindly but firmly, that it is important for all members of the therapeutic team to share any information that might contribute to his treatment. In addition, you might ask the client to explore why he is unable to trust the other members of the treatment team. As a student, you might try to understand the dynamics of how accepting and keeping the client's "secrets" separates you from the rest of the team.

Another crucial issue in psychiatric–mental health nursing is that of maintaining a "separateness" in the therapeutic role. You may hear this called "detachment," "objectivity," or

(Continues on p. 18)

"distance," but despite how thoughtfully this topic is discussed with you, you may bristle and think that others are suggesting that you develop an attitude of coldness. On the contrary, your values of compassion and empathy are not being challenged; indeed, it is virtually impossible to be therapeutic without those qualities. What experienced psychiatric–mental health clinicians recommend is that in order for you to use your knowledge and skills therapeutically, compassion and empathy must be expressed in a manner that leaves your personal life separate from the client's. Clients do not need us personally, as friends or companions, as much as they need us to teach them how to have (or why they don't have) friendship and companionship outside of treatment. Identifying your own feelings and attitudes and discussing them with an experienced clinician may help you develop as a professional who is both caring and effective in relationships with clients.

As you work with clients, keep in mind that, although you may provide an opportunity and an environment in which change may occur, you cannot make a client change. You cannot transfer your observations, knowledge, and assessment of what you believe is best for him into his awareness. Try to imagine, at times, what it would cost the client to make the changes you feel would benefit him.

Change is the client's choice. He may need our skills, knowledge, and a safe place to work; and although he may sometimes borrow our hope, he makes the choices, he does the internal work, and he needs to feel the pride and take the credit. He lives with the choices.

Clients' Views of Mental Health Care

The clients' views and feelings are likewise important to consider. Often, clients are frightened or relieved in response to being hospitalized in a psychiatric unit. They may fear that treatment will dehumanize them or that mental health care providers will overmedicate, discount, or neglect them.[7] Clients may also be suspicious of the new environment (if they are hospitalized for psychiatric treatment) and the strange, but seemingly well-intentioned, mental health professionals.

Clients seeking psychiatric treatment often expect that the care providers will be able to solve their problems for them. They may expect to play a passive role while the psychiatrist, nurse, psychologist, or social worker actively "cures" them. It is necessary for mental health care professionals to clarify these client perceptions and provide clients with straightforward information about the processes of mental health care and the expected behavior of the client as a member of the health care team. Chart 1-4, "The Mental Health Nurse As Person," explores the phenomenon of clients ascribing omnipotence to mental health care professionals and ways to deal with this occurrence.

Stress and Burnout Among Nurses

The pressures of psychiatric–mental health nursing are significant. Intervening daily with individuals whose behavior is disordered or maladaptive requires a great deal of personal and professional resources. The toll on the nurse can be heavy.

The nurse should be alert to certain warning signs of increasing job stress. These include job dissatisfaction, loss of enthusiasm and energy, fatigue, sleep disturbances, and escape activities (such as alcohol and drug use).[10]

More severe, chronic, or crisis symptoms of stress include exhaustion, chronic fatigue, physical illness that may become critical (such as a bleeding ulcer), loss of control of emotions, obsession with problems, withdrawal, moodiness, and increased use of escape activities.[10]

Positive coping with job stress and burnout requires a concerted effort by the nurse or other mental health care provider. Support systems, at work and away from work, are necessary to allow the nurse to ventilate feelings and help keep events in perspective. It is also useful if the nurse does not expect 100% satisfaction from her job, because this expectation is destined to failure. Taking frequent, brief vacations, or minivacations, has been found to be more refreshing and relaxing than infrequent, longer vacations. Positive imagery, such as imagining job success and satisfaction, is an effective use of fantasy and provides a mental minivacation.[10] Specific measures for preventing job burnout are described in Chart 1-4, "The Mental Health Nurse As Person."

Experience and Stress

A recent study examined the effects of therapists' experience levels on vulnerability to stresses associated with therapeutic work. Older, more experienced therapists found the work-related issues of maintaining the therapeutic relationship, scheduling, professional doubt, work overinvolvement, and personal depletion less stressful than inexperienced therapists. Level of experience, however, was not predictive of the stress

CHART 1-4
The Mental Health Nurse As Person

Jan W. Dalsheimer, M.S., R.N.
Formerly, Mental Health Nurse Consultant
Dallas, Texas

Entering mental health nursing may be a career choice that appears exciting and sometimes a little overwhelming. We may wish to understand all of the intricacies of human behavior to work more effectively with our clients, but a sometimes-overlooked fact is that people are complex. Even with many years of study and experience in the field of mental health, we cannot hope to comprehend every facet of being a person. We can, however, strive toward greater understanding of the people to whom we give care if we initially embody some concepts about people in general. Next, undertaking the complex task of understanding ourselves and our needs can further reduce the risk of relating to clients in less-than-effective ways.

It is helpful to remember that, as people, we share more similarities than differences. We all have concerns about our lives, our health, our relationships, and our well-being. As human beings, we experience happiness, anger, loneliness, joy—literally, a full spectrum of emotions. Within this framework of our thoughts and feelings, we then function with varying degrees of mental health.

Because mental health cannot be demonstrated at the cellular level, in order to examine this phenomenon, we must rely on theoretical constructs and symptoms reflected in behavior. How do we know when we have mental health? Is it an "all or nothing" condition? Mental health has been defined as the most appropriate adjustment a person can make at a particular time based on internal and external resources. This definition implies that mental health is like physical equilibrium—it is necessary to constantly adjust it in order to retain it. Continuous effort is needed to cope with new situations.[4]

When we are mentally healthy, we experience some of the following "inner signals":

Self-esteem; self-respect that prevails even in the face of discouragement, failure, or frustration
An open, flexible approach to life; the ability to experience a failure without berating ourselves or others
A spontaneous, outgoing temperament; the ability to enjoy others and the capability of giving and accepting love; the ability to express strong feelings appropriately
Minimal nervous tension; freedom from crippling worry and strain; the ability to face life in a relaxed, confident manner
Appropriate depression, anxiety, and anger under stress; a philosophy that facilitates the handling of frustration and pressure reasonably well.[1]

Needless to say, the complete and constant attainment of the above criteria is practically impossible. No one can be expected to cope with, or adapt perfectly to, every one of life's crises. Nevertheless, can we, as mental health professionals, help others if our own mental health is not perfectly intact? If we accept the fact that people are not perfect, and that we are likewise human, then part of our self-understanding is to accept thankfully that we can, indeed, fit into an imperfect world. Like everyone else, we are in the process of striving toward higher levels of mental health.

Despite our understanding of life's imperfections, a myth persists that mental health professionals are all-knowing or possess magical powers. This is a problem of "imbued omnipotence," a term referring to a complex of unrealistic beliefs held about mental health professionals by others outside of the profession.[5] Some of these "beliefs" may be that mental health professionals have the ability to read minds or predict the future. Mental health care providers may be regarded as people who should cope with and act appropriately in every situation or, even more unrealistically, as people who have no problems at all.

It is important to understand this external view of the mental health nurse in order to avoid the subtle trap of an omnipotent image. Inexperienced nurses who believe that they must produce a "magic" answer that will solve a client's problems, or who even believe that there is one such "magic" solution, will find this expectation terribly self-defeating. It is a self-expectation that will crush professional spirit and create insurmountable distance between nurses and their clients.

What, then, is the dividing line between nonhospitalized persons and those who are hospitalized with an emotional disorder? It is sim-

(Continues on p. 20)

ply the ability to cope at a given point in time—the ability to draw upon available resources and weather life's daily stresses.

When mental health is viewed within this framework, it is easier to recognize that, as creatures who are vulnerable, all of us face the possibility of needing professional help at some point in our lives. We, as mental health nurses, are in no way dramatically different from our clients. If we see our clients as "different" or as persons to be pitied, we are behaving defensively to protect ourselves. This stance may be antitherapeutic or unhelpful, for we are at risk of thinking and acting in ways that lack compassion and sensitivity to our clients' needs.

If, on the other hand, we adopt the philosophy that mental health, like physical health, is a matter of degree and is a fluctuating condition, we leave ourselves open to experiencing empathy, or *feeling with* our clients. Perhaps some of us may have developed an interest in mental health nursing after a personal experience with therapy, or we may find a need for therapy at some point in our careers. The self-understanding attained through therapy not only provides personal benefits, but it also facilitates further understanding of the process through which our clients travel. Remembering the feelings of pain and those of satisfaction that may be evoked in therapy can provide us with personal experiences from which to draw and can help us approach others with greater empathy.

In addition to understanding ourselves as people in the role of mental health nurse, we should also remember that the role itself has limitations. We often need the ideas of our colleagues, and we may need other disciplines. Collegial support can come from a clinical nurse specialist as well as from staff nurses. We should also feel free to consult the chaplain, social worker, occupational therapist, psychiatrist, and psychologist. Each specialty has much to contribute to the client's care, yet each has its own limitations. By working together as a team, we provide better care for the client.[2]

Finally, self-understanding means knowing how to take care of ourselves mentally and physically. Again, we must know our limitations and be kind to ourselves. We cannot perform emotionally draining work and ignore the importance of replenishing ourselves. A great deal of material has been written in recent years on the topics of stress and burnout. To remain effective as mental health professionals and to avoid becoming "burned out," it is important to incorporate strategies for coping with stress into our daily lives. The following suggestions will help prevent stress from turning into distress.

Take care of your body. This is a twofold process that involves paying attention to diet and exercising regularly. To avoid feeling overwhelmed while trying to change old patterns, set small goals and reward yourself for accomplishments. For example, if you have decided to cut down on refined sugar, you might decide to substitute fruit for candy during the next week. You might also think about several pleasurable activities that could be substituted for eating when a craving for sugar surfaces. In the area of exercise, it is important to pick an enjoyable activity, a form of exercise you will stick with. Setting a goal of walking around the block or campus every day may be just the starting point that is needed to embark on an exercise program. A balanced diet and adequate exercise are essential for an overall feeling of well-being.

Learn to play. We need to escape from the pressures of life and have fun on a regular basis. Resurrecting old board games from childhood, such as Monopoly, can be fun. It is important to pick an activity that is absorbing and enjoyable. Remember to use vacation time to get away, both physically and mentally, from work or school.

Make some friends outside of nursing and mental health. It is mentally refreshing to learn and talk about subjects other than work-related topics.

Learn to plan. Whenever possible, take on projects one at a time and work on them until they are completed. Making lists, rather than committing tasks to memory, aids organization tremendously.

Learn a substance-free method of relaxing. While they may be more socially acceptable than other habits, excessive eating, drinking, and smoking are health-damaging means to relaxation. More positive ways to relax include yoga, meditation, and progressive relaxation techniques.

Attempt to solve problems when at your best mentally and physically. Determining what time of day you feel most alert and functional may be helpful in getting difficult tasks completed.

Do something simple that can be accomplished

easily, something over which you have a high degree of control. Tasks such as washing clothes or sweeping the walk are nearly always available to undertake.

Break your routine by seeking new experiences. Give of yourself in a non-nursing area. Select a cause that is of genuine interest and volunteer your time.

Talk out your troubles. We need to remind ourselves that expressing concerns to an understanding friend or counselor is important. We set an example for our clients by not bottling up problems.[3,6]

By understanding and nurturing ourselves, we will become healthier and will strengthen our sense of well-being. Our clients, in turn, will benefit from this self-understanding by which we learn to identify commonalities among people. A mixture of theoretical knowledge about people and self-understanding allows us to bring to our practice the highest level of mental health nursing care.

References

1. Didato SV: Am I "Normal"? Parade, p 22, September 11, 1983
2. Lipkin GB, Cohen RG: Effective Approaches to Patients' Behavior. New York, Springer–Verlag, 1973
3. Robinson AM: Stress Can Make You—or Break You. RN 38: 73–77, 1975
4. Robinson L: Psychiatric Nursing as a Human Experience, 2d ed. Philadelphia, WB Saunders, 1977
5. Travelbee J: Intervention in Psychiatric Nursing: Process in the One-to-One Relationship. Philadelphia, FA Davis, 1969
6. Woolfolk RL, Richardson FC: Stress, Sanity, and Survival. New York, Monarch, 1978

experienced by the therapists as a result of working with particularly difficult patient behaviors such as negative affect, resistance, suicidal threats, psychopathological symptoms, and passive-aggressive behaviors.[21] Nurses who work as therapists or in other kinds of therapeutic positions with psychiatric clients therefore suffer the effects of personal depletion, the stress of maintaining the therapeutic relationship, work overinvolvement, and so forth, and are also frustrated by difficult patient behaviors.

Use of Nursing Models

There is some truth or usefulness to all models of nursing, given the diverse problems and needs of diverse clients in diverse settings.[9] Important issues to explore in various models include the following:

Who defines the client problems?
Is the client blamed for his problems?
Is the client expected to take responsibility for arriving at solutions to his problems?
Who evaluates the success or failure of the solutions?[5]

Providing people with increased responsibility for solving their own problems develops competence and independence. The medical model of helping, wherein the helpers decide the solutions to client problems, promotes the client's dependence on health care providers.

Roy's model of nursing aims to promote adaptation of the client to a changing environment. The nurse assesses the adaptiveness or maladaptiveness of client behaviors and plans interventions to modify maladaptive behaviors.[9]

The goal of nursing intervention may be regained stability for the client; that is, adaptation of the client to his environment. On the other hand, the goal may be more dynamic and change-oriented, related to an improved level of wellness or mental health.

The long-term nurse-patient relationship traditionally taught to nursing students is rooted in psychoanalytic and interpersonal theories. Many of today's treatment settings and situations, however, need to build their supporting structure on the theories of crisis intervention and brief psychotherapy.[34] Within these time-limited and here-and-now frameworks for therapy, the nurse learns to make rapid assessments, to formulate realistic plans, and to intervene swiftly and appropriately. This approach, by ridding itself of unrealistic goals and plans, may also reduce job frustration and burnout among psychiatric–mental health nurses.

The Nursing Process

The nursing process is a problem-solving approach to effecting change in client problems. The steps of the nursing process—assessment, nursing diagnosis, planning, intervention, and evaluation—allow a systematic method by which nurses deliver care to clients. The American Nurses' Association's Standards of Psychiatric and Mental Health Nursing delineate the scope of nursing practice (see Chart 1-5).

C H A R T 1-5

Standards of Psychiatric and Mental Health Nursing

American Nurses' Association
Division on Psychiatric and Mental Health
Nursing Practice, 1982

Professional Practice Standards

Standard I.   Theory
   The nurse applies appropriate theory that is scientifically sound as a basis for decisions regarding nursing practice.

Standard II.   Data Collection
   The nurse continuously collects data that are comprehensive, accurate, and systematic.

Standard III.   Diagnosis
   The nurse utilizes nursing diagnoses and/or standard classification of mental disorders to express conclusions supported by recorded assessment data and current scientific premises.

Standard IV.   Planning
   The nurse develops a nursing care plan with specific goals and interventions delineating nursing actions unique to each client's needs.

Standard V.   Intervention
   The nurse intervenes as guided by the nursing care plan to implement nursing actions that promote, maintain, or restore physical and mental health, prevent illness, and effect rehabilitation.

Standard V-A.   Intervention: Psychotherapeutic Interventions
   The nurse uses psychotherapeutic interventions to assist clients in regaining or improving their previous coping abilities and to prevent further disability.

Standard V-B.   Intervention: Health Teaching
   The nurse assists clients, families, and groups to achieve satisfying and productive patterns of living through health teaching.

Standard V-C.   Intervention: Activities of Daily Living
   The nurse uses the activities of daily living in a goal-directed way to foster adequate self-care and physical and mental well-being of clients.

Standard V-D.   Intervention: Somatic Therapies
   The nurse uses knowledge of somatic therapies and applies related clinical skills in working with clients.

Standard V-E.   Intervention: Therapeutic Environment
   The nurse provides, structures, and maintains a therapeutic environment in collaboration with the client and other health care providers.

Standard V-F.   Intervention: Psychotherapy
   The nurse utilizes advanced clinical expertise in individual, group, and family psychotherapy, child psychotherapy, and other treatment modalities to function as a psychotherapist, and recognizes professional accountability for nursing practice.

Standard VI.   Evaluation
   The nurse evaluates client responses to nursing actions in order to revise the data base, nursing diagnoses, and nursing care plan.

Standard VII.   Peer Review
   The nurse participates in peer review and other means of evaluation to assure quality of nursing care provided for clients.

Standard VIII.   Continuing Education
   The nurse assumes responsibility for continuing education and professional development and contributes to the professional growth of others.

Standard IX.   Interdisciplinary Collaboration
   The nurse collaborates with other health care providers in assessing, planning, implementing, and evaluating programs and other mental health activities.

Standard X. Utilization of Community
Health Systems
The nurse participates with other members of the community in assessing, planning, implementing, and evaluating mental health services and community systems that include the promotion of the broad continuum of primary, secondary, and tertiary prevention of mental illness.

Standard XI. Research
The nurse contributes to nursing and the mental health field through innovations in theory and practice and participation in research.

Assessment

Assessment, the first step of the nursing process, is the systematic collection of comprehensive data about clients and their problems and needs. Psychological, social, and cultural influences on the client's functioning are explored.

Nursing Diagnosis

The second step of the nursing process, *nursing diagnosis,* includes the organization of data into categories; the determination of actual and potential client problems; analysis of the causes of the problems, if possible; and the formulation of conclusions.

Planning

Planning, the third step of the nursing process, involves the determination, in cooperation with the client and his family, of goals and interventions to achieve the goals.

Intervention

Intervention, the fourth step of the nursing process, is the implementation of nursing activities designed to reach client goals.

Evaluation

Evaluation, the fifth and final step of the nursing process, is the determination of outcomes of nursing interventions. Evaluation of present services may demonstrate the need for additional services; Burgess and Holmstrom's work entitled Rape: Crisis and Recovery, for example, demonstrates the need for services to rape victims to prevent more serious disturbances later.[8]

Part Two of this text, The Process of Psychiatric–Mental Health Nursing, studies in depth each step of the nursing process.

Summary

This chapter introduced the reader to the basic principles of the psychiatric field of nursing. Some of the major emphases of the chapter include the following:

1. Mental health and mental illness are imprecisely defined states.
2. Satisfaction with one's characteristics, abilities, and accomplishments; effective and satisfying interpersonal relationships; effective coping or adaptation to one's life events; and personal growth characterize mental health.
3. The stigma attached to mental illness or disorder may hamper a person's willingness to seek treatment and his rehabilitation.
4. Problems hindering the progress of mental health care today are cost of treatment, separation of clients from their support systems, lack of governmental support of community mental health centers, and unequal access to care.
5. Stress is the nonspecific response of the body to any demand made on it.
6. Stressors, or stress-producing factors, whether physical or psychological, pleasant or unpleasant, elicit the same biologic stress response.
7. The General Adaptation Syndrome evolves in three stages—alarm reaction, stage of resistance, and stage of exhaustion.
8. Coping mechanisms, such as denial, rationalization, regression, fantasy, and so forth, protect the individual from anxiety.
9. Roles of psychiatric–mental health nurses include advocate, communicator, role model, member of the health team, and nurse–therapist.

10. Self-awareness, self-exploration, and working through feelings and reactions to disturbed behavior are necessary for nurses to intervene in therapeutic ways.
11. Job stress and burnout can be minimized through an early detection of symptoms of stress, regular attention to physical health and exercise, and involvement in non-nursing activities.
12. The nursing process—assessment, nursing diagnosis, planning, intervention, and evaluation—is a problem-solving approach by which nurses deliver care to clients.

References

1. Antonovsky A: Health, Stress, and Coping. San Francisco, Jossey-Bass, 1979
2. Bachrach LL: Dimensions of Disability in the Chronic Mentally Ill. Hospital and Community Psychiatry 37 (October): 981–982, 1986
3. Barash DA: Deflecting Suicide: A Clinical Case Report. Bulletin of the Menninger Clinic 50 (4): 367–378, 1986
4. Bloom BL: Focal Issues in the Prevention of Mental Disorders. In Preventing Stress-Related Psychiatric Disorders: Proceedings of a Research Planning Workshop, UCSF, Rockville, MD, National Institute of Mental Health, 1981
5. Bower EM: Prevention: A Word Whose Time Has Come. Am J Orthopsychiatry 57 (January): 4–5, 1987
6. Bruch H: Learning Psychotherapy: Rationale and Ground Rules. Cambridge, Harvard University Press, 1974
7. Burgess AW: Psychiatric Nursing in the Hospital and the Community, 4th ed. Englewood Cliffs, NJ, Prentice-Hall, 1985
8. Burgess AW, Holmstrom LL: Rape: Crisis and Recovery. Bowie, MD, Robert J Brady, 1979
9. Cronenwett LR: Helping and Nursing Models. Nurs Res 32 (November/December): 342–346, 1983
10. Dillon A: Reducing Your Stress: Six Experts Tell You How. Nursing Life 3 (May/June): 17–24, 1983
11. Dolan JA, Fitzpatrick ML, Hermann EK: Nursing in Society: A Historical Perspective, 15th ed. Philadelphia, WB Saunders, 1983
12. Dongier M, Wittkower ED (eds): Divergent Views in Psychiatry. Hagerstown, MD, Harper & Row, 1981
13. Douglas CJ, Druss RG: Denial of Illness: A Reappraisal. Gen Hosp Psychiatry 9 (January): 53–57, 1987
14. Flagg JM: Public Policy and Mental Health: Past, Present, and Future. Nurs Health Care 4 (May): 246–251, 1983
15. Freedman AM, Kaplan HI, Sadock BJ: Modern Synopsis of Comprehensive Textbook of Psychiatry. Baltimore, Williams & Wilkins, 1972
16. Friedrich O: Going Crazy: An Inquiry into Madness in Our Time. New York, Simon and Schuster, 1976
17. Garmezy N: Stress, Competence, and Development: Continuities in the Study of Schizophrenic Adults, Children Vulnerable to Psychopathology, and the Search for Stress-Resistant Children. Am J Orthopsychiatry 57 (April): 159–174, 1987
18. Glazebrook CK, Munjas BA: Sex Roles and Depression. J Psychoso Nurs Ment Health Serv 24 (December): 8–12, 1986
19. Haber J, Leach AM, Schudy SM, Sideleau BF: Comprehensive Psychiatric Nursing, 2d ed. New York, McGraw-Hill, 1982
20. Häfner H: The Concept of Disease in Psychiatry. Psychol Med 17 (February): 11–14, 1987
21. Hellman ID, Morrison TL, Abramowitz SI: Therapist Experience and the Stresses of Psychotherapeutic Work. Psychotherapy 24 (Summer): 171–176, 1987
22. Kalinowsky LB, Hippius H, Klein HE: Biological Treatments in Psychiatry. New York, Grune & Stratton, 1982
23. Kalisch PA, Kalisch BJ: The Advance of American Nursing, 2d ed. Boston, Little, Brown & Co, 1986
24. Kaslow FW et al: Supervision, Consultation, and Staff Training in the Helping Professions. San Francisco, Jossey-Bass, 1977
25. Kravetz D, Jones LE: Androgyny as a Standard of Mental Health. Am J Orthopsychiatry 51 (July): 502–509, 1981
26. Laing RD: The Facts of Life: An Essay in Feelings, Facts, and Fantasy. New York, Pantheon Books, 1976
27. Langner TS, Michael ST: Life Stress and Mental Health: The Midtown Manhattan Study, vol II. London, The Free Press of Glencoe, 1963
28. Lewis JM, Usdin G (eds): Treatment Planning in Psychiatry. Washington, DC, American Psychiatric Association, 1982
29. Looney JG, Blotcky MJ: Special Perspectives on Treatment Planning for Children. In Lewis JM, Usdin G (eds): Treatment Planning in Psychiatry, pp 289–336. Washington, DC, American Psychiatric Association, 1982
30. Luckey JW, Berman JJ: Effects of New Commitment Laws on the Mental Health System. Am J Orthopsychiatry 51: 479–483, 1981
31. Mallick M: Nursing Diagnosis and the Novice Student. Nurs Health Care 4: 455–459, 1983
32. Maslow AH: Toward a Psychology of Being, 2d ed. New York, Van Nostrand Reinhold, 1968
33. Morris MM, Myton CL: Ego Function: Enhancement Through Social Interaction. J Psychosoc Nurs Ment Health Serv 24 (December): 17–22, 1986
34. Nix J, Dillon K: Short-term Nursing Therapy: A Conceptual Model for Inpatient Psychiatric Care.

Hosp Community Psychiatry 37 (May): 493–496, 1986

35. Peplau HE: Interpersonal Relations in Nursing. New York, GP Putnam's & Sons, 1952

36. Rosenhan DL: On Being Sane in Insane Places. In Brink PJ (ed): Transcultural Nursing: A Book of Readings, pp 175–197. Englewood Cliffs, NJ, Prentice-Hall, 1976

37. Ruesch J: Therapeutic Communication. New York, WW Norton & Co, 1973

38. Rutter M: Psychosocial Resilience and Protective Mechanisms. Am J Orthopsychiatry 57 (July): 316–331, 1987

39. Satir V, Bernhard YM, Macdonald N: Using the Family Unit for Change. In Beiser M, Krell R, Lin T, Miller M (eds): Today's Priorities in Mental Health: Knowing and Doing, pp 35–39. Miami, Symposia Specialists, 1978

40. Schwab JJ, Schwab ME: Sociocultural Roots of Mental Illness: An Epidemiologic Survey. New York, Plenum Medical Book Company, 1978

41. Selye H: Stress Without Distress. New York: New American Library, 1974

42. Shires B: Nurses Need Nurturing, Too. Nursing Life 3 (January/February): 40–43, 1983

43. Shives LR: Basic concepts of Psychiatric—Mental Health Nursing. Philadelphia, JB Lippincott Co, 1986

44. Shore MF: Marking Time in the Land of Plenty: Reflections on Mental Health in the United States. Am J Orthopsychiatry 51 (July): 391–402, 1981

45. Smith WK: The Stress Analogy. Schizophr Bull 13 (2): 215–220, 1987

46. Toward a National Policy on Aging. Proceedings of the 1971 White House Conference on Aging, Vol II. Washington, DC, 1971

47. Westlake RJ (ed): Shaping the Future of Mental Health Care. Cambridge, Ballinger, 1976

48. Wilson HS, Kneisl CR: Psychiatric Nursing, 2d ed. Menlo Park, CA, Addison-Wesley Publishing Co, 1983

49. Zinman S: Self-Help: The Wave of the Future. Hosp Community Psychiatry 37 (March): 213, 1986

2 Conceptual Frameworks for Care

Judith A. Greene

The intimate union of theory and practice aids both.
Alfred North Whitehead

Chapter Preview

A *theory* is a conceptual system that describes and explains selected phenomena. In this way, theory serves as a tool to guide and shape human understanding and behavior. To the extent that theories apply to real events, they are considered useful. When theories apply to real nursing events, they serve to guide the understanding and behavior of nurses.

Nurses use theories of human behavior to understand clients and to intervene therapeutically. Theories used by psychiatric–mental health nurses fall into four categories:

Psychoanalytic theory
Behavioristic theory
Biologic theory
Systems theory

Each of these theoretical categories views humankind from a different perspective and thus emphasizes or accentuates one aspect of human existence over others. Nevertheless, all of these theoretical perspectives are equally useful to nurses.

Learning Objectives

On completion of this chapter, you should be able to accomplish the following:

1. explain the purpose of theoretical perspectives or frameworks
2. discuss the basic assumptions underlying the psycholanalytic, behavioristic, biologic, and systems theoretical perspectives
3. apply the selected theoretical perspectives to the nursing care of clients
4. compare the selected theoretical perspectives and their applications to nursing

The Psychoanalytic Theoretical Perspective

The psychoanalytic theoretical perspective is derived from the work of Sigmund Freud and his followers. Psychoanalytic theory is deterministic in nature and reflects a pessimistic attitude toward society's and humankind's potential for constructive change.[1,3] The basic assumptions underlying this theoretical perspective include the following:

1. All human behavior is caused and thus is capable of explanation. Slips of the tongue, accidents, dreams, artistic creations, and all other forms of human behavior have meaning and, therefore, can be explained.[6] In other words, human behavior, however obscure, does not occur randomly or by chance; rather, all human behavior is determined by antecedent life events.

2. All human behavior from birth to old age is driven by an energy called the *libido*. The goal of the libido is the reduction of tension through the attainment of pleasure. The libido is closely associated with physiological or instinctual drives (hunger, thirst, elimination, sex). Release of these drives results in the reduction of tension, which is experienced as pleasure; hence, the *pleasure principle* becomes operative when pleasure-seeking behaviors are employed.[10]

3. Human behavior that channels impulsive pleasure-seeking behaviors into creative pursuits (sublimation) is considered the highest form of human expression. Maturity is thus associated with the ability to invent and use substitutive or disguised forms of gratification.[10] This ability to delay pleasure in favor of more acceptable behavior is referred to as the *reality principle*.

4. The personality of the human being can be understood by way of three major hypothetical structures: id, ego, and superego.

The *id* represents the most primitive structure of the human personality; it houses the instincts. The id cannot delay the attainment of pleasure. Human behavior that originates from the id is impulsive, pleasure-oriented, disconnected from reality, and consequently often inappropriate. Thought processes deriving from the id are characterized by their illogic, confused form, and preverbal content.[10] Such thought patterns are referred to as *primary process*. Examples of primary process thought are often reflected in verbalizations of psychotic schizophrenic individuals (see Chap. 24).

The *superego* is the personality structure that contains the values, legal and moral regulations, and social expectations that thwart the free expression of pleasure-seeking behaviors. The superego thus functions to oppose the id. Society and the family determine the content of the superego and the kinds of limitations it places on the individual.[6]

The *ego* represents that part of the human personality that has greatest contact with reality. Unlike the id, the ego is capable of postponing pleasure until an appropriate time, place, or object is available. Unlike the superego, the ego is not driven to blind conformity with rules and regulations. Rather, the ego, acting as a mediator between the id and the superego, gives rise to more mature and adaptive behavior.[10]

With the id and superego constantly at odds with one another, the ego is faced with the task of maintaining control over instinctual impulses while simultaneously taking into consideration moral values and injunctions. Understandably, the human being from time to time experiences anxiety when confronted with situations that challenge the tenuous balance between the id and the superego. At these times, the ego employs defense mechanisms to ward off anxiety.[8] Among the defense mechanisms commonly used are repression, denial, regression, rationalization, reaction formation, undoing, projection, displacement, sublimation, isolation, and fixation.

5. The human personality functions on three levels of awareness: the conscious, preconscious, and unconscious. *Consciousness* refers to the perceptions, thoughts, and feelings existing in a person's immediate awareness. *Preconscious* content, on the other hand, is not immediately accessible to awareness. The person must make an effort to retrieve this content before it reaches awareness. Unlike both conscious and preconscious content, *unconscious* material remains inaccessible for the most part.[10]

6. The unconscious affects all three structures of the personality—the id, superego, and ego. Though the id's content resides totally in the unconscious, the superego and ego have aspects in all three levels of consciousness.[10] Through these three levels of consciousness, the ego maintains contact with reality as well as with the id and superego.

7. Human personality development unfolds through five innate stages referred to as *psychosexual stages*. The sequence of these stages corresponds to the changing manner in which the individual seeks pleasure. The stages are called psychosexual stages because the theory further assumes that all pleasure is essentially sexual in nature. These stages are the oral, anal, phallic, latency, and genital stages. While these stages extend throughout the lifespan, the theory also holds that the first six years of life determine the individual's long-term personality characteristics.[10] That is, early life events, especially with regard to parent-child experiences, determine the individual's behavior throughout life.

8. Despite this theory's deterministic and pessimistic view of human behavior, it assumes that human personality and behavior possess enough flexibility to progress toward change.[7]

Therapeutic Approaches

In keeping with these basic assumptions, the psychoanalytic view of human behavior relies on the therapeutic approach of *psychoanalysis*. This therapeutic approach is exercised by psychiatrists, psychologists, and psychiatric–mental health nurses who have undergone extensive education and training in its use. Psychoanalysis employs strategies such as hypnosis, dream interpretation, and free association (in which the client verbalizes every idea that comes to mind regardless of how trivial or shameful it may sound). The psychoanalyst attempts to maintain a relatively passive demeanor in order to create a neutral environment devoid of approval or disapproval and to encourage the client to be natural. When the psychoanalyst interacts with the client, it is usually to make an interpretation of the client's verbal or nonverbal behavior. No touching occurs between the client and psychoanalyst. Usually the psychoanalyst remains largely out of the client's sight.[7]

The primary goal of psychoanalysis is to create a permissive, yet safe, situation in which the client can recall past traumas and work through residual conflicts and emotions that have thwarted or fixated his growth and integration as a person. In short, the goal is to help the client release his full potential as a healthy, well-integrated human being.

Application to Nursing

Psychoanalytic theory has influenced psychiatric–mental health nursing in many ways. This theoretical perspective, perhaps more than any other, has helped mental health professionals understand psychopathology and stress-related behaviors. More important, this theory illustrates the importance of not taking human behavior at face value. That is, it helps the psychiatric–mental health nurse to discern and explore the meaning behind human behavior.

The Behavioristic Theoretical Perspective

The behavioristic theoretical perspective derives from the works of Ivan Pavlov, John Watson, and B.F. Skinner. Like psychoanalytic theory, the behavioristic theoretical perspective is deterministic in nature. But unlike psychoanalytic theory, the behavioristic theoretical perspective is concerned only with observable behavior, rather than with unconscious processes or the personality itself.[1] Several basic assumptions underlie the behavioristic theoretical perspective.

1. All human behavior is a response to a stimulus or to stimuli from the environment.
2. Human beings are passive organisms that can be conditioned or shaped to do anything if correct responses to specific stimuli are rewarded or reinforced.
3. Human beings can control or determine the behavior of others, whether or not they wish to be controlled.
4. The human personality is a mere pattern of stimulus–response chains or habits.
5. Both adaptive and maladaptive behaviors are learned and perpetuated through reinforcements.
6. Maladaptive behavior can be unlearned and replaced by adaptive behavior if the person receives exposure to specific stimuli and reinforcements for the desired adaptive behavior.[4,9]

Therapeutic Approaches

Several therapeutic approaches stem from the behavioristic theoretical perspective. *Token reinforcement* is one such approach. With this approach, the direct use of reinforcers is delayed through the administration of tokens. When desired adaptive behavioral responses are emitted, tokens are awarded. After a specific number of adaptive behavioral responses occur, then the tokens can be redeemed for actual reinforcers, such as an extra cup of coffee or a higher level of privileges.[10]

Shaping is another behavioral reinforcement technique used to condition close approximations of some desired adaptive behavior. In applying this technique, reinforcement of successively closer approximations occurs until the final adaptive behavioral outcome is reached.[10] Shaping requires careful observation and a great deal of patience to identify and reinforce desired behavior approximations.

Other behavior-change techniques derived from the behavioristic approach include relaxation therapy, aversion conditioning, implosion, flooding, and assertiveness training. In using these techniques, the therapist usually determines what behavior should be changed and what behavioral approach to use to effect that change.

Application to Nursing

Nurses with advanced psychiatric–mental health education often employ behavioristic techniques in working with chronically mentally ill clients in one-to-one as well as group situations. They may also manage psychiatric settings based on behavioral strategies. Nurses who work with physically disabled clients in rehabilitation settings may find behavioristic strategies useful.

The Biologic Theoretical Perspective

This theoretical perspective originated in the early era of psychiatric medicine as the result of an effort to explain the causes of maladaptive behavior. The following biologic factors are often offered as possible causes of maladaptive behavior:

Genetic factors. Defective genes due to heredity, mutation, or chromosome damage
Congenital factors. Defects present at birth due to intra-uterine damage or birth injuries
General health. Effect on mood, stress tolerance, energy level, and sensitivity to stimuli.
Specific physical conditions. Disease, endocrine or other hormonal imbalances, auto-immune reactions, or chemicals introduced into the human organism
Fatigue. Physical exhaustion associated with the lack of sleep, of relaxation, and of recreation

Much research has been and is being conducted into causal relationships between or among these factors and specific forms of mental illness.[1] To date, conclusive evidence of causal relationships between or among the factors and specific maladaptive behaviors has not been scientifically demonstrated. Nevertheless, this theoretical perspective is useful to psychiatric nurses and other mental health care providers in both its practical and its scientific applications.

The assumptions underlying the biologic theoretical perspective include the following:

Departures from normal adaptive behavior are due to either organic illnesses, structural or genetic defects, or biological imbalances affecting the central nervous system.
Restoration to adaptive mental health usually requires somatic therapy, such as psychotropic medications, psychosurgery, hormonal therapy, or electroconvulsive therapy.
Mental or psychological illnesses are like physical ill

nesses in that they can be either cured or controlled through medical or surgical treatments. Psychosocial or interpersonal processes play no real role in the etiology of maladaptive behaviors.[1]

Application to Nursing

While the biologic theoretical perspective places little emphasis on psychosocial etiologic explanations of maladaptive behavior, it does provide explanations for why some therapies control symptoms of maladaptive behavior. Critics of this theoretical approach, however, claim that it has unnecessarily resulted in the relabeling of a large number of human problems as medical problems. As a consequence of this relabeling process, potentially dangerous or addictive psychoactive agents are prescribed and administered to ever-increasing numbers of people.[1] For this reason, nurses assisting with somatic therapies must be constantly mindful of both the benefits and the detrimental effects of somatic therapies. More important, nurses must be careful to avoid viewing somatic therapies as easy answers to complex human problems, for, where human behavior is concerned, there are no easy answers.

The Systems Theory Perspective

This theoretical perspective derives chiefly from the works of Ludwig von Bertalanffy.[12,13] It has influenced the ways in which dyadic, group, family, and organizational behaviors have been analyzed and explained by other theorists of human behavior.[2,11] Some basic assumptions of this theory, as well as others derived from it, include the following:

1. The human being is a living, open system consisting of interrelated subsystems.[5,13]
2. These interrelated subsystems are components or parts of the total human organism.[5,13]
3. These subsystems in relation to each other tie the human system together forming a whole.[13]
4. Individual subsystems or subwholes possess attributes in common with each other and with the human system as a whole. Consequently, every part of the human system is so related to its fellow parts that a change in one part or subsystem will cause a change in the remaining parts or subsystems.[13]
5. Thus, the human system behaves not as a composite of independent elements, but coherently and as an inseparable whole.[5,13]
6. The human system is surrounded by a boundary that separates it from the surrounding environment. Information may cross this boundary in order to enter or leave the human system.[13]
7. The five sensory channels plus the verbal and nonverbal behavioral modes of the human system are the boundary separating the human system from the surrounding environment. Information that crosses this boundary provides sensory input to the human system. The human system then transforms this sensory input into useful, meaningful forms. This transformation process, referred to as thruput, involves feeding the sensory input through thoughts, feelings, memories, values, attitudes, intelligence, physiological structures, and so forth. In turn, the human system produces information (output) which can be fed back to the human organism itself or to the environment and other human beings through verbal and nonverbal behaviors. Output, also referred to as feedback, is not always equivalent or similar to input; consequently, output is not always predictable on the basis of input. The reason for this lack of predictability is that the transformation of input (the thruput process) is unique for each human system.
8. The human system tends to favor a steady state, in which there is an orderly exchange of information or input within the human system and between the human system and the environment.[5]
9. Disruption of stability results in stress on the total human system, and this stress affects the amount of energy available to activate or maintain the human organism. The amount of available energy in turn affects the quality and quantity of information processing. Lastly, the effect of stress and the accompanying change in energy level affect not only informational input and thruput processes but also the quality and quantity of the human organism's output; that is, of its verbal and nonverbal behavior.

Application to Nursing

According to systems theory, the goal of nursing care is to help clients maintain or regain a steady state. This theory also provides the nurse with a wholistic theoretical perspective from which to understand the human being. In other words, systems theory resolves the mind–body dispute by viewing the human organism from a matter–energy–information perspective.

Recognizing that human beings are not simple, passive organisms, this theory assists the nurse to ob-

Table 2-1.   **Conceptual Models of Treatment**

MODEL	SUBJECT	INTERVENTIONS
Psychoanalytic	Developmental events causing mental illness	Psychoanalysis Free association Dream interpretation Hypnosis
Behavioristic	Stimuli causing human behavior	Token economy Behavior modification Shaping Operant conditioning
Biologic	Physical illness or defect causing mental illness	Chemotherapy Psychosurgery Insulin coma therapy Electroconvulsive therapy
Systems	Whole system and subsystems	Interpersonal Environmental Physical treatment Social change Family treatment

serve and understand how clients affect and are affected by the environment, by other people, and by themselves. In providing such a wholistic viewpoint, systems theory allows the nurse to identify client strengths that can be used to overcome or compensate for weaknesses and limitations. Moreover, this theory views the human being as complex; it acknowledges that human behavior has multiple causes and meanings. In doing so, the systems theory performs its most valuable function—shedding light on the uniqueness and complexity of human life.

Summary

This chapter has examined various theoretical bases for understanding human behavior and intervening in maladaptive behavior (Table 2-1 summarizes the four types of theories discussed). Some of the major points of the chapter are as follows:

1. Psychoanalytic, behavioristic, and biologic theoretical perspectives emphasize that human behavior is largely determined by external forces or other factors outside the individual's control; that is, the human being is viewed as a passive organism.
2. Systems theory acknowledges the effect of external forces on human behavior, but maintains that the individual can either influence these outside forces or compensate for them; that is, the individual is viewed as an active and interactive human system.
3. Psychoanalytic, behavioristic, and biologic the-

oretical perspectives hold that human behavior is monocausal; in other words, it is determined by one cause.
4. Psychoanalytic theory holds that behavior is determined by early life events with parental figures.
5. Behavioristic theory holds that exposure to given stimuli and reinforcements determine how the human being learns to behave.
6. The biologic theoretical perspective holds that human behavior is determined by the individual's genetic and biologic constitution.
7. Systems theory holds that human behavior has multiple causes.
8. All four theoretical perspectives are useful to nurses in assessing, diagnosing, planning, implementing, and evaluating nursing care.

References

1. Bart PB: Ideologies and Utopias of Psychotherapy. In Roman PM, Trice HM (eds): The Sociology of Psychotherapy, pp 9–55. New York, Aronson, 1974
2. Boulding KE: General Systems Theory: The Skeleton of Science. In Modern Systems Research for the Behavioral Scientist, pp 3–10. Chicago, Aldine Publishing, 1968
3. Freud S: Civilization and Its Discontents. New York, WW Norton & Co, 1961
4. Hilgard ER, Bower GH: Theories of Learning, 4th ed. Englewood Cliffs, Prentice-Hall, 1975
5. Miller JG: General Living Systems Theory. In Freeman AM, Kaplan HI, Sadock BJ (eds): Compre-

hensive Textbook of Psychiatry/III, Vol. 1, 3d ed, pp 98–114, Baltimore, Williams & Wilkins, 1980

6. Nye RD: Three Views of Man. Monterey, CA, Brooks/Cole, 1975

7. Offenkrantz W, Tabin A: Psychoanalytic Psychotherapy. In Arieti S (ed): American Handbook of Psychiatry, Vol. 5, 2d ed, pp 183–205. New York, Basic Books, 1975

8. Roberts SL: Behavioral Concepts and Nursing Throughout the Life Span. Englewood Cliffs, NJ, Prentice-Hall, 1978

9. Snelbecker GE: Learning Theory, Instructional Theory, and Psychoeducational Design. New York, McGraw-Hill, 1974

10. Starr BD, Goldstein HS: Human Development and Behavior. New York, Springer, 1975

11. Sutherland JW: A General Systems Philosophy for the Social and Behavioral Sciences. New York, George Braziller, 1973

12. von Bertalanffy L: General System Theory. New York, George Braziller, 1968

13. von Bertalanffy L: General System Theory and Psychiatry. In Arieti, S (ed): American Handbook of Psychiatry, Vol. 1, 2d ed, pp 1095–1117. New York, Basic Books, 1975

3

Nursing Theory and Psychiatric–Mental Health Practice

Judith A. Greene

*To engage in theorizing means not just to learn by experience
but to take thought about what is there to be learned. To speak
loosely, lower animals grasp scientific laws but never rise to the
level of scientific theory. They learn by experience but not from
it, for from learning requires symbolic constructions which can
provide vicarious experience never actually undergone.*

Abraham Kaplan
The Conduct of Inquiry, 1964

Chapter Preview

An enormous and ever-increasing body of literature addresses the subject of nursing theory. These literary efforts have largely been directed toward the explication of nursing phenomena and the delimitation of nursing's philosophical, educational, practical, and research boundaries. As a result of these efforts, a wide array of published opinions currently exist with regard to nursing's essence and functions. This diversity is reflected in several conceptual schemes commonly referred to as nursing theories.

Learning Objectives

On completion of this chapter, you should be able to accomplish the following:

1. define the term "theory"
2. identify three types of theory
3. discuss the functions of theory
4. identify types of nursing theory applicable to psychiatric–mental health nursing
5. analyze selected nursing theories according to type and major conceptual components

Theory Defined

A theory is conceptual system consisting of interrelated propositions that describe, explain, and predict selected phenomena. As such, a theory functions to order knowledge about reality. No single theory, however, can address all aspects of reality. Rather, a theory orders knowledge about a specific aspect of the real world and suggests ways of further extending and refining that knowledge through scientific research.

All theories are tentative in nature and subject to change or even to obsolescence. The extent to which a theory is verified by scientific research determines its validity and usefulness. When a theory begins to falter under repeated scientific investigations, it is either changed or discarded. Thus, a theory does not represent an absolute truth but rather serves as a tool to increase understanding of the real world.

Types of Theory

Most theories can be classified as *deductive, inductive,* or *analogical* in nature. *Deductive theory* consists of a large group of propositional statements based on minimal sensory information that are developed and interconnected through deductive logic. Because deductive theory is based on minimal sensory information, it is assumed that it may contain faulty or incorrect theoretical details. It is further assumed, however, that these faults will be corrected through scientific research. Examples of deductive theory include psychoanalytic theory, quantum theory, and general system theory.

Inductive theory, on the other hand, consists of a modest group of summary statements or generalizations based on ample sensory information. Unlike deductive theory, inductive theory maintains a close connection between observation and conceptualization. Consequently, inductive theory uses deductive logic minimally and contains few inferential statements. A well-known inductive theory is Skinner's behavioristic theory.

Analogic theory differs significantly from both deductive and inductive theory. An analogic theory, more commonly referred to as a model, depicts or explains relationships between things, events, objects, or functions that are basically different yet share similar attributes. Statements of relationship articulated in this way may be based more on imagination than on reality, in that analogic theory relies chiefly on thinking of the "as if" variety. That is, analogic theory focuses primarily on discerning comparisons, correspondences, parallels, or associations that may or may not actually exist. For this reason, hypotheses derived from analogic theory seldom hold up to scientific investigation. Despite this fact, however, analogic theory can be useful in both theory construction and scientific research.

Numerous examples of analogic theory exist. Most notable among these in nursing literature is Roy's Adaptation Model. In constructing this theory, Roy used Helson's theory of learning and adaptation as a model to organize nursing concepts in a logical pattern. Roy believed not only that the logical pattern of Helson's theory corresponded to the logical sequence of events in nursing practice, but also that some content of Helson's theory applied to nursing.

Functions of Theory

Theory functions not only to organize knowledge, but also to suggest ways of validating and extending knowledge through scientific research. Theory also enables people to accurately predict future events; it can thus serve as a guide to human action. Most important, theory enables individuals to understand phenomena in relation to their unique situations. Through this understanding, individuals may be able not only to predict accurately the outcome of their actions, but also to gain some control over the course of future events.

Nursing Theory

The development of theory, rather than the standardization of roles and procedures, is necessary for the further development of nursing as a profession. Several nurse theorists have made significant contributions toward this goal. Some theorists, such as Peplau, Travelbee, and Orlando, have focused on the interpersonal relationship or interaction between the nurse and the client. Others, such as Roy, Orem, and Johnson, have focused on the behavioral effects of nursing. Still others, such as Neuman and Rogers, have attempted to address the entire field of phenomena associated with nursing from a systems perspective.

To a great extent, almost all current nursing theories can be classified as *interpersonal, behavioral,* or *systems-oriented* in nature. Some nursing theories, however, reflect mixed characteristics of these types. Nursing theories in each of these classes are useful in psychiatric–mental health nursing as well as in other nursing specialties. Furthermore, analyzing nursing theories according to classification, theory-type, and function assists in their application to psychiatric–mental nursing practice and research.

Analysis of Selected Nursing Theories

Peplau's Theory

Hildegard Peplau has been a pioneer in formulating nursing theory. Drawing on the works of Harry S. Sullivan and Rollo May and her own clinical experience, Peplau proposed an *interpersonal theory* applicable to nursing practice in general and to psychiatric–mental health nursing in particular. Peplau described the interpersonal aspects of nursing as a process.

This process consists of four phases. The first phase is the *orientation phase,* in which the nurse and client meet as strangers, exchange social amenities, and then proceed to clarify each other's roles. From this initial phase, the nurse and client enter the *identification phase*. During this phase the nurse assists the client to express his feelings and to correct or clarify misconceptions based on previous life and health care experiences. Through these transactions, the nurse and client begin to experience each other as unique individuals. As a result, the client experiences acceptance and a high degree of trust in the nurse.

The foundation provided by these first two phases prepares the nurse and client to enter the *exploitation phase*. During this phase, the client begins to derive the full value of the nurse-client relationship. The client begins to test alternative ways of coping with his health problems and to formulate goals for the future. As the client becomes more skillful in employing the problem-solving process, convalescence begins.

As convalescence progresses, the client and nurse enter the *resolution phase* of the nurse-client relationship. The groundwork for terminating the relationship was initiated during the orientation phase. It is during the resolution phase, however, that the nurse and client complete the work associated with terminating the relationship. Ideally, both nurse and client experience termination as a freeing process in which both of them experience fulfillment; the nurse feels fulfilled professionally while the client moves toward greater maturity.

While working with the client through these phases, the nurse assumes six roles, Initially, the nurse assumes the role of *stranger* because the nurse and client do not know each other. The tasks of forming trust and acceptance are most prominent at this time.

As the client's needs and limitations are assessed, the nurse assumes the role of *resource expert* in an effort to provide alternative ways of meeting client needs and to assist the client in reducing his limitations. Because the client may be incapacitated or immobilized physically and emotionally, the nurse may also need to assume the role of *leader* during the relationship to ensure that client needs are addressed.

Another role assumed by the nurse is that of *surrogate*. Because clients often regress during illness and have dependency needs associated with earlier developmental stages, they often unconsciously view nurses as parent substitutes. As the nurse assumes the role of *counselor*, the client is assisted to recall past experiences and traumas and to work through these. The role of *teacher* is also assumed in an attempt to assist the client to learn from present and past experiences and traumas.

Analysis of Peplau's Theory

As stated previously, Peplau's nursing theory can be classified as *interpersonal* in natural because it focuses primarily on the nurse-client relationship. Although the influence of Harry S. Sullivan, Rollo May, and other theorists is obvious, Peplau's is an *inductive theory* because it is based predominantly on her observations and clinical experience. Although this theory is logically developed, it lacks the intricate, formal logic characteristic of deductive theory. Additionally, it appears that Peplau has taken special care to keep the theory's generalizations closely attached to observable nursing situations.

Although Peplau's theory describes, explains, predicts, and to some extent permits control of the sequence of events occurring in the nurse-client relationship, it has some limitations. It is of minimal use in short-term, acute care nursing settings, in which hospitalizations last only for hours, or at most for a few days, precluding relationship development. Additionally, it is applicable only to dyadic nurse-client relationships. Nurse-client relationships in which the client is a group of individuals, a family, or a community are not addressed. Despite these limitations, however, Peplau's theory continues to apply to today's nursing scene, especially with respect to long-term care in ambulatory, home health, and in-hospital psychiatric–mental health care settings. In these settings, Peplau's work continues to stand the test of time.

Orem's Theory

Dorothea E. Orem also has been a pioneer in developing nursing theory. The theoretical origins of her theory are not readily recognizable. It appears that the development of her theory was based primarily on her own observations, particularly the self-care behavioral capacities of clients and required nursing care behaviors. Orem's theory can thus be typed as an *inductive theory* and classified as a *behavioral* nursing theory.

Orem's theory is based on the premise that persons need a composite of self-care actions in order to survive. Self-care actions consist of all behaviors performed by individuals to maintain life, health, and well-being. The capacity of the client and the client's family to perform self-care is referred to as *self-care agency*. Orem states that a need for nursing care exists if the client's *self-care demand* exceeds the client's self-care agency. Thus, the goal of nursing is to meet the client's self-care demands until he or his family is capable of doing so.

According to Orem's theory, there are three types of self-care: universal, developmental, and health deviation.

Universal self-care behaviors are required to meet physiologic and psychosocial needs.
Developmental self-care behaviors are required to undergo normal human development.
Health deviation self-care behaviors are required to meet client needs during health deviations.

The classification of self-care behaviors in this manner is for the purpose of making a complete assessment of the client's self-care agency.

Although Orem's theory does not specifically incorporate the standard nursing process, the following components of the nursing process are easily discernible: assessment, planning, and implementation. Assessment focuses on the client's self-care demand, self-care agency, and self-care deficits. Orem's theory does not specifically address nursing diagnoses derived from analysis of the assessment information. A plan, however, is formulated from the information obtained in the assessment.

The plan indicates the nursing approach needed to meet the client's needs. These plans can be categorized as follows:

Wholly compensatory, in which the client does not participate behaviorally in self-care.
Partially compensatory, in which both the client and nurse participate behaviorally in meeting the client's self-care needs.
Educative development, in which the client meets his own self-care needs with minimal nursing assistance.

To implement the required nursing approach, the nurse uses one of five behaviors:

1. Acting or doing for the client
2. Guidance
3. Supporting
4. Providing
5. Teaching

The nurse does not evaluate the effects or results of these behaviors, but rather evaluates whether the client still requires nursing care. According to Orem, the need for nursing intervention ceases when either the client or the client's family is able to meet the client's self-care demands.

Analysis of Orem's Theory

Orem's theory consists of a small group of summary statements or generalizations regarding nursing. These statements appear to be based on Orem's observations and analyses of nursing phenomena and are virtually devoid of deductive logic. Consequently, this theory can be typed as an *inductive theory*. Because Orem's work focuses primarily on self-care related behaviors, it can also be classified as a *behavioral nursing theory*.

The strength of Orem's theory lies in its emphasis on the capabilities rather than the limitations of clients. Additionally, the theory explains the necessity of the client's and his family's involvement in the nursing process. Furthermore, Orem's theory does not permit the client to be forced into a passive, dependent role.

The major weaknesses of Orem's theory are twofold. First, the theory's language is somewhat confusing and unnecessarily complex. For example, the term "self-care agency" could be more simply phrased as "self-care capacity."

The second and more important major weakness lies in the theory's failure to address the evaluation of the effects of nursing care behaviors. This failure precludes the use of the theory to guide evaluation research concerning the effectiveness of nursing care. This weakness, however, could be easily eliminated through further development of the theory with regard to nursing diagnosis and criteria for evaluating the results of nursing care behaviors.

Rogers's Theory

Martha Rogers, another pioneer in nursing theory development, proposed a theory concerning the nature of humankind from what she considered a unique nursing perspective. The theory has close ties to Bertalanffy's general system theory and physics. Because Rogers drew extensively on the content and deductive logical form of these two bodies of knowledge, her theory can be typed as both *analogical* and *deductive* in nature. It can also be classified as a *systems-oriented* nursing theory because of the strong influence of general system theory.

Rogers's theory is based on four major premises. The first premise is that the human organism is characterized by *openness* and, as a result, is in continuous mutual interaction with the environment. Secondly, the human organism is conceptualized as having an energy field which is in constant mutual interaction with the energy fields of the environment and of other human organisms. This dynamic mutual interaction can be perceived as wave patterns or auras. Third, the way in which the energy fields appear is characterized by organized patterns or designs. Fourth, human existence is four- rather than three-dimensional. Four-dimensionality, according to Rogers, is the human being's capacity to transcend conventional concepts of time-space interaction.

Rogers's three principles of homeodynamics rest upon these four premises. The first principle of homeodynamics asserts that human life proceeds in one direction along a spirallike course. Because human organisms are open systems with energy fields capable of continuous, mutual interaction with the environment and each other, *organized patterns*

emerge depicting the mutual interaction of human and environmental energy fields along a unidirectional spiral through time and space. The simultaneous mutual interaction of human and environmental energy fields is referred to as *complementarity*.

When complementarity between organisms and their environments encounters interference, the four-dimensional aspect of human existence comes into play. To reduce interference and restore order and complementarity, the individual has the capacity to transcend time and space; this transcendence results in paranormal experiences such as clairvoyance and other altered states of consciousness. These paranormal experiences may provide information needed by the individual to reduce untoward interference and restore balance and resonancy to his or her life. Rogers's theory accounts for these phenomena by suggesting that loops of the individual's unidirectional spirallike life trajectory—and their respective energy fields—come temporarily into close proximity, transcending time and space and permitting the occurrence of paranormal phenomena.

The goals of nursing, according to Rogers, are to maintain and promote the maximum health potential of clients, to prevent disease, to formulate nursing diagnoses, and to provide rehabilitative nursing care. From these goals, it is evident that Rogers believed that all individuals, sick or well, rich or poor, in all geographic locations, require nursing services. Rogers did not, however, delineate an operational framework for the nursing process to take place in administering these services.

Analysis of Rogers's Theory

The major strengths of Rogers's theory are twofold. First, the theory is holistic and takes into account the entire field of phenomena associated with nursing. The theory addresses the psychological, social, environmental, physiologic, and physical realms of human existence and attempts to relate these to nursing. Second, Rogers's theory addresses the spirituality of human existence by attempting to explain the four-dimensionality of the universe and the occurrence of paranormal experiences. In doing so, Rogers implicitly suggested that further study of these phenomena may eventually change the way psychiatric–mental health nurses and other similar professionals regard and treat what are now viewed as mental illnesses.

A major weakness of Rogers's theory lies in the fact that its terminology is overly complex. Additionally, the absence or weakness of logical bridges or transitions between or among its conceptual components obfuscates the theory's content. Nevertheless,

Rogers's theory has contributed and will contribute to nursing practice, theory development, and research because it broadens both the minds and imaginations of nurses and the field of nursing itself.

As stated previously, Rogers's theory has characteristics of both *deductive* and *analogical* theory. Rogers used a diagrammatical model of a spiral to depict the life trajectory of the human organism and to illustrate the ways in which energy fields emanate from the individual and the immediate environment; the use of this diagram is one example of the analogical component of her theory. Also analogical is Rogers's use of the logical framework of system theory and physics laws also reflects the analogical nature of her theory. Because it is organized using deductive logic and based on minimal observations, Rogers's theory may also be typed as a deductive theory.

Summary

This chapter has provided the reader with an overview and analysis of the concept of theory, the types and functions of theory, the application of theory to nursing in general, and selected nursing theories applicable to psychiatric–mental health nursing in particular. This chapter includes the following major points:

1. A theory is a conceptual system consisting of interrelated propositions that describe, explain, and predict selected phenomena.
2. All theories are tentative in nature and subject to change or obsolescence.
3. The extent to which a theory is verified by scientific research determines its validity and usefulness.
4. A theory is not absolutely true.
5. Theory can usually be classified as deductive, inductive, or analogical in nature.
6. Theory functions to organize knowledge and to suggest ways of validating and extending knowledge through scientific research.
7. Theory also permits prediction of future events and thus serves as a guide to human action.
8. The development of theory is necessary for the development of nursing as a profession.
9. Most current nursing theories can be classified as interpersonal, behavioral, or systems-oriented in nature.
10. Hildegard Peplau, Dorothea Orem, and Martha Rogers, all of whom are pioneers in nursing theory development, have formulated theories applicable to psychiatric–mental health nursing.

References

1. Brodbeck M (ed): Readings in the Philosophy of the Social Sciences. New York, Macmillan, 1968
2. Bush H: Models for Nursing. Adv Nurs Sci 1 (2): 13–20, 1979
3. Ellis R: Characteristics of Significant Theories. Nurs Res 17 (3): 217–222, 1968
4. Fitzpatrick J, Whall A, Johnston R, Floyd J: Nursing Models and Their Psychiatric Mental Health Applications. Bowie, MD, Brady Co, 1982
5. Hardy ME: Theories: Components, Development, Evaluation. Nurs Res 23 (2): 100–107, 1974
6. Hardy ME: Perspectives on Nursing Theory. Adv Nurs Sci 1 (1): 37–48, 1979
7. Hempel CG, Aspects of Scientific Explanation and Other Essays in the Philosophy of Science. New York, Free Press, 1965
8. Johnson DE: Development of Theory: A Requisite for Nursing as a Primary Health Profession. Nurs Res 23 (5): 372–377, 1974
9. Kaplan A: The Conduct of Inquiry. New York, Thomas Y. Crowell, 1964
10. Khun TS: Structure of Scientific Revolutions. Chicago, University of Chicago Press, 1965
11. McFarlane JK: Developing a Theory of Nursing: The Relation of Theory to Practice, Education, and Research. J Adv Nurs 2:261–270, 1977
12. Nagel E: The Structure of Science. New York, Harcourt, Brace, and World, 1961
13. Neuman B: The Neuman Systems Model: Application to Nursing Education and Practice. Norwalk, CT, Appleton-Century-Crofts, 1982
14. Orem D: Nursing: Concepts of Practice, 2d ed. New York, McGraw-Hill, 1980
15. Orlando I: The Dynamic Nurse-Patient Relationship. New York, GP Putnam's Sons, 1961
16. Peplau H: Interpersonal Relations in Nursing. New York, GP Putnam's Sons, 1952
17. Rogers M: Nursing Science: An Introduction to the Theoretical Basis of Nursing. Philadelphia, FA Davis, 1970
18. Roy SC: Adaptation: A Conceptual Framework for Nursing. Nurs Outlook, 18 (3): 42–45, 1970
19. Roy SC: Adaptation: A Basis for Nursing Practice. Nurs Outlook 19 (4): 254–257, 1971
20. Suppe F: The Structure of Scientific Theories, 2d ed. Chicago, University of Illinois Press, 1977
21. Sutherland JW: A General Systems Philosophy for the Social and Behavioral Sciences. New York, Braziller, 1973
22. Travelbee J: Interpersonal Aspects of Nursing, 2d ed. Philadelphia, FA Davis, 1971
23. Von Bertalanffy L: General System Theory. New York, Braziller, 1968

4 Communication

Juliann Casey Reakes

So healthy, sound, clear, and whole.
Alfred Lord Tennyson

Chapter Preview

Adaptation to the environment is one of the goals of productive living. The interpersonal process is an indispensable component of psychiatric–mental health nursing that facilitates the adaptation process. This chapter focuses on the experiences that assist the client to understand and learn new, adaptive ways of dealing with the environment and developing patterns of productive living.

Both the client and nurse make interpretations and evaluate each other's behavior in an interactive process.[6] This chapter emphasizes how nurses learn to become skillful communicators who extrapolate from both the nursing and communication processes to build a relationship with a client that is therapeutic for the client and professionally functional for the nurse.

Learning Objectives

Upon completion of the chapter, you should be able to accomplish the following:

1. define communication and the communication process
2. describe the nursing communication model
3. discuss the interrelationships of the components of the communication process
4. assess the communication needs and problems of clients
5. explain the nurse's use of listening and observation skills in the therapeutic communication
6. identify therapeutic uses of self-disclosure
7. apply the techniques of therapeutic communication, including the following:
   clarification
   reflection
   confrontation
   verification
   self-disclosure
   informing
   silence
   summarizing
   directing
   questioning
8. identify barriers to therapeutic communication
9. list goals for intervening in psychotic communication

Communication Process

Each person has a unique relationship with the environment that is manifested in behavior. The transport system for behavior is the process known as communication. *Behavior* can be thought of as a transmission or series of transmissions that take place when the individual interacts with the environment. Communication is the conveyor of these transmissions and is always present and occurring.[26] Even if an individual tried, he could never *not* communicate; his lack of verbalization, eye contact, and so forth would communicate something to others.

Communication is a personal, interactive system—a series of ever-changing, ongoing transactions in the environment. Transmissions are simultaneously received (or decoded), are sent (or encoded), and are influenced by the sum total of the experiences and perceptions of the receivers and senders.

Purpose of Communication

Interaction with others gives the individual a sense of identity and being. A person's concept of self and the relationship of this self to another individual, to a group of people, and to the world occur because of communication.

Communication System

Communication, whether verbal or nonverbal, includes three essential aspects:

1. The transmission of information
2. The meaning of the transmission
3. The behavioral effects of the transmission

The transmission of information is the sending and receiving of *messages*, or units of information. Through the feedback process, every person in the transaction is affected by the behavior of everyone else involved.

Communication Models

Communication models, or graphic representations of various approaches to communication, provide overviews or perspectives about communication. The following adapted model serves as a pattern that outlines the essential components of communication.[26]

A model of communication compatible with the nursing process is an adaptation of the Wenburg and Wilmot process model of communication.[26] This model is particularly useful for nursing application because it emphasizes the behavioral aspects of the communication process and the internal and external environmental variables that influence the process. Use of this model assists the nurse to explore the communication process and identify those elements pertinent to the communication and nursing processes.

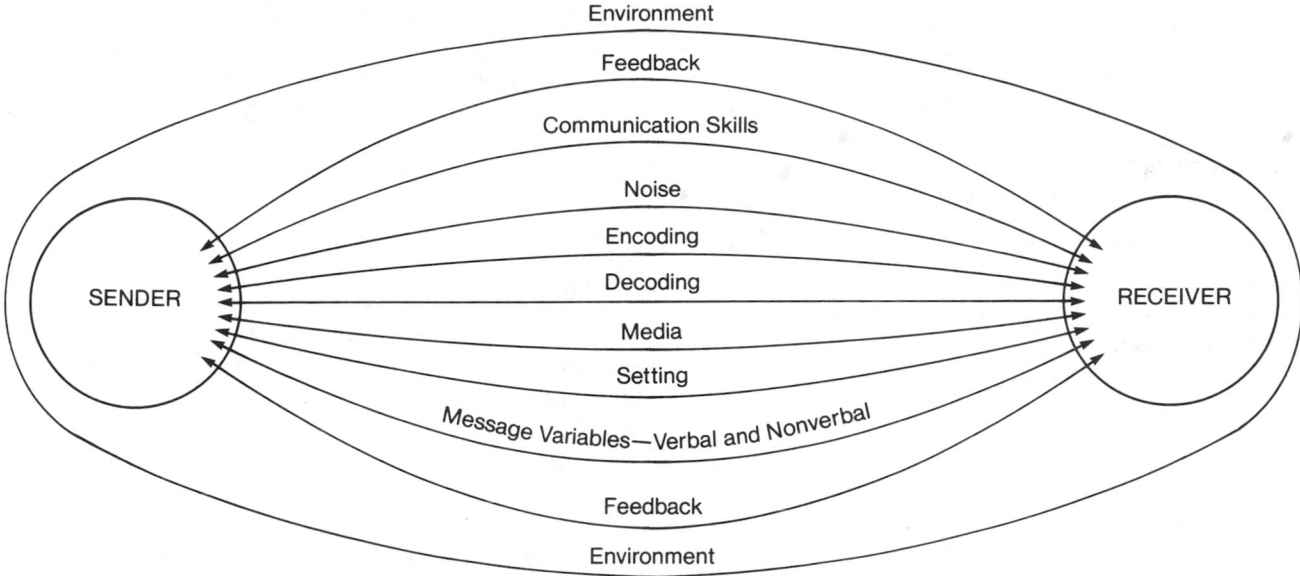

Figure 4-1. *Nursing communication model.*

◊Components of the Communication Process

Communication is an ongoing, ever-changing, infinite transmission system influenced by all the participants in the transmission. Components of the communication process include the sender, the receiver, the message, message variables (verbal and nonverbal communication), noise, communication skills, setting, media, feedback, and environment (see Fig. 4-1).

Sender

The sender is the encoder, the person who initiates the transmission. This event, the transmission of the message, is both verbal and nonverbal.

Receiver

The receiver of the message is the decoder. Encoding and decoding occur simultaneously and are activities of both sender and receiver. The past and present experiences of sender and receiver influence the transaction.

Message

The message is the unit of information received. A message is made up of many variables that can be verbal or nonverbal.

Message Variables

Message variables are selective verbal and nonverbal stimuli from the internal or external environment that give shape, direction, and focus to the message. The written and spoken language are examples of

verbal communication; gestures, smiles, and dress are examples of nonverbal communication.

Verbal Communication. Language is the expression of ideas according to society's shared format for sentence structure and grammatical rules.[15] Language is an acquired form of symbolization, a verbal behavior specific to humans.[28]

Although speech is ongoing social behavior, it frequently fails to explain behavior accurately. Speech itself is a complex activity involving the oral, respiratory, auditory, and nervous-system components of the body. Structural defects, malfunctioning due to disease, auditory and verbal impairments, sensory deprivation or overload, and learning disabilities may affect its use and decrease its transmission accuracy.

The schizophrenic person is characterized by his inability to abstract and use word symbolization to translate meaning that is reality-oriented. The stutterer experiences an interruption in the normal rhythm of speech sounds and he, too, is impaired in his ability to express his relationship with the environment. The mentally retarded child may be unable to learn language and is deprived of an expected social behavior. The autistic child exemplifies the individual who cannot symbolize with words.

In addition to attending to words and sounds, the nurse recognizes that nonverbal behaviors, such as voice pitch, voice quality (that is, harsh, weak, or strained), and voice amplification (that is, soft or loud) influence the message and are essential components of communication assessment. The choice of words, grammar, and understanding of language also influence the nature of the nurse–client relationship and are, therefore, included in the assessment.

Nonverbal Communication. Approximately 35% of the meaning of a communication transaction is due to verbal variables; the remaining 65% represents the impact of nonverbal communication. Nonverbal communication may do the following.

1. Contradict verbal behavior
2. Emphasize an emotional tone or mood
3. Complement verbal behavior
4. Control the environment
5. Be the communication of choice[10]

Many nonverbal behaviors are associated with messages. The familiar behaviors of crying, screaming, laughing, moaning, giggling, and sighing are examples of nonverbal communication. Other forms of nonverbal communication include facial expressions, body posture and gait, tone of voice, and gestures.

Noise

Noise refers to interferences within the communication system that hinder the accuracy of the transmission.

Communication Skills

Communication skills include the abilities of the sender and receiver in using message variables to observe, listen, clarify, and validate the meaning of the transmission.

Setting

The setting refers to the place or location where communication takes place.

Media

Media are the sensory channels that carry the message. Sensory channels include auditory, visual, touch, taste, and smell. A client's verbal message to the nurse for medication to relieve his anxiety will be carried via the nurse's auditory channel. The nurse, through the visual channel, sees tears in the client's eyes. The client leans forward and grasps the nurse's hand, emphasizing his need through touch. More than one sensory channel is involved in communication.

Feedback

Feedback is inherent in the communication system. Negative feedback functions to regulate the system to maintain the steady state, and positive feedback is responsible for change and disruption within the system. When applied to the communication system, feedback functions as a regulatory mechanism in the communication process. The receiver may see a sad or depressed expression on the sender's face but decide not to share this perception with the sender, thereby failing to clarify the communication. If the receiver had told the sender of his perceptions and the sender had explained that his sad expression had nothing to do with the present communication, a positive change might occur and the facial expression might change to reflect the ongoing transaction.

Feedback involves the continuous interpretation of responses of the sender and receiver as messages are simultaneously encoded and decoded. Private variables experienced by the sender and receiver are continually being communicated to each other and therefore influence the transaction.

Environment

The internal and external influences affecting the communication process make up the environment. Contextual cues affect the quality and sometimes the content of communication. Factors in the external environment are seen by everyone, but may be perceived differently by each individual. Room temperature, noise levels, smells, and lighting are examples of external environmental factors. Influences in the internal environment are known only to the individual and are not experienced in the same way by other people. Feeling tired, experiencing stomach discomfort, and feeling cold are examples of internal environmental factors.

Levels of Communication

A basic premise of the communication process is that it is intrapersonal in nature; all reactions to communication take place within one's self regardless of the number of people involved in the transaction. Communication occurs intrapersonally, interpersonally, in small groups, and in public or large groups. A characteristic of group communication is that the members are interdependent (*e.g.,* in social, therapy, or task groups). Public communication refers to the public-speaking setting in which one person sends a verbal message to a number of receivers. In psychiatric–mental health nursing, the main focus of interaction occurs at the interpersonal and group levels.

Interpersonal Needs

Individuals have interpersonal needs that include knowing that the self is personable, worthy, and able to interact with and use the environment satisfactorily. An individual whose interpersonal needs are not met adequately may be withdrawn, cold, and superficial in relationships. An overly friendly, possessive, and confiding individual may also be giving cues of a less-than-satisfying self-image. A loner, a shy and passive sort, as well as a talkative "attention getter" may present behaviors that display feelings of unworthiness.

Submissiveness, lack of confidence, inability to make decisions, as well as domination and aggressiveness, may indicate an inability to use and control the environment.[26] The communication process is a potent approach to assisting others in making adaptive changes to the environment.

Interpersonal Communication

Interpersonal communication is affected by the sensitivity of the participants to their own feelings and to the feelings of the other participants. Verbal and nonverbal communication may be spontaneous or calculated to affect the receiver. In therapeutic communication, for example, the nurse communicates to the client by arrangement of the environment, use of space, touch, voice inflection, dress, and so forth. Interpersonal communication is the most direct and pertinent form of communication, because it is through this transaction that needs are met.

Communication and the Nursing Process

Client problems may involve a variety of maladaptive patterns of communication. The nurse identifies these problems as objectively as possible and uses a systematic approach, utilizing listening skills and the nursing process to formulate tentative nursing diagnoses or to identify client problems. During the assessment interview, the interaction between the nurse and client is not designed exclusively for data collection purposes. The nurse's creation of an environment that is conducive to communication conveys to the client that she is attuned to his feelings and needs. Within a therapeutic atmosphere, change can occur and the client can be helped to identify and understand his behavior in a neutral, caring atmosphere.

Assessment of Communication

Congruence Between Verbal and Nonverbal Communication

A goal of the nurse in a therapeutic relationship is to assess the *congruence,* or agreement between the client's verbal and nonverbal communication. The client may not be aware that disharmony between his verbal and nonverbal communication exists.

If the client tells the nurse that he feels fine but has a sad facial expression and tear-filled eyes, his nonverbal communication does not agree with his words and the nurse is alerted to incongruent behavior. Assessment of nonverbal communication is an integral part of the communication assessment process. Facial expressions, motor activity, gestures, feeling tone, and congruence between verbal and nonverbal message variables are important categories for assessment (see Chart 4-1, "Communication Assessment Tool").

Use of Space and Territory

The use of space and territory is a form of nonverbal communication. The distance a person places between himself and another person or between himself and a group of people is a significant factor in interpersonal activities.

The concept of distance as a communication variable has been categorized as meeting public, social, and personal needs. The interpersonal aspects of public space involve the most distancing of people, while intimate personal space involves close contact. Personal (nonintimate) and social space are often reflected in informal gatherings, and interpersonal contact falls between the public and intimate distancing.

The goals and duration of the nurse–client relationship determine the space and distancing involved in the interaction. When designing a therapeutic milieu, the nurse assesses space and territorial needs of all clients.[12, 24, 27]

The nurse may observe certain behaviors that indicate a client's personal space and territory are being invaded. *Personal space* refers to the space preferred for interaction, whereas *social space* has a connotation of companionship.

Territory implies assigned space, such as a client's room, public room, or a specific seating arrangement. Territory is a designated place that implies ownership or personal possession. Intrusion or violation of someone's space or territory can distract and distort communication.[2]

Therapeutic Communication

Listening

Listening, or focusing on all of the behaviors expressed by a client, is the foundation of therapeutic communication. Listening requires energy in a form of concentration that does the following.

1. Minimizes distractions
2. Conveys objectivity
3. Is not evaluative in terms of agreeing or disagreeing with the communicator
4. Focuses on the client's behavior
5. Uses feedback objectively[13]

CHART 4-1

Communication Assessment Tool

Name_____ Age_____ Sex_____ Diagnosis_____

I. Sender or receiver impairments
 A. Structural deficit
 B. Sense deficits: hearing, sight, smell, touch, taste
 C. Loss of functions
 D. Disease
 E. Drugs
 F. Other

II. Message variables
 A. Nonverbal communication
  1. Facial expression
  2. Gestures
  3. Body movements
  4. Affect
  5. Tone of voice
  6. Posture
  7. Eye contact
  8. Voice volume, quality, pitch
  9. Other
 B. Verbal communication
  1. Content of message
  2. Communication patterns
   a. Blocking
   b. Slow
   c. Rapid
   d. Quiet
   e. Halting
   f. Aphasic
   g. Discontinuous
   h. Excessive
   i. Detailed
   j. Stammering
   k. Circumstantial
   l. Tangential
   m. Long silences
   n. Other

III. Noise

IV. Communication skills
 A. Openness, spontaneity
 B. Use of clarification
 C. Request for feedback
 D. Tolerance of silence
 E. Acceptance of confrontation
 F. Other

V. Setting
 A. Inpatient unit
 B. Community settings
 C. Other

VI. Media

VII. Feedback
 A. Precise
 B. Pertinent
 C. Goal-directed
 D. Informative
 E. Solicited
 F. Positive
 G. Negative
 H. Clarified
 I. Opportune

VIII. Environment
 A. External influences
  1. Temperature
  2. Physical arrangement
  3. Lighting
  4. Noise level
  5. Other
 B. Internal influences
  1. Beliefs
  2. Experiences
  3. Thoughts
  4. Attitudes
  5. Other

IX. Cultural influences
 A. Health practices
 B. Religious implications
 C. Language barriers
 D. Food preferences
 E. Other

Listening is an active process that focuses objective, empathic attention on the client. Maintaining eye contact, facilitating close proximity (if not threatening to the client), projecting a relaxed physical orientation and closeness, and speaking in a normal, audible voice are all characteristics of this process.[5,6,8]

The nurse attends to physical cues, such as room temperature and physical comfort. She tries to eliminate noise from the listening environment and tries to discontinue other media channels, such as the telephone, television or radio, in order to meet therapeutic listening goals and prevent interruption of the interaction.

Listening to another person requires the decoding of both the content and the feelings expressed in the message. Verbalizations, opinions, thoughts, and impressions make up the *content* part of messages. The *feeling* portion of a message is the emotional one, which may be described verbally (although this verbal description may or may not be accurate) or nonverbally.[24] A client who speaks in a relaxed voice may nevertheless reveal his anxiety by his nonverbal behaviors of chain smoking, clenching his hands, tense body posture or movement, and so forth. To individualize approaches to clients, the nurse notes congruence or incongruence between verbal and nonverbal communication and then validates her observations with the client. The anxiety or preoccupation of either nurse or client may be reflected in nonverbal communication that interferes with the therapeutic listening environment.

Observation

The nurse carefully observes for the client's communication of internal influences that may prevent the attentiveness needed for the therapeutic communication process (see Chart 4-2). The nurse, too, is influenced by internal variables and may be sleepy, hungry, thinking about a meeting with a supervisor, and so on. These kinds of influences can interfere with the nurse-client relationship and should be evaluated and modified, if necessary, to maintain an objective and empathetic environment conducive to the communication process.

CHART 4-2
Diagnosing Communication Needs

The nurse analyzes assessment data and formulates nursing diagnoses that may include the following:

The client's maladaptive behaviors, as manifested in
> Low self-esteem
> Poor self-concept
> Feelings of unworthiness
> Inability to express anger

The client's use of the communication process
> Inability to speak
> Limited understanding of language
> Nonassertive communication
> Distorted decoding
> Inability to send an accurate message
> Incongruence in verbal and nonverbal communication

The client's expression of feelings about his communication abilities
> Anxiety when talking to authority figures
> Withdrawal when involved in group communication
> Continuous talking when interacting with certain individuals

Self-Disclosure

One of the major goals of therapeutic communication is to use a planned, systematic approach to foster the client's self-disclosure so that he can make adaptive changes.[21,23] In our culture, we learn at an early age to control or conceal our authenticity—we disguise, hide, or deny our feelings.[13] Feelings are expressed in behavior, however, and the client can learn to recognize these inner experiences and express them as adaptively as possible.

> A 35-year-old woman was able to identify her promiscuous sexual behavior as a way of dealing with her self-deprecatory feelings resulting from an incestuous relationship with her step-father during early adolescence. Her suicide attempt, at the age of 14 years, symbolically ended the relationship, but her sexual behavior during adulthood continued to express her rage and low self-esteem.

Feelings form the bases for intervention that aims to deal with those feelings realistically.[14]

Cultural Influences. A person's culture influences how he expresses his feelings, and each culture has certain sanctioned verbal and nonverbal channels of expression. Whereas an American conceals his feelings, a member of an Eastern culture openly and loudly expresses his grief, anger, or joy. Communication is an integral part of the culture of a group, and the nurse must therefore understand how a specific culture uses it. Cultural variables, such as the perception of time, bodily contact, and territorial rights, also influence communication. The communication practice of different cultures affects their expression of ideas and feelings, decision-making, and communication strategies.[12]

The nurse is less concerned with the causes of behavior than with the effect of the client's behavior on the immediate environment. The "now," "how," and "what" of behavior are major areas of nursing assessment and intervention. The nurse's specific communication skills allow her to use the communication process as a vehicle for implementing the nursing process.[13]

Communication Techniques

Communication techniques include clarification, reflection, confrontation, informing, verification, self-disclosure, silence, summarizing, directing, and questioning.

The feeling and content components of communication are usually presented simultaneously in a transaction. The client's abilities to label feelings and to identify whether his behavior is adaptive or maladaptive represent therapeutic progress to the psychiatric–mental health nurse. When a feeling has been labeled, the nurse then uses a translating or paraphrasing technique to help the client focus on this feeling, correct his misperceptions, and alter the resultant maladaptive or distorted behavior. In this way, the client learns new interpersonal skills; he learns to explore his feelings and express them in an adaptive manner.[13]

The content portion of the message is also important because it enables the client to repeat or describe an experience from his point of reference. The nurse identifies similarities in themes or concerns of the client and develops an appreciation of the uniqueness of the client's situation. The following are examples of therapeutic communication techniques.

Clarifying Feelings. When clarifying the client's feelings,

1. repeat the feeling tone of the message in your own words, or restate an emotional word or a phrase used by the clients;
2. use an open, questioning tone of voice; that is, a nondirective and noninterrogating one;
3. wait until the client responds.

Marian, a 31-year-old married woman, is admitted to the unit because of depression and recent alcohol abuse.

Client (Marian): I don't know what happened—I left the children at the neighbor's and went to a bar just to see who was there. I woke up the next morning in a motel with a strange man (begins to cry, puts her clenched fists to her eyes).

Nurse: You're frightened and ashamed because you don't know what happened and you woke up in a strange place?

Client: It was so scary. I'm afraid it will happen again. I wouldn't leave even when my husband came for me. I feel so humiliated.

The nurse tried to help Marian label her feelings to create a clearer, more meaningful picture of her behavior. The nurse attended to the client's nonverbal cues and the feeling tone of her communication. Marian verified the message the nurse perceived.

Reflecting Feelings. When reflecting the client's feelings,

1. state your comprehension of the feeling message, using emotional and feeling descriptive words;

2. use a nonquestioning tone of voice;
3. wait until the client responds.

Client (Marian): I don't know who I am anymore (wipes eyes, lights a cigarette, talks in a whisper). I'm drawn to go to any barroom even though I tell myself it won't happen again.

Nurse: You feel frightened and ashamed that you're not in control of yourself.

Client: I can't seem to conrol my actions when these feelings come over me.

The nurse identified the feelings of shame and depression that Marian verified as being a part of her behavior and one of the reasons for her voluntary admission to the mental health unit. (For another example, see Chart 4-3.)

The nurse may use the clarifying technique to help the client label any other feelings she is experiencing, before reflecting on those feelings. The reflecting technique helps build a trusting nurse-client relationship because the client can express painful or uncomfortable feelings that are empathetically received by the nurse.

Clarifying Content. When clarifying the content of the client's communication,

1. repeat your comprehension of the thought or idea in your own words;
2. repeat a specific word or idea used by the client;
3. use an open, questioning tone of voice;
4. wait until the client responds.

Client (Marian): The man who brought me back to the motel was a gentleman.

Nurse: The man in the bar?

Client: Yes, the one I went with to the motel. I didn't even know him.

The nurse clarified the content part of Marian's message. This clarification acknowledged the client's recollection of her experience. The client needs to know and believe that the nurse has an accurate picture of her perceptions of the experience. Reflecting the content part of the message is another way of telling the client that the nurse is actively listening to obtain an accurate picture of his behavior.

Reflecting Content. When reflecting the content of the client's communication,

1. state your comprehension of the content message using descriptive or cognitive words;

CHART 4-3
Admission to a Mental Health Unit: Communication and Perceptions

Tom, an 18-year-old, is admitted to a mental health unit because of a chronic problem with "stomach ailments," insomnia, and anorexia. Tom was reluctant to enter the unit, but his physician had told him he would learn new ways of handling his stressful environment, which involved many family problems related to his divorced parents and drug-dependent brother and sister.

Tom was admitted at 3:30 P.M., experienced a 30-minute structured intake interview by the nurse, was oriented to the unit by another client assigned to this task, and went to his room. Thirty minutes into the dinner hour, the nurse realized that Tom hadn't been informed of the unit's dinner time. She escorted him to the dining room and asked a client Tom's age to help him.

Because Tom was admitted to the unit on a "pass day" for many of the residents (therefore, group activities were not being held), Tom went back to his room to read. Meanwhile, the nurse and other staff were busy admitting another new client and assisting clients with passes. Tom was given sleep medication at 9:30 P.M. and was asleep at 10:30 P.M.

The next day, Tom checked out against medical advice because, he said, "The unit wasn't what I expected." Tom's perception of this new environment was of a polite but uncaring, strange new environment that was not very different from the one he was trying to escape. The communication and behavior of the nurse and others in the environment reinforced Tom's perception of the unit and his low self-esteem.

2. use a nonquestioning tone of voice;
3. wait until the client responds.

Client (Marian): My brother is a diabetic and my sister has hypoglycemia problems. I read in a magazine that people who drink a lot may have trouble burning up sugar in their blood.

Nurse: You think because of the history of diabetes and your sister's glucose tolerance, you may have a glucose problem, too.

Client: Yes, I'm wondering if the doctor would check my blood.

The nurse informed Marian that a blood sugar test had been completed and the results were within normal limits.

Confronting Feelings.   When confronting the client's feelings,

1. describe the emotional message or feelings you are perceiving;
2. describe the client's ongoing behavior that is influencing your perceptions;
3. identify the contradictions using a questioning tone of voice;
4. wait for the client's response.

Marian has been less depressed since intensive therapy began 2 weeks ago. She is taking an antidepressant medication and is participating actively in the unit program.

The team has noticed incongruence in Marian's expression of feelings toward her husband. Marian discusses her feelings of love and need for closeness with her husband, but refuses his phone calls and does not open his letters. The team has decided to confront Marian with her behavior.

Client (Marian): I love my husband so much, and I know he understands why I go to bars when I'm upset.

Nurse: You feel your husband knows you love him so much that he accepts your behavior when you become anxious. Is refusing his calls and not opening his letters contrary to these strong feelings of love you say you feel for him?

Client: Sometimes I feel so confused. I hate him at times and then, at other times, feel overwhelming love for him.

Confronting Content.   When confronting the content of the client's communication,

1. describe the message you are perceiving, using cognitive terms;
2. describe the mixed-content messages you are perceiving using the specific cognitive terms of the client;
3. identify the contraindications using a nonquestioning tone of voice;
4. wait for the client's response.

Client (Marian): My husband isn't interested in visiting me. I know 50 miles is a long way to come, but he won't make the effort.

Nurse: You think your husband doesn't care about you because he hasn't visited you, but you told me you sent him a letter asking him not to come. I'm confused, Marian.

Client: Well, don't you think he should know I really didn't mean for him not to come?

Nurse: I'm sure he's trying to do what you want and not visit you if that's your request. He has called every day.

Verifying Perceptions.

When verifying or "checking out" your perceptions of the client's behavior,

1. describe your perceptions of the client's behavior, using terms similar to his own descriptions of content or feelings;
2. use an open, questioning tone of voice to enable the client to verify your perceptions;
3. wait for the client's response.

Client (Marian): I don't think I have a drinking problem. I think all my trouble stems from my parent's divorce when I lost my friends and home.

Nurse: You're having difficulty accepting the fact that you are an alcoholic, and it's easier to blame your parents for your problems.

Client: I feel so uncomfortable when I look at the other people at our meetings who are so open about being alcoholics—I guess I can't or don't want to accept the fact that I'm like them.

Self-Disclosure.

The nurse reinforces the genuine regard for, and respect of, the client by means of the therapeutic use of self. Self-disclosure may be used after the client describes a feeling or an emotional message. When self-disclosing,

1. clarify the client's message or feeling tone;
2. describe similar experiences or feelings of your own;
3. wait for the client's response.

Client (Marian): I'm very frightened to go to the employment agency and apply for a job.

Nurse: I think I know what you mean. I've always felt "scared" when I had to apply for a new job.

The nurse avoids asserting "I know how you feel" because this response may be interpreted by the client to mean that his experience is a common one or that the nurse is far superior to him. On the other hand, the nurse's self-disclosure helps the client realize that his feelings, thoughts, or behaviors are shared and appreciated by others. It reinforces the nurse's empathy and willingness to share an experience with the client.

Bear in mind that this technique and all techniques of therapeutic communication are designed to meet a specific goal, after which the nurse immediately refocuses on the client. The nurse uses the technique of self-disclosure judiciously and sparingly so that the interaction does not become one dominated by the nurse's disclosures.

Giving Information.

Communicating facts to the client is a frequent component of intervention. It is a cognitive, goal-directed function and meets an identified objective for the client. When giving information to the client,

1. state the purpose of an activity, procedure, or situation;
2. describe an activity, procedure, or situation;
3. identify the components of an activity, procedure, or situation.

Client (Marian): I signed some kind of a contract yesterday about drugs and passes, but I can't remember all the facts.

Nurse: Each client signs a contract with our unit within 24 hours of admission. This contract identifies the rules and regulations about drugs and 20-minute, free-time passes. The contract you signed stated the following.
1. I do not have any drugs with me nor will I take any drugs that are not a part of my treatment.
2. I will sign out when I leave the unit, identifying where I'm going in the hospital, and will return in 20 minutes.

The nurse removed Marian's contract from the chart to show her the contract and her signature.

Silence.

When using silence,

1. describe the behavior that needs the client's response;
2. use an open, questioning, or declarative tone of voice;
3. wait for the client's response.

Marian had signed a behavioral contract to attend Alcoholics Anonymous meetings, which were being held at another area in the hospital.

Nurse: You didn't attend the AA meeting last night.

Client (Marian): I—just...(Marian puts her head in her hands; silence followed for about 2 to 3 minutes. Marian had recently talked about her feeling that she was not an alcohol abuser. She then begins to cry.) It's so hard for me to see myself as an alcoholic. (Silence for about 1 minute) I feel so ashamed and even unclean when I go to those meetings.

Nurse: You feel humiliated and dirty.

Client: I know it's not the people there. It's accepting myself as I am and not the make-believe I've been living.

Although it is often uncomfortable for nurse and client alike, using silence therapeutically is a very effective measure to encourage the client's communication. Silence provides time for the client to contemplate a thought, feeling, or decision. If a client is not comfortable with or trusting of the situation, he may use silence as a way to resist the interaction.

Summarizing. When summarizing the interaction with the client,

1. review the interaction in specific terms;
2. wait for and listen to the client's response;
3. clarify any misunderstandings.

Nurse: Marian, during the last month you've said that you accept the fact that you abuse alcohol, you have complied with the behavioral contract, and you have attended two AA meetings a week for the past 4 weeks.

Client: I've gotten something out of them, too. I'll continue until my stay here ends, right?

Nurse: As I recall that is correct, but let's look at the behavioral contract.

Summarizing is an effective way to assist the client to examine themes in the interaction and to examine progress in general. It is also an appropriate technique for terminating a nurse–client counseling session, but may be useful at any time in the interaction to emphasize progress or focus on specific areas that are of concern to the client.

Directing. When directing the client's interaction,

1. use nonverbal or succinct, open-ended questioning, or declarative statements;
2. wait for client's response.

Nurse: You were saying—.

Client (Marian): I know that when my husband called last night, I wanted to be kind and considerate about the out-of-town trip he needs to take, but—.

Nurse: Please go on, Marian.

Directing encourages the client to explore and express his thoughts and feelings. It also communicates the nurse's interest and attentiveness. Expressions such as "you were saying," "you mentioned this previously," "please continue," "Mmm-hmmm," or a nod of the head function as cues for the client to continue. Allowing the client time to respond is an essential part of this therapeutic technique.

Questioning. Frequently, the nurse uses direct questions or indirect questionlike responses during therapeutic communication. A client, however, may become defensive or may intellectualize when asked the "why" of his behavior. Open-ended questions are helpful ways to elicit the "how," "what," "where," and "when" of the client's behavior. Questions such as "Will you elaborate?" "Will you give me an example?" and "Am I correct?" are examples of these responses. The nurse avoids asking questions that require an answer of "yes" or "no" and those that are probing and interrogative during therapeutic communication.[3,5,6,13]

Interviewing

Interviewing is a specific type of guided and limited intercommunication with an identified purpose. An interview is usually conducted to collect a data base for analysis and decision-making purposes. The nurse often employs structured assessment tools and questionnaires to gather and categorize data.[11,17]

Guidelines for interviewing include the following:

1. Conduct sessions seated in a private, comfortable area with adequate lighting and hearing distance.
2. At the beginning of each session, plan and discuss with the client the length and purpose of the session.
3. Observe, listen, and use facilitative communication techniques.
4. Convey a professional demeanor through dress and manner.
5. Summarize the interaction at the end of the session and make arrangements with the client for the next session.
6. Positively reinforce the client for his attention, effort, and so on.

(For more information about interviewing techniques, see Chap. 7.)

Barriers to Therapeutic Communication

Barriers to therapeutic communication inhibit or interfere with nurse–client communication (note italicized examples of barriers below). Lack of planning or inadequate preparation by the nurse during the communication process may result in failure to meet the client's identified goals. The goal of precise data collection directs communication assessment; *inadequate data collection* is a significant barrier to facilitative communication.

Nurse–client interaction is built on the development of a trusting relationship. *Lack of regard* for the other person in an interaction inhibits, or functions as a barrier to, therapeutic communication.

Other verbal and nonverbal communication of the nurse may cause disruption or cessation of the nurse–client interaction. *Changing the subject* indicates to the client that the nurse is uncomfortable with the present communication and has therefore introduced a new, and usually superficial, topic of conversation. The client may perceive the nurse's *probing questions* as morbid curiosity, threatening elements, and an intrusion into his privacy.

Advising the client, or telling him what he should do, what he should think, or how he should feel, is a dangerous trap into which any helping professional may inadvertently slip. To advise the client impinges on his individuality and his right to determine his own behavior.

Belittling the client, such as discounting his feelings, tells him that he and his feelings are not important or worthy of others' attention. *Defending* the hospital or agency, staff, therapy, or other aspect of treatment usually fails to respond to whatever the client is saying or asking, and it reduces the likelihood of continued communication with the client.

Closed-ended questions limit the client's responses to one- or two-word answers, such as answers of "yes" or "no." These questions inhibit the client's freedom to elaborate on his thoughts and feelings.

False reassurance is a common barrier to therapeutic communication. Telling the client that "everything will be all right," unless, of course, the nurse is absolutely sure that everything will end satisfactorily, is an attempt to give a pat solution to what may be complex questions or problems. This reassurance, arising out of habit rather than the facts of the situation, tends to eliminate the client's further elaboration of his thoughts and feelings and tends to terminate communication with the nurse.

Intervening in Psychotic Communication

The nurse does not reinforce the client's psychotic communication. Initial interaction with an individual demonstrating psychotic behavior involves showing interest in, and concern for, the client. A realistic approach to the client may be spending time with him in an activity, such as walking. (See Chart 4-4 for another example.)

The tasks of recognizing his feeling messages, decoding his content, and clarifying his feelings without causing him to be overstimulated by the interaction are difficult ones for the psychiatric–mental

---

C H A R T 4-4
Responding to Psychotic Communication

The following is an example of an interaction between a psychiatric–mental health nurse and a client who is using psychotic communication. The nurse has been meeting and spending time with the client since his admission a week ago and has been using various activities within the milieu during their sessions to develop a relationship.

Client: The voices are talking to me again and told me not to go with you on this walk today, but to stay in my room and talk to them.

Nurse: Are you confused about whether I want to be with you?

Client: The voices (puts hands to head) are mad at me, and they're saying awful things and using bad words because I'm with you.

Nurse: I look forward to our walks and getting to know you better.

Client: The voices tell me you're just saying that because you want to trick me.

Nurse: I care about you and want to be able to help you. I will be with you every day at this time for the next week.

The nurse was aware of the client's history of abuse by his parents and of spending his adolescence in foster homes. He was diagnosed as schizophrenic and has had repeated admissions to the psychiatric hospital. He has been in a rehabilitation–work program successfully for the past year but became psychotic again when he learned his mother died. Eventually, the nurse and client talked about his feelings of rejection and helplessness. The client was able to return to his rehabilitation–work program and outpatient care.

C H A R T 4-5

Process Recording

Applying Therapeutic Communication Techniques

A 24-year-old man is admitted voluntarily to a mental health unit.
The following recording is part of an admission interview.

Client's Verbal and Nonverbal Communication	Nurse's Verbal and Nonverbal Communication	Therapeutic Technique	Evaluation
	Will you tell me your reasons for admitting yourself to the unit (relaxed, open posture, maintaining eye contact)?	Clarifying content	The nurse asks the client to identify his reasons for seeking mental health treatment. The nurse is likely already to have completed introductions and the sharing of initial information about the purpose, length, and process of the admission interview. Instead of relying on the views or opinions of others, the nurse seeks information and perceptions directly from the client.
Well, my wife left me 2 weeks ago, and I (starts to cry, speaking between sobs) feel like my world has come to an end.			
	(She allows silence for 2 to 3 minutes.)	Silence	Although it is often tempting to say something to stop the client from crying, it is therapeutic to allow him free expression of his feelings and his thoughts.
I can't sleep or eat—I want her back and I know I've got to get my head together (holds head in hands, elbows resting on knees).			
	You're feeling sad and hurt right now (softer voice).	Clarifying feelings	The nurse tries to help the client identify his feelings, an important initial step before he can begin to cope with, or work through, them.
I've been feeling this way since she left. I love her so much, but I've never been able to tell her until the day she was packing to leave.			
	Not able to tell her you love her—	Reflecting feelings	The nurse focuses on the issue of the client's feelings, which are usually more difficult to express, or to deal with.
Betty and I have been together for 3 years—we lived together for 1½ years. Those were good times, and then we got married (looks away, fidgets with ring on finger).			

(Continues on p. 52)

Client's Verbal and Nonverbal Communication	Nurse's Verbal and Nonverbal Communication	Therapeutic Technique	Evaluation
	You were saying that you couldn't tell her you loved her (looks directly at client, nods).	Reflecting content	The nurse again tries to focus the interaction on what appears to be a significant issue for him—his inability or failure to express his love for his wife. This is also a useful technique when the client's communication is rambling or difficult to follow.
Yeah, see ever since we met, Betty thought I was a macho man, and I tried to be that kind of guy, and I'm not.			
	If you were macho, you couldn't tell her you loved her—is that what you're saying?	Clarifying content	
I thought she wanted the strong, silent type, but I seemed to drive her away (shakes his head from side to side, sad facial expression).			
	Go on (nods).	Directing	The nurse encourages the client to continue, verbally and non-verbally. She informs him that she is interested in what he is saying and how he is feeling.
Betty is just 19—we met when she was 16. She never went out much, and lately she's been going out with my sister—to the clubs to dance, and I felt it was OK because I go out with the boys.			
	Go on.	Directing	
She seemed always ready to go out but didn't pay attention to the house or meals—so I shook her and slapped her. I'm no good (starts to cry)—she was scared of me.			
	Scared of you?	Reflecting content	Reflection of a word, a phrase, or a sentence encourages the client to elaborate on his statements.
Yeah, scared and felt all I thought about was work—and I did. I wanted Betty to have things—she's had it hard.			
	You felt you could show Betty your love by giving her things.	Clarifying feelings	The nurse explores how the client feels about his wife and his pattern of relating to her; she also gives him
I played a role with her so long that I hated			

Client's Verbal and Nonverbal Communication	Nurse's Verbal and Nonverbal Communication	Therapeutic Technique	Evaluation
myself—and I took it out on her.			the opportunity to evaluate the accuracy of her clarification.
	You say you love her, but you slapped and shook her.	Confronting content	The nurse verbalizes the incongruence between the client's verbalizations (his love for his wife) and his actions (physically abusing her).
(He puts head in hands and begins to cry.) I'm no good—I love Betty, and I finally told her I wasn't a big tough guy, but just an ordinary person—			
	You're feeling down, and upset about your past behavior with Betty?	Reflecting feelings	Again the nurse reflects the client's feelings to help him identify and own them.
Oh, I am—even though I told her the truth, she still packed up.			
	(She remains silent for 1–2 minutes; looks at client.)	Silence	The nurse's use of silence offers client and nurse a time to reflect on what's been said and collect their thoughts for the next interchange.
	You said the 1½ years you two lived together were the good times.	Clarifying content	The nurse next returns to an earlier point in the discussion, encouraging the client to elaborate, if he wishes.
Yeah, we weren't around any family, and I didn't drink like I do now.			
	You abuse alcohol?	Verifying	In response to the client's communication about his drinking the nurse verifies this information which he has shared.
Yes, that's another problem I have.			

Discussion

A process recording is an analysis of an interpersonal interaction. It examines closely the verbal and nonverbal communication of the nurse–helper and the client seeking help. Specific therapeutic techniques are identified at each point of intervention during the interaction. Evaluation of the helpfulness of the interaction—both verbal and nonverbal communication—is an integral part of the recording.

health nurse. Frequent use of silence may increase the client's anxiety and his hallucinatory behavior. Saying "I can't follow your thinking" to the client who evidences psychotic communication is a way to introduce him to the reality of interpersonal communication.

Listening for and clarifying themes or needs with the psychotic client is difficult and often perplexing for the nurse. The client who needs time to develop a trusting relationship with another may continue to use psychotic communication and behavior to test the relationship. The nurse continuously evaluates the relationship and the effectiveness of communication with the client.

Summary

This chapter has explored the purposes, systems, and models of communication. Other emphases of the chapter include the following:

1. The components of the communication process are the sender, receiver, message, message variables, noise, communication skills, setting, media, feedback, and environment.

2. The communication and nursing processes interweave to provide the nurse with a foundation to assist clients' progressions toward optimal adaptation.

3. Empathy enables the nurse to view the client in a caring and objective manner and to interact with him in a planned, systematic way.

4. The techniques of therapeutic communication—clarification, reflection, confrontation, verification, self-disclosure, informing, silence, summarizing, directing, and questioning—are the nurse's tools to elicit helpful or facilitative interaction with the client.

5. Barriers to therapeutic communication—such as defending, lack of regard for the other person, and advising—interfere with, or inhibit, communication between the nurse and client.

6. Therapeutic communication is one of the most powerful tools of the psychiatric–mental health nurse.

References

1. Applebaum R, Anatol KW, Jenson O, Porter RE, Mandel JE: Fundamental Concepts of Human Communication. San Francisco, Canfield Press, 1973

2. Ardrey R: The Territorial Imperative. New York, Atheneum, 1966

3. Authier J, Authier K, Lutey B: Clinical Management of the Tearfully Depressed Patient: Communication Skills for the Nurse Practitioner. J Psychiatr Nurs Ment Health Serv 17 (February): 34–41, 1978

4. Berne E: Games People Play. New York, Grove Press, 1964

5. Brammer LM: The Helping Relationship. Englewood Cliffs, NJ, Prentice-Hall, 1973

6. Carkhuff RR: The Art of Helping, IV, 4th ed. Amherst, Mass, Human Resources Development Press, 1980

7. Crouch L: Disturbance in Language and Thought. J Psychiatr Nurs Ment Health Serv 10 (May–June): 5–8, 1972

8. Dominick AB (ed): How to Make People Listen to You. Springfield, IL, Charles C Thomas, 1971

9. Doona ME: Travelbee's Intervention in Psychiatric Nursing, 2nd ed. Philadelphia, FA Davis, 1979

10. Edwards BJ, Briehart JK: Communications in Nursing Practice. St Louis, CV Mosby, 1981

11. Enelow AJ, Swisher SN: Interviewing and Patient Care. New York, Oxford Press, 1972

12. Hall, ET, Whyte WF: Intercultural Communication: A Guide to Men of Action. In Brink PJ (ed): Transcultural Nursing, pp 44–62. Englewood Cliffs, NJ, Prentice-Hall, 1976

13. Headington BJ: Communication in the Counseling Relationship. Cranston, RI, Carroll Press, 1979

14. Longo DC, Williams RA: Clinical Practice in Psychosocial Nursing: Assessment and Intervention. New York, Appleton-Century-Croft, 1978

15. Miller GA: The Magical Number Seven, Plus or Minus Two: Some Limits on Our Capacity for Processing Information. In Silverstein A et al (eds): Human Communication: Theoretical Explorations, pp 81–97. New York, John Wiley & Sons, 1974

16. Ong WJ: The History and the Future of Verbal Media. In Silverstein A et al (eds): Human Communication: Theoretical Explorations, pp 165–183. New York, John Wiley & Sons, 1974

17. Peplau H: Basic Principles of Patient Counseling, 2nd ed. Philadelphia, Smith, Kline & French Laboratories, 1964

18. Phillips LW: Language in Disguise: Nonverbal Communication with Patients. Perspect Psychiatr Care 4 (July–August): 18–21, 1966

19. Pryser PW: The Psychological Examination: A Guide for Clinicians. New York: International Universities Press, 1979

20. Rickelman B: Bio-Psycho-Social Linguistics. Nursing Research 20 (September–October): 398–403, 1971

21. Ruesch J: Therapeutic Communication. New York, WW Norton, 1961

22. Sielski LM: Understanding Body Language. Per-

sonnel and Guidance Journal 57 (January): 238–242, 1979

23. Smitherman C: Nursing Actions for Health Promotion. Philadelphia, FA Davis, 1980
24. Vance B: Human Relationships in Nursing. Provo, Utah, Brigham Young University, 1979
25. Watzlawick P: Pragmatics of Human Communication. New York, WW Norton, 1967
26. Wenburg JR, Wilmot WM: The Personal Communication Process. New York, John Wiley & Sons, 1973
27. Wilson JS: Deciphering Psychotic Communication. Perspect Psychiatr Care 18 (November–December): 254–256, 1979
28. Wolfgang A (ed): The Teacher and Nonverbal Behavior in the Multicultural Classroom. Nonverbal Behavior, Application and Cultural Implication, Part 3, pp 159–174. New York, Academic Press, 1979

5

Therapeutic Relationships

Patriciann Furnari Brady

How strange is the lot of us mortals! Each of us is here for a brief sojourn; for what purpose he knows not, though he sometimes thinks he senses it. But without deeper reflection one knows from daily life that one exists for other people—first of all for those upon whose smiles and well-being our own happiness is wholly dependent, and then for the many, unknown to us, to whose destinies we are bound by the ties of sympathy. A hundred times every day I remind myself that my inner and outer life are based on the labors of other men, living and dead, and that I must exert myself in order to give in the same measure as I have received and am still receiving.

Albert Einstein,
Ideas and Opinions

Chapter Preview

During hospitalization and many other health care experiences, the nurse is the primary person accessible to the client to meet his physical and psychological needs. To maximize effectiveness in communication and intervention, nurses strive to develop therapeutic relationships with their clients.

This chapter focuses on the therapeutic relationship—what it is and what it is not, its purposes and phases. The attitude of the nurse helper and the measures that facilitate growth are examined as critical issues affecting the development of the therapeutic relationship.

Learning Objectives

After studying this chapter, you should be able to accomplish the following:

1. define therapeutic relationships
2. differentiate between social, intimate, and therapeutic relationships
3. describe the characteristics of a therapeutic relationship
4. identify the anxieties of the nurse and client in a therapeutic relationship
5. discuss the expectations of the nurse and client in a therapeutic relationship
6. discuss the impact of the attitude of the nurse helper on a therapeutic relationship
7. describe ways in which the nurse facilitates the growth of clients

Dynamics of the Relationship

Definition and Purposes of Relationships

A *relationship* is a state of being related or a state of affinity between two individuals. Clients and nurses have an affinity for each other or are related to each other within the health care system.

Nursing is a dialogue—a human-to-human event.[23] Clients enter the health care system with an awareness of their expected role behavior and with certain expectations of the nurse. Most of these behaviors focus on the "ill client" and the "nurse caregiver" roles. Explicit in the nurse caregiver role is the provision of physical care; implicit in the role is the meeting of client's psychological needs and the facilitation of growth. The development of a therapeutic relationship enables the nurse to meet client needs and intervene in client problems.

Hildegard Peplau describes nursing as an educative instrument—a maturing force—that aims to promote forward movements of personality in the direction of creative, constructive, productive personal, and community living.[31] Nurses provide for clients the opportunity for an honest relationship. The care dimensions in such a relationship promote human growth through empathic understanding in an atmosphere conducive to the client's self-exploration.[1]

Types of Relationships

In relationships with clients, the temptation to see the person as a friend may arise. The nurse who says, "I feel so close to the client, I feel he is my friend" is altering the implied focus of the interaction between the professional and the one seeking help. Three possible types of relationships—social, intimate, and therapeutic—are observed between individuals.

Social Relationship

The *social relationship* is the one we experience most commonly in our everyday lives. Both individuals are equally involved in this relationship and are concerned with meeting their own needs through the relationship. There is neither a predetermined goal or focus in the social relationship, nor is the continuation of the relationship determined at its outset.

Intimate Relationship

An *intimate relationship* is a relationship between two individuals committed to one another, caring for and respecting each other. Intimacy is usually exclusive to those involved and implies that they love each other.

According to Erikson, the ability to develop an intimate relationship with an adult of the opposite sex is highly dependent on completing developmental tasks.[9] The intimate relationship forms the basis for the procreation of future generations.

Therapeutic Relationship

A *therapeutic relationship* is one in which the nurse and client work together toward the goal of assisting the client meet his needs and facilitate growth. The interaction is purposefully established, maintained, and carried out with an anticipated outcome of assisting the client obtain new coping and adaptation skills. The most basic assumptions underlying the therapeutic relationships are as follows:

The client's difficulties are expressed in the relationship.

The previous, learned difficulties of former relationships are amenable to change in this relationship.[12]

The nurse-client relationship is a helpful, purposeful interaction between an authority in health care (the nurse) and a person or group with health care needs.[28] The one-to-one psychiatric nurse–client relationship is an interpersonal relationship between a psychiatric–mental health nurse and a client for the purpose of brief counseling, crisis intervention, or psychotherapy.[23]

Phases of a Therapeutic Relationship

Initial or Introductory Phase

The *initial phase* or introductory contact between a client and nurse can occur in a variety of settings. The initial admission procedure or provision of technical care for the client offers opportunities for an initial interaction. Often, nursing students ask "What do I say first?" The nurse should acknowledge the client by name and should then introduce herself. Establishing the frequency and length of contact and establishing a reason for the contact assist the client to clarify the purpose and particulars of the relationship.[14] Structuring the interaction avoids the client's misunderstanding or misinterpreting the relationship, and it helps the nurse and client establish goals for the relationship.

During this phase of a therapeutic relationship, the nurse must demonstrate acceptance of the client's behavior, must establish rapport, and must provide an opportunity for the client to begin to develop trust. Frequently, clients test the nurse's commitment by missing appointments or by exhibiting acting-out behavior. In this phase of the relationship, the client's problems are identified, nursing diagnoses and goals are determined, priorities are set, and plans are formulated to achieve the goals.

During this initial interaction, the nurse and client may also establish a contract to formalize the terms of their relationship. The contract may include designating a time and place to meet, finding alternatives for initially contracted goals, keeping appointments, exploring problems, maintaining confidentiality, and re-evaluating the expectations at any point in the relationship (see Chart 5-1 for a sample treatment contract).

The nurse and client must recognize and differentiate what types of problems are amenable to intervention. When setting goals with clients, the nurse also recognizes that, because patterns of behavior are not developed in a short period of time, brief or short-term interventions may not be appropriate for "deep-rooted" problems and behavior.

The nurse informs the client when his desired goals are beyond her realm of expertise or the duration of the interaction. Failure of the nurse to share this information with the client in an open and honest manner will interfere with the establishment of trust and the ultimate outcome of the relationship.

The nurse and client affect each other; the nurse should recognize the effect she has on the client and his effect on her. The nurse strives to care for the client in such a manner that a sense of trust and confidence develops. Therapy begins when the nurse and client progress beyond exchanging information and the client begins to share subjective content underlying his behavior.[6]

During the initial phase of a relationship, the nurse also gathers data about the following:

1. How the client views himself and his problems
2. Problematic areas of interpersonal relationships
3. Problematic areas the client denies[32]

Before moving to the next phase of the relationship, the nurse and client evaluate the initial phase and assess whether the following tasks have been accomplished:

1. Security is being established through continued development of trust.
2. The client is being assisted to verbalize thoughts and feelings.
3. Areas of inadequate stress adaptation are being identified.
4. Strengths and weaknesses are being assessed.
5. Goals for the relationship are established.

Middle or Working Phase

The *working phase* of the relationship occurs when the client and nurse are actively involved in meeting the goals established during the initial phase of the relationship. The client may fluctuate between dependence and independence in an attempt to acknowledge the painful and unpleasant aspects of his life and begin to try out healthy, adaptive behavior.[28] The nurse encourages the client to express his feelings and attempt new adaptation approaches without danger of punitive treatment; she also reinforces his effective problem-solving.

In this phase of the relationship, the client is also likely to feel more secure and will openly discuss topics that he was unable to discuss previously. The client is more likely to successfully learn new behaviors because his anxiety level decreases when trust is reinforced through the nurse's acceptance. The nurse and client continue to discuss his problems and conflicts and the nurse encourages him to try new ways of resolving his conflicts.[26]

The *therapeutic tasks* of the working phase of the nurse-client relationship include the following:

CHART 5-1
Treatment Contract

Formalizing Expectations and Consequences

John W., 24 years old, was admitted to a psychiatric hospital with a diagnosis of antisocial personality 2 weeks prior to his initial contact with Ms. G., who was assigned as his primary nurse. John was having difficulty following the routines of the ward, was missing group therapy, was frequently demanding the nurses' and doctors' attention, and was borrowing cigarettes and money from other clients.

In their initial contact, John and Ms. G. decided to meet weekly to assist him to follow his treatment plan and discuss problems he was having during his hospitalization. After identifying together his areas of concern and what privileges he hoped to attain, they established the following contract:

"I, John W., agree to follow this contract outlining the expected behavior and will then receive the privileges listed below.

1. Attend meals as scheduled
2. Shower and change clothes daily
3. Attend group sessions on time, as established in my treatment plan
4. Participate as an active member in group therapy
5. Meet Ms. G. at 10:00 A.M., Wednesdays, on the Unit

6. Not ask other patients for cigarettes or money
7. Ask nurses for assistance with problem areas and leave the nurses' station when requested
8. Make an appointment to see the physician, when needed, and not try to talk to him without an appointment unless permission is given by ward nurses
9. Report to the ward staff prior to leaving the ward"

John W. agreed to abide by the contract immediately, and when he demonstrated the expected behavior for three days, the following schedule of privileges was established.

John W. will be permitted the following:

1. One hour off ward every shift for 1 week
2. Two hours off ward every shift for 1 week
3. Four hours off ward every shift for 1 week
4. May be off ward at all times except during therapy time and must report to nursing staff prior to meals

John W. and Ms. G. discussed the consequences of his failure to follow one of the expected behaviors and decided that, in that instance, he would lose his current privilege level and would be moved back to the previous privilege level.

---

1. Increase awareness and perception of the reality of specific personal experiences.
2. Develop realistic self-concept and promote self-confidence.
3. Recognize areas of discomfort and verbalize these feelings.
4. Attempt to make comparisons between the ineffective behavior within the relationship and the ineffective behavior outside the relationship and draw conclusions regarding these comparisons.
5. Encourage a plan of action, implement the plan, and evaluate the results of the plan to alter the client's behavior.
6. Assess readiness for, and provide opportunities for, independent functioning.[21]

Termination Phase

The *termination phase* of the therapeutic relationship is bound by the time restriction established during the initial phase. As time of termination draws near, the nurse reminds the client (or the group of clients) of the agreed-upon duration of the relationship and assists him to socialize with others.

The termination of the relationship represents possible traumatic difficulties for the client. The nurse recognizes his imminent loss and helps him adapt to this stressor.[14,29,41] If the client feels rejected, insecure, and unloved at the time of termination, he may regress. The nurse recognizes that termination provokes stress; she supports the client's coping behaviors; and she is sensitive to his individual needs. Other members of the mental health team also help the client deal with termination issues.

Tapering off contact with the client is a helpful way to encourage his independence. The nurse summarizes the client's progress toward attaining his goals and freely expresses her own feelings regarding the termination.

Termination means dissolving a relationship.

The primary tasks for the nurse during termination include the following:

1. Space contacts with each client further apart and begin to decrease the amount of time of each contact.
2. Establish a more relaxed, less intense interaction.
3. Focus on the future.
4. Discourage cues that lead to new areas of exploration.
5. Provide necessary referral to others in the health care team.[21]

Dimensions of a Therapeutic Relationship

Conceptual Framework

For clients with emotional problems, nursing provides a unique opportunity to deal with problems of living. "Emotional illness is a pattern of living—of thinking, feeling, and behaving—that a person adopts in an attempt to lessen his anxiety and solve his problems of relating to others."[15] Although this pattern of adaptation may temporarily relieve stress for the individual, it merely postpones the resolution of problems. As an active member of the treatment team, the nurse provides opportunities for the development of a relationship with the client that can be close enough to deal with his special fears, symptoms, and interpersonal problems.

In a therapeutic relationship, the nurse and client purposefully strive to establish goals. The kinds of interactions in which nurses participate vary from assisting a client to eat to undertaking individual, group, or family therapy with him. The nurse recognizes that, although not all contacts with clients are therapy sessions, each contact with a client has the potential for being therapeutic, for promoting interpersonal growth, for changing behavior, or for benefiting the client in some way. Nurses identify the adaptive skills a client uses to relieve his stress, assess the effectiveness of such skills, and help him develop new adaptive skills.

The communication that is developed and nurtured by the nurse and client should be carefully planned and implemented so that the client feels protected, recognizes that he is accepted, and attempts further communication with the helper. This communication, in turn, becomes the vehicle for progress and behavior adaptation.[17]

Characteristics of the Therapeutic Relationship

The core of nursing is the relationship between the nurse and the client. This therapeutic relationship is a goal-directed relationship that helps the client develop more appropriate coping skills and offers him the potential for growth.

Carl Rogers has described the benefits of a helping relationship in these words:

> If I can provide a certain type of a relationship, the other person will discover within himself the capacity to use that relationship for growth and change and personal development will occur.[36]

The nurse's behaviors and attitudes affect the client's view of himself. Her effectiveness depends on the qualities of genuineness, honesty, and authenticity. The nurse cares about the humanism and dignity of the client. Mentally disturbed clients often misinterpret reality; they lack interpersonal skills; and they interpret a nurse's aloofness as rejection. Therefore, the nurse maintains constant self-awareness of both verbal and nonverbal behavior. Consistency in approach fosters the development of trust, particularly when the client tests the relationship.

The client's behavior is his best adaptation to stress. Unconditional acceptance of him as a person reinforces his worth and dignity. If the client must perform ritualistic behavior, for example, care is planned to allow him time to complete his rituals.

One of the client's rights is to be involved in his own care. Together, the nurse and client determine the goals of the relationship, although the primary responsibility for maintaining the relationship falls within the nurse's realm. The nurse acknowledges the potential for growth and movement toward mental health. Her hopefulness and faith support the client's newly learned coping skills.

The various steps of the nursing process can be associated with a therapeutic relationship. During the initial phase of the nurse-client relationship, the nurse and the client begin to develop a trust relationship. Once the nurse and client have described and clarified the experience, they are ready to progress to the next phase of the relationship, which involves exploration.[30] Together the nurse and client put together the pieces of subjective and objective data.

During the working phase of the relationship, the nurse and the client assess the data, plan an action, and begin to evaluate the action. If the evaluation demonstrates that the new behavior is ineffective, the nurse and client together need to identify and develop a new course of action.[30] The relationship ends

CHART 5-2
How Can I Create a Helping Relationship?

Self-understanding is the nurse's responsibility in a nurse-client relationship. The following questions may help the nurse examine the relationship:

1. Can I *be* in some way that will be perceived by others as trustworthy, dependable, or consistent?
2. Can I be expressive enough as a person so that what I am will be communicated unambiguously?
3. Can I let myself experience positive attitudes toward this other person—attitudes of warmth, caring, liking, interest, respect?
4. Can I be strong enough as a person to be separate from the other?
5. Am I secure enough within myself to permit him his separateness?
6. Can I let myself enter fully into his world of his feelings and personal meaning and see these as he does?
7. Can I receive him as he is?
8. Can I act with sufficient sensitivity in the relationship so that my behavior will not be perceived as a threat?
9. Can I free him from the threat of external evaluation?
10. Can I meet this other individual as a person who is bound by his past and my past?

(From Rogers CR: On Becoming a Person. Boston, Houghton Mifflin, 1961)

during the termination phase, as the action has been evaluated as effective.

Anxieties of Nurse and Client

In a therapeutic relationship, both nurse and client are involved in a stress-producing situation. The openness and honesty inherent in the relationship make them vulnerable to its impact.

Dealing with the client's dependency needs requires a great deal of skill and self-awareness. Dependency needs may elicit within the nurse a feeling of having the sole solution to the client's problems. If the nurse does not recognize the potential or actual growth of the client, perhaps because it does not match her expectations, a relationship may develop that meets the nurse's needs instead of the client's needs. It is always a temptation to try to make the other person into a reflection of ourselves or our ideals rather than to help him develop his individual potential.[16] The nurse constantly re-evaluates her feelings, thoughts, and behavior within a relationship.

When the client does not meet the ideals of the nurse—for example, when he does not appear to be gaining insight into his behavior—the nurse may view the relationship as lacking progress. In turn, the client feels internal stress trying to please the nurse and may test her commitment to the relationship. At this point, the nurse may realize that she cannot meet all the client's needs and may seek assistance from others in the health care team.

The nurse and client may also need to discuss honestly the course of the relationship. Perhaps the goals of the relationship should be re-evaluated. The nurse must be able to tolerate, accept, and redirect the anxiety that accompanies the recognition of possible failure. The tension required to produce action must be differentiated from the hostility resulting from frustration.[16]

The client and nurse may elicit in each other feelings that are hard to admit. Testing the nurse and the relationship may indicate that the client is unable to express his feelings. Likewise, a difficult situation exists when the nurse experiences feelings of anger and frustration. An inability to verbalize these feelings by either member of the relationship places a strain on the relationship and affects trust and honesty. The nurse strives to become aware of her own feelings and to help the client identify and deal with his feelings.

Expectations of the Client and Helper

Clients seeking medical or psychiatric treatment expect to experience the relief of anxiety. This can result from the health care team's response to the client's physical or emotional stress.

The nurse who strives to understand the client's behavioral needs must be aware of implicit, explicit, rational, irrational, and symbolic patterns of behavior.

The nurse initiates a relationship with a client in which he is free to verbalize needs; as the relationship progresses, he also verbalizes fears and anxieties. The nurse urges him to evaluate his adaptive pattern and the consequences of his defensive behavior. The therapeutic relationship provides the client with the opportunity to test new adaptive skills. As the client receives positive feedback within the relationship and experiences growth and increased self-esteem, he is able to relinquish ineffective behavioral patterns. As the relationship leads to termination, the nurse encourages the client to use healthier skills in interactions outside the relationship. The ultimate goal is one of independence for the client.

Family and friends of the client have expectations of treatment as well. The nurse acknowledges the family unit as a significant part of the treatment process. At times, however, the family and friends of the client may encourage, elicit, or reinforce his inappropriate or maladaptive behavior. The client must determine what type of relationship, if any, he wants to continue with his family. Frequently, nurses believe that union with one's family is the ultimate goal of healthy adaptation, but this is not always true.

Issues in a Therapeutic Relationship

Attitudes of the Nurse Helper

Our attitudes, developed at a young age, determine our behavior. Each attitude is a signal of a need present in the individual. To facilitate growth in an individual, nurses first identify attitudes present within themselves. Mentally disturbed clients are often viewed by our society as hopeless and helpless individuals. The presence of these attitudes, either consciously or unconsciously, prevents the nurse from intervening in ways that encourage the client's independence. Feelings of hopelessness are particularly evident when working with clients who have long-term emotional disorders. Nurses and other care providers may question, "What is the use of working with these individuals when they are not likely to return home ever again?" Failure to recognize and modify their own attitudes results in failure to provide quality nursing care to clients.[19]

The nurse offers hope that the client will lead a productive life within his environment. Regardless of the client's present level of adaptation, growth is possible. Assisting a client to move from one level of functioning to another is progress, although it may seem minimal to the observer. For example, a withdrawn client who establishes even brief periods of eye contact with the nurse demonstrates a beginning trust level.

Each client, regardless of his status or place within our environment, has worth and dignity. Respect for the individual is an essential component of nursing. When respect from others is lacking, the client experiences worthlessness, anxiety, and disturbed behavior.

The difference between tolerance of behavior and acceptance of behavior is an often-misunderstood concept. Tolerance is a passive activity; no action is required of the nurse. Acceptance is an active process that requires recognition of the client's behavior as meeting a need and representing his best adaptation at the time. Respecting the human dignity of the individual, hoping for potential growth, and accepting the client's behavior are beginning steps in facilitating growth for the client.

Facilitating Growth

An important objective of therapeutic intervention is to provide the client with opportunities to recognize the needs his behavior meets and to develop more effective attitudes and behaviors. The approach of the nurse in the therapeutic relationship should be one of consistency. The nurse's behavior and approach give the client feedback about the appropriateness of his behavior. When the nurse makes a promise, care should be taken to ensure adequate follow-up. Casual remarks are often taken seriously.[2]

The nurse's consistency also provides the client with security. In this environment, he is free to deal with problems and develop adaptation skills. When the client experiences inconsistency in the nurse's behavior, he often focuses his attention on pleasing the nurse, rather than on his own personal growth.

To encourage the client to try out new adaptive behaviors, the nurse provides emotional support by assisting him to pay attention to his feelings, to link his feelings to his troublesome behaviors, and then to explore alternative behaviors. The nurse creates a relationship in which the client shares decision-making and validates his perception of the outcome of his decisions. This offers the client an opportunity to try his new behavior without penalty (wherein he can receive feedback from others and can evaluate the outcome of his behavior) as he develops a new set of adaptation skills that are less destructive than those he used previously. During the client's growth process, the nurse supports and reinforces the healthy aspects of his personality, assesses the client's movement toward independence, and encourages him to assume more responsibility for himself.

Interpersonal Skills

Carl Rogers states, "... the degree to which I can create a relationship which facilitates growth of others as a separate person is a measure of the growth I have achieved myself." Self-awareness is an essential component of effective therapeutic relationships. The nurse also takes responsibility for examining her own behavior and for making the necessary changes in behavior when that is indicated. To function as a healthy adult role model, the nurse must demonstrate sufficient emotional maturity to be able to postpone the satisfaction of her own needs and allow the client's needs to take precedence.[16]

The nurse's most basic and important therapeutic tool is herself, her own personality. Many physical, cultural, psychological, social, and environmental factors interact to create a unique personality; the nurse's awareness of these factors increases her insight into her own and others' feelings and behavior. Objectivity and empathy grow out of the nurse's self-awareness, emotional maturity, responsibility, and insight, and these tools prevent misinterpretation of the client's needs through interference of the nurse's own needs.

Transference and Countertransference

The client who is functioning at a regressed level may misinterpret or unconsciously displace onto the nurse his earlier feelings about important persons, such as his parents. This misinterpretation or unconscious displacement of feelings is termed *transference*. Transference distortion, based on unconscious conflict, is the inevitable consequence of human encounter.[39]

The nurse recognizes and accepts that the client is responding to her on the basis of a previous relationship. Lack of recognition of the transference would lead the nurse to respond to the client's behavior in ways that may negate its effectiveness.

Countertransference is the helping person's distorted or inappropriate responses to clients due to the helper's unconscious conflict.[39] A nurse, for example, may displace feelings for her younger brother onto a young male client for whom she is caring. Nurses should attend to the feelings they experience when interacting with clients, particularly when they differ from usual feelings. If the nurse identifies or suspects that transference or countertransference is occurring, she may solicit the aid of clinical supervisors or other mental health team members to help her develop objectivity in the relationship.

Summary

This chapter has presented the dynamics and dimensions of a therapeutic relationship, as well as the issues that may arise in such a relationship. It has also included the following points:

1. A therapeutic relationship is one in which the nurse and client participate and work toward the goals of meeting the client's needs and facilitating his growth.

2. There are three possible types of relationships—social, intimate, and therapeutic.

3. Therapeutic relationships progress through initial or introductory, middle or working, and termination phases.

4. The core of nursing is the relationship between the nurse and the client.

5. The nurse recognizes that the client's behavior is his best possible adaptation to stress at the time.

6. The therapeutic relationship provides the client with an opportunity to examine unsuccessfully adaptive (or maladaptive) behaviors, and to explore and try out new adaptive skills.

7. The nurse's self-awareness, responsibility, emotional maturity, objectivity, and empathy are powerful tools of intervention.

References

1. Aiken L, Aiken JL: A Systematic Approach to the Evaluation of Interpersonal Relationships. Am J Nurs 73 (May): 863–866, 1973
2. Bailey DS, Cooper SD, Bailey DR: Therapeutic Approaches to the Care of the Mentally Ill. Philadelphia, FA Davis, 1984
3. Bailey DS, Dryer S: Therapeutic Approach to the Care of the Mentally Ill. Philadelphia, FA Davis, 1971
4. Campaniello JA: The Process of Termination. J Psychiatr Nurs Ment Health Serv (February): 29–32, 1980
5. Carser DL: Primary Nursing in Milieu. J Psychiatr Nurs Ment Health Serv 19 (February): 35–41, 1981
6. Carter FM: Psychosocial Nursing, 3d ed. New York, Macmillan, 1981
7. Clemence M, Sr: Existentialism: A Philosophy of Commitment. Am J Nurs 66 (March): 500–505, 1966
8. Egan G: The Skilled Helper. California, Brooks/Cole, 1982
9. Erikson EH: Childhood and Society, 2d ed. New York, WW Norton, 1964
10. Fagin CM: Psychotherapeutic Nursing. Am J Nurs 67 (February): 298–304, 1967
11. Fitzpatrick JJ, Whall AL, Johnston RL, Floyd JA: Nursing Models and Their Psychiatric Mental Health Application. Bowie, MD, John J Brady, 1982
12. Grace HR, Camilleri D: Mental Health Nursing, 2d ed. Dubuque, IA, Wm C Brown, 1977
13. Haber J et al: Comprehensive Psychiatric Nursing. New York, McGraw-Hill, 1978
14. Hale JS, Richardson J: Terminating the Nurse-

Patient Relationship. Am J Nurs 63 (September): 1116–1119, 1963

15. Hays JS, Larson KH: Interacting with Patients. New York, Macmillan, 1964

16. Irving S: Basic Psychiatric Nursing, 2d ed. Philadelphia, WB Saunders, 1978

17. Janosik EH, Davis JL: Psychiatric Mental Health Nursing. Boston/Monterey, Jones and Bartlett Publishers, 1986

18. Jensen HN, Tilloston G: Dependency in the Nurse-Patient Relationship. Am J Nurs 61 (February): 81–84, 1961

19. Johnson MM: Self-Disclosure: A Variable in the Nurse–Client Relationship. J Psychiatr Nurs 18 (January): 17–20, 1980

20. King I: A Conceptual Frame of Reference for Nursing. Nurs Res 17 (January–February): 27–31, 1968

21. Kriegh HZ, Perko JE: Psychiatric and Mental Health Nursing: A Commitment to Care and Concern. Reston, VA, Reston Publishing, 1979

22. Lamonica EL: The Nursing Process: A Humanistic Approach. Menlo Park, CA, Addison-Wesley, 1979

23. Lego SM: The One-to-One Patient Relationship. Perspect Psychiatr Care 18 (March/April): 67–88, 1980

24. Leininger M: Caring, A Central Focus of Nursing and Health Care Services. Nursing and Health Care 1 (Oct): 135–143, 1980

25. Long L, Prophit P, Sr: Understanding/Responding: a Communication Manual for Nurses. Belmont, CA, Wadsworth Health Science Division, 1981

26. Manfreda M, Krampetz SD: Psychiatric Nursing, 10th ed. Philadelphia, FA Davis, 1977

27. McCann J: Terminating of the Psychotherapeutic Relationship. J Psychiatr Nurs 17 (October): 37–39, 1979

28. Murray RB, Zentner JP: Nursing Concepts for Health Promotion, 2d ed. Englewood Cliffs, NJ, Prentice-Hall, 1979

29. Nehren J, Gillian NR: Separation Anxiety. Am J Nurs 65 (January): 190–112, 1965

30. Pasquali, EA et al: Mental Health Nursing: A Holistic Approach. St. Louis, CV Mosby, 1985

31. Peplau H: Interpersonal Relations in Nursing. New York, GP Putnam's Sons, 1952

32. Rector C: Content in the Initial Therapeutic Patient Interview. Perspect Psychiatr Care 3 (March): 33–35, 1965

33. Robinson L: Psychiatric Nursing as a Human Experience, 2d ed. Philadelphia, WB Saunders, 1977

34. Robinson, L: Psychological Aspects of the Care of the Hospitalized Patients. Philadelphia, FA Davis, 1984

35. Rogers CR: Client-Centered Therapy. Boston, Houghton Mifflin, 1951

36. Rogers CR: The Characteristics of a Helping Relationship. Personnel and Guidance Journal 37 (September): 6–16, 1958

37. Rogers CR: On Becoming a Person. Boston, Houghton Mifflin, 1961

38. Schoffstall C: Concerns of Student Nurses Prior to Psychiatric Nursing Experience: An Assessment and Intervention Technique. J Psychiatr Nurs Ment Health Serv 19 (November): 11–14, 1981

39. Schwartz LH, Schwartz JL: The Psychodynamics of Patient Care. Englewood Cliffs, NJ, Prentice-Hall, 1972

40. Sene B: Termination in the Student–Patient Relationship. Perspect Psychiatr Care 8: 39–45, 1969

41. Taylor MC: Mereness' Essentials of Psychiatric Nursing, 11th ed. St Louis, CV Mosby, 1982

42. World Health Organization: Expert Committee on Psychiatric Nursing, First Report. World Health Organization technical report series, No 105, July, 1956. In Hays JS, Larson KH (eds): Interacting with Patients. New York, Macmillan, 1964

43. Yura H, Walsh M: Human Needs and the Nursing Process. New York, Appleton-Century-Croft, 1978

6 Sociocultural Aspects of Care

Margie N. Slaughter

If we are to achieve a richer culture, rich in contrasting values, we must recognize the whole gamut of human potentialities, and so we are a less arbitrary social fabric, one in which each diverse human gift will find a fitting place.

Margaret Mead

Chapter Preview

Many ethnic groups presently call America home. In addition, members of ethnic minorities continue to arrive daily from other countries. Psychiatric–mental health problems increase in relation to unemployment, economic decline, and interpersonal alienation. An individual's culture encompasses many factors that influence his perceptions of health and illness and whether he seeks assistance from mental health care professionals.

This chapter is written to help the health care provider understand and appreciate how a person's culture affects his perceptions of, and reactions to, health and illness, emotional problems, and disorders. The overview of culture focuses on the specific aspects of ethnicity, lifestyle, religion, and family influences. The nursing process—assessment, nursing diagnosis, planning, implementation, and evaluation—is applied to psychiatric–mental health clients of different cultures.

Learning Objectives

Upon completion of the chapter, you should be able to accomplish the following:

1. define culture
2. discuss the influence of culture on the health beliefs and practices of individuals
3. recognize the existence of racial and cultural diversity in American society
4. recognize and discuss feelings and behaviors that influence your ability to interact with individuals of another culture
5. apply the nursing process to clients of different cultures:
   assess clients of different cultures
   formulate nursing diagnoses for clients of different cultures
   identify nursing goals and actions designed to alleviate the problems of clients and families of different cultures
   formulate nursing care plans for clients and families of different cultures
   evaluate the effectiveness of nursing interventions

Culture

Culture is man's basic roadmap for living.[23] Specific cultural beliefs include an individual's values and patterns of living, and these beliefs have always been a part of human existence. A person's reactions to illness, health maintenance, daily activities, food preferences, interpersonal relationships, patterns of action, beliefs, and feelings are all culturally linked.

Culture is learned behavior—dynamic and everchanging. Culture is transmitted from one generation to another through socialization practices that are reinforced by cultural and social interactions. As an individual matures, he may accept or reject certain portions of his culture, thereby inducing cultural changes.

Subculture and Ethnicity

A *subculture* is a group of people who may be distinguishable by ethnic background, religion, social status, or other similar characteristics; at the same time, they may share certain features with larger social segments.[20] Nevertheless, although some of these features are shared, certain differences exist due to ethnic background. An *ethnic group* is a group of people with a common origin who hold basically similar values, beliefs, and means of communication.[34]

Why Study Culture?

The concept of culture provides a comprehensive framework for care providers to understand and appreciate the cultural differences and similarities essential to providing quality patient care. Being knowledgeable about cultural similarities enables care providers to appreciate common human behaviors and bonds. Failing to appreciate cultural differences leads to ineffective communication and relationships between clients and care providers and limits the providers' ability to work effectively with members of other cultures.

Culture is a patterned way of life with special meaning to the individual members of the culture. To develop a therapeutic plan of care, the health care provider needs to be aware of the client's way of thinking, feeling, and responding. Knowledge of the client's background helps health professionals understand cultural factors related to health care, their role in working with clients and families of different cultures, and approaches they might take in order to facilitate changes in health practices.

Multiethnicity of the United States

For many years, people in the United States have lived with the myth of the "melting pot," or cultural homogeneity. According to this myth, various European people immigrating to the United States were absorbed into America's mainstream.[9] This process of assimilation required that the particular European ethnic groups relinquish those behavioral practices that failed to fit into their new culture. Although some European ethnic groups, such as the Italians, Irish, Jews, and Polish, were persecuted for certain beliefs, practices, and behaviors, they were nevertheless absorbed into the main culture. This was not true, however, of all ethnic groups.

Ethnic groups of color, those with yellow, brown, black, or red skin, have never been totally assimilated into the main culture. Their color, as well as other distinctive racial characteristics such as facial features, body build, and hair texture, made it impossible for them not to be noticeable. Ethnic groups of color have been, and still are, oppressed and discriminated against.

A new ethnicity movement that began in the early 1970s focused on the multiethnicity of the United States and attempted to dispel the melting-pot myth. This movement encouraged ethnic awareness, ethnic traditions, and the practice of specific ethnic customs. The movement further stressed that it was not necessary to relinquish all cultural differences to become totally assimilated into American society.[41]

American Cultural Values

Cultural values are powerful forces that govern an individual's behavior.[20] Many times, people are not fully aware of American cultural values and their effect on the individual's manner of thought and behavior.

The white middle-class American represents the norm of behavior for the people of the United States. Growth and development theories pertaining to family structure and function, personality development, and physiologic and anatomic characteristics are based on this norm of white America.[20]

American culture stresses the values of automation, time, success, cleanliness, and optimal health.[27] Health care providers are also members of a subculture and influenced by the overall American culture; the values of the dominant culture are reflected in the administration of health care.

Automation

Modern technology has hurled American society toward increasing automation. Some of the positive results of technology are improvements in the quality of life by early detection of certain diseases of adults, children, and the unborn. On the other hand, today's technology has provided us with the ability to annihilate life.

Through automation, jobs that were formerly held by human beings may be performed faster and more efficiently by machines. Automation has altered the job market and has caused many people to seek career changes. The need for career changes, and the rise in unemployment when jobs are unavailable, increase stress in individuals, families, and communities.

Modern technology has also had its impact on nursing. Nurses and other health care providers use computers in the processes of gathering and categorizing client data and administering health care services. They operate sophisticated, efficient machines in the treatment of selected diseases. Some subtle dangers exist when health professionals use and rely on particularly advanced machinery. One growing concern is the tendency of people to relate more readily to machines than to other humans. Health care providers may become so involved in technical skills that the client and his stresses, anxieties, and fears are overlooked.

Time

Time is valuable and not to be wasted in America. Time dominates work, sleep, and play. Time influences economic, political, and social values. Time also stimulates emotional reactions in people who are influenced by its power. For example, an individual may feel guilt if he believes he is wasting time, fear or stress if he fails to be on time for an appointment, and anger or frustration if he has to wait for another person who is not on time.

Many other cultures of the world do not view time as such a high-priority consideration as we do in the American culture. Some countries have no clocks; many depend on the sun and moon to influence their actions and activities. The failure or the need to adhere to a time schedule does not seem to create a problem for these cultural groups.[38]

Success

Successful people are perceived as those who keep busy, work hard, and strive to reach the top. Americans continue to push themselves to greater achievements, to compete, to increase their salaries, and to become more successful socially, economically, and politically. Having the power to control others is equated with success. In conjunction with this continual push for upward mobility, Americans are resorting to more over-the-counter medications, illegal drugs, prescribed drugs, and alcohol to alleviate their daily stresses and problems.

Nursing is likewise influenced by the cultural value of success. Nurses are perceived by others as achievers and are measured by their ability to perform. Nurses themselves often measure their success by their ability to complete tasks. Nursing education in the past stressed actions and tasks; nursing students were rewarded for their task performance, and often not for being active listeners or for being independent, critical thinkers. In more recent years, however,

C H A R T   6-1
Dealing with Cultural Differences Among Psychiatric Clients
Cheryl Taylor-Walton, M.N., R.N.
Assistant Professor of Nursing
Louisiana State University School of Nursing
New Orleans, Louisiana

Conveying an attitude of acceptance of the client is an integral component of the therapeutic relationship. The nurse's attitude of acceptance and ability to hold her own preconceptions in abeyance are even more important when providing care to a client who is culturally different.

During the assessment phase of the nursing process, it is essential for the nurse to examine her own thoughts and feelings about the client who is culturally different from her. Often the nurse is unfamiliar with clients' personal values; furthermore, the nurse may find some of the values of culturally different clients to be repulsive or abnormal. For example, the religion and spirituality of the African American client may be central to, even the core of, his being. A nurse who does not recognize this as a value in her own life may overlook it in the client's experience or perceive it as an abnormal occurrence requiring a diagnostic label, rather than viewing it as the stabilizing force of the cleint's life.

One critical factor during the assessment phase is to accept the client as a person while avoiding misperceiving his cultural heritage as a part of his diagnosis. Another important guideline of client data assessment is to become familiar with the cultural norms of various ethnic groups. This familiarity requires background reading and discussion about the world views, values, and practices of specific cultures, such as black American, Spanish-speaking American, and Asian American. The client who is experiencing an emotional imbalance should not be expected to teach the nurse about his culture in order to receive competent care.

Members of ethnic minorities, because of their historical relationship with the dominant culture, have had many opportunities to learn about the dominant culture's values and experiences. For many years they worked as maids, butlers, and in other domestic roles in the homes of members of the dominant culture; this experience provided the minorities with direct exposure to many aspects of the white culture. The reverse, however, is not true; consequently, members of ethnic minorities have been incorrectly viewed as having one-dimensional personalities.

While analyzing client data, the nurse should base the formulation of nursing diagnoses on objective assessment data, not on subjective, stereotyped assumptions. Phrases such as "passive Oriental male" and "attractive black female" should be avoided. The planning and implementation phases of the nursing process pose creative challenges to the nurse who is working with a culturally different client. Utilizing client strengths and incorporating and engaging client values into the planning and intervention phases are essential components of effective treatment. The client must never be deterred from his own cultural experience in order to participate in treatment.

Knowing oneself is critical for the nurse who is working with culturally different clients. Self-knowledge and self-awareness help the nurse to recognize her own anxieties, stereotypes, biases, and prejudgments about culturally different clients. Further experience, introspection, and study empower the nurse to appreciate the strengths of other cultures. While concurrently planning and intervening in a manner sensitive to the client's cultural issues, the nurse evaluates the client's freedom to offer open, honest feedback, to disagree, or to confront real or perceived problems without being penalized by means of chemical restraints or withdrawal of staff attention.

In the clinical setting, you should avoid the following behaviors:

1. Distance behavior, such as staying in the nurses' station or clustering in staff groups, with culturally different clients
2. Patronizing culturally different clients by extolling the virtues of one person you know who is a credit to their race or ethnic background ("I have a black/Asian/hispanic friend who is so smart...")
3. Talking as if "people are people and color doesn't matter" while acting in subtle, nonverbal ways that clearly say that color does matter
4. Addressing culturally different persons on a first-name basis without their permission

5. Expecting total trust and self-disclosure from the culturally different client and using that occurrence as a determinant of whether you will help the client
6. Trivialization of the client's experience as a hispanic, black, Asian, or native American with health professionals and others of the dominant culture
7. Thinking that there is something inherently wrong with people who are different from yourself
8. Expecting one member of a specific culture to be an expert on the behaviors of the entire culture
9. Condemning or prejudging an entire cultural group based on your negative experience with, or media hype about, one individual of that cultural group

Suppose that you, as a student or novice nurse, are assigned to the subacute unit of a psychiatric hospital. You enter the treatment facility, walk into the unit, and discover that the clients are predominately male and black (if you're anglo or hispanic or Asian or native American), anglo (if you're hispanic or black or Asian or native American), and so on. What do you do?

Step 1. Try not to look as if you were just tossed into a terrorist camp.

Step 2. Remember that there is a wide range of beliefs and behavior patterns in every culture.

Step 3. Relax and initiate the nursing process.

the nursing profession has emphasized the need for nurses to be thinkers, planners, and assessors of health care.[28]

Cleanliness

Bathing, using deodorants, and wearing clean clothes are stressed through media advertisements, through health education in school, and through education by parents and others. Americans spend billions of dollars on body soaps, washing powders, house cleaners, and other products that promote optimum cleanliness and physical aesthetics. During toilet training, children quickly learn that it's not okay to get soiled; children are often reprimanded for dirtying their clothes.

America's cultural attitude toward cleanliness often conflicts with the attitudes of other cultures. Some cultures feel that exposure to dirt enhances health. Other cultures do not believe that deodorants should be used and do not find the body odor offensive. Some cultures do not think that it is necessary to wash as frequently as Americans do and believe that frequent washing wastes valuable water. Many of these attitudes and values of other cultures are difficult for health care providers to understand and accept because they conflict with their own beliefs about cleanliness.

Nurses strive to maintain a clean, orderly, and relatively germ-free environment for the patient. They spend an enormous amount of time keeping the patient and his environment tidy and clean. The nurse's personal cleanliness is effected by her wearing clean uniforms and maintaining an odor-free body.

American culture stresses that a patient should feel better when he is clean. Assessment of an individual's emotional status includes an evaluation of his physical appearance. For example, are his clothes clean? Is he unkempt; that is, is his hair dirty, does he have body odor, or does he have an unwashed body? Lack of cleanliness often indicates to mental health professionals that the individual is experiencing some type of emotional upset or disorder. Lack of attention to one's personal appearance is frequently interpreted, according to American cultural values, as a sign of depression or decompensation.

Optimal Health

The maintenance of health is held as a human right, as well as a civil right, by health officials and by national, state, and local governments. According to middle-class norms, the culturally disadvantaged and deprived experience poor health practices. Senior citizens on fixed income and low-income families who fail to consider health a primary goal are identified as part of these culturally disadvantaged.

Members of many cultures do not view health maintenance as a primary need as long as they are free of pain and have no symptoms that indicate a need to seek health care. The members of some cultures, when interacting with health care providers, may subtly or overtly receive a message that their health practices are unacceptable. Many of these patients will listen politely and then choose either to ignore the information or simply not return to the health care facility. Health care providers may inadvertently attempt to impose their own health practices on members of other cultures without realizing that each individual has health norms and practices that are governed by his own culture.[36]

Process of Enculturation

Enculturation is the process by which an individual learns the expected behavior of the culture. These behaviors incorporate that culture's specific values, beliefs, sanctions, and constraints.[27] The primary goal of enculturation is to provide the individual with the skills needed to function within a given community. This community may consist of people of the same or a different ethnic group.

Agents of Enculturation

It is the responsibility of the agents of enculturation to convey values and a sense of belonging, warmth, and cohesion within a culture. The family, neighborhood, religion, and educational system are agents of enculturation.

Family

The family is the earliest and most effective agent of enculturation. Each unique family interaction conveys to its members communication patterns, role behavior, values, beliefs, and views of the world. Within the family, the individual learns fear, love, hatred, and hope. He develops his aspirations, even those of an intense and deeply personal nature, within the family, and is both positively and negatively affected by others' perceptions of who and what he is.

A family, particularly a minority family, transmits not only what is valued by the group, but also clues regarding how members of the group are likely to be perceived and received by others outside the group.[4] For minority groups and those suffering the effects of discrimination, ethnic identity and its transmission serve to protect their members from the larger world.[7] The larger world belittles or demeans the members of minority groups, often out of ignorance and frequently intentionally. Ethnicity protects against the insinuation that, if the members abandon their ethnic group identity or related behaviors, discrimination against them will cease. This insinuation has proved to be false; blacks or hispanics who have chosen to abandon subtle, but characteristic, speech patterns still experience job discrimination in certain areas of America.

Neighborhood

The neighborhood is another agent of enculturation. Neighborhoods consist of shops, church, school, taverns, and many members of a social network. An ethnic group residing together over a long period of time develops a strong sense of belonging and community. This social network helps members develop and structure relationships outside the home and maintain endangered values, customs, and beliefs when individual members of the ethnic group begin to move into mainstream America.

Neighborhood networking varies according to geographic locations and different ethnic groups. For example, in large urban areas, only pockets of stable neighborhoods may be found. Many inner-city neighborhoods are being destroyed by vandals, are sold to land developers, or are slowly deteriorating due to neglect. When neighborhoods change rapidly, the stability of the social network is threatened or lost. In some cases, when mothers and fathers both work outside of the home, members of the neighborhood may offer the primary means of socialization and protection for children. From these neighbors, children may learn how to protect themselves from strangers and criminal elements in the community.

Religion

Religion plays an important role in the life of many ethnic groups. Some people look to religion for answers to their questions about why certain events, such as illness or injury, occur in their lives. Religion also affects the way in which people interpret the signs and symptoms of illness. Religious beliefs often influence the course of the illness and the person's willingness to seek medical care. For example, members of religions that promulgate a belief that God ultimately controls all that happens on the earth and teach that man should accept with humility and resignation the fate to which he has been assigned, may tend to avoid the use of medical services.[19]

Church attendance provides spiritual involvement for some and a basis of social life for other members of the church community. Religious groups also act as enforcers of ethnic values, customs, and behaviors. Through their church participation and involvement, some church members gain status that is self-affirming and confers on them the respect and honor of the community.[27]

Educational System

Within the schools, children begin to relate with others outside of their immediate environment. Often, the school environment provides the child with his first opportunity to encounter someone from a different ethnic group. The teacher becomes a critical figure to the child. The child's ability to adjust to school progresses effectively when the child is able to relate with a teacher of the same ethnic group or with a teacher who is culturally sensitive and supportive.

Busing has probably contributed to the problem of maintaining ethnic identity. In the pursuit of better educational opportunities for all children, many children coming from schools and teachers who promote adjustment to the process of formal education are bused to other schools and teachers who are not sensitive to cultural differences. A teacher may be unsuccessful in interacting with children of different ethnic groups due to the lack of educational preparation in working with children of different cultures, the fear of not being an effective teacher of the child, the mistake of "trying too hard" to help the child succeed in school, the fear of identification with the child, and the bigotry and prejudices that the teacher may be unable to deny. The child quickly learns that the teacher is the authority figure. If a child receives negative responses from the teacher or other person in the authority role, he may react to them strongly; that is, negative responses may have profound effects on him and his behavior.

Process of Acculturation

Acculturation is the process in which groups with different cultures and backgrounds meet and live together. Efforts to understand and accurately describe acculturation were triggered by the mass migrations of Europeans to the United States, by the importation of slaves, and by the contacts between the original settlers and the American Indians.

Cultural change takes place gradually and in many degrees. Acculturation makes one group's culture the point of reference and focuses upon the events and processes by which that group responds to continuous contact with another group.[34] The group may accept, reformulate, or reject elements of the other culture.

During the process of acculturation, the ethnic group may adopt only the major themes or behaviors of the dominant society, such as its language, or the ethnic group may establish even deeper relationships with the dominant society, such as through intermarriage. Many ethnic groups value their traditions and differences and actively attempt to prevent total assimilation into the dominant culture, while at the same time they seek social and economic equality.[41] On the other hand, not all members of an ethnic group necessarily believe or practice all aspects of that culture. One reality to bear in mind is that, because of intermarriage within different cultures, there are few people who can be considered culturally pure.[43]

Aspects of Cultural Learning of Specific Ethnic Groups

Each ethnic group has a unique history with respect to oppression and discrimination, the value attached to academic pursuits, the roles of men and women, the value of the family, and the translation of religious teachings into dicta for daily living.

The traditions transmitted by the family, the special inflection of language, and even the foods a person eats let him know that he is with his own. For the lower-class white, as well as for ethnic groups of color, the reality of cultural distinctions has also perpetuated continuing and persistent discrimination in jobs, in housing, in schooling, in the reception received in the work place, and often in institutions providing health care.[16]

The term *ethnic people of color* has been designated to persons belonging to the four large minority groups in the United States. These four minority cultures have been defined by the federal government and include the Spanish-speaking, American Indian or native American, Asian American, and black American. The following discussions of these four minority groups are, of necessity, generalized. It should be noted that subcultures exist within each of the ethnic groups discussed. Care must be taken to avoid overgeneralization. Specific nursing actions and implications related to each ethnic group are also discussed.

Spanish-Speaking Americans

Spanish-speaking Americans have their origin in a number of countries—Spain, Mexico, Cuba, Puerto Rico, and other nations of Central and South America. The majority of the Spanish-speaking people in America are Mexican-Americans. Although each of the Spanish-speaking subcultures is distinctive in origin and characteristics, they share some commonalities in relation to health practices, attitudes toward health care providers, the use of healers, and so forth.

Health Practices
In the Spanish-speaking culture, a sick person remains within his group or family. The danger of illness or harm is perceived as coming from outside the patient, such as from the impersonal physical world or from the unknown.

Generally, an older family member within the home, usually the grandmother, treats mild illnesses by means of various herbs and home remedies. Illness, harm, and the hazards of the unknown are prevented by men and women wearing certain objects, such as copper pennies, cloves of garlic, or a "deer's eye," or by performing certain rites. A piece of red cloth may be worn over the heart to prevent angina. The health care provider should not remove these objects unless their removal is absolutely necessary, because they provide comfort and security to the Spanish-speaking patient. Men and women may believe that by observing the ritual calendar, by being a good Catholic, and by being a respected member of the community, a person is able to maintain balance in his or her life.

Attitudes Toward Health Care Providers

Many Spanish-speaking patients are uncomfortable when treated by a physician. They often perceive the doctor's professional approach as being indifferent to personal needs.[32] Spanish-speaking women may feel embarrassment and bashfulness in the presence of male physicians or medical students and may prefer to have a female conduct the interview or examination. A male would prefer, likewise, not to be cared for by a female health provider. In the hospital, the fear of surgery, the impersonality of the doctors and nurses, the infringement on one's modesty, and the possibility of death contribute to the anxiety of being hospitalized.

Healers

It is important for the health care provider to be aware that a Spanish-speaking patient may consult both a faith healer and a physician. Many times, the patient may be referred to a physician by a healer who determined that the patient was too critically ill for him to treat.

Two kinds of healers are involved in folk medicine. The *curandero* (male) or *curandera* (female) is seen when a person is ill. The curandero or curandera uses rituals, massages, and herbs to combat the illness, and he or she involves the patient and his family in the treatment. These healers are believed to be chosen by God to heal natural folk illnesses.[32] (See Chart 6-2, "Curanderismo.")

The second healer is known as the *epiritualisto* (male) or *epiritualista* (female). The spiritualist is usually consulted when there is a need to remove hexes or communicate with the dead, or a desire to predict the individual's future.[41]

Social and Kinship Ties

The family is a cherished institution among Spanish-speaking people, probably second only to God and the church. Typically, the father is the patriarch whose authority is recognized and exercised. He is responsible for providing guidance and leadership to the family and for making all major decisions.

The mother is subordinate to her husband or to the head of the household. The mother's interests primarily include bearing children and caring for her family, home, and close kin.

Respect is accorded to members of the family on the basis of age and sex. The old are accorded more respect than the young, and men more respect than women.

Religion

Religion is an important influence because the Spanish-speaking peoples believe that religion unifies and integrates their life in the family and the community. The predominant religion is Roman Catholicism.

A strong belief among Spanish-speaking people is that God gives health and allows illness for a reason. They also believe that faith in God is necessary for recovery from illness.

The priest continues to be recognized as a spiritual leader, even though some of the religious activities of the Catholic church are changing. The priest also serves as a counselor in temporal, religious, and community matters.

Language

Many Spanish-speaking patients and families experience their language as a barrier to health care in institutions that expect an individual to be proficient in English. The language difference further isolates Spanish-speaking clients from organizations and services that could help improve their living conditions.

Mental Illness

Research has demonstrated that there is less incidence of mental illness among Spanish-speaking people than in the general population, in part because there are fewer role conflicts; that is, the rules of behavior of the culture are clearly defined.[32] The family also serves as a buffering mechanism that allows members to share, and thereby reduce, anxiety and stressful situations. Their view of the world enables them to blame external forces for failures, and this further reduces guilt. Spanish-speaking people are also likely to be averse to hospitals and are reluctant to seek treatment for mental illness.

Implications for Nursing Actions

1. Recognize and attend to the role of the nuclear and extended family in Spanish-speaking cultures. Illness of the Spanish-speaking patient tends to be a social, family, and, oftentimes, a community matter rather than an isolated illness state of one person.
2. Provide explanations that take into account

CHART 6-2
Curanderismo

Juanita Zapata Flint, M.S., R.N.
Coordinator/Instructor, Nursing
El Centro College
Brookhaven College Satellite
Dallas, Texas

Curanderismo is the practice of folk healing that evolved from European medical practices of the 15th and 16th centuries and that continues today within the Mexican-American community. The Aztecs, Mayas, and other Indian groups left these folk beliefs and curing practices to the Spanish Catholics in Mexico. Curanderismo has persisted as a tradition in the Mexican-American culture because of that culture's members' rural background, illiteracy, poverty, and distrust of the modern medical care system.[2]

Curanderos and *curanderas,* or folk healers, are usually women who believe they are endowed with curing powers from God. The healer comes to hold this belief by experiencing a dream or a vision or by being involved in the care of a sick person who recovers. Curanderos are sincere in their belief that they were chosen by God and therefore do not usually charge fees for their healing services. They believe that if they expected or demanded payment, their divine gift of healing would be taken away. Recently, however, it has become common for curanderos to develop a fee system, although their charges are minimal.[3]

The diseases treated by the curandero are thought to be due to the will of God or to witchcraft. *Susto,* or fright, is a condition that follows an emotional upset and is characterized by depression, restlessness, loss of strength, and anorexia. If the patient suffers from susto, the curandero will be asked to intervene, because curanderos are the only ones believed to have the power to perform the necessary healing rituals.[4]

Mal ojo, or evil eye, is thought to be caused by envy, covetous expressions, or attention paid by one person to another. For example, telling a mother that her child is attractive, but failing to touch the child after making that statement, will cast the spell of mal ojo and the child will become ill with fever. The person complimenting the child should touch him, thereby breaking the spell of mal ojo.

The belief in mal ojo is widespread. Mexican-Americans may take preventive measures, such as wearing amulets, gold earrings, snakes' fangs, garlic, or oil crosses on the head, to deflect the mal ojo.[1,5]

These diseases, mal ojo and susto, are only two of the many folk diseases that the nurse might encounter when caring for the Mexican-American patient. The nurse should not assume that, because a patient is educated or acculturated, he does not hold these beliefs in curanderismo.

For example, when I was pregnant with my son, there was a death in the family. I planned on going to the funeral, but when making arrangements with my mother, she told me that I could not go to the funeral due to my pregnancy. It seemed very odd to me that she would say this, because she never seemed to hold much faith in some of the Mexican-American cultural beliefs. When discussing this further with my grandmother and mother, they told me that the embalming fluid would be in the air around the body, causing "mal aire," and this could cause my baby to be born with deformities or make me very ill. They told me that I could very possibly miscarry if I came to the funeral. I did go to the funeral, but in respect for their wishes, especially my grandmother's, sat in the back and did not view the body. (Several months later I delivered a healthy boy.)

A patient's perceptions of health and illness are influenced strongly by his cultural beliefs; health care services must acknowledge and understand those cultural beliefs to provide optimal care to Mexican-American patients.

References

1. Henderson G: Transcultural Health Care. Menlo Park, CA, Addison-Wesley, 1980
2. Ingham JM: On Mexican Folk Medicine. American Anthropologist, 1970
3. Kiev A: Curanderismo: Mexican-American Folk Psychiatry. New York, Free Press, 1968
4. Madsen W: The Mexican-American of South Texas. New York, Holt, Rinehart, and Winston, 1964
5. Orque, SM et al: Ethnic Nursing Care: A Multicultural Approach. St. Louis, CV Mosby, 1983

(Continues on p. 74)

6. Rodriguez J: Mexican Americans: Factors Influencing Health Practices. The Journal of School Health 53 (February): 136–140, 1983

7. Spector RE: Cultural Diversity in Health and Illness, 2d ed. Norwalk, CT: Appleton-Century-Crofts, 1985

8. Swafford-Gonzalez MJ, Gutierrez MG: Ethno-Medical Beliefs and Practices of Mexican Americans. Nurse Practitioner 8 (November–December): 29–34, 1983

the extent to which the client and his family are acculturated.

> Define and clarify any technical or professional terms.
>
> Use audiovisual aids whenever possible.
>
> Obtain an interpreter or bilingual health care provider if needed.

3. Avoid cultural labeling, which might contribute to degrading attitudes toward the patient and family.

4. Accord respect by using proper forms to address Spanish-speaking patients, instead of using first names.

5. Listen attentively to the comments and responses of client and family and validate with them their perception of the communication.

6. Recognize that ritual acts and health practices are important to the Spanish-speaking patient and his family.

7. Recognize that modesty and privacy are valued; provide as much privacy as possible.

Native Americans

There are more than 200 American Indian, or native American, tribes in the United States; the greatest portion of these reside in Oklahoma, Alaska, Arizona, California, and New Mexico.[2] More than one half of these tribes reside on reservations. In recent years, increasing numbers of native Americans are migrating from reservations to the larger cities in search of educational and employment opportunities. Although each of these tribes has its own language, customs, beliefs, and practices, there are some commonalities that guide the nurse in working with the native American. Nevertheless, caution needs to be exercised when making general statements about the Native American culture.

Family Structure and Roles

The native American family includes both the nuclear family and the extended families and the community. Each family member has rights and specific duties. The native American family is child-oriented and all family members participate in the childrearing process.

Food, shelter, and survival are supported on a community basis.[40] Adoption rituals are performed within tribal ceremonies to prevent a family's loss of ties due to death and to ensure that the individual will always have a family. When an individual member of the culture becomes hospitalized, family members and friends may travel a great distance to visit him.

Native American families of many tribes are experiencing serious disorganization. This has been attributed to the changes in the native American's way of life on the reservation and to his difficulties in adapting to the expectations of the dominant society.[40]

Food

Food has both religious and social value to native Americans. Food is incorporated into religious ceremonies. It is also an integral part of any social gathering. Good, plentiful food increases a family's reputation in its tribe.

Time

The native American's life is not governed by a clock. Rather, actions are initiated and develop, not according to a time schedule. Time is viewed as a continuum without a beginning or an end.[2] Native Americans are often more concerned about the completion of a task than being on time.

Religion

The members of native American tribes hold a holistic view of life and believe that God is the giver of life. Illness is perceived in association with religion. An individual who becomes ill is likely to seek intervention from a medicine man and subscribe to religious rituals to remove the illness.

Values

Some of the values upheld by native Americans on the reservations are in transition for those who are moving to the city. An important value of the native

American is that of sharing, rather than possessing, material objects.

Healers and Health Practices

Many native Americans view the world through the realm of the supernatural and seek assistance from the medicine man or *shaman*. Although most native Americans recognize the value of modern medicine, they may continue to use native healers in addition to medical intervention.[40] The native healers' use of herbs, plants, and other healing techniques has been proven effective.[43]

Healing ceremonies usually take place in the home and involve the participation of family members and other members of the tribe. It is not unusual for a hospitalized native American to desire to use a native healer. The family of the hospitalized member may want to leave certain objects in the patient's room, objects which they believe caused the illness and can also effect the cure.

Mental Illness

The impoverishment of native American life has contributed to the high incidence of such health problems as tuberculosis, communicable diseases, malnutrition, and high maternal and infant mortality rates.[43] There are, among native Americans, high rates of suicide, alcoholism, and homicide.[40] There is also a high rate of automobile accidents, which many researchers suspect are actually undocumented suicides.[2]

The native American community experiences social and personal disorganization as a result of the dominant society's insistence that the Indian community relinquish its culture and religion. This leads to a loss of an integrated value system, leaving the individual with feelings of hopelessness, despair, and anger as he attempts to cope with everyday problems.

Though geographically different, the Alaskan native American experiences similar difficulties trying to live in two different cultures. There are no native reservations in Alaska. The Alaskan native American's villages are located within the interior of Alaska. The only means of transportation to some of these villages is by air. Many Alaskan natives experience anger and frustration about the changes in their villages and way of life, and they experience depression and helplessness about their dependence on the dominant society.

Implications for Nursing Actions

1. Remember that the family and community play important roles in the care of the individual native American.

2. Do not prevent the hospitalized patient and family from seeking treatment from a native healer. Using a healer may reduce some of the client's feelings of alienation in the health care system and may therefore contribute to his psychological well-being.

3. Be aware that native Americans may perceive hospitals as places that isolate them from their major cultural and social group.

4. Recognize that time does not have the same value for native Americans as it does for the dominant society and that an individual who keeps an appointment at a health clinic or hospital may not necessarily be on time.

5. Listen attentively to the native American's words; he often speaks softly and expects the listener to pay careful attention.

6. Observe and assess nonverbal behavior of native American clients; they are likely to watch the health care provider but say little or nothing.

7. Avoid note-taking and the extensive use of questions during the history-taking process. The native American resents excessive questioning and believes that writing while he is talking shows disrespect.

8. Break eye contact with the client intermittently when interacting with him; maintaining continuous eye contact is perceived by the native American as an invasion of privacy.

Asian Americans

The numerous cultures from eastern Asian countries include the Chinese, Japanese, Philippine, Korean, and Vietnamese peoples. Although each culture has distinct differences, there are some similarities that help the health care provider administer quality health care.

The Family

The family plays a significant role in all of the Asian cultures. Asian American families are controlled by the father who has total authority over the members. The traditional wife may or may not speak English and is responsible for maintaining the home life.

The family assumes greater importance than the individual; family loyalty binds the individual to his home. For most Asian Americans, emotional security and economic well-being depend on the family. The individual will compromise other personal obligations in the interest of family ties and the family unit.

Socialization

Family members of the Asian American cultures convey their caring for each other with less verbalization than the dominant society. Parents expect that their child will submit to their guidance without disagreement, hesitation, or questioning. "Back-talk" from a child is shocking and distressing to adults and marked independence of the child is discouraged. Although the main responsibility for a child's socialization rests with the parents, extended kin actively participate in helping the child become a respected and wanted person in society.

In the traditional Asian home, the child learns from his parents to respect, admire, and fear the family ancestors, whose strength and virtue are extolled.[38] The child is encouraged to follow the example of his ancestors for moral, ethical, and social behavior.

Food

Asian cultures believe that it is necessary to eat a balanced diet of foods containing the properties of yin and yang. The forces of yin and yang are believed to control nature and the body. Yin is the negative force—dark, cold, and empty; yang is the positive force—light, warm, and full.[43]

Members of Asian cultures believe that too much of the wrong foods could lead to illness and that certain illnesses can be cured by proper foods. When an imbalance of food exists, an increase in the opposite force is needed to bring the body back into harmony. Vegetables are mixed together to balance yin and yang forces. Diets consisting entirely of high-protein foods, raw fruits and vegetables, or extremely cold or hot foods are viewed unfavorably by Asian Americans. The classification of yin and yang foods is traditional and passed down through generations.

Health Practices

Asian medicine is based on the concept that the universe and man are susceptible to the laws of five elements—fire, earth, metal, water, and wood. Every organ of the body is believed to possess the properties of taste, emotion, sound, odor, season, power, climate, and other elements. Health is perceived as the balance of yin and yang; imbalance leads to dysfunction and disease.

Folk medicine practitioners, or herbalists, practice widely and actively in Asian American homes. Other Asian Americans may use spiritual healing, the transfer of psychic healing energies from the person administering care to the one who is ill.

Implications for Nursing Actions

1. Remember that Asian Americans may experience language difficulties.

   Request a bilingual staff member or interpreter.

   Use creativity to develop alternate means of communication when an interpreter is unavailable.

2. Recognize that members of Asian cultures may be upset by the drawing of blood, because blood is viewed as the source of the body's life.

3. Be aware that Asian Americans may be reluctant or unable to express feelings of anger, frustration, or pain.

4. Realize that the patient may refuse surgery unless under critical circumstances, because he believes it is best to die with an intact body.

5. When familiarizing Asian American patients with the hospital, be sensitive to their perception of the hospital as an alien place and to their feeling of isolation from the rest of the family.

6. Intervene by fostering communication between patient and physician. Members of the Asian culture may perceive the physician as the authority and be reluctant to complain or inform him of their problems. Talking to a physician about their concerns may be perceived as disrespect.

7. Plan meals for Asian American patients according to a balance of foods containing yin and yang properties and appealing arrangement and taste.

Black Americans

Black Americans originated in Africa from a culture that reflected skill in agriculture, government, scholarship, and the fine arts.[15] The largest importation of slaves to the United States occurred in the 1700s. Once brought to this country, blacks were unable to preserve their customs, religion, or family traditions because the institution of slavery actively discouraged enculturation.

All blacks can probably trace their heritage to some part of Africa. The slave trade dispersed them throughout America. Isolated and faced with an alien environment, each group of blacks was forced to develop its own language, folklore, music, and religion.

Within the United States, there are considerable differences between blacks in the upper class, blacks in the middle class, and blacks who are poor. Nevertheless, their similarities, including a commonality of suffering, are stronger than the differences. The nurse is cautioned, however, to refrain from generalizing about the black American culture.

When a group of people are in a subjugated

position in a culture, they will, in order to survive, band together and form a subculture. Therefore, to survive in a dominant society that has historically and repeatedly ignored them, blacks have developed, as a means of identification, different ways of living, eating, dressing, and, in some cases, different ways of speaking. Continued discrimination has been a chief factor in the confinement of blacks to ghettos and in their inability to become a part of the dominant society.

The Family

The concept of the family as an important unit has been traced to ancient Africa. The union between two people benefited both families economically, politically, religiously, and socially.[3] During the era of slavery, men and women were perceived as commodities to be bought and sold by their owners as they deemed necessary and marriages between two slaves were therefore often not recognized. Members of the extended family, which may include uncles, aunts, boyfriends, girlfriends, and other members of the community, participate in and influence childrearing.

Language

Language is one of the most important means of comprehending reality. For the black culture, language has presented a reality of insults, confusion, and depression. Black language has been denigrated by whites, contributing to self-deprecation and insecurity among some blacks.

Historically, black language evolved for a definite purpose. Slaves borrowed or adapted language forms from their white masters to deceive or make fun of their masters, to communicate secretly with each other, and to plan revolts and methods of escape.[22]

The black slaves soon learned that whatever they said to each other or to their masters must be couched in words with double meanings, in half-truths, and in other forms that would not endanger their own safety. As a result, black slaves became adept at verbal survival mechanisms.

The reasons for the development of black language have changed with the times. The language spoken by black Americans varies according to socioeconomic status as well as geographic areas. Even educated blacks who speak perfect standard English can speak the black language when the situation demands it. This does not hold true, however, for a person who has not been exposed to the black culture.

Religion

Religion has been a source of strength for black Americans in times of trouble or stress. A strong religious orientation has provided a strong foundation for the development, survival, and stability of the black family. The predominant religion of the black American is Baptist.

It is not unusual to see some members of a religious congregation of blacks come together to pray for a hospitalized patient. The meeting may include prayer, singing, and religious readings. This support is comforting to black Americans during stressful times.

The black minister is a significant member of the black community and often serves as a counselor for members of his community. The church provides emotional and often financial support to members of the community in need.

Food

Food habits of black Americans are influenced by both heritage and by socioeconomic factors. Hogs, chicken, corn, and beans were food products of the early United States, particularly the southern region. Parts of hogs that were not considered good enough for the plantation master to consume, such as the head, brains, intestines (chitterlings), stomach (maw), and feet were fed to the slaves. These parts of the hog, as well as greens, yams, and other foods, are considered "soul food." Many blacks still prefer to eat these parts of the hog due to their low price. Although this type of food is preferred by many black Americans, it would be incorrect to assume that all black Americans enjoy and eat the same kinds of food.

Health Practices

Many black Americans will not seek health care assistance until the health problem is a serious one. Some of the factors that influence this behavior include fear of health care providers and hospitals, fear of death, refusal or inability to consider health maintenance a priority, and the belief that home remedies will cure the problem. Other blacks may rely on healers to restore their health.

Mental Illness

The greatest proportion of clients in mental institutions are black.[10] There are many factors contributing to this phenomenon. Fewer blacks can afford a private physician and, therefore, do not seek treatment until their psychiatric–mental health problem reaches a state requiring hospitalization.[37] Some black Americans fail to develop the kinds of qualities, such as extensive verbal skills and adequate insight, needed by people in order to respond appropriately to psychotherapeutic assessments.[28] Because they have not developed these skills, blacks receive custodial forms of care more frequently than members of the dominant culture.[37]

Implications for Nursing Actions

1. Use nonverbal behavior carefully designed to convey an accurate message. Black Americans are skilled at assessing others' nonverbal behavior and may be particularly observant when interacting with health care providers.

2. Speak to the patient with courtesy and respect. Do not address him by first name unless he has asked you to do so.

3. Ask food preferences rather than assuming that black Americans prefer the same kinds of food.

4. Plan interventions to reduce the hostility and suspiciousness that patients may demonstrate within the health care setting. People who have been lonely or rejected by others over long periods of time or during their formative years, such as black Americans, are frequently not brave enough to risk the possible pain of new human relationships.

5. Attend to client and family communication, which may be extremely difficult and frustrating for the health care provider. Many black Americans will assume an exaggerated air of indifference or ignorance in the health care environment and this behavior may result in cultural mislabeling.

6. Avoid attempting to impress black Americans by talking about other blacks you know. This may be interpreted by blacks as a means of hiding insecurity and discomfort by the interviewer.

Culture and the Nursing Process

Assessment of Cultural Factors

Although most nurses recognize the need for cultural sensitivity, many experience frustration when developing this awareness and sensitivity. Some of the factors related to this frustration are lack of knowledge regarding different cultures and fear of offending a person of a different ethnic group. One cannot be expected to know everything about every ethnic group. People of the same ethnic group do not know everything about their own ethnicity. Neither should one pretend to know about a different cultural group when interacting with members of that group. A more honest approach is to admit lack of knowledge and carry out an assessment that encourages rapport between client and health professional and that gathers information needed to formulate nursing care plans.

The assessment and analysis of cultural factors include the client's language skills, behavior related to health care, taboos and prohibitions, and coping behaviors.

Languages

Language differences between staff and patients, and even between staff members themselves, are significant barriers to communication in the health care environment. Language differences may create or further complicate health care problems. Even individuals who speak the same language but are members of different cultural groups may have difficulties understanding each other. For example, a health care provider from the North may experience difficulty in understanding a patient from the South whose speech patterns may be slower and who may pronounce certain letters and words less clearly.

Another language difficulty may occur when different age groups or generations within the same culture do not understand each other. For example, young black Americans may use a slang word or idiom that an older black health care provider does not understand.[15]

Nurses and other health professionals may overestimate how much language a member of another cultural group understands. They may also fail to appreciate the degree of fear and anxiety a patient feels when he is unable to understand what is being said to him. One bilingual nurse described the feelings of Asian patients who recently immigrated to the United States.

> Nothing is more frightening and frustrating than to be in a foreign country and to visit the doctor and not understand what is being said. That is frequently one of the reasons why some patients are hesitant to go to the doctor. First, they have to find someone to go with them to translate. It is a frightening feeling to go to a hospital of any type where no one understands or speaks the same language.[20]

Some patients may feel so ashamed that they are unable to speak the language expected of them that they pretend to understand when they do not. Some are afraid to admit that they do not understand the language for fear of being labeled "dumb" or "ignorant."

Health care providers often unconsciously treat patients, families, and other staff members who are unable to speak their language in an insensitive manner. When health care providers try to communicate with an individual who speaks a different language, they may experience anger and exasperation.

Assessing Barriers to an Effective Nurse–Client Interaction. Barriers to effective interaction between the health care provider and the client are influenced by many factors. These factors include cultural beliefs and practices, education, sex, socioeconomic status, and values. For effective communication, these barriers must be overcome.

Problems of communication often arise during the process of history-taking and, consequently, diminish the effectiveness of the nurse's clinical expertise. Problems with communication may prevent the patient from even reaching the examining room. A nurse practitioner in an American Indian health service hospital related the following incident.

> The nurses would call out each patient's name as he was to see the physician. Many of the patients were not only old and hard of hearing, but also were not accustomed to the anglicized version of their names. Quite often, the patient failed to respond unless a younger member of the family who understood English was present and responded to the name.
>
> Often the patient's name was just skipped over when the patient did not respond immediately. Consequently, a patient might sit in the waiting room the entire day unless the waiting room personnel noticed this patient's continual presence or the patient got up and left.[35]

What to Assess

1. How do members of the family communicate with each other?
2. Which languages are used in the home? Outside of the home?
3. How much English do the patient and family understand?
4. Do the patient and family speak English well enough to communicate their needs?

Taboos and Prohibitions

The areas of conversation that are sensitive or even taboo vary according to geographic locations, customs, values of the culture, and values of the individual. In one culture, a person may be forbidden to mention certain animals; in another, certain secret words may be prohibited. In a third culture, certain political issues or particular types of illness are forbidden topics for discussion.

Prohibitions against discussion of bodily functions and display of parts of the body are more pronounced in some cultures than in others. In some cultures, an individual is not permitted to discuss issues related to the family outside of the family system.

What to Assess

1. What are the norms of confidentiality?
2. Are there certain health topics about which patients may be sensitive or unwilling to talk?
3. Are there behaviors expected in the health care setting that may be embarrassing or unacceptable to the patient?
4. How might the nurse best approach sensitive-but-necessary topics?

Coping Behaviors

Individual coping behaviors are culturally influenced. The emotions of anger, love, frustration, and embarrassment are universal, but the indications of their presence and the manner of their expression vary in each culture.

Health care professionals must be aware of cultural differences regarding the display of emotions and expression of feelings. Understanding how a particular culture expresses feelings and displays emotions helps health care providers behave in ways that are consistent with those values. In the following situation, the mental health caregivers did not provide care consistent with the client's values.

> Mrs. Lu, an Asian American, visited a local mental health center with the complaint of inability to communicate with her husband. The mental health center staff, however, were uninformed regarding the cultural values and expected behavior of the Chinese people. Mrs. Lu's therapist encouraged her to express her anger directly and also to express her affection for her husband openly through such behaviors as holding his hand.
>
> When Mrs. Lu tried out these new behaviors, her husband became distraught and feared that his wife was losing her mind because her behavior was unfamiliar and unacceptable. The Chinese community neither understands nor accepts the open expression of anger or of warm feelings by holding hands.[27]

What to Assess

1. How does the client show approval or disapproval? Agreement or disagreement?
2. How are anger, embarrassment, love, and other emotions expressed?
3. What are the cultural norms concerning raised voices, arguments, expressions of humor, and so forth?

Analysis of the assessment data allows the nurse to classify and categorize client information and formulate nursing diagnoses that then direct nursing care planning.

Nursing Diagnosis

After the client data are assessed, the nursing diagnosis for an individual patient is formulated. The cultural influences of the client's ethnicity, race, environment, religious background, and so forth may lead to any number of variables in the diagnosis process. Examples of possible nursing diagnoses follow:

Impaired verbal communication (the person experiences, or could experience, a decreased ability to speak appropriately or to understand the meaning of words) related to language barrier

Ineffective individual coping (the person experiences, or is at risk of experiencing, an inability to manage internal or environmental stressors adequately because of insufficient resources) related to changes in physical environment, disruption of emotional bonds, or inadequate psychological resources

Alterations in family processes (a normally supportive family experiences a stressor that challenges its previously effective functioning ability) related to an illness of a family member and secondary to cultural conflict with reality

Fear (the person experiences a painfully uneasy feeling that is related to an identifiable source or stimulus which the person perceives as dangerous)

Alterations in health maintenance (the person experiences, or is at risk of experiencing, a disruption in his present state of wellness because of inadequate preventive measures or an unhealthy lifestyle) related to cultural belief

Powerlessness (the person perceives a lack of personal control over certain events or situations) related to hospitalization and secondary to social isolation, relocation, or lack of explanations from caregivers

Social isolation (the person experiences a need or desire for contact with others but is unable to make that contact) related to moving into another culture

Planning

After implementing the first two steps of the nursing process (assessment and nursing diagnosis), the nurse begins planning nursing care that will meet the identified health care needs of the client and family. This planning process must incorporate the goals of the individual and his family. The health care provider attends to such factors as who stays with the patient in the hospital or health care agency and who is the spokesperson. In some cultures, the male speaks for the female; in other cultures, the elder or another respected member of the family may speak for the patient. This situation may be particularly uncomfortable for the health care provider if her culture dictates that each individual has the right to speak for himself.

The nurse or other health professional may request the help of clergy or another influential person outside of the family to assist the client and family

adapt to the available health care services. Acceptance of the patient and family without imposing more hospital rules or regulations than necessary will foster effective nurse–client relationships.

The health care provider should communicate honestly with others when she lacks knowledge of the behaviors, rules, values, and lifestyles of other cultures. Seeking information from the patient and family about their culture is an effective tool. To pretend to be knowledgeable about different cultures only alienates people and induces fear and distrust of the health care system.

Developing a quality plan of care takes time. When health care providers lack the time needed to make adequate plans, they experience stress, which the culturally different patient and family perceive as frustration directed at them personally.

Intervention

After assessing the patient and family, formulating nursing diagnoses, and identifying goals, the care provider identifies nursing interventions to meet identified health needs and to resolve patient problems. Cultural awareness and sensitivity should guide the nurse's implementation of each stage of the nursing process. Intervening with clients and families of different cultural groups also requires that the nurse examine her own biases, fears, and prejudices. Specific nursing actions have been outlined in the discussion of the four large minority groups in the United States.

Evaluation

The effectiveness of the plan of care is evaluated by observing, interacting with, and reassessing the patient and family and their problems and needs. The nurse collects further data from other health professionals who are involved with the patient and family. The patient's and family's participation in their own care and their volunteering of information beyond what is requested by the caregiver may indicate that nursing intervention has been effective. The evaluation process is continuous, but ever-changing, as the health care provider reassesses and redefines the needs of the patient and family.

Attitudes, Values, and Prejudices of the Health Care Provider

The health care provider is a product of an ethnic group that has its own set of values and attitudes and that has influenced the development of prejudices.

Case Study 6-1

Cultural Implications of Therapeutic Planning

Presenting Information

Mrs. P., a 36-year-old black woman and mother of three children (ages 6, 9, and 11½), was seen in a psychiatric treatment setting for the first time. She was described as being out of touch with reality and mumbling about the "judgment day" when she would be punished. She was diagnosed as paranoid schizophrenic, acute onset. Her family refused to admit her to a psychiatric institution. She was placed on high doses of Thorazine and her family was instructed to bring her for daily therapy. Her husband was also instructed to attend therapy.

Discussion
1. What goals had been developed for Mrs. P. and her family?
2. Who developed these goals?

Continuing Problems

Mrs. P. was very depressed when she returned to the mental health clinic. She remained uncooperative with the assigned therapist. Her affect was described as flat and she did not establish eye contact with the therapist. The therapist observed that Mrs. P. became agitated when the discussion turned to Mr. P. or their children, particularly their 11½-year-old son. She also noted that Mr. P. failed to accompany Mrs. P. to her therapy sessions.

The therapist, who was white, expressed her frustration and inability to establish rapport with Mrs. P. to other health team members. She expressed doubts that Mrs. P. could remain functional in her home and community. Furthermore, Mrs. P. was not taking the medication prescribed for her.

Discussion
1. Why did Mrs. P. and her husband not cooperate with the therapist?
2. Describe the therapist's feelings.
3. What is the significance of Mrs. P.'s agitation?

New Information

The therapist decided to discuss Mrs. P. at the next staff meeting and seek others' suggestions. The staff physician believed that Mrs. P. should be admitted to an inpatient treatment unit where her medication regimen would be followed. He predicted that she would become increasingly nonfunctional without the medication. Some of the therapists questioned the sincerity and committment of the husband who failed to attend the therapy sessions with Mrs. P. A black therapist expressed interest in Mrs. P. and her situation and volunteered to work with her. A few therapists questioned the effectiveness of any therapeutic approaches to Mrs. P. because she was obviously seriously mentally ill. Nevertheless, Mrs. P.'s case was reassigned to the black therapist.

At subsequent meetings, the newly assigned therapist was able to supply additional information regarding Mrs. P. and her life. Mrs. P. informed the therapist that she stopped taking her medication because it made her feel sleepy and unable to care for her son, who was severely retarded as a complication of meningitis at the age of 5 years.

Mrs. P. believed that it was her fault that her child was retarded because she had taken him to the state where the meningitis outbreak occurred. She stated that God was punishing her for being so careless with her child's life and she must therefore suffer the burden. She was totally responsible for caring for her son during the day and part of the night, 7 days a week, and the care included diaper changing and gastrostomy feedings. Her son also needed suctioning via his tracheostomy and his need for suctioning had increased within the last few months.

The doctor had told Mrs. P. that her son would not live to be older than 12 years of age. The child would become 12 years old 2 months from the day Mrs. P. suffered her apparent psychotic break.

Mrs. P. further related that her husband worked two jobs and that they "just didn't talk about" their son's illness. After she began to talk about her son and his special needs, she no longer seemed delusional. The therapist described the behavioral changes as marked. Although she still spoke in monosyllables, Mrs. P. displayed a wider range of affect and sometimes established eye contact. Mrs. P. defined "judgment day" as her son's 12th birthday and her "punishment" as his death.

What Was Done

The therapist and Mrs. P. worked out an acceptable agreement regarding the issue of her
(Continues on p. 82)

medication. Mrs. P. agreed to continue attending and participating in therapy; she also agreed that if she or the therapist observed that her emotional well-being was endangered, they would again consider the resumption of medication.

The therapist focused on helping Mrs. P. accomplish the following:

1. Identify positive qualities in herself
2. Set realistic goals regarding what she could and could not do for her son
3. Seek outside sources of help with her son's care (Mrs. P.'s devotion to her son was her "penance" for her "sin.")
4. Develop effective communication with her husband (Mrs. P. saw herself as self-sufficient and needing no one; to tell him of her feelings, she felt, may make her "weak and beholding to him.")
5. Deal with her grief and work on anticipatory grief

It is possible that mental health care providers may overlook the cultural implications of a client's problems. Health care workers must be aware of their own behavior, feelings, and values when interacting with members of different ethnic groups. The client's behavior may represent coping with what is perceived as a hostile environment. The nurse responds, without labeling, to the client's behavior within its context.

Nursing education may serve as a vehicle to enlighten an individual about different ethnic groups and about the importance of being culturally sensitive and aware.

The assessment of cultural sensitivity starts with the self. What makes you who you are? What do you value most? About which group or groups of people do you feel prejudice? All of us have prejudiced feelings about something or someone. These feelings may be mild (*e.g.*, we'd rather not be with a certain person) to strong (*e.g.*, we feel great hostility toward, and fear of, a certain person). Prejudices, biases, and fears are less likely to interfere with a care provider's ability to administer quality patient care when she is aware of these feelings, admits their presence, and fills in her knowledge gaps with information about the feared cultural groups.

Members of minority groups may have never had the opportunity to experience what is taken for granted by the dominant culture. Nevertheless, they want neither the pity of members of the dominant society nor their apologies for being who they are or who they desire to become. Cultural conflict develops when one culture attempts to impose its values on another.

People of different ethnic groups, particularly minority groups, are not patterned after people of the dominant western civilization. They are people who have distinctive histories, who have a set of distinctive life experiences, who deserve a distinctive place in American society, and who are capable of making a distinctive contribution to the wider society.[41]

If the health care provider has negative or unresolved feelings related to her own cultural background, she may be unable to take a genuine interest in assisting the client of any culture. It is difficult to work with a client who activates your own unresolved feelings.

Another difficulty may be encountered when a health professional is expected to be an expert about her own culture and is also expected to relate well with every client of the same culture. The interaction of two people of the same culture will not guarantee the development of a therapeutic relationship, just as the fact that two individuals belong to different cultures will not prevent its development. Many factors, including goals of care, nature of the health problem, interpersonal skills, and degree of enculturation influence the development of an effective nurse–client relationship when the two are members of different cultures.

Summary

This chapter has focused on the concept of culture, cultural similarities and differences, the health care needs of clients of different cultures, and nursing intervention designed to meet those needs. The major ideas of the chapter include the following:

1. Culture is learned behavior that is transmitted from one generation to another.
2. Culture governs an individual's patterns of action, beliefs, and feelings.
3. Awareness of cultural similarities allows health care providers to appreciate common human behaviors and bonds; failure to appreciate cultural variations results in ineffective communi-

cation and ineffective relationships between the client and the health care providers.

4. Health care providers are members of a subculture influenced by the values of their (in our case, American) culture, and these values are reflected in the administration of health care.

5. Enculturation is the process whereby an individual learns the expected behavior of a culture; acculturation is the process whereby two cultural groups come into contact with each other.

6. Each ethnic group has a unique history.

7. The four large minority groups in the United States are Spanish-speaking Americans, native Americans, Asian Americans, and black Americans.

8. No form of behavior can be judged normal or abnormal outside of its cultural context.

9. The nurse recognizes that the quality of communication between health care provider and client directly affects the quality of health care.

10. The health care provider needs to be aware that, in some cultures, the family assumes greater importance than the individual.

11. Failure to identify the decision-maker in the client's family may result in sabotage of the plan of care.

12. Nursing intervention is planned with sensitivity to the client and family's unique health needs and cultural influences.

13. Knowledge of cultural similarities and differences is essential in the delivery of quality health care.

References

1. Atkinson D, Morten G, Sue DW: Counseling American Minorities: A Cross-Cultural Perspective. Dubuque, IA, Wm C Brown, 1979

2. Beuf AH: Red Children in White America. Philadelphia, University of Pennsylvania Press, 1977

3. Billingsley A: Black Families in White America. Englewood Cliffs NJ, Prentice-Hall, 1968

4. Blumberg P: The Impact of Social Class. New York, Thomas Cromwell, 1972

5. Branch MF, Paxton PP: Providing Safe Nursing Care for Ethnic People of Color. New York, Appleton-Century-Crofts, 1976

6. Brownlee AT: Community, Culture, and Care: A Cross-Cultural Guide for Health Workers. St Louis, CV Mosby, 1978

7. Bullough E, Bullough M: Ethnic Identity and Health Care. New York, Appleton-Century-Crofts, 1972

8. Carpenito LJ: Nursing Diagnosis: Application to Clinical Practice. Philadelphia, JB Lippincott, 1983

9. Carter FM: Psychosocial Nursing: Theory and Practice in Hospital and Community Mental Health. New York, Macmillan, 1976

10. Cheek D: Assertive Black, Puzzled White. San Luis Obispo, CA, Impact Publishers, 1977

11. Chohen E, Eames E: Cultural Anthropology. Toronto, Little Brown, 1982

12. Cleckly H: The Mask of Sanity. St Louis, CV Mosby, 1976

13. Cogdell R, Wilson S: Black Communication in White Society. Century Twenty-One, 1983

14. De La Garza, R et al: The Mexican American Experience: An Interdisciplinary Anthology. Austin, University of Texas Press, 1985

15. Delaney AJ: Black Task Force Report. New York, Family Service Association of America, 1979

16. Devore W, Schlesinger EG: Ethnic-Sensitive Social Work Practice. St Louis, CV Mosby, 1981

17. Eaton J, Weil R: Culture and Mental Disorders. New York, Free Press, 1955

18. Erikson EH: Identity, Youth and Crisis. New York, WW Norton, 1960

19. Fish S, Shelley J: Spiritual Care: The Nurse's Role. Downer's Grove, IL, Inter Varsity Press, 1978

20. Folta JR, Deck E: A Sociological Framework for Patient Care. New York, Wiley Medical Publications, 1979

21. Glazer N, Moynihan P: Beyond the Melting Pot. Cambridge, Harvard University Press, 1963

22. Haskins J: The Psychology of Black Languages. New York, Barnes and Nobles, 1973

23. Henderson G, Primeaux M: Transcultural Health Care. Menlo Park, CA, Addison-Wesley, 1981

24. Howze B: Black Suicides: Final Acts of Alienation. Human Behavior (February): 10–15, 1979

25. Jones RL: Black Psychology. New York, Harper & Row, 1972

26. Kearns FE: Black Identity: A Thematic Reader. New York, Holt, Rinehart and Winston, 1980

27. Keesing FM: Acculturation: A Dictionary of the Social Sciences. New York, Macmillan, 1974

28. Leininger M: Cultural Diversities of Health and Nursing Care. Nurs Clin North Am 12 (March): 5–18, 1977

29. Longo DC, Williams RA: Clinical Practice in Psychosocial Nursing. Connecticut, Appleton-Century-Crofts, 1986

30. McDonald M: Not by the Color of Their Skin: The Impact of Racial Differences on the Child's Development. International Press, 1970

31. Moore BM: Cultural Differences and Counseling Perspective. Texas Personnel and Guidance Association Journal, pp 39–44, 1974

32. Murillo N: The Mexican American Family. In Martinez RA (ed): Hispanic Culture and Health Care: Fact, Fiction, Folklore. St Louis, CV Mosby, 1978

33. Orque M, Bloch B, and Morroy L: Ethnic Nursing Care: A Multicultural Approach. St. Louis, CV Mosby, 1983

34. Pasquali EA, Alesi EG, Arnold HM, DeBasio N: Mental Health Nursing: A Bio-Psycho-Cultural Approach. St Louis, CV Mosby, 1981

35. Primeaux MH: American Indian Health Care Practices. Nurs Clin North Am 12 (March): 55–65, 1977

36. Saunders L: Cultural Differences and Medical Care: The Case of the Spanish Speaking People. New York, Russell Sage Foundation, 1959

37. Seham M: Blacks and American Medical Care. Minneapolis, University of Minnesota Press, 1973

38. Spector RE: Cultural Diversity in Health and Illness. New York, Appleton-Century-Crofts, 1979

39. Tripp-Reimer T, Brink P, Saunders J: Cultural Assessment: Content and Process. Nursing Outlook (March–April): 78–82, 1984

40. Westmeyer J: The Drunken Indian: Myth and Realities. In Unger S (ed): The Destruction of the American Indian Family. New York, Association of American Indian Affairs, 1974

41. White EH: Giving Health Care to Minority Patients. Nurs Clin North Am 12 (March): 27–39, 1977

42. Williams RL: The B.I.T.C.H. Test (Black Intelligence Test of Cultural Homogeneity). Black Studies Program, St. Louis, Washington University, 1974

43. Wolff L, Weitzel M, Zornow R, Zshohar H: Fundamentals of Nursing. Philadelphia, JB Lippincott, 1983

PART 2

The Process of Psychiatric–Mental Health Nursing

7 Psychosociocultural Assessment

Sharon Byers

Even as a melody is not composed of tones, nor a verse of words, nor a statue of lines—one must pull and tear to turn a unity into a multiplicity—so it is with the human being I say You. I can abstract from him the color of his hair or the color of his speech in the color of his graciousness; I have to do this again and again; but immediately he is no longer You.
Martin Buber,
I and Thou, 1958

Chapter Preview

Psychosociocultural assessment is the first step of the nursing process employed in psychiatric–mental health care. It is a holistic assessment process that is designed to provide efficiency, reliability, and adaptation to the needs of the client and nurse. The conceptual framework for this approach is based on the nursing process, Selye's stress–adaptation model, and Maslow's formulation of the hierarchy of needs. This chapter emphasizes the nurse's relationship skills as the most critical assessment tool. To facilitate the novice interviewer's development of competence and confidence, client expectations of assessment interviewers are behaviorally defined and described. The hypothesis approach to structuring the interview presents a multidimensional and comprehensive system of assessment.

Learning Objectives

On completion of this chapter, you should be able to accomplish the following:

1. define psychosociocultural assessment
2. distinguish the types and purposes of assessment used in clinical situations
3. describe various tools of psychosociocultural assessment
4. discuss the importance of the relationship aspect of the interview in the assessment process
5. describe the role and expectations of the nurse interviewer
6. identify stages and other structural aspects of the interview
7. apply the hypothesis approach to structure a psychosociocultural assessment
8. compare methods of recording assessment data

Assessment: First Step of the Nursing Process

The effectiveness of the nursing process depends on the accurate completion of each step of the process. Assessment begins this process and is therefore the foundation. *Nursing assessment* is defined as the gathering, classifying, categorizing, and analyzing of client information and forms the basis of nursing care planning. A nursing assessment is a holistic assessment; that is, all areas of the client's life are examined as possible sources of important assessment data. The recovery of a surgical patient, for example, is enhanced by basing his nursing care on a solid understanding of his cultural background, sexual beliefs and fears, spiritual needs, social activities, and psychological status.

The nurse exercises professional judgment to determine the depth of the assessment of each area of client functioning and to choose the methods of gathering needed data, especially data that include sensitive or emotionally laden topics. The nurse also uses assessment information gathered by other psychiatric–mental health professionals, when possible, to protect the client from frequent and repetitious interviews.

Conceptual Frameworks

The use of theoretical models to form a conceptual framework of the nursing assessment process allows a more precise definition of that process. Accordingly, Maslow's hierarchy of needs and Selye's stress–adaptation syndrome form a framework for assessment that focuses on the needs of the individual, the adaptation resources of the individual, and the methods by which the nurse may facilitate both the individual's meeting those needs and his adaptation process.[14] Although this chapter will emphasize the assessment of the psychological, sociologic, and cultural aspects of the client's life, it is understood that the processes of adaptation on both physiological and psychological levels are intertwined and inseparable; they are, therefore, equally important for examination.

Assessment in Various Health Care Settings

The setting of a nursing assessment does not necessarily determine the focus of the assessment. In the medical areas of a hospital, as in a psychiatric treatment center, it is essential to attend to the psychosocial needs of the individual. In the nursing care planning of a patient experiencing postoperative psychosis or sensory deprivation delirium, for example, careful assessment of psychosociocultural aspects of the patient's condition will facilitate intervention in responses that can be life-threatening.

It cannot be assumed that psychosocial needs and problems of clients are readily apparent to the nurse in any health care setting. Studies show that clients and their family members are reluctant to report "nonmedical" problems or fears, because they do not believe these are within the realm of concern for the nurse or physician.[13] A purposeful, comprehensive psychosociocultural assessment should be conducted in all health care settings and should include the collecting and analyzing of information not always identified as problematic for the client at that time.

Analysis of Assessment Information

Following data gathering and an ongoing exploration of client problems, an analysis of the data should be completed. During the *analysis,* the second step of the nursing process, assessment information is examined and categorized according to the goals of "making sense" of the data and clarifying a picture of the client as a whole person.

The nurse records the information obtained during the assessment process according to the policies of the health care facility and professional nursing judgment. Formulation of a *nursing diagnosis* or diagnoses is based on the nurse's assessment and analysis of client data, which, in turn, form the basis for planning nursing care (see Chaps. 8 & 9).

Types of Assessment

Problem Identification

The type of assessment employed is usually determined by the nature of the client's problem and needs. Various purposes, goals, objectives, and methods distinguish assessments. In a crisis or emergency, the purpose of the assessment is to identify the problem, formulate a brief, clear statement of the problem, form a working hypothesis regarding the nature, intensity, and cause of the problem, and begin some type of therapeutic intervention. The goal of a crisis assessment is to furnish some measure of relief to the client and family in acute distress. This necessitates delaying a comprehensive data gathering. A suicidal and intensely disturbed client who presents himself in the psychiatric emergency room of a hospital is an example of a person in need of crisis assessment and intervention.

Problem Clarification

If a problem has been identified but is of a less urgent nature, the purpose of the assessment is clarification of the problem. The nurse systematically assesses the client concerning his perspective of the identified problem and his psychosocial and cultural history. A client who presents himself at a community mental health center to receive treatment for stress-related dysfunctions of eating and sleeping is an example of a person in need of problem clarification. In attempting to clarify the problem, the assessor's questions focus on the following elements:

The nature and intensity of the disruption caused by the problem

The time and context, or circumstances, wherein the problem was first noticed

Situations in which the problem is most and least disturbing

Specific fears concerning the problem and the changes it has caused in the client's life

In addition to clarifying the problem, the assessment usually includes a search for potential problems, strengths, resources, and normal habits of living in healthy and disrupted times. This kind of information about a client might assist in planning nursing interventions that would prevent a health disruption or that would facilitate client adaptation to a major change in role, image, or social space.

Special Considerations: Age, Cultural Background, and Physical Health Status. Priorities in the assessment process vary according to client factors that represent special needs, such as age, cultural background, and physical health condition. Briefer assessment tools are used when assessing the elderly client, with greater emphasis placed on observation of the client rather than on information obtained during the interview. Assessment of children requires increased attention to observation of the child's interaction, communication, and play.

The client's sociocultural group also determines priorities in assessment. *Client norms,* or expected behavior and experience in particular life situations, guide the nurse's assessment, analysis, and diagnosis of client problems and needs. The assessment process discussed in this chapter primarily focuses on the adult client in the middle years, although the nurse may apply this basic approach to any client by taking into consideration the client's special needs. (Also see chapters that deal with special populations—children, adolescents, aged.)

In particular, the cultural background of the client may greatly affect his responses to questions in the interview, in psychological exams, or on the mental status exam. Words are used differently in different cultures. Priorities and values differ as well, and these differences affect clients' answers in areas such as judgment, insight, and general interpretations. Clients from some cultures appear more passive than the nurse might expect, yet are within the normal range for their cultures. In general, the nurse must be cautious when deriving conclusions without the benefit of consultation with someone familiar with the client's culture.[10] Psychological tests and psychiatric rating scales are developed for the "white-Anglo-Saxon-Protestant" client for the most part.

Holistic Assessment

Hypothesis Approach to Assessment.   Based on an understanding of the holistic nature of people, the nurse assesses all aspects of the client's life and experience. According to the hypothesis approach to assessment, the nurse considers key and probable questions about the client's life in each of the areas of biologic, psychological, social, cultural, cognitive, and behavioral experience.[3,9] Consideration of these hypotheses guides the nurse's questioning during the interview process. This guidance assures that the as-

CHART 7-1
Guide to Client Assessment

Demographic Data

Name
Age
Sex
Marital status
Religion
Height
Weight
Date of admission
Admitting diagnosis

Client's Perceptions and Expectations

How does the client define "the problem" and
   its cause?
What are the client's expectations of treatment?
What is the length of time client expects to be
   involved in treatment?
What are the client's discharge plans?

History

Social and Cultural Data

Occupation
Educational background
Race/national origin
Who lives with the client?
Availability of family or significant others
Client's view of society/world
Recent loss or change in social space, role,
   habits
Leisure-time activities
Use of tobacco, alcohol, and other drugs

Sexual

Is client satisfied with his sexual activity and
   identity?
What is the effect of current problems on
   sexual functioning?

Medical

Allergies
Previous major illnesses, surgeries, and
   hospitalizations
Medications taken regularly

Review of systems
   Sensory
   Musculoskeletal
   Circulatory
   Integumentary
   Respiratory
   Gastrointestinal
   Urinary
   Reproductive
   Neurologic
      Mental status
      Thought content and form

Basic Needs

Dietary preferences, habits, allergies, and
   restrictions
Rest/sleep/comfort
Personal hygiene
Eliminatory habits and needs
Psychosocial

General Observation

Appearance
   Posture
   Gait
   Dress
   Jewelry, makeup
   Facial expression
Behavior
   Motor activity
   Eye contact
   Purposeful or goal-directed actions
Communication
   Verbal (rate, pace, flow of speech)
   Nonverbal (gestures, body language)
   Clarity of communication
   Communication of feelings
   Communication with family and significant
      others

Summary

Client functioning and problems
Identified needs and resources
Suggested interventions

sessment is comprehensive, complete, and directed by the needs of the client. The following discussion includes hypotheses that address many possible etiologies of, and explanations for, the client's behavior.

Psychological Hypotheses. Psychological hypotheses are explored through various psychological assessment tools, such as psychological tests, the mental status exam, history taking, and the interview. The assessor evaluates the results of these examinations and considers certain psychologic theories during the client interview.

The client's problem, according to psychological hypotheses, is related to, or caused by, the following factors:

1. The client's personality style and pattern of response to others (ask the client about identifiable patterns of problems in relationships)
2. The dynamics of unresolved conflicts, such as early relationships, self-image, interaction with significant people (ask the client about ambivalence regarding self or in relationships with others, perceived losses, unresolved anger or grief, ongoing conflicts with parents or others)
3. A maturational or situational crisis (ask about life changes, potential or real stressors, changes in self-image, expectations of self or the world)
4. Psychodynamic issues, such as impaired or weak ego functioning (ask the client about any changes in cognitive functioning; assess his ability adequately to test reality; ask him about content of thought and unusual perceptions)
5. Self-image, body image, or sexual identity (ask the client about thoughts and feelings about his body and sexual identity and about self esteem in general)

Social Hypotheses. The nurse assessor gathers social information about the client, including socioeconomic status, social habits, social skills, and social values. Data should also be collected to explain how the client views society, socialization, and significant others with whom he interacts. The assessor must also understand how the client is, in turn, viewed by society, by social groups significant to him, and by those individuals who constitute his significant relationships.

The client's problem, according to social hypotheses, is related to, or caused by, the following factors:

1. A change in the client's social space, such as role, support system, and social relationships (ask about changes in the client's role assumed at home or work, changes in social support, losses or changes in relationships with friends, changes in ability or opportunity to be close with others)
2. Social isolation (ask about recent withdrawal from others by choice or circumstances, as in a geographic move or a job change)
3. The impact of the client's behavior, attitudes, or lifestyle on society or significant social groups (ask how the client sees other people responding to him, how accepted he feels)
4. His communication of a social statement, such as a form of rebellion or refusal to cooperate with society (ask the client about his view of society, and consider if his behavior is, at least in part, intended to make a statement to society or to someone; if this seems a possibility, discuss this with the client)

Biologic Hypotheses. Biologic hypotheses refer to assumptions that the client's behavior is partially due to some biologic factor (*e.g.*, a disease process, neurochemistry, endocrine activity, physical dependence on some substance, or a biologic reaction to an internal or external environmental event). Methods of gathering data about biologic problems of the client include laboratory tests, x-rays, general physical examinations, and neurologic assessments.

The client's problem, according to biologic hypotheses, is related to, or caused by, the following factors:

1. An affective disorder caused by a biologic imbalance or dysfunction (ask the client about family history of similar problems; assess the client's mood and flow of thought; assess changes in his pattern of eating, sleeping, and general activity; assess changes in his perceptions of self and others, his level of hope and confidence)
2. A schizophrenic disorder caused by a biologic problem (ask the client about family history of similar problems; assess his content of thought, reality-testing, perceptual changes, unusual experiences, bizarre affect or mannerisms, changes in ability to function or in level of anxiety)
3. An organic disease (ask the client about physical symptoms, changes in sensorium, sudden changes in cognitive functioning, or memory or intellectual changes)
4. Stress (ask the client about recent changes or losses in life or pressures to perform and about symptoms such as headaches, backaches, sleep disturbances, increased irritability, or appetite changes)

5. Physical dependence or abuse of alcohol or other drugs (ask the client about use of mood-altering chemicals and any problems related to chemical use)
6. Response to a psychotropic agent or other chemical taken as part of a therapy regimen (ask the client about current medications used and related effects; consider both side effects and problematic drug interactions)
7. An allergic response to some environmental substance (ask about occurrence of headaches, dizziness, skin eruptions, and sensitivity to odors if this seems a likely possibility)

Behavioral Hypotheses.   Behavioral hypotheses focus on the assumption that the client's maladaptive behavior is socially learned and can therefore be "un-learned" and replaced with more adaptive behavior. Target behaviors—that is, the particular maladaptive response patterns—are identified and manipulated by the therapist. To increase the client's repertoire of responses, the therapist teaches him adaptive behaviors.

The client's problem, according to behavioral hypotheses, is related to, or caused by, the following factors:

1. Learned undesirable behavior patterns or emotional patterns (ask the client if there are any specific behaviors that consistently cause problems for him, such as compulsive behaviors or anxiety-related behaviors, and whether these are behaviors he would like to change)
2. Inattention to, or misperception of, cues in the environment (observe the client's sensitivity to normal social behaviors, ability to interpret nonverbal communication, and understanding of others' expectations of him)
3. Deficits in learning or skills (observe the client's social skills, hygiene skills, communication skills, and ability to benefit from experience)

Cognitive Hypotheses.   Cognitive hypotheses are based on the assumption that the client's thoughts or thinking processes result in the identified problem. Underlying this assumption is the belief that an individual's perceptions and images of self and others, messages to self, and perceptions of the world are learned and may be identified as incorrect or maladaptive; they also may be replaced by more positive thoughts.

The client's problem, according to cognitive hypotheses, is related to, or caused by, the following factors:

1. The client's negative perception of self (ask the client how he feels and thinks about himself, how he views himself with others, how he compares himself with his self-expectations or expectations he perceives from others)
2. The client's negative statements to self that increase his anxiety, fear, hopelessness, and maladaptive behavior (ask the client about self-talk, what he tells himself about himself and his place in the world, how he interprets events and experiences in his world, automatic thoughts that may be irrational but may silently reinforce negative self-perceptions)
3. The client's maladaptive view of others, the world, and others' expectations of him (discuss the client's sense of hope and his belief in a potential for good in the world or in others; look for unusual cynicism or irrational ideas about the world and other people)
4. The client's faulty expectations of others (ask about the client's expectations from others and relationships, and assess how realistic or rational these are)
5. Inconsistency of the client's thoughts, values, and attitudes, which creates confusion and may create a perceived inability to act (assess the consistency of the client's thoughts, values, and attitudes, looking for areas in which the client may feel strongly about something but somehow act the opposite, or may hold values that have not been reviewed in accordance with changes in the client's other thoughts)

Cultural Hypotheses.   The nurse assessor accurately evaluates client behavior as adaptive, maladaptive, or disturbed in relation to cultural norms, expectations, and beliefs of the client's reference group. The cultural reference group refers to the group of people with whom the client most closely shares beliefs, behaviors, and attitudes. This group determines norms and values with and for the client, and is, in effect, the "in group" by whom the client wishes to be accepted.

Cultural beliefs and values affect how an individual interprets the behavior of a health care provider. Cultural conflicts and pressures explain client behavior that may otherwise be misunderstood by the mental health professional. The cultural beliefs and values of the health care provider, in turn, influence his or her understanding and acceptance of the client. (Further discussion of the cultural aspects of psychiatric–mental health care may be found in Chap. 6.)

The client's problem, according to cultural hypotheses, is related to, or caused by, the following factors:

1. The culture into which the client was born, or in which he grew and developed
2. The adoption of a cultural pattern different from, or in addition to, the culture of origin
3. An identifiable conflict between the client's culture of origin and his adopted culture (ask the client about the problems with differing sets of expectations from his older family and friends who belong to the culture of origin and from new friends or more "americanized" family living in the adopted culture)
4. Norms, values, and expectations of the client's reference group (ask the client about his values as they compare with those of significant people in his world, and assess how well the client is aware of his own values and attitudes, or whether he is unconsciously controlled by the values and attitudes of people close to him)
5. The cultural reference group's view of the world and the group's place in, and treatment by, the world at large (discuss how the client feels as a member of a minority group, if this is the case, or whether he feels he is an entitled member of a superior or majority group and has unrealistic expectations or resentments secondary to these ethnocentric beliefs)
6. Cultural taboos and myths (discuss with the client how he views his problem or mental illness in the content of his culture of origin, or whether taboos or myths in his belief system necessitate some behavior in him that creates problems)
7. Acceptance, encouragement, discouragement, and prohibition of variations of group members' behaviors (discuss the client's perceptions of such pressures from his cultural reference group)
8. Rituals practiced in response to events of transition within, separation from, and incorporation into the cultural group (discuss rituals practiced by the client's cultural group)
9. The cultural group's definition of health and illness
10. The cultural group's practices of caring, nurturing, and healing (you will benefit from gaining general information about the client's culture from a variety of sources; discuss with the client how he and his culture make sense of his current problem and how people of his

culture respond to crises, problems like his, and illnesses)

Spiritual Hypotheses. The nurse gathers information about the client's spiritual beliefs, values, and expectations. Moral and ethical beliefs and values are also of importance to the nurse assessor. The nurse can better understand the client by knowing how the client views himself in relation to the universe, the larger scheme of the cosmos, and a higher power in the client's belief system. The nurse assesses this area in the interview, generally with broad questions, maintaining sensitivity to the client's ability to discuss this material with comfort. With some clients, a trusting relationship is a better context for this discussion than the initial interview.

According to spiritual hypotheses, the client's problem may be related to or partially caused by the following factors:

1. A discrepancy between the client's behavior and his spiritual beliefs, possibly resulting in guilt or shame (after gathering data about the client's spiritual beliefs and related values, discuss the client's behavior in crucial areas of value judgment, taking care to avoid direct confrontation of the discrepancy so as not to provoke a shame response)
2. A transition in which the client's values or spiritual beliefs are changing and creating anxiety and identity confusion (ask the client if he feels comfortable or clearly set in his spiritual beliefs or values; if not, discuss the client's ambivalence and perhaps in this manner discover the point of transition, which can then be discussed in greater detail)
3. A conflict between the client's spiritual beliefs and related expectations of the world and his actual observations and experiences in the world (ask the client how he feels about the world; discuss any disappointments he may feel)
4. The client perceives himself as missing or having lost a supportive relationship with his higher power and feels disappointed and abandoned or alienated (discuss the client's relationship with his higher power and the anger or disappointment he experiences)

Tools of Assessment

The nurse gathers assessment information using a variety of structural approaches and perspectives of inquiry, which are called *assessment tools*. A comprehensive psychosociocultural assessment necessitates the use of several tools; a variety of perspectives are provided by an interdisciplinary mental health team. Within the team that is functioning, the nurse administers some of these assessment tools, interprets the results, formulates a list of client problems and nursing diagnoses, and plans and evaluates nursing interventions. The psychologist administers psychological tests, analyzes the test results, and formulates a diagnostic impression from his disciplinary perspective. Other disciplines also use certain assessment tools to gather essential client data.

Gathering Historic Information

The client's historic data are collected in a holistic assessment. The depth of the history is determined by the problem area and the purpose of the assessment. The history's functions are to form a background against which current client functioning may be measured and to gain an understanding of the client's past, present, and potential.

Objectives of the history-taking include the following:

To describe adaptive and maladaptive patterns of behavior

To formulate priorities of care

To identify client problems and analyze client data in the proper context

To consider the client's probable responses to potential therapeutic interventions

To analyze the client's perception of the world, health, and illness

The history format chosen by a discipline is generally consistent with its philosophy and approach. A nursing history, for example, focuses on the problems and needs of the client and gathers information to assist in nursing care planning in health and illness adaptation. Medical histories are often oriented toward the client's symptoms and the diagnosis of an illness state. A psychiatric history, for example, centers on the client's psychodynamics, or internal conflicts, conflict resolution, and previous psychiatric difficulties.

A nursing history form is a vehicle for organizing and recording client information prior to, during, and following the interview. The sample questions and general categories of examination should be adapted to the client's personality, needs, wishes, and level of communication.[10] (See Charts 7-1 and 7-2, "Guide to Client Assessment" and "Summary of Nursing History: Mr. S. G.")

Psychological Testing

Psychological testing is a structured and systematic process of observing and describing specific behaviors through the use of a numeric or category system.[7] The usefulness of such tests depends on their proper administration and the accurate interpretation of the test results. The significance of psychological test results depends, in turn, on the degree of agreement of several assessment tools (*e.g.*, a battery of psychological tests administered in conjunction with a diagnostic interview and history-taking). There are three general categories of psychological tests—projective tests, personality inventories, and intelligence tests (see Table 7-1 for examples and uses of a variety of psychological tests).

Projective Tests. The projective test is designed to reveal the structure of the client's mind by focusing on his verbalized projections onto ambiguous figures. Although these projections have been shown reliably to identify patterns of thinking, they only represent potential states and not the client's current or highest level of functioning. Projective tests are not standardized, objective, or predictive of behavior in actual situations.[7]

Personality Inventories. Personality inventories are standardized, objective tests (usually in the form of a questionnaire) that measure attitudes, inhibitions, and action tendencies. The liabilities of personality inventories lie in the limited response choices offered by these tests and the artificial nature of the situation in which the questions are asked. Nevertheless, these tests have been shown to be reliable indicators of thought patterns and potential behavior.

Intelligence Tests. Intelligence tests measure intellectual functioning on verbal and nonverbal levels. These tests are standardized according to age but usually do not take into account sociocultural influences on the individual's vocabulary and reasoning. The purpose of administering intelligence tests to a psychiatric–mental health client is to determine the role of intellectual functioning in the development and existence of his problem.

Mental Status Exam

The mental status exam is an assessment tool that was developed primarily from the medical model perspective. This examination aims to identify psychopathologic symptoms and also assesses the current mental status of the client (*i.e.*, his intellectual and emotional functioning). The tool is useful for identifying acute psychotic features of the client quickly and for distinguishing functional conditions from organic conditions.

As with all assessment tools, the significance of the results of the mental status exam can only be un-

CHART 7-2
Summary of Nursing History: Mr. S. G.

Mr. S. G. is a 26-year-old married male admitted to the psychiatric–mental health unit with a diagnosis of *schizophrenia, paranoid type*. His weight is 160 pounds, height is 5 feet 11 inches. The client is a practicing Catholic from Center City, admitted for the first time to this facility. He has no history of previous admissions to any psychiatric facility, but he has been seen in outpatient therapy for 6 years by his admitting psychiatrist, Dr. R. B.

S. G. stated his reason for admission is to "hide until the heat is off," referring to his apparently delusional belief that he is being searched for by the mafia. This fear has recently caused S. G. to quit his job, following 2 weeks of absenteeism. S. G. does not expect the hospital to help with his fear, but he does feel he will be protected here.

S. G. is an attorney who graduated from law school in Minnesota and has been practicing law for 1 year at the Office of Legal Services. He is white, of middle-class background, and comes from the midwestern United States. He lives with his wife and 6-month-old son in an apartment complex near his office. He generally enjoys tennis and jogging.

He states that he does not smoke tobacco but does drink alcohol moderately—about one to two drinks or beers, about once or twice weekly. He denies the use of other drugs.

S. G.'s wife is frightened by her husband's behavior but appears supportive and concerned. S. G.'s parents have also expressed support and concern and are now staying in town, although they live in Texas. S. G. has had many changes in his life in the past 2 years—graduation from law school, accepting his first full-time job, marriage, and a child.

S. G. does not have any physical complaints. He has had no major illnesses, nor does he have any allergies. His sexual interest has decreased recently in relation to the increase in his fear and anxiety, but he has expressed no anxiety regarding his sexual identity.

S. G. is alert and attentive to the interviewer. He is disoriented to the situation at times, believing he is being interviewed for acceptance into a refugee camp. Memory, retention, judgment, and intellectual ability are all appropriate upon questioning. His affect is intense, labile, and indicative of anxiety and fear. His behavior appears normal for the situation. He relates to the interviewer in a somewhat friendly manner.

S. G. described his self-image by saying, "I am a failure. I've lost it all to the mafia." His body image appears normal. The client believes people are watching him and that he is usually being followed. No abnormalities of speech are assessed. His flow of thought appears to be racing at times, and the client agrees with this description. The client's thought content is obsessed with fear of the mafia.

Review of systems is, otherwise, unremarkable. Eating and drinking habits are normal for the client. He expresses no special diet preference and has had no trouble with his appetite since the delusional system developed, but has had difficulty sleeping, with early morning waking. Hygiene habits appear normal for the client's situation—clean, neat, casually dressed. Eye contact is good. The client states that he has no problems communicating his feelings to others, and that marital communication is "excellent"; however, eye contact between the client and his wife during the admission interview appeared, at times, to indicate tension and avoidance of conflict.

The client is an intelligent, 26-year-old man who appears his stated age and is functioning normally except for overwhelming fear and obsession related to a delusion of persecution. He responds to this delusion with anxiety, sometimes panic, and withdrawal from normal activities. His marital relationship appears to be a supportive factor, as does the presence of his parents and other family and friends in the area.

His strengths include intelligence, family support, understanding coworkers (his boss called to express support), and a history indicative of strong previous coping skills and interpersonal relations. His needs include control of anxiety, reinforcement of reality, acceptance of therapeutic relationships with staff, and exploration of stressors that resulted in this apparent psychotic break. Stressors evident at this time include several changes in the life space of the past 2 years—graduation, marriage, new job, new baby, new location. Further assessment of the marital relationship is warranted.

Diagnostic Impression

Disturbance in mood related to delusional thought content
Poor anxiety control related to delusional thought content
Disturbance in motivation related to delusional thought content
Disturbance in thinking related to inadequate coping with environmental stressors

Table 7-1.   **Psychological Tests**

PSYCHOLOGICAL TEST	CATEGORY	AREA ASSESSED	DESCRIPTION	PURPOSE
Rorschach	Projective	Pattern of thinking; level of development of thinking, reasoning and association	The client interprets ambiguous figures (inkblots)	To rule out psychosis; to determine potentialities of personality
Thematic Apperception Test (TAT)	Projective	Pattern of thinking; responses to hypothetic situations	The client interprets ambiguous figures (drawings)	To rule out psychosis; to predict social response patterns
Draw-a-Person Test	Projective	Pattern of thinking; self-image and image of others	The client draws self or another person, or an anonymous human figure	To rule out organic impairment; to determine image of self or others; to rule out psychosis
Bender–Gestalt	Projective	Cognitive abilities; pattern of perception; coordination of intellectual, perceptual, and psychomotor functions	The client is asked to copy nine designs from memory or with design in sight	To rule out organic brain syndrome; to differentiate some psychotic states
Sentence Completion/Word Association	Projective	Prominent themes and patterns of thinking; areas of thought that are threatening to client	The client is asked to respond spontaneously to a stated or written word or phrase with an associated word or phrase	To identify areas of fear, preoccupation, and image of self and others; to rule out psychosis; to rule out personality disorder
Minnesota Multiphasic Personality Inventory (MMPI)	Personality inventory; objective	Personality patterns; characteristic responses to stress	Paper-and-pencil standardized test	To rule out dangerous personality patterns, such as suicidal or homicidal thinking, or bizarre psychotic states; to identify general response patterns
Tennessee Self-Concept Scale	Personality inventory; objective	Personality patterns; image and concept of self in relation to others and the environment	Paper-and-pencil standardized tests	To rule out dangerous personality patterns or potentials of behavior; to predict behavior in social situations; to define feelings about self
Wechsler Adult Intelligence Survey	Intelligence test	Intelligence; cognitive abilities	The client completes 11 tasks that give overall information about intelligence	To assess current intellectual functioning, as compared to potential; to rule out organic impairment; to rule out intellectual impairment due to functional psychosis
Sanford–Binet Intelligence Test	Intelligence test	Intelligence; cognitive abilities	This paper-and-pencil test is accurate only for clients under age 16	To assess current intellectual functioning, as compared to potential; to assess ability to learn in a structured setting

derstood in relation to the client's history, sociocultural status, and physical condition. A hearing impairment, religious belief or custom, or subcultural jargon may cause the nurse assessor to misinterpret the client's response as evidence of psychopathology, when the response actually represents normal behavior for him.

Level of education, degree of social interaction, and environmental stimulation at home are other factors that influence client responses. The assessor evaluates test results and the client's current level of functioning in relation to these factors and compares the client's responses to the average responses of a person of similar age, religion, ethnic group, and past experiences. (See Chart 7-3, "Mental Status Exam," for the categories and approaches to explore each area of client functioning.[6])

Self-Assessment

Ever since the civil rights movement of the 1960s, people have been increasingly aware of their personal rights, including the rights to understand one's body and mind and to determine one's own health care. The nursing profession has fostered this self-help movement by emphasizing client education and support, rather than labeling and directing the client.

This self-help trend is also evident in the assessment process. Today's professional nurse may encourage the client to assess himself through the use of such tools as life-stress scales and assertiveness scales.[12] Many self-assessment scales center on the client's wellness and strengths and help him identify and interpret his own personality, perceptions, anxieties, coping patterns, and needs.

C H A R T 7-3
Mental Status Exam

The following general categories should be explored during the mental status exam. Suggestions for pursuing each area are included.

Appearance. General appearance, grooming, motor behavior, mannerisms, posture, gait (assess through general observations and record as a general impression)

Behavior. Speech patterns, tone of voice, use of slang, flow of speech, eye contact, body language, general behavioral responses to others and environment (assess through general observation; compare findings to the client's usual behavior)

Orientation. Awareness of reality of person, place, time, situation, relationship with others (assess through direct questioning)

Memory. Immediate recall, recent memory, remote memory (assess through direct questioning)

Sensorium. Ability to attend and concentrate; perception of stimuli—internal and external (assess through direct questioning)

Perceptual Processes. Processing of information received through sensorium; includes awareness of self and one's thoughts, reality, and fantasy (assess by asking questions about delusions, illusions, and hallucinations)

Mood and Affect. Mood refers to the prevailing emotion displayed; affect refers to the range of emotion displayed, (happy, sad, unchanging); emotion refers to subjective physiological changes in response to thoughts and perceptions (assess through observation and judge the appropriateness of the behavior in relation to the client's usual behavior)

Intellectual Functioning. General fund of knowledge; cognitive abilities, such as the ability to calculate simple arithmetic problems; ability to abstract, or think symbolically and according to categories of association (assess through direct questioning, such as requesting the client to solve simple math problems or interpret a simple proverb or analogy)

Thought Content. Recurrences of topics of thinking, themes of conversation (assess by observing what the client discusses spontaneously in conversation)

Thought Processes. Stream of conscious or mental activity, as indicated in speech (observe for rate, flow, associations made, and ability to pursue a topic logically)

Insight. Awareness of one's own responsibilities and abilities, especially regarding the current area of concern; ability to analyze problem with objectivity (ask the client to explain the current problem)

Judgment. Decision-making abilities, especially regarding delaying gratification for an ultimate gain; describe the style as impulsive, rational, methodological, or "trial-and-error" (assess by asking the client what he would do in dilemmas requiring important decisions involving personal welfare, such as if he inherited a large sum of money or smelled smoke in a theater)

(Taken from Crary WG, Johnson CW: The Mental Status Exam. In Johnson CW, Snibbe JR, Evans LE (eds): Basic Psychopathology: A Programmed Text, pp 50–89. New York, Spectrum, 1975. Also taken from Margolin C: Assessment of Psychiatric Patients. J Emerg Nurs 6 (July–August): 30–33, 1980)

Another tool of self-assessment is called the algorithm, which offers a structured decision-making method for self-assessment, self-diagnosis, and evaluation of need for further assessment and treatment.[2] The algorithm is sometimes referred to as a "decision-making tree." Individuals may use the decision-making tree to help them reach sensitive, personal decisions as objectively as possible, while considering the possible results of each option (see Fig. 7-1). Algorithms provide a model for understanding such an abstract concept as a diagrammatic definition.[16]

The liabilities of these self-assessment approaches concern the apparent simplification and generalization of very complex and individually specific situations. In addition, the value of all self-help assessment techniques depends on the client's insight, self-awareness, and motivation. These approaches assume that, with appropriate education and support, the individual has the potential for accurate self-assessment, self-diagnosis, and self-improvement.

The Interview

The most important assessment tool is the interview process. The hypothesis method of structuring the interview ensures that no essential information is overlooked; it also gives the client an opportunity to "tell his story" in response to open-ended questions.

The findings of social research have defined the qualities, appearance, and attitudes of an effective interviewer.[11] The interviewer's sensitivity and skill can be developed through training. The critical element in the psychiatric–mental health interview is the human element—spontaneity, warmth, and caring. The goal of an interviewer is to develop these qualities to such an extent that they become a part of her, so that they flow with the qualities she has always owned.

Conducting the Interview. The interview is a purposeful, goal-directed interaction between two people.[11] A powerful implication in this definition is that both participants share actively in the process,

Figure 7-1. *Algorithm for fear and phobia.*

and each is influenced by the other. The relationship-building interaction of nurse and client determines the success or failure of the interview as an assessment tool.

Professional therapeutic relationships differ from social interaction. The professional interview has a select purpose, unlike the casual nature of social interaction. The professional interview also has unity, progression, and thematic continuity. The roles of interviewer and client in the interview do not reflect the equality seen in most social situations; the client may, in fact, view the interviewer as the "expert" and feel in awe of her. Spontaneity, always present in human interaction, may be less evident during the interview. Social taboos, which usually demand that a person avoid the discussion of unpleasant facts and feelings, do not apply during a professional interview.

In a professional relationship, therapeutic rapport must progress from a superficial to an intimate level in a brief period of time to enable the client to feel comfortable in self-revelation. The image of the nurse as a professional facilitates the client's acceptance of such an unusual situation. To foster the development of this relationship, the nurse maintains a nonjudgmental attitude and responds to self-disclosure with honesty, support, and acceptance.[8] The client discloses at his own rate and in whatever manner is comfortable for him. The professional nurse usually limits self-disclosures to demographic data and here-and-now perceptions.

The Role of the Nurse Interviewer. Either in an overt or subtle manner during the interview, the content, or factual aspect, of the interaction is related to the process, or relational aspect, of the interaction. The nurse interviewer must continuously observe both major levels of interaction—process and content—that take place. The nurse's subjective emotional responses often serve as a barometer to assess these two levels of interaction.[5] The nurse's experience of comfort during the interview probably reflects the client's feeling of security; her experience of anxiety or fear probably indicate that he is uneasy or lacking control of angry impulses. Maturity and self-awareness help the nurse distinguish between personal conflict and an honest sharing of the client's experience.

The nurse assumes a participant–observer role during the interview. On one hand, the nurse empathizes and imagines the client's experience and the expectations placed on him by self and society. On the other hand, the nurse observes the progression of the relationship, the client's patterns of interaction, the information he discloses, and her subjective responses to him. Therefore the nurse participates actively in the interaction of the interview while still observing it. It is necessary to attend to the client's cues that indicate his preferences for timing (when to discuss what topic), pacing (how fast or slow to proceed with the data gathering), and his expectations and needs.

Skills of the Nurse Interviewer. A client usually prefers an active, friendly interviewer who verbalizes minimally and uses effective communication techniques.[7] The functions of communication techniques during the interview are to assist the client make transitions in his thinking, label amorphous experiences, and gain a clearer understanding of the situation. The key elements in facilitative communication include the following:

Careful listening
Attending
Demonstration of sincere interest in the importance of the client's words

The nurse interviewer expresses the quality of attentiveness through eye contact, body language, verbal feedback, and the appropriate use of silence.

Other techniques of facilitative communication are concreteness (*i.e.,* the interviewer's specificity of communication) and persistence in requesting the client to describe feelings and events in specific, rather than vague or abstract, terms.

Immediacy, a critical skill, refers to the interviewer's ability to recognize feelings and thoughts of immediate importance to the client and to deal with those issues first. Immediacy also facilitates data gathering, because the client distracted by strong emotion cannot concentrate on the interview.

Experiential and didactic confrontations are also techniques that facilitate authentic relationships. A didactic confrontation occurs when the interviewer objectively offers the client relevant information to correct misinformation. Experiential confrontation involves the nurse's consistently pointing out discrepancies and generalizations in the client's conversation as they occur; this provides first-hand and immediate feedback.[11] (See Chap. 4, "Communication.")

Client Expectations of the Interviewer. Client expectations influence the interview process. At least initially, clients respond more positively to interviewers who meet their expectations and preferences.[7] The preferred image of the nurse interviewer is that of an expert who is confident in personal and professional roles. The client prefers the professional who conveys warmth and authentic concern and, simultaneously, maintains emotional objectivity. This quality of *emotional objectivity* is the ability to express feelings and responses about the client in a professional and nonjudgmental manner.[1]

The nurse is expected to be competent at starting an interview and keeping the flow of conversation moving. Clients tend to feel uncomfortable during lengthy pauses in conversation, unless the silence is obviously allowing the client to reflect on a question or response.

The client expects the nurse interviewer to be knowledgeable about human behavior and to interpret *his* behavior, in particular, within the proper context. The client also expects the interviewer to realize that the client is an "expert on himself."[1] The nurse should recognize her powerful position, the client's relative dependency, and the importance of ethics and self-responsibility in accepting the client's trust.

The effects of an interview may be therapeutic or deleterious. A personal and professional code of ethics guides the nurse's actions in the following ways:

The nurse does not engage in social, physical, or business contacts with the client.

The nurse respects the client's right to confidentiality.

The nurse determines when it is necessary to refer a client to another professional.

The nurse accepts the role of client advocate and teaches and supports the client regarding his rights.

Finally, the mental health professional is aware that clients seldom fit the ideal image (*i.e.*, the energetic, verbal, motivated partner in the interview process). To work effectively with an uncooperative client, the mental health care provider must find his areas of motivation and nurture them.

Stages of the Interview

Introductory Stage. The introductory stage of the interview consists of the client and interviewer introducing themselves, stating their goals and expectations, and discussing the purposes of the interview. This stage is crucial because it allows the client to dispel or maintain his expectations and establishes the rules and roles of the interview relationship. For example, the interviewer informs the client how long the interview will last. During this initial stage, the interviewer "scans" the client, gathers superficial information about the problem, and makes general observations of the client.

Working Stage. The second stage of the interview is the middle or working phase. This stage begins when the client permits a serious pursuit of the problem, to which the interviewer responds with therapeutic skills of problem identification or clarification. During this phase, the nurse interviewer focuses in depth on the emergence and development of the problem, the extent of disruption caused by the problem, and the client's approaches to the problem thus far. The nurse also assesses the strengths and resources of the client and begins to consider possible intervention strategies.

During the working phase, the nurse and client influence each other; a process of change occurs in both. This is the enactment of the participant–observer role.[5] The middle stage of the interview concludes with an exploration of all potential problems not previously examined.

Termination Stage. The termination stage of the interview begins with a reminder to the client that the interview will soon be ending. This reminder should be given 5 to 10 minutes before the interview is scheduled to end or 5 to 10 minutes before termination at the interviewer's discretion based on the client's responses. The interviewer then reviews and summarizes what has been accomplished and asks the client to add, clarify, or correct information reviewed. The need for follow-up sessions or referrals to other professionals is suggested at that time.

Finally, in recognition of the difficulty the client endures in revealing so much of himself and his past experiences, the nurse interviewer informs the client that she appreciates his cooperation and intrinsic worth. This should consist of a positive and entirely truthful statement that gives the client something to go away with and helps him to feel better because of the interview.

Professional Handling of Client Data.

The information gathered in a nursing assessment should be treated as vital and strictly confidential material, even if it does not seem to be of a "private" nature.

Recording Interview Data. Recording of data gathered during the interview can be completed in a variety of ways, depending on the needs and wishes of the client and nurse. One method is for the interviewer to keep a verbatim written recording. This method, although allowing accuracy, disrupts the flow of the interview process. Sometimes, students of mental health professions use this method as a learning experience to examine communication patterns.

Another method of recording is to use a third-person nonparticipant to record the verbatim interview conversation and to note, as much as possible, the nonverbal communication. The presence of the third person, however, may significantly alter the dynamics of the interview, particularly trust, and may be perceived as a violation of psychological privacy.

Probably the most widely used approach is the recording of brief notes throughout the interview or the making of "mental notes," followed by the writing of a summary of verbal and nonverbal client data later. Although this method offers greater comfort for the client, it may not provide optimal accuracy.

CHART 7-4
Interview Guide

The following sample questions are intended to aid the nurse in posing appropriate questions during the interview. The nurse relies on overall understanding of the client and the context of the interview to determine specific wording for questions. Remember that open-ended questions will facilitate the interview with higher-functioning clients. However, the more disorganized client may be more comfortable, as well as more cooperative, with closed-ended questions, "yes or no" questions, or short-answer ones. A closed-ended question can introduce a subject as pertinent for the client and be followed by a "tell me about it" question to gain more information.

Introductory Phase

What do you see as the primary problem that brought you here? Why did you decide to seek help at this particular time?

What areas of your life are particularly stressful and what areas are easy for you now?

What kinds of support do you have now? Do you see friends or family regularly? What do they say about the current situation, or your coming here?

Are finances a problem now?

What goals do you have for your life in general and for your experience here?

What do you expect from a counselor (or from a hospitalization or treatment experience)?

How do you expect us to go about helping you?

Working Phase

Psychological

Have you been having problems thinking clearly lately?

How does this problem relate to other problems you've had in the past? Is there a pattern? Is this similar to conflicts with parents in the past?

Have there been a lot of changes in your life lately?

How do you see yourself now? Has this situation affected your self-esteem?

Social

Are you spending as much time with other people as usual?

Are other people responding to you differently now?

Have your most significant or intimate relationships changed lately?

How do your friends feel about your situation now?

Biologic

Have any family members had this kind of problem? Has anyone in your family been hospitalized for a psychiatric illness?

Have your eating and sleeping habits changed lately? Have you been feeling unusually sad or happy lately?

Have you had unusual experiences that were hard to explain to others? Do your thoughts seem to be moving more slowly or faster than usual? Have there been some thoughts you can't seem to control?

How are you feeling physically?

Are you feeling pressured by expectations of others?

How often (and how much) do you drink alcohol? Do you use any other drugs? Do you have any drug- or alcohol-related problems?

What prescription drugs are you on now?

Behavioral

Are there any specific behaviors that always cause you problems? Are there any behaviors you cannot seem to control but would like to stop? Do you feel compelled to do some behaviors you really don't want to do?

How do other people seem to respond to you? Does it seem easy for you to make friends?

Cognitive

Do you tend to fuss at yourself in your head? What kinds of things do you tell yourself about this situation? Are you pretty critical of yourself?

What do you think about your ability to get along in this world today? How do you think things are going in the world today?

Do you feel other people are responsible for your problems today?

Does it seem like you act according to your values or other influences?

Cultural

How is your life now different from your parents' lives when you were growing up? Do your family and older friends have trouble understanding you now?

(Continues on p. 102)

How do people from your former culture respond to this sort of problem? How do they explain or make sense of this sort of situation?

Spiritual

Do you believe in a higher power or supreme being? What's your relationship with this being or power like?

How does your religion make sense of problems in the world today? Or of your situation now?

Mental Status Exam

Orientation

Have you been having trouble realizing where you are or what's on around you? Would you tell me where you are now?

Memory

Can you remember what you had for breakfast today?

What did you do yesterday?

Can you remember what I said my name was?

What was the name of the high school you graduated from?

Sensorium

Do you have trouble concentrating or focusing your thoughts? Can you watch a movie or read a book and follow it through?

Do you have trouble keeping up in conversations?

Perceptual

Are there things that you can see or hear that other people cannot know are there?

Do you have unusual abilities or experiences often now?

Are there things you believe that other people say are all wrong? Do you believe there are people trying to hurt you?

Does it seem easy lately to mistake one thing for another, like a shadow for a man?

Mood and Affect

What's your mood been like lately? Are you more or less emotional than usual now?

Intellectual Fund

What's the governor's name? Can you think of one big item in the news lately?

Would you please subtract 7 from 100 and keep going with that until I ask you to stop?

What does it mean when people say "Don't cry over spilled milk"?

Thought Content

Are there certain subjects you think about a lot or almost all the time lately?

Thought Processes

Are your thoughts moving more slowly or quickly than usual?

Does it seem as if your mind just goes blank lately?

Do you have trouble keeping up with your thoughts or understanding your thoughts?

Insight

What do you think the real problem is that resulted in your being here today?

How do you make sense of this whole situation now?

Judgment

What would you do if a policeman stopped you for speeding?

What would you do if you received a $10,000 check in the mail, just for you to use?

History

How many brothers and sisters do you have? Where were you born? What were your parents like when you were a young child? What's your earliest memory?

Did you enjoy grade school? How were your grades? Did you play with other children a lot? What was it like at home?

What was it like in junior high? What kinds of things did you like to do? Were your grades okay? Did you get into any trouble at school?

What were you like in high school? Did you date? How were your grades? Any chemical use? Did you get into trouble a lot? How was it at home? Did you keep your friends from grade school?

What did you do after graduation? When was your first significant intimate relationship? When was your first real job?

What kinds of jobs have you had? How did you do with your jobs?

Have you ever had this sort of problem before? Any other emotional problems severe enough to warrant seeking help? Any hospitalizations?

Do you have contact with family now? Do any family members have any history of psychiatric illness?

Termination Phase

Are there any other things you would like to tell me that would help me understand you better?

Do you have any responses to this interview? Can you tell me what this was like for you?

What questions do you have for me?

Audio- and video-tape recordings are the most reliable methods of recording during the interview. Videotaping allows a review of the session and gives the most complete information about the client's communication within the environmental context. Audiotaping, however, is usually seen as a less formidable recording method than videotaping. Before planning to tape record an interview, the nurse must ascertain that institutional policies permit taping and that the client has given his approval by signing a permission form. The permission form should clearly state the purpose of the taping, who will have access to the tape, and when and how the tape will be destroyed or erased. Problems related to taping an interview include client discomfort, irritation, and suspicion.

Regardless of the method of recording chosen, a concluding summary should complete the report. The summary should consist of the following.

1. A demographic description of the client, such as age, sex, and so forth
2. Major patterns of behavior
3. A comparison of the client's behavior to accepted norms
4. Suggestions for further assessment, referral, or intervention strategies
5. Subjective impressions of the client, identified as such
6. Client strengths and resources, as well as problem areas of functioning
7. A reasonable approach to the client's situation

Recording of assessment information, including a thorough client history, description of the problem, and the client's abilities and potential sources of motivation, allows for an accurate analysis of the data. Gathering client-assessment data enables the nurse to formulate accurate diagnoses, which form the bases for nursing care plans.

Summary

This chapter has discussed the first step of the nursing process and has examined its characteristics, components, and structure. The major emphases of the chapter have included the following points:

1. Nursing assessment is the gathering of client data, which is then classified and categorized in the analysis step of the nursing process.
2. Nursing assessment explores the needs, problems, and adaptive resources of the individual and the means by which the nurse may help the client move to a higher level of health.
3. Identification and clarification of the client's problems are major purposes of nursing assessment.
4. Through the hypothesis approach to assessment, the nurse interviewer explores client functioning in the psychological, social, biologic, behavioral, cognitive, cultural, and spiritual areas of his life.
5. A variety of assessment tools should be used to conduct a comprehensive assessment of the psychiatric–mental health client.
6. The communication and relationship skills of the nurse constitute the most essential element of the assessment interview.

References

1. Bernstein L, Bernstein RS, Dana RH: Interviewing: A Guide for Health Professionals, 4th ed. New York, Appleton-Century-Crofts, 1985
2. Blattner B: Holistic Nursing. Englewood Cliffs, NJ, Prentice-Hall, 1981
3. Burgess AW, Lazare A: Community Mental Health. Englewood Cliffs, NJ, Prentice-Hall, 1976
4. Coler M, Vincent K: Psychiatric–Mental Health Assessment. Archives of Psychiatric Nursing 1, (August): 258–263, 1987
5. Francis G, Munjas B: Manual of Socialpsychologic Assessment. New York, Appleton-Century-Crofts, 1976
6. Hagerty BK: Psychiatric–Mental Health Assessment. St. Louis, CV Mosby, 1984
7. Hersen M, Turner S (eds): Diagnostic Interviewing, New York, Plenum Press, 1985
8. Longo D (ed): Clinical Practice in Psychosocial Nursing: Assessment and Intervention. Norwalk, CT, Appleton-Century-Crofts, 1986
9. Lazare A: The Psychiatric Examination in the Walk-In Clinic: Hypothesis Generation and Testing. Arch Gen Psychiatry 33 (January): 96–102, 1976
10. Lego S (ed): The American Handbook of Psychiatric Nursing. Philadelphia, JB Lippincott, 1984
11. MacKinnon R, Yudofsky S: The Psychiatric Evaluation in Clinical Practice. Philadelphia, JB Lippincott, 1986
12. McCandless-Glimcker L et al: Use of Symptoms by Schizophrenics to Monitor and Regulate Their Illness. Hosp Community Psychiatry 37 (September): 929–933, 1986
13. Nishiura E, Whitten C, Jenkins D: Screening for Psychosocial Problems in Health Settings. Health Soc Work 5 (August): 22–28, 1980
14. Orem D: Nursing: Concepts of Practice. New York, McGraw-Hill, 1971
15. Sullivan HS: The Psychiatric Interview. New York, WW Norton and Co, 1970
16. Vickery DM, Fries JF: Take Care of Yourself: A Consumer's Guide to Medical Care, 2d ed. Reading, MA, Addison-Wesley, 1981

8 Nursing Diagnosis

Sharon Byers
Diane M. Snow

It has been said and written scores of times, that every woman makes a good nurse. I believe, on the contrary, that the very elements of nursing are all but unknown.

Florence Nightingale,
Notes on Nursing: What It
Is and What It Is Not

Chapter Preview

Analysis is a cognitive process using skills of critical thinking. The second step of the nursing process focuses on analysis of the data so that a nursing diagnosis may be established. The nurse uses theoretical knowledge to cluster the data together, identify strengths and resources, determine motivational readiness, and use the resulting problem list to arrive at the nursing diagnosis.

The formal step of analysis, or nursing diagnosis, follows the initial step of assessment and is critically important in guiding the next steps of planning, intervention, and evaluation. A taxonomy is often used to organize and categorize the data into appropriate, care-guiding diagnoses. In the interdisciplinary setting of psychosocial nursing, the Diagnostic and Statistical Manual, Third Edition Revised (DSM-III-R), is an important tool for understanding the signs and symptoms of the medical diagnosis; it provides a communication tool for the team to use in understanding the client's problems. Nursing can use this knowledge of the medical diagnosis as part of the basis for evaluating the client's response to the health problems during the analysis phase of the nursing process.

Learning Objectives

On completion of this chapter, you should be able to accomplish the following:

1. identify the steps of analysis leading to the nursing diagnosis
2. formulate a patient problem list based on analysis of patient data into clusters or categories, on review of strengths and resources, and on motivational readiness
3. discuss the importance of nursing diagnosis to the development of nursing knowledge
4. define nursing diagnosis and various ways to write the diagnosis
5. explain the use of a taxonomy in writing an accurate nursing diagnosis
6. explain the use of the five axes of the DSM-III-R classification of psychiatric diagnoses

Analysis of Assessment Data

The analysis phase of the nursing process involves examining the data that has been collected during the assessment phase. This step in the nursing process assists the nurse in arriving at the most accurate and definitive nursing diagnoses. It involves the cognitive process of clustering pieces of data together to look for patterns; addressing the resources and strengths available to the client and his family; identifying the motivational readiness of the client to make recommended changes in his behavior, lifestyle, responses to his family, and coping patterns; identifying problem areas as well as potential problem areas of functioning; and, finally, arriving at the nursing diagnosis.

Examining and Clustering Data

By examining the data, the nurse begins to look for patterns of behavior that reflect certain problem areas or potential problem areas for the client. The data, which consist of nursing history, mental status assessment, developmental data, and assessment of physical, psychological, sociocultural, and spiritual strengths and needs, are analyzed for factors that form groupings reflecting known variables that nursing can diagnose and treat. Data are compared with the client's stated problem and the nurse's initial clinical impression. Analysis of this type is often done during nursing rounds, when staff members contribute observations of both client and family behavior and the possible reasons for these behaviors. An initial treatment plan is often necessary before the nurse has enough data to validate the "hunches" or emerging patterns. Examples of patterns at this stage of analysis might be the presence of religious ideation, refusal to eat, refusal to take medication, pacing around the unit, and lack of personal hygiene. These all "fit" together, and they will probably lead to a nursing diagnosis as more information is received and analyzed.

Strengths and Resources

Next, the data from the client and his family are assessed to identify strengths and available resources. It is a well-known principle in working with people that there are healthy parts of any personality; these *strengths* should be identified and listed so that they can be accessed to help the client cope with his situation. When the client is able to participate in this process, the nurse can help him identify these assets for himself. This is often a therapeutic move that helps signify both a sense of self-value and a sense of hope because there is strength. When the client is unable to participate because of the difficulty with thought processes, the nurse can gain this information from the family and from daily observations of the client. For example, the client whose behavior clustered in a suspicious pattern in the above section may, in fact, have high-level intelligence, good physical health, a stable job, and a positive body image.

CHART 8-1
Identifying Strengths and Resources

Examples of Personal Strengths	Examples of External Resources
Intelligence	Family support
Physical health	Friendships
Valuing health	Financial resources
Hope for future	Transportation
Physical features	Living arrangements
Ability to hold job	Church affiliation
Concern for others	Self-help groups
Generosity	School affiliation
Self-care	Social clubs
Spiritual practices and values	Rehabilitation training and vocational help
Parenting skills	Current job
Working with hands; skill in music, art, sports	Mental health clinics
	Community agencies such as Meals on Wheels, telephone crisis lines, parenting clinics

These strengths may be the balancing factors that enable the client to move quickly along the mental health–mental illness continuum toward mental health. They may be the factors that give the client a sense of self-esteem and mobilize hope for recovering from this episode of illness.

The *resources* available to the client are important to his overall coping. These are external factors that may include support networks, such as family and friends, financial resources, transportation, community resources, church or school support, and other favorable environmental supports. Family support is extremely important and may include communication and closeness of family members for mutual support, a sense of unity of the family, and healthy family members who can be taught to help the client and other family members cope with the situation. The client's history of use of the various potential resources is important so that nursing interventions can be planned to help the client gain access to these resources. (See Chart 8-1, "Identifying Strengths and Resources.")

③ Motivational Readiness

The nurse cannot assume that either the client or the family is ready to make any changes in their lives. Patterns of coping develop over time, and it is unrealistic to expect the client to want to change something that is so familiar that it is actually more comfortable to continue the behavior than to change it. Even behavior that is self-destructive or obviously harmful to those people who are important to the client will often

be continued. This can be extremely frustrating to the nurse, who naturally assumes that all people value health and want to improve their lives. The client, in reality, may be dealing with the issue of survival in a world that is perceived as threatening and painful. He has difficulty learning because the focus for behavior is on coping with the pain of living. This involves high levels of anxiety, which narrows the perception of events and causes the client to be preoccupied with certain fears. These concerns must be the focus of nursing care until the client feels a degree of safety and security that can result from a trusting, caring nurse–client relationship. Paradoxically, it is important to remember that pain is a powerful motivator. The effort to instill hope by empowering the person to strive for survival, to have the will to live and "make it," is critical for any type of therapy to be effective.

Through an analysis of the assessment data, the nurse determines potential sources of motivation for the client. These are aspects of the client's life that seem important to him and could be sources of power to give him an increased sense of personal control and self-esteem. In attempting to access these sources of motivation, the nurse is encouraging the client to give up the resistance to change, the forces that restrain the client from forward movement toward wellness. These restraining forces must also be identified in order to reduce them or to change them into motivational factors.[30] (See Chart 8-2, "Motivational Readiness.")

Whereas the client may be motivated by a desire to return home and be with his family, he may experience an equal restraining force based on a previous experience in a health care setting, such as being placed in seclusion. This experience may have left the client fearful of a recurrence. The nurse's action must then involve reducing the fear or perhaps redefining it. The fear of being placed in seclusion could be reframed as a desire to stay in control, and the nurse could offer assistance to the client to maintain control. With this restraining force reduced, the nurse would continue to search for additional motivations and to value these with the client. For the client who is able to delay gratification, these may include such things as a desire to decrease medication, a desire to become more independent, a desire to find new friends, or a desire to improve a relationship. Or, for the client who is unable to delay gratification and needs short-term reinforcement, the desire may be to get his "teeth fixed" or a "warm bed and a hot meal." Whatever the motivation, the nurse needs to recognize it as important to the client and thus important to the overall plan of care. If the nurse responds to the need with either negative reinforcement or withdrawal from the client, the client's negative self-image and anxiety, which are not conducive to learning or to adaptive, lasting behavior change will be reinforced.

A feeling of powerlessness often prevents the client who is mentally ill from wanting to change. If a person does not believe that what he desires is within his control, often his response is to increase efforts to control the environment.[40] This may confound the problem because he may be unable to control most aspects of living. By trying to control the environment, the client is attempting "to get control back." The suspicious client uses projection and blame, the alcoholic client uses denial and rationalization, the depressed client uses self-defeating behavior, and the violent client uses aggression—all in an attempt to feel valuable. These may be the only ways perceived by the client to achieve some control. Nursing can play an important role in helping the client tap a new source of power.[40] For example, an external source of power might be identification with a group, such as Alcoholics Anonymous, a social club for clients with schizophrenia, or the other clients in the milieu environment. Or it may be an improved relationship with a significant other. An internal source of power could be increased knowledge through formal or informal education, increased self-control through stopping a negative pattern such as abuse, or an improved body image from loss of weight.

Problem List

Analysis of the focus of care for the psychiatric–mental health client includes evaluation of all the collected information and inferences about the problematic behaviors, strengths and resources, and sources of motivation in order to form a problem list within a holistic nursing framework. Family and related community problems as well as individual problems should be included in the problem list. The family's level of motivation for change is as important as the client's. If the family is dealing with the death of a family member or the loss of economic security, this affects the client. The whole family is suffering and needs the support of the nurse, who is often the one health care person who has access to the concerns of the family.

Community resources and other environmental concerns are important as well. The client who lives alone in a rural area where there are no close neigh-

---

C H A R T 8-2
Motivational Readiness

Sources of Motivation	Restraining Forces
To get well	Fear of confinement
To return home	Loss of freedom
To feel safe	Mistrust
To find new friends	Fear of abandonment
To stay sober or "straight"	Anxiety
To solve problems	Fear of responsibility
To have relief from physical pain	Fear of independence
To stay in control	Fear of reality
To improve a relationship	Lack of knowledge
To decrease medication	Lack of purpose in life
To be more productive	Fear of rejection

CHART 8-3

Suggested Nursing Diagnoses and Client Problem List

Each category below represents the first part of a diagnostic statement, and the phrases that follow are examples of problems seen in association with that diagnosis. The second part of the diagnostic statement begins with "related to" and represents, in some way, an etiology of the syndrome described in the first part of the diagnostic statement. The complete diagnosis represents a syndrome that is disruptive to the health or adaptation of the client.

Disturbance in Self-Concept

Potential for self-injury
Withdrawn behavior
Poor hygiene habits
Ruminations

Ineffective Coping

Acting out
Ruminations
Withdrawn behavior

Impaired Thought Processes

Acting out
Social isolation
Restless behavior
Fear
Poor social skills

Lack of Social Skills

Acting out
Aggressive behavior
Limited self-care abilities

Limited Communication Abilities

Acting out
Disorganized speech
Social isolation

Potential for Injury

Inability to communicate
 impending seizure

Note that some problems appear under several diagnostic statements. A phrase listed as a problem in one situation may be listed as a diagnostic syndrome statement in another situation. Making these distinctions carefully and accurately is important when planning nursing interventions. Such decisions must be based on thorough knowledge of the client's problem, of the client as a diagnostic entity, and of the client as a person with a set of behavioral responses.

bors to call on for help has special needs. These needs must be addressed. Similarly, the client who has the support of a prayer group or numerous "telephone friends" will have resources that are available and accessible.

Since nurses espouse a philosophy of holism and self-determination, the client's perception and validation of the areas of concern are most helpful in formulating a problem list. Life-threatening problems are the exception and are of greatest concern. Examples of such problems include suicidal ideation, homicidal ideation, fluid and electrolyte imbalance, threatening hallucinations, and violence. These are problem areas that the nurse determines from the data and that may or may not be validated by the client. Labeling certain areas of concern as "prob-

lems" may not be appropriate if they are adaptive for the client. The context of the problem and the personality of the client are dimensions to be considered before labeling something a problem. For example, a low IQ may be the main reason an adolescent client does not do well in a school program. This then is not a problem for nursing to address. The effects of the low IQ on the client's self-esteem, however, may be a problem that nursing can address.

Nursing Diagnosis

There has been increasing interest in developing a taxonomy for nursing diagnosis and in assisting nurses to make accurate diagnoses in their clinical

Case Study 8-1: Ms.

Analysis of Assessment Data

Examination

Ms. Deborah K., R.N., is a 30-year-old unmarried woman and a chiropractic student in her second year of school. She presented herself at the community mental health center, complaining of anxiety attacks, withdrawal from significant relationships, headaches, sleep disturbances, and "feeling like I'm falling apart." These symptoms, of 5 weeks' duration, lack a clearly identified precipitating factor. She stated that her primary affect is anger that is unfocused and pervasive. She reported the ending of a romantic relationship 3 months prior to the appearance of her symptoms; the termination of the relationship, she stated, was in response to a mutual decision and acceptable to her. She also reported anxiety over finances and grades, compounded by her difficulty finding a job that would fit her demanding schedule.

Deborah is the middle child of a large Polish Catholic, upper-middle-class family. Most of her siblings are successfully employed, financially secure, and in stable marital relationships. There is no history of psychiatric disturbances of the client or other family members. The client has had successful intimate relationships.

By means of analysis, the nurse recognized the need for ongoing assessment throughout the development of a therapeutic relationship. Certain topics may be explored more openly and thoroughly after the nurse and client have established rapport and the client's symptoms have been somewhat controlled. The reduction of anxiety would allow introspection and learning.

Synthesis

There seems to exist a relationship among Deborah's anxiety attacks, physical complaints, and feelings of impending loss of control. Anger may or may not be related to frustrations experienced in school, financial worries, and the loss of a significant relationship, which may be perceived as a failure by the client. Anxiety may be related to her need for achievement and the high expectations set by herself and her family. No relationships among data seem to indicate severe psychopathology at this point.

This client has successfully dealt with responsibilities, intimate relationships, and normal living demands and has been viewed as a high achiever. Single marital status is described as her choice due to her many personal goals and to her not having found a partner who would fit in that personal goal pattern.

Categorization

An appropriate descriptor of this client's experience, including her complaints of sleep disturbance, anxiety attacks, headaches, and "feeling like I'm coming apart," is *anxiety reaction*. This anxiety may also be placed in another category of *perception of loss of control*, as seen in the many obstacles to goal attainment in the client's life and the implications of her expectations of achievement and success. The subjective feeling of "coming apart" may be an indicator of this perceived loss of control.

The client's angry affect and withdrawal in relationships may be seen as "stress reactions" in response to a variety of frustrations.

It can be assumed by the previous personal and family history that the client's self-concept includes an achievement orientation in all areas of her life, which would be threatened during this period of mental and physical distress. This *threat to self-image* would result in anxiety, and might also lead the caregiver to place this problem in the category of *unrealistic or overly rigid expectations for self*. Considering the stress of graduate-level education, the expense and financial burden incurred in professional tuitions, and the overall impact these factors have on lifestyle and relationships, an expectation to succeed at all endeavors during this time could be termed *unrealistic*.

Evaluation

In this situation, the nurse working with Deborah K. would identify the need for further questioning and would identify the need for further exploration in the areas of goals and expectations of self, perceived need for control, previous experiences with disappointment, family relationships and expectations, and the recent romantic relationship. The impeding factor in this process seems to be the client's lack of insight, which is incongruent with her history and accomplishments. Further exploration of the client's prior experiences with failures, crises, or losses is indicated.

(Continues on p. 110)

Problem List for ▮Ms. Deborah K.▮

Strengths

1. Youth and physical health
2. No history of psychiatric disturbances of self or family members
3. Previous successful employment
4. Previous successful intimate relationships
5. Intelligence
6. Ambition and motivation
7. Short-term duration of symptoms
8. Adaptability to lifestyle changes
9. Generally high self-esteem and self-confidence
10. Previous positive experiences with health care system
11. Pleasant appearance and manner

Resources

1. Large, supportive, involved family
2. At least three concerned, close friends
3. School counselors and resource people
4. Ability to earn money (if work can be scheduled around school commitments or in the event that she has to withdraw from school)
5. Community mental health center near her home

Motivations

1. Goal of becoming a chiropractor
2. Interest and belief in feedback from others
3. Goal of self-actualization

Problems

1. Overwhelming anxiety and lack of experience with, and knowledge of, coping skills
2. Withdrawal from friends
3. Possible unrealistic expectation of self and need to compete with family members
4. Lack of significant other to provide support
5. Real concerns and problems in meeting goals, possibly due to external causes
6. Possible grief or guilt over recent failure of romantic relationship
7. Apparent lack of insight regarding relationships between symptoms or origin of feelings

practices. The American Nurses' Association (ANA) Social Policy Statement of 1980 gave a clear mandate toward this development through its definition of nursing as "the *diagnosis* and treatment of human responses to actual or potential health problems."[1] In addition, the 1982 revised Standards of Psychiatric and Mental Health Nursing Practice, which guide the practice of psychiatric nursing in any health care setting, include a standard (#3) that clearly states that the nurse "utilizes *nursing diagnosis* and standard classification of mental disorders to express conclusions supported by recorded assessment data and current scientific premises."[2] The categorization scheme and the method of assigning names to phenomena that nurses treat through their own prescriptions of care are still the focus of much research and remain practice issues of the nursing profession. Accountability for the practice and the definition of that practice are critical to the practice of the psychiatric nurse. The way to a mature, autonomous profession is in defining what our knowledge base is, both in our diagnosing and in our intervening, to assist the client toward wellness.[8]

A nursing diagnosis is a statement of the client's response pattern to a health disruption. It is a concept, which means that it is an abstract, broad definition of phenomena. The nurse uses it to help the client explore—and change, if he has sufficient motivation. The purpose of the diagnosis is to direct the intervention toward altering the influencing factors, or etiology, associated with the diagnosis. Thus, the diagnosis is a critical component of the nursing process. The client's status is expected to improve if the correct etiology is identified during assessment and if the intervention actually helps alter the causative factors. The mechanism for evaluation is the change in the behaviors or symptoms that initially were clustered to arrive at the diagnosis. The goals that are the predicted changes in behavior serve as the outcome criteria for this evaluation.[8]

Nursing diagnoses imply decision-making. The psychiatric nurse must make informed decisions as part of clinical nursing. Through an accurate assessment of the individual, family, and community, the nurse clusters the data according to how the pieces fit together.[36] This implies making inferences about the significance of the data to the person and the family. It means prioritizing the most important needs of the client and family. Diagnoses can be ranked, with life-threatening needs first and areas of deficit after these needs.

The nurse assesses the physical, the psychologi-

C H A R T   8-4
Standard III, Standards of Psychiatric and Mental Health Nursing Practice

Diagnosis

The nurse utilizes nursing diagnoses and/or standard classification of mental disorders to express conclusions supported by recorded assessment data and current scientific premises.

Rationale

Nursing's logical basis for providing care rests on the recognition and identification of those actual or potential health problems that are within the scope of nursing practice.

Structure Criterion

In the practice setting, opportunities are provided for validation of diagnosis by peers and for exchange of information and research findings regarding the scientific premises underlying nursing diagnosis among peers.

Process Criteria

The nurse—
1. identifies actual or potential health problems
   a. self-care limitations or impaired functioning whose general etiology is mental and emotional distress, deficits in the ways significant systems are functioning, and internal psychic and/or developmental issues
   b. emotional stress or crisis components of illness, pain, self-concept changes, and life process changes
   c. emotional problems related to daily experiences, such as anxiety, aggression, loss, loneliness, and grief
   d. physical symptoms that occur simultaneously with altered psychic functioning, such as altered intestinal functioning and anorexia
   e. alterations in thinking, perceiving, symbolizing, communicating, and decision-making abilities
   f. impaired abilities to relate to others
   g. behaviors and mental states that indicate the client is a danger to self or others or is gravely disabled
2. analyzes available information according to accepted theoretical frameworks
3. collects sufficient data to verify a diagnosis
4. makes inferences regarding data from phenomena
5. formulates a nursing diagnosis subject to revision with subsequent data

Outcome Criteria

1. Nursing diagnoses are validated with the client when validation has a therapeutic purpose and is not clearly impossible or contraindicated. If illness precludes this capacity in the client, affirmation of the nursing diagnosis is sought from the client's significant others and/or the nurse's peers.
2. Nursing diagnoses are recorded in a manner that facilitates nursing planning and research.

Source: American Nurses' Association, Standards of Psychiatric and Mental Health Nursing Practice, Kansas City, MO: ANA, 1982.

cal, the social, and the spiritual dimensions as one theoretical framework for collecting data. The results of the mental status exam provide much information, including cognitive, affective, motor, language, insight, and judgment data. Also, the nurse uses the results of the nursing history to help formulate the diagnosis. For example, in the physical dimension, the client may complain of insomnia and early wakening, while the mental status exam yields a depressed mood and feelings of hopelessness for the affective

---

C H A R T   8-5

North American Nursing Diagnosis Association (NANDA) Approved Nursing Diagnoses

Activity intolerance	Incontinence, total
Activity intolerance, potential	Incontinence, urge
Adjustment, impaired	Infection, potential for
Airway clearance, ineffective	Injury, potential for: (specify) suffocation, poisoning,
Anxiety	trauma
Aspiration, potential for	Knowledge deficit (specify)
Body temperature, altered, potential	Mobility, impaired physical
Bowel elimination, altered: Constipation	Noncompliance (specify)
Colonic constipation	Nutrition, altered: Less than body requirements
Perceived constipation	Nutrition, altered: More than body requirements
Bowel elimination, altered: Diarrhea	Nutrition, altered: Potential for more than body
Bowel elimination, altered: Incontinence	requirements
Breastfeeding, ineffective	Oral mucous membrane, altered
Breathing pattern, ineffective	Parental role conflict
Cardiac output, altered: Decreased	Parenting, altered: Actual
Comfort, altered: Pain	Parenting, altered: Potential
Comfort, altered: Chronic pain	Post trauma response
Communication, impaired: Verbal	Powerlessness
Coping, family: Potential for growth	Rape trauma syndrome
Coping, ineffective family: Compromised	Role performance, altered
Coping, ineffective family: Disabling	Self-care deficit: Feeding, bathing/hygiene, dressing/
Coping, ineffective individual	grooming, toileting
Defensive coping	Self-concept, disturbance in body image, self-esteem, role
Ineffective denial	performance, personal identity
Decisional conflict (specify)	Self-esteem disturbance
Disuse syndrome, potential for	Chronic low self-esteem
Diversional activity, deficit	Situational low self-esteem
Dysreflexia	Sensory perceptual alteration: Visual, auditory, kinesthetic,
Family process, altered	gustatory, tactile, olfactory
Fatigue	Sexual dysfunction
Fear	Sexuality patterns, altered
Fluid volume altered: excess	Skin integrity, impaired: Actual
Fluid volume deficit, actual	Skin integrity, impaired: Potential
Fluid volume deficit, potential	Sleep pattern disturbance
Gas exchange, impaired	Social interaction, impaired
Grieving, anticipatory	Social isolation
Grieving, dysfunctional	Spiritual distress (distress of the human spirit)
Growth and development, altered	Swallowing, impaired
Health maintenance, altered	Thermoregulation, ineffective
Health-seeking behaviors (specify)	Thought processes, altered
Home maintenance management, impaired	Tissue integrity, impaired
Hopelessness	Tissue perfusion, altered: Cerebral, cardiopulmonary,
Hyperthermia	renal, gastrointestinal, peripheral
Hypothermia	Unilateral neglect
Incontinence, functional	Urinary elimination, altered patterns
Incontinence, reflex	Urinary retention
Incontinence, stress	Violence, potential for: Self-directed or directed at others

From North American Nursing Diagnosis Association Classification of Nursing Diagnosis: Proceedings of the Eighth Conference, Philadelphia, JB Lippincott, 1989 component. These facts, combined with a reported history of a suicide attempt and a series of losses over the past year, as well as the nurse's theoretical understanding of depression, suggest that the behaviors cluster around a sleep-pattern disturbance, hopelessness, and a potential for suicide, all of which are areas that nursing can treat. The known etiological factors (there may be several) are the series of losses and the tendency toward self-destructive behavior. These factors then become the focus of nursing intervention, which is aimed at helping the client work through the grieving process and learn more effective coping skills to deal with strong emotions.

Development of Taxonomy

The development of a taxonomy for nursing diagnosis is a mechanism to provide nursing with a listing of the major areas that nurses treat. To be valid and reliable, such a list needs to be tested by nurses in clinical practice and revised as new diagnoses are found to be important aspects of nursing practice. The danger of such a list is that it discourages the use of intuition and may not include the vast range of responses that nursing addresses.[38] The most recent taxonomy is "Nursing Taxonomy I," the first official taxonomy of nursing diagnoses.[33] It was endorsed by the Seventh National Conference General Assembly of the North American Nursing Diagnosis Association (NANDA) in April 1986, replacing the alphabetic list used since 1982 (see Chart 8-5). The conferences are held by this group every 2 years to update and further develop its work.[2] Nurses are being asked to implement this system of classification, or they may choose a system developed by a particular institution. Such systems usually are computerized listings with defining characteristics and common etiological factors.

The organizing scheme for the current NANDA taxonomy is called "human response patterns." This includes the broad patterns of exchanging, communicating, relating, valuing, choosing, moving, perceiving, knowing, and feeling.[33] Under each of these are the subcategories of "alterations," such as "alteration in socialization" under relating and "alteration in coping" under choosing. A still lower level of categorization increases the specificity of the concern, such as "social isolation" under alteration in socialization and "ineffective individual coping" under alteration in coping. Some of the new diagnoses added to the list are especially useful in psychosocial nursing; these include impaired adjustment, developmental delay, hopelessness, altered patterns of sexuality, impaired socialization, and posttrauma response.[33] Qualifiers

can be chosen that apply to the individual patient, including the following:[33]

decreased	excessive
depleted	increased
deficient	acute
impaired	chronic
dysfunctional	intermittent
disturbed	actual
ineffective	potential

An additional taxonomy which addresses the phenomena of concern in psychiatric–mental health nursing practice has been constructed through the work of an ANA task force (see Chart 8-7).

The general format for writing a nursing diagnosis is the category or concern from the list, followed by the etiology and the defining characteristics (signs and symptoms or clarifier). Or the defining characteristic may be listed after the concern as a "clarifier" of the concern. A nursing diagnosis should be concrete and descriptive enough to accurately label a client's condition and give direction for intervention. It may be helpful in psychosocial nursing to use the subcategories, such as hopelessness, confusion, fear, grieving, and powerlessness.[5] Then the etiology or causative factors could be specific influencing factors, such as series of losses, change in environment, and loss of belief in higher power. In general, the causative factors are such things as family influences, past experiences, and current environmental factors. When the diagnosis is a "potential for" diagnosis, the etiological factors could be the risk factors involved. The defining characteristics are the "evidenced by" behaviors. For social isolation, the defining characteristic might be "verbalized or observed discomfort in social situations."[41] These are derived from the actual subjective and objective data of the assessment phase of the nursing process.

The most important aspect of writing a nursing diagnosis is to remember that the focus becomes the aspects of daily life affected by the problems, not necessarily the problems themselves.[5] Nursing cannot change a person's thought problem if he is delusional, but it can help him decrease the anxiety associated with the thought problem, the fear that accompanies the delusion, and the problems with hygiene and safety that may be present because of the disordered thinking. In this way, using a diagnosis helps nurses communicate with each other about client concerns in a systematic, orderly, coherent manner. The future will then bring an orderly, systematic collection of nursing interventions to accompany the diagnoses.

C H A R T   8-6
Errors in Writing Nursing Diagnoses

Error	Example
Use of medical diagnoses, pathologies, treatments, or diagnostic procedures	Hallucinations related to schizophrenia
Wording nursing diagnostic statements in terms of nursing problems or client needs, goals, inferences, or symptoms	Need for constant attention related to insecure ego
Phrasing the etiologic statement so that it essentially repeats the problem, rather than stating the etiology	Sexual dysfunction related to inability to maintain an erection
Use of judgmental statements or statements implying legal responsibility in the nursing diagnosis	Fluid volume excess related to inadequate monitoring of IV fluids by nursing staff

(From Carpenito LJ: Nursing Diagnosis: Application to Clinical Practice. Philadelphia, JB Lippincott, 1983. Also from Marriner A: The Nursing Process: A Scientific Approach to Nursing Care, 3d ed. St Louis, CV Mosby, 1983)

Nursing Diagnosis and Medical Diagnosis

The psychiatric–mental health nurse works closely with other disciplines to arrive at the most appropriate plan of care for the client and his family. The physician's responsibility is to make a medical diagnosis when there is sufficient support to determine that a psychiatric problem is present. The taxonomy used to make the medical diagnosis is the Diagnostic and Statistical Manual, Third Edition, Revised (DSM-III-R) of the American Psychiatric Association.[3] This taxonomy uses a biopsychosocial perspective but is considered to be atheoretical, so that it can be readily accepted and used by all who diagnose the psychiatric client. The nurse can assist in this process by sharing important information about the client from the nursing history and mental status assessment, as well as from daily observations of the client. A working knowledge of the DSM-III-R is important in maximizing the team effort to help the client, and knowledge of the criteria for deciding on a particular medical diagnosis found in the DSM-III-R may help the nurse in making a clinical decision about a nursing diagnosis (see Chart 8-8).

Axes of DSM-III-R

The DSM-III-R is a multiaxial system. The diagnostic criteria are inclusive for each diagnosis and allow room for individual differences within a pattern of behavior. This is accomplished by including lists of several signs and symptoms that constitute the criteria for each diagnosis and suggesting that only a certain number must be present to make the diagnosis. Also, the duration is specified, as in schizophrenia, where the symptoms must be present for 6 months or more for the client to receive a diagnosis of schizophrenia. Five axes constitute the format for a complete psychiatric diagnosis. A five-digit coding system is used for the first three axes. Axis I contains the major mental disorders, such as schizophrenia, bipolar illness, and substance abuse disorders. A disorder of this nature is usually the main reason the client is seeking help. Axis II contains the personality disorders and developmental disorders. It is then feasible to separate the patterns of lifestyle and coping that have developed from childhood from the more acute manifestations of behavior in the major mental disorders. When criteria for a personality disorder are not met, it may be indicated as "Deferred" and given a specific code number. A person may have more than one diagnosis

CHART 8-7
Classification of Human Responses of Concern for Psychiatric–Mental Health Nursing Practice

01. Human response patterns in activity processes

01.01 Altered motor behavior
  01.01.01 Bizarre motor behavior
  01.01.02 Catatonia
  01.01.03 Impaired coordination
  01.01.04 Hyperactivity
  01.01.05 Hypoactivity
  01.01.06 Muscular rigidity
  01.01.07 Psychomotor retardation
01.02 Altered recreation patterns
  01.02.01 Inadequate diversional activity
01.03 Altered self-care
  01.03.01 Altered eating
  *01.03.02 Altered grooming
  01.03.03 Altered health maintenance
  *01.03.04 Altered hygiene
  01.03.05 Altered participation in health care
  *01.03.06 Altered toileting
01.04 Altered sleep/arousal patterns
  01.04.01 Difficult transition to and from sleep
  01.04.02 Hypersomnia
  01.04.03 Insomnia
  01.04.04 Nightmares
  01.04.05 Somnolence
01.97 Undeveloped activity processes
01.98 Altered activity processes not otherwise specified
01.99 Potential for altered activity/processes

02. Human response patterns in cognition processes

02.01 Altered decision making
02.02 Altered judgment
*02.03 Altered knowledge processes
  02.03.01 Agnosia
  02.03.02 Altered intellectual functioning
  *02.03.03 Knowledge deficit
02.04 Altered learning processes
02.05 Altered memory
  02.05.01 Amnesia
  02.05.02 Distorted memory
  02.05.03 Long-term memory loss
  02.05.04 Short-term memory loss
02.06 Altered orientation
  02.06.01 Confusion
  02.06.02 Delirium
  02.06.03 Disorientation
02.07 Altered thought content
  02.07.01 Delusions
  02.07.02 Ideas of reference

  02.07.03 Magical thinking
  02.07.04 Obsessions
*02.08 Altered thought processes
  02.08.01 Altered abstract thinking
  02.08.02 Altered concentration
  02.08.03 Altered problem solving
  02.08.04 Thought insertion
02.97 Undeveloped cognition processes
02.98 Altered cognition processes not otherwise specified
02.99 Potential for altered cognition processes

03. Human response patterns in ecological processes

03.01 Altered community maintenance
  03.01.01 Community safety hazards
  03.01.02 Community sanitation hazards
03.02 Altered environmental integrity
*03.03 Altered home maintenance
  03.03.01 Home safety hazards
  03.03.02 Home sanitation hazards

04. Human response patterns in emotional processes

04.01 Abuse response patterns
  *04.01.01 Rape-trauma syndrome
04.02 Altered feeling patterns
  04.02.01 Anger
  *04.02.02 Anxiety
  04.02.03 Elation
  04.02.04 Envy
  *04.02.05 Fear
  *04.02.06 Grief
  04.02.07 Guilt
  04.02.08 Sadness
  04.02.09 Shame
04.03 Undifferentiated feeling pattern
04.97 Undeveloped emotional responses
04.98 Altered emotional processes not otherwise specified
04.99 Potential for altered emotional processes

05. Human response patterns in interpersonal processes

*05.01 Altered communication processes
  05.01.01 Altered nonverbal communication
  *05.01.02 Altered verbal communication
05.02 Altered conduct/impulse processes
  05.02.01 Aggressive/violent behaviors

(Continues on p. 114)

05.02.01.01 Aggressive/violent behaviors toward environment
05.02.01.02 Aggressive/violent behaviors toward others
05.02.01.03 Aggressive/violent behaviors toward self
05.02.02 Dysfunctional behaviors
05.02.02.01 Age-inappropriate behaviors
05.02.02.02 Bizarre behaviors
05.02.02.03 Compulsive behaviors
05.02.02.04 Disorganized behaviors
05.02.02.05 Unpredictable behaviors
05.03 Altered role performance
05.03.01 Altered family role
05.03.02 Altered leisure role
*05.03.03 Altered parenting role
05.03.04 Altered play role
05.03.05 Altered student role
05.03.06 Altered work role
05.04 Altered sexuality processes
05.05 Altered social interaction
05.05.01 Social intrusiveness
*05.05.02 Social isolation/withdrawal
05.97 Undeveloped interpersonal processes
05.98 Altered interpersonal processes not otherwise specified
05.99 Potential for altered interpersonal processes
*05.99.01 Potential for violence

06. Human response patterns in perception processes

06.01 Altered attention
06.01.01 Distractibility
06.01.02 Hyperalertness
06.01.03 Inattention
06.01.04 Selective attention
*06.02 Altered comfort patterns
06.02.01 Discomfort
06.02.02 Distress
06.02.03 Pain
06.03 Altered self-concept
*06.03.01 Altered body image
06.03.02 Altered gender identity
*06.03.03 Altered personal identity
*06.03.04 Altered self-esteem
06.03.05 Altered social identity
06.03.06 Undeveloped self-concept
06.04 Altered sensory perception
*06.04.01 Auditory
*06.04.02 Gustatory
06.04.03 Hallucinations
06.04.04 Illusions
*06.04.05 Kinesthetic

*06.04.06 Olfactory
*06.04.07 Tactile
*06.04.08 Visual
06.97 Undeveloped perception processes
06.98 Altered perception processes not otherwise specified
06.99 Potential for altered perception processes

07. Human response patterns in physiological processes

07.01 Altered circulation processes
07.01.01 Altered vascular circulation
*07.01.01.01 Tissue perfusion
*07.01.01.02 Altered fluid volume
07.01.02 Altered cardiac circulation
07.02 Altered elimination processes
*07.02.01 Altered bowel elimination
*07.02.01.01 Constipation
*07.02.01.02 Diarrhea
*07.02.01.03 Incontinence
07.02.01.04 Encopresis
*07.02.02 Altered urinary elimination
*07.02.02.01 Incontinence
*07.02.02.02 Retention
07.02.02.03 Enuresis
07.02.03 Altered skin elimination
07.03 Altered endocrine/metabolic processes
07.03.01 Altered growth
07.03.02 Altered hormone regulation
07.03.02.01 Premenstrual stress syndrome
07.04 Altered gastrointestinal processes
07.04.01 Altered absorption
07.04.02 Altered digestion
07.05 Altered neurosensory processes
07.05.01 Altered levels of consciousness
07.05.02 Altered sensory acuity
07.05.03 Altered sensory processing
07.05.04 Altered sensory integration
07.05.04.01 Learning disabilities
07.06 Altered nutrition processes
07.06.01 Altered cellular processes
07.06.02 Altered systemic processes
*07.06.02.01 More than body requirements
*07.06.02.02 Less than body requirements
07.06.03 Altered eating processes
07.06.03.01 Anorexia
07.06.03.02 Pica
07.07 Altered oxygenation processes
07.07.01 Altered respiration
07.07.01.01 Altered gas exchange

*07.07.01.02 Ineffective airway
clearance
*07.07.01.03 Ineffective breathing
pattern
07.08 Altered physical integrity processes
*07.08.01 Altered skin integrity
*07.08.02 Altered tissue integrity
07.09 Altered physical regulation processes
07.09.01 Altered immune responses
07.09.01.01 Infection
07.10 Altered body temperature
*07.10.01 Hypothermia
*07.10.02 Hyperthermia
*07.10.03 Ineffective thermoregulation
07.97 Undeveloped physiological processes
07.98 Altered physiological processes not
otherwise specified
07.99 Potential for altered physiological
processes

08. **Human response patterns in valuation
processes**
*08.01 Altered meaningfulness
*08.01.01 Hopelessness
08.01.02 Helplessness
08.01.03 Loneliness
*08.01.04 Powerlessness
08.02 Altered spirituality
*08.02.01 Spiritual distress
08.02.02 Spiritual despair
08.03 Altered values
08.03.01 Conflict with social order
08.03.02 Inability to internalize values
08.03.03 Unclarified values
08.97 Undeveloped valuation processes
08.98 Altered valuation processes not
otherwise specified
08.99 Potential for altered valuation
processes

*NANDA diagnosis.

(From ANA Classification of Individual Human Responses by M. Loomis, A.
O'Toole, M. Brown, P. Pothier, P. West, H. S. Wilson. Copyright 1986. Published by
the American Nurses' Association and reprinted with permission. This classification
is based on previous work of the Phenomenon Task Force and the Advisory Panel
on Classifications for Nursing Practice of the American Nurses' Association.)

on these two axes. Axis III indicates the related physical disorders and conditions that may be affecting the client's response to the psychiatric problems. These may include asthma, gastric ulcer, diabetes, and the like. Axis IV indicates the severity of the psychosocial stressors over the past year, with a ranking from 1 to 6. A rank of 6 is used for catastrophic stressors, such as a natural disaster; 1 represents no recognized events. Examples or circumstances are delineated for both adults and children/adolescents (see Tables 8-1 and 8-2 for the ranking of stressors). Axis V represents the global assessment of functioning over the preceding year, which means a rating of psychological, social, and occupational functioning on a continuum from mental illness to mental health. The DSM-III-R indicates that 81 to 90 means good functioning in all areas; 1 to 10 meaning persistent danger of severely hurting self or others, persistent inability to perform minimal personal hygiene, or a serious suicide act with clear expectation of death.[3] (See Chart 8-9, "Global Assessment of Functioning Scale.")

Particularly important for nursing directives are Axes IV and V, both of which nurses can use in planning care. If a client has not been functioning well for the past year, the nursing interventions will be individualized to the client's realistic capabilities. In addition, if the stressors have been overwhelming, as in a loss of several family members in a short period of time, the nursing care will be more supportive and less focused on helping the client make major life decisions. Psychiatric nurses are often asked to make these two diagnoses, which are another form of nursing judgment. An additional axis has been suggested but not yet implemented; it would be called the "nursing adaptation evaluation."[32] This proposed axis would assess overall functioning and levels of functioning in the areas of nutrition, solitude, social interaction, grooming, activity, and elimination on a 1 to 4 rating scale for each category.

Interface of Nursing Diagnosis and DSM-III-R

Another helpful way to interface the DSM-III-R with nursing is to consider common concerns of clients with certain medical diagnoses. Several institutions are looking at the most common nursing diagnoses they treat in order to allocate nursing resources in the most productive way (staffing, equipment, and so

(Text continues on p. 123)

C H A R T 8-8
Psychiatric Diagnoses Using DSM-III-R

Example: Complete Psychiatric Diagnosis using DSM-III-R (for adult)

Axis I
296.32 Major depression, recurrent, moderate
303.90 Alcohol dependence

Axis II
301.83 Borderline personality disorder

Axis III
Obesity
Hypertension

Axis IV
3 Moderate: family arguments, decrease in income

Axis V
50 Serious symptoms: suicidal ideation, difficulty with job, impaired
    social functioning.

Example: Complete Psychiatric Diagnosis using DSM-III-R (for child)

Axis I
314.01 Attention-deficit hyperactivity disorder
296.22 Major depression, single episode, moderate

Axis II
315.80 Developmental expressive writing disorder

Axis III
None known

Axis IV
5 Extreme: sexual abuse

Axis V
30 Severe acting-out episodes of aggressiveness toward others, abusive
    to self and own possessions.

Table 8-1.   **Severity of Psychosocial Stressors Scale: Children and Adolescents**

CODE	TERM	EXAMPLES OF STRESSORS	
		Acute Events	*Enduring Circumstances*
1	None	No acute events that may be relevant to the disorder	No enduring circumstances that may be relevant to the disorder
2	Mild	Broke up with boyfriend or girlfriend; change of school	Overcrowded living quarters; family arguments
3	Moderate	Expelled from school; birth of sibling	Chronic disabling illness in parent; chronic parental discord
4	Severe	Divorce of parents; unwanted pregnancy; arrest	Harsh or rejecting parents; chronic life-threatening illness in parent; multiple foster home placements
5	Extreme	Sexual or physical abuse; death of a parent	Recurrent sexual or physical abuse
6	Catastrophic	Death of both parents	Chronic life-threatening illness
0	Inadequate information or no change in condition		

(From American Psychiatric Association: Diagnostic and Statistical Manual of Mental Disorders, 3d ed, rev. Washington, APA, 1987.)

Table 8-2.   **Severity of Psychosocial Stressors Scale: Adult**

CODE	TERM	EXAMPLES OF STRESSORS	
		Acute Events	*Enduring Circumstances*
1	None	No acute events that may be relevant to the disorder	No enduring circumstances that may be relevant to the disorder
2	Mild	Broke up with boyfriend or girlfriend; started or graduated from school; child left at home	Family arguments; job dissatisfaction; residence in high-crime neighborhood
3	Moderate	Marriage; marital separation; loss of job; retirement; miscarriage	Marital discord; serious financial problems; trouble with boss; being a single parent
4	Severe	Divorce; birth of first child	Unemployment; poverty
5	Extreme	Death of spouse; serious physical illness diagnosed; victim of rape	Serious chronic illness in self or child; ongoing physical or sexual abuse
6	Catastrophic	Death of child; suicide of spouse; devastating natural disaster	Captivity as hostage; concentration camp experience
0	Inadequate information or no change in condition		

(From American Psychiatric Association: Diagnostic and Statistical Manual of Mental Disorders, 3d ed, rev. Washington, APA, 1987.)

C H A R T   8-9
Global Assessment of Functioning Scale (GAF Scale)

Code	Psychological, Social, and Occupational Functioning
81–90	Absent or minimal symptoms (*e.g.,* mild anxiety before an exam), good functioning in all areas, interested and involved in a wide range of activities, socially effective, generally satisfied with life, no more than everyday problems or concerns (*e.g.,* an occasional argument with family members)
71–80	If symptoms are present, they are transient and expectable reactions to psychosocial stressors (*e.g.,* difficulty concentrating after family argument); no more than slight impairment in social, occupational, or school functioning (*e.g.,* temporarily falling behind in schoolwork)
61–70	Some mild symptoms (*e.g.,* depressed mood and mild insomnia) OR some difficulty in social, occupational, or school functioning (*e.g.,* occasional truancy or theft within the household), but generally functioning pretty well, has some meaningful interpersonal relationships
51–60	Moderate symptoms (*e.g.,* flat affect and circumstantial speech, occasional panic attacks) OR moderate difficulty in social, occupational, or school functioning (*e.g.,* few friends, conflicts with co-workers)
41–50	Serious symptoms (*e.g.,* suicidal ideation, severe obsessional rituals, frequent shoplifting) OR any serious impairment in social, occupational, or school functioning (*e.g.,* no friends, unable to keep a job)
31–40	Some impairment in reality testing or communication (*e.g.,* speech is at times illogical, obscure, or irrelevant) OR major impairment in several areas, such as work, school, family relations, judgment, thinking, or mood (*e.g.,* depressed man avoids friends, neglects family, and is unable to work; child frequently beats up younger children, is defiant at home, and is failing at school)
21–30	Behavior is considerably influenced by delusions or hallucinations OR serious impairment in communication or judgment (*e.g.,* sometimes incoherent, acts grossly inappropriately, suicidal preoccupation) OR inability to function in almost all areas (*e.g.,* stays in bed all day; no job, home, or friends)
11–20	Some danger of hurting self or others (*e.g.,* suicide attempts without clear expectation of death, frequently violent, manic excitement) OR occasionally fails to maintain minimal personal hygiene (*e.g.,* smears feces) OR gross impairment in communication (*e.g.,* largely incoherent or mute)
1–10	Persistent danger of severely hurting self or others (*e.g.,* recurrent violence) OR persistent inability to maintain personal hygiene OR serious suicidal act with clear expectation of death

(From American Psychiatric Association: Diagnostic and Statistical Manual, 3d ed, rev. Washington, APA, 1987.)

CHART 8-10
Using NANDA Nursing Diagnosis Taxonomy 1986 in Psychiatric Nursing: Fitting DSM III-R Medical Diagnosis with Nursing Diagnosis

Medical Diagnosis	**Related Nursing Diagnosis**
Mental Disorders	**Physical (add #23)**
Schizophrenia	1. Alteration in nutrition: less than body requirements related to mistrust, fear, and disorganized thinking
Paranoid	
Disorganized	2. Alteration in self-care: hygiene and grooming related to low self-esteem, fear, and confusion
Catatonic	
Undifferentiated	3. Alteration in activity: activity intolerance related to withdrawal, effects of psychotropic drugs
Residual	
	4. Alteration in rest: sleeping pattern disturbance related to anxiety and fears, environment distractions, ritualistic behavior
	Psychological
	5. Alteration in coping: ineffective individual related to poor self-concept, lack of social support system, poor impulse control, difficulty managing feelings
	6. Alteration in participation: noncompliance related to lack of knowledge, poor motivation, memory deficit, disorganized thinking and mistrust
	7. Alteration in thought process: delusions and loose association related to loss of control and coping mechanisms, low self-esteem, internal conflict
	8. Alteration in self-concept: disturbance in self-esteem related to repeated negative experiences, inadequate interpersonal relationships, lack of coping strategies
	Social
	9. Alteration in socialization: social isolation related to mistrust of others, dysfunctional family relationships, low self-esteem, fear of closeness
	10. Alteration in role: difficulty with work performance related to mistrust, low self-esteem, poor communication skills, difficulty in interpersonal relationships
	11. Alteration in activities of daily living: impaired home maintenance management related to poor motivation, cognitive disturbance, financial concerns, lack of family support
	Spiritual
	12. Alteration in spiritual state: spiritual distress related to loss of hope
	13. Alteration in meaningfulness: powerlessness related to repeated failures, lack of perceived control, poor sense of identity
Mood (affective) Disorders	**Physical**
Bipolar disorder	Alteration in rest (see 4)
Major depression	Alteration in activity (see 3)
Dysthymia	Alteration in self-care (see 2)
Cyclothymia	Alteration in nutrition (see 1)

(Continues on p. 122)

Medical Diagnosis	**Related Nursing Diagnosis**

Mood (affective) Disorders

Physical

14. Alteration in physical integrity: potential for suicide related to loss of hope, anxiety, fear of future, feelings of inadequacy

Psychological

Alteration in coping (see 5)
Alteration in thought process (see 7)
Alteration in self-concept (see 8)

15. Alteration in emotional integrity: grieving related to series of losses, difficulty managing feelings, internalized anger

Social

Alteration in socialization (see 9)
Alteration in role (see 10)
Alteration in activities of daily living (see 11)

16. Alteration in role: sexual dysfunction related to low self-esteem, lack of psychic energy, poor communication, side effects of psychotropic drugs

Spiritual

Alteration in spiritual state (see 12)

17. Alteration in meaningfulness: hopelessness related to lack of perceived purpose in life, series of losses, negative thinking

Personality Disorders

Antisocial
Borderline
Narcissistic
Dependent
Obsessive-compulsive
Passive-aggressive
Histrionic
Schizotypal
Schizoid
Paranoid

Any of above 17 diagnoses plus:

18. Alteration in coping: manipulation related to need for power and control learned behavior style, lack of concern for others, low self-esteem
19. Alteration in emotional integrity: potential for violence related to poor impulse control, threatened self-concept, anger

Substance Abuse

Alcohol abuse
Alcohol intoxication
Alcohol withdrawal delirium
Alcohol hallucinosis
Alcohol dependence
Opioid dependence
Cocaine abuse
Amphetamine abuse
PCP abuse
Hallucinogen abuse
Cannabis abuse

Any of above 19 diagnoses plus:

20. Alteration in comfort: pain related to withdrawal effects from drugs or alcohol
21. Alteration in emotional integrity: fear related to loss of substance as coping mechanism, awareness of need for lifestyle changes
22. Alteration in knowledge: deficit in knowledge of substance use effects related to denial, projection rationalization
23. Alteration in sensory-perceptual: tactile, auditory, or visual hallucinations related to drug withdrawal
24. Alteration in thought process: confusion and blackouts related to lack of adequate nutrition, loss of control of drinking

Medical Diagnosis	Related Nursing Diagnosis
Childhood and Adolescent Disorders	
Attention deficit hyperactivity disorder	Any of above 24 diagnoses:
Conduct disorder	**25.** Alteration in coping: family related to lack of knowledge of parenting skills, chronic stress in home, financial concerns, lack of stable family unit
Separation anxiety disorder	
Avoidant disorder	**26.** Alteration in participation: family related to fears, guilt, lack of motivation
Overanxious disorder	
Oppositional defiant disorder	**27.** Alteration in role performance: deficit in parenting related to lack of knowledge, lack of motivation, learned patterns
Identity disorder	
Anorexia nervosa	
Bulimia nervosa	
Autistic disorder	
Pervasive developmental disorder	

forth), as well as to identify the roles of psychiatric nurses.[7] Nurses who are just beginning their work in psychiatric nursing or those who are not well versed in diagnosis terminology will benefit from a list of common nursing diagnoses that seem to "fit" with certain DSM-III-R diagnoses. These links to the medical diagnosis come from the signs and symptoms that are common to both. In addition, the focus in the mental health field is interdisciplinary, meaning that several disciplines work together with the client and often with the family to arrive at the nature of the concerns that need attention from the various disciplines. In most settings, the DSM-III-R is the language of choice for the various disciplines. It seems logical that the nursing diagnoses could flow from the knowledge of the client's medical diagnosis, if known. However, nursing looks at many additional variables that are of concern primarily to nursing; DSM-III-R diagnoses alone should not be used to determine nursing diagnoses. Also, certain nursing diagnoses may occur in almost all DSM-III-R categories; these include ineffective coping and potential of harm. Thus, it would not be advisable to limit certain nursing diagnoses to particular DSM-III-R diagnoses. The danger is the loss of individuality in determining the concerns that are the focus of care for a particular client.

In addition to identifying common themes in nursing diagnoses by specific medical diagnoses, nursing diagnoses may be specifically age-related, *e.g.,* child-related, adolescent-related, young adult–related, middle adult–related, and older adult–related. Also, nurses who work in addictions nursing need specific nursing diagnoses for their particular clients. Another distinction is whether the diagnosis is individual-, family-, or community-focused. Child and adolescent psychiatric nurses especially need family-focused nursing diagnoses because the philos-

ophy of these specialities is to assist the whole family to make a positive adjustment, which includes changing family patterns of coping as well as altering individual patterns. Those nurses who work in the outpatient setting especially need to make accurate community-focused diagnoses.

Chart 8-10, "Using NANDA Nursing Diagnosis Taxonomy," identifies a few of the more common nursing diagnoses that may correspond with medical diagnoses. Chart 8-11, "Schizophrenia and Bipolar Disorders," shows how these diagnoses can be used to make a partial care plan for the client, with short- and long-term outcomes or goals, interventions, and evaluations demonstrating whether or not a change in behavior has occurred.

Summary

This chapter has discussed the second step of the nursing process as the phase in which the nurse analyzes client assessment data, looks for clusters of data that fit together in patterns, identifies strengths and resources of the client and family, determines the motivational readiness of the client and family for change, formulates a problem list, and writes the diagnosis. Some of the major points in the chapter have included the following:

1. Analysis of the assessment data gathered for a client culminates in the determination of the most important, clearly written, definitive nursing diagnoses.
2. Clients have a varying level of motivation for change and may need help from the nurse to reduce the restraining forces and increase the

(Text continues on p. 126)

C H A R T   8-11
Schizophrenia and Bipolar Disorders

Schizophrenia

Psychological

Sensory-perceptual alteration: auditory hallucinations related to high anxiety, poor communication, withdrawal coping patterns, fear of relatedness, mistrust of others

Outcomes

Short-term Goals

1. Client will admit to hallucination by the end of today
2. Client will identify type of hallucination (auditory, visual, tactile) by end of week
3. Client will describe nature of hallucination (kind, threatening, commanding)
4. Client will participate in one reality-based activity today.

Long-term Goals

1. Client will connect feeling with hallucination by discharge
2. Client will accept need to decrease hallucinatory behavior by discharge
3. Client will use one thought-stopping technique by discharge
4. Client will recognize the ability to control the hallucination
5. Client will recognize environmental aids to prevent hallucinations
6. Client will connect withdrawal from others with hallucinations by discharge

Nursing Plan

1. Ask client when suspect hallucinations are occurring

Sociological

Alteration in socialization: social isolation related to mistrust of others, low self-esteem, fear of closeness, poor social skills, coping pattern of withdrawal

Outcomes

Short-Term Goals

1. Client will sit in day room for 10 minutes today
2. Client will speak to one staff member today
3. Client will speak to one patient today
4. Client will eat in day room today
5. Client will participate in one activity in 2 days

Long-Term Goals

1. Client will interact with primary nurse 5 times a week for 20 minutes each time by discharge
2. Client will participate in social activities on unit by discharge

2. Ask client to describe the experience and type of hallucination
3. Reassure client of help to diminish hallucination
4. Administer antipsychotic drug as ordered, explain that drug will help decrease hallucinations
5. Remind client that experience is his, not nurse's
6. Encourage reality-based activity, participate with client
7. Assist to connect anxiety event with onset of hallucination
8. Offer control techniques when client states desire to end hallucinations
9. Reinforce client's need to involve self in activities with people as much as possible
10. Give sleep aid information if hallucination is worse at night, encourage to keep radio or TV on to diminish fear
11. Teach mechanism of projection causing hallucination when client is ready
12. Call client by name and involve in one-on-one communication daily

3. Client will identify activities involving people for participation by discharge
4. Client will attend group therapy 3 times a week without leaving by discharge
5. Client will identify feelings about social relatedness by discharge
6. Client will connect patterns of childhood with current social behavior
7. Client will identify need for people
8. Client will identify purpose of withdrawal as way of coping
9. Client will initiate activity with peer by discharge

Nursing Plan

1. Provide consistent, predictable, gentle accepting care

2. Accept client's fears as need for safety and security
3. Protect client from threatening events on unit
4. Reinforce positive social behavior
5. Assist with physical needs
6. Contract for one-on-one interaction daily
7. Accept client's difficulty with verbal interaction

8. Invite client to activity and attend with him
9. Discuss fears with client, nudge to try new behavior
10. Teach coping skills (getting away from as one), teach coping skills to replace this
11. Introduce to other clients and encourage activity and interaction

Psychological

Alteration in thought process: delusions and loose associations related to loss of control and coping mechanisms, low self-esteem, internal conflict, high anxiety, fear of closeness

Outcomes

Short-Term Goals
1. Client will discuss one reality-based event by end of day
2. Client will identify name of one nurse by end of day
3. Client will communicate one need by end of day

Long-Term Goals
1. Client will maintain reality-based communication by discharge
2. Client will identify relationship between anxiety and thoughts and perception
3. Client will use/tolerate group activity (one) by discharge
4. Client will express one feeling by discharge
5. Client will learn three relaxation methods by discharge
6. Client will initiate one activity by discharge

Nursing Plan
1. Use concrete, clear, simple communication
2. Call patient by name

3. Listen for reality-based communication and respond to this
4. Listen for clues as to meaning of delusions (theme of rejection, anger, abandonment, loss of control) and acknowledge this with client in gentle manner
5. Establish one-to-one relationship with one consistent person (primary nurse)
6. Acknowledge client anxiety and need for safety
7. Reassure client of safety and help available
8. Watch for signs of increased ability to tolerate group activity, go with client to activity, increase gradually
9. Teach need to keep ideas (paranoid ideation) to share with nurse and not with others
10. Gently present reality-based interpretations of events
11. Introduce to peers on unit who can build trust and friendship
12. Help discuss fear of closeness and accept this in client, helping client to build positive experiences with people

Bipolar Disorders

Physical

Alteration in rest: sleep pattern disturbance related to hypersensitivity to environmental stimuli, denial of depression

Outcomes

Short-Term Goals
1. Client will sleep 2–4 hours by the end of this week
2. Client will sleep 6–8 hours by the end of the hospital stay

Long-Term Goals
1. Client will sleep 6–8 hours each night.
2. Client will recognize need for sleep and develop sleep-enhancing activities.

Nursing Plan
1. Provide reduced environmental stimu-lation (soft lighting, low noise level, re-duced activity with groups, minimizing new people in the environment)
2. Provide one consistent care giver to set limits on activity
3. Provide opportunity for frequent short naps
4. Provide sleep aids (warm milk, sedatives when necessary, reassurance of concern and acceptance of client, warm bath, quiet room)

(Continues on p. 126)

Evaluation

Evaluate number of hours slept per 24-hour shift, number of hours rested, and response of client to environmental stimulation, including groups

Physical

Alteration in nutrition: less than body requirements related to increased physical activity, lack of perception of needs, delusional thinking (grandiose)

Outcomes

Short-term Goals

1. Client will eat 1000 calories today
2. Client will drink 1000 cc. liquid today

Long-term goals

1. Client will gain 2 pounds per week for the next 6 weeks
2. Client will maintain normal weight

Nursing Plan

1. Provide finger foods, quick high-calorie snacks
2. Weigh client every 2 days
3. Observe for diaphoresis, compulsive eating patterns, opportune times for nourishment
4. Teach patient nutritional needs, foods with high protein, need for increased fluid intake (especially with lithium therapy)

Evaluation

Evaluate weight gain, eating patterns, knowledge of nutrition

---

motivating forces for change, increasing the client's sense of personal control.

3. Reviewing the client's strengths and resources helps determine his ability to cope with his problems and assists in directing the decision regarding nursing diagnoses.

4. The nursing diagnosis is a statement of a client's response pattern to a health disruption and guides the planning and intervention phases of the nursing process.

5. The medical diagnosis is made using the criteria set in the Diagnostic and Statistical Manual-III-R. The nurse can use this information in the decisions regarding nursing diagnoses.

6. The Diagnostic and Statistical Manual-III-R is an atheoretical multiaxial classification system that fosters a holistic approach to the client; it includes specific behavioral criteria for each diagnosis.

7. The current NANDA taxonomy of nursing diagnoses contains useful diagnoses for psychosocial nursing.

Case Study 8-2: Ms. Ella C.

Nursing Diagnosis

An Assessment Report

Ella C., a 30-year-old woman appearing slightly older than her stated age, was admitted for the first time to City General Hospital Mental Health Unit. The client was accompanied by her sister, Mrs. Sadie R., who appeared concerned but reluctant to obligate herself. Ms. C. has had no previous psychiatric admissions or treatment. Mrs. R. described her sister as "a loner" who has, in the past 6 months, appeared increasingly withdrawn, neglectful of her appearance, preoccupied, and disinterested in her environment. Ms. C.'s stated reason for admission was "I just can't go on." Mrs. R. stated that her sister lives alone in a rooming house and was employed by a shoe factory for 11 years, until 4 months ago, when she was "laid off," along with several hundred other workers. Ms. C. is currently on unemployment compensation, and has no insurance or cash savings.

Methods of Assessment

A mental status exam, a personal history, and an open-ended interview were used in the assessment process. Ms. C.'s sister was present during most of the history-taking. Ms. C. was interviewed according to hypotheses of psychological, social, biologic, cultural, and behavioral theories of the etiology of her problems.

Results of Assessment: Mental Status Exam

Ms. C. is a thin, poorly nourished, poorly groomed woman who states she has not eaten in 4 days. Her explanation for this behavior was "I don't care." Ms. C.'s gait, posture, and mannerisms are those of a much older woman and convey an attitude of defeat. Ms. C. is oriented in all five spheres, is alert when spoken to, exhibits normal attention and concentration, denies any unusual experiences, sensations, morbid thoughts, suicidal thoughts, and complains only of extreme fatigue. Her memory appears intact on all three levels. Her mood is of despair, with physiologic complaints indicative of grief. Her affect is sad, with limited affective response to the environment. Intellectual functioning appears normal for the client's educational and occupational status. She was able to subtract by 3's from 100, although slow in her responses. Abstraction abilities are normal; she is able to compare apples and oranges, cats and trees; she can explain the proverb "A rolling stone gathers no moss." Ms. C. speaks in a soft voice, and psychomotor retardation is notable. Recurring themes of conversation are fatigue and sadness. Her judgment appears appropriate. She responded normally for her sociocultural group to the question, "What would you do if you inherited $10,000?" Her insight appears poor; the client blames herself for the loss of her job, although this was clearly due to economic problems within the company.

Social History

Ms. C.'s parents were described by the client's sister as "uninvolved." The mother and father were of middle-income status, and both were killed in a car accident when the client was 8 years old. The client and her sister, then 16 years old, were taken in by the maternal grandmother, who was described as "moody, always angry" by the client. The grandmother was reportedly of middle income, unemployed, and supported by her deceased husband's retirement.

The client's sister stated that Ms. C. had few friends while growing up but appeared happy. The client was reportedly punished frequently by the grandmother (especially for loud or "excessive" talking) by being sent to the basement or a similar place of isolation for over an hour. The client's sister feels this method of discipline increased Ms. C.'s shyness and social isolation.

The client's grandmother died suddenly of a "heart attack" when the client was 17 years old. Ms. C. and Mrs. R. lived in the grandmother's house for 2 years, until the client's sister's marriage, at which time the client moved out into a rooming house and began working for a shoe factory, where she was employed for 11 years.

Summary of Interview Findings

Although the client related in a distant fashion throughout the mental status exam and history, eye contact and mannerisms indicated increasing trust and comfort in the interview, as well as responsiveness to the interviewer. Ms. C.'s withdrawn behavior appears somewhat related to social learning from parents and grandmother and was reinforced by multiple losses. Ms. C.

(Continues on p. 126)

believes she was mistreated by her grandmother and appears to hold some anger toward the deceased grandmother, although she denies any anger. The client appears to believe she has been defeated by life and is perhaps communicating her need to be dependent, nurtured, and given attention now as she has not been treated in her past. The vegetative signs of depression warrant consideration for psychotropic medication. Ms. C. denies suicidal thoughts, but she is obviously apathetic about her welfare. Although no disorder in thinking was noted, a schizophrenic condition cannot be ruled out at this time, in view of a lifelong pattern of isolation and withdrawn behavior. Ms. C. has an obvious deficit of social skills, is retarded in emotional development, and appears aware that she is different from most 30-year-old women, which is perhaps another source of stress. Ms. C.'s response to the interviewer indicates a potentially successful response to one-to-one counseling of an educative and supportive nature at this time.

Summary and Suggestions

Ms. C. is a 30-year-old woman admitted to the Mental Health Unit for depression with no history of psychiatric admissions or treatment. She has a lifelong pattern of withdrawal and isolation. She has no friends and, although accompanied to the hospital by her sister, does not appear to have a substantial support system. The client is recently unemployed due to economic cutbacks. She is, perhaps, feeling victimized by multiple losses since childhood—of her parents, grandmother, home, relationship with sister, and now, job. There is evidence of poor adaptation to these crises. Ms. C. has appeared to be unsuccessful in completion of developmental tasks since the death of her parents, 22 years ago. Ms. C.'s immediate needs concern

her anorexia and apathy about her own welfare. She will be referred for psychological examination to rule out a psychotic condition, and will be assessed for possible medication intervention. Ms. C. was assigned a primary nurse and will meet with the undersigned clinical nurse specialist in daily one-to-one sessions. A support network assessment will be considered, if approved by the client, involving interviews with the client's landlady, seemingly involved neighbors, and the client's sister's family. No group interactions are suggested at this time.

Diagnoses

Nursing Diagnoses
These are to be modified as appropriate following further observation.

1. Alterations in self-concept, related to multiple losses and unresolved grief
2. Limited social skills, related to social isolation
3. Potential for organic injury, related to anorexia and apathy regarding self-welfare

Diagnostic and Statistical Manual, Third Edition, Revised, Diagnoses
Axis I—269.33 Major depression, recurrent, with melancholia (Provisional: R/O schizophrenic condition)
Axis II—301.82 Avoidant personality disorder
Axis III—Poorly nourished, dehydrated state due to anorexia
Axis IV—Psychosocial stressors: Loss of job and economic security. Severity: 5, severe
Axis V—Highest level of adaptive functioning past year: 5, poor

References

1. American Nurses' Association: Nursing: A Social Policy Statement. Kansas City, MO, ANA, 1980
2. American Nurses' Association: Standards of Psychiatric and Mental Health Nursing Practice. Kansas City, MO, ANA, 1982
3. American Psychiatric Association: Diagnostic and Statistical Manual of Mental Disorders, 3d ed rev. Washington, APA, 1987
4. Barnard MKE: Nursing Diagnosis: A Descriptive Method. Matern Child Health Nurs 8: 223, 1983
5. Berry KN: Let's Create Diagnoses Psych Nurses Can Use. Am J Nurs 87(May): 707–708, 1987
6. Briar S: Toward Autonomous Social Diagnosis. Bull Menninger Clin 40: 593–601, 1976
7. Brown P et al. Linking Psychiatric Nursing Care to Patient Classification Codes. Nursing and Health Care 8:156–164, 1987
8. Bulechek G, McCloskey, JC: Nursing Interventions: What They Are and How to Choose Them. Holistic Nursing Practice 1 (May): 36–43, 1987
9. Carpenito LJ: Nursing Diagnosis: Application to Clinical Practice. Philadelphia, JB Lippincott, 1983

10. deChesnay M: Problem Solving in Nursing. Image 15 (Winter): 8–11, 1983
11. Doenges ME, Moorhouse, MF: Nurse's Pocket Guide: Nursing Diagnoses with Interventions. Philadelphia, FA Davis, 1985
12. Dossey B, Guzzetta C: Nursing Diagnosis: Framework, Process, and Problems. Heart Lung 12 (May): 281–291, 1983
13. Estes J et al: Nursing Diagnosis of the Alcoholic Person. St. Louis, CV Mosby, 1980
14. Gordon M: Manual of Nursing Diagnosis. New York, McGraw-Hill, 1985
15. Gordon M, Sweeney MA: Methodological Problems and Issues in Identifying and Standardizing Nursing Diagnosis. Adv Nurs Science 2 (October): 1–15, 1979
16. Henderson B: Nursing Diagnosis: Theory and Practice. Adv Nurs Science 1 (October): 75–83, 1978
17. Iyer PW, Taptich BJ, Bernocchi-Lossey D: Nursing Process and Nursing Diagnosis. Philadelphia, WB Saunders, 1986
18. Kelly MA: Nursing Diagnosis Source Book: Guidelines for Clinical Application. East Norwich, CT, Appleton and Lange, 1985
19. Kim MJ, Moritz DA (eds): Classification of Nursing Diagnosis: Proceedings of the Third and Fourth National Conferences. New York, McGraw-Hill, 1982
20. Kritek PB: Commentary: The Development of Nursing Diagnosis and Theory. Adv Nurs Science 2 (October): 73–79, 1979
21. Kritek PB: Diagnostics: The Struggle to Classify Our Diagnoses. Am J Nurs 86 (June): 722–723, 1986
22. Jauron GD, Mundinger MO: Developing a Nursing Diagnosis. Nurs Outlook 23 (February): 94–98, 1975
23. Loomis ME: Phenomenon of Concern for PMH Practice. ANA Pacesetter 10 (October): 1–5, 1983
24. Loomis ME, O'Toole AW, Brown MS, Pothier P, Wilson HS: Development of a Classification System for Psychiatric/Mental Health Nursing: Individual Response Class. Arch Psychiatr Nurs 1 (February): 16–24, 1987
25. Lunney M: Nursing Diagnosis: Refining the System. Am J Nurs 82 (March): 456–459, 1982
26. Mallick J: Nursing Diagnosis and the Novice Student. Nursing and Health Care 4 (October): 455–459, 1983
27. Marriner A: The Nursing Process: A Scientific Approach to Nursing Care, 3d ed. St. Louis, CV Mosby, 1983
28. Matthews C, Gaul A: Nursing Diagnosis from the Perspective of Concept Attainment and Critical Thinking. Adv Nurs Sci 2 (October): 17–26, 1979
29. McFarland G, Wasli E: Nursing Diagnosis and Process in Psychiatric–Mental Health Nursing. Philadelphia, JB Lippincott, 1986
30. McGovern WN, Rodgers JA: Change Theory. Am J Nurs 86 (May): 566–567, 1986
31. McLane A: Classification of Nursing Diagnosis: Proceedings of the Seventh Conference. St. Louis, CV Mosby, 1987
32. Morrison E et al: NSGAE: Nursing Adaptation Evaluation. J Psychosoc Nurs Ment Health Serv 23 (August): 10–13, 1985
33. North American Nursing Diagnostic Association: 21 New Diagnoses and a Taxonomy. Am J Nurs 86 (December): 1414–1415, 1986
34. Perry A: Nursing Diagnosis Research. J Neurosurg Nurs 14 (April): 108–111, 1982
35. Porter EJ: Critical Analysis of NANDA Nursing Diagnosis Taxonomy I. Image 18 (Winter): 136–139, 1986
36. Putzier DJ, Padrick KP: Nursing Diagnosis: A Component of Nursing Process and Decision-Making. Topics in Clinical Nursing 5 (Jan): 21–29, 1984
37. Schultz JM, Dark SL: Manual of Psychiatric Nursing Care Plans, 2d ed. Boston, Little, Brown & Co, 1986
38. Shamonsky S, Yanni C: In Opposition to Nursing Diagnosis: A Minority Opinion. Image 15 (Spring): 47–50, 1983
39. Shoemaker J: How Nursing Diagnosis Helps Focus Your Care. RN 42 (August): 56–61, 1979
40. Smith FB: Patient Power. Am J Nurs 86 (May): 1260–1262, 1986
41. Townsend MC: Nursing Diagnoses in Psychiatric Nursing: A Pocket Guide for Care Plan Construction. Philadelphia, FA Davis, 1988
42. Walker LW: Nursing Diagnosis and Interventions: New Tool to Define Nursing's Unique Role. Nursing and Health Care 7 (June): 322–326, 1986
43. Williams AB: Rethinking Nursing Diagnosis. Nurs Forum 19: 357–363, 1980
44. Williams J, Wilson H: A Psychiatric Nursing Perspective on DSM-III. J Psychosoc Nurs Ment Health Serv 20 (April): 14–20, 1982

9 Planning

Anne Warner Toothaker

Hold fast the time! Guard it, watch over it, every hour, every minute! Unregarded, it slips away, like a lizard, smooth, slippery, faithless, a pixywife. Hold every moment sacred. Give each clarity and meaning, each the weight of thine awareness, each its true and due fulfillment.

Thomas Mann,
The Beloved Returns, 1940

Chapter Preview

Through planning, the third step of the nursing process, the nurse determines from client data and diagnosis what needs to be accomplished, in what order it needs to be done, how it will be done, who will do what, and who is responsible for seeing that the plan of care is completed. The client entering the mental health arena is trying to find order in a chaotic existence; his world is awry and a change is necessary.

The nurse, through assessment and analysis, examines the client's physical and mental health, his social and economic stressors, and his functioning in his family, work setting, and community. Planning is the ordering of that information and the use of it, in collaboration with the client and the other members of the treatment team, in order to deal effectively with the client's mental health needs and problems.

Learning Objectives

On completion of the chapter, you should be able to accomplish the following:

1. define the planning process
2. differentiate between long-term and short-term goals
3. discuss your own ability to accept the values and goals of the client and his family
4. formulate a nursing care plan including
     client problems or nursing diagnoses
     client outcomes
     deadlines
     nursing orders or approaches
5. explain the use of standardized nursing care plans and the balanced service system in psychiatric–mental health care

Planning and the Nursing Process

This chapter is about planning—how to devise a plan, how to write a plan, how to rewrite a plan. Despite its commonality and universality, planning is a learned procedure. We learn to plan each day. Time-management and self-improvement courses devote much attention to the topic of planning. But what is it? *Planning* is the structuring of needs and problems in an orderly manner to achieve an end or a goal. A plan provides a map of how to reach a certain point and also provides reference markers to allow us to observe and evaluate progress along the way.

Organization

Planning is common to everyone; however, that very universality obscures its difficulty. If everyone can plan, why are some people more organized than others? The organization of a plan determines its workability. Through ordering or structuring, one chooses not to be chaotic, because chaos serves to defer decision-making, responsibility-taking, and choice.

Nursing care planning is intrinsic to the profession. A nursing plan provides structure to care-giving and measures what a nurse thinks and does. Just as the student plans for school work, the student nurse learns to plan care for and with the client. Planning is also a growth-producing experience because one's choices in weighing and selecting alternatives, in prioritizing, and in assigning values are, inherently, judgments. The plans of the nurse must reflect the choices of the client. Growth occurs as the nurse reflects, "Whose choices are these? Whose plan is this? Whose values does this plan reflect?"

Purposes of Planning

After a need is recognized or determined, and a goal (or goals) has been established, planning begins. The purposes of planning are twofold:

1. To establish the process or direction of change
2. To measure progress during the change

Process of Planning

Planning is a learned activity. It necessitates the establishment of limits to determine how much detail is necessary and when detail becomes awkward, cumbersome, and constricting.

The writing of a plan enhances its workability and usefulness, because the concreteness of words on paper clarifies one's thinking. A written plan solidifies choices, keeps the planner on track, and serves as a reminder of where the planner has been and is heading.

Goal Setting

A long-term goal is determined when a need for change is established. Short-term goals provide direction and concreteness to change. (See Chart 9-1, "Long-Term and Short-Term Goals.") They are determined by prioritizing, or choosing the order in which changes will occur. Completion of short-term goals is an indication that one is on the way to the accomplishment of long-term goals. The time frames that determine long-term and short-term goals depend on the end one wishes to achieve. A freshman student with a career goal measures short-term goals in terms of semesters or courses. A person facing

CHART 9-1
Long-Term and Short-Term Goals

Changes require goal setting. Long-term goals are oriented toward the future, whereas short-term goals are the markers of achievement that one attains along the way toward a goal. Goals are observable and measurable by others.

Long-Term Goals	Short-Term Goals
To achieve independence through employment	To graduate from high school or pass equivalency exam To graduate from an appropriate vocational or collegiate program To apply for and attain a job
To increase ability to cope with stress, as demonstrated by decreased angry outbursts	To seek counseling or self-help group and attend meetings regularly To identify one coping strategy and "try on" that coping method for 1 month
To improve organization and promptness	To organize and list responsibilities of home, work, school, children To prepare general schedules based on prioritizing or responsibilities To prepare individual daily schedules with daily tasks, appointments
To increase self-esteem by altering body image	To achieve ideal body weight To improve body tone through daily exercise To assess and redo wardrobe

spring house cleaning measures short-term goals in hours and days. Short-term and long-term goals are not inflexible time determinates.

Another important use of time is determining when a step in a plan will be completed or reviewed. A college student may set a long-term goal of graduation, but his short-term goal is passing a particular semester with a grade average of "B"; his daily study sessions are check points. Learning to plan is learning time management. Dealing with smaller time increments provides the manageability to achieve short-term goals and, eventually, long-term goals.

Client Outcomes
The formulation of specific, behavioral client outcomes provides the nurse and other members of the mental health team with a precise means of measuring the client's movement toward treatment goals. A client outcome states *what* the client will do, how often or when he will do it, under what conditions he will do it, and in what time period he will do it. The client outcome describes, in specific, behavioral terms, the outcome or result of the client's long-term and short-term goals.

For example, a client's long-term goal might be "to maintain sobriety following discharge from a chemical dependency treatment facility." One of his short-term goals might be "to seek an AA sponsor and attend AA meetings regularly." One of his outcomes might be "client will attend an AA meeting at First Methodist Church every day for the first 90 days following discharge from the Chemical Dependency

Unit of Brookside Hospital." Client outcomes, therefore, spell out in unambiguous terms the exact behavior desired as a result of treatment.

Method

Finally, the planner determines what will be necessary to accomplish the goals (*i.e.*, what method or approach will be needed). The method is a list of instructions one writes to oneself in order to complete the step. A junior student planning study time would not necessarily include on his list "bring pens, scratch pads, and calculator"; however, a freshman student might need those specifics in order to not waste study time. The method may be as individual as the planner. It is important to strive for detail and not take too much for granted.

Nursing Care Planning and Change

The nursing care plan is a remarkable document—a reflection of the professionalism of the nurse. It allows everyone to learn what nursing is and does and helps define nursing's relationship to other disciplines. The nursing care plan in the treatment of the mental health client is a fluid document. Treatment may be crisis-oriented, continuous, or both. Therefore, the plan reflects the current problems and goals identified by the client. This is a crucial aspect of psychiatric–mental health nursing. The plan is created *with* the client, not *for* the client. The essence of mental health treatment is change, and change is unlikely unless the client and his family believe it is necessary.

Change is demanded and expected when the client seeks professional assistance. The circumstances surrounding the client become increasingly uncomfortable and intolerable. The client or family usually demand a very general change. "Change her," or "I can't control him anymore," parents may say about a troubled child. "I can't take it anymore," a woman may declare. The changes involved in psychiatric–mental health treatment are not unilateral. The changes in behavior made by the client affect his relationships and threaten his social structure.

Nurses teach, counsel, nurture, and facilitate change. Their ability to understand and appreciate other disciplines places nurses in facilitator roles between clients and various therapeutic modalities. Nursing incorporates into the treatment plan all members of the mental health team. This liaison role assists the client and those close to him during the changing process.

When the client enters a mental health facility, the goals that are established must be understandable and acceptable to all those associated with the client. These objectives are established by the client, the family, and the treatment team; they also take into account the mores and support systems in the community. When many people are involved in the goal-setting process, negotiations leading to acceptable long-term objectives are imperative. (See Chart 9-2, "Negotiating Goals: A Case Example.")

Hidden Agenda

Sometimes, a goal is not stated directly or even alluded to, but is a "hidden agenda," a secret. For example, before exposing a family secret or directly confronting a hidden rationale for therapy, the nurse carefully evaluates what purpose will be served by exposing the "secret." In this delicate situation, the benefit of discussing or exploring the hidden agenda must clearly outweigh the pain the client and family will endure. Because mutual trust and respect are critical for successful therapy and change, the nurse builds rapport and trust before approaching these problems.

Accepting Others' Values

The goals that are established in treatment planning must be acceptable to the client and his family. This requires that the nurse be familiar with, and accept, differing cultures and values. Learning about different cultures and examining one's own values are growing experiences and responsibilities of psychiatric–mental health nurses.

Formulating the Nursing Care Plan

Nurses use nursing care plans throughout their professional lives, from student to practitioner. The purposes of the care plan vary. During the educational process, the care plan helps the student identify health care problems and effective ways to deal with them. The nurse practitioner uses the care plan to communicate data about the client and therapeutic approaches to other members of the treatment team.[20]

Format of the Plan

A nursing care plan includes assessment data, nursing diagnosis, short-term and long-term goals, expected client outcomes, deadlines, and nursing orders.

The purpose of the care plan is to communicate information and rationale clearly, effectively, and quickly. For this reason, care plans are written in columns. Reading horizontally, the nurse can readily

CHART 9-2
Negotiating Goals: A Case Example

A 15-year-old boy, John, is brought to a mental health clinic for counseling because of his continued drug addiction and delinquent behavior. John is well known to the courts and juvenile detention authorities and is brought to the clinic by his probation officer. John's parents have previously requested that the state assume his custody due to his uncontrolled behavior. The state has been reluctant to fulfill their request because of lack of funding. The probation officer has been meeting weekly with John, but there have been no changes in his drug addiction and truancy.

At the completion of the assessment, the treatment team identified the following objectives of each of the people involved with John:

John's goal: to be "left alone"
State's goal: to minimize the amount of money that will be spent for John
John's parents: to control John's behavior, "make him a good boy"
John's probation officer: to remove John from his case load
John's therapist: to eliminate John's drug addiction

The therapist is working with John individually, not with any family members. The overall treatment goal is written to reflect John's desire for independence and is stated as a positive, concise, measurable goal.

Treatment Plan Goal: Increasing independence through responsible behavior as demonstrated by graduation from high school or obtaining a G.E.D.

Increasing independence allows John a means so that he can be "left alone." High-school graduation or the equivalent provides the means for measurement of his change. Allowing John to choose treatment outcomes permits him an active role in his treatment. Studying for his classes and exams will provide structure for John. His graduation from high school will promote future employment and meet the state's goal of spending less money. John will be meeting regularly with his counselor, which should reduce the amount of time he spends with his probation officer. The nurse in this situation acts as a liaison and communicates the treatment goal and rationale to all members of the mental health team.

identify problems, goals, approaches, and deadlines, thereby expediting daily care.

Defining the Nursing Diagnosis
It is important that the nurse state the nursing diagnosis so that it conveys the same meaning to many people. The use of the simple declarative sentence insures that the team will begin at the same point. Defining the cause of the problem focuses the team in one direction. Establishing a causal tone also allows all members the freedom to address their areas of expertise and bias.

The problem statement or nursing diagnosis contains a "related to" clause. (See Chart 9-3, "Examples of Nursing Diagnoses.") These words define the nurse's analytic ability. The observable problem is generally an indication of a more serious difficulty that also must be addressed. This statement reflects the effectiveness of the assessment and analysis processes and direct nursing approaches.

Defining Expected Outcomes
When defining outcomes, the nurse is actually stating specific behavioral results of the treatment goals. The

outcome statement requires a measurable action by the client that is observable by other persons. Outcomes are client-related and the nurse reflects, once again, "Is this best for the client? Whose choice is this?" (See Chart 9-4, "Examples of Client Outcomes.")

Defining Deadlines
Time clarifies, solidifies, and anchors a plan. Without deadlines for completion or evaluation, a plan is an idea. Deadlines are not absolute, but serve as a reminder for the nurse. Deadlines may be instructions of when to evaluate or record progress as is illustrated in Chart 9-5, "Example of Deadlines." Frequently, deadlines structure the type of care the nurse provides for a client.

Delineating Nursing Orders or Approaches
Nursing orders or approaches define what nurses do—their judgments, actions, and choices. Included in the nursing orders may be statements of activities performed by other members of the mental health team, as shown in Chart 9-6, "Examples of Nursing Orders or Approaches."

CHART 9-3

Examples of Nursing Diagnoses

Nursing Diagnosis	Discussion
1a. Self-care deficit: bathing/hygiene	If a person is unwashed and dirty, nursing care is directed by the cause. A brain-damaged client may never be independent in his self-care. A person preoccupied with differentiating reality from fantasy will require guidance with hygiene. A depressed client may lack the energy to wash himself or change his clothes.
1b. Self-care deficit: bathing/hygiene related to low self-esteem	The treatment is now directed by the client's lack of self-interest and self-respect. A change in this behavior indicates a change in self-perception.
2a. Sensory-perceptual alteration	The nursing approaches to a client who is hallucinating decidedly differ if the cause of the hallucination is chemical, physiological, or psychological.
2b. Sensory-perceptual alteration related to lack of sleep	The nursing care is now directed toward creating an environment in which the client can rest.

The mental health nurse is in a unique position to be familiar with many aspects of the client's treatment plan—medical, psychological, and social. The challenge to the nurse is to include in the care plan orders, which are client-centered, approaches that may be directed by other disciplines, yet still reflect nursing care.

Standardized Nursing Care Plans

The use of standardized nursing care plans allows the nurse to achieve the goals of communicating objectives of care and efficient planning. The acknowledgement of behavioral similarities permits more time for nurses to recognize and deal with the client's uniqueness. (See Sample Nursing Care Plans 9-1, 9-2, and 9-3 for standardized nursing care plans.)

Purposes of Standardized Care Plans

Standardized nursing care plans serve several functions in assisting the nurse to maintain high-level care. Standardizing of care plans acknowledges the similarities of symptoms and evaluates current nursing

practice within a particular treatment setting. These care plans also serve as educational and orientation tools for new employees of an agency. Standard care plans serve to insure comparable levels of nursing care within a treatment setting. The standardization of plans allows the nurse time to focus on the individual problems, needs, and goals of the client. Finally, the standard care plan is utilized to communicate information about client problems and therapeutic approaches when clients move from one treatment setting to another.

Forms of Standardized Care Plans

Standard nursing care plans are drafted according to medical or nursing diagnoses and generalized treatment goals. Client problems, for example, may be differentiated as actual, potential, possible, and unusual problems. *Actual problems* are those behaviors or symptoms usually seen in that category or diagnosis. Examples of usual problems are listed below.

Depression: low self-esteem and poor hygiene
Manic behavior: loud, rapid speech; grandiosity

C H A R T   9-4
Examples of Client Outcomes

Nursing Diagnosis
Self-care deficit: bathing/hygiene related to low self-esteem

Client Outcome
His hygiene improves

Discussion

Which aspect of hygiene—washing hair, wearing clean clothes? Who measures improvement? Whose idea is it to wash? The vagueness of this outcome statement does not give direction to treatment activities.

Nursing Diagnosis
Self-care deficit: bathing/hygiene related to low self-esteem

Client Outcome
The client initiates and follows through with washing hair and wearing clean clothes

Discussion

Clean hair and clothing are readily observable and measurable. If the client initiates bathing and changing of clothes, it is meaningful behavior. Conversely, if the client performs these actions to comply with a staff member's request, his behavior may express no more than his reluctance to argue. A person with low self-esteem may interpret the staff's suggestion as further proof of his inherent worthlessness.

Nursing Diagnosis
Sensory-perceptual alteration related to lack of sleep

Client Outcome
The client sleeps

Discussion

How does one determine whether another is sleeping unless the person is deliberately awakened? If the client states that he has slept well, how does the nurse diagnose hallucinatory behavior?

Nursing Diagnosis
Sensory-perceptual alteration related to lack of sleep.

Client Outcome
The client verbalizes that he is no longer hallucinating

Discussion

The outcome is now measurable; the client reports a change.

C H A R T   9-5
Example of Deadlines

Nursing Diagnosis	**Client Outcome**	**Deadline**
Self-care deficit: bathing/hygiene related to low self-esteem	The client initiates and follows through with washing hair and changing clothes	Observe client daily at 2 P.M.

Discussion

Reviewing the care plan early in the day, the nurse knows that observation and documentation are required regarding the progress of the client in performing his self-care.

C H A R T 9-6
Examples of Nursing Orders or Approaches

Nursing Diagnosis	Client Outcome	Deadline	Nursing Orders
Self-care deficit: bathing/hygiene	The client initiates and follows through with washing hair and changing clothes	Observe daily at 2 P.M.	Beginning treatment 1. a. In the morning, schedule shower time b. Assist the client as needed 2. Observe clothing and condition of hair in morning; note any changes throughout the day

Discussion

These nursing approaches are readily applied in psychiatric–mental health care settings.

Nursing Diagnosis	Client Outcome	Deadline	Nursing Orders
Impaired social interaction related to diminished sense of self-worth	The client identifies one person as a friend	Client discharge from in-patient facility	1. Involve the client in group therapy daily (led by group therapist) and note the client's reaction after the group 2. Provide activities through occupational therapy; note where the client sits and whether he interacts with anyone 3. Seek the client out during "non-prime-time" hours and engage him in superficial, social conversation

Discussion

The nursing orders provide an overview of the treatment program. Although two of the activities are directed by other team members, the nurse is able to observe and measure outcomes during and after these therapies.

Potential problems are those behaviors or symptoms that might occur when a client has that particular diagnosis; the nurse should observe for their occurrence and take preventive measures. Examples of potential problems are listed below.

Depression: potential suicidal ideation related to low self-esteem; potential malnourishment related to anorexia

Manic behavior: potential violent outbursts related to emotional lability

Possible problems are those behaviors or symptoms that may or may not occur. Possible problems are the "rare quirks" of a diagnosis that are sometimes forgotten in the day-to-day concerns of nursing. Possible problems are reminders that a particular problem, although rare, is related to the client's diagnostic classification.

Sample Nursing Care Plan 9-1

STANDARD NURSING CARE PLAN #
ALTERATION IN COPING

Initiated by: _____

_____
Client name or Addressograph

COMPLETE AS APPROPRIATE

DATE	NURSING DIAGNOSIS	EXPECTED OUTCOME	TARGET DATE	NURSING ORDERS AND CHECKING INTERVALS
	1) Ineffective individual coping, 2°	1a) Verbalizes positive statements about self		1a) Teach client positive reinforcement
		b) Demonstrates insight into needs and problems		b) Assist client with identification and seeking realistic solutions
		c) Increased appropriate behavior		c) Encourage client to accept responsibility for own behavior

Consider also:
Noncompliance
Family coping, ineffective
Parenting, alteration in
Alteration in nutrition

(Reprinted with permission from Saint Alphonsus Regional Medical Center, Boise, ID)

Examples of possible problems are listed below.

Depression: Possible auditory and visual hallucinations related to sleep disturbances
Manic behavior: Possible suicidal attempt related to grandiosity; possible legal difficulty related to excessive buying

Finally, the standardized nursing care plan provides blank spaces labeled *unusual problems,* which are the identified problems unique to the client. A blank column is also provided for dates and initials, which notify the mental health team when problems are identified and nursing approaches are initiated.

Balanced Service System

Mental health care is a team approach, and the team members are often public and private sector agents of health care delivery—social workers, psychologists, physicians, nurses, clinics, hospitals, schools. Treat-

Sample Nursing Care Plan 9-2

STANDARD NURSING CARE PLAN #
CLIENT WITH DISTURBANCE IN AFFECT

Initiated by: _____

Client name or Addressograph

COMPLETE AS APPROPRIATE

DATE	NURSING DIAGNOSIS	EXPECTED OUTCOME	TARGET DATE	NURSING ORDERS AND CHECKING INTERVALS
	1) Self-concept, disturbance in _____ _____ _____ _____ 2° _____	1) Participates in therapies a) _____ b) _____ c) _____ d) _____ e) Socialization Specify _____		1a) Assist client in developing realistic goals and plans involved _____ b) Involvement in unit activities _____ c) Type of participation/ frequency _____ d) Provide client education _____
	2) Violence, potential for _____ _____ 2° _____	2) Will not hurt self or others		2) Provide safe environment _____ _____
	3) Injury, potential for _____ 2° _____	3) Will not injure self		3a) Develop realistic controls _____ b) Safety precautions ____ _____
	4) Grieving, dysfunctional, 2° _____ _____	4) Expresses normal grieving _____		4a) Help client understand grieving process b) Identify present stage of grieving _____ c) Intervene appropriately _____

Consider also:
  Sleep pattern disturbance
  Self-care deficit
  Bowel elimination, alteration in
  Spiritual distress
  Sexual dysfunction
  Diversional activity, deficit
  Alteration in nutrition

(Reprinted with permission from Saint Alphonsus Regional Medical Center, Boise, ID)

Sample Nursing Care Plan 9-3

Depression

Overall criteria for discharge:
1) Sleep pattern approximates normal
2) Affect brighter
3) Verbalizing no suicidal concerns

Please circle appropriate problem number and orders.

Date	Nursing Diagnoses	Expected Outcome	Checking Intervals	Nursing Orders
	I. Usual client behaviors Core symptoms of depression related to the interaction of: Blunted flat affect Repetitive, ruminative thoughts Hopeless, helpless feelings Psychomotor retardation			
	1) Alteration in nutrition: less than body requirements Lack of activity Flat affect Preoccupation with disturbing thoughts	1a) Client maintains weight b) Eats 75% of all meals	Tues. & Fri.	1a) Accompany client to meals b) Do not make eating a major issue c) Weigh Tues. and Fri. d) Record appetite
	2) Sleep pattern disturbance: Difficulty falling asleep and/or Early morning awakening (EMA)	2) Client sleeps in his predepression pattern	Nightly	2a) Assess client's normal sleep pattern—insomnia remedy if has developed one b) Encourage light, non-stimulating activity before bedtime c) Contract with client: No daytime naps unless medically contraindicated
	3) Social isolation related to negative attitude evidenced by withdrawal from other clients	3a) Participates in basic unit social activities b) Controls negative outlook so that he does not talk about his hopelessness around other clients	Daily	3a) Discourage client from using room *excessively* to avoid social contact b) Encourage participation in social activities c) Make time to discuss with client problems he has in social situations d) Try to lead conversation away from

Date	Nursing Diagnoses	Expected Outcome	Checking Intervals	Nursing Orders
				totally negative pre-occupation; try physical, food, occupational therapy, or game activity
				e) Do not try to argue patient out of negative attitude.
	4) Ineffective individual coping evidenced by a) Somatic complaints related to preoccupation with self and anxiety (headache, backache, nausea) b) Inability to make decisions related to lack of concentration and ambivalence	4) After medical testing has ruled out physical cause, the client is able to state that symptoms may be a result of stress	Daily	4a) Give medication as ordered in a non-punitive manner; do not comment or criticize b) Offer some time to talk with the client about physical complaints
		5a) Rejects decisions made for him b) Demonstrates ability to make appropriate decisions from simple to complex	Daily	5a) Assign primary staff member to plan with the client a simple daily schedule, with short-duration activities at which he can succeed b) Do not ask the client to decide activities if he is unable—rather, make decision and tell him, "it is time for..." or "you can have your bath at 9 or 10...do you have a preference?" c) Discourage major decision-making d) Make fewer decisions for client as he begins to reject them
	II. Potential Problems 1) Constipation and/or urinary retention related to inadequate fluid intake, lack of activity	1a) Bowel movement at normal pattern for client b) Voids q shift c) Drinks at least 8 glasses fluid/24 h (if no fluid volume problems)	Daily	1a) Assess and record the client's normal bowel, bladder routine b) Encourage fluids at meals—q2h. c) Encourage physical rather than sedentary activity
	2) Suicide related to feelings of helpless-	2a) No suicide gestures or actions	Every 15–30 minutes	2a) Be aware of possibility of suicide as

(Continues on p. 142)

Date	Nursing Diagnoses	Expected Outcome	Checking Intervals	Nursing Orders
	ness, hopelessness, or as a manipulation or in response to hallucinations	b) Verbalizes rather than acts out desires for suicide		client gets "better," is more spontaneous, energetic b) Make sure client swallows all prescribed medicines (to prevent hoarding) c) If client is giving suicide "clues," ask him if he is indeed thinking about suicide, if he has made any plans, what the plans are d) Do not be afraid to approach subject of suicide with client (usually it is a relief for him to be able to talk about it) e) Room search with client in attendance may be necessary, looking especially for hoarded over-the-counter or other medicines, sharps, long belts, cords f) Notify client's physician g) Check client every 15–30 minutes or be in constant attendance if necessary h) May ask client to sign in at nursing station as often as checks are ordered
III.	Possible Problems 1) Sensory-perceptual and thought processes alterations are coping mechanisms with anxiety	1) See SNCP Schizophrenia section: impairment in reality testing		
IV.	Unusual Problems 1) Social isolation related to family's inability to communicate effectively	1) Client reports to nurse a conversation between herself, husband, and children	Discharge	1a) Allow the family to visit at times convenient to them b) Nurse visit with family, observe interaction, do social group leading

(Reprinted with permission from Saint Alphonsus Regional Medical Center, Boise, ID)

Case Study 9-1A: Planning Care for the H. Family

Carol H. is a 34-year-old mother of two children: Amy, 10, and Justin, 7. She has been married 13 years to Henry H., a 35-year-old salesman. While Henry has been moderately successful at his job, Carol has remained at home to raise the children.

Presently, Carol is hospitalized following a suicide attempt. The nursing assessment reveals a woman who has been increasingly "homebound" for 3 years, since Justin started school. She has many recriminations that her suicide attempt failed and declares, "That proves I can't do anything right." She has no hobbies or interests outside of the home and says, "My house keeps me busy."

Henry expresses bewilderment that his wife is unhappy and has attempted suicide. Henry is a firmly voiced, positive man. He informs the nurse that he and his wife do little together "because I'm selling." The house is generally clean and "that counts, or at least, that's what I thought." Henry believes there must be a marital problem, but doesn't know what it is.

Amy is having trouble in school paying attention. Justin is "perfect"; his school work is immaculate and he is overly polite and cooperative at school and at home.

A team conference is held to formalize care planning for Carol. Carol's therapist has determined that the conference would be too overwhelming for Carol to attend. She is unable to make decisions and this is further eroding her self-esteem. Henry would like to know the options he has to "get his family back the way it was before 'this' happened." An initial plan is formulated that states that when Carol verbalizes that she is no longer suicidal, has an alternative to suicide when she feels hopeless and helpless, and has met twice with her after-care

counselor, she will be evaluated for discharge. To facilitate Carol's recovery, she will be given antidepressant medication. Recognizing the impact of a suicide attempt upon children, plans are made to notify Amy's and Justin's teachers. A hospital plan and a system plan are initiated to monitor progress and to coordinate treatment efforts.

As Carol's hospitalization progresses, Henry becomes less positive and asks for more direction in caring for the children. He continues to ask for help to "fix the family...make it the way it was." A conference of the treatment team, including Carol and Henry, is held. Options for after-hospitalization treatment are discussed and the decision is made to begin marital counseling and family therapy. The system plan is amended to reflect these additions. Appointments with the therapists are made so that marital counseling can begin prior to Carol's discharge. The nurse facilitator coordinates these efforts.

Carol will continue her antidepressants and marital counseling after discharge from the psychiatric facility. When Carol is discharged, the school teachers and counselors continue to be actively involved in monitoring the children's behavioral reactions to the changes at home. Goals are established to increase Amy's attention span and for Justin to become less "perfect." These goals are communicated to the school nurse, who then incorporates them in the systems plan.

Use of the Balanced Service System Plan helps to coordinate the H. family's treatment. Each agency uses both its own detailed plan and a system plan to ensure that they do not duplicate efforts.

ment may take place in an inpatient or outpatient setting.

The client seeking help dealing with mental health problems is often overwhelmed by the number and diversity of agencies available to him and involved with him. Although the goals of treatment are continuity and consistency, these goals are not always met. A client may enter an inpatient facility, be discharged, and continue therapy in an unrelated outpatient clinic. As treatment progresses, the client may be referred to other agencies to assist in rehabilitation, such as agencies involved with vocational training, housing, and foster-child services. Each agency em-

ploys professionals with their own philosophies and biases. Each professional feels responsible for knowing all aspects of the client's situation and status. Consequently, there are overlaps of information and, often, a time-wasting repetition of history-taking. The client is constantly beginning again.

The *balanced service system* permits the professionals to know what aspects of the client's problems are being handled and by whom. It dignifies the client by allowing him to progress.[14] The balanced service system also allows the members of the team to focus on their areas of expertise, thereby reducing the duplication of services. Time is used more efficiently

Case Study 9-1B: Balanced Service System—The H. Family

Goal: To increase H. family's self-awareness and awareness of each other as measured by depression of mother

Date	Nursing Diagnosis	Outcome	Modality	Deadline	Approach
4/14	1. Carol (mother) suicidal related to ↓ self-esteem and ↑ deep depression evidenced by verbalization of feelings of hopelessness and helplessness	Verbalize alternatives to suicide ↓ depression as demonstrated by ↑ in activity level and return to "presuicide attempt" dress: clean clothes, make-up, hair washed and set	Hospitalization: St. Georges Antidepressant, as prescribed by Dr. Jones	Weekly Discharge from hospital	a. Standardized Nursing Care Plan: Depression St. Georges (M. Allen to coordinate) b. Routine medication education to be done by R. Rose c. Establish rapport with client, collaborate with husband, record d. Monitor activity level on unit's record
4/14	2. Potential school behavior problems of children related to anxiety caused by mother's suicide attempt	Children verbalize fear re suicide attempt	School	Weekly Monthly	a. Inform school teacher and counselors and record response; to be done by M. Allen b. Identify and record on System Plan name of teachers and counselor
4/26	3. Lack of individual understanding between Carol and Henry related to ↓ communication and time spent together	Verbalize new information about each other	Mental health clinic	Weekly	a. Marital counseling by R. Smith weekly to begin prior to discharge from hospital
4/23	4. Ineffective family coping related to ineffective communication among family members	Family interactions ↑ as measured by spontaneous conversation	Family therapy at mental health clinic	Every 2 weeks	a. Family therapy: R. Smith (therapist)

because one therapist knows with whom to speak at another agency.

Clients are frequently overwhelmed when entering new agencies or meeting new therapists. Using a balanced service system, clients and therapists can arrange introduction prior to therapy times, and the responsibilities of everyone involved in the client's care become clear. The treatment plan is truly the client's. (See Case Study 9-1.)

Summary

This chapter has explored the third step of the nursing process. Planning is a structuring of needs and problems in an orderly manner so that a goal may be achieved. Some of the important points of the chapter include the following:

1. When a client seeks therapy, he is mandating change that will affect all his relationships.
2. The writing of a plan clarifies the planner's thinking and details the choices available to him.
3. Establishing time frames within the plan provides guidelines for review and evaluation of the plan.
4. Nursing care plans provide structure for care and define nursing.
5. Nursing care plans contain the nursing diagnosis, long-term and short-term goals, outcomes, deadlines, and nursing orders or approaches.
6. Standardized nursing care plans acknowledge the similarities of behavior and therefore allow the nurse in the workplace to focus on the client's uniqueness.
7. Consistency and effectiveness of care are promoted by a system of care planning that identifies the responsibilities of each team member.

References

1. Altschul AT: Psychiatry Under Review—1: The Care of Mentally Disordered: Three Approaches. Nursing Times 76 (March 13): 452–454, 1980
2. Altschul AT: Psychiatry Under Review—3: The Role of Professionals. Nursing Times 76 (March 27): 555–556, 1980
3. Bachrach L: The Challenge of Service Planning for Chronic Mental Patients. *Community Ment Health J* 22 (Fall): 170–174, 1980
4. Baker BW, Kastelic FA: Patient Care: Four Steps to Increasing Positive Interactions Between Hospital Staff and Patients. Hosp Forum 23 (April–May): 12–15, 1980
5. Cady JW, Freshman DJ, Nroby RB: Taking the Pain Out of Care Planning. Medicus Systems Corp, 1975
6. Fowler G: A Needs Assessment Method for Planning Alternatives to Hospitalization. Hosp Community Psychiatry 31 (January): 41–45, 1980
7. Frances A, Greenwald B, Denicoff K, Meyerson AT: Chronic Patient Has Numerous Changes in Drugs, Therapists Makes Only Limited Gains. Hosp Community Psychiatry 36 (March): 233–235, 1985
8. Gallup R, Wynn F: Difficult Young Adult Chronic Patients: Re-evaluating Short-Term Clinical Management. Psychosoc Nurs Ment Health Serv 24 (March): 29–32, 1986
9. Giovannetti P: Understanding Patient Classification Systems. J Nurs Admin 9 (February): 4–9, 1979
10. Gladstone TU, McKegney FP: Relationship Between Patient Behavior and Nursing Staff Attitudes. Supervisor Nurse 2 (June): 32–35, 1980
11. Glazer WM, Aaronson HS, Prusoff BA, Williams DH: Assessment of Social Adjustment in Chronic Ambulatory Schizophrenic. J Nerv Ment Dis 168 (August): 493–497, 1980
12. Greig S, Miller J, Rolb J, McGillvray J: Putting Theory into Practice. Nurs Times (November 27): 28–30, 1985
13. Hessler I: Psychiatry Under Review—2: Roles, Status and Relationships in Psychiatric Nursing. Nursing Times 76 (March 20): 508–510, 1980
14. Huey K: Conference Report: Patient Reentry into Community. Hosp Community Psychiatry 31 (January): 52–55, 1980
15. Johnson MN: Self-Disclosure: A Variable in the Nurse-Client Relationship. J Psychiatr Nurs Ment Health Serv 18 (January): 17–20, 1980
16. Joseph B, Ryan CF, Boudveault TM: Evaluating the Impact of a Continuity-of-Care Program on Discharged Inpatients. Hosp Community Psychiatry 32 (August): 574–575, 1981
17. Kelly JA, Patterson J, Laughlin C, Urey J, Snowden EE: Objective Evaluation and Prediction of Client Improvement in Mental-Health Aftercare. Soc Work Health Care 5 (Winter): 187–202, 1979
18. Krispin AL: Nursing—A Role in Multidisciplinary Treatment Planning. J Psychiatr Nurs Ment Health Serv 18 (April): 14–17, 1980
19. Lang E, Mattson M: The Multidisciplinary Treatment Plan: A Format for Enhancing Activity Therapy Department Involvement. Hosp Community Psychiatry 36 (January): 62–68, 1985
20. Mayers MG: A Systematic Approach to Nursing Care Plan. New York, Appleton-Century-Crofts, 1972
21. McEnany G, Tescher B: Contracting for Care. J Psychosoc Nurs 23 (April): 11–18, 1985
22. Newberry P, Weissman MM, Myers JK: Working Wives and Housewives: Do They Differ in Mental

Status and Social Adjustments? Am J Ortho-psychiatry 49 (April): 282–291, 1979

23. Okin R, Dolnick J: Beyond State Hospital Unit-ization: The Development of an Integrated Mental Health Management System. Hosp Community Psychiatry 36 (November): 1201–1205, 1985

24. Pardue S, Dick C: Patient Classification. J Psychosoc Nurs 24 (December): 23–30, 1986

25. Parsons PJ: Building Better Treatment Plans. J Psychosoc Nurs 24 (April): 9–14, 1986

26. Reinke B, Greely JR: Organizational Analysis of Three Community Support Models. Hosp Community Psychiatry 37 (June): 624–629, 1986

27. Ritter S: Primary Nursing in Mental Illness. Nursing Mirror 160 (April 24) 16–17, 1985

28. Schain W: Patients' Rights in Decision Making: The Case for Personalism versus Paternalism in Health Care. Cancer (Supplement) 46 (August 15): 1035–1041, 1981

29. Skodel AE, Plutchik R, Kardsu TB: Expectations of Hospital Treatment: Conflicting Views of Patient and Staff. J Nerv Ment Dis 168 (February): 70–74, 1980

30. Standard Nursing Care Plan: Depression. Saint Alphonsus Regional Medical Center, Boise, Idaho, 1981

31. Syson-Nibbs L: Progress Through a Planned Approach. Nursing Mirror 150 (February 14): 41–44, 1980

32. Torrey EF: Continuous Treatment Teams in the Care of the Chronic Mentally Ill. Hospital and Community Psychiatry 37 (Dec): 1243–1247, 1986

33. Tsuang MT, Dempsey M: Long-Term Outcome of Major Psychoses, Parts One and Two. Arch Gen Psychiatry 36 (November): 1295–1304, 1979

10   Intervention

Patricia N. Mahon

If the wrong man uses the right means, the right means work in the wrong way.

Ancient Chinese Proverb

Chapter Preview

This chapter presents an eclectic, developmentally based approach to the process of psychiatric–mental health nursing. Each developmental stage and its needs and associated tasks are discussed in relation to adult psychiatric problems and the approach to their treatment. Nursing interventions, specifically helping relationships, are explored; the value of such relationships is also discussed.

Learning Objectives

On completion of the chapter, you should be able to accomplish the following:

1. identify the role of the psychiatric–mental health nurse
2. discuss the assumptions underlying an eclectic approach to psychiatric–mental health nursing
3. summarize the developmental tasks and issues of each stage of development
4. explain the developmentally based nursing approaches for various psychiatric–mental health disorders
5. describe the usefulness of an eclectic approach to mental health care

Role of the Psychiatric–Mental Health Nurse

The psychiatric–mental health nurse is an active, respected member of the mental health team in a variety of treatment settings. Definitions of the role of the psychiatric nurse have become increasingly blurred over the years. As their therapeutic skills and education grow, nurses are assuming the role of primary therapist in addition to their more traditional roles. The focus of therapeutic nursing intervention is not the personality disorder, psychosis, depression, or any other diagnostic category; it is the individual with specific needs and developmental tasks. The individual's disorder does not arise as a phoenix from an obscure niche of the unconscious; it is formed in the totality of a person's life experiences and interactions.

Many theories and techniques of psychotherapeutic treatment have been utilized as if each one were the only theory or technique in existence. These individual schools of thought speak only to a small part of the whole person and his needs and purport a narrow etiologic view. Nurses assess the needs of the individual client and employ the appropriate approach for meeting the identified needs. This process and a holistic orientation imply the need for more than a single theoretical and therapeutic approach to client care. In addition to learning appropriate approaches for holistic individualized care, we must keep in mind the individual nurse's personality. Self-awareness and understanding form the basis of our psychiatric–mental health nursing practice (see Chart 10-1, "A Historical Perspective").

Assumptions Underlying an Eclectic Approach

Any approach to psychotherapeutic treatment presupposes a certain underlying philosophy and set of beliefs. The following are beliefs or assumptions about human individuals, interactions, growth, maturity, and behavior that underlie an eclectic approach to psychiatric–mental health nursing.

Individuals develop and make choices about their life experiences.

An individual constantly interacts with his environment and assumes a major role in determining the types of experiences he eventually integrates. Each person's environment presents a plethora of situations from which he can select experiences. Selecting experiences that are meaningful can create situations that engender growth experiences. The greater the individual's developmental maturity, the more this selection process is under his control.

Individual personality growth is aided by significant human interactions.

Interpersonal relationships constitute the center of our life experiences. The types of relationships we choose change or differ according to our level on the developmental ladder. Therefore, the quality, depth, and appropriateness of interpersonal interactions become the determinants of our growth.

For example, to a newly born individual, a relationship engendering security inherently provides a growth potential for the infant. On the other hand, a relationship offering self-acceptance or "belongingness" offers nothing for growth at this stage of development.

Immaturity is the main impetus for seeking emotional treatment.

Psychopathology may be defined as the difference or gap between the existing emotional developmental level of an individual and the expected emotional developmental level that corresponds to his chronological age. If one accepts this premise, emotional

CHART 10-1
An Historical Perspective

Psychiatric Nursing in 1920

From the publication of the first psychiatric nursing textbook, Nursing Mental Diseases (Bailey H, R.N., New York, Macmillan) in 1920, psychiatric nursing has maintained and refined its active role in the treatment of clients. The role of the psychiatric nurse, at the time of its formal academic beginning, included the skills of observation (the most important nursing activity, according to Bailey), recognition of symptoms, limit setting, and the use of "sympathies of the heart." Nursing intervention during that era was based on the observation of symptoms and the inherent needs of the client that were communicated through those symptoms. "While signs are the province of the doctor," said George H. Kirby, M.D., in 1920, "symptoms are in a peculiar way that of the nurse." Growth and development were approached from a purely neurophysiological stance rather than from the standpoint of developmental tasks.

In this historic book, Bailey also described the qualifications that she believed were necessary for a nurse working with clients with mental disorders. To function in this area of nursing, she said, is "a task which calls for the full use of all the powers of the mind, sympathies of the heart, and skill of hand." Bailey's expectations of the effective psychiatric nurse are contemporarily expressed in familiar terms—self-knowledge, self-understanding, emotional maturity, and strength of personality. She emphasized not only the importance of the special knowledge and skill acquired by the nurse's training, but also the benefits of culture, social accomplishments, and "reading, study, and travel in the broader school of life."

A list of the expectations of the psychiatric nurse in 1920 declared that the individual must

Be intelligent (because no form of nursing makes such a constant appeal to the intellect)
Possess observational skills
Possess accurate reasoning
Possess the ability to make quick judgments
Have the mastery of her own emotions
Have more than ordinary capability
Be versatile
Be resourceful
Be mature
Be educated

---

disturbance may be equated with developmental immaturity. It is important, then, that the nursing process be based on an accurate assessment and analysis of the individual's level of emotional maturity and the corresponding needs. The planning of care calls for a relationship that is consistent with the assessed level of functioning in order to provide the interpersonal experience necessary for optimum developmental and emotional growth.

Developmental Issues, Needs, and Tasks

To use an eclectic approach to psychiatric–mental health nursing, the nurse must have an understanding of the developmental levels and their inherent relationship needs. The developmental stages are presented in the familiar hierarchical order and each stage is discussed in relationship to the needs, issues, and tasks.

Infancy

The first 2 years of life, or infancy, are designated as the *oral period*, in which the personality structure of the individual is centered around the issue of impulsivity. Until the infant begins to develop speech, his behavior and interpersonal relationships are autistically motivated. The ego is still in a primitive stage, with its minimal strengths and abilities focused on the management of impulses and impulse gratification. Impulse identification and communication of a need (for example, crying for a bottle, fussing when wet) are the important developmental tasks during this early period. Successful mastery of this developmental period includes the expression and gratification of impulses.

The infant experiences security through interaction with parental figures who create a protective and secure atmosphere, which is necessary for growth to take place. Crucial aspects of this stage of development are the effectiveness of the mother figure and the establishment of trust.[9]

Toddlerhood

Late infancy, or toddlerhood, which may extend from 2 years of age to 3 or 4 years of age, is referred to as the *anal period*. The core needs during this period are for support in the appropriate expression of feelings and the control of impulses. During this period, the child is involved in the development of social, emotional, and physiological control, such as bowel and bladder control. A major task is learning that there is not only an appropriate time and place to defecate, but that other types of feelings can also be modulated and expressed at appropriate times and in an appropriate manner.

The child's ego functions begin to take root during the battle for control of impulsivity. The pleasure principle is slowly being displaced by the reality principle and the child begins to relate and deal with the world in a new way.[12] The child responds to the world in terms of societal demands and expectations. During this stage, the superego is born.

The parents' role of providing security seems to be less important than providing support in impulse control. The child experiences feelings such as shame, guilt, and depression during this stage and needs parental support to begin to face superego demands.

Preschool Years

From the ages of 3 or 4 to 6 years, the child is in the *oedipal stage* of development. During this stage, the child's dominant developmental needs are to deal with sexual and aggressive impulses and to come to terms with parental and societal demands. The development of the ego is of primary importance during the preschool years. The child engages in a struggle between sexual impulses and their appropriate expression.

This stage is one in which one parent is seen as an unobtainable love object due to the threat of the more powerful and potent parent of the same sex. An unconscious decision, the only feasible way out of the threatening dilemma, is to become as much like the parent of the same sex as possible; that is, to identify.[15] The child identifies with the parent of the same sex in order to cope with the impossible, internal interaction between the id, ego, and superego, and the external family situation. Growth and healthy identification require a healthy dependency on the same-sexed parent, the parent with whom the child identifies.

A successful resolution of this developmental stage increases ego strength and assists the child in changing his or her role within the family unit. The evolution of certain life skills and the realization that gratification of impulses involves a time-delay factor are significant hallmarks of learning during this stage of development.

Early School-Age

The years from 6 to 9, identified as *early latency*, constitute a stage in which learning, the acquisition of knowledge, and the development of the social role outside the protection of the home and family take place. During the earlier stages of development, the child established some peer relationships, although the primary relationships were focused on the "all-important" family. During the early school-age years, however, the child begins to make his way into the world and develop relationships with significant adult and authority figures such as neighbors. The child's control over the environment increases greatly as he acquires knowledge and new learning.

At this developmental stage, the self-concept is still in a primitive, rudimentary form. The self is the *perceived self*; that is, the individual as he observes himself operating in the larger world and in varied situations. The child now possesses the beginning ability to "step outside" of, and observe, himself in various situations. With growth come the ability and power to modify or change behavior. The prime developmental task during this stage is to relate specific "self" concepts to specific interactional situations with others and the environment. The ability to differentiate the self and the ego is a necessary skill in the process of interaction. The "self-sets" that begin to form are the forerunners of an integrated, adult sense of self.

The early-latency-age child needs guided experiences from reliable adults in authority. Guidance from the father or mother figure as a social representative within the family setting is necessary; guidance is also necessary from a teacher, coach, neighbor, or other important adult outside the nuclear family.

Late School-Age

Latency, the period that precedes adolescence, stretches from the ages of 9 to 12 years. The harmonization of various aspects of the differentiated self-concept occurs during this time, although several areas of the self, including sexual, vocational, and scholastic development, are neither owned nor integrated. The integration of these facets of the self is slowed because they inherently carry with them the threat of independence and separation from the family. The continuing need for dependency is transferred from family to peer relationships. In the process of forming peer relationships, experiences with independence are accumulated through new self-concept structures that carry very little or no threat at all (sports teams, Boy and Girl Scouts, clubs), while those that pose the greatest threat (sex, vocation) are denied and avoided.

Adolescence

The stage of adolescence brings with it the physiological changes of puberty, the full blown emergence of the self-concept, and the integration of the biopsychosocial aspects of the individual. The young adolescent who is just beginning to integrate a sense of self may swing violently from viewing self as completely inadequate to the opposite end of the continuum, that of pridefulness and being puffed up over a sense of adequacy. The underlying theme of adolescence is a sense of striving, a need for a feeling of adequacy, and the search for an opportunity to test out the "self."

Equipped with the psychological skills for adult maturity, the adolescent must distance himself from the child–parent–family relationships and move toward adult relationships in the larger world. The intellectual choices made for adulthood must be actualized and the associated responsibilities must be accepted in this stage.

The major developmental tasks during adolescence are making a commitment, working through the commitment, and solidifying the personality structure so that the self is viewed as a participant in the larger world. This is a painful, but necessary, process in the movement up the developmental ladder to adulthood.

The adolescent's need to prove himself as a person in his own right, as an adequate and independent human being, gives rise to conflicts with parents and authority over power issues. This conflict is usually the rule rather than the exception.

Adulthood

The successful completion of adolescence, which is a difficult task for many, can lead to what has been referred to in modern times as the *existential crisis*. The individual, at this point in development, is no longer in need of the family constellation for self-identity. The person is faced with life, in the form of aloneness, the absurdity of existence, and all the responsibilities inherent in his attained freedom. The standards and structures by which the adolescent had previously structured his life are no longer seen as meaningful. A reorganization of the meaning of life, along with the blatant knowledge that he is no longer a child in an adult world, confronts the individual. The "adult" must be an active, productive participant in the activities and responsibilities of the larger, nonprotective world. The emotional development of the human be-

ing is not at all completed at this stage. During adulthood, various issues, problems, and stresses arise; confronting them is another, separate phase of development.

Developmental Framework for Nursing Intervention

Knowledge and understanding of the stages of development and the issues, tasks, and needs of each period form the framework within which the planning of nursing intervention takes place. For example, the drives of infancy center around impulsivity and immediate need gratification. These issues are eloquently discussed by Harry Stack Sullivan, whose theoretical discussion centers on impulse gratification, maternal empathy, and autism. These psychological factors provide an understanding of behavior dominated by the primary process, as in schizophrenia.

If the individual's emotional needs are not met and the tasks of a developmental stage are not completed, "lags" in maturity may be identified. Such deficits at various developmental levels result in emotional fixations that halt the natural movement through the remainder of the developmental stages and, hence, result in immaturity. As a result, psychopathology, or emotional disorder, arises from the fixation at a specific stage of development. Certain disorders can, in fact, be linked to fixations at these specific stages. The following are examples.

Schizophrenia—Infancy

Schizophrenic individuals function at the level of extreme dependence and are preoccupied with the fulfillment of their basic security needs. The impetus behind schizophrenic behavior is the gaining of greater security experiences from the world around. One finds that schizophrenic clients become intensely involved with their therapists and those who are identified as significant to them in an attempt to gain security. Security is also found within the hospital setting, in which the basic needs of the individual are met by another.

The schizophrenic's life revolves around the meeting of basic security and dependency needs. When these basic, infantile needs are not fulfilled, the individual engages in delusional and hallucinatory behavior. The symbolism of the delusional and hallucinatory material usually reflects impulses and needs that center on dependency and security.

Manic Depression—Toddlerhood

Problems revolving around the issue of impulse control can be traced to the anal phase of development. Primitive attempts at impulse control by a child in the anal period of development can also be similarly observed in the individual with a diagnosis of manic–depressive disorder.

An individual with this affective disorder is torn between the expression and the avoidance of aggression, impulse, and feelings. The major objective of the professional mental health caregiver, in working with this client, is to create a learning environment in which the client can learn how to express his impulses and feelings appropriately.

Neurotic Disorder—Preschool Years

Ego development emerges out of the process of dealing with the aggressive and sexual impulses that arise during the oedipal period of development. The preschool child becomes an enigmatic challenge for his parents because, if he is limited too severely, he may develop a punitive superego that restricts and punishes him and limits his effectiveness as an adult with adult ego functioning. This may be observed in the individual exhibiting neurotic or maladaptive behavior.

The neurotic personality is laden with unacceptable impulses that must be severely restricted and controlled or the individual becomes overwhelmed by anxiety. The individual attempts to maintain internal homeostasis of impulse control and restriction by continuing an overdependency on parental figures or on some significant individual who is placed in a parental role.

Neurotic disordering that begins early in the oedipal stage may result in obsessive-compulsive behavior. The obsessive-compulsive conflict of the adult is closely associated with anality, in which depression and repressed aggression exist. The hysterical neurotic personality is fixated at a later oedipal stage and focuses more on concerns with sexuality. The obsessive-compulsive individual utilizes the defense of denial in a primitive manner to attempt to rid the self of threatening, unacceptable impulses. The hysterical individual, more mature on the developmental scale, utilizes more sophisticated defenses, is easier to interact and develop a relationship with, and is easier to treat.

Personality Disorder—Early School-Age

The demands of a formal education and of society are issues that must be dealt with in the early latency or school-age period. In the process of functioning and judging that functioning, in the world larger than the family, the child's ego and superego merge into what has been termed the *developing self*. Individuals with personality disorders, which represent a fixation at the early latency stage, are continually struggling with their unsuccessful transition from the ego mechanisms that controlled impulses during the oedipal period to the expression of the self in a world viewed as confusing.

A successful transition into the larger world requires the individual to compile and index the self-images that have been tested in the larger world of peers and adult authority. The person discovers acceptable channels for the expression of impulses and incorporates them into his repertoire of behavior. The pathology of a personality disorder is expressed by the rejection of cultural systems and values (as in antisocial individuals) or by the identification with a subculture that possesses its own values different from those of the large society (as in members of street gangs). Both of these pathologic expressions are found in clients who desire the gratification of impulses as their end; therefore, both types of clients attempt to manipulate the world to attain this end.

Behavior Disorder—Late School-Age

The individual with a behavioral disorder is viewed as being fixated late in the latency period of development. During this period, the individual's self-concept is being integrated into the personality. Fixations at this level of development are characterized by very adequate functioning in all areas of life, with the exception of one area. Not unlike a preadolescent child, an individual with a behavioral disorder utilizes certain symptoms to maintain dependency and avoid the impending conflict of dependency-independency; that is, he tries to avoid growing up! Individuals with behavioral disorders use avoidance behaviors to relate with others. "Gamesmanship" is easily observed as their mode of operation in relationships and in the avoidance of the decisions and choices needed to move toward maturity.

The individual with a behavioral disorder does not typically seek help until he reaches a point of being overwhelmed by his symptoms. He seeks out peer relationships that protect and reinforce his avoidance of maturity. Generally, such individuals get along well with others, function at a satisfactory level, maintain friendships, work and do superficially well in their life . . . with the exception of never achieving what is needed to "move on" in life, such as finishing school, achieving job promotions, and so on. If asked how things are going for them, their usual response is, "Everything is fine . . . just great." When verbally confronted with their behavior in regards to achievement, they usually respond by stating, "Sure, everything is great, except that," and then proceed to avoid the problem. Such individuals possess an unlimited catalog of rationalizations to explain why they haven't succeeded at any particular time or in any particular endeavor. They possess extensive knowledge about a variety of topics—cars, stereos, hobbies, the stock market, and others—but never use that knowledge for their own movement to a more mature, responsible level of development.

The behavior of the individual diagnosed with a behavioral disorder is used to prevent progress toward maturity and the responsibilities inherent in adult roles. The individual may be well-versed in the responsibilities that he is avoiding and is conscious of his avoidance behaviors. He copes with the independence-dependence conflict by maintaining the dependence of a more immature level of development. Those individuals who appear to be frightened by success and those who become dependent on chemical substances (drugs and alcohol) are identified in this developmental fixation.

Adolescent Reaction—Adolescence

The problem for the adolescent is twofold—conflict between independence and dependence, and the growing sense of awareness of the self's operation within the larger world of adulthood. In the attempt to attain and maintain a sense of social adequacy, the individual faces the feared possibility of finding the self adequate and acceptable. Many of the symptoms observed in the adolescent reaction are the social and behavioral reflections of an attempt to gain a sense of social adequacy and acceptance. Adolescents are frequently plagued with feelings of inadequacy when their accomplishments do not meet their unrealistic expectations of themselves.

During adolescence, the individual is expected to choose goals in life and move actively toward attaining these goals. The growing of sexual and social adequacy along with the commitment to grapple with the problems of life are the areas that need to be supported during this stage of development. Fixation at the adolescent level of development produces an individual who is neither able to move forward with a decision nor able to carry through with it energetically once a decision has been made.

At the adolescent stage of development, a fairly high level of personality development has been achieved and the superego and ego have been integrated into the personality. The identified needs of an individual fixated at the adolescent phase of development are acceptance and support during the decision-making process, and the peer group is naturally sought out to meet these needs.

Existential Crisis—Adulthood

With the successful attainment of maturity and the confrontation of the self with the idea of freedom of choice, the individual must then deal with the meaning of life and aloneness. Inherent in this phenomenon is the concept of a *transcendental self,* a self that exists beyond one's individual self-image, or a self in relation to the larger universe.

The developmental crisis during this period includes profound anxiety, depression, and exploration of the meaning of death and its finality. The crisis is intense and the associated painful emotions are exquisitely experienced. An individual experiencing such a crisis needs mature relationships that provide an environment in which to interact, react, and act on choices made. At this developmental stage, a meaning in life can only be ascribed by the individual.

Nursing Interventions

Helping Relationships

At the foundation of a helping relationship is a basic belief that individuals grow as a result of positive interpersonal interactions. Therapeutic relationships are sought because of earlier developmental needs that have not been satisfactorily met. A helping relationship that identifies developmental needs and provides the appropriate behavioral learning leads to developmental and emotional growth.

The therapeutic aspect of nursing care is the relationship shared by the professional and client. This relationship is an intense involvement in which resistance and defenses are lifted and in which direct, honest communication occurs. The relationship is based on trust and involves individualized nursing approaches according to the identified developmental needs of the client.

Eclectic Therapeutic Approach

Theorists have conceptualized therapeutic approaches from specialization with diagnostic categories of clients; such specializations have included Sullivan's work with schizophrenic individuals, Freud's work with neurotic clients, and Rogers' work with individuals with adolescent reactions. Each of these therapists conceptualized a framework that was applicable to a specific group of clients and developed appropriate interventions that met identified needs.

Nursing calls for an eclectic understanding and

approach to treatment based on the specific needs of the client, rather than on any one specific framework. A developmental approach provides the nurse with a framework for assessment, analysis, planning, and implementation of care based on the individual client's developmental needs. The initial interviews call for the nurse's assessment of the individual and his family and the generation of a series of questions or hypotheses about his developmental level and needs. Based on this assessment, the nurse then applies the theoretical approaches and interventions that appropriately meet the identified needs, as discussed in Chart 10-2, "Guidelines for a Developmental Approach to Interviewing."

For example, the schizophrenic individual relates to others and the world in terms of security and need fulfillment. These communications are seen in his concrete thinking, dream-like fantasy (hallucinations), and demands upon the nurse to assume a maternal role. Basically, the schizophrenic message is that others, including the nurse, are not providing motherly care. In the relationship, it is necessary to search out the meaning of the client's symbolic expressions, as a loving mother must, in order to "understand" the needs of her child. The most imperative aspects in working with a schizophrenic patient are to accept the commitment that is necessary in the relationship, to take the risks involved, and to meet the client's oral-dependent needs in a therapeutic and growth-producing manner.

The behavioral cycles in the affective disorders, such as manic depression, are attempts at impulse control utilizing an archaic ego structure. Delusional systems and primary thought processes can be observed in this pathological fixation. During the normal anal period, the mother meets needs for superego control and shares in ego functioning with the child. This is done while providing the support needed as the child attempts to develop self-control and higher ego functioning. Similarly, the nurse's role with the manic-depressive individual focuses on supporting the existing ego strength while providing external limits and protection.

The phenomenon of transference within helping relationships aids in the resolution of turbulent, neurotic interactions based in oedipal fixations. Interpretation, another psychotherapeutic technique, is an advanced skill that is important for the resolution of intrapsychic and developmental conflicts and movement toward greater maturity.

In a helping relationship with an individual with a personality disorder, the nurse is viewed as a societal representative of authority and must possess a clarity of her own values to help the client develop healthy behaviors for dealing with the world. Theoretically,

ego psychology, neoanalytic approaches, and group therapy are appropriate treatment approaches for the individual fixated in early latency.

The helping interpersonal relationship needed to treat a person with a behavior disorder calls for a less intensive, peer-type relationship in which exploration may occur. Because of a more highly developed personality structure, the client is agile in avoiding situations that pose a threat. Appropriate nursing interventions focus on exploring the effectiveness of specific behaviors used to maintain pathology and on examining the "games" used in gaining "payoffs." Such approaches open the door to the formation of peer relationships needed for the movement toward growth.

The relationship needs of an individual with an adolescent reaction are minimal and are most appropriately met with a nondirective approach encompassing a permissive atmosphere and the reflection of feelings, genuineness, and unconditional positive regard. The client-centered approach of Carl Rogers is the appropriate interpersonal approach for an individual fixated at the adolescent stage of development.[29]

A therapeutic helping interaction with an individual experiencing an existential crisis involves two individuals (client and professional) who are able to share their common struggles and find meaning in their existence. Therapists such as May, Frankl, and other existential theorists and philosophers present extensive conceptualizations regarding the existential crisis.[10,23,24] The nurse, in this type of helping relationship, must be armed with a vast, organized body of understanding, knowledge, and maturity from which to interact, evaluate, and treat the individual experiencing an existential crisis.

Summary

This chapter has explored the role of the psychiatric—mental health nurse and the developmental issues, needs, and tasks of each stage of development on which nursing interventions are based. Some of the emphases of the chapter include the following:

1. In the treatment of psychiatric—mental health clients, it must be remembered that individuals do not move from their fixation, or pathology, to maturity in one leap, but move from one level of fixation to the next-higher level toward maturity.
2. Underlying helping relationships is the basic belief that individuals grow as a result of positive interpersonal interactions.

C H A R T   10-2
Guidelines for a Developmental Approach to Interviewing

The following are suggested guidelines for an interview of a client using the developmental approach. The proposed areas of exploration will aid in the collection of data during the first session. The nurse should phrase questions as ambiguously as possible, so that the client can respond in a manner that is meaningful to him and reveal through this any patterns of defense or pertinent issues. In addition, when the queries are of equal strength, any increase in anxiety or defensiveness in one area or another may be a revelation of diagnostic import.

It is imperative that the nurse keep in mind that the client will be responding not only to interview questions but also to the interviewer. Questions that flow in a smooth pattern, rather than serendipitously, aid in the comfort of the client and elicit data which will present a Gestalt of his story and concerns. To gain deeper information in any area of the interview, especially where anxiety issues are evident, the nurse must be nondirective and nonthreatening. A simple query such as "Tell me more about that..." or "How do you feel about...?" will allow the client to move into these areas without experiencing undue pressure.

A preliminary profile of the client and his needs may be compiled after the following five areas have been explored:

1. The client's perspective or view of his problem
2. The client's family relationships (past and present)
3. The client's peer relationships (male and female)
4. The client's self-concept
5. The client's image of the future (wishes, hopes, plans)

What is the *client's view* of the problem? The nurse may open with questions such as, "What was happening in your life that you decided to come here?" or, "What is it that brings you here; what was happening in your life?"

In exploring the area of family and *family relationships*, the nurse may ask, "How are things at home?", "Tell me about your mom (dad, brother, sister, wife, husband, children), "What's your mom's (dad's, wife's) feeling about (your job, you going to school, coming for help)?" Such questions give not only the interviewer but also the client the freedom to pursue any problem areas in more depth.

The third area of *peer relationships* will not only provide information on the interpersonal interactions and skills of the client but will give clues to the amount of isolation or overextension in his life. Requests such as "Tell me about your friends", "What kind of activities are you involved in?", "Tell me about your leisure time (hobbies, interests)" may aid in this exploration.

Self-concept, the fourth area of importance (especially the client's self-concept in relation to others and the world) must be attended to also. Requests such as "Tell me about yourself", "How would your best friend describe you?", "Would you agree with that description?", and "What kind of person are you?" can be the jumping-off points in the most difficult area of self-concept.

Last, but not least important, is the area of *future*. What are the client's plans for his life? Does he see a future? How does he imagine or visualize the future? Is he suicidal? Leading questions such as "How do you see yourself in 2, 5, 10 years?", "Other than working, what will you be doing?", "Where will you be living?" may be used to explore this area. An individual who cannot visualize his future has little hope and may be communicating covert suicidal messages.

During the interaction, be aware of how the client focuses the problem areas, how he is handling the problems, and the specific areas of concern that surface. Ask yourself, "What does the client want from me, need from me?", "What kind of relationship does the client need?" During the interview, the nurse may have a heightened sensitivity so that these questions may begin to be answered.

To plan adequately interventions for each client, the nurse must first have arrived at a diagnosis of needs through an interview that allows free expression. The word "diagnosis" comes from the roots *gnosis* (knowledge) and *dia* (through and through). That is, it refers to thorough knowledge of the client.

The first and most important aspect of all treatment is an interested effort to know the client fully, in all the happenings of his life that have shaped, formed, and led him through the years to his present situation. This is a challenge to the nurse or to any health care professional, for our own and others' pains are difficult to face. Just as we all prefer to take shortcuts to our goals, we also would like to offer ad-

(Continues on p. 156)

vice, counsel, and treatment to others without having to know fully the wounds that need healing.

It is in the willingness to know the client fully that we can reach out to heal. The relationship then must be formed around an empty, but friendly space, where those who are hurting can relate their stories to someone who will listen with a sincere and educated attention. True listening is an art that must be developed and that calls for individuals to be truly present to each other.

Intervention also includes allowing the clients to become sensitive to their own stories. The nurse must then become the "student" who wants to learn, and the client the "teacher". Teachers best learn and master their material during preparation and ordering of their ideas for presentation; likewise, the client learns his own story and gains insight by relating it to another who truly listens. Listening to know is the most essential aspect of the helping relationship.

Thus intervention, at its root, is the receiving and full understanding of the client's story. The story may be hard to tell, filled with disappointments, frustrations, hurts nestled in deviations and stagnations, but it is the only story the client has, because it is his own. There will be little hope for his future if the story remains untold, unreceived, or misunderstood. Most often it is our fear of the hidden times in our own past that keeps us paralyzed and unlistening.

The major issue in a relationship is not "What to say" or "What to do" but "How to develop that special inner space where a story may be received and listened to?" We, as helpers, must offer safe boundaries where painful pasts may be unveiled and a new search may begin— a place where pain and suffering may be exposed without fear or judgment.

3. The helping person has a responsibility to be knowledgeable in varied theoretical and conceptual approaches, in order to be consistent with the growth of the client.

4. The developmental eclectic approach should ultimately provide a framework to help individuals resolve developmental fixations and reach the level of a mature, fully functioning person.

References

1. Alexander F, Eisentein G, Grotjahn M: Psychoanalytic Pioneers. New York, Basic Books, 1966
2. American Psychiatric Association: Diagnostic and Statistical Manual of Mental Disorders, 3d ed. Washington, DC, American Psychiatric Association, 1980
3. Berne E: Games People Play. New York, Grove Press, 1964
4. Berne E: Transactional Analysis in Psychotherapy. New York, Grove Press, 1961
5. Brenner C: Psychoanalysis. New York, Doubleday, 1957
6. Brill A: Psychoanalysis. New York, Washington Square Press, 1960
7. Bruch H: Learning Psychotherapy. Cambridge, Harvard University Press, 1974
8. Ellis A: The Rational Emotive Approach. New York, Julian Press, 1973
9. Erikson E: Childhood and Society. New York, WW Norton, 1963
10. Frankl V: Man's Search for Meaning: An Introduction to Logotherapy. New York, Washington Square Press, 1971
11. Freud A: Normality and Pathology in Childhood— Assessments of Development. New York, Internal University Press, 1965
12. Freud S: Beyond the Pleasure Principle. New York, Bantam Books, 1959
13. Freud S: Character and Culture: General Psychological Theory. New York, Collier Books, 1963
14. Freud S: Dora: An Analysis of a Case of Hysteria. New York, Collier Books, 1963
15. Freud S: Early Psychoanalytic Writings. New York, Collier Books, 1963
16. Freud S: New Introductory Lectures on Psychoanalysis. New York, Norton Press, 1965
17. Fromm-Reichman F: Principles of Intensive Therapy. Chicago, University of Chicago Press, 1950
18. Goffman I: Asylums. New York, Anchor Books, 1959
19. Hartman H: Essays on Ego Psychology. New York, Internal University Press, 1964
20. Horney K: Collected Works of Karen Horney, David Rapport (ed). New York, Basic Books, 1967
21. Luchins AS: Group Psychotherapy. New York, Random House, 1967
22. Luft J: Group Process. California, National Press Books, 1970
23. May R: Courage to Be. New York, Norton Co, 1975

24. May R: Power and Innocence. New York, Harper & Row, 1972

25. Patterson CH: Relationship Counseling and Psychotherapy. New York, Harper & Row, 1974

26. Perls F: Gestalt Therapy. New York, Dell Publishing, 1951

27. Perls F: Gestalt Therapy Verbatim. New York, Bantam Books, 1970

28. Perls F: In and Out of the Garbage Pail. New York, Bantam Books, 1971

29. Rogers C: On Encounter Groups. New York, Harper & Row, 1970

30. Rosenbaum M, Berger M: Group Psychotherapy and Group Function. New York, Basic Books, 1963

31. Sullivan HS: Interpersonal Theory of Psychiatry, Helen Perry (ed). New York, Norton Books, 1953

11 Evaluation

Susan Kah

Institutions are weighted with the past; the individual is on the side of vitality and the future.

John W. Gardner,
In Common Cause

158

Chapter Preview

Evaluation is the process of determining the value of something in the attainment of preset goals.[13] Evaluation of nursing practice is an essential component of professional accountability. Nurses are answerable to clients and their families. They are also answerable to themselves, to others who participate in the client's care, to the agencies in which they practice, to the community, and to the profession of nursing—which, in turn, is accountable to society.[15]

One focus of this chapter is the exploration of the process of evaluation as an essential component of the nursing process. The chapter also addresses the broader issue of self-regulation to assure quality in professional performance. The evaluation of client progress and nursing care in a psychiatric–mental health setting is discussed. Also included in the chapter are descriptions of various approaches to evaluation and the components of quality assurance programs in nursing.

Learning Objectives

On completion of the chapter, you should be able to accomplish the following:

1. define the process of evaluation
2. explain the relationship of the evaluation phase to the other phases of the nursing process
3. discuss the difficulties that the nurse may encounter when evaluating the care of clients with psychiatric–mental health problems
4. compare three different, but interrelated, approaches to evaluation—structure, process, and outcome
5. describe how the phases of the nursing process—assessing, diagnosing, planning, implementing, and evaluating—provide data or input for quality assurance programs in nursing

Evaluation: A Component of the Nursing Process

Evaluation is the fifth component of the nursing process and should follow the implementation of actions designated by the nursing care plan.[18] The nursing process is cyclic; evaluation serves as the catalyst for modifying the other components of the care plan. (The dynamic nature of the nursing process and the significance of evaluation are illustrated in Fig. 11-1.)

Evaluation has two targets:

1. The changes experienced by the client as a result of the actions of the nurse
2. The quality or effectiveness of the nursing care itself

The nurse compares the changes experienced by the client with the client-centered objectives specified in the care plan. These objectives are the criteria for evaluation. For example, the nurse may assess a withdrawn client as being disoriented and specify "client awareness of time and place" as an objective of nursing care. Subsequent nursing actions may include visual clues placed in the client's environment, such as a clock and calendar, and verbal reinforcement of time and place. The nurse accompanies and follows these actions with observations of the client's behavior.

Does he keep appointments?
Is he present at activities he is expected to attend?
Are his eating and sleeping patterns fairly regular?

If the client's behavior does not change, then the nurse must review and modify the assessment, planning, and implementation phases of care.

Review and modification of the care plan provide nurses with important information about their practice. Was the original assessment of the client complete? Was the nursing diagnosis correct? Was the identified problem a problem for the client or for the nurse? Were the objectives realistic for the client? Did new problems cause a change in the client that was not recognized? Did the client participate in the planning of care? Were the nursing actions appropriate for the identified problem? Is documentation of care available? Is the client's response described completely enough to provide a basis for evaluation? Finding the answers to these and other similar questions engages nurses in the problem-solving that is essential to accountable practice.

Evaluation of the Client with a Mental Health Problem

It is often difficult, for a variety of reasons, to appraise changes experienced by the client and to determine which resulted from nursing intervention. Nurses in psychiatric–mental health care settings assess clients who have difficulty with thinking, feeling, and behaving rather than with more objectively measurable changes in physical status, such as vital sign changes. Thinking and feeling are subjective processes; behavior has multiple causations and is frequently open to many interpretations. Detecting changes in another person's self-image and perceptions of reality requires not only knowledge of human behavior but sensitivity and skillful communication as well.

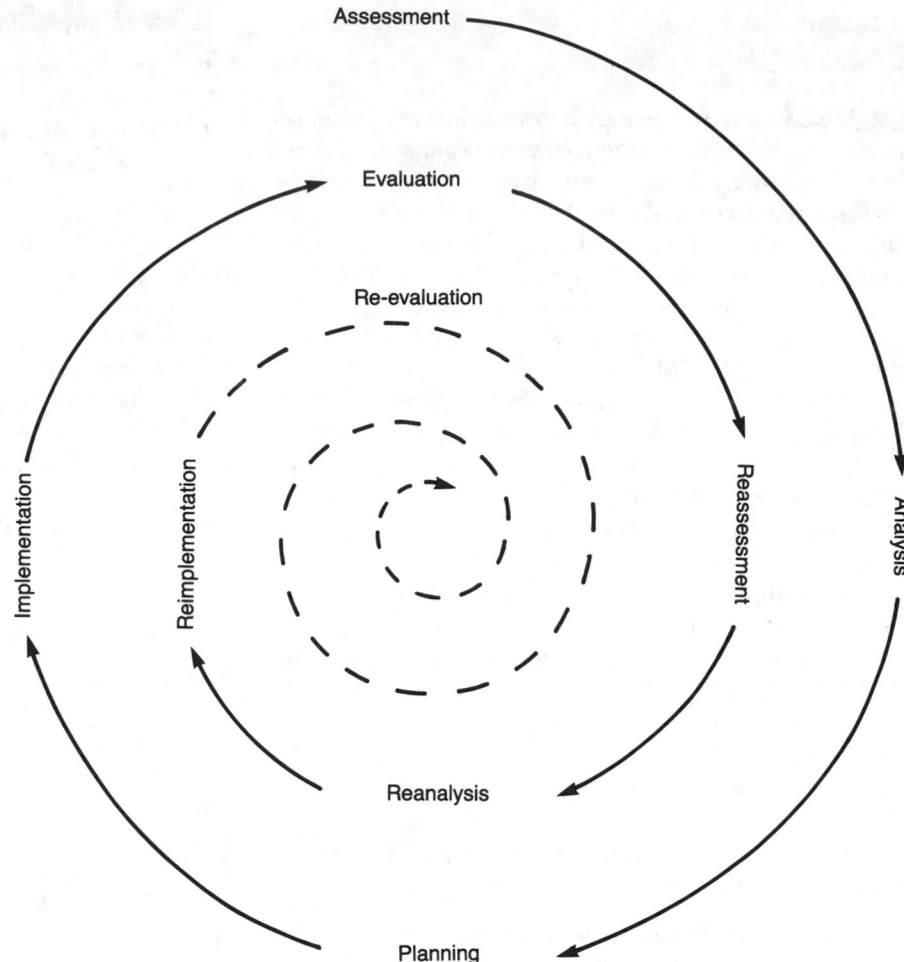

Figure 11-1. *The nursing process.*

Another difficulty in evaluating changes in the client's condition stems from the nature of mental illness. Clients with mental health problems usually do not recover quickly, and they may never be completely free of problematic behaviors. If nurses are not perceptive of minor changes in the client's condition, they may overlook progress. A client's decision to eat with others or to join a therapy group may be a milestone in his recovery. Sometimes, clients take three steps toward health and two backward before they continue on again. This regression is not uncommon. After examining possible reasons for this regression, the nurse must be sufficiently patient to recognize the progress that is occurring.

The nurse must also take care to maintain realistic expectations when formulating objectives of care for, and with, the client. Client care resources must be considered. The level of staffing of a psychiatric unit is frequently a limitation. The nurse must also maintain an awareness that some clients will not be able to reach a high level of achievement or functioning. When beginning nurses recognize this possibility, they are more likely to see clients as they really are.

Evaluation of Psychiatric–Mental Health Nursing Practice

Evaluating nursing practice itself can be as difficult or elusive as evaluating changes in the client's condition. One reason for this difficulty is the multidisciplinary and closely collaborative nature of client care. Nurses usually function as part of a health care team, each member contributing to the client's recovery. The client may receive medication, psychotherapy, and occupational therapy; he may live in a therapeutic environment; and he may interact with significant others as well as with nurses. Nurses participate in and influence many of these therapies and also make their own unique contribution to client care; however, it is frequently impossible for nurses to determine that a particular change in client behavior resulted from a specific nursing action or series of actions. Nursing research may lead in this direction, but nurses caring for clients with mental health problems must be able to derive satisfaction from a collaborative role and must not underestimate their own significance.

Another factor that makes care evaluation difficult is the predominance of psychosocial nursing approaches or actions employed in the care of a client with mental health problems. The nature of an interaction with a client is very difficult to quantify, describe, or reproduce. The psychiatric–mental health nurse practices an art as well as a science. In order to modify an action or approach, nurses must be able to define what they are already doing. This is a goal worthy of pursuit.

Evaluation: A Broader View

Although novice nurse practitioners are not expected to assume administrative or nursing management responsibilities, they practice within a system that they must be familiar with. Nursing managers, as well as others responsible for the effectiveness of health care delivery systems, are experiencing increasing pressures to demonstrate commitment to improved client care. As a result, evaluation has become "an open-ended and continuous variable aiding growth and change in outcomes," rather than remaining a closure for a process.[9] Because nurses are becoming increasingly accountable for their practice, as in primary care, a broader view of evaluation is necessary.

Approaches to Evaluation

A view of nursing evaluation that addresses and goes beyond changes in the client's condition encompasses three approaches: structure, process, and outcome.[7] These three approaches are reflected as evaluation criteria in the Standards of Psychiatric and Mental Health Nursing Practice enunciated by the Division on Psychiatric and Mental Health Nursing Practice of the American Nurses' Association.

Structure

An evaluation of structure includes a consideration of the purpose of the health care facility, organizational characteristics, fiscal resources and management, qualifications of health care personnel, physical facilities and equipment, and the facility's status regarding accreditation or approval by appropriate bodies. The public usually assumes that these structural attributes are related to the quality of client care; however, this assumption does not obviate the need to evaluate the care clients actually receive.

Nurses have traditionally been more involved in process-and-outcome evaluation than in structure evaluation. Nevertheless, structural attributes, such as written policies and procedures, job descriptions, and the availability of supervision, consultation, and continuing education, have a very strong influence on the nature of nursing care provided in a facility.

Process

Evaluation of the process of care entails an appraisal of all major and significant minor steps in the care of the client. In this type of appraisal, the standards of practice of the profession serve as the basis for judgments of quality.[15] The American Nurses' Association has established general Standards of Nursing Practice to fulfill the nursing profession's obligation to provide and improve practice in any setting.[1] The Standards, utilizing a systematic approach to nursing practice, provide a means for determining the quality of nursing care received by the client.

The Division on Psychiatric and Mental Health Nursing Practice of the American Nurses' Association has also identified Standards of Psychiatric and Mental Health Nursing Practice. They too reflect the steps of the nursing process and are accompanied by rationale and lists of structure, process, and outcome criteria that are useful in measuring the achievement of each standard. The Standards of Psychiatric and Mental Health Nursing Practice are presented in Chart 11-1.

Whether nurses use these standards or develop their own guidelines for practice, a process approach to evaluation reflects the assumption that the process of care (*e.g.*, discussing client-related data and reviewing clinical practice with peers) is directly related to general or specific outcomes of care for clients.

Outcome

Evaluation of the outcomes of care centers on the end results of care.[15] Outcomes are, in fact, the ultimate validators of care.[7] Evaluation of outcomes focuses on the status of the client following assessment, diagnosis, and a specific period of nursing and other health care intervention. As discussed earlier in this chapter, it is often difficult to specify those nursing activities that are directly related to client care outcomes, such as the client's acquisition of knowledge and self-care activity. Nurses are challenged, nevertheless, to analyze and document nursing actions that make a difference in the client's situation or condition.

Quality Assurance in Nursing

Quality assurance is the delivery of health care to all individuals at the optimum level of excellence and the persistent endeavor to obtain continued improvement.[13] Quality assurance focuses on what should be done to achieve desired objectives. The American public has become increasingly concerned that health care be appropriate and acceptable, as well as available and accessible. Federal legislation, which is intended to prevent the unnecessary utilization of costly resources, has reflected this concern for quality. The

CHART 11-1
Standards of Psychiatric and Mental Health Nursing Practice

Standard I. Theory

The nurse applies appropriate theory that is scientifically sound as a basis for decisions regarding nursing practice.

Standard II. Data Collection

The nurse continuously collects data that are comprehensive, accurate, and systematic.

Standard III. Diagnosis

The nurse utilizes nursing diagnoses and standard classifications of mental disorders to express conclusions supported by recorded assessment data and current scientific premises.

Standard IV. Planning

The nurse develops a nursing care plan with specific goals and interventions delineating nursing actions unique to each client's needs.

Standard V. Intervention

The nurse intervenes as guided by the nursing care plan to implement nursing actions that promote, maintain, or restore physical and mental health, prevent illness, and effect rehabilitation.

Standard V-A. Psychotherapeutic Interventions

The nurse (generalist) uses psychotherapeutic interventions to assist clients to regain or improve their previous coping abilities and to prevent further disability.

Standard V-B. Health Teaching

The nurse assists clients, families, and groups to achieve satisfying and productive patterns of living through health teaching.

Standard V-C. Self-Care Activities

The nurse uses the activities of daily living in a goal-directed way to foster adequate self-care and physical and mental well-being of clients.

Standard V-D. Somatic Therapies

The nurse uses knowledge of somatic therapies and applies related clinical skills in working with clients.

Standard V-E. Therapeutic Environment

The nurse provides, structures, and maintains a therapeutic environment in collaboration with the client and other health care providers.

Standard V-F. Psychotherapy

The nurse (specialist) utilizes advanced clinical expertise in individual, group, and family psychotherapy, child psychotherapy, and other treatment modalities to function as a psychotherapist and recognizes professional accountability for nursing practice.

Standard VI. Evaluation

The nurse evaluates client responses to nursing actions in order to revise the data base, nursing diagnoses, and nursing care plan.

Standard VII. Peer Review

The nurse participates in peer review and other means of evaluation to assure quality of nursing care provided for clients.

Standard VIII. Continuing Education

The nurse assumes responsibility for continuing education and professional development and contributes to the professional growth of others.

Standard IX. Interdisciplinary Collaboration

The nurse collaborates with interdisciplinary teams in assessing, planning, implementing, and evaluating programs and other mental health activities.

Standard X. Utilization of Community Health Systems

The nurse (specialist) participates with other members of the community in assessing, planning, implementing, and evaluating mental health services and community systems that include the promotion of the broad continuum of primary, secondary, and tertiary prevention of mental illness.[2]

Standard XI. Research

The nurse contributes to nursing and the mental health field through innovations in theory and practice and participation in research.

(Reprinted with permission from the American Nurses' Association)

Social Security Amendments of 1972 mandated professional review of health care delivered to recipients of Medicare, Medicaid, and Maternal and Child Health Programs through Professional Standards Review Organizations.

Professional Standards Review Organizations (PSROs) were created to serve as external control mechanisms for quality assurance. The PSROs involve local practicing physicians in ongoing review and evaluation of health care services; they reflect the belief that effective peer review at the local level is the best method for assuring the appropriate use of health care resources and facilities. Although a review of nursing care is not a specific legal mandate, the implications are present. Professional Standards Review Organizations are expected to provide evidence over time that nonphysician health care practitioners have become involved in the development of standards for their areas of practice, peer review mechanisms, and continuing education that reflect evaluation of care. Nurses and nursing care must be an integral part of any quality assurance program.

Quality assurance in nursing is an effort requiring the time and commitment of nurses. The exact process will be unique to the health care facility and the individuals who practice there. Generally, several steps must be taken:

1. Identifying desirable outcomes for defined populations of clients
2. Relating the nursing process to these outcomes
3. Using established guidelines to assess the care actually given

Nurses have already developed tools and methods designed to assure the quality of nursing care.

Components of a Quality Assurance Program

The tools and methods used by nurses to assure the quality of nursing care generally provide for either concurrent evaluation or periodic retrospective evaluation. *Concurrent evaluation* takes place while the client is receiving care; *periodic evaluation* occurs retrospectively, or after the fact, such as monthly or quarterly.

Concurrent evaluation, which focuses on both processes and outcomes of care, continually compares the planned for, or expected, result with what is actually being accomplished.[13] Bases for concurrent evaluation include, but are not limited to, nursing histories, nursing care plans, problem-oriented records or other nursing notes, nursing rounds, and client feedback. One retrospective evaluation tool is the nursing audit. The *nursing audit* is a method for evaluating quality of care through appraisal of the nursing process as it is reflected in the client care records for discharged clients. Both concurrent and retrospective evaluation methods or tools may be combined in a systematic manner to become a quality assurance program. Each method will be briefly discussed in relation to its quality control function. Froebe and Bain conceptualize a quality assurance program (QAP) "package" that is shown in Fig. 11-2.

Nursing History

The inclusion of the nursing history in a quality assurance program is necessitated by the fact that it provides the base for other components in the program. This logical data gathering technique culminates in an original nursing assessment of client problems from which the problem-oriented record or care plan develops. Clients, families, other health care team members, and earlier records are major resources for the nursing history. The nursing history should be concise and comprehensive; data should clearly support the identified problems.

Problem-Oriented Records

Kerr asserts that "the primary reason for the existence of the hospital chart is to record problems and solutions, *i.e.,* that care of the client."[12] *Problem-oriented records* (POR), a concept that is implemented by all persons contributing to the client's care, have four components:

1. A defined data base
2. The problem list
3. The initial plan
4. The progress notes[13]

The nursing history provides information for the data base, from which client problems are identified. Additional problems are added to the list as they are identified. Problems may be socioeconomic and physical, as well as psychosocial. The problem-oriented method of charting assures that the client is viewed holistically by all members of the health care team. All data, health care interventions, and client responses can be found in one place on the client's record (*i.e.,* the progress notes) that are documented by the nurse, physician, and other health care professionals. These notes, written in the SOAP format (Subjective data, Objective data, Assessment, and Plan) reflect the client's response to care as well as the reasoning process for the plan of care. This systematic form facilitates both concurrent evaluation of client care and the retrospective evaluation of auditing the client's record. (See Chart 11-3, "Problem-Oriented Record.")

CHART 11-2
Advances in Computer Technology Ensure Quality

Sophisticated automated information systems can now enhance and streamline the quality assurance process in a health care facility. These systems provide a mechanism for assuring individual accountability, for tracking care activities for individual clients, and for comparing these activities with well-defined standards. An on-line, real-time medical record that can be manipulated by standard data processing tools quickly provides accurate data to health team members.

According to Mowry and Korpmann,[1] rapid and accurate data retrieval and concurrent quality analysis are possible with hospital information systems that use the following design principles:

1. Data should be entered at the source— terminals should be in the clients' rooms as well as at the nursing station.

2. Systems should be integrated, using a single, hospital-wide data base.
3. Systems should scan all normal client data to ensure performance and documentation and automatically flag abnormal or unexpected data for human intervention.

These design principles result in a client-based quality assurance approach that enables care givers to avoid problems, not to uncover them.

Advances in computer technology must be embraced to control health care costs and ensure quality. Effective automation will be not a luxury but a necessity for quality client care management in the future.

1. Mowry, MM, Korpmann RA: Automated Information Systems in Quality Assurance. Nursing Economics (September–October): 237–244, 1987

Nursing Rounds

"*Rounds,* by definition, are planned, purposeful excursions by administrators into a work area to experience and to see first hand the climate and interactions of staff within the client care delivery areas."[9] Direct encounters with clients and their care, as well as with the staff, provide nursing managers with feedback about the quality of care and the overall achievement of nursing goals.

Nursing rounds can also be made by nurses to formulate the client's plan of care. The nurse visits and interacts with each client to validate the plan, ask questions, answer questions, clarify misunderstandings, and evaluate progress. "There is nothing as reassuring as a nurse who takes the time with the rest of the nursing team to visit each client to update the nursing care plans...."[5] This reassurance is especially meaningful to clients with mental health problems.

Nursing Care Plans

A well written plan provides a central source of information about the patient and a description of his nursing needs....A nursing care plan does not insure optimal patient care, but it will never be attained without a plan.[11]

Care plans are an effective measure of accountability in nursing. Unfortunately, the use of care plans has not always been embraced by nurses. A well-written care plan takes time and intellectual effort and reflects continual practice. Nurses, for many reasons, do not always have these to give. Unless the situation is remedied by nurses, they may find it increasingly

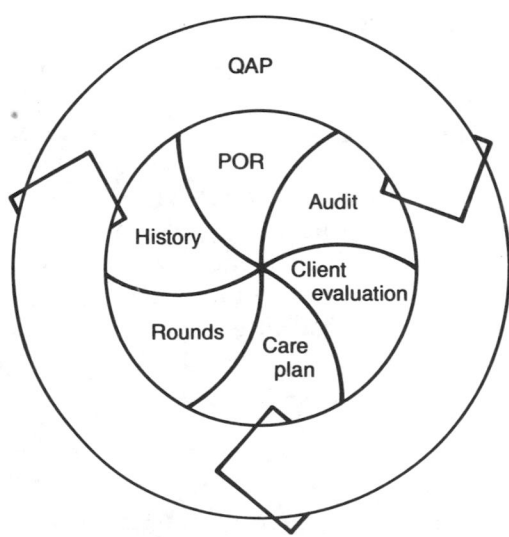

Figure 11-2. *Quality Assurance Program package concept.* (From Froebe DJ, Bain RJ: Quality Assurance Programs and Controls in Nursing. St Louis, CV Mosby, 1976)

CHART 11-3
Problem-Oriented Record

Problem List

Date	Problem #	Problems	Date Resolved
5/06/88	1	Self-destructive behavior related to rejection by husband and guilt associated with abandonment of children	
	2	Low self-esteem related to childhood rejection and unrealistic expectations of self	
	3	Inability to express anger related to fear of rejection	

Progress Notes

5/10/88	6:00 A.M.	#1 Self destructive

S—She says she is unable to sleep because she hates herself so much

O—Pacing in the hall; hair disheveled; in night clothes; talking to self at intervals

A—She is experiencing high level of anxiety, which may indicate an increase in suicide risk

P—Stay with the client and encourage verbalization of feelings; continue assessment of suicidal risk

Signature, R.N.

difficult to overcome the task-oriented image that has plagued the profession of nursing for so long. Nurses caring for clients with mental health problems must substantiate how they use a therapeutic milieu, the surrogate parent role, their knowlege of somatic therapies and related clinical skills, health teaching, and psychotherapeutic intervention in order to solve these problems.

Client Feedback

An accepted fact is that any successful business, to maintain its success, must know whether it is satisfying its consumer. Any business receiving its direction from sources other than its customers may be led to false conclusions and ultimate disaster.[9]

Nursing rounds have already been mentioned as one way of eliciting client feedback. Other methods

Nursing Care Plan 11-1

Evaluating Nursing Interventions

Nursing Diagnosis	Client Outcome	Intervention	Evaluation
Moderate anxiety possibility related to agitation and hospitalization The client was admitted with agitated depression, was unable to sit during the interview, and was fidgeting with clothes and necklace.	The client will verbalize her feelings concerning hospitalization.	Observe for behavioral symptoms of anxiety that may be expressed as muteness, hyperactivity, swearing, striking out, complaining, or crying. Observe for physiological symptoms of anxiety, such as tachycardia, increased blood pressure, increased respirations, decreased peristalsis, vasoconstriction, sweating, dry mouth, or dilated pupils. Use therapeutic communication techniques. Explain the unit routine to the client and enlist participation in all aspects of care. Encourage visits from significant others. Include family in the provision of care, when possible, and as they express a desire to participate.	Outcome is not met; client has less interaction with health care team since initial assessment, speaks only when spoken to, frequently stares out the window, and cries during the evening. Continue interventions. Additional nursing actions: Observe for an increase in depression (apathy, decreased ability to concentrate, insomnia, fatigue, anorexia). Spend at least 15 to 30 minutes with the client in am and pm. Specifically use techniques of silence, directing, reflection, and clarification during interactions Show acceptance by encouraging free verbalization of anger and other feelings.
Possible nutritional deficit due to anorexia The client is on a regular diet; weighs 115 lbs., is 5'5".	The client will attain adequate nutritional intake by eating at least half of each offered meal.	Offer small frequent feedings with supplemental high-protein nourishments. Encourage oral hygiene before and after meals. Maintain an attractive environment during meals.	The outcome is currently met; client is maintaining weight. Continue interventions and stay with client during meals.

can be used as well. A well-structured questionnaire given to clients and their families can formalize opinions so they are not lost to those who could do most with the information. Meetings with groups of clients can be held to explore client perceptions regarding all aspects of care and to address issues as they arise. Discharge interviews and suggestion boxes on psychiatric–mental health units can also be used to elicit feedback.

Nurses who ask for client feedback are risk-takers. They may get more than they bargained for; they may also be pleasantly surprised. Most important, they may learn how to improve client care. Feedback is not used to assign blame but to appraise care and identify areas for improvement. Defensiveness in response to client feedback is a confusing message, one that is especially inimical in a psychiatric care setting.

Nursing Audit

The nursing audit is a means of looking into the charts of discharged clients to appraise the type of care they received. For this reason, it may be difficult to determine whether deficiencies in nursing care lie in the documentation of the care or in the actual care. The nursing audit centers on professional standards or processes that have been developed internally or adopted and, perhaps, adapted from an external source. The American Nurses' Association, the National League for Nursing, and the Joint Commission for Accreditation of Hospitals have all developed guides for periodic nursing audits.

The focus of the nursing audit is on the client and his nursing care. Nurses or peer reviewers make the final appraisal of the "extent to which nursing care has measured up to the characteristics that are specified."[8] The nurses' records and care plans are examined to determine the completeness and accuracy of all phases of the nursing process. To exemplify the client care focus, six points are included in the audit plan of the Joint Commission of Accreditation of Hospitals:

1. Establishment of criteria for patient care
2. Comparison of criteria and actual practices
3. Analysis of actual practice findings
4. Corrective action
5. Follow-up studies to determine whether the corrective action was effective
6. Report of the results of the audit activity to those to whom one is accountable, with accompanying notations describing the actions of the governing body in response to all the foregoing[10]

In addition to delineating professional responsibility, the nursing audit has other uses. It can serve as an educational tool and team builder within and across professional disciplines. The criteria developed by those practicing in the facility determine definite goals for client progress. A final use of the nursing audit is the way in which audit criteria become the focus for uniformity of planning and recording.[3]

Summary

Evaluation has been presented as an essential but sometimes elusive component of the nursing care provided for clients with mental health problems. The information presented in this chapter includes the following:

1. The manifestations and long-term nature of mental illness, as well as the artful and collaborative qualities of psychiatric care, work against "cause and effect" appraisals.
2. The broader and timely issue of self-regulation aims to assure quality in professional performance.
3. Approaches to evaluation—structure, process, and outcome—are related to quality assurance programs, the goal of which is improvement in health care.
4. Nursing histories, problem-oriented records, nursing rounds, nursing care plans, client feedback, and nursing audits all are tools or methods that can be used by nurses to maintain quality of care.

References

1. American Nurses' Association: Standards of Nursing Practice. Kansas City, MO, American Nurses Association, 1973
2. American Nurses' Association: Standards of Psychiatric and Mental Health Nursing Practice. Kansas City, MO, Division on Psychiatric and Mental Health Nursing, 1982
3. Betts V: Using Psychiatric Audit as One Aspect of a Quality Assurance Program. In Kneisel C, Wilson H (ed): Current Perspectives in Psychiatric Nursing, Vol II, pp 202–208. St Louis, CV Mosby, 1978
4. Blackwell BL, Bolman WM: The Principles and Problems of Evaluation. Community Ment Health J 13 (February): 175–186, 1977
5. Bower FL: The Process of Planning Nursing Care: A Theoretical Model. St Louis, CV Mosby, 1972
6. Debski-Himberger A: A Quality Assurance Pro-

gram for Psychiatric Nursing. Supervisor Nurse 11 (November): 25–26, 1980

7. Donabedian A: A Guide to Medical Care Administration, Vol II. New York, American Public Health Association, 1969

8. Donabedian A: Some Issues in Evaluating the Quality of Nursing Care. Am J Public Health 59 (October): 1833–36, 1969

9. Froebe DJ, Bain RJ: Quality Assurance Programs and Controls in Nursing. St Louis, CV Mosby, 1976

10. Joint Commission on Accreditation of Hospitals: Accreditation Manual for Hospitals. Chicago, The Commission, 1970

11. Kelly N: Nursing Care Plans. Nursing Outlook 14 (May): 61–64, 1966

12. Kerr AH: Nursing Notes, That's Where the Goodies Are. Nursing, 75 (February): 34–41, 1975

13. Kron T: The Management of Patient Care, 5th ed. Philadelphia, WB Saunders, 1981

14. Miller TW, Lee LI: Quality Assurance: Focus on Environmental Perceptions of Psychiatric Patients and Nursing Staff. J Psychiatr Nurs 18 (December): 9–14, 1980

15. Phaneuf MC: The Nursing Audit: Profile for Excellence. New York, Appleton-Century-Crofts, 1972

16. Phaneuf MC: The Nursing Audit: Self Regulation in Nursing Practice. New York, Appleton-Century-Crofts, 1976

17. Ryan LJ, Gearhart MK, Simmons S: From Personal Responsibility to Professional Accountability in Psychiatric Nursing. J Psychiatr Nurs 15 (June): 19–24, 1977

18. Yura H, Walsh M: The Nursing Process: Assessing, Planning, Implementing, Evaluating, 3d ed. New York, Appleton-Century-Crofts, 1978

PART 3

Intervention Modes

12   Milieu Therapy

Judith A. Greene

Once from a big, big building,
When I was small, small
The queer folk in the windows
Would smile at me and call.

And in the hard wee gardens
Such pleasant men would hoe:
"Sir, may we touch the little girl's hair!"
It was so red, you know.

They cut me coloured asters
With shears so sharp and neat,
They brought me grapes and plums and pears
And pretty cakes to eat.

And out of all the windows,
No matter where we went,
The merriest eyes would follow me
And make me compliment.

There were a thousand windows.
All latticed up and down.
And up to all the windows,
When we went back to town,

The queer folk put their faces,
As gentle as could be;
"Come again, little girl!" they called, and I
Called back, "You come see me!"

Edna St. Vincent Millay,
A Visit to the Asylum

Chapter Preview

This chapter defines concepts related to the creation and maintenance of a therapeutic milieu in the hospital setting. Components, characteristics, and goals of a therapeutic milieu are described, and functions of the mental health team are delineated. Furthermore, the role of the nurse and the use of the nursing process in milieu therapy are discussed. Some basic guidelines for managing and coordinating a therapeutic milieu, or milieu therapy, are introduced and then illustrated with case examples.

Learning Objectives

On completion of this chapter, you should be able to accomplish the following:

1. discuss concepts related to the creation and maintenance of a therapeutic milieu
2. identify the components, characteristics, and goals of a therapeutic milieu
3. describe the functions and humanistic attributes of a mental health team
4. discuss the nurse's role and functions within the therapeutic milieu
5. apply general guidelines for facilitating a therapeutic milieu.

Therapeutic Milieu Defined and Described

Milieu is a French word meaning "middle place." In the English language, milieu means "environment" or "setting." As used in psychiatric—mental health nursing, it refers to the people and all other social and physical factors in the environment with which the client interacts.

More specifically, a *therapeutic milieu* is a 24-hour environment designed to provide a secure retreat for individuals whose capacities for coping with reality have deteriorated. The therapeutic milieu gives them opportunities to acquire adaptive coping skills. By offering secure, comfortable physical facilities for sleeping, dining, bathing, and engaging in recreational, occupational, social, psychiatric, and medical therapies, the therapeutic milieu does the following:

1. Shelters clients physically from what they perceive as painful, terrifying stressors
2. Protects clients physically from discharges of their own and others' maladaptive behaviors
3. Supports the physiological existence of clients

4. Provides pleasant, attractive sensory stimulation to clients
5. Educates clients and their families about adaptive, effective coping

To accomplish the preceding goals, the therapeutic milieu must contain caring, concerned, intelligent persons who can work together effectively as a mental health team. A mental health team is composed of nurses, occupational and recreational therapists, social workers, psychiatric nurse clinical specialists, psychologists, psychiatrists, pastoral counselors, paraprofessionals, and other mental health workers. All these people working together create a therapeutic milieu—a healing environment.

Characteristics of a Therapeutic Milieu

The overall goal of the mental health team within a hospital setting is to maintain and create a therapeutic milieu characterized by eight elements.

Individual Treatment Programs

A therapeutic milieu is tailored to the client's individual needs as much as possible without infringing on the needs and rights of other clients and mental health team members. Nevertheless, a definite structure, schedule, overall guidelines, and social controls are set forth to provide organization and predictability.

Self-Governance

To avoid the cultivation of dependence and regression, a therapeutic milieu must provide some formal mechanism whereby clients participate in decision-making regarding milieu issues. Structured community meetings, client-team meetings. or client-team committee meetings held at regularly scheduled intervals are examples of approaches used to elicit client involvement in milieu decisions. Furthermore, involving clients in such approaches enables them to exert a therapeutic influence upon the environment and each other.

Progressive Levels of Responsibility

In a therapeutic milieu, clients are expected to assume a responsible role in the maintenance of the environment. The degree of responsibility expected of clients is commensurate with their capabilities. Matching expected responsibilities with client capabilities promotes feelings of self-responsibility in clients.

A variety of approaches may be used to assist clients in becoming self-responsible. One approach is to use a level system, designating what clients must do to earn a specific set of privileges. This approach is a form of behavior modification in that it rewards and reinforces adaptive behavior. Assignment of clients to levels is primarily the responsibility of the mental health team; however, comments from clients during community meetings about their peers' readiness for changes in levels of responsibility are taken into consideration in making level assignments. Table 12-1 presents a sample level system.

A Variety of Meaningful Activities

To minimize social withdrawal and regression, a therapeutic milieu must provide each client with an individual activity schedule. Such activities may include structured exercise classes, jogging, training in interpersonal skills (*e.g.,* assertiveness training, listening, parenting), grooming classes, arts, crafts, relaxation training and stress management classes, dance classes, cookouts, and work and occupational therapies.

Links with the Client's Family

In addition to providing refuge to clients, a therapeutic milieu also provides opportunities for clients to re-enter the mainstream of family life at their own pace. Links with the family may be accomplished in several ways. Family visits can be incorporated into the overall therapeutic milieu program by including family members in selected milieu activities. Involving family members in this manner may necessitate "on-the-spot" family counseling from time to time to help clients and their families work through the conflicts and problems that inevitably arise during visits. This brief, "on-the-spot" family counseling is directed toward helping clients and their families acquire more adaptive modes of relating to each other.

Including family members in selected milieu activities, such as mental health classes, interpersonal skills classes, and medication classes, enables mental health team members to observe family dynamics and to model adaptive interpersonal behaviors to both clients and their families. It is to be hoped that providing such links with the family will decrease the likelihood of clients' becoming institutionalized to the hospital, while also helping clients and their families interact more effectively.

Links with the Community

Activities occurring outside the structured milieu, such as shopping trips, picnics, hikes, camping trips, visiting museums and zoos, and attending concerts,

Table 12-1. Progressive Levels of Responsibility According to Client's Self-Care Capacity

CLASSIFICATION LEVEL	*Characteristics of Clients Assigned to This Level*	*Requirement(s) for Progression to Next Level*
Severely limited self-care capacity	Display injurious behavior Disoriented as to time, place, and person Unable to function in group therapy Exhibit poor personal hygiene	No longer exhibit severely limited self-care capacity
Level I	Do not display dangerous behavior Know the current date, time, and place Attend at least one therapeutic group daily Attempt to maintain good personal hygiene and grooming	Know the names of their primary nurse, physician, and at least three names of other mental health personnel Attend at least three assigned activities
Level II	Successfully complete requirements for progression to this level and consistently maintain this level of performance	Attend all therapeutic activities Participate actively in community meetings and serve on at least one client committee Develop a self-directed behavior plan to change or resolve a personal problem Know the names of all medications and the times they are due Participate in a family session
Level III	Successfully complete requirements for progression to this level and consistently maintain this level of performance	Take an active role in assisting other clients to gain level changes Demonstrate willingness to serve as an officer on the client committee Assume a leadership role in the community, act as a positive role model, and ensure that other clients are prompt in their attendance of regularly scheduled activities and group meetings Initiate with the mental health team discussions concerning discharge planning

plays, and movies, serve to link clients to community life. Participating in such activities with mental health team members helps clients develop the social skills and confidence needed to re-enter the community. Additionally, such activities provide clients with opportunities to acquire or rekindle enjoyable leisure-time or cultural interests. Establishing links with the community demonstrates to clients that they can once again be active participants in the world about them.

Effective Working Relationships Among Mental Health Team Members

Interpersonal conflict occasionally occurs in any group of people. A mental health team, like all groups, experiences such conflicts. Consequently, mental health team members must have the ability to resolve interpersonal conflicts effectively and promptly. If mental health team members cannot do so, then the effectiveness of the therapeutic milieu may decline to the point where clients are placed in serious jeopardy. When mental health team members can engage in effective conflict resolution, they are more likely to trust each other and to act and interact as a mental health team and not as "lone therapists." Furthermore, mental health team members who can resolve interpersonal conflicts are effective role models for clients.

Humanistic Mental Health Team Members

For a therapeutic milieu program to be effective, mental health team members need to possess high degrees of the following attributes:

Optimistic attitudes toward people in general

The ability to inspire hopefulness in clients and team members

Creativity in working toward more effective ways of involving clients and team members in the environment

Lack of fear or prejudice when confronted with persons exhibiting unconventional or aberrant behaviors

Willingness to maintain frequent personal contacts with clients on a daily basis[9]

The ability to set limits on their own behavior and the behavior of others in a nonpunitive manner

Willingness to share control and decision-making with team members and clients

The belief that controls and limits should be provided by people to the greatest extent possible, rather than by locked doors, physical restraints, or psychochemotherapeutic agents.

Facilitating a Therapeutic Milieu: Milieu Therapy

Components of a Therapeutic Milieu

Comfortable, secure physical facilities, the mental health team, and the therapeutic milieu program are the three essential components of a therapeutic milieu. These essential components enable the milieu to exert a therapeutic influence upon clients. In other words, the total milieu, not just one component or mental health team member, is the therapeutic agent. The total milieu acting as the primary therapeutic agent is referred to as *milieu therapy*.

Milieu therapy is a group therapy approach that uses a total living experience—recreational, occupational, psychosocial, psychiatric, nursing, and medical therapies, plus mental health team–client relationships—to accomplish therapeutic objectives.[6,12] These therapeutic objectives in the broadest sense include helping clients to achieve the following goals:

1. Correct or redefine their perceptions of stressors
2. Correct maladaptive coping behavioral patterns
3. Develop adaptive coping behavioral patterns[6]
4. Acquire interpersonal and stress management skills in order to conduct themselves more effectively in the environment and strengthen or correct their coping abilities
5. Generalize what they learn about themselves, other people, and adaptive coping behavior to situations they encounter upon leaving the therapeutic milieu

Facilitating a therapeutic milieu that helps clients reach these objectives requires management of the environment and coordination of the mental health team's collaborative efforts.

It is important for the therapeutic milieu, which is a microcosm of society, to match the client's cultural background. The absence of such a match can create even greater cognitive dissonance or conflict within the client. Therefore, before recommending milieu therapy, mental health team members must ascertain that the therapeutic milieu is, to some extent, compatible with the client's cultural background. For example, it would be more destructive than helpful to recommend a milieu therapy program reflecting the religious values of the Roman Catholic Church to a client who is a devout Orthodox Jew. Similarly, a therapeutic milieu needs to reflect to a great extent the socioeconomic values held by its clients and mental health team members.

CHART 12-1
Managing and Coordinating the Therapeutic Milieu

Direct Client Care

Manages the day-to-day care of individual clients
Assists in contributing to the formulation and implementation of
    individualized treatment plans for clients: assessment, diagnosis,
    planning, implementation, and evaluation, including plans for dis-
    charge and re-entry into the community

Indirect Client Care

Maintains ongoing communication with other mental health team
    members
Enforces rules, policies and regulations of the therapeutic milieu
Maintains cooperative, supportive working relationships with other
    mental health team members
Schedules, assigns, manages, and evaluates clinical work
Conducts quality assurance studies to improve client care and the
    effectiveness of the therapeutic milieu

Nursing in the Therapeutic Milieu

Applying the Nursing Process

Traditionally, nurses have assumed responsibility for managing and coordinating milieu activities.[11] Viewing clients from a holistic, rather than fragmented, frame of reference enables nurses to fulfill these responsibilities. In other words, unlike many other mental health team members, nurses possess the knowledge and skills to help clients meet their physiological, psychosocial, and spiritual needs. Furthermore, because nurses maintain 24-hour contact with clients, they have greater opportunities to assume management and coordination responsibilities than do other mental health team members (see Chart 12-1).

To manage and coordinate a therapeutic milieu effectively, nurses use the nursing process to assess clients within the milieu, plan and implement milieu strategies, and evaluate client as well as milieu outcomes. More specifically, nurses assess the physiological and psychological states of each client within the milieu. Making these assessments on a continuing basis enables nurses to play a major role in the individualization of clients' treatment plans and activity schedules. Assessing the influence of the milieu on each client and the influence of each client on the milieu is another important aspect of the nursing role in the therapeutic milieu. Such assessments are invaluable in helping the mental health team understand the group dynamics of the milieu and select and implement appropriate milieu strategies and activities. Other ways in which nurses contribute to the management and coordination of the therapeutic milieu include the following:

Providing physical and safety care
Administering medication
Providing psychosocial care
Teaching mental health

Providing Physical and Safety Care. To meet physical care needs, nurses assess the extent to which clients are able to engage in daily living activities—eating, eliminating, bathing, dressing, and so forth. For example, some clients may require considerable assistance with daily living activities; other clients, however, may be entirely self-sufficient in these tasks. In any event, nurses are responsible for assessing client abilities in this area and implementing, directly or indirectly, an individual treatment plan designed to reinforce or promote client independence in performing daily living activities. Another important nursing care function is assessing the physical status of clients in order to detect signs of physical illness or adverse physical reactions to rigorous activity schedules (see Charts 12-2, 12-3, and 12-4).

To meet safety care needs, nurses assess the extent to which clients display self-destructive or other destructive behaviors. Clients who have these tendencies require unobtrusive surveillance by nurses. Unobtrusive surveillance involves visually observing the client at least every 15 minutes until the destructive tendencies are no longer present. Additionally, nurses are responsible for ensuring that the physical environment is safe for clients with such tendencies.

C H A R T 12-2
Providing Physical Care: Hygiene and Self-Care

Nursing Diagnosis	Goal	Desired Client Outcome	Nursing Action
Alteration in physical hygiene pattern, due to low self-esteem and social withdrawal	To become independent in hygiene and self-care	Bathe daily Brush teeth at least twice daily Wear clean clothes each day Do washing and ironing Comb hair neatly Shave daily	Teach the client hygiene and self-care skills by means of formal or informal classes Gently confront the client regarding hygiene and self-care behaviors Offer kind, consistent encouragement to the client in attempts to become more independent in self-care Act as a role model by following appropriate hygiene and grooming habits Guide the client verbally and nonverbally, with gradual withdrawal of assistance until client becomes independent in self-care Use peer group pressure as appropriate Positively reinforce signs suggestive of progress in hygiene and self-care

Administering Medication. In the therapeutic milieu, as in other hospital settings, nurses manage the administration of medications. Some of the methods used to administer medications, however, differ significantly from those used in other hospital settings. For example, in the therapeutic milieu, nurses are often expected to gain the client's informed consent prior to administering psychotropic medications. This process involves explaining in general terms the desired and undesired effects of the psychotropic drugs to be administered as well as the dose, frequency, time, and route of administration. The client is encouraged to ask questions about any aspect of medication administration and may, in fact, decline to take prescribed psychotropic medication.

Approaching medication administration in this manner not only shows respect to the client but also provides a logical point for medication teaching to begin. More importantly, using this approach is more likely to gain clients' acceptance of their medication because they are allowed to participate actively in this important aspect of treatment.

Another way in which medication administration differs in the therapeutic milieu is that clients are often expected to approach the nurse for their medication at specific times and places. In some progressive settings, capable clients are given responsibility for administering their own medications. For example, a responsible client may be given a 24-hour supply of medication to take independently in the milieu setting. Successful completion of this assignment would thereby demonstrate the client's readiness to assume self-care with regard to medication administration. Whatever methods are used, however, the goal is to help clients assume responsibility for taking their own medications. Nurses can assist clients to

C H A R T   12-3
Providing Physical Care: Nutrition

Nursing Diagnosis	Goal	Desired Client Outcomes	Nursing Action
Alteration in nutritional pattern related to client's paranoid ideation, as evidenced by client's 10-pound weight loss and belief that his food has been poisoned	To establish adequate dietary intake	Eat at least 75% of each meal Cease stating that the food is poisoned Gain one pound each week until he reaches his desired body weight	Serve meals buffet style Point out that all plates are filled from the same containers Taste client's food to demonstrate that it is safe to eat Unobtrusively observe client's intake and output and assess actual and potential weight loss Invite client to assist with community cookout

C H A R T   12-4
Providing Physical Care: Sleep

Nursing Diagnosis	Goal	Desired Client Outcome	Nursing Action
Alteration in sleep-wakefulness cycle, as evidenced by client's insomnia for 4 consecutive nights	To establish adequate sleep pattern	Sleep 4 to 5 hours without waking for seven consecutive nights and without use of sedative/hypnotics	Provide a restful, quiet environment free of external stressors Encourage a warm bath before bedtime Encourage client to read soothing, inspirational literature Provide relaxation therapy before bedtime Provide bedtime snack high in natural amino acid, L-tryptophan, *i.e.,* warm milk or cheese slice (if not taking MAO inhibitor) Allow the client to stay up, if indicated, and provide quiet activities

reach this goal by providing a caring and human approach to medication administration and medication teaching.

Providing Psychosocial Care. Providing psychosocial care to clients consumes the greatest proportion of nursing time and effort in a therapeutic environment.[3] To provide such care, nurses engage in a variety of helping behaviors. One area of helping behavior involves reducing stressors that may be perceived as psychonoxious by some clients. To illustrate, loud voices, televisions or radios, unsightly visual stimuli, and crowded spaces may be psychonoxious to schizophrenic clients who are hypersensitive to external stimuli.[1] Reducing the frequency and intensity of perceptual stressors experienced by such clients may be helpful.[7]

Encouraging clients to express their problems and conflicts, to attempt to understand them, and to experiment with new ways of handling problems and conflicts constitutes another form of psychosocial care offered by nurses in the therapeutic milieu. To provide this care, nurses may use informal group interventions such as community meetings and structured or unstructured group therapy sessions to assist clients with problems in their current life situations.

Conducting brief, "on-the-spot" counseling with clients and families to help them deal with problems arising during visits is another important aspect of the nursing role. Periodically, nurses may also need to engage in limit-setting in order to help clients deal with behaviors destructive to the self, others, or the environment (see Chart 12-5). Other helping behaviors important to the nursing role include helping clients use their time productively for leisure and work, involving withdrawn clients in the milieu, encouraging clients who have low self-esteem to value themselves, and serving as a role model by demonstrating interpersonal effectiveness in relating to clients and other mental health team members.

One-to-One Therapy. Another important aspect of the psychosocial care provided by nurses in a thera-

---

C H A R T   12-5
Providing Psychological Care: Limit-Setting on Maladaptive Group Behavior

Nursing Diagnosis	Goal	Desired Client Outcomes	Nursing Action
Dysfunctional group behavior, as evidenced by conspirant manipulative behavior: A group of clients conspired to receive extra privileges by requesting them from various mental health team members; they then attempted to pit staff members against each other by repeating different versions of staff responses	To become more functional as a group, evidenced by honest and open interactions	Trust staff, as evidenced by direct communications Able to dissent in a responsible manner Tolerate denial of requests with no passive–aggressive reactions	Initiate a mental health team meeting to discuss the problem and arrive at a group decision regarding milieu strategy Initiate a community meeting to share mental health team's assessment of the problem Inform the group that each client will be assigned to one specific team member and that seeking extra privileges from other team members will not be allowed Confront client every time he or she attempts to revert to former behavior pattern Initiate subsequent mental health team and community meetings if inconsistencies arise

peutic milieu is one-to-one therapy. Clients in a therapeutic milieu may have one or more one-to-one therapy sessions daily with the nurse assigned to their care. The purpose of one-to-one therapy is to help clients achieve the following objectives:

- Clarify and correct their perceptions of current stressors
- Identify their thoughts and feelings
- Examine how their thoughts and feelings influence their behavior
- Evaluate the extent to which their coping behaviors are adaptive or effective
- Identify alternative adaptive coping strategies
- Test identified alternative coping strategies in the therapeutic milieu

Working with clients in this manner allows them to experience empathetic understanding on a deep and meaningful level while developing the adaptive coping skills needed to re-enter their families and communities successfully.

Group Therapy. Nurses work with clients in small therapeutic groups on a daily basis to help them gain self-awareness about how they behave in groups. Clients also have the opportunity to develop and refine their social skills in therapeutic groups. More important, group therapy gives clients the opportunity to learn to trust others and to view themselves as trustworthy. By providing this form of psychosocial care, nurses help clients learn adaptive group roles and behaviors that can be generalized to group situations outside the therapeutic milieu. (For more information on this topic, see Chap. 14, "Groups and Group Therapy.")

Attitude Therapy. Psychosocial nursing care in the therapeutic milieu also includes the use of *attitude therapy*. This therapy is based on five fundamental attitudes:

1. Active friendliness, with which the client is helped to move out of his social withdrawal
2. Passive friendliness, when the nurse is available for interaction but makes no friendly overtures and merely waits for the client to make the first move
3. Kind firmness, by which the nurse directs the client into rewarding behaviors in a kind, yet persistent, manner
4. Matter-of-factness, or responding to the client in a calm, casual manner
5. No-demand, used especially when the client is in a state of panic or disintegration; nothing is expected of the client.[5]

Before attitude therapy is applied, each client's predominant behavioral style is identified. Then, nurses and other mental health team members jointly decide which of the preceding attitudes should be prescribed for each client. For example, passive friendliness might be prescribed for a highly suspicious client, whereas active friendliness might be used to draw out a client immobilized by feelings of worthlessness.[7] Although collaborative efforts by the mental health team are essential to implement attitude therapy effectively, the nursing role is the mainstay of this therapeutic approach (see Chart 12-6).

Mental Health Teaching. Mental health teaching is another important function of the nursing role in the therapeutic milieu. Mental health teaching that centers on psychotropic medications or methods of coping with psychiatric illnesses is often provided by nurses to clients and their families in order to increase their understanding of, and compliance with, treatment plans. Nurses and other mental health team members also teach classes focusing on interpersonal effectiveness (*e.g.*, assertiveness training, communication, problem-solving skills, parenting skills, and so forth) to clients and their families. Such classes help clients relate more effectively to others in the milieu and also help them prepare for their return to families, friends, and community. Similarly, involving families in such classes assists them to cope with and adapt to the client's changed behavior, and therefore prepares the family for the client's re-entry into the home and community.

A newer area of mental health teaching offered by nurses as well as by other mental health team members is stress management. In the therapeutic milieu, stress management focuses on helping clients learn to cope with stress through physical exercise, relaxation therapy, and enjoyable leisure-time pursuits. Engaging in these activities not only fosters a sense of well-being in clients but also cultivates self-confidence, self-control, and increased self-esteem. Added benefits of physical exercise include improved body image, weight loss, increased muscle tone, poise, and balance. In some instances, these activities also promote positive client-other social interactions.

Relaxation therapy, another useful method of coping with stress, is especially helpful for clients with psychiatric disorders characterized by maladaptive anxiety, *e.g.*, chemical dependence, anxiety and stress-related disorders, depressive reactions, and so forth. For example, progressive muscle relaxation, visual imagery, soothing auditory experiences, or massage, may produce favorable relaxation responses in clients.[2]

Relaxation therapy techniques can be taught in individual or group sessions. Usually, a mental health team member demonstrates the technique and then

C H A R T   12-6
Attitude Therapy

Client Behavior	Attitude Prescription
The client refused to do finger painting prescribed by the art therapist	The nurse used kind firmness by directing the client in activity; eventually the client complied
The client ran to his own room when he was enrolled in the mediation class	The nurse slowly followed the client to his room and then matter-of-factly told him to join the class; the client responded immediately
A tearful, dependent, depressed client continually criticized her self-care abilities	The nurse used a matter-of-fact approach in expressing the expectation that the client would perform self-care; avoided sympathizing with the client; the client became self-sufficient in self-care
A suspicious client refused to attend community meetings	The nurse used passive-friendliness by telling the client the time and place community meetings occurred; she told the client that she could come when she decided to do so; later, the client began attending community meetings on her own initiative

coaches clients in using it. The use of audio or video training cassettes to teach relaxation therapy techniques is common. Furthermore, the use of audiovisual aids gives clients who are skilled in the techniques the opportunity to practice relaxation on their own as needed.

Other Nursing Considerations

Depending on the organizational structure of the milieu, nurses may be responsible for developing individual nursing care plans, rather than contributing assessment data to an overall interdisciplinary treatment plan. In either case, however, nurses must function within the context of the total mental health team in order to manage and coordinate milieu activities in an effective, harmonious manner. Failure to do so can result in clients' pitting mental health team members against one another, thereby sabotaging the therapeutic milieu's effectiveness.

Usually, nurses are also responsible for making assignments for nursing and paraprofessional personnel. In making these assignments, nurses must re-

main cognizant of the overall purposes of the therapeutic milieu program, the client's individual needs, and the needs and capabilities of personnel. As much as possible, nurses need to avoid assigning personnel to clients who have exaggerated forms of problems similar to those that the mental health team members have and as yet have not identified and resolved. For example, a psychiatric–mental health nurse whose spouse has a substance abuse problem may tend to perceive and react to clients with similar problems as she does to her spouse. In this situation, the nurse would not only fail to respond to the client's uniqueness but also may tacitly support the client's substance abuse lifestyle. This type of perceptual distortion may be referred to as *countertransference.*

Moreover, although it would be ideal for personnel to be able to work with all clients, such an expectation is extravagant, if not totally unrealistic. Nurses and other personnel of the mental health team are human and therefore subject to many of the same life stressors and strains that affect clients. For this reason, nurses may find the following guidelines use-

CHART 12-7
Nursing Behaviors for a Therapeutic Milieu

Encourage clients to help and support each other individually and as a group.

Assist clients to understand each others' feelings and problems.

Conduct community meetings in which clients have the opportunity to discuss their concerns with each other and the mental health team, and if appropriate, give them the opportunity to determine group actions and rules.

Support community/group rules and actions by assisting clients to work through or overcome specific difficulties (*i.e.*, noncompliance with community or group decisions or rules; issues such as stealing, pranks, excessive noise).

Participate freely in milieu activities (*i.e.*, exercise, art, craft classes, social functions).

ful in implementing their role in the therapeutic milieu and in creating and maintaining the therapeutic milieu itself:

— Cultivate self-awareness through self-evaluation and the evaluations of supervisors and peers

— Relate to the emotionality of clients, team members, and the social climate of the therapeutic milieu without becoming overly involved or taking sides

— Be sensitive to the needs of all yet sensible enough to recognize your limits in attempting to meet the needs of others

— Communicate clearly and do not hesitate to seek clarification of others' communications, while always recognizing the possibility of miscommunication

— Always expect the unexpected, despite the best efforts and plans

Summary

This chapter has described the components of a therapeutic milieu, the milieu's role as the primary therapeutic agent, and the functions nurses perform in creating and maintaining a therapeutic milieu. The following information has been discussed:

1. From a stress-adaptation framework, clients may require milieu therapy in a hospital setting as a result of a decreased ability to cope with, and adapt to, life stressors.

2. The therapeutic milieu provides a temporary, safe haven from these life stressors, while offering clients opportunities to acquire adaptive coping behaviors; that is, the therapeutic milieu affords asylum, in the truest sense of the word, while simultaneously extending an invitation to clients to return to the mainstream of living and being in the world.

3. Essential characteristics of a therapeutic milieu include individual treatment programs, links with the client's family and community, effective relationships among members of the mental health team, and humanistic attributes of the mental health team members.

4. Milieu therapy is a group therapy approach that uses the client's total living experience as the primary therapeutic agent.

5. Nurses have traditionally assumed the responsibility for managing and coordinating therapeutic milieu activities; they also serve as a link between clients and the socially constructed reality of everyday life.

6. One important nursing function in the therapeutic milieu is mental health teaching (*e.g.*, information about psychotropic medications, psychiatric disorders, interpersonal and communication skills, stress management, relaxation therapy, and so forth).

7. Nurses in the therapeutic milieu must communicate by their every action and word, "Come, come join us in the world, you are welcome here."

References

1. Arieti S: Interpretation of Schizophrenia, 2d ed. New York, Basic Books, 1974

2. Bulechek GM, McCloskey JC: Nursing Intervention. Philadelphia, WB Saunders, 1985

3. Carleton EJ, Jonson JC: A Therapeutic Milieu for Borderline Patients. In Mereness D (ed): Psychiatric Nursing, Vol 1, 2d ed, pp 288–293. Dubuque, WC Brown, 1971

4. Gunderson JG, Will DA, Mosher LR (eds): Principles and Practice of Milieu Therapy. New York, Jason Aronson, 1983

5. Hayden LK, Hannah HD, Cozart NR: Attitudes in Action. Am J Nurs 69 (December), 2693–2695, 1966

6. Holmes MJ: Psychiatric Mental Health Nursing. In

Arieti S (ed): American Handbook of Psychiatry, Vol 5, 2d ed, pp 652–665. New York, Basic Books 1975

7. Jacobs AM, Brotz CA, Gamel NN: Critical Behaviors in Psychiatric–Mental Health Nursing. In Psychiatric–Mental Health Nursing, Vol. 2. Palo Alto, American Institutes for Research, 1973

8. Janosik EH, Phipps LB: Life Cycle Group Work in Nursing. Monterey, 1982

9. Linn L: Occupational Therapy and Other Therapeutic Activities. In Freeman AM, Kaplan HI, Sadock BJ (ed): Comprehensive Textbook of Psychiatry/III, Vol 2, 3rd ed, pp 2382–2390. Baltimore, Williams & Wilkins, 1980

10. Luker RF (ed): Partial Hospitalization. New York, Plenum Press, 1979

11. O'Toole AW: Psychiatric Nursing. In Freeman AM, Kaplan HI, Sadock BJ (eds): Comprehensive Textbook of Psychiatry/III, Vol 3, 3rd ed, pp 3001–3004. Baltimore, Williams & Wilkins, 1980

12. Robbins LL: The Hospital as a Therapeutic Community. In Freeman AM, Kaplan HI, Sadock BJ (eds): Comprehensive Textbook of Psychiatry/III, Vol 3, 3d ed, pp 2362–2368. Baltimore, Williams & Wilkins, 1980

13

Individual Psychotherapy

Joy. Randolph Davidson

With them it is as though an artist were to gather the hands, feet, head and other members for his images from diverse models, each part excellently drawn, but not related to a single body, and since they in no way match each other, the result would be a monster rather than man.

Copernicus,
De revolutionibus orbium
caelestium

In each of us, there was, like unused muscle and organs of the Spirit, courage and energy and responsibility never employed in our time in the world. The blessed one was he who confronted with a crisis in life was driven to call upon those resources, to use them to survive, even triumph over life itself. One so challenged and so triumphant had won the only prize that counted...the prize of the Maker of the spirit...the rebirth of a withering soul, and, as such, a Homeric victory over life's disaster.

Author Unknown

Chapter Preview

Psychotherapy is a method of facilitating change in a person's feelings, attitudes, and behaviors. For most of us, this is both intriguing and disturbing. The idea that major changes can be brought about by talking with another person seems almost like magic; it brings out hopes and fears in everyone.

People hope for more happiness and less pain. They fear changes in themselves and in the people they love. How will change, no matter how desirable it may be, affect important relationships? What does it mean in terms of time, effort and responsibility for the individual? What will the person have to do in therapy, and how can the habits and feelings of a lifetime be altered?

This chapter discusses how people can change in therapy by becoming able to use their own hopes, dreams, and strengths. Emphasis is placed on the origins of therapy, the evolution of therapeutic techniques, and the qualities that are necessary for effective therapy. Certain commonly used terms are defined and discussed in relation to the specific meanings and concepts they convey about the nature of human behavior.

Although psychotherapy is based, in large part, on Freudian theory, it is now viewed as a mixed discipline, the result of many contributions from many areas. Therapy is an open-ended process that continues throughout a person's life. New ways of perceiving, relating, and being are learned as life situations change and as the individual reaches new developmental stages.

Learning Objectives

On completing this chapter, you should be able to accomplish the following:

1. discuss the purposes of individual psychotherapy
2. describe levels and stages of psychotherapy
3. contrast social and therapeutic relationships
4. identify the qualities of an effective therapist
5. compare client and therapist expectations of therapy
6. discuss concepts of psychotherapy

What Is Psychotherapy?

Psychotherapy is the use of a group of techniques to modify feelings, attitudes, and behavior in people. The therapist uses both verbal and nonverbal means of communication to build a relationship with the client. The basic concept of therapy involves understanding—both self-understanding and being understood by another, to achieve relatedness and to relieve emotional pain.

Psychotherapy may be a treatment choice for a variety of reasons—to treat an emotional disorder, to deal with problems in people who would not be described as emotionally ill, to gain insight and self-knowledge, and to train people in the helping professions. Still other indications for therapy are the reduction of stress and the treatment of medical problems, especially those illnesses with psychosomatic features.

How does psychotherapy work? An onlooker might look at a therapy situation and see that two people meet and talk to each other very regularly over a period of time. One of the two people might seem to be very emotional—angry, happy, crying at times, and sometimes in despair. Nevertheless, these brief meetings, only an hour long, would appear to have profound effects on both the person and his family.

In therapy, two people come together in an encounter that is specifically designed for the purposes of relieving emotional pain, treating mental illness, and facilitating growth. The dialogue between them is focused on issues of great importance to the client. To enter therapy, most people must have a strongly perceived need to understand themselves, to make some kind of change in themselves, or to get relief from pain. Often, more than one of these factors motivates the client to enter therapy. In a therapy situation, one person is designated as the helping person and the other is called the client (*i.e.*, the person who is seeking help).

Specificity of purpose of the interaction, identification of the roles of therapist and client, and the use of primarily verbal means of communication mark the differences between psychotherapy and other human relationships. Nonverbal techniques used in therapy include the use of silence, body language, and facial expression, and respect for personal space.

Levels of Psychotherapy

The abilities, needs, and motivation of the client and the resources available to him help determine the level of psychotherapy in which he participates. These levels of therapy are generally classified as supportive, re-educative, and reconstructive.

Supportive Therapy

Supportive therapy allows the client to express feelings, explore alternatives, and make decisions in a safe,

CHART 13-1
Students and Therapy

Students sometimes work with psychiatric–mental health clients on a one-to-one basis in inpatient and outpatient settings. The students usually function as members of a treatment team and participate in carrying out a plan of care.

Members of the treatment team have input in planning and implementing client goals, and regularly provide feedback on client and team interaction. Within this setting, the nursing instructor acts as a resource person and supervisor to the student. Together, the treatment team and instructor provide direction and support for the student.

The central, or most important, element of therapy is the ongoing process that involves the client, the student, and the staff. By the term *process*, we mean the experience of self-discovery, understanding, and relating. This process extends to everyone involved and, in a truly therapeutic setting, leads to growth and self-actualization.

Students have a great deal to contribute to clients; they bring interest, concern, and caring to the clinical setting. Clients respond to this and often feel less threatened by students than they do by the professional staff.

Problems may arise because of the students' vulnerability and tendency to become over-involved with a client. Both of these tendencies are also related to the students' therapeutic qualities. Without empathy and concern, little therapy could occur.

As the clinical experience progresses, students often begin to realize that they and their family and friends are really not very different from the client. There is a common humanity and most human problems are similar. It is difficult for the student in the sense that she begins to question long-held values and beliefs and to wonder just how healthy she is. The student's personal problems often become more visible.

Over-identification with the client seems to be related to this awareness that we are not very different from each other. As increased self-awareness, recognition of similarities, and empathy occur, the student may develop very intense emotional ties with the client. Furthermore, the emphasis on congruence and positive regard will affect the student as it does the client. A staff member who has these qualities brings out feeling, and the student experiences a therapeutic environment in action.

The student needs to realize that her feelings and concerns are not "wrong" or "bad," but need to be shared with the nursing instructor and staff. This openness will keep the student–client relationship in a therapeutic framework and will help to relieve the student's anxiety.

A large part of the anxiety many students feel stems from the fear of harming the client. They often express this fear as "What if I say the wrong thing?" or "Do you think I said the right thing?" The student's fear or anxiety, therefore, relates to both the self and the client.

A student may want or need to work further on personal problems and may be referred for counseling. A need for counseling does not have to be considered a weakness. Insight, empathy, and therapeutic concern are typical of people in helping professions. Working out one's own problems allows for personal and professional growth.

---

caring relationship. It may be needed briefly or over a period of years. In supportive therapy, there is no plan to introduce new methods of coping; instead, the therapist reinforces the client's existing coping mechanisms.

Re-educative Therapy

Re-educative therapy involves learning new ways of perceiving and behaving. The client explores alternatives in a planned, systematic way, which requires a longer period of time. Often, the client enters into a contract that specifies desired changes in behavior. Changing a behavior may change the way in which the client perceives himself. Talking about alternative ways of coping opens up new options that the client may then try. Examples of re-educative therapy include short-term psychotherapy, reality therapy, cognitive restructuring, and behavior modification.

Reconstructive Therapy

Reconstructive therapy typically involves deep psychotherapy or psychoanalysis; it may take 2 to 5 or more years of time; and it delves into all aspects of the client's life. Emotional and cognitive restructuring of the self takes place. Positive outcomes of reconstructive therapy include greater understanding of self and others, more emotional freedom, development of potential abilities, and heightened capacity for love and work. The focus of this chapter is long-term, reconstructive therapy.

Stages of Psychotherapy

Introductory Stage

The introductory stage is the stage in which the client and therapist meet and begin to work together. This stage usually involves taking a history of the client's life, including any medical problems. It is important to realize that many physical illnesses resemble emotional problems and that the opposite is also true. Referrals or consultations may be indicated at this time to understand the problem.

The exploration of the client's background and problems should include any precipitating factors or events that caused him to seek help. The client should discuss his perceptions of his problems and needs and his expectations of therapy.

The therapist, during this introductory stage, forms some preliminary ideas about the client and his needs. Together, client and therapist discuss issues such as the length of time therapy will require, meeting dates, fees, and so forth. These issues are more fully described later in this chapter, in the section on client and therapist expectations.

During the introductory phase, the client and therapist also begin to form some ideas about each other regarding personality compatibility, whether there is mutual respect or liking, and whether they can work together. The ability to work together and to be invested emotionally in the task of therapy is known as the *treatment alliance.*

The introductory phase may last from a few weeks to 2 or more years in a situation with an extremely withdrawn, defended, or psychotic person. The goal of this first stage of therapy is to establish a degree of trust that will allow the client to give up his defenses as he enters into the second, or working, stage of treatment.

Working Stage

As the client becomes able to trust and to disclose more about himself in the *working stage* of therapy, the client and therapist begin to explore the thoughts, feelings, and behaviors that have caused him pain or problems. This exploration may take months or years to accomplish. Often, the client reworks material previously explored as his level of trust deepens. Deeper trust allows the client to experience greater recall and insight and to express his previously repressed feelings. As the client comes to understand and function more effectively, the last stage, working through, is reached.

Working Through Stage

In the final stage of therapy, the *working through stage,* the client understands much more about himself and his relationships and begins to try out new ways of perceiving, thinking, feeling, and behaving. As he interacts with others and uses his newly acquired coping skills, changes occur, both in the client and the people around him. In other words, his inner emotional changes are reflected in his external behaviors and in his interactions with others. The client may need a great deal of support and encouragement and may rework emotional material during this stage. *Termination* of therapy may be viewed as a kind of separation. The client becomes more autonomous and ready to live his own life.

Client and Therapist

During individual psychotherapy, the client explores issues of such an intimate and personal nature that they can only be discussed with a person who is felt to be trustworthy. Trust is a necessary condition for growth and change. Let's examine how trust comes about.

Many of us have experienced change in our own lives—it probably happened because someone was therapeutic at a time of need. Looking back, we remember a grandparent, a parent, a friend, or maybe a teacher or minister who had a profound effect on our lives. Somehow, the presence, the understanding, or the example of that person helped us to understand, to feel better, or to make a needed change. Some quality in that person met our own need to find meaning or direction in life.

Our own change and growth may have resulted from a love that made no demands and set no conditions. Or, we may have responded to another's acceptance or ability to see worth in another human being. Perhaps it was the integrity of mind and spirit that made it safe to confide in him or her. We say of such people, "he always loved me and believed in me," "she understands me, she was always there when I needed her," "he is solid as a rock."

These qualities that are so powerful in our personal lives are the qualities that are effective in therapy. In therapy, there is a person, the client, who is in conflict or in a process of growth and change. The client is experiencing enough pain or discomfort to cause him to perceive a need for help. Another per-

CHART 13-2
Nursing Process and Individual Therapy

The nursing process is a form of problem-solving. The steps of collecting and analyzing data, identifying problems, formulating goals, planning actions, and evaluating progress are also those of the process of therapy.

It is important to remember that the major focus of therapy is how the process is carried out. In a team approach, physicians, nurses, psychologists, social workers, occupational therapists, mental health technicians, and nursing students work in collaboration to meet the client's needs. Students work with the staff and with clinical nursing supervision in interaction with clients; these interactions may be on a one-to-one basis with inpatients or outpatients.

Client goals need to be jointly determined by the client, therapist, and staff. Goals and outcomes should be simple, measurable, and stated in behavioral terms.

An example of this process applied to a withdrawn adolescent client follows:

Problem:	Fourteen-year-old Mary has difficulty in forming relationships with peers. She neither talks with them nor joins in their activities.
Goal:	Mary will relate more effectively to her peers.
Nursing Diagnosis:	Social isolation related to depressed mood and feelings of worthlessness, evidenced by sad, dull affect, uncommunicative behavior, absence of supportive significant others.
Client Outcomes:	Mary will talk with at least two peers daily for a minimum of 10 minutes each. Mary will use "I" messages to express feelings and thoughts.
Evaluation:	Mary has been able to carry out the actions planned this week. The "I" messages are difficult for her, but the result of using this method has been the expression of more feeling. Her speech is less flat. Peers have been more responsive to her.

son, the therapist, has the essential qualities to provide that help.

Why is it necessary to go to a therapist to get help? Why can't we achieve the same results by talking to the people who are important in our lives? All of us have families, friends, doctors, teachers and ministers available to us in time of need. Even the poorest and most lonely have some available resources.

Many people can, and do, use these resources. One of the goals of therapy is to learn to relate more effectively to others to meet more of our own, and their, needs. Another goal is to grow so that we have more strengths and are able to give more of ourselves to others.

For many people, however, the realities of living and relating to others have been difficult and painful. Perhaps the person has grown up in a family that was conflicted, chaotic, or dysfunctional to a greater extent than most families. Perhaps family members were locked into constricting roles; there were hidden agendas, unclear communication patterns, or incidents of physical and emotional abuse. Ways of relating and expressing feelings may have been distorted, causing painful, unproductive encounters with the people most important to the client as a child. Perhaps they were not able to understand the child or give him what he needed.

Early ways of relating and early experiences are

carried from the past into the present. Often, faulty or unproductive ways of relating are modified by other experiences and other relationships. Relearning and emotional repair take place. These processes are normally seen as children enter school and form friendships; adolescence is also a time of major reworking and relearning. This reworking and relearning is what therapy is designed to do. The client experiences emotional relearning in a safe relationship.

In therapy, the client relates to the therapist and behaves in the same way as he does with the significant other people in his life. Patterns of client behavior become evident as the process of therapy continues. In traditional psychotherapy, a great deal of emphasis is placed on the client's memories of childhood relationships and events. In present-oriented therapies, the emphasis is on the client's behavior in current relationships. In both kinds of therapy, however, distortions or problem areas in interpersonal relations are identified and become the foci of therapy.

Therapist Versus Family or Friends: Whom to Choose?

When faced with a problem, the client may consult any helping person—a family member, friend, minister, or therapist; he may choose a therapist because of his *objectivity.* The therapist is not related to, or involved with, the client outside the therapy situation. This is one of the therapist's important ethical responsibilities. The therapist should not engage in a social relationship, and particularly not in a sexual relationship with a client. If this should occur, the relationship can no longer be considered therapeutic. Obviously, people may consult friends or those who are already known to them for therapy. In this situation, it is important that the therapist discuss the need for objectivity with the client and, if there is a conflict, refer him to another therapist. Often, however, a friend or acquaintance is able to be both objective and therapeutic.

The therapist provides a *different perspective* for the client and offers him alternative ways of perceiving, thinking, feeling, and behaving. Often, a client is locked into one mode of being, like "being in a rut" and unable to get out. The therapist is not limited by the client's special set of circumstances.

The therapist also brings *specialized knowledge* to the relationship with the client. The specialized knowledge is in the area of human behavior and includes understanding problems and problem-solving techniques. In addition, the therapist brings a background in medicine, nursing, psychology, social work, the ministry, or counseling.

Because of these qualifications—objectivity, perspective, and specialized knowledge—the therapist operates outside the framework of the client's life and within the context of stated goals designed jointly by client and therapist for the client's benefit.

Qualities of the Therapist

Carl Rogers identified the qualities that promote a therapeutic relationship.[17] Rogers believes that therapist attitudes provide "necessary and sufficient conditions" for therapeutic change. These attitudes are congruence, unconditional positive regard, and accurate empathetic understanding.

Congruence, or genuineness, means that the feelings, thoughts, and behaviors of a person are consistent. To be congruent, the therapist needs to understand himself, to be aware of his feelings, and to be free of deceit or misleading behaviors. This does not imply that the therapist expresses or acts on every thought or feeling; awareness, rather, allows for a choice of behaviors.

Clients are often incongruent; that is, they are not aware of their feelings or thoughts. They may express feelings and ideas that do not match what is really felt or thought. Congruence in the therapist allows the client to become aware of his true feelings and thoughts and to feel free to express them.

Unconditional positive regard involves being able to feel concern and caring for the client without making any value judgments. This means being able to accept both positive and negative statements made by the client and being able to have faith in his potential as a human being. This attitude allows the client to accept and value himself, and to move toward realizing his potential.

Accurate empathetic understanding involves feeling and experiencing with the client "almost as if" the therapist were having those feelings and experiences. This empathy allows the client to become more aware of his feelings and to feel validated. Someone, he realizes, has heard what he is trying to express and understands him.

The therapist, because of what he or she is, facilitates growth and development in the client. It is not a matter of giving to, or doing for, someone; rather, it is a way of reaching the client's energies and potentials and freeing them for use.

Client Expectations

The energies and potentials of the client are powerful. The wishes, hopes, and dreams of our lives have great emotional energy invested in them, and this provides a key to understanding what motivates people to go into therapy. To understand themselves or to change behavior in even small ways, people must have a strongly perceived need to change, the hope that change is possible, and at least some belief that someone can help.

Usually, the client realizes that something in his life is causing so much emotional pain that something needs to be done. The need must be strong enough to cause the client to risk self-disclosure and to continue in therapy even when it is painful and embarrassing.

Sometimes, the client seems to expect the therapist to solve all his problems. This may not be a conscious thought; however, it is a very human one and probably a wish that all of us have had at one time or another. We wish that someone would love us, take care of us, and make things right.

The therapist usually makes it clear from the beginning that therapy is a joint effort in which the client will come to understand what the problems are and what he needs to do. To "help" or "do for" the client would take away from the growth and autonomy that therapy is designed to accomplish.

The client can expect confidentiality, specialized knowledge, and skill from the therapist. In addition, he needs to know how often therapy will take place, the probable length of treatment, and how much it will cost. He should know how to contact the therapist in case of an emergency or a change in plans. Usually, there is some formulation of the situation and an explanation of how therapy will be conducted.

Therapist Expectations

The major expectation of the therapist is that the client will be as open and honest in discussing his situation as he is consciously able to be. This is sometimes referred to as the *therapeutic contract.*

Other therapist expectations include keeping appointments on time and being paid for services. The therapist should arrange ways in which the client can contact him in case of need. He should also schedule holidays and vacations in such a way as to let the client know well in advance and provide for another therapist to take care of any problems that arise.

Usually, the therapist will use a collaborative approach in planning therapy, identifying problem areas, and setting goals. This may take several sessions or may evolve as therapy continues and a better understanding of the situation comes about. Therapy is almost always a process of verbal interaction between the client and the therapist. Sometimes it is difficult to put feelings into words, but this is a very valuable kind of learning, because it allows other people to understand one another and helps to clarify feelings for the client.

Physical acting out of loving or hostile feelings

between client and therapist is inappropriate and this should be clarified with the client if any confusion or misunderstanding is present.

The therapist may also expect rewards such as receiving pleasure from facilitating growth and change, or from understanding more about human behavior. The therapeutic relationship is always maintained within the orientation of a professional person working with a client to meet the client's needs. Personal and social needs of the therapist are properly met through family, friends, and the community.

The therapist has a further obligation—that of protecting the client who is suicidal or likely to harm another person. In this situation, it may be necessary to hospitalize the client. Taking steps to protect the client is often reassuring to him, even though he is angry and protests. Hospitalization, for example, supplies external control at a time when the client feels out of control. Being out of control or feeling out of control is very frightening for both the client and the people around him.

Sometimes, people use threats of suicide to get attention or to manipulate others. The nurse must realize that, even when the client threatens suicide for these reasons, the possibility of suicide is real. This kind of behavior also provides fertile ground for exploring the client's need to manipulate others and the feelings that would lead to such behavior.

How client problems are defined and what kind of therapy is engaged in depends to a great extent on the therapist's orientations. The therapist forms a theoretical framework of values and beliefs, or concepts, derived from his education and life experiences. The next section of the chapter will discuss how some of the concepts used in individual therapy came about.

Origins and Development of Psychotherapy

There is a tremendous amount of information available dealing with human behavior. Some of it is old, some is new. Contributions to the study of human behavior have come from medicine, psychiatry, psychology, and biology. A particularly interesting area has been that of ethology. Studies of animal behavior have inspired much of the current research on human behavior. Such seemingly diverse areas as Harlow's work with monkeys and studies of imprinting in animals have helped us to understand ourselves.[9] Studies of social behavior have also broadened our conceptions of how people develop and relate to each other. Many of the original ideas of Freud and his colleagues about individuals and therapy are still in use; others

C H A R T   13-3
Research Update: The Ineffectiveness of Psychotherapy

People involved in psychotherapy feel a great deal of pleasure and gratification in seeing clients grow. As clients become less focused on pain and unhappiness, they become pro-active— able to act effectively on behalf of themselves and others. They become able to be responsible, that is, able to respond emotionally. Most of us feel that the worth of therapy is evident. Demonstrating this worth is not always easy, however; and published reseach has been the subject of a great deal of controversy.

One of the difficulties encountered in psychotherapy is that of evaluating results. Confidentiality is a necessary condition for therapy. This means that the client and therapist are the only people who have access to all of the exchange of information in each session. Even video and audio tapes, if permitted, may not convey all the nuances of feeling present in the therapy situations. To review the work of years would take as much time as the analysis itself, so at best, samples can be used to show progress or problems.

Probably this method, the use of tapes with evaluation by professional independent reviewers, is the most effective one at present. Self-reports and the reports of therapists are useful but fall farther from scientific methodology.

Another difficulty in evaluating the outcomes of psychotherapy is the presence of so many variables. Each person's life contains many different factors unique to that person that determine how he or she perceives the self, other persons, and the nature of the world in general. These unique perceptions, in turn, determine how the person structures and defines problems.

Of course, a person's perceptions may not be the same as, or even similar to, the perceptions of significant others or of people in general. A lot of what we call normal or even "real" is only what a number of people have agreed to identify in those ways. Trying to mold people to some kind of imaginary norm is dangerous. Much of what we think of as learning or progress depends on creativity and unique perceptions in individuals.

Scientists, of course, stick to what is measurable and reproducible, and get good (relatively accurate) results. This allows them to base further studies on their data. However, the more one gets away from the physical and chemical sciences, the harder it is accurately to account for and decribe all the variables and to state a problem or hypothesis in a measurable and meaningful way. What is a good description of a successful outcome in psychotherapy? Freud fell back on the ability to love and to work, saying also that ordinary human misery is not the province of psychoanalysis.

Despite these difficulties, there is a stubborn belief that therapy works. Some promising ideas are being studied, and preliminary results are exciting. New scanning technology and the study of neurotransmitters offer an opportunity to demonstrate changes as a result of both psychotherapy and drug therapy. If psychotherapy alone can cause changes in metabolic functions of the brain or in the balance or production of adequate amounts of neurotransmitters, and if these changes can be correlated with behavioral change, we may have a means of measuring therapy more effectively.

As an example, positron emission scanning using a tagged glucoselike substance is being used to demonstrate normal brain metabolism. The brain requires a large blood supply and is very metabolically active, using large amounts of glucose and oxygen. The radioactive tagged substance is taken up by the normal brain and utilized, showing all areas of the brain and allowing for comparison among different levels of activity in waking, sleeping, active problem-solving, and so on. There are differences between the brains of people in good states of health and people who are depressed, schizophrenic, or have medical illnesses with identifiable pathologies, such as brain tumors or strokes. In depression, changes toward normal metabolic activity can be demonstrated as the client improves.

Neurotransmitter functions have been the object of intense research for at least 40 years. Many transmitters have been identified, and the general functions of some major transmitters are fairly well understood. The balance of these transmitters in the nervous system, the lack or oversupply of one or another transmitter, and the changes in different systems in response to physical and emotional change are much harder to study. At present we can say that an increase or decrease of norepinephrine, serotonin, or dopamine, for example, can be related to depression or schizophrenia. Much of the research has been done in relation to drug therapy; as a result, more is known about the working of the central nervous system, and at least a little has been learned about the emotions.

The next generation may see some interesting changes. Perhaps a means will be developed of validating the effectiveness of what we call "the talking cure," the strongly held belief that human relatedness and caring make the major differences in human behavior.

References

1. Bachrack HM, Weber JJ, Solomon M: Factors associated with the outcome of psychoanalysis: Report of the Columbia Psychoanalytic Center Research Project: IV. Int Rev Psychoanal 12(4), 1985

2. Kantrowicz J, et al: Affect availability, tolerance, complexity, and modulation in psychoanalysis: followup of a longitudinal, prospective study. J Amer Psychoanalytic Assn 34(3), 529–559, 1986

have been modified as new information and new perspectives became available.

As we review some of the thinking and major concepts that have shaped the development of therapy as we know it today, it is important to keep in mind that all theories and concepts are formed within the context of a historical period. They arise in a given culture out of the general level of knowledge of that time. That is one reason why theories change over time as the culture changes. Another reason for ongoing change in theories is that research techniques are constantly being improved and each period of active research provides us with more accurate information. Theories, or hypotheses, are ideas that try to explain how or why something occurs. By understanding behavior, we can predict it and can, perhaps, make changes.

Theories or concepts are formed by individuals. The therapist shapes his beliefs and values out of his own experiences within the larger cultural framework. For example, a person who had difficulty forming a warm, close relationship with parents during infancy might grow up to form a theory that interpersonal difficulties during infancy may cause or contribute to mental illness. Research on infant attachment, in fact, tends to support this belief.[1,3,4,5] Self-understanding helps the therapist to understand others.

In therapy, both the client and therapist are involved in trying to understand and form ideas as to what causes problems, and are trying to find solutions to those problems. To do this, they must explore the client's beliefs and values.

Freud's Theories

Sigmund Freud, who is known as the father of psychiatry, certainly was affected by his culture and the state of knowledge at that time. His genius was his ability to transcend culture and, from his observations of his patients, develop ideas that are still influential in therapy.

He studied in Vienna, which was the world center for medical education at that time. He could be described as a middle-class, Jewish, professional male who had access to the new knowledge of that day. There was a tremendous amount of work being done in all the sciences in the Victorian era and in the first part of the 20th century. Application of the scientific method, the use of the microscope and telescope, and the new theory of evolution had opened up whole new areas for investigation.

Freud was a neurologist. He was interested in applying the scientific method to his work. At that time, people in the sciences were engaged in describing, classifying, and labeling their discoveries. Mental illness and the workings of the mind could be studied, described, labeled and classified. The medical model originated in this way and proclaimed that mental illness is a disease manifested by symptoms. This was a radical idea at the time and represented a significant change from older ideas that mental illness was caused by sin or constitutional inferiority.

Freud became convinced that the mind was a major factor in mental illness when he observed that patients suffering from amnesia or from hysterical paralysis became symptom-free under hypnosis. The patient was able to remember, or was able to use the previously paralyzed body part, thereby demonstrating that the illness was not an organic impairment, but a functional one. This distinction is still utilized in health care. Organic illness can be demonstrated by alterations in the anatomy or physiology of the body; in functional illness, an organic cause cannot be demonstrated. (Note: with improved diagnostic studies such as Positron Emission Tomography, Nuclear Magnetic Imaging, and the Dexamethasone Suppression Test, these classifications may change.)

As Freud talked with patients and they told him

about their lives and experiences, some interesting things happened. The patients often remembered previously forgotten experiences. Talking allowed them to express some of the painful thoughts and feelings attached to those experiences and, sometimes, their physical or emotional distress would be relieved; that is, they became free of symptoms. Freud began to try to understand and account for what he experienced. In time, he called this work *analysis* or *psychoanalysis*, a study of the workings of the mind. From his experiences with patients and his self-analysis, Freud formed major concepts about mental functioning.

Concepts of Psychotherapy

Insight

A person is said to gain *insight* when he becomes consciously aware of the odd, painful, angry, or socially unacceptable thoughts or feelings that he had repressed. *Intellectual insight* is an understanding of the origins and consequences of a symptom or behavior. *Emotional insight* involves both understanding and re-experiencing the very painful, frightening, or angry feelings that are associated with that symptom or behavior. This re-experiencing, also called *catharsis*, frees a person's fixed emotions and allows for emotional growth.

Repression

The concept of repression is central to Freudian theory. Through the mechanism of *repression*, feelings, thoughts, and experiences that are too painful or threatening to the person to be allowed to remain in conscious awareness, or to become conscious, are pushed back into the unconscious part of the mind. *Unconscious* means, literally, not available to consciousness. Repression is an unconscious phenomenon; that is, the person does not try to forget. Instead, events or ongoing situations that threaten the ego integrity (*i.e.,* the person's self-image or safety) are too painful to realize. Sometimes, there is partial repression. For example, knowledge of a situation may be in a person's awareness, but the feelings about the situation are repressed.

Repressed knowledge and feelings exert powerful influences on people that come out in all kinds of ways. Freudian slips or "slips of the tongue" occur. Sometimes, a word or phrase that seems funny or inappropriate in the context of a sentence makes very good sense in expressing the person's real feelings.

Dreams also provide a way of getting at repressed thoughts and feelings. People in therapy often have vivid, and sometimes recurring, dreams. In fact, recurring dreams may be present for a long time and may represent the client's attempt to solve a problem. It is fairly common to have vivid dreams or to remember more dreams when we are anxious or excited. Therapy represents both a form of stress that causes anxiety and an emotionally secure situation. The security offered by the therapist allows for weakening of repressions and access to emotionally important material. The client's emotional content may be disguised in dreams.

Originally, therapists attempted to analyze both manifest and latent dream content; that is, they believed that a specific kind of dream had a specific meaning. Now, therapists believe that the most productive use of dream material comes from the client's discussion of his thoughts and feelings and what the dreams mean to him.

Free Association

Free association is the free expression of thoughts and feelings just as they come to mind. This method encourages the lowering of the client's defenses. It is the primary method of treatment in psychoanalysis and in much of psychotherapy.

Resistance

Resistance means that the client resists recalling information or recalling feelings. It often occurs as *blocking*, wherein a client will suddenly "blank out" and be unable to finish a thought or idea. He may suddenly change the subject without any cue or obvious reason to do so. In blocking, there is not only repression of painful knowledge and feelings, but also resistance to recall and understanding.

Techniques such as having the client lie on a couch and face away from the therapist are used in psychoanalysis to avoid influencing the client as to what he should say. These are ways of trying to decrease resistance. Therapeutic attitudes of being accepting and nonjudgmental are also ways of decreasing resistance and allowing the client to express his thoughts and feelings.

Maslow helps us to understand resistance through his assertion that people have both a need to know and a fear of knowing.[13] Knowing and understanding may imply action and change. In therapy, the therapist supports the client's need to know. This support is needed because the knowledge that has been repressed is literally unthinkable, the feelings are too painful to feel. Therapy, then, represents both threat and opportunity.

What is so terrible that it cannot be thought or felt or said? Each of us has secrets, things we would not want other people to know because they would disapprove, reject us, stop loving us, or be very angry.

In unconscious material, the fear that drives or mediates the repression is so strong that it is experienced as a threat to the person's existence—a fear of total rejection, abandonment, loss of existence, or intolerable feelings of being worthless or bad.

Infants and small children are literally dependent on significant adults, usually parents, for survival in both a physical and an emotional sense. Lack of love, disapproval, or an inability to accept the child and love him as he is is a threat to that child's survival.

Sometimes, a family will place adult burdens of emotional responsibility on a child and expect that child to meet the dependency needs of the parents. Each family also has standards of behavior for children that include which feelings may be expressed and how they may be expressed. If a child learns that it is not safe to express pain and anger or that it is not safe to express love, tenderness, and vulnerability, then repression is the price the child pays for surviving in that family. The effects of that repression may include shame and guilt.

Reworking

Through *reworking,* children learn other ways of behaving as they grow and develop. Other family members, peers, and people outside the immediate family model different ways of feeling and behaving. Adolescents, especially, rework earlier developmental stages and modify earlier feelings, beliefs, and attitudes.

To a great extent, this *emotional relearning* is what happens in psychotherapy. Early therapists believed that the personality was fairly rigid and could only be modified slightly. Now we believe that there is far more plasticity and potential for change, even in middle age or old age.

Transference

Transference is a major tool or technique—a powerful force—in psychotherapy. In therapy, the client transfers feelings and attitudes held toward significant others onto the therapist. The client then reacts toward the therapist in the same ways he reacts, or reacted, toward the important people in his life. There may be different sets of feelings and attitudes for each person in the client's life. At times, for example, he may behave as if the therapist is mother, father, brother, or sister. The sex of the therapist doesn't seem to make much difference. In *transference,* the client is deeply involved with the feelings and experiences of his own life and projects these experiences onto the therapist. The transference may be *positive,* in which all good qualities are transferred onto the therapist, or it may be *negative,* in which the therapist becomes all bad. A positive transference may become negative as the client gets in touch with his feelings of pain and anger and hurt. A negative transference may become positive as the client begins to establish trust with the therapist and work through his hurt and anger.

The term *significant others* seems very pale and weak; these are, after all, the people who have profound importance in our lives. We love, hate, fear, want, and depend on them. We are often almost as concerned with their feelings and needs as our own.

In transference, the client realizes, as therapy continues, that the therapist is not like the significant others in his life. The projection or transference allows both client and therapist to understand the feelings, attitudes, and behaviors that the client has learned. An important part of emotional relearning is the client's realization that other people do not possess the stereotyped or punitive reactions that have been present in his relationships in the past. The client also realizes how he or she contributes to, or feeds into, present relationships to maintain the faulty, incongruent, or inappropriate perceptions and behaviors. The experience of being valued and understood allows the client to have new perceptions and form new perspectives.

Countertransference

In *countertransference,* the therapist sometimes experiences a transference of his or her feelings for significant others onto the client. Usually, something about the client—appearance, tone of voice, mannerisms, or behavior—will trigger countertransference. An unusual like or dislike of the client is a clue to the therapist that countertransference is operating. This clue can be very useful if it alerts the therapist to analyze the reaction. If not detected, countertransference can cause problems. Therapists will often consult with a colleague or request supervision to deal effectively with this kind of situation. Consultation or supervision allows for working through both client's and therapist's feelings in a therapeutic way with benefits for both.

Ambivalence

Ambivalence is the experience of two strong, opposing feelings or wishes toward the same object, or person, at the same time. It could equally well be described as the conflict experienced when strong approach/avoidance tendencies are present. Dollard, Miller, and others were able to create ambivalence in laboratory rats by giving them an electric shock while they were eating. A strong drive or need (hunger) caused approach to food; the painful shock caused strong avoidance tendencies.[7]

In human beings, the opposite feelings or needs are almost always love/hate, love/fear, or some combination. Anger usually results when strong drives or needs are frustrated; that is, not allowed appropriate expression. Another outcome of this frustration may be what is called *learned helplessness,* which is believed to be a major component of depression.[18]

Ambivalence, then, causes a great deal of conflict that may be expressed as feelings of distress, anxiety, tension, or an inability to make decisions or to move at all. In extreme states, this would be called panic, if it manifested as anxiety, or immobility, if the client were frozen in conflict.

Ambivalence is present in all of us. We have differing feelings toward people that vary with the amount of closeness in the relationship and with different situations. A small child expresses feelings very directly and can say, "I hate you" when frustrated, and a few minutes later say, "I love you" with equal intensity. Both feelings are real and, as the child grows up, he comes to realize that being angry at a person does not mean not loving the person also.

In a "good enough" family, children are taught to own their feelings and to label them correctly. The family functions to meet the child's needs for love and security and socializes the child by teaching him to get his needs met in socially acceptable ways.

Problems arise when parents are unable to fulfill these necessary functions for their children. Parents who cannot allow a child to separate and become autonomous contribute to ambivalence over dependence/independence and love/hate issues. If being dependent means being loved and being independent means being emotionally abandoned, a tremendous amount of conflict and anger will be generated within the child.

Parents who have difficulty allowing feelings of anger, aggression, or sexuality may react to the child's expression of these feelings in such a punitive way that these feelings are repressed. In our culture, it is particularly true that girls repress angry, aggressive, and sexual feelings. Boys are more likely to repress feelings of love, tenderness, and dependency. By repressing strong feelings, we not only inhibit emotional development in regard to the feelings repressed, but we also inhibit the appropriate expression of its opposite feelings.

Ambiguity

Ambiguity describes the experience of uncertainty. One measure of emotional competence is how well a person is able to tolerate living with a degree of uncertainty. An element common to many people in therapy is difficulty in tolerating ambiguity, which indicates a strong need for certainty and stability. Most of us would like to live in what has been referred to as a reasonably predictable environment.

We need to feel that we have some control over our lives. Children who live in a chaotic or deprived environment and children who never experience stability in their lives will be at risk in the world. Often, when they become adults, they will cling to very rigid ideas to feel secure.

Tolerating ambiguity means that we are able to perceive the world and the people around us in a way that allows for shades of meaning and also allows for many feelings about a given person or situation. Sometimes, we think it would be easier or safer to live in a world where things could be categorized as good or bad, either this or that. Perhaps, though, there would be fewer possibilities and our experiences would not be as rich in meaning. Part of becoming adult is the ability to accept in each of us, the subtle shifting of complex thoughts and feelings toward other people in our lives.

Object Constancy

The feeling of security or stability in our lives is known as *object constancy* or *object permanence.* It is a general feeling that people are reliable and that the world is a pretty good place. Several influences during an individual's growth and development help to establish this feeling.

One very useful concept is that of the "good enough mother" and the expansion of that to the idea of the "good enough" family. No family is perfect and no mother could possibly be all-loving and all-giving. Most of us, in fact, would be pretty uncomfortable with perfection, having not quite achieved that state for ourselves. Nevertheless, families, and mothers in particular, do some very important things.

Object constancy comes about partly as the result of a secure maternal–infant attachment.[1,3,4,5] A secure maternal–infant attachment has survival value for the infant and for the human species. It is manifested by the infant's maintenance of proximity to the mother in times of stress and by his exploration from a safe base (mother) in times of security.

Maternal qualities that foster attachment are sensitivity to the infant's needs, warmth, and nurturance. The infant both initiates and limits interaction with the mother or primary caregiver. This is done by eye contact or vocal cues (*i.e.,* crying or vocalizing). Mother cues in to the baby's signals, mirrors, and selectively emphasizes the behavior. The first faint twitch of the baby's lips is identified as a smile and positively reinforced by mirroring the behavior.

Accurate empathetic mirroring reinforces desired social behaviors. The sensitive mother is aware that her baby is tired when he ends eye contact. This is a signal to end the interaction. Soon after birth, the parents identify the baby's cries as indicating hunger, pain, or a cry for attention. This concern and care for the infant's needs and individuality insures that the infant's needs will be met and that he can depend on his mother or father to do this. Babies seem to be genetically programmed to prefer the human face and their eyes focus best at a distance of about 9 inches in early infancy. Babies quickly learn to recognize and prefer mother. After about 7 months, the baby begins to discriminate and prefer mother, father, and known others to strangers, and to be anxious with strangers. Distinctions made between self and others and between known people and strange people are precursors of a clear sense of self or identity.

As the baby becomes more mobile, we can observe the gradual processes of separation and individualization. Babies love games. In peek-a-boo, the very young baby loves the experience of hiding and then being seen. A young baby will hide his or her eyes. The belief seems to be that if the baby can't see, then he can't be seen! If a person or an object can't be seen, does it exist? The fun of peek-a-boo and hide and seek is finding that people do still exist even though we can't see them for a little while. As the baby becomes a toddler, we can watch him play happily for a while, go to another room, come back to his parent, and then return to play. The parent, the infant discovers, still exists even if he or she is in another room.

The ability to say "No" and to control bowel and bladder functions also reinforces the experience of being autonomous. This experience further emphasizes the distinction between what is I and mine and what is you and yours.

As these processes of identification, separation, and autonomy occur, there is a corresponding internalization of the feelings, attitudes, and behaviors of the parents or significant others. This internalization is known as *introjection.* The infant incorporates aspects of significant others as part of the self. At the same time, he internalizes constructs, or conceptions, of the significant others or object. This internal representation of others supplies object constancy. Later in life, even when death occurs, we continue to carry a realistic conception of those we love; they remain constant for us as they were experienced. The feeling of being loved and being able to depend on others to meet accurately our needs for both security and autonomy allows for a sense of self-identity and a sense of the identity, or object permanence, of others.

In therapy, clients may need to achieve object constancy and may need to separate from a fused sense of identity with a parent or other person. This may require a considerable amount of work and sometimes involves multiple types of therapy, utilizing an inpatient milieu structure.

All of these aspects of therapy sound simple, as though therapy follows an outline or sequence of mental or emotional events. That is the plan, but not at all the usual situation. Each success of the client's is reinforcing and leads to more work, but the repressed material is both painful and powerful. Resistance is seen in other forms.

Acting In

Acting in is the kind of resistance that circumvents therapy through blocking, forgetting, changing the subject, or trying to elicit the therapist's approval or disapproval while trying to recall or express feelings. Consciously, the client is earnestly trying to express everything as it comes to mind.

Acting Out

In *acting out,* the client substitutes some kind of action for feeling or thinking. As memories, feelings, and thoughts begin to reach awareness, a kind of reflex substitution of action occurs. The painful awareness is not allowed to reach consciousness.

The defenses seen in acting out are learned ones and the client may show a pattern of defensive acting out. Common defenses are the use of alcohol or drugs, getting involved in fights, running away, or the compulsive or promiscuous use of sexual activity. Even ordinary activities like work or exercise can be used or overused as defenses, instead of thinking or feeling.

Sometimes in therapy, a client will get married, divorced, form new friendships, and so on as a "short cut" to getting support or getting dependency needs met. This is another way of avoiding the more difficult task of becoming aware of one's feelings and understanding one's self. The therapist may ask the client to sign an agreement or contract to postpone major lifestyle changes during therapy until a better self-understanding exists.

Interpretation

Interpretation appears very exciting in movies in which the analyst arrives at a brilliant interpretation of the patient's problem. The patient would say, "Aha! That explains everything!"

Actually, the important aspect of *interpretation* is the client's understanding of his feelings and behavior. The client's insight is the therapeutic element. A therapist may make beautiful formulations of the client's problems and their origins and causes, but

Case Study 13-1: Using Individual Psychotherapy to Foster Lifestyle and Behavioral Changes

Ms. Jane V. is an attractive young woman in her early twenties. She is slender, of average height, well-developed, and well-nourished. Her posture is erect. She seems a little overactive, perhaps due to anxiety.

"I came to see you because my family doctor recommended you," she said during her first interview with a therapist. She added that since her engagement ended recently, she has been unable to sleep and has had suicidal thoughts.

When the therapist asked her to talk more about her feelings, she stated, "I feel like my world has ended. I've been abandoned again. I just want to die. This always happens—everytime I love someone, I lose. At first everything is so wonderful, but it doesn't work out. They just can't meet my needs."

The therapist then asked Jane how she handles disappointments. "Well," she responded, "I have wondered if I drink a little too much. Sometimes I smoke a joint—just to relax, you know—or maybe a Valium will help. That scares me, though. I cut myself once—see my wrists. Maybe the Valium makes it worse."

The therapist also learned that Jane has done well in school and is now a junior in college, but has no clear idea of what she wants to do for a career.

Jane is the third child of a highly achievement-oriented family. An older brother has just finished law school, her sister is a graduate student in business, and a younger brother is interested in computer science. Her father is an attorney and her mother is a homemaker.

Jane described her father as distant, but demanding, and her mother as very protective and with few interests outside the family. She related that she had asthma when she was a child, and that her mother has "always babied" her. (Later, in therapy, Jane expressed her difficulty in identifying with her weak but manipulative mother, and her own poor self-image as a woman.)

At times, Jane tried to hold summer jobs, which she always left because of personality differences with her employers. While talking about these experiences, she became quite angry and expressed that people had been unfair to her. She became tearful at this point in the interview and said, "You know I always try so hard, but everything goes wrong. No matter what I do, it falls apart. I feel so helpless! Sometimes I think things will never be better."

Subsequent therapy sessions tended to confirm the therapist's impressions that Jane has a borderline personality disorder. Jane's specific problems include the following:

1. An overly close, dependent relationship with her mother
2. A distant and hostile relationship with her father
3. Lack of a clear sense of self, especially in relation to gender identity and self-esteem
4. Indecisiveness about a career choice
5. Habitual use of alcohol or drugs to cope with emotional pain
6. A pattern of unstable relationships
7. Depression, evidenced by self-mutilation and feelings of helplessness and hopelessness.

Jane and the therapist set up these initial goals:

1. To form a treatment alliance
2. To involve the family in the therapeutic process

The treatment alliance requires that Jane attend therapy sessions and express her feelings openly and honestly.

Family involvement is expected as Jane and her family meet every 2 weeks with a family therapist to work on the family's definition of itself and its problem areas. The therapist explains that Jane might need 2 or more years of therapeutic work and suggests that two therapy sessions per week would be useful at this time to deal with her severe depression.

The purposes of the treatment alliance are to reduce Jane's extreme dependency on her mother and encourage exploration of her problems from the safe base the therapist provides. The difficulty in these tasks occurs because of the symbiotic state that exists between Jane and her mother. Jane's mother rewards her dependency (*i.e.*, she responds to Jane's dependency with love and approval). Jane's efforts at becoming independent have, in the past, been punished by the withdrawal of her mother's love and approval—in essence, abandonment.

Jane has learned to get her needs met primarily by manipulating her mother and other people. She also has a feeling of "entitlement," which means that she feels special and deserves special privileges.

Jane also has a number of strengths that

have allowed her to experience some successes. Her compulsiveness has helped her to do well in school and to finish tasks. She has talent in painting and has sold a little of her work. She is intelligent and tries to understand and make sense of her life.

Family therapy will relieve some of the pressure from Jane as the identified patient. The pattern of an over-functioning but emotionally distant father and an over-emotional but under-functioning mother can be addressed. Therapy will redefine Jane's privileged and emotionally damaging position in the family. Her brothers and sister can also learn to relate better to each other and to redefine themselves.

As therapy progresses, Jane will become aware of her role in the dependent, too-close and too-distant relationships with her parents. Jane and the therapist first address the hostile relationship with her emotionally distant father and the distress and anger she feels about it. Later, they examine both Jane's anger at her all-powerful mother and her own dependent and manipulative behaviors.

Giving up dependency means taking on responsibility for one's own feelings and behavior. This is a difficult task and small gains need to be repeated. The therapist might encourage Jane to decide on an area of study and finish college. Another goal might be to form friendships with peers to provide a supportive network and meet some of the needs previously met by her mother.

Success is highly reinforcing. As Jane succeeds in mastering the smaller goals, she will become able to attempt greater tasks. Self-understanding and mastery will help to improve her self-esteem and provide feelings of self-worth.

Gender identity is achieved partly by modeling or identifying with women whom one would like to emulate. Feelings of mastery and achievement also help to change the idea of being helpless and dependent to feeling good about being a woman.

Relationships also solidify as a result of therapy. The experience of the therapist as a dependable person helps to relieve fears of abandonment. Through this therapeutic relationship, achievement and independence are rewarded.

Feelings of depression and fears of abandonment should decrease as Jane improves. Friends and social activities can replace alcohol and other drugs as more effective ways to get her needs met. When Jane begins to place greater value on herself, her relationships with family and friends will strengthen.

Major tools of individual psychotherapy are the setting of firm, consistent limits and the use of confrontation. In addition, clients like Jane may need hospitalization with the use of an entire milieu to provide support and emotional relearning. Other clients may be able to take advantage of outpatient care. Jane was able to make changes in herself and within her family.

Questions for Discussion

1. Can you identify client problem areas other than those listed?
2. What are the purposes and tasks of the therapeutic alliance?
3. Goals are identified for Jane during the introductory stage of therapy; what goals would you formulate for the working and working through stages of Jane's therapy?
4. Explain Jane's perceptions of her problems and needs. Are these consistent with expected behavior of a client with a borderline personality disorder?

this is not helpful unless the client arrives at self-understanding.

Sometimes, the therapist will offer a tentative explanation or ask whether it is possible that a particular feeling or experience is connected to another. Questions such as this are best asked infrequently and with respect for the client's anxiety and need for his defenses. Even a cautious and accurate comment may arouse a good deal of anger or denial. Interpretation of this kind is useful when the client is ready to deal with this aspect of himself and when his awareness is just below the surface.

Working Through

Working through comes in the last phase of therapy. At this point, the client has reached a fairly good understanding of the feelings and patterns of behavior that have caused him distress. The client has more emotional energy available and is able to perceive more of the world around him and to form new perspectives.

Working through means that the client's insights have to be discussed and reworked over a period of time. The long repressed pain, guilt, anger, shame, grief, or sadness must be expressed—not just once, but many times—in order to be owned and integrated into the self. This takes a lot of work and there are often periods of regression, discouragement, or acting out. At the end, however, the pain is gone.

Part of the process of working through is the knowledge that therapy will eventually end. A relationship that has been of great importance will gradually become less important and then end, usually by agreement of the therapist and client.

Translating

Translating insight and understanding into new behaviors is the final aspect of working through. Discussion is not enough; success in trying new behaviors is highly reinforcing. As the client feels less angry, vulnerable, or frightened, he feels more freedom to try new ways of behaving. The client becomes more autonomous, more aware of options. Feelings are often more vivid and more consciously experienced. The client is better able to live with tensions, ambivalence, and ambiguity.

The process of emotional re-education is now internalized so that, as time goes on, the client's emotions become more congruent, and a greater choice of behaviors are available to him. Psychotherapy then becomes a process of being—a process of learning, trying out, and adapting that continues through the client's life.

Summary

This chapter has discussed how people change their feelings, attitudes, and behaviors through therapy. Some of the important points discussed in the chapter are as follows:

1. An individual may choose to engage in the process of psychotherapy to treat an emotional disorder, to deal with his problems, or to gain insight and self-understanding.
2. Various levels of psychotherapy—supportive, re-educative, and reconstructive—describe the depth of therapy and the degree of change undertaken by the client.
3. During each of the three stages of individual psychotherapy, the client and therapist have certain tasks to accomplish, such as exploring the client's history and current problems and needs during the introductory stage.
4. Because of his objectivity, perspective, and specialized knowledge, a therapist can generally be more effective than a person's family or friends in helping him deal with problems and growth needs.
5. The client and therapist need to clearly communicate their expectations of each other and of therapy.
6. The important concepts of psychotherapy, such as insight, repression, resistance, and reworking, are explored and applied to the client involved in individual psychotherapy.

References

1. Ainsworth MD, Blehar MD, Waters E, Wall S: Patterns of Attachment: Assessed in the Strange Situation and at Home. Hillsdale, NJ, Lawrence Erlbaum, 1978
2. Arieti S: On Schizophrenia, Phobias, Depression, Psychotherapy and the Farther Shores of Psychiatry. New York, Brunner/Mazel, 1978
3. Bowlby J: Attachment, Vol I. New York, Basic Books, 1969
4. Bowlby J: Separation, Anxiety and Anger, Vol II. New York, Basic Books, 1973
5. Bowlby J: Loss, Sadness and Depression, Vol III. New York, Basic Books, 1980
6. Carkhuff RR, Truax CB: Training, Counselling and Psychotherapy: An Evaluation of an Integrated and Experiential Approach. J Consult Psychol 29:333–336, 1965
7. Dollard J, Doob LW, Miller N, Mowrer OH, Sears RR: Frustration and Aggression. New Haven, CT, Yale University Press, 1939
8. Fromm-Reichman F: Principles of Intensive Psychotherapy. Chicago, The University of Chicago Press, 1950
9. Harlow HF, Zimmerman RR: Affectional Response in the Infant Monkey. SCIENCE 130:421–432, 1959
10. Korchin SJ: Modern Clinical Psychology: Principles of Intervention in the Clinic and Community. New York, Basic Books, 1976
11. Kvarnes RC, Parloff GH (eds): A Harry Stack Sullivan Case Seminar. New York, WW Norton, 1976
12. Mahler MS, Bergman A, Pine, F: The Psychological Birth of the Human Infant. New York, Basic Books, 1975
13. Maslow AH: The Need to Know and the Fear of Knowing. J Gen Psychol 68:111–124, 1963
14. Masterson JF: The Narcissistic and Borderline Disorders: An Integrated Developmental Approach. New York, Brunner/Mazel, 1981
15. Meninger K: The Vital Balance, pp 79–152. New York, The Viking Press, 1967
16. Rioch MJ, Coulter WR, Weinberger DM: Dialogues for Therapists. San Francisco, Josey Bass, 1976
17. Rogers C: On Becoming a Person. Boston, Houghton Mifflin, 1961
18. Seligman MP: Helplessness: On Depression, Development, and Death. San Francisco, WH Freeman, 1975
19. Sullivan HS: Interpersonal Theory of Psychiatry. New York, WW Norton, 1953

14 Groups and Group Therapy

Barbara G. Tunley Crenshaw

No man is an island, entire of itself;
every man is a piece of the continent,
a part of the main; ...
any man's death diminishes me,
because I am involved in mankind;
and therefore never send to know for whom
the bell tolls;
it tolls for thee.

John Donne,
Devotions XVII

Chapter Preview

We live and work in groups. Each of us is born into a family, we attend school with groups of our peers, we enter into friendship and work-related groups, and we establish our own groups of family or significant others. In psychiatric–mental health and other areas of health care, nurses interact with groups of students, faculty, professional colleagues, and clients and their families. An understanding of group dynamics and their application is essential to effective functioning.

The family may be defined as the individual's primary group. The characteristics of this primary group influence how the individual is socialized into future groups, and how he adopts various roles within groups.

This chapter discusses group process, dynamics, theory, group norms, roles, decision-making, and outcome. It examines various types of groups and the advantages and disadvantages of group therapy. An overview of theoretical frameworks for group therapy, such as Rogerian, Gestalt, Transactional Analysis, and T (training)-groups are also presented. The chapter focuses on nursing intervention through the media of group process and therapy.

Learning Objectives

On completion of the chapter, you should be able to accomplish the following:

1. identify the characteristics of a group
2. explain group norms and how they are developed and enforced
3. compare styles of group leadership and their effects on group members' functioning
4. describe the process of structuring a group
5. define three major categories of group roles
6. discuss the purposes, advantages, and disadvantages of group therapy
7. discuss the curative factors of group therapy
8. compare the various types of therapy and self-help or growth groups
9. describe the stages of group development
10. apply therapeutic interventions to groups of clients
11. identify process communication in group behavior

Group Process

What Is a Group?

A *group* is three or more persons with related goals. These goals of group members are influenced by many forces—intrapersonal, interpersonal, need, the physical environment, and the unique interaction of the group.

The physical environment is one factor that affects group development. For example, the physical environment or climate in some countries is so severe that the survival of the individual depends on his relationship to other individuals. The individuals form bonds of relationship that develop into groups. These groups develop structure, characteristics, and roles. The further creation of systems and subsystems leads to the development of more complex societies that display certain characteristics called culture.

Characteristics of Groups

Characteristics of groups include the following:

The size of the group
The homogeneity or heterogeneity of group members
The stability of the group
The degree of cohesiveness, or "bonding power," between members
The climate of the group (*i.e.,* warm, friendly, cold, aloof, and so forth)
The group's conformity to group norms
The degree of agreement of the leader's and the group's norms
The group's ability to deal with members' infractions
The goal-directedness and task orientation of the group's work

Types of Groups

Groups may be primary or secondary, formal or informal. Members of *primary groups* have face-to-face contact. They have boundaries, norms, and explicit and implicit interdependent roles. An example of a primary group is a family.

Secondary groups are usually larger and more impersonal than primary groups. Members of secondary groups do not have the relationship bonds or emotional ties of members of a primary group. An example of a secondary group is a political party or a business.

A *formal* group has structure and authority. Authority in a formal group usually emanates from above and interaction in the group is usually limited.

A faculty meeting is an example of a formal group. *Informal* groups provide much of a person's education and contribute greatly to their cultural values. The members of an informal group are not dependent on each other, such as in friendship groups and hobby groups.[4]

Group Norms

A *group norm* is the development, over a period of time, of a pattern of interaction within a group to which certain behavioral expectations are attached. Group norms affect the scope and functioning of a group. Norms also help to structure role expectations. Norms provide sanctions, taboos, and reference power to the group.

To explain group norms, let us examine a nursing team meeting, designed to discuss both client care planning and communication among the nursing staff. A role expectation norm is that the team leader will chair the meeting. A norm of the membership is that the members will be on time and will, possibly, sit in certain places. There may be a formalized norm called an agenda of the meeting, which states that communication among nursing staff members will occur before the discussion to plan client care. Other group norms may be universal with regard to the task role of one member, such as the role of the secretary who records the minutes of the meeting. Group members who present their client's history and assessment accurately, clearly, and with organization receive sanction. A group taboo is to fall asleep and snore while another member is talking. When a group member falls asleep and snores during meetings, especially if this occurs numerous times, he is viewed as a deviant. A deviant may eventually be isolated by the group. Members neither speak to him nor listen when he speaks. They may physically isolate him by not sitting next to him. Therefore, punishment, formal or informal, is metered out to the deviant along with criticism.[73]

Norms exert a controlling element over groups by setting the boundaries of group activities. To promote the growth and stimulation of group members, it is important that groups learn to change their norms when they are no longer functional for the group. A group remains more creative if each member becomes a "change agent" for norms no longer needed (see Group Nursing Care Plan 14-1, "Interventions in Group Process and Group Therapy.")

Group Leadership

To become an effective group leader, the nurse must understand the concepts of leadership and the forces, scope, and limitations inherent in each concept. The three concepts of influence, power, and authority have an impact on leadership.[76] *Power* is the perceived ability to control appropriate reward, therefore lending *influence* to the leader. The nurse leader gains *authority* through influence, power, and her knowledge or expertise. The leader also understands that there are effective ways of using authority and she decides to what extent she will expand or limit her authority.

The effective leader also decides to what extent her authority will be autocratic; (*i.e.*, centralized) or democratic (*i.e.*, decentralized). The leader reaches this decision, in part, according to the type of group. For example, the leader may relinquish authority readily in a training group. The purpose of the T-group (or training group) is to improve the group members' ability to communicate or relate to others in the group. The members, however, generally possess a certain degree of knowledge and experience in relating to others and are therefore capable of imparting their skills to other group members.

In psychoanalytic groups, where members are likely to exhibit high degrees of personality disorganization and faulty communication and interpersonal skills, the leader may exercise centralized authority. In other types of therapy groups, such as Gestalt groups, which deal with the "here and now" and whose members are generally healthy, the distribution of power within the group may depend on the age and emotional maturity of the group members.

Styles of Group Leadership

Leadership styles are influenced by several factors, including the following:

The philosophy of treatment
The personality of the leader
The traits and characteristics of the group
The purpose of the group
The degree of mental, emotional, or cognitive impairment of the group members

The nurse group leader alters her style of group leadership according to the demands of the therapeutic situation. The three basic styles of group leadership are as follows.

1. Autocratic style
2. Democratic style
3. Laissez-faire style

An *autocratic* leader is one who exercises significant authority and control over group members, who rarely, if ever, seeks or uses input from the group, and who does not encourage participation or interaction of the group.

In some circumstances, such as in emergencies,

(Text continues on p. 206)

Group Nursing Care Plan 14-1

Interventions in Group Process and Group Therapy

Group Problem	Outcome	Intervention
Fear of authority, resulting in timid, hostile, aggressive, or withdrawn behavior	Group members will deal with authority directly and openly	Use nonverbal and verbal communication techniques; listen to the client and encourage him to share and explore his feelings
		Reassure the client that the nurse-therapist will not respond punitively when he expresses his feelings
		Respond in an understanding manner when the client presents his feelings (even when they are hostile)
		Role-play various patterns of authority to determine which ones cause the client to become defensive or uncomfortable
		Provide the client with "desensitization" problem-solving situations related to his specific problem (*e.g.,* record conversations with persons of authority and analyze them for problematic areas, themes, patterns, and other situations resulting in the client's discomfort or maladaptive behavior)
		Help the client develop problem-solving strategies around the identified problem situations
Initial anxiety in a group, displayed by silence, fidgeting, nervous movement, and selective hearing	Group members' anxiety will be lessened so they can function more effectively in a group	Give "strokes" for positive interaction
		Help the client establish a role in the group related to his skills
		Share with the client that discomfort in the initial stage of group development is not uncommon
		Meet the client's dependency needs
Hidden agenda	Group members will express communication and action in an open manner	Identify the source of individual and group anxiety causing the hidden agenda

Group Problem	Outcome	Intervention
		Explore the hidden agenda with the group and its meaning and effect on the group's functioning
Subgrouping	Unproductive subgroups will be eliminated	Establish clarifying goals and purpose of the group (thereby lessening the group's anxiety and aiding in elimination of subgroups)
		Direct subgroup interest toward the goals of the group, thereby lessening subgroup preoccupation with outside themes
		Shorten the group's "fight and flight" stage through the use of independent members as catalysts to speed up the group process
Difficulty in giving and receiving information in a group	Group member will become more comfortable in giving and receiving information	Help the client explore his feelings about receiving objective data about himself
	Group members will learn techniques of giving and receiving feedback	Help the client to connect the feedback he is giving and receiving with a specific incident to lessen ambiguity and distortion
		Help the client explore the advantage of giving feedback at the proper time
		Help the client learn how to validate his feedback with others for accuracy and tact
Feeling threatened to the point of defensiveness and verbal outbursts	Group members' anxiety will decrease	Reduce the anxiety of the group by reassuring the client
		Assess the group's level of anxiety to determine its effect on the client
		Assess your own level of anxiety to determine its effect on the client's feeling of threat
		Explore the topic being discussed in the group to see what meaning this topic holds for the client (*i.e.,* is the topic a "high impact" one?)
Discomfort with established group norms	Group members will adapt to group norms	Help the client evaluate the purpose of the norm (*i.e.,* why

(Continues on p. 204)

Group Problem	Outcome	Intervention
		it is developed and how it represents group standards)
		Help the client understand the result of breaking the group norm, such as increased anxiety of the group
		Help the client learn methods of changing norms (present the change to the group, state rationale for change, allow discussion by the group, and so forth); remind the client that there is a definite risk in violating a current norm in order to challenge its desirability
Deviant behavior	Members' deviant behavior will be modified	Identify deviant behavior and discuss it with the client
		Identify sources of discomfort in the environment that affect the client
		Explore with the client whether or not he identifies his behavior as deviant
		Help members of the group identify deviant behavior
		Help the client explore how his behavior affects his relationship in the group
		Use group pressure to help the deviate change or conform to group norms
		Help the group identify which behavior is destructive and which might foster group growth
Indecision	Group members' decision-making ability will improve	Help the client develop assertive communication skills
		Help the client explore methods of decision-making in a group
		Help the client implement conflict resolution strategies in the group to arrive at the most productive decision for the group
		Help the client explore all aspects or data related to the decision, thereby reaching a broader view of the issue before coming to closure

Group Problem	Outcome	Intervention
Overdependency	Members will demonstrate appropriate independence in accomplishing the group's task	Provide a leadership void to make the client more independent
		Explore with the client his feelings about dependency and how it affects the group's growth
		Share specific techniques with the client, such as a list of the group's tasks and requesting that he volunteer for the job for which he is most suited
Role confusion or lack of clarity of membership activity	Members will exhibit increased understanding of own role in the group and understanding of group norms relating to specific roles within the group	Ask the client to express his ideas about his perception of roles in the group
		Help the client express how he perceives his role in the group in relationship to other client–members' roles
		Clarify distortions of interpretation about role and role-taking
Lack of interpersonal closeness or trust Feeling frightened when he shares himself with others	Members will demonstrate increased ability to trust lessened fear of selves and others	Display consistent behavior as the group leader
		Listen to the client's fears
		Explore with the client the reality of his fears
		Show respect, dignity, and caring when the client discusses closeness
		Reassure the client that closeness is possible
		Time interventions involving closeness carefully
Resistance to therapy (*e.g.*, grunting, moaning, staring into space, overresponding to situations, changing the subject)	Members will demonstrate increased acceptance of, and participation in, therapy	Explore with client his resistant behavior
		Confront the client with his actions and behavior, utilizing an understanding approach
Competition that stimates group progress	Members will demonstrate increased skill and comfort with competition, compromise, and cooperation	Help the client learn how to gain recognition for his effort in socially acceptable ways
		Explore the concepts and goals of competition, compromise, and cooperation with client

(Continues on p. 206)

Group Problem	Outcome	Intervention
Termination of the group, resulting in increased anxiety and self-defeating behavior	Members will accept group termination and grow from termination experience	Help the client identify his accomplishments while he has been a member of the group
		Help the client work through feelings of loss during termination (*i.e.,* feelings of anger, depression, euphoria, rejection)
		Help the client express both positive and negative feelings about the group and evaluate the group experience realistically
		Plan a termination activity that allows expression of group members' feelings

the autocratic style of leadership may be the most effective; it conserves time and energy and dictates roles and responsibilities to members. On the other hand, constant use of an autocratic leadership style may cause hostility, scapegoating behavior, dependence on the leader, and limitation of growth potential for group members.

The *democratic* style of leadership encourages group interaction and participation in group problem-solving and decision-making. A democratic group leader values the input and feedback of each group member, seeks spontaneous, honest interaction among members of the group, and creates an atmosphere in which members are rewarded for their contributions. The group's opinions are solicited and the group's work is tailored to their common goals. A group with a democratic leadership style may require more time and effort than an autocratic group to accomplish its goals; however, the group's efforts are more productive and cohesive and instill in members a sense of participation in decision-making.

In a *laissez-faire* style of leadership, group members are free to operate as they choose. This style of group leadership may be effective if the members are highly knowledgeable, task-oriented, and motivated. On the other hand, the laissez-faire approach is time-consuming and often inefficient in the accomplishment of group tasks.

Decision-Making

Decision-making is a necessary component of leadership, power, influence, authority, and delegation of authority. In formal groups, specific guidelines determine which decisions will be made by the leader and which decisions will be decentralized—that is, delegated to group members.

The ability to make effective decisions depends on the following:

The group's knowledge of the subject
The group's ability to choose appropriate methods to solve specific problems
The group's ability to test and evaluate problem-solving decision-making, after a decision has been put to the test
The group's maturity and its ability to reverse or modify a decision that has proved to be unwise, unfair, or otherwise unacceptable

Decisions may be made by consensus, majority vote, or minority decision. In a *consensus,* all members of the group agree on a decision. Although consensus may prove to be time-consuming and costly, especially in a large group, it gives more satisfaction to the total group. The democratic leader uses consensus whenever possible.

Majority vote is a form of decision-making in which the issue is decided by the larger number of group members. This method is often used by democratic leadership when it is not possible to reach a consensus.

A *minority decision* may be formulated by a self-delegated subgroup or a group appointed as a subcommittee to explore the situation in greater depth and reach a decision.

CHART 14-1

Responsibilities of Group Leaders and Members

Sandra Carter Patterson Chandler, M.S., R.N.
Nursing Instructor
El Centro College
Dallas, Texas

Group leaders' responsibilities to members include the following:

1. Ensuring the psychological safety of group members
2. Establishing and maintaining group norms
3. Role-modeling relationship skills
4. Commenting on group process

To receive gratification from group membership, members must do the following:

1. Introspect
2. Self-disclose
3. Nurture others
4. Express their feelings
5. Contribute to the maintenance of the group

Structuring the Group

The group leader is instrumental in establishing and maintaining cohesiveness in the group. She selects and orients new group members in both beginning and continuing groups. An effective leader ensures that the structuring process for the group defines group norms, clarifies expectations, sets standards for group performance, and works to maintain cohesiveness as new members are introduced into the group. The leader discusses some of these issues with new members before introducing them to the group. An example of such a discussion follows.

Leader: Jane, welcome. I am Ms. C., the group leader. I always meet with new members to share with them the goals and expectations of the group. (pause)

Leader: The group will have eight members, including you. We will meet from 1 to 2 pm each day in the Blue Room. Members will enter and leave the group as their behavior and needs change. (pause)

Jane: What are we expected to do?

Leader: Group members are expected to share their problems and their feelings about those problems with other members of the group.

Jane: Is that all?

Leader: No, it is also my expectation that group members will discover techniques of problem-solving through exploring these problems and feelings and that, eventually, when members learn to relate more effectively to each other, they will transfer these newly acquired skills to other relationships.

Jane: That sounds difficult and frightening.

Leader: Changing and growing have a certain amount of pain.

The leader therefore structures the group by determining its size, homogeneity of group members, and leadership style. The group's purpose and goals define its scope, limitation, and hoped-for accomplishments.[17]

Roles in Groups

The functions of group leaders and members are interdependent. Member roles can enhance the effectiveness of a group leader and vice versa.

Roles observed in groups are categorized as follows:

Group task roles
Group building and maintenance roles
Individual roles

Group task roles identify group problems and select methods to solve those problems.[46] Problem-solving helps the group to reach its goal or mission. Some examples of group task roles are as follows:

1. The initiator-contributor, who suggests or proposes to the group new ideas or different ways of regarding the group problem or goal
2. The information seeker, who asks for clarification
3. The opinion seeker, who does not ask primarily for facts of the case, but for a clarification of values pertinent to what the group is undertaking
4. The information giver, who offers facts or generalizations that are "authoritative" or who shares his own experience in relation to the group problems
5. The opinion giver, who states his ideas and values about group suggestions
6. The elaborator, who develops the meaning of suggestions offered to the group
7. The coordinator, who shows or clarifies how ideas can work
8. The orienter, who keeps the group on target by defining where the group is in relationship to its goal

9. The evaluator-critic, who sets standards by evaluating the accomplishment of the group in relation to its task, using previously set standards of group functioning
10. The energizer, who arouses the group to greater productivity by prodding members
11. The procedural-technician, who speeds up group movement by doing things such as handing out material and so forth
12. The recorder, who is the "group memory," who writes down productive discussions and group decisions[46]

Group building and maintenance roles are oriented toward the functioning of the group as a whole. They are designed to alter or maintain the group's way of working to strengthen, regulate, and perpetuate the group as a group. Some examples of group building and maintenance roles are as follows:

1. The encourager, who gives acceptance to the contributions of others
2. The harmonizer, who reconciles differences between group members
3. The compromiser, who admits his error to maintain group harmony and meets the person with an opposing idea halfway
4. The gate-keeper, who facilitates the contributions to others, thereby keeping communication open through his encouraging remarks about these contributions
5. The standard-setter, who sets group goals to be achieved and evaluates the functioning of the group
6. The group-observer, who notes what is occurring in the group and feeds it back to the group with his evaluation or interpretation of the group's procedure
7. The follower, who goes along with the ideas of other members, assuming more of an audience role[49]

Individual roles are roles that meet only the needs of the group member, not of the group. They do not enhance, rather they hamper, group functioning. They support individual needs and goals, not group needs and goals. Some examples of individual roles are as follows:

1. The aggressor, who deflates the status of individual and group accomplishment
2. The blocker, who resists progress by arguing or disagreeing beyond reason
3. The recognition-seeker, who calls attention to himself through boasting and pointing out his achievements
4. The self-confessor, who expresses feelings and

ideology not related to the group, but uses the group as an audience
5. The play-person, who "horses around," demonstrating his lack of involvement
6. The dominator, who asserts his authority and superiority in manipulating the group or certain members of the group
7. The help-seeker, who tries to elicit sympathy from the group or individual members
8. The special interest pleader, who tries to have his own biases and prejudices accepted through the use of others

All of these roles are observed in group behavior. Individually oriented behavior, which often grows out of personal anxiety, detracts from and temporarily stymies the group and its progress, whereas task, maintenance, and building roles promote group growth and productivity.[49]

Group Therapy

Purposes

One of the purposes of group psychotherapy is to intervene in psychopathology. Group therapy offers multiple stimuli for distortions in interpersonal relationships to be revealed, examined, and resolved.

The purpose of a group is related to its goals and expected outcomes. For example, a training group's purpose is to help members improve their present styles of relating to others. An individual needing to develop or heighten these skills would join a T-group instead of a psychotherapy group.

Advantages and Disadvantages

Group therapy, as a form of treatment for psychiatric–mental health clients, has advantages and disadvantages. The advantages of group therapy include the following:

1. A greater number of clients can be treated in group therapy, making the method cost-effective.
2. Members profit by hearing other members discuss their problems. This discussion decreases the member's feelings of isolation, alienation, and uniqueness, and encourages him to share his feelings and problems.
3. Group therapy provides an opportunity for clients to explore their specific styles of communication in a safe atmosphere where they can receive feedback, and can undergo change.
4. Members learn multiple ways of solving a

problem from other group members, and group exploration may help them discover new ways of solving a problem.

5. Members learn about the functional roles of individuals in a group. Sometimes, a member shares the responsibility of the co-therapist. Members become culture carriers.

6. The group provides for its members' understanding, confrontation, and identification with more than one individual. The member gains a reference group.[52]

There are also disadvantages of group therapy. An individual's privacy may be destroyed; for example, when a conversation shared within the group is repeated outside of the group. This behavior obstructs confidentiality and hampers complete and honest participation in a group.

Clients may experience difficulty exposing themselves to a group or believe that they lack the skills to communicate effectively in a group. Some clients may use these factors as resistance; others may be reluctant to expose themselves to the group because they do not want to "change."

Group therapy will not be a helpful form of therapy if the therapist conducts the group as if he is giving individual therapy. Such a therapist may see dynamics and group processes as incidental or antagonistic to the therapeutic process. The effective group leader must be skilled in techniques and interventions that foster group interaction and shape group behavior and growth.

Curative Factors of Group Therapy

Yalom described ten curative factors of group therapy:

1. Imparting of information
2. Instillation of hope
3. Universality
4. Altruism
5. Corrective recapitulation of the primary family group
6. Development of socializing techniques
7. Imitative behavior
8. Interpersonal learning
9. Group cohesiveness
10. Catharsis[75]

Imparting of information is the use of information in a planned, structured manner, such as didactic instruction given in a lecture format. These lectures may be accompanied by audiovisual and other teaching aids. The topic of the lecture or didactic presentation is clear.

Instillation of hope helps the client maintain faith in the therapeutic modality. The client is optimistic; he believes that he will get better.

Universality prevents the client from feeling unique and different. Within the group, he begins to feel less isolated and more like other people. This feeling is strengthened by the client's learning that others in the group have problems, thoughts, and feelings similar to his own.

Altruism is the process of clients' aiding or helping each other. The act of giving to others becomes therapeutic for the giver, which increases the self-esteem of the giver.

Corrective recapitulation of the primary family group means that the client is influenced in therapy group by his history. Initially in group therapy, the client usually perceives the behavior of other members as being like his siblings', and the behavior of the leader (or therapist) as being like his parents'. When neither the members nor the leader respond to him as his siblings or parents have in the past, the client begins to gain insight into his own behavior.

Development of socializing techniques occurs in group therapy. Social skills are related to interpersonal success in our society. Feedback and role-playing of social events are two techniques employed in group therapy that develop social skills. It is expected that clients will terminate their group therapy experience with greater social skills than they previously had. Clients with regressed behavior may learn elementary social skills, such as not belching during group, whereas clients in higher functioning groups may learn to attend to feedback about styles of communication such as rushing one's words, repeating oneself, and interrupting other members when they are speaking.

Imitative behavior is a powerful therapeutic tool through which a group member identifies with the healthier aspects of the other members and the leader. Imitating the behavior of an assertive group member or leader, for example, demonstrates growth.

Interpersonal learning results from therapy groups because the groups are, in effect, microcosms of society. Learning from a therapy group can be transferred to other groups. The client learns to profit from the therapeutic use of anxiety. When anxiety is minimized, the client relates more openly, he learns to trust, to expose himself, to give of himself, to expect from others, to test reality, and therefore to experience growth.

Group cohesiveness relates to bonding or solidarity, the feeling of "we" instead of "I." Cohesiveness is demonstrated through group attendance and the ability of the group to communicate positive and negative expressions to each other without the group disintegrating. In cohesive groups, members try hard to impress one another, are accepting of each other, and enter and leave the group with minimal disruption of the process.

Catharsis is the expression of feelings, especially those that involve deep emotions. Expression of feelings is particularly important in the curative process.[68]

Nurses and Group Process and Therapy

Historically, nurses have used groups and group process in hospitals and other health care settings. As nursing progressed from functional assignments to the team approach, many studies were undertaken to gather information on the most effective ways to use the team's task and maintenance roles. The search for this information led nurses to collaborate with colleagues in examining group theory, group dynamics, and group functioning in various health care delivery systems. Psychiatric–mental health nurses have specifically explored the use of groups as a teaching method, a therapeutic tool with clients, and a form of peer group supervision.

Nurse educators have employed group seminars as part of the teaching-learning process to enable nursing students to participate in groups, to learn group roles, and to learn the function and dynamics of the student-participant role. Instructors delegated a certain amount of authority to the nursing students, yet also served as democratic leaders, structuring the course to a certain degree and defining expectations of the class. This methodology of experiential learning sparked an exciting involvement in learning group theory, enabling students to transfer their knowledge of, and experience in, group dynamics to other arenas of therapy, such as milieu, client groups, and supervision groups. Often, these seminars served as prerequisites for advanced courses in group therapy in graduate nursing programs.

Psychiatric–mental health nurses learned group therapist and co-therapist roles and responsibilities. Dr. Hildegard Peplau, an early authority on psychiatric nursing specialist programs, augmented nurses' involvement in group therapy through "experiential learning." Nurses developed increasing skill in the techniques of group therapy; psychiatric nursing clinical specialists became highly skilled in group intervention.

The Mental Health Revolution, sponsored by President John F. Kennedy, demanded greater numbers of health professionals to administer formal and informal group therapy in community mental health centers. Responding to this need, psychiatric–mental health nurses, and, particularly, psychiatric clinical nurse specialists, became more active in group leader roles in therapeutic communities, outpatient settings, and private therapy, and also became more active as liaison psychiatric nursing consultants in general hospital settings.

Psychiatric–mental health nurses participate as leaders or co-leaders in many formal and informal group therapies, including revitalization, resocialization, re-education, supportive therapy, insight, psychoanalytic therapy, transactional analysis, family therapy, couples therapy, adolescent therapy, T-groups, and prevention groups in the community.[12]

Types of Therapy Groups

Growth Groups and Psychotherapeutic Groups

In the past three decades, numerous forms of growth groups, such as self-help groups and group counseling, have developed. Guidelines to determine the maximal therapeutic benefit of a growth or therapy group for an individual participant include the following:

1. The extent of personality disorganization of the participant
2. The effect of personality disorganization on interpersonal functioning, as a family member, provider, productive citizen, and so on
3. The degree of functional ability and role success or failure of the participant
4. The participant's ability to harness his impulses in stressful group situations; for example, does the member become verbally or physically disruptive or destructive in anxious situations?
5. The member's purpose or goals in joining a group, both articulated goals and hidden agendas
6. The participant's ability to share and support others in problem-solving tasks
7. The participant's ability to use the material produced in group to problem-solve his own situation

There are different functions of the leader in psychotherapeutic and self-help groups. The leader in the psychotherapy group assumes more responsibility for the group than does a leader of a self-help group. In the psychotherapy group, the group members or clients may have limiting neurotic or maladaptive-to-severe emotional disturbances. The member may be referred to the group from individual therapy, where he was seen in an initial crisis state but is now able to tolerate the group setting. Clients in a therapy group do not become the therapist, and the therapist never assumes the client's role in the group. The leader may also provide more support for members of a therapy group who may have less tolerance for stress.

In a growth or self-help group, such as a T-group, both leader and members have attained a certain degree of emotional stability and one does not observe a great discrepancy between their functioning by the end of the growth group experience. The group initially uses the leader to provide guidance and clarification; however, toward the end of the group experience, he becomes a part of the group and several of his functions may be performed by the group members. In a growth group, the members may receive less support from the leader while dealing with their anxiety, but there is conflict resolution by the end of the group.

Psychoanalytic Group Psychotherapy

In a psychoanalytic group, the therapist holds a prominent position. Each client in the group has a relationship with the therapist. Group communication is focused on the three levels of unconscious, semiconscious, and conscious material. The group focuses on interpretation of dreams, free association, and other latent content produced in the group. The therapist turns these experiences into conscious, healthy learning experiences for the client. This process is accomplished by transference to the therapist and multitransferences to group members.

Transactional Analysis (TA)

The three ego states of the individual—the parent, the child, and the adult—are examined in transactional analysis groups. A goal of TA groups is that individuals in the group will communicate from the proper ego state for the situation and the responses of others, thereby lessening conflict and promoting mature relationships.

Rational–Emotive Therapy

Based on the theory of Albert Ellis that human beings, although subject to powerful biologic and social forces, still have the capacity for being rational, rational-emotive group therapy aims to maximize a person's rational thinking. People, says Ellis, tend to overgeneralize situations when they are anxious. If they do not employ thinking and reasoning at this point, they become irrational. The therapist designs activities to rid the members of the group of their irrational ideas.

Rogerian Group Therapy

In a Rogerian group, the therapist's goal is to help the members express their feelings toward one another during group sessions. The therapist's role is one of encouraging this expression of feelings, clarifying these feelings with clients, and accepting clients and their feelings nonjudgmentally. Through this process, the client learns to accept his own feelings, a first step toward self-acceptance. The client gains positive self-regard through his relationship with the therapist.[12] Inherent in Rogerian theory is the belief that change and growth can take place at any age.

Gestalt Therapy

Fritz S. Perls pioneered the techniques of Gestalt therapy. Gestalt theory emphasizes the "here and now"; that is, it emphasizes self-expression, self-exploration, and self-awareness in the present. Clients and therapist focus on everyday problems and try to solve them. The individual becomes aware of his "total self" and "the world" that surround him; awareness of the problem renders him capable of change. The leader's role in Gestalt therapy groups is to help members express their feelings and grow from their experiences.

Interpersonal Group Therapy

Interpersonal theory development is attributed to Harry Stack Sullivan, who also worked extensively with Peplau to introduce interpersonal theory into nursing. Anxiety is the focus of interpersonal therapy—how the individual develops anxiety and how he resolves it. Anxiety has the potential to hamper, distort, or enhance relationships between individuals. Interpersonal group therapists explore the members' anxiety and stress and their effects on the individual.

It is believed that anxiety arises from interpersonal relationships and is reduced or relieved through interpersonal support. One of the main goals of interpersonal group therapy is to promote the individual's comfort with others in the group, which then transfers to other relationships.

Psychodrama Groups

Psychodrama in the United States has its origin, implementation, and direction in the work of Jacob L. Moreno. He promoted this method of group therapy with individuals, small groups, and large groups. He even tried to help the citizens of America resolve their guilt over John F. Kennedy's assassination through sociodrama.

Psychodrama can be used as a form of group psychotherapy that explores the truth through dramatic methods. During *psychodrama,* the subject (or client) produces a topic to be explored. The director (or therapist) directs the subject through role-playing of scenes related to the topic and incorporates the use of auxiliary egos (or therapeutic aides) in the action. The audience experiences the feelings and identifies with the action on the stage. A catharsis occurs for the subject and also for the audience.

Bion Method

Also termed the Travistock conference, the *Bion method* emphasizes experiential learning that is translatable into action in work and community life. The group provides a setting in which experience can be studied and partially understood as it occurs. The group examines transactions, boundaries, the function of leadership, and attitudes toward authority.[8]

Marathon Groups

The term *marathon group* refers to the amount of concentrated time the participants spend together as a group. Marathon groups are similar to each other, not by virtue of the leaders' theoretical orientations or techniques, but because each is a single uninterrupted session. These sessions may last from 12 hours to 2, 3, or more days, allowing short periods away from the group for sleeping and eating. These groups have a clearly stated goal of personal change or growth of the participants.

Encounter Groups

The purpose of an encounter group is personal change, often as a result of deeply felt experiences. The differences between marathon and encounter groups are minimal, and the theoretical orientations of group leaders are diverse.

Examples of themes of encounter groups are "The Challenge of Change, Danger, and Fulfillment"; "Closeness, Can It Hurt?"; and "Marriage, How to Survive It."

T-Groups

The *T-group* is the oldest and best known therapeutic method coming out of the sensitivity training group movement. The first T-group conference was held in Bethel, Maine in 1946. The goal of each T-group conference is to verify experimentally the T-group method. This involves the study of group norms, roles, communication distortions, and the effects of authority on behavior patterns, personality, and coping mechanisms. Group members receive feedback by exposing themselves to others in the group, and they also experiment with new and more productive behavior.

Other sensitivity groups may have similar objectives, such as interpersonal skill groups, discussion groups, self-analytic groups, and process groups. All of these groups focus on the growth process of the individual through the help of the leader and the group.

Community Support Groups

Numerous support groups have emerged under the category of mental health community psychiatry. Some were founded to lend continued or added support to previously hospitalized psychiatric clients. Other groups have been formed as a result of the needs of individuals in the community. Self-help groups have been developed by lay persons to address specific needs shared by group members. Community support groups, of which there exist more than 500 examples, may be classified in various ways, including the following (which are discussed in more detail in Chart 14-2):

Community violence support groups
Birth anomaly support groups
Acquired diseases support groups
Chronic illness support groups for patients and families
Developmental adjustment groups from birth to death
Grief education and resolution groups
Interracial and biracial support groups
Self-help improvement groups
Family structure support groups
Work-related stress groups

The main purpose of community support groups is to provide identification, clarification, understanding, role-modeling, feelings of togetherness, and group cohesion. They help prevent the individual member from feeling lonely and isolated. Some groups evolve into educational models that enhance communication, self-image, body image, problem-solving, decision-making, and growth processes.

Most community support groups help their members decrease levels of stress and increase levels of self-acceptance. With the help of the group, the member is better able to deal with the problems that he brought to the group. The outcome of this process is rewarding; the member develops new or more effective patterns of behavior.

Although community support groups have structures similar to those of other groups, they may be larger than therapy groups. Leadership in community support groups may be shared among the members, *i.e.,* "leadership as a process." Senior members are expected to provide direction and structure and help establish norms.

Stages of Group Development

Initial Stage

The initial stage of group development is likely to involve superficial, rather than open and trusting, communication. The members are becoming acquainted with each other and are searching for similarity between themselves and other group members. Members may also be unclear about the purposes or goals of the group. A certain amount of structuring of group norms, roles, and responsibilities takes place (see Chart 14-3, "Stages of Group Development").

CHART 14-2

Community Support Groups

Community Violence Support Groups

These groups are formed to support individuals and families that have been physically or emotionally battered or abused. Examples include Safe House groups, rape trauma groups, and battered children groups.

Birth Anomaly Support Groups

These groups are formed to support individuals and families with birth defects and congenital anomalies. Examples include groups for families with a member who has Down syndrome or cerebral palsy.

Acquired Diseases Support Groups

These groups are formed to support individuals and families coping with, and adjusting to, diseases originating after birth that are not inherited or innate. Examples include groups for families with a member who has leukemia, AIDS, or diabetes.

Chronic Illness Support Groups

These groups are formed to support individuals and families in which there is an illness of long-term duration, slow progression, and often little change in the symptomatology. Examples include groups to support persons with chronic obstructive pulmonary disease, cancer, or arthritis.

Developmental Adjustment Groups

These groups are formed to support individuals and families with physical or emotional development that deviates from the norm. Examples include groups to support persons with autistic

children, members with cretinism, or runaway teens.

Grief Education and Resolution Groups

These groups are formed to support individuals and families with physical and emotional loss. Examples include groups to support those who have suffered the death of a significant person or lost a child to SIDS.

Interracial and Biracial Support Groups

These groups are formed to support individuals and families of interracial siblings, children, spouses, parents, and neighborhoods. Examples include groups to support Amerasian families and children and the Greater Park Hill Neighborhood Association.

Self-help and Improvement Support Groups

These groups are formed to give support and offer perspectives on change (behavior change, attitude change) to members. Examples include assertiveness groups, Weight Watchers, Alcoholics Anonymous, Al-Anon.

Family Structure Support Groups

These groups are formed to support individuals and families of nontraditional (nonnuclear) family structure. Examples include step-parenting groups, Parents Without Partners, Lucky Mother's Club.

Work-related Support Groups

These groups are formed to support workers who experience job-related stress. Examples include burnout groups and Friday evening sessions.

Working Stage

During the working stage of group development, the real "work" of the group is accomplished. Because members are already familiar with each other, with the group leader, and with the group's rules, they are free to approach their problems and to attempt to solve their problems. Conflict and cooperation surface during the group's work.

Characteristics of a Mature Group. The mature group demonstrates the following characteristics:

1. The group develops workable norms and a group culture.
2. Conflict exists but resolution follows; when it occurs, conflict arises due to issues of importance, not emotional issues.
3. Members evaluate their own work and assume responsibility for their work.
4. Members are accepting of each others' differences without placing value judgments on them.
5. Role assignment is sanctioned by members of the group.

CHART 14-3
Stages of Group Development

Stages	Characteristics of Stages
Initial stage	Getting acquainted with group leader and members Dependency on the leader Searching for meaning and purpose of the group Restricted content and communicational style Search for similarity among members Giving advice
Working stage	Solving some of the problems of working together Conflict between members or between members and leader Working on issues of dominance, control, and power within group Cooperating to accomplish the group's work
Termination stage	Evaluating and summarizing the group experience Exploring positive and negative feelings about the group experience

(Adapted from Clark CC: The Nurse as Group Leader. New York, Springer-Verlag, 1977; also from Yalom ID: The Theory and Practice of Group Psychotherapy. New York, Basic Books, 1970)

6. Topics are discussed and decisions are made by means of rational behavior, such as sharing information and open discussion.
7. The group provides a feeling of "we" for the leader and members.
8. The group has cohesion.
9. The group is willing to validate itself; it has a "group image."[10]

Termination Stage

During termination, the group evaluates the experience and explores members' feelings about it and the impending separation. The termination of the group may be an opportunity for group members who have difficulty with "good-byes" to learn to deal more realistically and comfortably with this normal part of human experience, separation. (Chart 14-4 further illustrates the stages of group development.)

Group Communication and Nursing Intervention

Therapeutic Interventions with Groups

The use of therapeutic communication techniques with groups requires that nurses possess considerable preparation and skill in group work, as is shown by Chart 14-5, Therapeutic Intervention. Some of these therapeutic group interventions include the following:

Approval—condoning or encouraging an attitude, feeling or action

Acceptance—an attitude or a relationship that recognizes the worth of a person without implying either approval of particular behaviors or personal affection

Clarification—restatement by another, in what is hoped to be clearer terms, of the substance of what the client has said

Exploration—a shift from considering one aspect of a situation to considering another

Identification—delineating specific factors for the purposes of understanding or clarifying

Interpretation—finding or explaining the meaning or significance of the information

Information-giving—stating facts about a problem

Encouraging expression of feelings or ideas—indicating in some way that it is permissible or desirable to talk about feelings or ideas

Reassurance—offering the client confidence of a favorable outcome through suggestion, through persuasive arguments, or through comparing similar cases

Support—giving comfort, approval, or acceptance

C H A R T   14-4
Stages of Group Development: A Basketball Team

Group growth, functioning, and development can be compared to a basketball team. The team has appointed members designated to play certain roles, a leader (coach), and a co-leader (captain or point guard).

The team enters its *initial stage* of group development when the team members become acquainted. The leader (coach) *structures* the group by informing members of the frequency and time of practice and the expectations of the team, such as, "team members will work together to develop a winning team." Another group *norm* is that members (players) respect each other and their contributions.

Players are instructed to be on time for practices and for games; a player who persists in arriving late becomes a *deviant.* Together, players and coach decide that chronically late members will not be permitted to play the next game (sanctions).

The group learns to depend on the leader for guidance and instruction in certain skills. The leader uses the didactic method and group participation exercises to effect the skills of basketball during the *working stage*.

The coach and team study and practice different plays. They change plays, however, if they do not achieve the *goal* of winning basketball games. The coach functions as a "change agent" because his *interventions* impact the direction of the team and promote growth.

The captain or point guard may be the team's *co-leader* who brings in the plays from the coach to the team during the game or calls the plays in the role of "playmaker."

The team guards work at *maintenance and building roles,* while the team forwards work at the *task roles* of scoring points. *Individual roles* are observed when players make fouls and tempers flare.

The team demonstrates both competition and cooperation. The coach strives to build cohesion and a feeling of "we." Members symbolically show this identification through team uniforms, team colors, and team mascot.

Toward the end of the basketball season, the team enters its *termination stage*. Players and coach evaluate and summarize their group and individual performance for the season. Players also evaluate the coach's leadership skills. They express feelings of happiness and sadness. Because the team is an open-ended group, senior players face leaving the team at the end of the school year and younger players are added to the squad. Farewells and good wishes are spoken; an awards ceremony or party may mark the goodbyes.

Intervention—an action that directs or influences the client's behavior

Understanding—indicating verbally or nonverbally that you know or comprehend what is being communicated by the client and what he is feeling

Reflection—repeating back to the client what he has said, mirroring his statement

Listening—concentration on the client's communication without interruption

Teaching—helping the client learn specifics in relation to events and behavior

Silence—the use of no verbal or spoken words

Structuring—shaping the content of the group meeting

Limit-setting—deciding how far group members and the group may go before the therapist ceases or restricts, to a point, the behavior, activity, or verbal expression of members

Latent and Manifest Communication

Groups use both latent and manifest communication. *Latent content* is that content which is not discussed, that which occurs on a feeling level and is seldom verbalized, such as hidden agendas; *manifest content* involves spoken words (see Fig. 14–1). Groups are most effective when their latent content and manifest content are similar. The further apart these levels of communication are, the more problems in communication are experienced by the group.

A group may not solve its problems readily, due to the interference of latent content. Hidden agendas hinder group communication. For example, if a group member feels that he would be punished if he verbalized his opinion in the group, especially if he disagrees with the leader, his latent communication would influence his overt behavior and interfere with group growth. (Text continues on p. 218)

CHART 14-5

Therapeutic Intervention in Groups

Reflection

Mr. B: "All this talking is really a pain in the neck."

Nurse: "This talking is a pain in the neck."

Interpretation

Mr. B: "All this talking is really a pain in the neck."

Nurse: "Mr. B, you seem annoyed at all the talking."

Encouraging Expression of Feelings

Mr. W: "It takes me about 10 or 15 minutes to get oriented again in the morning and then I'm all right."

Nurse: "Are there others who feel this way?"

Ms. S: "I always get up to eat and have some coffee. Then I feel more like facing others."

Offering Support

Marty: "Well, I don't know. My busted arm has played heck with me. Getting anything for it has been a federal case. And I am not one who shows pain easily."

Nurse: "This must be pretty infuriating."

Marty: "Well, it really bugs me."

Structuring

Frank: "I'm going home soon."

Mrs. C: "Really?"

Nurse: "Maybe you would like to talk about going home?"

Teaching

Abel: (to the nurse) "You were irritated at me, weren't you, but we were able to talk about it and work it out."

Nurse: "Yes, we did, Abel. I was irritated because I felt you were not listening. And we did talk about it."

Understanding

Marty: "Nurse, I feel frightened about discharge."

Nurse: "I can understand your feeling frightened. Leaving the hospital is not always easy."

Exploration

Frank: "My son decided to leave the business."

Nurse: "Tell me how that came about."

Clarification

Abel: "I feel hopeless, no way out."

Nurse: "You feel you have no way out?"

Interpretation

Abel: "I feel hopeless, no way out."

Nurse: "You sound suicidal."

Giving Information

Marty: "All the staff write notes in the charts after the group meeting and put their own interpretation on what we say, don't they?"

Nurse: "I can only speak for myself. I write notes in the chart, but I try hard not to misinterpret what members state in the group."

Approval

Frank: "I decided to move to a new apartment."

Nurse: "You made a wise decision."

Reassurance

Frank: "I was afraid to move at first."

Nurse: "Frank, we are always here to listen to your fears and try and help you work them out."

Limit-setting

Marty: "I feel we need to cancel our therapy session next week since the next day is a holiday and we need a long weekend to travel."

Nurse: "Holiday weekends are difficult; however, we will not cancel our group session."

Acceptance

Marty: "Nurse, I was angry at you for not cancelling the session."

Nurse: "It's all right for you to get angry at me, Marty."

Levels of communication in groups

Figure 14-1. *Communication diagram: "the group mind."*

Content and Process Communication

Content and process are other ways of observing group communication. When we observe the group's discussion, we are focusing on the *content*. When we observe how the group is handling its communication, then we are focusing on *process*. Who talks to whom, what is said, and what is left unspoken are examples of process.[32] An example of content and process communication follows:

Content	Process
1. Discussing how a mother does not take care of her children may mean...	the leader or therapist is not meeting the dependency needs of the group.
2. Talking about the fighting of sisters and brothers at home may mean...	there is a lot of conflict and fighting in the therapy group.

C H A R T   14-6
Group Case

Theme: The group theme is "authority," or, more pointedly, transference. Our therapist is punitive to the group, like our mothers, if we disagree.

Countertransference

Therapist I, Mrs. A (angry): "You are rebellious and don't want to listen to reason. I am particularly angry at Marty because she started this...

Resistance

Three-fourths of the group did not attend the next meeting.

Interpretation

Therapist II, Mr. B (at a later session): Marty, when you stated we were like your mother, it sounded as if you were angry.

Acceptance

Marty: Yes, and afraid.

Exploration

Therapist I, Mrs. A: Marty, I wonder if you felt your weekend pass being cancelled was related to you disagreeing with me in group?

Acknowledgement

Marty: Yes.

Consensual Validation

Group: "You know, Mrs. A, we all thought that."

Insight

Group: "Later we realized that there was no connection between the cancellation of Marty's pass and the group meeting."

Problem-solving

Group: "We decided next time we would check out the situation before coming to a conclusion."

The co-therapist, in this example, listened for latent and manifest content to identify the group theme and used techniques of communication to help the group solve the problem.

An effective group leader brings the group's attention to the issues of process and their meaning.

Transference and Countertransference

Transference occurs when a client attributes characteristics and behavior of a family member or significant other to the therapist, thereby causing himself to respond to the therapist in a certain manner.[73] The clarification of this distortion with the client helps to create a therapeutic process of learning. *Countertransference* occurs when the therapist responds in a negative manner to the client's transference, further complicating communication.

Themes

The group leader observes for themes in the group's communication that recur or relate one group session to another and then explores the meanings of these themes. Through therapeutic communication, the leader may help the group uncover and problem-solve the issue. Group functioning is also evaluated by observing changes in members' behavior, such as their ability to apply these new techniques to problem-solving future tasks. Chart 14-6, "Group Case," illustrates how communication themes are used.

Higher functioning groups or those with less overt psychopathologic symptomatology will work through problems with minimal hidden agendas and symbolic language. The therapist can encourage the group to deal with "here and now" material and can manage anxiety more readily than in a group that communicates on a symbolic level.

Summary

This chapter has discussed group process and theory and their application to therapeutic needs. Some of the major foci of the chapter have included the following:

1. A group is three or more persons with related goals.
2. Groups vary according to their size, homogeneity of membership, climate, norms, and goal-directedness.
3. Group norms are the patterns of interaction that develop over time within a group.
4. A group leader designs the group's structure, style of leadership, and decision-making policies.
5. Roles in groups are task, building and maintenance, and individual roles.
6. The advantages of group therapy include its effectiveness and efficiency in time and cost.
7. Nurses participate as leaders and co-leaders in multiple formal and informal groups.
8. Most therapeutic group experiences can be categorized as psychotherapy or growth groups.
9. The three stages of group development are the initial, working, and termination stages.
10. Nurses and other group leaders employ a variety of therapeutic interventions with groups; they identify and explore latent versus manifest communication and process versus content communication.

References

1. Bach G: Intensive Group Psychotherapy. New York, Ronald Press, 1954
2. Battery R, Schill S, Durking HE, Friedmann A, Krasner T, La Hullier D: The Challenge for Group Psychotherapy: Present and Future. New York, International Universities Press, 1974
3. Benne KD, Sheats P: Functional Roles of Group Members. Group Development (Selected Series Number I), pp 51–59. Washington, DC, National Training Laboratories, National Education Association, 1961
4. Benne K (originally presented by), Bennett TR (revised by), Thornton R (further abbreviated by), Gertz B (final revision): Examples of Decision Making. Unpublished handout of National Training Laboratories Workshop, Washington DC, 1972
5. Berne E: Transactional Analysis in Psychotherapy. New York, Grove Press, 1961
6. Berne E: Principles of Group Treatment. New York, Oxford University Press, 1966
7. Bingham A, Bargar J: Children of Alcoholic Families: A Group Treatment Approach for Latency Age Children. J Psychosoc Nurs Ment Health Serv 23 (December): 13–15, 1985
8. Bion WR: Experiences in Groups and Other Papers. New York, Basic Books, 1961
9. Birckhead L: The Nurse as Leader of Group Psychotherapy with Psychotic Patients. J Psychosoc Nurs Ment Health Serv 22 (June): 24–30, 1984
10. Bradford L, Gibb J, Benne K: T-Group Therapy and Laboratory Method, 2d ed. New York, John Wiley & Sons, 1964
11. Braier M: Group Therapy with Parollees in a Community Mental Health Center. J Psychosoc Nurs Ment Health Serv 20 (February): 27–30, 1982
12. Burgess AW: Psychiatric Nursing in the Hospital and the Community, 3d ed. Englewood Cliffs, NJ, Prentice-Hall, 1981
13. Cathcart RS: Small Group Communication: A Reader, 2d ed. Dubuque, IO, WC Brown, 1974
14. Cartwright D, Zander A: Group Dynamics, 3d ed. New York, Harper & Row, 1968

15. Clark CC: Teaching Nurses Group Concepts: Some Issues and Suggestions. Nurse Educator 1 (January–February): 17–20, 1978

16. Clark CC: The Nurse As Group Leader. Springer Series on the Teaching of Nursing, Vol 3. New York, Springer-Verlag, 1977

17. Crosbie P: Interaction in Small Groups, p 2. New York, Macmillan, 1975

18. Dinnauer L, Miller M, Frankforter M: Implementation Strategies for an Inpatient Women's Support Group. J Psychosoc Nurs Ment Health Serv 19 (August): 13–16, 1981

19. Douglass LM: The Effective Nurse Leader and Manager, 2d ed. St Louis, CV Mosby, 1984

20. Durald MM, Hanks D: The Evaluation of Co-Leading a Gestalt Group. J Psychosoc Nurs Ment Health Serv 18 (December): 19–23, 1980

21. Eaton MT, Peterson MH, Davis JA: Psychiatry, Medical Outline Series, 3d ed. New York, Medical Examination Publishing, 1976

22. Edmands M: Overcoming Eating Disorders: A Group Experience. J Psychosoc Nurs Ment Health Serv 24 (August): 19–25, 1986

23. Fisher BA: Small Group Decision Making: Communication And The Group Process. New York, McGraw-Hill, 1974

24. Forsyth D, Cannady J: Preventing and Alleviating Staff Burnout Through a Group. J Psychosoc Nurs Ment Health Serv 19 (September): 35–38, 1981

25. Foulks SH, Anthony ET: Group Psychotherapy: The Psychoanalytic Approach. Baltimore, MD, Penguin Books, 1965

26. Gallese L, Trenting E: Help for Rape Victims Through Group Therapy. J Psychosoc Nurs Ment Health Serv 19 (August): 20–21, 1984

27. Gazda GM: Basic Approaches to Group Psychotherapy and Group Counseling. Springfield, IL, Charles C Thomas, 1971

28. Gazda GM: Innovations to Group Psychotherapy. Springfield, IL, Charles C Thomas, 1968

29. Goldberg AA: Group Communication: Discussion Processes Application. Englewood Cliffs, NJ, Prentice-Hall, 1975

30. Goldberg C: Encounter: Group Sensitivity Training Experience. New York, Science House, 1970

31. Glassman SM: Some Considerations in Building an Effective Group. Journal of the Fort Logan Mental Health Center 3 (Fall): 47–60, 1965

32. Glassman SM, Schiff S: Basic Concepts in Group Psychotherapy. Unpublished paper presented at Fort Logan Mental Health Center, Denver, CO, 1972

33. Glassman SM, Wright TL: A Conceptual Framework for Group Therapy. Unpublished paper for classroom presentation, 1974

34. Glassman SM, Schiff S: Large and Small Group Therapy in a State Mental Health Center. Int J Group Psychother 19 (April), 1969

35. Haber J, Leach A, Schudy S, Sidelean BF: Compre-

hensive Psychiatric Nursing, 2d ed. New York, McGraw-Hill, 1978

36. Hardin S, Durham J: First Rate: Exploring the Structure, Process, and Effectiveness of Nurse Psychotherapy. J Psychosoc Nurs Ment Health Serv 23 (May): 8–16, 1985

37. Hill J: Power in Therapy. Unpublished paper presented to the Fourth Annual Alumni Meeting of Graduate Psychiatric Nursing Specialists, University of Colorado Health Science Center, 1980

38. Hoover R, Parnell P: An Inpatient Education Group on Stress and Coping. J Psychosoc Nurs Ment Health Serv 2 (February): 17–22, 1984

39. Hunka A, O'Toole A, O'Toole R: Self-help Therapy in Parents Anonymous. J Psychosoc Nurs Ment Health Serv 23 (July): 24–33, 1985

40. Hurley EA: An Investigation of Therapeutic Intervention as Practiced by Four Psychiatric Nurses in Group Work With Selected Psychiatric Patients. Masters Thesis. University of Colorado, 1960

41. Jackson EN: Group Counseling: Dynamic Possibilities of Small Group. Philadelphia, Pilgram Press, 1969

42. Johnson R, Richardson J, Lindgren K: The Professional Support Group: A Model for Psychiatric Clinical Nurse Specialists. J Psychosoc Nurs Ment Health Serv 20 (February): 9–13, 1982

43. Jones M: The Therapeutic Community: A New Treatment Method in Psychiatry. New York, Basic Books, 1953

44. Kaplan-Koehne N, Levy K: An Approach for Facilitating the Passage Through Termination. J Psychosoc Nurs Ment Health Serv 16 (June): 11–14, 1978

45. Kassaz D: The Development of a Psychiatric Team in the Light of a Group Development Theory. Journal of the Fort Logan Mental Health Center 2:101–115, 1965

46. Kozier B, Erb G: Fundamentals of Nursing Concepts and Procedures, 2d ed. Menlo Park, CA, Addison-Wesley Publishing Co, 1983

47. Larkin A: What's a Medication Group? J Psychosoc Nurs Ment Health Serv 20 (February): 35–37, 1982

48. Levitt D, Freeman E, Sondheimer S, Rickel K: Group Support in the Treatment of PMS. J Psychosoc Nurs Ment Health Serv 26 (January): 23–27, 1986

49. Lippit GL, Seashore E: Leadership in Nursing Theories: The Professional Nurse Looks at Group Effectiveness. Washington, DC, Leadership Resources, 1966

50. Loomis ME: Group Process for Nurses. St Louis, CV Mosby, 1979

51. Luft J: Group Processes: An Introduction to Group Dynamics, 2d ed. Palo Alto, CA, National Press, 1970

52. Marram GD: The Group Approach in Nursing Practice. St Louis, CV Mosby, 1973

53. Moreno JL: Common Grounds for All Group Psychotherapists: What Is a Good Psychotherapist? Group Psychother 15:263–264, 1962

54. Moreno JL: Who Shall Survive the Foundation of

Sociometry, Group Psychotherapy and Sociodrama? 2d ed. New York, Beacon House, 1978

55. Morris KT: A Handbook of Non-Verbal Group Exercises. Springfield, IL, Charles C Thomas, 1975

56. Morris KT: A Handbook of Verbal Group Exercises. Springfield, IL, Charles C Thomas, 1974

57. Mueller A, Metzbaugh C: Nursing Home for Student Learning. Nurse Educator 3 (January–February): 14–16, 1978

58. Murray RB, Huelskoetter MW: Psychiatric/Mental Health Nursing. Englewood Cliffs, NJ, Prentice-Hall, 1983

59. Napier RW, Gersherfield MK: Groups: Theory and Experience. Boston, Houghton Mifflin, 1973

60. Newton G: Self-Help Groups. J Psychosoc Nurs Ment Health Serv 22 (July): 27–31, 1984

61. Nixon HL: The Small Group. Englewood Cliffs, NJ, Prentice-Hall, 1979

62. Pasquali EA, Alesi E, Arnold H, De Basio N: Mental Health Nursing: A Bio-Psychocultural Approach. St Louis, CV Mosby, 1981

63. Patterson CH: Theories of Counseling and Psychotherapy. New York, Harper & Row, 1966

64. Reed G, Sech E: Bulimia: A Conceptual Model for Group Treatment. J Psychosoc Nurs Ment Health Serv 25 (May): 16–23, 1985

65. Robinson L: Psychiatric Nursing as a Human Experience. Philadelphia, WB Saunders, 1977

66. Roich MJ: Dialogues for Therapies: Dynamics of Learning and Supervision. San Francisco, Jossey-Bass, 1976

67. Singerman B, Higgins C, Warring B: An Evening Diversional Activity Program for Psychiatric Patients. J Psychosoc Nurs Ment Health Serv 18 (December): 28–31, 1980

68. Stuart G, Sundeen SL: Principles and Practice of Psychiatric Nursing. St Louis, CV Mosby, 1979

69. Trousley MM: The Use of Family Therapy in Terminal Illness and Death. J Psychosoc Nurs Ment Health Serv 20 (January): 17–22, 1982

70. VanServellen MG, Dull VL: Group psychotherapy for depressed women: A model. J Psychosoc Nurs Ment Health Serv 19 (August): 25–31, 1982

71. Veninga R, Fredland D: Teaching the Group Approach. Nurs Outlook 22 (June): 373–376, 1974

72. White EM, Kahn ME: Use and Modifications in Group Psychotherapy with Chronic Schizophrenic Outpatients. J Psychosoc Nurs Ment Health Serv 2 (February): 14–20, 1982

73. Wilson H, Kneisel C: Psychiatric Nursing, 2d ed. Menlo Park, CA, Addison-Wesley, 1983

74. Witt J: Transference and Countertransference in Group Therapy Settings. J Psychosoc Nurs Ment Health Serv 20 (February): 31–34, 1982

75. Yalom ID: The Theory and Practice of Group Psychotherapy, 3d ed. New York, Basic Books, 1985

76. Yura H, Ozimek D: Nursing Leadership: Theory and Process, 2d ed. New York, Appleton-Century-Crofts, 1981

77. Zander A: Motives and Goals in Groups. New York, Academic Press, 1971

15

Families and Family Therapy

Christina R. Hogarth

...And what of Marriage, Master?
You shall be together when the white wings of death scatter your days.
Ay, you shall be together even in the silent memory of God.
But let there be spaces in your togetherness,
And let the winds of the heavens dance between you.
Love one another, but make not a bond of love:
Let it rather be a moving sea between the shores of your souls.
...Sing and dance together and be joyous, but let each one of you be alone.
Even as the strings of a lute are alone though they quiver with the same music.
Speak to us of children...
...They are the sons and daughters of Life's longing for itself.
They come through you but not from you.
And though they are with you yet they belong not to you.
You may give them your love but not your thoughts.
You may house their bodies but not their souls,
For their souls dwell in the house of tomorrow, which you cannot visit, not even in your dreams.
You may strive to be like them, but seek not to make them like you:
For life goes not backward nor tarries with yesterday.
You are the bows from which your children as living arrows are sent forth.

Kahlil Gibran,
The Prophet,
1923

Chapter Preview

Fairy tales, television, and the wedding industry would have us believe that marriage is finding the prince or princess and living happily ever after. In recent years, however, "happily ever after" has given way to unprecedented rises in divorce, child and spouse abuse, substance abuse, adolescent suicide, crime, teenage pregnancy, and heavy reliance on social welfare and mental health services. During these troubled times, many families have lost hope and control over their own destinies, but others have organized to avoid becoming one of these alarming statistics. For many years, sociologists, anthropologists, psychiatrists, psychologists, social workers, and, to some extent, nurses have studied the family and have explored the structure and form of the family. More recently, they have examined the dynamics and interactions of the family as a system. Initially, systems theorists studied families that had a schizophrenic member, but they have now focused on the less disturbed and, importantly, successful families.

Stress and change are present in the lives of all families. How the family adapts to these stresses and changes depends on the ability of the adults to love and care for each other, while providing a caring atmosphere for children to learn and grow to capable adulthood. Parents are indeed, as Kahil Gibran says, "the bow from which [their] children as living arrows are sent forth."[20] The static fairy tale is truly a myth.

This chapter presents the major theories of family functioning, with particular emphasis on the family systems approach, common stressors and changes that affect families, an assessment methodology based on Beavers's and Satir's work with families, family therapy approaches, and other nursing interventions used when working with families who fall on the continuum from optimum to troubled.

Learning Objectives

On completion of the chapter, you should be able to accomplish the following:

1. define family
2. describe four theoretical approaches to the study of family
    developmental theory
    structure and function analysis
    communication theory
    systems theory
3. identify the characteristics of living systems
4. discuss eight variables of the family that are instrumental in producing competent individuals
5. discuss the historical, developmental, role-related, and environmental stressors affecting families
6. apply the nursing process to healthy and dysfunctional families:
    identify assessment criteria for optimal, adequate, midrange, and troubled families
    formulate nursing diagnoses for dysfunctional families
    list goals for nursing interventions with families
    describe interventions of nurses who work with midrange to troubled families and of nurse therapists
    identify evaluation criteria of family functioning
7. describe characteristics and skills essential to psychiatric–mental health nurses who work with troubled or dysfunctional families

Family Theories

Defining Family

Most definitions of family describe the traditional nuclear family. There are, however, many types of family structures that need to be included in a comprehensive definition. A *family* is a "culturally produced social system," made up of two or more people in a primary group. The persons in this primary group may be related by blood, marriage, adoption, or mutual consent; they may interact through certain familial roles; and they may create and maintain a common subculture.[49]

Family functions include at least two of the following:

1. Maintenance of a common household
2. Rearing of children
3. Companionship and mutual support among members
4. Sexual relationship between one or more pairs of adults
5. Financial cooperation
6. Enculturation of members[49]

These components of a definition of a family take into account varying compositions of family members, such as the traditional nuclear family, homosexual couples, elderly persons not related by blood living together as a family group, and variant family forms, such as single-parent families and extended family groupings. Although the form or structure of the family is changing considerably, the family persists as the most important force in providing economic necessities, socialization, and companionship for people of all ages.

Although families are small in size, they are typically complex and difficult to analyze. Anthropologists, sociologists, and mental health professionals and researchers have studied the family from various theoretical perspectives including developmental stages, structure-function analysis, communication theory, and systems theory.

Developmental Stages of the Family

Development refers to an orderly evolution of events moving from simple to more complex. Human development has been studied extensively in all spheres of human experience including biologic, psychological (*i.e.,* cognitive and emotional), social, and spiritual realms. The family is both a group of people in varying stages of development and a family group in a stage of development.

Duvall has described the basic tasks and development stages of families. The eight basic tasks of families are as follows:

1. Physical maintenance
2. Allocation of resources—meeting family needs and costs; apportioning goods, facilities, space, authority
3. Division of labor
4. Socialization of family members
5. Reproduction; recruitment and release of family members
6. Maintenance of order
7. Placement of members into the larger society
8. Maintenance of motivation and morale—encouragement and affection, meeting personal and family crises, refining a philosophy of life and sense of family loyalty through rituals[17]

The eight stages of family development are as follows:

1. Beginning families (married couple)
2. Early childbearing families (oldest child infant to 30 months)
3. Families with preschool children (oldest child 2½–5 years)
4. Families with school children (oldest child 6–13)
5. Families with teenagers (oldest child 13–20)
6. Launching center families (children leaving home)
7. Families of middle years (empty nest through retirement)
8. Family in retirement and old age (retirement to death of both spouses).[18]

Chart 15-1 describes stage-critical family developmental tasks based on critical issues facing the couple or oldest child.

Stevenson has identified four stages of family development based on the length of the couple's relationship.

Stage I—emerging family
Stage II—crystallizing family
Stage III—integrating family
Stage IV—actualizing family[49]

The *emerging family* encompasses the first 7 to 10 years of the relationship. The couple is initiating work and career paths, and children often enter the family during this stage. Both developments—career and children—are stressful events, as are the beginning stages of the relationship. By the end of this period of the emerging family, patterns of family life are established.

The *crystallizing family* stage extends from 10 to 25 years of cohabitation. This period of family life is usually calm until children reach adolescence. There is also considerable contact between children and parents before the children are launched from the family. The adults continue to grow and begin to participate in community life.

The *integrating family* stage lasts from about the 25th year of the relationship until the 40th. Usually, the children are young adults by this time and the couple or adults who lead the family renew and enhance their relationship. Although work roles continue to be important, humanistic tendencies appear and leisure is significant to the couple during this stage. The grown children may need to make adjustments to aging parents.

The *actualizing family* period encompasses the years past 40 years of living together. The couple continues to grow, hopefully, or, if one partner dies, the remaining partner grieves and continues to grow. Family members deal with aging, chronic illness, dying parents, and death.

Family Structure and Function

Structure refers to the organization of the family. Structure includes type of family (*i.e.,* nuclear or extended) and the value system of the family, which in turn dictates roles, communication patterns, and power distribution within the family.[18] The value system includes basic beliefs about man, nature, the supernatural, time, and family relationships. Value systems tend to cluster by socioeconomic status or ethnic group.

C H A R T   15-1
Stage-Critical Family Developmental Tasks Through the Family Cycle

Stage of the Family Life Cycle	Positions in the Family	Stage-Critical Family Developmental Tasks
Married couple	Wife Husband	Establishing a mutually satisfying marriage Adjusting to pregnancy and the promise of parenthood Fitting into the kin network
Childbearing	Wife–mother Husband–father Infant daughter or son or both	Having, adjusting to, and encouraging the development of infants Establishing a satisfying home for both parents and infant(s)
Preschool-age	Wife–mother Husband–father Daughter–sister Son–brother	Adapting to the critical needs and interests of preschool children in stimulating, growth-promoting ways Coping with energy depletion and lack of privacy as parents
School-age	Wife–mother Husband–father Daughter–sister Son–brother	Fitting into the community of school-age families in constructive ways Encouraging children's educational achievement
Teenage	Wife–mother Husband–father Daughter–sister Son–brother	Balancing freedom with responsibility as teenagers mature and emancipate themselves Establishing postparental interests and careers as growing parents
Launching center	Wife–mother–grandmother Husband–father–grandfather Daughter–sister–aunt Son–brother–uncle	Releasing young adults into work, military service, college, marriage, and so on with appropriate rituals and assistance Maintaining a supportive home base
Middle-aged parents	Wife–mother–grandmother Husband–father–grandfather	Rebuilding the marriage relationship Maintaining kin ties with older and younger generations
Aging family members	Widow/widower Wife–mother–grandmother Husband–father–grandfather	Coping with bereavement and living alone Closing the family home or adapting it to aging Adjusting to retirement

(From Duvall E: Family Development, 4th ed, p 151. Philadelphia, JB Lippincott, 1971)

Families of lower-class status, for example, tend to have a present-time orientation and view themselves as subjugated to the environment and supernatural (fate). Family relationships tend to be disrupted by desertion of spouses and early emancipation of children due to severe economic difficulties. Families cope, however, by taking in other extended family members' children and often by the grandmother's provision of direct assistance to family members. Power is usually authoritarian or not exerted.

Middle-class families espouse the Protestant work ethic prevalent in this country. This ethic dictates the importance of work and planning for the future, and the belief that man is somewhat evil but changeable by hard work. Financial stability and success are viewed as rewards for hard work. Family relationships center around the nuclear family with socialization among work-related or neighborhood friendships. Power is more egalitarian in middle-class than in lower-class families, but it becomes more male-dominated as the economic level of the family rises. Middle-class families see themselves as able to control, and work for mastery over, the environment. These statements are broad generalizations of social class values and do not account for cultural differences. Many ethnic groups, for example, place great importance on extended family relationships, rather than on the individualism valued by middle-class Americans.

Functions of the family include procreation and socialization of children, maintenance of a household, affection, health and illness care, adapting to change within and from outside the family, and providing necessities for family members.

Family Communication Theory

The family communication theory developed from research at the Mental Research Institute in Palo Alto, California, in the 1950s. Jackson, Watzlawick, Haley, Beaven, and Satir have contributed to a theory of family dynamics in schizophrenia and double-bind communication and have pioneered still relevant efforts in family therapy. These researchers and practitioners stated that the child learns and develops by responding to verbal and nonverbal communication. The child's interpretation of himself and the environment depends on messages received from parents. The messages are powerful because the child depends on his parents for survival. Communication, says Satir, is the way members "work out to make meaning with one another." In nurturing families, communication is congruent, "direct, clear, specific and honest." Self-worth is high in nurturing families; the family members have positive feelings about themselves. Rules are norms for how people in the family should think and act. In nurturing families, the rules are "flexible, human, appropriate, and subject to change." Links to society are the ways family members relate to the community. The linking in nurturing families is "open and hopeful." Satir views families as peoplemaking factories with the parents as engineers or architects of the family.[44] Communication, self-worth, rules, and links to society are assessed by observing interactions among family members. Communication is the focus of intervention in the family.

Family Systems Theory

The family systems theory developed during the 1950s on both the East and West coasts of the United States. The West coast group of Jackson, Haley, and associates in Palo Alto explored the notions of communications theory (*i.e.,* cybernetics and feedback loops) and homeostasis applied to the family with a schizophrenic member.[4,45,55] In Washington, DC, Bowen based his family systems concepts on a biological systems model.[8] In Philadelphia, Minuchin utilized the systems model in his research with families exhibiting psychosomatic disorders.[33] Most recently, Lewis and Beavers have explored not only disturbed families, but also healthy families, from a systems viewpoint.[5,29]

A system is a whole that consists of more than the sum of its parts. Although a system can be divided into subsystems, the subsystems are not representative pieces of the whole. Human beings are complex organisms who respond, grow, and change in the context of relationships with others and in response to the environment. To study family research, theory, and therapy, one must understand the basic characteristics of living systems.

Characteristics of Living Systems

Boundaries are limits, or imaginary lines drawn to define the limits, beyond which one should not intrude. Boundaries pertain to the system as a whole, as well as to subsystems within it. Concrete examples of boundaries are the use, or nonuse, of bedroom doors. Boundaries exist between individuals, between subsystems, and between the family system and the environment. The family's values, style, and self-worth determine the permeability of the boundary to outside influences, such as the media, friends, school, church, and so forth. Boundaries may be clearly defined but open to change and input, or so poorly defined that confusion and chaos exist, or so rigid that little input can permeate.

Negentropy is a tendency toward openness to the environment, both inside and outside the family. Living, open systems tend to increase in complexity over time; this increase in complexity is called *differentiation*. An example of differentiation is human growth and development. The child grows from a dependent infant to a child with concrete thinking and a short attention span who feels safe at home to a young adult with abstract thinking and a lengthy attention span who is capable of living on his own in a complex environment. *Entropy* is the tendency of a system to be closed to the environment. If a person remains closed to feedback from others, he tends to develop distorted and peculiar perceptions, thoughts, and feelings.

Time is an important entity in families because systems change with the passage of time, as people age and children are born and leave home. *Stresses* and strains impinge on and occur within family systems. Stress is normal and inevitable as change occurs. Adolescence is an example of a common developmental stressor. *Conflict* often results from stress and change and is also a normal and common phenomenon. A family's ability to manage change and conflict is termed *adaptation*. Adaptation may range from failure to adapt to mere survival to growing and changing into a more highly differentiated system.

It is useful to view families on a continuum from most negentropic to most entropic, or from more growth-oriented to less growth-oriented. Families that are most negentropic, or more open and growth-oriented, are those that produce the most personally and interpersonally capable people. Families that are more entropic, or less open and growth-oriented, produce less capable people who often come to the attention of health care workers, mental health care providers, educators, and law enforcement personnel.

Producing Competent People

Beavers describes eight variables that are critical for producing competent people.[5] Optimal families have an *open system orientation*. This orientation assumes that an individual needs a group from which he derives satisfaction and personal definition, and that life is complex, with experience flowing not from a single cause, but from multiple factors.

These optimal families have *permeable boundaries*. The family views the world outside of itself positively, utilizes input from society and the environment to enrich their lives, and discards input that they do not value. The boundaries between subsystems within the family, such as the subsystems of parents and children, permit privacy and aloneness, but allow for the inclusion of others.

The optimum family experiences *contextual clarity*, which means that verbal and nonverbal communication are congruent and clear and that generational lines are clear, with a strong parental coalition. Oedipal issues in these families are resolved appropriately.

Power in optimal families is shared and flows from the parental couple. The parental pair have an egalitarian partnership that consists of complementary role behaviors. Roles are not shared, but complement one another; for instance, one partner relates as the more aggressive one and the other relates as the more supportive. These complementary roles

exist without sexual stereotyping, but follow the prevalent social patterns of the time. Sex does not define overt power in optimal families. Neither do people in these families lose their power by becoming close and intimate. Children do not assume parental responsibilities; parents use authoritarian approaches, if needed.

Optimal families encourage *autonomy*. They consciously believe that children are being prepared to leave the family and live interdependently, and progressively encourage independent thinking and behaviors. Each member's views are respected and each member claims responsibility for, and communicates clearly, his or her thoughts, feelings, and actions. People from optimal families possess a high degree of initiative and performance.

The *affective tone* in optimum families is caring, warm, empathetic, and hopeful. Members ask about and attend to feelings; they are involved with one another. Conflict, which is inevitable, is dealt with and resolved. The family members believe that they are able to survive difficult or unpleasant situations and occurrences. Their management or resolution of conflict strengthens their relationships and increases their confidence in the relationships.[2] *Negotiation and task performance* are accomplished with input from all members and attention to the developmental capabilities of children. No one is excluded. Parents lead the negotiations, typically in family meetings.

The optimum family has *transcendent values;* that is, the family has a belief system that tolerates and transcends the pain of loss and change. This belief system may be in part based on conventional religious beliefs, but is usually an intrinsic belief that love is a worthwhile risk even though the loved one may be lost. The family has an altruistic bent toward society. Children, of course, cannot conceptualize these notions until they are nearing adulthood. Nevertheless, mature parents set the tone for the family with their own abilities to transcend the inevitability of loss, death, and change.

Change

It is evident that the concept of change is central in the family systems theory. Western, particularly American, views about marriage and family are influenced by fairy tales and the media, wherein the hero and heroine find each other and live "happily ever after." The couple soon finds, however, that living happily ever after is, indeed, a fairy tale. They discover, instead, that their lives and the environment are constantly changing. If children enter the family, change and conflict are inherent. Every system, though, works to maintain homeostasis; that is, some kind of stability that provides a balance between what is valued and desired and the changes that impinge on and disrupt that homeostasis or steady state. Change causes stress within the system.

Stressors and Their Impacts on Families

Historical Development

During this century and particularly during the past 30 years, enormous technological and social change has occurred in the United States. Following the sacrifices and pain of World War II, families settled into a conservative pattern of the nuclear family, wherein the wife-mother gave up her job in the factory to the returning veteran and stayed home to raise the children while the husband-father went to work. In greater numbers, families moved away from the city to suburban areas, a sign of increasing affluence and materialism. The adults of the 1950s were children of the depression who feared economic deprivation and wished to spare their children the pain of poverty.

During the 1960s, tremendous, indeed revolutionary, changes took place. The civil rights movement and college-age children's rebellion against the materialistic society and the United States' increasing involvement in Vietnam disrupted the long-accepted values of patriotism and the work ethic. Humanitarian social values became prevalent; minority groups in the United States insisted on their rights to participate in the affluent life of the middle-class American. Their insistence took place through political influence, through passive tactics (*e.g.,* civil disobedience), or through violence. The rights of the individual became paramount in education, health care, hiring practices, housing, and business opportunities.

The 1970s brought the women's movement and emphasis on self-awareness and fulfillment. Divorce rates skyrocketed and the family, in its normal configuration of homemaker-mother, breadwinner-father, and children, was threatened. Individual freedom was important. Inflation was rampant.

By the end of the 1970s, the dual-earner family was the predominant family form and half of the mothers in the work force had preschool children.[7,59] Violent crime, sexual promiscuity, adolescent pregnancy, substance abuse, mental health problems, and suicide were epidemic, particularly among adolescents. The era of self-fulfillment appeared to have exacted a high toll among the youth of the country. The emergence of ultra-conservative groups, such as the "moral majority," and increased membership in fundamentalist churches signaled a swing of the pendulum toward more traditional values.[58] Universities raised standards and were unwilling to provide tutorial services to substandard students. High schools began to reinstitute stiff discipline. The public demanded heavier penalties for crime.[53]

The families of the 1980s have the challenge and opportunity of choosing those values and lifestyles that best meet the needs of the adult and child members. The forging of competent selves remains the mission of family life, with the parents providing competent leadership within the family. Assisting families with this monumental task is the focus of nursing intervention in numerous health care settings.

Developmental Stressors

In addition to developing as a unit in the context of historical events, the family undergoes changes related to the growth and development of its members. The birth of the first child, whether unplanned and unwanted or planned and anticipated with joy, is a significant stressor. The physiological and emotional changes of pregnancy test the couple's ability to be supportive of one another. Lifestyle changes related to nausea or fatigue may also be difficult for the couple. The birth of the child is now usually a shared experience for the couple and often a peak experience in their lives. The demanding infant, however, soon commands a central position in the family by requiring a great deal of energy, time, and emotional investment. The couple must learn to meet the baby's needs without neglecting their own, a task that persists through the childhood and adolescence of their children.

The adolescent period is a highly stressful time for families. The teenager's ambivalence about dependence versus independence and his resultant limit-testing are frightening and frustrating experiences for parents. Finding a balance between giving the child freedom to grow and learn, while protecting him from harmful experiences until his judgment is sound, is a difficult job, requiring time, energy, careful thought, and sensitivity. Open communication centered on the teenager's thoughts and feelings regarding issues important to him, such as money, rules, school achievement, sex, love, career choice, and friends, is critical. Parents of the adolescent need to know his friends and his whereabouts, and they need to set appropriate, fair limits with consequences for the breaking of rules. On the other hand, every aspect of the adolescent's life should not be subjected to scrutiny, probing, and checking up. Trust should be established through childhood and early adolescence, and opportunities for role-taking, examining moral-ethical issues, and developing good judgment should be provided *with* the child.[21]

The middle years present two major crises, the mid-life crisis and dealing with aging parents. The crisis of mid-life begins when the middle-ager confronts the fact of his own mortality, often triggered by the appearance of wrinkles or competition from younger people at work. The middle-aged person confronts his or her own limitations and hopes for success, and comes to terms with accomplishments in life thus far, including work, family relationships, sexuality, and hopes for children. This is a painful time for the adult and often coincides with the presence of teenagers in the family. Diminished health and death of parents leave the middle-ager responsible for two generations, a considerable burden.[47,49]

The older adult must cope with the loss of work, friends, spouse, and often economic resources. He also looks back on his life and concludes that it has been a meaningful experience with which he is satisfied, or that it has not been meaningful, which leads to despair.

Role Development and Change

Role development and change cause considerable challenges or difficulties for families. Since the late 1970s, the predominant family structure has been the *dual-earner family,* in which there are often preschool children. The physical and emotional care of children, maintenance of the household, participation in children's activities, providing transportation to children's activities, as well as maintaining and developing the self and the relationship with a spouse dictate a full, interesting life or a frustrating, exhausting one. Women in these families experience more role strain and stress and spend more hours on household chores than men. Household help is expensive to hire.[7] Child care facilities are often inadequate in quantity or quality and are rarely available at the workplace.

The skyrocketing *divorce* rate profoundly affects the families involved. Self-esteem of the spouses suffers a severe blow, and the children become angry and confused, are often forced to choose the parent with whom they will live, and feel they are to blame for the breakup of their parents' marriage. Most families cannot recover from divorce without counseling, usually instigated by the mother-wife's pain or by the acting-out behavior of the children. Serious economic setbacks occur when one household becomes two households with the same income. Women usually earn less money than their male counterparts and are more likely to receive custody of the children than men. Child support payments may or may not be paid reg-ularly. Children of divorce undergo moves to new schools, loss of friends and activities, and loss of the parent who does not have custody. The grief process may be prolonged because of the proximity of the spouse-parent; that is, the parent without custody.[12]

Loss of a family member through death or desertion is not uncommon. The family may grieve the loss of the parent, spouse, or child and move on. Economic conditions in these families vary according to socioeconomic class, whether the lost member was a breadwinner or the sole breadwinner, and whether the death was due to catastrophic illness.

The *single-parent* family is at risk because of its limited financial resources and the parent's limited time and energy. Because one parent is absent from the home, that parent's role-modeling is not available for the children.[24]

An increase in remarriages has resulted in the *blended* family. Putting two families together, particularly if there are children in the families, takes time and patience.[64] The adoptive family of an older child must have considerable patience and love for the child, who has often been in a succession of foster homes.[11]

Another increasing phenomenon is the *adolescent parent.* A dramatic rise in teenage pregnancy, with large numbers of teenage mothers keeping their babies, has resulted in increasing numbers of teen-aged parents. The adolescent girl may choose marriage or may choose to live at home and finish school. Either way, adolescent parents have not reached adulthood themselves, but have the responsibility for a baby for which they are emotionally and financially ill-equipped. In addition, the adolescent mother and her infant are often at physiological risk.

Environmental Influences on the Family

Although descriptions of the family primarily refer to middle-class families or those with middle-class values, a variety of cultures are represented in the United States. The family cannot be adequately assessed or effectively treated without an understanding of the ethnic group from whence it came. Different cultures have different orientations to time and relationships that the health care provider must comprehend and appreciate in order to assist the family in maximizing its potential.[10,34,38,43,51,52] For further exploration of this topic, examine Chapter 6, which deals with cultural variations.

Poverty is an overwhelming obstacle for many families. The struggle for existence in terms of obtaining food, clothing, and shelter, all substandard and far from the American dream, occupies the family's time and energy and depletes its dignity. Frustration

C H A R T   15-2
Surviving Divorce: The Children

In addition to the already strenuous developmental tasks of childhood and adolescence, children of divorce must master six more psychological tasks, according to Judith Wallerstein, who has conducted a longitudinal study of children of divorce. This study has produced some sobering data.

The process of recovery from divorce is a lengthy one, lasting through late adolescence or early adulthood. Even when the psychological tasks of coping with divorce are mastered, the child of divorce experiences "some residue of sadness, of anger and of anxiety about the potential unreliability of relationships...." The tasks of coping with divorce include the following.

Task I, *acknowledging the reality of the marital rupture,* is usually completed within a year, although usually accompanied initially by considerable regression. Younger children have more difficulty with this task because of their inability to conceptualize time, space, and the nature of relationships.

Task II, *disengaging from parental conflict and distress and resuming customary pursuits,* is also usually completed by the child within a year or two of the divorce. In the year following the divorce or separation, the child often has difficulty in learning and has other school problems. Some children become involved in sexual activity or stealing. All children must distance themselves from their upset parents and overcome their own depression and anxiety. After the initial upset, most children resume their usual activities.

Task III, the *resolution of loss,* takes many years. In addition to grieving the multiple losses that the divorce precipitates, the child strives to recover from an overwhelming sense of rejection. This sense of rejection is diminished by frequent, reliable visiting arrangements and by the development of the relationship with the noncustodial parent.

Task IV, *resolving anger and blame,* also takes many years to accomplish. Usually in late adolescence, the child begins to understand the parents and the reasons for the divorce. Typically, the child forgives the parents and, perhaps, himself or herself.

Task V, *accepting the permanence of divorce,* is a gradual process during which the child wishes intensely for and fantasizes the restoration of the family. It is not uncommon for mature adults to continue to wish for and fantasize the reconciliation of their parents.

Task VI, *achieving realistic hope regarding relationships,* is a normal task of adolescence, but for the child of divorce, it is complicated by fears of rejection and failure based on his earlier experience.

Clearly, the child of divorce faces a dilemma—to learn to trust in his own lovability, in his capacity to love, in his self-worth, and in the reliability of relationships.

Findings from a 10-year follow-up of 38 youngsters now 16 to 18 years old, whose parents divorced during the children's early latency, suggest that separation from families and the transition into young adulthood are burdened by fear of disappointment in love relationships, lowered expectations, and a sense of powerlessness. A need for the father, especially among boys, appears to burgeon at middle and late adolescence.

(From Wallerstein JS: Children of Divorce: Report of a Ten Year Follow-up of Early Latency Age Children. Am J Orthopsychiatr 57 (April): 199–211, 1987)

is high, desertion and violence are common. Reliance on public assistance is demeaning and undermines individual initiative.

Television and other media have been significant influences on families during the past 20 years. The ubiquitous presence of the TV set has contributed to unprecedented materialism, increase in violent crime among young people, irresponsible sexual behavior, sapping of creative thinking, undesirable dietary practices, and lack of communication between family members.[21,32] Family members eat many dinners in the 25-inch, full-color presence of murder and mayhem. One may wonder whether Americans can face each other without the television intervening.

The changing *values* of society have an impact on schools and churches. Schools at all levels have been concerned with students' rights and with providing curricula for the development of the whole self, which inadvertently resulted in a decline in college entrance exam scores and serious discipline problems, particularly in high schools. As funding shrinks and conservative values return, high schools are raising academic standards and adopting stricter discipline policies. Church membership has decreased overall since 1970, but an increase of 1% was noted in 1980, with increases among Catholics, Mormons, and Southern Baptists.[53]

The rise in violent crime and in the incidence of *family violence* is staggering. The cluster of factors contributing to the occurrence of family violence includes low income, unemployed husband, husband and wife under age 30 and married less than 10 years, higher-than-average levels of conflict in the family, excessively high number of stressors, non-white racial group, lack of church membership, parental disagreement over children, presence of verbal aggression, residence in neighborhood less than 2 years, and abusiveness of the couple's parents.[50]

The presence of *chronic illness* or *handicap* in a family member taxes physical and emotional energy, time, and economic resources of both the ill or handicapped person and of the other members of the family.

Alcoholism and other *chemical dependencies* are major stressors for families. About one in ten persons in the United States is an alcoholic. There is increasing evidence that this disease is genetically transmitted and mediated by environmental factors.[46] Families of alcoholics are characterized by intense conflict, shame, lack of trust, denial, and physical illness.[56] Family members take on roles that help to stabilize this distressed family but ultimately result in increased problems for the family and actually enable the deterioration of the alcoholic and the family (see Table 15-1).

Although these stressors are significant and prevalent, a critical variable in whether the family survives and produces capable people is the self-esteem of the parents. The family can tolerate and cope with a great deal of stress if parents feel satisfied with themselves and their relationship. Low self-esteem is a stressor to the family.

Application of the Nursing Process to the Family

Assessment

The assessment framework presented in this chapter incorporates a number of variables found to effect the development of competent people and a category related to health.[26] (See Chart 15-3, "Guide to Family Assessment.")

People are continually subjected to stress and change; it is how one manages stresses that determines one's relative wellness. Individuals' ability to adapt and grow stems directly from their experiences in family life. Families' levels of adaptation fall on a continuum from optimal to midrange to severely disturbed functioning.[5] Families may also be described as nurturing or troubled.[44] (See Chart 15-4, "Family Mental Health Continuum.")

Optimal Families

The optimal family has been described earlier in this chapter in the section dealing with systems theory and the development of competence in people. The *optimal family* also has little physical illness and usually practices high-level health care, including excellent

Table 15-1.   Roles and Dynamics of an Alcoholic Family

| ROLE | MOTIVATING FEELING | IDENTIFYING SYMPTOMS | PAYOFF | | POSSIBLE PRICE |
			For Individual	*For Family*	
Dependent	Shame	Chemical use	Relief of pain	None	Addiction
Enabler	Anger	Powerlessness	Importance; self-righteousness	Reponsibility	Illness; "martyrdom"
Hero	Inadequacy; guilt	Overachievement	Attention (positive)	Self-worth	Compulsive drive
Scapegoat	Hurt	Delinquency	Attention (negative)	Focus away from dependent	Self-destruction; addiction
Lost Child	Loneliness	Solitariness; shyness	Escape	Relief	Social isolation
Mascot	Fear	Clowning; hyperactivity	Attention (amused)	Fun	Immaturity; emotional illness

Wegschieder S: Another Chance: Help and Hope for the Alcoholic Family, Palo Alto, CA: Science and Behavior Books, 1981.

CHART 15-3
Guide to Family Assessment

1. *Open-system orientation*
   Multiple causation of events
   Need for each other and other people
2. *Boundaries*
   Touching
   Interaction between family members
   Allocation of space in household
   Links to society
3. *Contextual clarity*
   Oedipal issues resolved
   Clear generational lines
   Strong parental coalition
   Communication
     Clear, direct, honest, specific
     Congruent
4. *Power*
   Flows from parental coalition
   Delegated to children appropriate to age
   Clear role definition
   Not sex-defined
   Rules
5. *Encouragement of autonomy*
   Differentness accepted

6. *Affective issues*
   Warmth–caring
   Empathy
   Feelings attended to
   Amount of conflict
   Resolution of conflict
   Self-esteem of members high
7. *Negotiation and task performance*
   Input from all members
   Led by parents
   Little amount of conflict
8. *Transcendent values*
   Expect loss
   Recover from and prepare for loss
   Hopeful
   Altruistic
9. *Health measures*
   Healthy diet
   Freedom from drugs and chemicals
   Regular exercise and recreation
   Concern for the environment
   Abstinence from dangerous activities
   Family history of health

nutrition and abstinence or near abstinence from alcohol, drugs, tobacco, caffeine and saccharine; the family also participates in regular exercise and recreation, avoids dangerous activities, and demonstrates concern for the environment. The optimal family is, indeed, the ideal family. Most families function in the adequate and midrange area and a smaller proportion of families function in the troubled range.

Adequate Families

Adequate families produce people who do not have mental health problems. The adequate family maintains an open systems orientation; the family is flexible and open, does not believe causation of events is linear, and expresses need for each other and other people. The intrasystem boundaries are clearly defined but open. Members of the family respect each others' privacy, but there is considerable face-to-face interaction and touching.

The family's links to society are numerous and viewed positively. The societal links are likely to include work, schools, church, friends, extended family, family physician, and community service organizations. The family is not likely to have connections with social welfare agencies. Contextual clarity is present in these families. Oedipal issues are resolved appro-

priately according to the ages of the children. The parents provide strong leadership and maintain their relationship as a couple. Communication is clear, direct, honest, specific, and congruent.

Power in adequate families flows from the parents, who use authoritarian measures when necessary. Parents delegate responsibility to children as it is deemed appropriate for their age and stage of development. Roles are clear; that is, family members know and agree on their functions and performance of activities. Family members understand and generally respect family rules. Power and authority are not ascribed by sex, although the mother in the family generally has less power than her husband for two reasons—she earns less money and she is more likely to set aside her goals, including her employment responsibilities, to meet the needs of children.[7] It is rare to find a truly egalitarian couple with children with equally divided family and work responsibilities. Achievement of an egalitarian relationship necessitates an enormous output of energy, and probably occurs with paid help or extended family providing some of the nurturing of children and household chores.[40, 41] For children's needs to be met in an adequate or optimal manner, at least one of the marital partners must sacrifice some aspect of self-realization

C H A R T   15-4
Family Mental Health Continuum

Family:	Troubled	Midrange	Adequate	Optimal
Children evidencing:	Process schizophrenia Severe behavior disorder Borderline personality disorder	Neuroses Behavior disorders	No obvious pathology	Unusual individual competence

(Adapted from Beavers RW: Psychotherapy and Growth: A Family Systems Perspective. New York, Brunner/Mazel, 1977)

and, at present, that person is most likely to be the mother.

Adequate families encourage autonomy by encouraging children and adults to try new activities and express their ideas, even when they are divergent with the families' values. Family members are valued for their differences as well as their similarities with others. Idiosyncrasies are tolerated with good humor.

The affective tone in adequate families is warm and caring. Members are empathetic, often at early ages. Members consider and ask about others' feelings. Although there is more conflict in the adequate family than in the optimum family, it is resolved without loss of self-esteem. Self-esteem is high in these families; however, the mother may experience more stress, loneliness, or depression than other family members.

Negotiation and task performance are accomplished with considerable ease, but not as easily as in optimal families. Decisions are often reached at family meetings; parents lead the discussions and have the final say in decisions. Some conflict over household work exists and the mother is likely to assume a disproportionate share of the work, which may be self-imposed or may be due to the many activities in which the other family members engage. Nevertheless, the adequate family can usually work out ways to prevent the overload of one person. Family members are competent and excel in some areas. The family is less likely to be an entire group of superachievers than the optimal family. There exists no significant deviance in performance in school or work or in relationships with others.

Transcendent values include a hopeful, positive outlook, the expectation and preparation for loss of children, retirement, and so forth, and an altruistic bent toward neighbors. These families also practice adequate health measures and do not suffer significant health problems.

Midrange Families

Midrange families produce people who evidence mental health problems. The "identified patient" in the family is likely to be neurotic or behaviorally disordered, depending on the family style. Family members may also have physical illnesses. Although family members are reasonably effective, they are restricted. An open-system orientation is absent in these families; family members need others but under certain conditions. The family tends to believe that there are causes for events, but they are not sure what they are. They continuously strive to find answers and to do well.

Boundaries remain fairly clear in these families, although, when under pressure, the family will solidify its boundaries and turn inward (*i.e.*, keep the trouble inside) or lose its boundaries and spill into the environment. Interaction between family members (intrasystem interaction) is restricted.

Links to society are present, but they disrupt when the family is under unusual pressure. Families who tend to externalize trouble (*i.e.*, push it into the environment) have contact with law enforcement agencies.

Midrange families also have difficulty with contextual clarity. Oedipal issues are not resolved because expressions of sexuality are stereotyped and stifled. The parental coalition is present but weak, and other coalitions develop that undermine the effectiveness of the parents. Communication in these families is generally clear, but expressed with fear, guilt, or anger.

Power is the central difficulty in midrange families. The family confuses love and power. Love is a feeling that moves one to care about the life and growth of another.[19] Midrange families often believe that caring is controlling the life of another and, by means of overt or covert coercion, applying a system of "oughts" and "shoulds." The "shoulds" are often sex-stereotyped. The parents believe in doing the "right" thing and are constantly struggling for control of the children through discipline, money, and so forth. Children become powerful by manipulating the parents, not by learning to assume power and responsibility. Family roles are defined by sex or by other beliefs about the family member, such as "she's so good and never causes any trouble," or "Johnny's the athletic one." The family behaves as if there is someone judging the goodness or badness of the family's actions, thoughts, and feelings.

Encouragement of autonomy is not found in midrange families; on the contrary, children are expected to adhere to the family's norms. The constant power struggles and repression of feelings and ideas within the family sap family members' creativity. Children tend to stay in the parental home well into adulthood or leave home very early in a kind of pseudo-autonomy.

The affective issues that characterize midrange families are depression, anxiety, and anger. The enormous resultant conflict may be overtly expressed in angry exchanges or repressed through submission to the "oughts" and "shoulds." As a result, members display little empathy, conflict over rules and norms, considerable frustration, and caring that is controlling rather than growth-producing. The self-esteem of the family members is low, and the identified patient has very low self-esteem.

Negotiation and task performance are accomplished by coercion because the parental team cannot agree on who does what. Nevertheless, the work of the family is accomplished. These families do not hold family meetings.

Transcendent values of hope and altruism are lacking in midrange families. The family eventually accepts change and loss, but with a great deal of pain, anger, and frustration. They look toward the future as if to say, "What difficulty will present itself?" Martyrdom is not an unusual stance for members of these families.

Health problems in midrange families include excessive use of alcohol, prescription tranquilizers, and other drugs for relief of the pain of daily living. The stressful existence of midrange families produces some psychophysiologic illnesses, such as headaches, ulcers, obesity, and so forth. Because the family is concerned with doing the "right" thing, they meet their basic health needs. The family attempts recreation and exercise, but the conflict that surfaces during the planning of events reduces their pleasure. In some families, the presence of a great deal of anger leads to dangerous activities, such as hitting, driving at excessive speeds, and running away. The midrange family is too preoccupied with daily events to explore health promotion and wellness activities.

Troubled Families

Families who function on the more entropic end of the family health continuum tend to produce people who exhibit antisocial disorders, borderline personality disorders, or psychotic disorders. *Troubled families* display qualities that are the opposite of the optimal family's characteristics. The family tends to be very rigid or disordered, rather than open and flexible.

The boundary issues in troubled families are problematic. The family system boundary is rigid with minimal links to society. The links are tentative and mistrustful and input from the larger society is limited. Troubled families may also have diffuse boundaries, which means that family business tends to spill over into the environment. Interpersonal boundaries in these families are also diffused, resulting in family members' global response to input. Distancing between people is prevalent.

Contextual clarity is blurred in troubled families. Due to a weak parental coalition, cross-generational clinging occurs and oedipal issues remain unresolved. The parents deal with their pain of disappointment in each other by reaching across generational boundaries for comfort or control of the situation. Often this cross-generational clinging takes the form of a triangle; that is, mother and son form a coalition against father. Often, there is covert or overt incestuous behavior. The child who is "triangled" is usually the symptom-bearer in the family. This child (or young adult) responds to these pressures with mental disorder, physical illness, or delinquent behavior.

Communication in troubled families is not clear, congruent, specific, direct, or honest. Because people in troubled families have low self-esteem, they fear rejection from others and are embarrassed about it. To "cover up" their fear of rejection, members of troubled families tend to use the four following patterns of communication described by Satir:

1. Placating, or doing anything to prevent others from getting angry
2. Blaming, or attempting to look strong and reject first
3. Computing, or treating the others as if they were insignificant by using big words
4. Distracting, or eliminating the possibility of rejection by changing the subject or talking in a "crazy" way[44]

CHART 15-5
Family Assessment Guidelines

1. *Open system orientation*
   What do you believe are the reasons for the difficulty?
   What do you think the solution is?

2. *Boundaries*
   (Notice who touches whom, who talks to whom, presence of eye contact.)
   (Notice whether the touching is parental, kind, loving, seductive, rough, or violent.)
   Where does everyone sleep?
   Do you all have time alone?
   How do you get along with Johnny's teacher? Scout leader? Other significant people in Johnny's life?
   How do you like Johnny's friends? Are you in touch with Johnny's friends' parents?

3. *Contextual clarity*
   Who's in charge in this family?
   Who gets along best with whom?
   Who does what around the house?
   (Notice whether parents agree on what is happening.)
   (Notice whether there is unusual closeness between child and opposite-sex parent.)
   (Is communication clear, honest, specific—do members make "I statements" or blaming "you statements"?)
   (Can the interviewer get an answer to a question? Can family members get an answer?)
   (Can the interviewer follow the family conversation?)
   (Are verbal and nonverbal communications congruent?)
   How much is your TV turned on?

4. *Power*
   (Do the parents set the tone for the interview, set limits on children's behaviors? Are the limits reasonable, not just talk or punitive?)
   (Does one person control the group by talking or distracting?)
   (Does everyone talk or at least seem involved?)
   Tell me your rules. What happens if they are broken?
   What are everyone's jobs at home?

5. *Encouragement of autonomy*
   If you, Sue, like to stay home and read and you, Bob, like to go to parties, how do you deal with these different desires?
   (Are members stereotyped as "the angel," "the wild one," "just like his Uncle Joe," and so on?)
   What kinds of things are you, Johnny, interested in?
   How are you different from your sister?

6. *Affective issues*
   (Can the interviewer feel warmth and caring, or does the interviewer feel uncomfortable, fearful?)
   (What do you think Johnny is feeling? What are you feeling as you listen to Johnny?)
   (Notice whether family members seem ashamed or embarrassed.)
   (Are conflicts resolved?)
   What do you do when you get angry?

7. *Negotiating and task performance*
   Do you argue about household chores?
   (Can the family solve a problem with parents having final say in the issue?)
   Do you have meetings?

8. *Transcendent values*
   (Do family members believe that problems can be solved?)
   What do you think and feel about Johnny going to camp? Getting married? And so on?
   What do you (parents) do for fun?
   (Do family members accept that life is complicated, difficult, joyous, routine?)
   What kinds of community activities are you involved in?
   (Do family members laugh at themselves, have a sense of humor?)

9. *Health measures*
   When and where do you eat meals? Do you eat one meal each day together? What kinds of things do you eat?
   How often do you have a drink? Does anyone take medications?
   Tell me how you have fun.
   Do you participate in sports or other exercise? What do you do to relax yourself?
   What illnesses have family members had? Grandparents, aunts, uncles?
   Any suicide, mental illness, drug or alcohol addictions?

Another characteristic of communication in troubled families is the lack of congruence between the content of what is said and the feeling beneath it (*i.e.,* incongruence between verbal and nonverbal communication); for example, smiling when talking in an angry tone of voice. *Double-bind communication* occurs when an incongruent message is sent that includes a direction to do something with a nonverbal message to do the opposite, and, furthermore, the receiver of the message is not permitted to comment on it. For example, a father says to his child, "Come here and let me hug you. You know Daddy loves you" (in angry tone of voice). The child answers, "You sound mad." The father responds, "I don't know what you're talking about." The child is then faced with the dilemma of choosing to which communication he will respond. A child faced with continuous double-bind communication is unable to determine the true meaning of verbalizations or to identify and name normal feelings. As the child's ability to test reality becomes impaired, he may invent his own language and peculiar explanations for events; that is, the child becomes schizophrenic. In some troubled families, anger is communicated through hitting and other forms of assault.

Another communication difficulty found in troubled families is disqualifying. *Disqualifying* takes place when an individual fails to attend to another's message by silence, ignoring, or changing the subject. Evasiveness in communication is also common in these families.

Power is diffuse in the troubled family and does not flow from the parents. Autonomy is discouraged, rather than encouraged. In fact, the troubled family does not tolerate differentness. Paradoxically, the family tends to view one of its members as "different" and the cause of its trouble; this process is called *scapegoating.*

The affective tone in troubled families with diffuse boundaries tends to be exaggerated. The members react inappropriately to threats or one member's difficulties. In families with rigid boundaries, the affective tone is restricted, depressed, and despairing, there is a lack of empathy, and great distance exists between the members. Undue attention, which is confusing, smothering, or rejecting, is paid to one member. Self-esteem in troubled families is low, and hate, inability to respond empathetically to others, loneliness, and hopelessness predominate. Negotiation is not accomplished and performance of tasks varies widely. Conflict may be a constant, overt, and unresolved presence in families with diffuse boundaries; this conflict is denied, not commented on, and unresolved in families with rigid boundaries. Transcendent values are absent. The inability of troubled families to tolerate loss or differences leads to a cynical, hopeless outlook, rather than an altruistic, hopeful one. The stresses of unhappy family life often produce serious physical illness, usually in one member.

Nursing Diagnosis

The formulation of nursing diagnoses can be applied to the family and its functioning or adaptive abilities. The following nursing diagnoses are appropriate descriptions for altered and disturbed family interactions:

Family coping: potential for growth
Ineffective family coping: compromised
Ineffective family coping: disabling
Alteration in family process
Alteration in parenting: actual or potential

The formulation of these and new nursing diagnoses assists the psychiatric–mental health nurse in planning interventions for the family whose less-than-optimal coping methods or responses to stress and crisis prevent it from attaining its goals. Often the nurse uses family-focused nursing diagnoses, in addition to individual-centered diagnoses, when working with child, adolescent, and chemically dependent clients. Incorporating family diagnoses, however, may be appropriate during the application of the nursing process for any client exhibiting emotional or behavioral problems.

Planning

The optimal and adequate families are not likely to present themselves for assistance at traditional mental health care settings. These families are found at church activities, PTA meetings, community functions, adult education centers, and other such events. They read newspapers, magazines, and books and select television programs. Therefore, the nurse plans to reach optimal and adequate families in nontraditional health care settings. These families do, however, participate in preventive and health maintenance programs where nurses come into contact with them. Family members may be enriched in four areas: enhancement of existing strengths, anticipatory guidance, parenting education, and holistic health measures.

Enhancement of existing strengths may be as simple as a word of praise or as complex as a series of structured, goal-directed activities. Providing encouragement and praise for the successful performance of parental functions develops trust and increased self-esteem. Anticipatory guidance refers to teaching parents and families what to expect next, particularly in terms of developmental events and crises. Childbirth education is an example of anticipatory guidance. Classes on adolescence and aging parents are also very useful. Parenting programs may be formal or informal.[13,14,15,16,22,37,39] There is currently a need for parenting programs adapted to the teenage years. Holistic health principles, including nutrition with natural foods, exercise, and stress management techniques, are still unknown to, or are not practiced by, many people.[59] Stress management focuses on relaxation techniques, meditation, and leisure activities.

Midrange families utilize mental health facilities and interact with nurses in community health settings. The midrange family with school-age children is likely to come in contact with the school nurse.[6,30] These families benefit from enhancement of their strengths and parenting programs. The nurse may help the family with problem-solving, conflict management, and education of the family about normal growth and development, especially as it relates to their present difficulties. The nurse may also refer the family for family therapy if problem-solving and education approaches fail to relieve the family problems.

Troubled families require family therapy for resolution of their difficulties. Family therapy is available through therapists in private practice, community mental health centers, and psychiatric inpatient units. Networking is often essential for troubled families, particularly if economic problems exist, if protection for one or more members is needed, or if there is involvement with the legal system. The therapist, nurse, social worker, or other health care professional responsible for service to the family seeks sources of support for the family and assists them in arranging for these services. Some examples of these services are churches, social welfare agencies, emergency pantry service, Red Cross, voluntary agencies, hospices, and community health services. Another source of assistance to families is multiple family group therapy.[23,35]

Intervention

Characteristics and Skills of the Nurse

To work effectively with families, the nurse must possess self-awareness, empathy, therapeutic communication skills, and knowledge of family theory. The nurse expands her understanding of family life through formal education, self-directed learning, observation, and supervised practice.

Self-awareness is critical for understanding the behaviors of others. One must be able to identify and "own" one's own thoughts, feelings, and biases before understanding others' feelings and behaviors. The psychiatric–mental health nurse pursues personal growth as part of ongoing education. The nurse must also become aware of her own family dynamics, roles,

and values so that she will not confuse, compare, or impose her own family style upon others.

Another critical characteristic of the psychiatric–mental health nurse working with families is *empathy*. The nurse interacts and intervenes with many different families who possess varying problems and strengths. The ability to experience the family's trouble "from their shoes," and then step back to analyze and intervene, is essential for helping relationships of all kinds, including those with the family. Empathy is essential to building trust.

Therapeutic communication skills are essential for health care providers working with families. The nurse serves as a role model of clear, open, direct, honest, and congruent communication and as a clarifier of the family's unclear communication. The nurse who works with families possesses certain beliefs about families. These include the beliefs that families are functioning as well as they are able, that no one is to blame, that parents want very much to do a good job, and that people behave in nonproductive ways because they are in pain. The nurse, empathizing with the family's pain, works from the position of their strengths and assists them, primarily through communication skills, to learn that the problem is a family problem and that there are more satisfying ways to live as a family, and as people.

There are additional skills that nurses utilize in caring for families. Skillful use of the nursing process, particularly taking adequate time to define the problem accurately, leads to a more productive plan with successful outcomes. So-called "noncompliance" is usually a result of failure of the nurse or other health care provider to discover underlying issues that result in nonresolution of the problem. Knowledge of various *teaching* strategies, an understanding of *learning* principles, and the ability to make adequate *referrals* for other services are important.[57] The nurse actively assists the family through the steps to assure entry into the desired system. The nurse may refer to self-help groups such as Al-Anon, Toughlove, and Parents Anonymous.[25,60] (Chart 15-6 lists self-help groups and resources for families.)

Collaboration is working with others, as an equal, toward a common goal. The nurse serves as a peer on the mental health team and strives to provide the best service to clients by utilizing the contributions of other disciplines in the interest of the family.[3] Nurses also serve as *consultants* on family health in the community by serving on advisory boards, committees, and school boards, and by communicating with legislators and candidates about the needs of families.

The development of *personal coping* skills is essential to the well-being of the nurse who works with families. The intensive nature of family health nurs-

---

C H A R T   15-6
Self-Help Groups and Resources for Families

Al-Anon—Alateen
P.O. Box 182
Madison Square Station, NY 10159

Alcoholics Anonymous
P.O. Box 459
Grand Central Station, NY 10163

Families Anonymous
P.O. Box 528
Van Nuys, CA 91408

M.A.D.D.
669 Airport Freeway, Suite 310
Hurst, TX 76053

Nar-Anon Family Groups
P.O. Box 2562
Palos Verdes, CA 92704

Narcotics Anonymous
N.A. World Service Office, Inc.
P.O. Box 622
Sun Valley, CA 91352

National Alliance for the Mentally Ill
1901 N. Fort Meyer Drive, Suite 500
Arlington, VA 22209

National Federation of Parents for
   Drug Free Youth
8730 Georgia Avenue
Suite 200
Silver Springs, MD 20910
1-800-554-KIDS

Parents Anonymous
7120 Franklin Avenue
Los Angeles, CA 90046

Parents Without Partners
7910 Woodmont Avenue
Bethesda, MD 20814

PRIDE
(National Parents' Resource Institute for
   Drug Education, Inc.)
100 Edgewood Avenue
Suite 1002
Atlanta, GA 30003
1-800-241-7946

Stepfamily Association of America
28 Allegheny Avenue, Suite 1307
Baltimore, MD 21204

Toughlove
P.O. Box 1069
Doylestown, PA 18901

(For a complete directory of self-help organizations, see Gardiner N, Borman L:
The Self-Help Source Book. Denville, NJ, St. Clares-Riverdale Medical
Center, 1986)

---

ing, especially psychiatric–mental health nursing, requires that the nurse obtain sufficient rest, exercise, relaxation, and nurturance and support from colleagues, friends, and significant others in her personal life. Adequate *clinical supervision* from an experienced clinician promotes objectivity, continued professional growth, and support of the nurse.

Family Therapy

Family therapy is undertaken by clinicians of various disciplines, including nurse therapists, who have undergone formal training in family therapy during graduate or post-graduate education. Sometimes, nurses without graduate education practice family therapy under close supervision, although graduate preparation is preferred and usually required for family therapy.

Family therapy is a specific intervention mode based on the premise that the member with the presenting symptoms signals the presence of pain in the whole family. This pain arises from the disappointment of the marital partners with each other. Their unhappiness, anger, and hurt are expressed overtly or covertly in a number of ways, such as triangling, scapegoating, psychophysiological illness, mental illness, and substance abuse. Whatever the presenting diagnosis, the therapist works in similar ways to assist the family to identify and express their thoughts and feelings, define family roles and rules, try new, more productive styles of relating, and restore strength to the parental coalition.

Taking the Family's History. Initiation of family therapy necessitates exploring the family's history, starting with the beginning of the relationship of the parents. This strategy starts the process of focusing on the couple as leaders of the family and takes the pressure off the "identified patient." During the history-taking, each person in the family is identified and recognized in chronological order, thereby acknowledging each member's uniqueness and defining his role(s).

Another historical approach to family therapy is through the use of the genogram (see Chart 15-7). The genogram is a three-generation map of the family structure and relationships.[19] As the therapist draws the map, she questions the family about significant events and identifies family roles. The therapist and family gain an enormous amount of knowledge about the family through the genogram. The genogram is a nonthreatening technique that may be used for diagnosing the family's problems and for helping the family members understand that their present structure, roles, values, and entire system evolved from the past. The use of the genogram is an excellent approach for nurse therapists and other psychiatric–mental health professionals who work with dysfunctional families (see Fig. 15-1 and Case Study 15-1).

Communication Techniques in Family Therapy.
Family therapy may be initiated by asking the family to talk together about the trouble and "monitoring the family conversation."[2, 27] The therapist intervenes in the family's conversation by clarifying, by interpreting double-level, double-bind, and nonverbal communication, and by assisting members to own their own thoughts, feelings, and actions and to communicate them clearly and congruently to others. The therapist deals with anger by talking about it openly and nonjudgmentally, by interpreting anger as hurt, by handling emotionally loaded issues through moving from the least to most emotionally loaded material, and by tying feelings to the facts.[45] The therapist uses humor and empathy, points out positive aspects of the individuals, never blames anyone, and assumes good will even when it is expressed poorly.[45]

Experiential Activities. Other therapeutic techniques available to the nurse family therapist and the family are homework assignments, paradoxical injunction, and sculpting. Homework assignments might require family members to engage in one recreational activity together during the next week, to eat one third of their meals together, or to verbally reinforce each family member once each day. Paradoxical injunctions are instructions to perform the opposite of what is intended, also called the therapeutic bind.[28] Sculpting is a technique wherein the

---

CHART 15-7
How to Prepare a Three-Generation Genogram

General Instructions

Divide the paper sideways into three levels.
Begin in the middle, with husband on left.
Males are in squares; females are in circles.
Place birthdates below symbol, prefaced by a "b."
Place deathdates below symbol, prefaced by a "d."
Place marriage date, preceded by "m" on the paired solid line. Separation = "s." Divorce = "d."
Adoption date is "a."
For first generation (the grandparents), indicate the sibling structure by "oldest of ____," or "youngest of ____," and so on.
Indicate occupation and ethnicity of the first generation along with symbols.
Indicate the occupation of the middle generation.
Indicate the school year or occupation of the third generation (children of major couple).

Notations

(Illustrated on genogram and marked as 1/, 2/, and so forth)
1/ Solid paired line indicates marriage.
2/ Broken paired line indicates non-marriage relationship.
3/ Solid vertical line indicates children of the couple.
4/ Date of doing genogram and clinician's name.

(Adapted from Smoyak S: Family Systems: Use of Genograms as an Assessment Tool. In Clements IW, Buchanan DM (eds): Family Therapy: A Nursing Perspective. John Wiley & Sons, 1982)

---

family enacts an experience without words, then "freezes." The sculpture expresses the feeling tone without word games and is a powerful device for assisting families to understand their relationships. The therapist instructs a particular member to arrange the sculpture as he or she would like it to be, thereby initiating change with action.[36]

Evaluation. Successful outcomes of work with families can be measured by comparing family func-

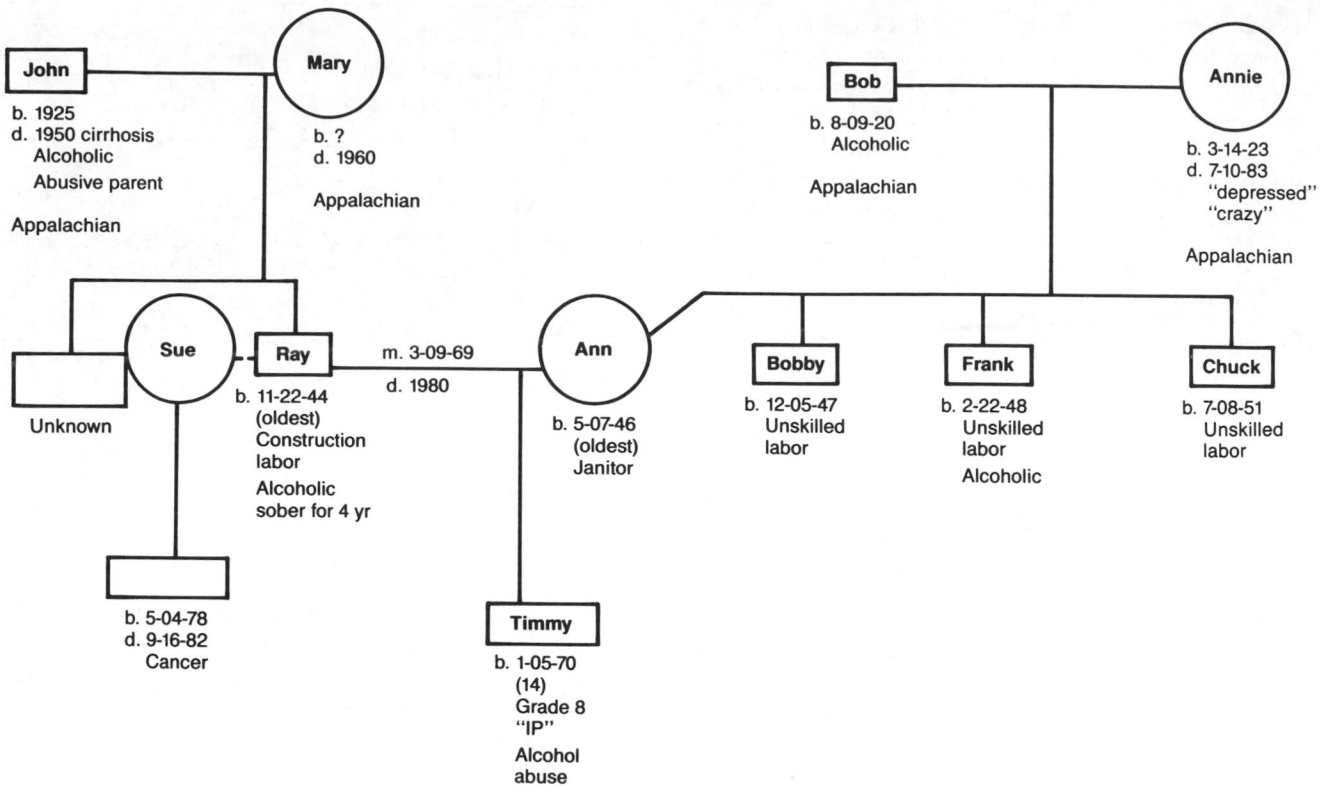

Figure 15-1. *Genogram for the M. family.*

tioning to the assessment criteria described in this chapter. The family who functions optimally has an open systems orientation, clear boundaries, positive links to society, contextual clarity with clear and congruent communication, a strong parental coalition, appropriate power distribution, autonomous people, a warm, caring, affective tone with high self-esteem of members, efficient negotiation and task performance, and transcendent values of hope and altruism. As Satir summarizes, "Family therapy is terminated when everyone in the family can use the first person singular followed by an active verb and ending with a direct object."[45] At that point, family members are free to express feelings and thoughts without fear of loss of self-esteem.

Summary

This chapter provides an overview of theories of family development, roles, structure, and functioning. Some of the critical points discussed in this chapter include the following:

1. A family is a culturally produced social system made up of two or more people in a primary group.

2. Stages of family development may depend on the adult members or the oldest child as an index of family development.

3. According to the family systems theory, the whole (the family) is more than the sum of its parts (the members of the family).

4. Living systems possess clear, but open, boundaries, negentropy, differentiation, and adaptation.

5. Successful families produce competent people through mature leadership of parents.

6. Historical, developmental, role-related, and environmental stressors influence today's family.

7. Assessment of families includes examination of the family's open system orientation, boundaries, contextual clarity, power, encouragement of autonomy, affective tone, negotiation and task performance, transcendent values, and health.

8. Goals planned for optimal to troubled families are enhancement of existing strengths, anticipatory guidance, parenting education, and holistic health measures.

9. Nurses working with families need to possess

(Text continues on p. 246)

Case Study 15-1: the M. Family

Assessment

Fourteen-year-old Timmy called the adolescent inpatient facility saying he wanted to "get off drugs and alcohol" and that he could not get along with his parents. An appointment was made with him and his family. Timmy and his mother, Ann, came for several appointments. When outpatient family therapy failed to assist the family, and the potential for violence increased, inpatient admission was arranged.

Timmy is the only child of Ann and Ray M. They were divorced years ago and are now "getting back together." The couple have known each other from childhood. Ann is a small, obese, woman who wore the soiled jacket from her janitor's uniform on every occasion that the therapist saw her. Ann talks continuously in a low voice and tells her "story" at every opportunity, whether or not it is relevant. Ann is a high-school graduate. She is one female of four siblings of an alcoholic father and a "mental case" mother. Two brothers are alcoholics. She describes her childhood as working very hard at keeping house, studying, and later working as a nurse's aide at an early age. She was, and remains, ashamed of her family or origin and is angry and ashamed that her son, whom she had hoped would be President of the United States, has been drinking for 2 years, cursing, skipping school, and generally not meeting her expectations.

Ray is angry that his son is in the hospital and believes that, with some reasonable rules, Timmy can behave and quit drinking. Ray quit drinking 4 years ago. Ray's father was an alcoholic and physically abused him and his siblings until about age 6; then his father died. His mother was ineffectual, and Ray left home in early adolescence. He was befriended by, and lived with, Ann's family. He learned to drink with her father and brothers.

Several years ago, Ray became involved in an affair during which a child was born. The child became ill with cancer and died. He has ended the relationship with the child's mother and is attempting to reestablish his marriage. He has maintained regular contact with his son throughout the separation and divorce.

Ray has a sixth-grade education. Both parents work two jobs and neither parent is in the home after 4 P.M. on weekdays or before 4 P.M. on weekends. The jobs are needed to provide necessities, but both parents work extra, in part, to buy Timmy a moped, computerized video games, and other expensive items. They do this so he will not have the childhoods they had. Ray also works so that he won't drink and because he cannot tolerate his wife's unpredictable behavior: her "telling her story" and blaming him for his affair. Ray tried to leave or end the assessment interview when he became upset. Ann works because it raises her self-esteem, and she knows no other way to accomplish this. Timmy was cared for by his maternal grandmother, who died 6 months ago after a year's illness. He was then supervised by his alcoholic grandfather.

Timmy is a very pleasant youth who is working hard on his goals in the program and is determined to stop drinking and maintain sobriety. He finds the treatment program's privilege level system logical and helpful. He is outgoing and friendly but angers quickly. He has average intelligence. He complains about his mother's overprotectiveness and says he has to leave the house during his parents' arguments.

This family has deficits in all nine areas of assessment and is described as a midrange family with some characteristics of a troubled family.

Open Systems Orientation

Ann believes the family's problems are unilaterally her son's failure. Initially, Ray stated that the problems are Ann's fault, but quickly decided that placing Timmy with his alcoholic grandfather for care, buying him too many things, and failing to set rules with logical consequences are errors. Timmy believes that being with his alcoholic grandfather and his parents' fighting are the problems. All family members imply or express a need for others in their lives.

Boundaries

No touching was noted during the assessment interview. Interaction occurs between parent and child with very little between parents. Ann has very few relationships outside the family.

Contextual Clarity

The parental coalition is absent. Ann uses her son, rather than her husband, for companionship and support. Ray behaves in a parental role but is unavailable to both his wife and Timmy because of his long work hours and his inability to negotiate with his wife. The parents

(Continues on p. 242)

use blaming patterns of communication and communicate with each other through their child. Only Ray is able to make "I statements."

Power

Ray and Timmy are essentially powerless. Although Ann is very passive superficially, she manipulates her family by not communicating in any other way than "telling the story," thereby inducing guilt and frustration. Her manipulations are a result of her very low self-esteem, shame, and loneliness. Role definitions are based on each individual's perception. Ann's role with her husband is that of a punitive parent; with her son, she assumes a peer role and expects her son to behave like an adult. Ray has a parental role but no husband role. Timmy wishes he were treated like an adolescent son, which his father does but his mother does not. Apparently, his grandmother fulfilled the role of parent for Timmy, but this was offset by the grandfather's treating Timmy as a peer.

Ann and Ray have different sets of expectations that are not clearly defined. Ann expects Timmy to stay at home at all times and bring his friends to their home; however, she does not approve of his friends. When Ray directs Timmy to perform a household chore without consulting Ann, she then tells Timmy not to do it. Timmy, in turn, becomes angry and confused, leaves the house, and drinks.

Encouragement of Autonomy

Although family members identify differences in each other, they are unable to accept them and they hold distorted, unrealistic, and unexpressed expectations of each other.

Affective Issues

Although this family has intense, painful conflicts, the very intensity indicates their concern about losing each other. Both parents care deeply for their son, who reciprocates the feeling. The parents were seriously hurt by their experiences in their families of origin and in their experiences with each other. The family earnestly desires to be together as a family but has been unable to negotiate the changes

needed. Self-esteem is low in all three members of the family with Timmy having the highest levels.

Negotiation and Task Performance

This family is unable to negotiate.

Transcendent Values

This family is in a great deal of pain and not hopeful because Timmy's drinking has upset their hopes for him to have a better life than the parents had.

Health Measures

Although the family has a regular dinner daily, other meals are irregular and unplanned. Timmy abuses alcohol and marijuana. Ann is obese. Ray has regular recreation with his friends, but Ann and Timmy do not. There is no family recreation at all. Ann's and Timmy's recreation together is watching soap operas.

Although there are deficits in all nine assessment areas, several major themes emerge as appropriate areas for nursing intervention. These are expressed as nursing diagnoses. Because the parental coalition is the critical factor in family functioning, the therapy is directed toward the couple.

Nursing Diagnoses

1. Alteration in parenting, ineffective, related to parental conflict
2. Family conflict related to ineffective communication patterns
    Ann "telling the story"
    Ray not talking, then leaving
    Timmy talking angrily, then leaving; being "in the middle" of the parents
3. Ineffective family coping: compromised, related to excessive work hours, low self-esteem, and fear of intimacy
4. Ineffective individual coping, related to alcohol abuse (Timmy)

Goals and Interventions

(See Family Nursing Care Plan 15-1)

Family Nursing Care Plan 15-1

The M. Family

Nursing Diagnosis	Goal	Intervention	Evaluation
2/1 Alteration in parenting, ineffective, related to parental conflict	1. Ray and Ann will determine a list of expectations for Timmy with consequences for unmet expectations by 2/7	1–3. Family therapy sessions with T. Robbins, R.N., M.S., Tuesdays and Thursdays from 12 to 1 P.M., discussion of goals achieved through homework assignments	1. Goal was met by 2/7
	2. Ray and Ann will decide what age-appropriate recreation activities they will permit their son to participate in by 2/14		2. Goal was met by 2/14
	3. Ray and Ann will adjust their work hours so that each parent is more available during non-school hours by 2/14		3. Ray changed hours to be home by 10 P.M. and more weekend hours. Ann plans to stop her weekend job.
	4. Timmy will experience success and/or consequences in levels system by 2/14	4. Milieu supervised by C. Smith, R.N., primary nurse, daily, and in privilege levels meeting Tuesday and Friday, 3:45 P.M.	4. Timmy kept all rules and met daily goals by 2/14
2/1 Family conflict related to ineffective communication patterns	1. Ann will say what she wants specifically from her husband and from her son by 2/21	1–3. Family therapy sessions with T. Robbins, Tuesdays and Thursdays, 12 to 1 P.M. for 3 weeks	1. Ann said specifically what she wanted from her son by 2/16 but not her husband
	2. Ray will stay in the sessions and say what he thinks and feels by 2/21	a. Therapist will direct family members to use "I statements" and eye contact	2. Ray refused to come to sessions after 2/14
	3. Timmy will stay in the sessions and say what he feels and wants without cursing by 2/21	b. Therapist will direct family to stay in "here and now"	3. Timmy was able to stay in sessions, state feelings, and not curse, with coaching, by 2/21

(Continues on p. 244)

Nursing Diagnosis	Goal	Intervention	Evaluation
		c. Therapist will emphasize (praise) family members' goodwill, attempts to change, and successes	
		d. Therapist will name feelings, etc., as concretely as possible	
	4. Parents will stop communicating through Timmy by 2/14	4. Therapist will redirect communication a. Primary nurse will direct parent communication to family therapist b. Primary nurse encourages verbalization of feelings and insight into his "being in the middle"	4. Parents attempted to communicate through the therapist and school teacher; they talked to each other on the phone
2/1 Ineffective family coping: compromised, related to excessive work hours, low self-esteem, and fears of intimacy	1. Ann will reduce her work hours and find one social activity outside the home by 2/21 2. Ann and Ray will spend 1 hour per day in household without arguing 3. Ray will reduce work hours so that there is time for family activity and time with Ann alone by 2/21	1–3. Therapist will facilitate couple's talking together about positive aspects of their long relationship; therapist will explore with couple and family possible fun activities	1. The family did not meet these goals

Nursing Diagnosis	Goal	Intervention	Evaluation
2/21 Ineffective individual coping, related to alcohol abuse	1. Timmy will maintain sobriety through 2/21	1. Participate in chemical dependency program a. Group 10:30–11:30 A.M. Monday through Friday, A. Budd, M.S., therapist b. Education and Big Book discussion 1–2 P.M., Monday through Friday with B. Brown, C.A.C. c. AA meeting, Friday, 6 P.M. at Good Samaritan Youth Services	1. Timmy did maintain sobriety including weekend day passes
	2. Family will verbalize understanding of family dynamics that contibute to Timmy's drinking by 2/21	2. a. Family sessions will include a discussion of this problem; therapist will point out dynamics as they occur b. Adolescent group therapy 2–3 P.M., Monday through Friday, T. Poffer, M.S.	2. Parents verbalized understanding of some contributing factors
	3. Parents will verbalize commitment to attend Al-Anon (Ann) and AA meeting with Timmy (Ray) once weekly by 2/21	3. Discharge planning in family session	3. Ray verbalized commitment but did not follow through

self-understanding, empathy, therapeutic communication skills, and knowledge of family theory.

10. The family therapist helps the family identify and express their thoughts and feelings, define family roles and rules, try more productive styles of relating, and restore strength to the parental coalition.

References

1. Alvino J: Parents' Guide to Raising a Gifted Child. New York, Random House, 1985

2. Andrews E: The Emotionally Distrubed Family. New York, Jason Aaronson, 1977

3. Aradine C, Pridham KF: Model for Collaboration. Nurs Outlook 21 (October): 655–657, 1973

4. Bateson G, Jackson D, Haley J, Weakland J: Toward a Theory of Schizophrenia. In Jackson DD (ed): Communication, Family, and Marriage. Palo Alto, CA, Science & Behavior Books, 1968

5. Beavers WR: Psychotherapy and Growth: A Family Systems Perspective. New York, Brunner/Mazel, 1977

6. Berkowitz I: The Role of Schools in Child, Adolescent, and Youth Suicide Prevention. In Peck M., Farberow N (eds): Youth Suicide. Litman R, New York, Springer, 1985

7. Bohen HH, Viveros-Long A: Balancing Jobs and Family Life. Phialdelphia, Temple University Press, 1981

8. Bowen M: Family Therapy in Clinical Practice. New York, Jason Aaronson, 1978

9. Brallier L: The Nurse as Holistic Health Practitioner. Nurs Clin North Am 13 (December): 643–655, 1978

10. Braxton E: Structuring the Black Family for Survival and Growth. Perspect Psychiatr Care 14 (October/November/December): 165–173, 1976

11. Brockhaus J, Brockhaus R: Adopting an Older Child: The Emotional Process. Am J Nurs 82 (February): 288–291, 1982

12. Collison C, Futrell J: Family Therapy for the Single-Parent Family System. J Psychosoc Nurs Ment Health Serv 20 (July): 16–20, 1982

13. Dinkmeyer D, McKay G: Systematic Training for Effective Parenting. Circle Pines, MN, American Guidance Service, 1975

14. Dinkmeyer D, McKay G: Systematic Training for Effective Parenting: Teen. Circle Pines, MN, American Guidance Service

15. Dobson J: The Strong Willed Child. Wheaton, IL, Tyndale House Publishers, 1978

16. Dreikurs R, Soltz V: Children: The Challenge. New York, Duell, Sloan & Pearce, 1964

17. Duvall E: Family Development, 4th ed. Philadelphia, JB Lippincott, 1971

18. Friedman MM: Family Nursing: Theory and Assessment. New York, Appleton-Century-Crofts, 1981

19. Fromm E: The Art of Loving. New York, Harper & Row, 1956

20. Gibran K: The Prophet. New York, Alfred A. Knopf, 1968 (original copyright, 1923)

21. Glenn SH, Warner JW: The Developmental Approach to Preventing Problem Dependencies. Bethesda, MD, Family Development Institute

22. Gordon T: Parent Effectiveness Training. New York, PH Wyden, 1970

23. Guerin PJ, Pendagast EG: Evaluation of Family System and Genogram. In Guerin PJ (ed): Family Therapy. New York, Gardner Press, 1976

24. Horowitz J, Perdue B: Single-Parent Families. Nurs Clin North Am 12 (September): 503–511, 1977

25. Hunka CD, O'Toole A, O'Toole R: Self Help Therapy in Parents Anonymous. J Psychosoc Nurs Ment Health Serv 23 (July): 24–32, 1985

26. Kelly A: Evaluating and Improving Family Health: The Holistic Health Handbook. Berkeley, CA, And/Or Press, 1978

27. Kempler W: Principles of Gestalt Family Therapy. Salt Lake City, Deseret Press, 1974

28. Lantz JE: Family and Marital Therapy. New York, Appleton-Century-Crofts, 1978

29. Lewis JM, Beavers WR, Gossett JT, Phillips VA: No Single Thread: Psychological Health in Family Systems. New York, Brunner/Mazel, 1976

30. Liebow PR: The New Look School Nurse. J Psychosoc Nurs Ment Health Serv 22(3): 37–41, 1984

31. Manatt M: Parents, Peers and Pot. Rockville, MD, National Institute on Drug Abuse. (DHHS Publication No. (ADM) 82–812) 1982

32. McCown D: TV: Its Problems for Children, Pediatr Nurs (March/April): 17–19, 1979

33. Minuchin S: Families and Family Therapy. Cambridge, Harvard University Press, 1974

34. Murray R, Zentner J: Nursing Concepts for Health Promotion, 2d ed. Englewood Cliffs, NJ, Prentice-Hall, 1979

35. O'Shea MD, Phelps R: Multiple Family Therapy: Current Status and Critical Appraisal. Fam Process 24 (December): 555–581, 1985

36. Papp P: Family Choreography. In Guerin PJ (ed): Family Therapy. New York, Gardner Press, 1976

37. Perkins WM, Perkins NM: How to Raise Drug Free Kids in a Drug Filled World. Center City, MN, Hazelden, 1986

38. Prattes O: Beliefs of the Mexican-American Family. In Hymovich D, Barnard M (eds): Family Health Care. New York, McGraw-Hill, 1973

39. PRIDE: Starting a Parent Group, Atlanta, PRIDE, 1982

40. Rapoport R, Rapoport R: Dual-Career Families. Baltimore, Penguin Books, 1971

41. Rapoport R, Rapoport R: Dual-Career Families Re-examined. New York, Harper Colophon Books, 1976

42. Richardson DB, Thornton J, Gest T, Wellborn S: End of the Permissive Society? U.S. News and World Report, pp 45–48, June 28, 1982

43. Rozendahl N: Understanding Italian American Cultural Norms. J Psychosoc Ment Health Serv 25(2): 29–33, 1987

44. Satir V: Peoplemaking. Palo Alto, CA, Science and Behavior Books, 1972

45. Satir V: Conjoint Family Therapy. Palo Alto, CA, Science and Behavior Books, 1977

46. Schuckit MA: Biological Vulnerability to Alcoholism. J Consult Clin Psychol 55(3): 301–309, 1987

47. Sheehy G: Passages: Predictable Crises of Adult Life. New York, Bantam Books, 1976

48. Smoyak S: Family Systems: Use of Genograms as an Assessment Tool. In Clements IW, Buchanan DM (eds): Family Therapy: A Nursing Perspective. New York, John Wiley & Sons, 1982

49. Stevenson J: Issues and Crises during Middlescence. New York, Appleton-Century-Crofts, 1977

50. Straus M, Gelles R, Steinmetz SK: Behind Closed Doors: Violence in the American Family. Garden City, NY, Anchor Books, 1980

51. Sue S: Asian-Americans: Psychological Perspectives Ben Lomond, CA, Science and Behavior Books, 1973

52. Tripp-Reimer T, Friedl M: Appalachians: A Neglected Minority. Nurs Clin North Am 12 (March): 41–54, 1977

53. U.S. News and World Report Tomorrow. pp 11–12, June 28, 1982

54. Visher EB, Visher JS: Step Families: A Guide to Working with Step Parents and Stepchildren. New York, Brunner/Mazel, 1979

55. Watzlawick P, Beaven J, Jackson D: Pragmatics of Human Communication. New York, Norton, 1967

56. Wegschieder S: Another Chance: Help and Hope for the Alcoholic Family. Palo Alto, CA, Science and Behavior Books, 1981

57. Wolff I: Referral: A Process and a Skill. Nurs Outlook 10 (April): 253–256, 1962

58. Yankelovich D: Stepchildren of the Moral Majority. Psychology Today (November): 5–10, 1981

59. Yankelovich, Skelly and White, Inc.: Family Health in an Era of Stress: The General Mills American Family Report, 1978–1979. Minneapolis, General Mills, 1979

60. York P, York D: Toughlove. Doylestown, PA, Toughlove, 1984

16 Behavioral Approaches

Juliann Casey Reakes

We are controlled by the world in which we live, and part of that world has been and will be constructed by men. The question is this: are we to be controlled by accident, by tyrants, or by ourselves in effective cultural design?

B. F. Skinner,
Freedom and the Control of Men,
1955

Chapter Preview

This chapter discusses principles of behavior therapy, strategies of learning theory, and the application of these principles and strategies in assisting clients to replace maladaptive behavior with adaptive behavior.

Learning refers to that process that brings about a change in behavior. For example, if a client stops abusing alcohol after serving 90 days in jail and seeks counseling after his release, learning may be inferred from his behavior.

Behavior therapy has proven to be a practical, efficient, parsimonious way of assisting clients and families to change their behavior by the application of learning theories. Behavior therapy is the essence of behaviorism. Behaviorism is a philosophical approach to life, as well as a psychological discipline built on a precise scientific orientation to the problems of man and other living organisms. Behaviorism represents reality and therefore views behavior that is outside of the expected social norm as maladaptive, not as a symptom of disease, a form of deviance, or a deficit. The cause of maladaptive behavior is not a relevant issue, because the focus of behavior therapy is to assist a person to adapt objectively to the real world by learning ways to change his responses to the internal and external environments.

The components of both the nursing process and the process of behavior analysis and application are similar. Assessment, nursing diagnosis, planning, intervention, and evaluation by means of specific outcome criteria are inherent in both methodologies. The goals of nursing and behavior therapy are also parallel—to help people deal more effectively with reality.

Learning Objectives

On completion of the chapter, you should be able to accomplish the following:

1. Define terms specific to behavior therapy
2. Apply principles of behavior therapy to nursing practice and client problems
3. Discuss the goals of behavioral therapeutic approaches
4. Differentiate between classical conditioning, operant conditioning, cognitive therapy, and other forms of behavior modification
5. Discuss the use of various forms of behavioral intervention
6. Apply the steps of the nursing process to the process involved in behavior therapy

Principles of Behavior Therapy

The term *behavior* implies an open and wide range of overt and covert responses that include emotions and verbalizations.[29,46] The contemporary use of behavior therapy refers to a group of diversified approaches for dealing with maladaptive behavior. Maladaptive behavior either may be learned or may be a result of a failure to learn adaptive behavior (see Chart 16-1, "Describing Adaptive and Maladaptive Behavior."). The basic premise of behavior therapy is that most behaviors are learned. This, however, does not rule out the biologic implications of maladaptive behavioral responses; that is, biochemical, genetic, or cellular disturbances.[10]

In behaviorist terms, maladaptive behavior is a way of dealing with stress. Obvious or overt responses are measured; hidden or covert responses are subjective, but can be described in behavioral terms and changed. Mediating processes or cognitions (*i.e.*, thoughts, feelings, and attitudes) are subjective variables and, similar to objective variables or events that are situation-specific (*i.e.*, birth, marriage, and job), they can be described in behavioral terms and influenced to effect behavioral change.[6]

The process of behavior therapy is a precise approach to bringing about behavioral change. Concepts, thoughts, or subjective representations (*e.g.*, anxiety, guilt, depression, anger, joy, and hope) are described in specific behavioral terms to present a detailed, finely tuned approach to client needs.[17]

The work of John B. Watson, an early 20th-century psychologist, formed the foundation for behavior therapy and for applying objective methodology to solving maladaptive behavioral problems. Learning, or behavioral change, occurs because of experiences that, over a period of time, result in conditioned response learning or classical conditioning, as described by Ivan P. Pavlov.

Classical Conditioning

In Pavlovian learning, an *unconditioned stimulus*, food, elicits an *unconditioned response*, salivation, in a hungry dog. When a bell, a *conditioned stimulus*, is paired with the food, an unconditioned stimulus, over a period of time the conditioned stimulus results in salivation in the dog, a *conditioned response*. The unconditioned stimulus, food, is a reinforcer for the conditioned stimulus and the conditioned response. This type of learning is affected by events that occur before the behavior. The preceding events elicit a certain response. The unconditioned stimulus may be rewarding or pleasant (*e.g.*, a smile from the nurse) or un-

CHART 16-1

Describing Adaptive and Maladaptive Behavior

Thorough data collection, thoughtful analysis, and specific behavioral descriptions result in accurate problem identification.

These are some descriptions of maladaptive behavior identified for a client:

1. Continually tells anyone who listens that she talks on the phone every day to the President of the United States
2. Sits in a chair in activity room with head bowed and hands tightly clasped in lap
3. Drinks only liquids on meal tray
4. Throws food on the floor at every meal
5. States continual preoccupation with thoughts of her son's death
6. Paces the length of the floor in her room
7. Complains of feeling a "tight, narrow band" around her head
8. Stares at the floor or ceiling when talking with other clients or staff members

Descriptions of a client's adaptive behavior include the following.

1. Completes assigned ceramic activities
2. Initiates conversation with group members
3. Volunteers to obtain equipment for outdoor games
4. Explains decision in an assertive manner to husband
5. Requests help in seeking solutions to a problem
6. Contracts with the staff to complete daily goals
7. Speaks with reality orientation and realism
8. Expresses angry feelings about marriage failure

Note that these descriptions of behavior do not imply judgment, that is, "good" or "bad" or "positive"or "negative" behavior. They are simply objective verbal or written pictures of behavior observed.

pleasant, noxious, painful or aversive (*e.g.*, as a drug that induces nausea). Aversive therapy has been used to treat alcoholism by pairing the drinking of alcohol with a nausea-producing drug.

There are many examples of classical conditioning in health care. Fear of injections may be conditioned by the nurse's white uniform or by the sight of the needle or syringe. The nurse's uniform, as unconditioned stimulus, elicits discomfort or fear, the unconditioned response. The needle becomes a conditioned stimulus, and fear, a conditioned response. For example, fear of arguing or fighting may result from an association with a traumatic event that involved arguing or fighting. When a child receives a toy after each visit to the doctor and is told by the doctor, nurse, and his mother how well he behaved, eventually praise alone is sufficient to elicit his positive behavior.

More than one stimulus not originally associated with a response may reinforce this learning by serving as a link in binding a response to a series of stimuli. By the process of chaining, more than one unconditioned stimulus may become a conditioned stimulus and higher-order conditioning, or learning, can result. For example, a child receives a toy at the doctor's office when he responds favorably to the doctor's examination and treatment. The office nurse verbally praises the child and hands him a toy while giving him a hug or a pat on the back. At the same time, the child's mother tells him his reward is a stop at McDonald's for a special treat because he was such "a good boy." The toy is a primary reinforcer for the child's behavior in the doctor's office; the praise, pleasant physical contact (touch), and the treat at McDonald's are successive reinforcers. Many emotional responses, such as an unfounded fear of objects, may become a conditioned response due to a higher order conditioning, despite the fact that there may have been no direct association with the feared object. Words, which can be symbols of experiences or events, may become conditioned stimuli that trigger respondent behavior or that signal dangerous or feared situations.[6]

The classic example of respondent conditioning is the work of psychologist John B. Watson and nurse Rosalee Rayner of John Hopkins Hospital. Albert, an 11-month-old child, was conditioned by noise association with a white rat and other white furry objects. This illustrates the behavioristic view that phobias are conditioned fears learned when a stimulus is paired with a feared object or event.[57]

Several years later, in 1924, Mary Cover Jones, a psychologist, used clinical conditioning theory to counter conditioned fear to furry objects experienced by a young boy. Pairing food eaten by the child in various distances from a rabbit, representing the class of feared objects, the child was able eventually to eat with the rabbit sitting on his table and his lap.[23]

In 1952, H. J. Eysnick conducted a survey of neurotic patients following psychotherapy and concluded that about two-thirds of the patients would have recovered eventually from their illness with or without psychiatric treatment. A few years later, Eysnick suggested a new approach for dealing with maladaptive behavior—behavior therapy. Behavior therapy is not concerned with dialogue as a treatment, as is traditional psychotherapy. On the contrary, behavioral therapy deals with changing the individual's maladaptive behavior by a planned, objective approach, such as respondent conditioning and counter-conditioning techniques.[15]

A contemporary of H. J. Eysnick, Joseph Wolpe, built on the theory of classical conditioning to demonstrate clinically that learned anxiety may be inhibited by another behavioral response. When behavioral responses—such as muscle relaxation, assertive responses, and sexual arousal responses—occur in the presence of cues that originally triggered anxiety, anxiety is lessened. These responses eventually become associated with the cues and weaken the anxiety response. Wolpe called this counter-conditioning process *reciprocal inhibitiion*.[58] For example, the person who experiences unsatisfactory job interviews and becomes anxious may become conditioned to employment situations because of encounters with similar cues and stimuli. The anxiety that is evoked may result in the avoidance of job situations. Learning to deal assertively with this situation in the presence of these cues can reduce his anxiety. Assertive responses, sexual responses, and muscle relaxation are associated with the parasympathetic nervous system; increased activity of this system decreases anxiety responses associated with the sympathetic nervous system, such as dilated pupils, increased blood pressure, heart rate, and increased blood supply to voluntary muscles.[58] Systematic desensitization based on reciprocal inhibition theory has been effective with a broad group of client problems including phobias, obsessive-compulsive disorders, sexual disorders, psychosomatic disorders, and alcoholism.[10]

In 1962, Lazarus and Abramovitz applied the principles of systematic desensitization to treat children's fears. A child's phobic behavior toward a dog was eliminated in a short 5-week session. A pleasant wished-for scene imagined by the child and the gradual introduction of the phobic object dissipated the anxiety originally associated with the dog.[30]

Operant Conditioning

Until B. F. Skinner and a colleague introduced a specific type of behavior therapy, operant conditioning, in 1954, classical conditioning was the force of behaviorism. Operant or instrumental behavior (such as eating or writing) refers to activity strengthened or weakened by its consequences (such as weight loss or weight gain). Operant behavior is under the control of the individual who can use behavior to change or modify the environment.

Operant conditioning is also called operant reinforcement theory. A *reinforcer* is anything that increases the probability of a response. In respondent conditioning, the unconditioned stimulus, paired with the conditioned stimulus, is the reinforcement that brings about specific behavior. In operant conditioning, reinforcement strengthens the emitting of a wide range of behaviors. The client learns to duplicate the response. The criteria for reinforcement are that the reinforcer meet a need and be goal-directed. Food, for example, may not always elicit an adaptive behavior if hunger is not a priority need for the individual.[53] A positive reinforcer, or reward, strengthens a behavior; the removal of a negative reinforcer strengthens or facilitates adaptive behavior when the client is able to evade or avoid the harmful reinforcer.

Both positive and negative reinforcers are specifically defined with regards to prior impact on the behavior to be changed. Punishment is not a negative reinforcer because it is designed to eliminate a behavior, whereas true negative reinforcement produces adaptive behavior.[53] Punishment often suppresses the maladaptive behavior, but does not eliminate it from the client's behavioral pattern.[14] If the individual is not offered a specific alternative, he may respond with a behavior that is more maladaptive than the original behavior. Regressive behavior or generalization to other situations may also occur if an alternative behavior is not available.[46] For example, a child may be punished for eating "junk food" at home and may, therefore, learn to eat his "junk food" at fast-food stands. Children often become enuretic when punished, whereas adults may resort to overeating, drinking alcoholic beverages, or retaliating with aggressive behavior toward spouse or children.

Operant conditioning has been successfully used with many clinical and behavioral problems that have not responded to other treatments. By means of negative and positive reinforcement, speech was successfully restored in a schizophrenic client who had not spoken for 30 years. Candy, cigarettes, magazines, books, and praise were successfully used as positive reinforcers to increase verbal communication in mute chronic schizophrenic clients.[4]

Free Operant Conditioning

In addition to operant conditioning, Skinner demonstrated a type of instrumental conditioning called free operant conditioning. Skinner also used this method, termed *free operant study*, to study behaviors. A response easily emitted is selected to be measured while other emitted behavior is also studied.

To study the effect of a drug on hallucinatory behavior, a hospitalized psychotic male was the subject of a free operant study. Two behaviors were first measured, hallucinatory behavior and the specific activity of pulling a plunger that was intermittently reinforced. A psychotropic drug was given to the client for the experimental phase and the same activities by the client were recorded. It was found that, when the plunger activity was decreased, the hallucinatory behavior increased. The experimenter concluded that the drug actually increased the hallucinatory behavior rather than decreasing it.[32] In a similar free operant study, a researcher found that a chronic schizophrenic client responded more positively following therapeutic interactions with a nursing student than from psychotropic drug therapy.[31]

Operant Control of Verbal Behavior

According to Skinner, verbal behavior is also under operant control. Verbal behavior is influenced by its relationship to the behavior of other people. Like other operant conditioning, verbal behavior is influenced by its outcome. It influences personal interaction and is maintained by social behavior. Verbal behavior translates other behavior into word symbols but, as in any translation, there is subjectivity in the interpretation. Words, when reinforced and under similar contingencies, become maintained as behavior patterns.[53] For example, the psychotic verbal behavior of one long-term schizophrenic client was eliminated by positively reinforcing rational verbal behavior with cigarettes and by withholding cigarettes when the client demonstrated irrational verbal behavior.[2]

Generalization

Adaptive behavior specific to one situation may occur in similar situations because of a phenomenon called *generalization*. Rational verbal behavior learned in a client–health team interaction may generalize in client–family and client–friend relationships.

Discrimination

Discrimination refers to a specific response occurring in a given situation. The client who is positively reinforced for completing an activity task and who is ig-

nored when the task is not completed, who then consistently completes his assigned work, is making a differential or a discriminating response.

Extinction

Extinction is the withholding of reinforcers and reducing the probability of the response occurring. If the staff ignore the client's attention-seeking behavior and positively reinforce group-participating behavior, the former behavior may be extinguished by the increase in the latter response.[54]

Prompting and Fading

Prompting and fading refer to creating conditions that facilitate or accentuate the reinforcer. *Prompting* is a cuing process; *fading* is the gradual reduction of this process. Enunciating a word carefully for an aphasic client who is learning to identify objects again following a stroke may be eliminated or faded as soon as the client begins to name the object without cuing by the nurse.

The following example illustrates the application of fading and prompting. A program was initiated to emphasize the need for client compliance with a prescribed daily activity program. The client was instructed to notify a staff member hourly when an activity was completed. The staff member prompted the client to check the schedule and reinforced the client's actions with praise when the task was completed. After a 3-day compliance with this plan, the hourly check was expanded to 2 hours for another 3-day period, 4 hours for the next 3 days, and as compliance increased, the schedule was checked once a day.

Shaping

Shaping behavior refers to the patterning of a group of actions by the continued reinforcement of responses essential to the desired target behavior.[10] A neat, clean physical appearance is targeted as the priority behavior to be achieved by the client. When the client is consistently rewarded with verbal praise and attention from the health team when his hair is combed, teeth are brushed, nails are trimmed and clean, the overall target behavior—a neat, clean physical appearance—is often achieved.

Reinforcers

The choice of reinforcers, as well as the timing, is important for adaptive change. When the response or operant occurs and is recognized by the individual as bringing about a desired action or modification in the environment, the client has discovered a potent tool for change.[26] *Social reinforcers* may include praise, attention, touch, or interest. *Material reinforcers* may include food, prizes, redeemable tokens, or money. *Activity reinforcers* may include watching television, attending plays or movies, attending dances, playing cards, or shopping.

Reinforcement Schedules

Reinforcement may be associated continuously with a specific target behavior or may occur at fixed or varying intervals.[46] Designing reinforcers and schedules of reinforcement for a specific client requires careful planning of the nurse. All of the staff involved in the client's 24-hour care must be consistent and must follow the schedule according to the protocol set for the client.

Reinforcement schedules may be of the following three types:

1. Continuous—every expected response is reinforced
2. Intermittent—every expected response is not reinforced; only selected responses are reinforced

    Fixed ratios—every certain response is reinforced, such as the third, eighth, or tenth response

    Variable ratio—the responses being reinforced are changed at certain times; at first, the third response may be reinforced and the next day the sixth response may be reinforced

3. At intervals—variable or fixed ratios that are defined by the time between reinforcement.[46]

Nursing Process and Behavior Therapy

Assessment

Collection of Data

The first step in both the nursing process and the application of behavioral principles is assessment. Assessment includes the collection of objective and subjective data. Objective data are data that can be measured, observed, or validated. Subjective data are data that reflect the client's feelings, perceptions, and "self talk" about his problems.

Information about the client's problem may be obtained from the following:

Nursing history
Systems review
Physical examination findings
Psychosocial, cultural, or mental status findings, including developmental data, demographic

data, and the duration, frequency, and extent of the presenting problem
Description of the behavior and situation before and after the problem
Consequences of the problem behavior
Client resources—likes, dislikes, support systems, and interests
Client expectations and motivations

The nurse may identify other problem areas that the client does not recognize, but that influence the presenting problem. For example, the nurse may perceive that the client has poor verbal communication skills, which may be directly related to his presenting problem of feeling anxious in situations with strangers. Cultural influences may have a direct effect on the presenting problem and cultural data should be included in an assessment.

Listening to the client is as necessary as the accurate recording and validating of data. Observation of the client during the interview, examinations, and testing situations contribute valuable information in identifying the following:

1. The problem behavior
2. The situations in which the behavior occurs
3. The consequences of the behavior
4. The parameters of the problem
5. The client's perception of the problem[15]

Problem Identification

The behavior or target problem should be clearly identified. Problems might include inadequate social skills, overwhelming anxiety when talking with strangers (as seen by perspiring, headache, dizziness, faltering speech), or the inability to use family resources, when necessary, without feeling guilty.

Planned observations by the members of the psychiatric–mental health team may disclose the modifying of a favorable response other than the target behavior. An unplanned event may become a reinforcer. For example, smiling associated with verbal praise, the primary reinforcer, may strengthen the target behavior when used alone. Withdrawing a reinforcer to bring about a desired behavior is an excellent intervention in many client management situations. Sending a disruptive client to a "time-out" area may increase a targeted behavior.

Chance Reinforcement

Chance reinforcement may also result in strengthening maladaptive behavior. When the nurse gives immediate attention to the client who refuses to eat by spoon-feeding him, even though extra cigarettes might be given to the client for eating without help, the nurse may be unknowingly reinforcing the non-eating behavior.

C H A R T   16-2
Therapeutic Dialogue

Identifying the Client's Perception of the Problem

The following dialogue between the nurse and client illustrates the importance of the client's identification of the problem:

Nurse: Tell me in your own words your feelings about what's happened.

Client: I've been laid off again. This is the second time in 6 months. My parents are elderly and barely making it financially. My brother and sister send them $50 a month and I can't even send $5. My son blames me for using his college money to keep the family going. He went into the service to get away from me. My brother refuses to talk to me. My wife and daughter ignore me—nobody listens to me.

Nurse: You're feeling very alone and sad, but angry that no one listens to you.

Client: They all hate me and blame me for their problems.

Nurse: You're feeling...

Client: It's like I told you. It's my mistakes. Yes, I feel sad and responsible. Why can't I stop crying—a grown man?

Nurse: You've felt this way before?

Client: Even in grade school when my friends were not happy, I always felt it was me. When things didn't go right at work, I would feel the same way. I was demoted 6 months ago and would have been let go but I took a lower-paying job. I wanted to try something different—I like carpentry but I was afraid...

Nurse: You've been afraid a lot?

Client: Well, when my wife had to go back to work and I couldn't continue helping my parents (begins to tear again and voice trembles)...

Nurse: You feel responsible for your wife, your parents, and your children?

Client: Yes, I feel I have lost control over life. I feel hopeless and responsible but I know I can't take care of everybody. I guess it's my "head trouble."

Discussion

The client is beginning to identify his irrational belief that he should be responsible for his wife, children, parents, and other family members. The nurse's therapy plan will be to assist the client in using the problem-solving process to identify the problem specifically, realistically, and logically, and identify adaptive ways to cope with the problem. Problem-solving is an essential intervention for clients who lack these skills or for those who are reluctant to use the process when faced with problems.

Secondary Reinforcement

Secondary reinforcers or conditioned responses are as influential in changing behavior as primary reinforcers.[20] Participation with others by playing bingo, the primary reinforcer, may become a secondary reinforcer for increasing verbal communication and illustrates the application of the Premack Principle. The *Premack Principle* states that a high-probability behavior can reinforce a low-probability response. For example, a client who likes to watch television may be allowed to watch his favorite program if he attends his occupational therapy activity. Another example of this principle occurs when anorexic clients are rewarded for weight gain by being permitted to participate in desired activities.[34]

Behavior includes aspects of both operant and respondent conditioning, and behavior can be modified and adapted by the use of a variety of techniques. The modification of a response requires data about the behavior's frequency of occurrence and the specific situation in which it occurs. The choice of effective reinforcers, the selection of a reinforcement schedule, and a precise plan to initiate behavioral techniques are essential.

Nursing Diagnosis

During the second step of the nursing process for psychiatric–mental health clients, the nurse examines the data gathered in the client assessment and formulates nursing diagnoses that will guide the planning and implementation of nursing interventions. The client's nursing diagnosis, for example, may be "social isolation related to depressed mood and lack of trust in others, evidenced by sad, dull affect, uncommunicative behavior, preoccupation with own thoughts, and absence of supportive significant others." Each part of this diagnosis provides the nurse and other mental health team members with a wealth of specific client behaviors to be modified by means of behavioral techniques.

Planning

Planning of behavioral interventions occurs as a cooperative effort of the psychiatric–mental health team. Objectivity of team members is a necessary component of planning behavioral methods; subjectivity affects the evaluation of clients' behavioral progress and treatment planning.[9]

Goal-Setting

Based on the assessment and analysis of client behavior, treatment goals are identified. These goals may include the following:

1. To provide a safe physical environment
2. To increase a defined behavioral performance
3. To promote self-care and independence
4. To implement competent, individualized care
5. To select learning methods

A treatment plan format for each client may incorporate the following elements:

Client's name
Purpose of the behavior modification program
Goals of the program
Place where the behavior occurs
Target behavior (see Chart 16-3)
Reinforcement schedule
Staff objectives (how to record behavior, reinforcement protocol, and so forth)
Time the behavior is to be observed or is to occur
Data-collection methods[49]

Intervention

Following the observation and recording of baseline data, the nurse employs the fourth step of the nursing process, intervention. Intervention includes compli-

---

C H A R T   16-3
Adaptive (Target) Behavior Protocol

Maladaptive behavior:

Frequency—

Duration—

Intensity—

Adaptive behavior desired in specific behavioral terms:

ance with reinforcement schedules, manipulations of the environment, and other treatment activities.

Self-Management Programs

Nurses have directed self-management programs with clients motivated for behavior change in the areas of weight control and smoking control. Self-management programs follow the same format as other modification programs; observing and recording one's own behavior are additional reinforcers.[12]

Contracting

The nurse has many interventions to use in behavior therapy programs in addition to reinforcement applications. *Behavioral contracting,* an agreement with a client for a specific behavior, is often used in self-control programs. Contracting may be an oral or a written agreement. If it is written, the contract is usually dated, behavior or other criteria are identified, and it is signed by the nurse and the client (see Chart 16-4).

Other Behavioral Activities

Positive or negative reinforcement of behavior, *prompting* (cues), *fading* (removing cues), extinction (ignoring a behavior), *time out,* and *revoking privileges* are activities that may be included in the nursing plan (see Chart 16-5). Teaching the client to *discriminate* (make a certain response) or *generalize* (apply a response to other situations) may also be goals of a treatment plan. The use of *over-correction* (another behavior is added to one that the client is repeating in an acceptable way) or *simple correction* (a repeat of the acceptable behavior) are examples of interventions that may be useful in treatment planning.

Cognitive Therapy

The goal of cognitive therapy is to decrease subjective distress and increase productive, rewarding behavior. Clients who benefit from this approach are those individuals who are able to learn the association of counterproductive beliefs, distorted thinking, self-defeating feelings and behaviors, and their logical fallacies. These illogical ideations include the following:

1. Personalization
2. All-or-nothing thinking
3. "Awfulization"
4. Overgeneralizations
5. Perfectionism
6. Fault-finding
7. "Wants," "oughts," and "shoulds" self-talk
8. Negating positive thoughts

The main foci of cognitive restructuring are using logical thinking to evaluate situations by recog-

---

C H A R T   16-4
Contract

Date _____

_____ and _____
(client's name)   (nurse's name)

agree that on _____ and ending on _____
(date)   (date)

the following agreement is made:

Client will:

Nurse will:

_____
Client's signature

_____
Nurse's signature

---

nizing the criteria that emphasize irrational and distorted thoughts, and neutralizing the situation so that rational thought is initiated. The client learns to change behavior and decrease subjective distress by initiating relaxation exercises, thought stopping, visualization activities, modeling, facilitative self-talk, and a variety of self-modeling techniques. The emphasis of cognitive therapy is on identifying alternative, creative, logical thinking to offset distorted thinking. Assertivness training, an integral part of this approach, teaches the importance and rights of the self.

CHART 16-5
Time Out Record

Behavior Before Intervention	Time Out Begins	Ends	Behavior During Intervention	Behavior After Intervention

The use of homework assignments is fundamental to this approach, because the client must learn to monitor his own behavior. Homework assignments may take the form of monitoring and recording dysfunctional thinking, prescribing activities to alter environmental variables, and countering distorted cognitions. Other valuable tools include writing an autobiography and composing letters (not necessarily to be sent) in which a conflicting issue is explored and feelings expressed. To counter the client's resistance and help him perceive the reality of his siutation, it may be helpful to prescribe activities that emphasize specific situational events and other eventual characteristics that reinforce distortions.

There are a variety of ways to teach clients to monitor feelings and thoughts. When preoccupation with these dysfunctional thoughts overwhelms the client, using a rubber band on the wrist, clapping the hands to emphasize thought stopping, or using self-talk "stop" is helpful. A slow increase in activities often increases the client's efficiency and can be a positive reinforcement to show progress.

Reframing or shifting illogical labeling helps the client to utilize a problem-solving and positive approach that facilitates the countering technique. The client can also use self-talk and visualization techniques to create a hierarchy to dissipate the anxiety that comes from irrational thinking. Countering techniques include the following:

1. Decrease subjective distress (calm self, visualize a pleasant scene, use relaxation techniques)
2. Utilize thought stoping (say word, "stop"; see red stop light; clap hands; snap rubber band on wrist)
3. Allow self to become neutral (rid self of distractions, distorted thoughts, preoccupations)
4. Visualize a mental white screen
5. Visualize self countering own distorted thinking

The following situations illustrate the use of countering techniques:

A 40-year-old engineer loses his job of 15 years. He has a son starting college in the fall and two school-age children and a wife whom he supports financially.

His interpretation is, "I'm a failure and I'll never get another job; my family will be in need."

Countering techniques might include the following:

1. "I've been thinking of changing jobs, as that one's no longer a challenge."
2. "I turned down two jobs a few years ago and was told to call when I was ready to change jobs."
3. "My company has lost a lot of money recently and its change in philosophy disturbs me."
4. "My wife and I have been unhappy with our current lifestyle."

A 30-year-old man who has been on Xanax for a number of months because of panic attacks decreases his medication at the order of his doctor.

His interpretation is to begin to feel anxious and think that his panic attacks are beginning again.

Countering techniques might include the following:

1. "These feelings are normal because I'm decreasing this medication."
2. "I've been under stress lately because of a business deal, and these feelings could be due to this situation."

3. "I want to come off all medication and know that the other techniques I've learned will help."
4. "I've been keeping long hours at work and only sleeping a few hours each night. I'm overworked."

Cognitive therapy, therefore, encompasses the use of relaxation exercises, assertiveness training, and a variety of other means to counter irrational thinking. Self-monitoring techniques reinforce the client's sense of control. Reality orientation and accurate perception of the client's real world are target behaviors.

Rational Emotive Therapy. One form of cognitive therapy is rational emotive therapy (RET). Rational emotive therapy is also built on the premise that an individual's values and beliefs control his behavior. Many beliefs and assumptions are illogical and irrational. People often evaluate their behavior by using these faulty illogical thoughts. Some of these false assumptions include the following:

1. A person should be loved and approved by all.
2. A person should be competent and talented and prove himself.
3. A person has little control over his life, and pressures make one feel angry, hostile, and depressed.
4. Dangerous and threatening situations should be feared.
5. Past experiences are the most important influence on present behavior.
6. Order and understanding of the world are necessary for well-being.
7. Dependency on stronger individuals or a supernatural power is necessary for living.
8. Understanding of the world is necessary for a happy life.
9. Performing well and being liked are necessary to feel adequate as a person.
10. Being depressed, angry, or anxious is giving in to situations or feelings that should be faced.
11. Beliefs of society and authority figures should not be questioned; if they are, punishment will follow.

The following example illustrates the RET model (see also Fig. 16-1).

A 42-year-old engineer is admitted to the hospital because he is experiencing severe anxiety, diarrhea, a "pounding" feeling in his chest, difficulty breathing, insomnia, a sensation of suffocation, and difficulty swallowing. His behavioral pattern occurred after his 17-year-old daughter told him and his wife that she was pregnant and wanted an abortion (A).

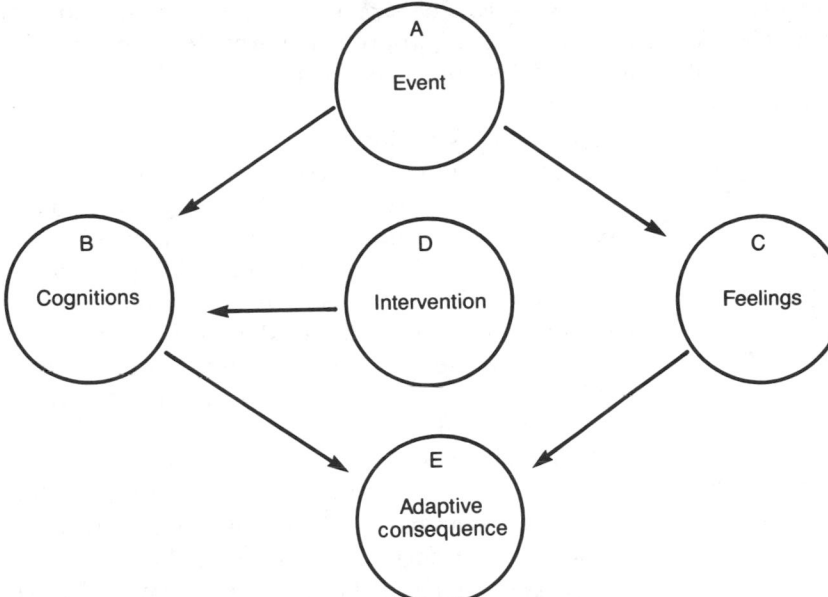

Figure 16-1. *The rational emotive therapy model. Rational emotive therapy uses the model above to illustrate a therapeutic approach to faulty assumptions or beliefs.*
A—the external event
B—the cognitions associated with A
C—the feelings and emotions associated with A
D—the interventions that modify B
E—the adaptive consequences
(From Ayllon T, Houghton E: Modification of Symptomatic Verbal Behavior of Mental Patients. Behav Res Ther 2:87–97, 1964–1965)

The client told the nurse that he is "no good" and a "harsh disciplinarian," that his wife and children do not love him, that he is to blame for his daughter's problems, and that he is worthless (B).

This father is experiencing anxiety, guilt, depression, and anger (C). The nurse focuses with the client on his self-talk, or assumptions, and the validity of these beliefs (D). The client is helped to discriminate between information that is rational and logical and information that is distorted and negative. The nurse and the client focus on his feelings that he is "no good" and worthless because he is to blame for his daughter's pregnancy.

The client realized his thinking was illogical, and that it would not be catastrophic if his family did not love him. The client was able to think logically and realize that he is not responsible for his daughter's behavior. He also realized that he quickly assumed responsibility for all family problems, which excluded his family from responsibility (E).

Cognitive methodologies involve the client and nurse in approaches whereby specific objectives and structured interventions apply learning principles to increase the client's problem-solving, social skills, and assertive communication. Self-assessment, self-monitoring, behavior reversal, role playing, modeling, visual imagery, and thought stopping, as well as interventions with operant and respondent conditioning, are included in this diversified approach to meeting clients' needs.[21]

Cognitive therapy has been successful in treating individuals with depressive behaviors. Based on the assumption that people are depressed because of inadequate social skills, lack of positive social reinforcement, and negative environmental events, emphasis is placed on increasing the client's social skills through assertive training, assessing events that may reinforce his negative feelings, setting goals, and rehearsing new social skills. The depressed person interprets cues and data illogically, thereby depreciating affirmative information and enlarging negative data.[25]

Thought Stopping. *Thought stopping*, developed by Wolpe, has been successful in treating individuals with depressive behaviors.[19,39,55] Behaviors that are irrational, of a brooding type, and anxiety-provoking are inhibited by a specific therapy approach. By shouting the word "stop" after he expresses his illogical behavior, the client realizes he can control his own thoughts.[58] Another approach to thought stopping is to request the client to substitute a positive thought for a negative, distorted thought.[56]

Thought stopping has been reported to be useful in treating obsessive–compulsive disorders. The word "stop" initiated by the therapist is often followed by an oversized stimulus, such as a loud noise or by the client's loudly echoing the word "stop." The troublesome thought is interrupted or blocked by counterconditioning principles.[50]

Modeling

Learning through another's performance, even if the behavior is not practiced or rewarded, is a principle of social learning theory. *Modeling*, or imitation, is a method of behavior change. Individuals learn vicariously by observing others' behavior or by verbal descriptions of a desired behavior, which serve as cues for initiating new responses. Both aggressive and non-aggressive behavior may be demonstrated by modeling techniques. For example, in one study, children who watched aggressive actions by real-life models on film and by cartoon characters displayed more aggressive behavior than children exposed to non-aggressive behavior or children in a control group.[7] Modeling strategies have also been effective in reducing children's fears. Brief, filmed experiences showing a child overcoming fear in certain situations, such as visiting a dentist's or physician's office or interacting with a feared animal, were shown to children who then rehearsed their own responses to the feared situation.[7]

Many studies have used modeling to promote adaptive behaviors in adolescents. To illustrate, peer modeling has helped teach young offenders to postpone rewards, and has helped mentally retarded boys use questions in a learning situation.[37]

Imagery

Imagery is an adaptable therapeutic approach used to facilitate positive self-talk. Mental pictures under the control of, and initiated by, the client may correct faulty cognitions.[29] The client pictures past significant memories and present events that, combined with relaxation therapy and role-playing, increase his awareness of situational events and other variables resulting in maladaptive behavior.

Imagery techniques have been used with a couple with severe marital problems. The marital partners complained of being depressed, anxious, unable to sleep, and sexually dysfunctional. Both were unable to express anger. The partners were asked to picture the parent of the opposite sex, imagine their spouse standing next to the parent, and note characteristic similarities. They therefore identified characteristics in each other they remembered in their parents, with whom they had poor interpersonal relationships. When their perceptions of each other were changed, their relationship improved.[36] Imagery is also an important aspect of systematic desensitization and has been successfully used with clients experiencing phobias.[40]

Behavior Rehearsal

Behavior rehearsal, or role playing, is a therapy approach used in conjunction with modeling. Clients rehearse new responses to problem situations after learning new adaptive responses portrayed through modeling. The nurse's specific attention to detail reinforces characteristics of assertive behavior, such as eye contact, clear and audible vocal tone, posture, and gait.[29]

Behavior rehearsal is advantageous in group settings for teaching social skills and for meeting specific therapy goals. The sharing of simulated situations as well as modeling approaches provides opportunities for participation by the group members.[17]

Assertiveness Training

Role playing is the technique most often used in *assertiveness training.* Assertiveness training deconditions anxiety arising from interpersonal relationships, because assertive behavior is an interfering emotional process free of anxiety.[58] Assertive behavior is expressive, spontaneous, goal-directed, and self-enhancing.[1]

Assertiveness training increases self-esteem and confidence, teaches ways to accept criticism and make it productive, helps an individual learn to cope appropriately with stress, and teaches the effectiveness of positive self-talk for self and others (see Chart 16-6, "Assertive Techniques"). Often, in their early years, people are punished for expressing their authentic selves. As nonassertive behavior has been, and is, rewarded, people become unassertive about their rights as human beings. Poor role models, lack of opportunity, and cultural differences discourage assertiveness. Assertiveness, however, is an alternative to personal powerlessness and manipulation.

Assertiveness training has been successful with a variety of client populations.[11,41,44,48] One nurse therapist used behavior rehearsal, modeling, imagery techniques, and reports of self-monitoring behavior in assertiveness training with women over 60 years of age. The following are examples of material discussed in the third session of the assertiveness training group. The objectives were to model, rehearse, and discuss these situations.

Telling a relative you do not want to vacation with her

Telling your daughter or son something positive about him or her

Telling a grocery clerk that you were overcharged for an item you bought the previous day

Talking to a group of women about volunteering for the local hospital

Modeling, role-playing exercises, and sharing experiences with practicing assertive responses were incorporated into each group session.[44]

Problem-Solving

Behavioral goals include increasing adaptive behavior and learning problem prevention and problem-solving.[27] *Problem-solving* involves the following phases:

1. A general approach to the problem
2. A specific definition of the problem and its parameters

CHART 16-6
Assertive Techniques

Evaluate the situation, then do the following:

Identify the legitimate rights and responsibilities of the people involved
Identify the short- and long-term consequences
Determine how you will behave

1. Express your own views, using "I" statements.
2. Maintain eye contact.
3. Assume a relaxed posture.
4. Use humor when appropriate.
5. Keep your nonverbal behavior congruent with verbal behavior.
6. Listen and wait for other people to respond.
7. Use reflecting and clarifying techniques.
8. Recognize your right to repeat assertive statements.
9. Acknowledge criticisms.
10. Use a firm, but empathetic, voice tone.

Counter nonproductive, illogical thoughts by reversing these irrational thoughts. Acknowledge that these are illogical thoughts and that subsequent negative feelings and maladaptive behaviors evolve from these thoughts. Then utilize thought-stopping techniques to initiate the countering procedure. When countering, be creative but logical.

The following questioning self-talk will help you to identify illogical thoughts.

Are your expectations unrealistic?
Are your thoughts aligned with cognitive distortions?
Do you have objective data to support these thoughts?
Do you acknowledge the "shoulds," "oughts," and "musts" that support maladaptive behavior?

References

1. Burns D: *Feeling Good.* New York, New American Library, 1980
2. Galassi M, Galassi J: *Assert Yourself: How to Be Your Own Person.* New York, Human Sciences Press, 1977

---

3. Generation of possible solutions and implications
4. Selection of a solution
5. Testing and evaluation of the solution

A lack of problem-solving skills is often associated with maladaptive behaviors and interpersonal problems.[17,21] In conjunction with other cognitive therapy methods, the client is taught to identify the situational and personal aspects of the problem that may be inhibitory to the problem-solving process.[26]

Problem-solving has been effective in helping parents adapt successfully to childrens' needs and problems. In one study, parents identified a need for assertive communication with their children by self-monitoring their interactions with their children. Children, both pre-school and school-age, were taught and practiced problem-solving skills.[21]

Progressive Muscle Relaxation
Muscle relaxation is a potent treatment strategy for dealing with a variety of client problems such as psychophysiological distress, chronic sleeplessness, and so forth. Anxiety lessens when muscles relax.[46]

More than 40 years ago, Edmund Jacobson recognized that muscle relaxation was a therapeutic tool for stress-related problems. After studying the physiological and psychological effects of muscle relaxation, he comfortably positioned clients and taught them to tense and relax the main muscle groups of their bodies. He then shared the monitoring information with the clients who were eventually able to use only passive activity to relax.[22]

Wolpe demonstrated that progressive muscle relaxation, combined with mental pictures (images) of a feared situation or increased association with the feared object in graduated increments, could desensitize phobic clients. Muscle relaxation is physiologically incompatible with the anxiety-evoking response.[58] Natural childbirth practices are based on muscle relaxation to decrease anxiety and facilitate delivery.[28]

The following guidelines are suggested when using relaxation therapy:

Keep the environment as quiet as possible and request that the client sit comfortably in a chair or lie down to facilitate muscle relaxation. Tell the client that he is learning a technique that may help him reduce tension and anxiety. Encourage him to close his eyes and let his thoughts focus on pleasant, quiet scenes, as he tenses and relaxes various muscle groups.

The nurse may demonstrate the technique and may emphasize that muscles should not be strained, but should be tensed to about 75% of their potential. In some client situations, a doctor's order and a careful physical assessment may be necessary to reduce the risk of any complications of this procedure. Use a ratio of a 5-to-10-second cycle of tension followed by a 20-second cycle of no tension.

Instruct the client in a quiet, calm way to "tense his hands by making a fist and then relax"...You may suggest that the client feels he is "letting go" and becoming very relaxed and comfortable. The biceps, triceps, shoulder, neck, mouth, tongue, eyes, back, midsection, thighs, stomach, calves, feet, and toes are tensed and relaxed in the same manner.

Breathing in a deep relaxing way and "letting it all out" is usually the final relaxation technique. It is important that the client not overexert the breathing exercise and cause hyperventilation.[17,46]

Evaluation

Objectives of behavioral change, which are stated in specific performance terms or in terms of detailed and precise outcome criteria, are measurable. Although careful monitoring is necessary to validate the desired behavioral outcome, evaluation is more simplified than in client situations with highly subjective descriptions of behavior.

During assessment, behavior is measured over time until a clear response is identified. An intervention is then applied and the behavior measured again for a specific period of time. If there is a change in behavior, the intervention is removed to validate that the intervention was responsible for the behavioral change. (It is not always possible to use this type of evaluation when working with people because of infringement or interference with therapeutic goals.) This technique is called the *reversal technique*. Is a daily recording of weight associated with the client's small, but continual, weight loss, or does a weight change occur when the recording is eliminated?

Multiple base line recording is another technique for both assessing and evaluating interventions. Through this technique, a number of behaviors are measured over time and an intervention is applied to one of these behaviors until a change in the behavior is noted. Little or no change may occur in the other behaviors. The intervention is then applied to one of the other behaviors to determine if there is a change (see Chart 16-7 and Figs. 16-2 and 16-3). Tidy dress, combed hair, and weight loss may be three base line behaviors recorded; recording weight may continue to be an intervention, although tidiness of dress or combed hair is now noted instead of weight change.[5]

The importance of evaluation cannot be overemphasized, because the effect of interventions may be unique to one targeted behavior or may influence other behaviors. Revising treatment plans and recognizing the need for modifications help to individualize care for psychiatric–mental health clients.

C H A R T   16-7
Base Line Recording

Hallucinatory Behavior

Time	M	T	W	TH	FRI	SAT	SUN
8 A.M.–10 A.M.	—	—	—	—	—	—	—
10 A.M.–12 NOON	—	—	—	—	—	—	—
12 NOON–2 P.M.	11	11	1	—	—	—	11
2 P.M.–4 P.M.	11	11	1	1	—	1111	111
4 P.M.–6 P.M.	1111	111	11	1	—	111	111
6 P.M.–8 P.M.	11	11	11	1	1	11	111
8 P.M.–10 P.M.	11	1	1	1	1	1	1
Total Records	12	10	7	4	2	10	12

Base line intervention

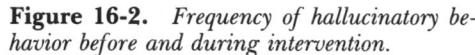

Figure 16-2. *Frequency of hallucinatory behavior before and during intervention.*

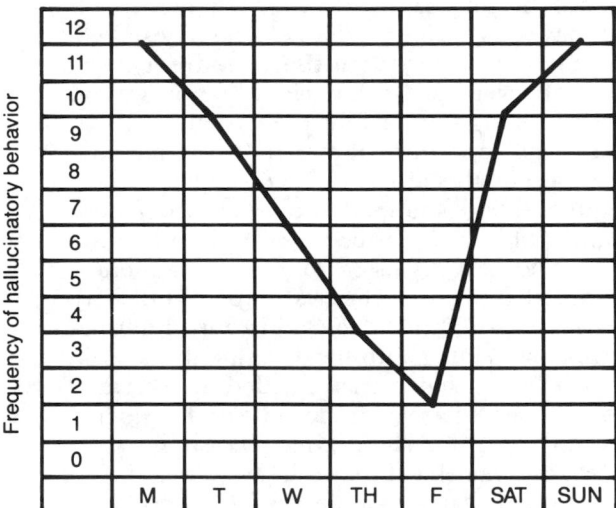

Figure 16-3. *Graph of hallucinatory behavior.*

Summary

Twenty years ago, the psychiatric nurse was described as a behavioral engineer who has a unique position to assist clients to learn adaptive behaviors.[3] The goals of nursing intervention and behavior therapy are both concerned with predicting behavior and providing accurate interventions for client problems. Some of the major points of this chapter have included the following:

1. Following a complete data collection, which includes health history, physical and mental status examinations, laboratory tests, and client and family interviews, objective observation of the maladaptive behavior for a period of time is essential for accurate behavioral assessment.
2. The health team documents the observation period and the frequency of the behavior.
3. Specificity, a key factor in behavioral analysis, results from objective systematic approaches to client problems.
4. Descriptions of both adaptive and maladaptive behavior and behavioral outcomes must be detailed in performance expectation to allow precise measurement and evaluation.
5. Behavioral interventions, including behavioral contracting, cognitive therapy, modeling, imagery, assertiveness training, and progressive muscle relaxation, are powerful approaches to client problems and needs.

Case Study 16-1

Behavior Therapy with a Suspicious Client

Marian Spivak, a 38-year-old housewife and part-time graphic artist for a building firm, is admitted to the psychiatric unit with the diagnosis of paranoia. Marian has two children—a boy 15 years old and a girl 17 years old. Marian was working full-time until a year ago when she felt her co-workers were talking about her. Her husband stated that, at that time, she was very hostile, both at home and at the office, "flying off the handle" when there was no provocation or logical reason. Marian decided to work part-time because she couldn't tolerate the "mean looks" and "laughing" that were going on around her.

Dave, her husband, an accountant who works for the same company, realized Marian was not herself. "Things came to a head," said Dave, "when Marian locked herself in her room and would not eat anything that she did not prepare"; she said that Dave and the children as well as her parents were against her.

Marian was unable to function at work, refused to do anything at home, and neglected her appearance because she had to be "on guard." She had not slept for 3 days before admission to the treatment facility and had barricaded herself in her room refusing to answer the phone or allow anyone in. Marian was an avid reader of mystery and historical novels, and she spent all day and night reading books she had stockpiled.

After a complete assessment, the nurse identified the following maladaptive behaviors:

Sits rigidly in large chair with hands clenched and held tightly to body; head and neck rigid; eyes shifting rapidly from side to side; legs bent and knees drawn close to body	Tension in body
Hair uncombed and snarled; cotton shirt wrinkled and collar ripped; slacks unpressed; tennis shoes unlaced and dirty	Unkempt appearance
Refuses to eat any food unless she prepared it herself from unopened packages or cans	Controls her eating
Verbalizes that the staff is laughing at her and she cannot leave her room because they intend to harm her	Suspicious of others
Verbalizes that the newscaster on the television told her to stay in her room and not to eat anything she has not prepared	Illogical thinking

Marian was placed on fluphenazine (Prolixin) while the identified behaviors continued to be observed and measured by the staff over a 7-day period. A staffing conference was arranged to discuss a treatment plan for Marian.

During the conference, the following information was shared among team members. Marian began sleeping through the night on her 4th day of admission. The behaviors observed initially were recorded at the same frequency by the staff over the 3-day period. Marian was observed calling the staff into her room and she drank milk and juice at mealtime and at bedtime, although she still refused solid food. She requested books to read and asked if her husband could bring her books from home.

The staff discussed Marian's treatment plan and explained what was expected of her. Marian was told that she could control her behavior by helping with her treatment plan. The staff believed that Marian needed to receive positive behaviors from the staff and residents, they believed that she needed to examine the effect of her behavior on other people, and they hoped that she would realize that other people could have pleasant and rewarding effects for her.

Because Marian was an avid reader of historical and mystery novels and had requested books to read, the treatment team selected books as the primary reinforcer and reading as the secondary reinforcer. Marian was placed on a token program, and when she participated in activities or completed a goal that indicated adaptive behavior, she earned tokens that could be redeemed for reading material and time to read. Refusing to eat, suspicious behavior, illogical thinking, body tension, and unkempt appearance were identified as priority target behaviors to be changed.

Reinforcers—tokens earned to be redeemed for historical and mystery novels and reading time on a
   daily basis:
   Three tokens—30 minutes reading   11 A.M.
   Six tokens—30 minutes reading   11 A.M.; 2 P.M.
   Eight tokens—30 minutes reading   11 A.M.; 2 P.M.; 7 P.M.
   Ten tokens—45 minutes reading   11 A.M.; 2 P.M.; 7 P.M.; 9 P.M.
   Twelve tokens—60 minutes reading   11 A.M.; 2 P.M.; 7 P.M.; 9 P.M.
   Fifteen tokens and over—anytime when planned activities are not involved

Refusing to eat—Marian was allowed to serve her food, under supervision, from the main food carts
   (food was served family-style at small tables seating six residents). Marian was to receive the
   following tokens immediately after eating:
   One token for eating one half of the main course
   One token for drinking 6 oz of liquid
   Three tokens if she ate all of the food and drank liquid (excluding dessert); no tokens
   awarded for dessert

The illogical thinking and suspicious self-talk were to be ignored by the staff. The staff was instructed to leave Marian immediately when she began to talk in a suspicious or illogical manner, such as if medication needed to be administered. When Marian's verbal behavior was logical, her tone of voice normal, and her behavior not indicative of unfounded suspiciousness, the staff was instructed to interact with her and praise her behavior. After a week, Marian began to eat most of the food on her tray. She redeemed her tokens for books and reading time. Her suspicious and illogical thinking decreased, although at stressful times (*e.g.,* following a visit with family, dialogue with her therapist, and psychological testing), suspicious behavior would increase for 2 or 3 hours.

The following week, Marian's unkempt appearance was targeted for change. Marian had requested phone privileges, and the staff decided tokens could be redeemed for phone privileges when her appearance improved.

Unkempt appearance: Marian was to receive
   one token for combing her hair, one token
   for wearing make-up, and one token for
   wearing suitable attire and shoes.
   One token—could be used for a
      3-minute call
   Two tokens—could be used for a
      5-minute call

Three tokens—could be used for a
   10-minute call

The staff was also instructed to praise Marian for her improved appearance. At the end of the 4th week, Marian was eating satisfactorily, suspicious behavior and illogical thinking had not been observed, and Marian was interacting with the staff and seeking out other residents.

Marian still displayed body tension, and she was assigned to a relaxation therapy group led by a resident of the treatment unit who initially had been taught relaxation therapy and who was supervised by a staff member. This group met daily for 30 minutes and members were encouraged to practice the relaxation exercises on their own during the day.

Marian was assigned to assist the personnel in food service. There, she helped serve the food to other residents of the unit and helped to plan table decorations and special parties that were held weekly under the supervision of the unit's activity director.

Marian continued to improve and was discharged to outpatient treatment after a 60-day period. Family therapy was begun and Marian attended the day hospital activities from 9:00 A.M. to 3:00 P.M. 5 days a week. Marian eventually returned to work, after an additional 3 months of outpatient treatment. Family therapy continues.

References

1. Alberti RE, Emmons ML: Your Perfect Right, 2d ed. San Luis Obispo, CA, Impact, 1974
2. Ayllon T, Houghton E: Modification of Symptomatic Verbal Behavior of Mental Patients. Behav Res Ther 2: 87–97, 1964–1965
3. Ayllon T, Michael J: The Psychiatric Nurse as a Behavioral Engineer. J Exp Anal Behav 2 (October): 323–334, 1959
4. Baer DM, Wolf MM, Risley TR: Some Current Dimensions of Applied Behavior Analysis. J Appl Behav Anal 1: 91–97, 1968
5. Baker R: The Use of Operant Conditioning to Reinstate the Speaking Mute Schizophrenics: A Progress Report. In Burns LE, Worsley JL: Behavior Therapy in the 1970s. Bristol, John Wright & Sons Ltd, 1970
6. Bandura A: Principles of Behavior Modification. New York, Holt, Rinehart and Winston, 1969
7. Bandura A, Walters RH: Social Learning and Personality Development. New York, Holt, Rinehart and Winston, 1963
8. Beck AT, Rush AJ, Shaw BJ, Emery G: Cognitive Therapy of Depression. New York, The Guilford Press, 1979
9. Buckholdt DR, Gubruin JF: The Underlife of Behavior Modification. Am J Orthopsychiatr 50 (April): 279–290, 1980
10. Burns LE: Introduction. In Burns LE, Worsley JL (eds): Behavior Therapy in the 1970s, pp 1–3. Bristol, John Wright & Sons, 1970
11. Butler P: Assertive Training: Teaching Women Not to Discriminate Against Themselves. Psychotherapy: Theory, Research and Practice 13 (Spring): 56–60, 1976
12. Carignan ST: Self-Motivation and Self-Control in Operant Conditioning. Perspect Psychiatr Care 13: 36–41, 1974
13. Ellis A, Grieger R: Handbook of Rational-Emotive Therapy. New York, Springer-Verlag, 1977
14. Estes WK: An Experimental Study of Punishment. Psychological Monographs 57, 1944
15. Eysenck HJ: The Effects of Psychotherapy: An Evaluation. J Consult Clin Psychol 16: 319–324, 1952
16. Fallon IH, Lloyd GG, Harpen RE: The Treatment of Social Phobia. J Nerv Ment Dis 169: 180–184, 1981
17. Goldfried MR, Davison G: Clinical Behavior Therapy. New York, Holt, Rinehart and Winston, 1976
18. Graziano AM, DeGiovanni S, Garcia K: Behavioral Treatment of Children's Fears: A Review. Psychol Bull 86: 804–830, 1970
19. Hackmann A, McLean C: A Comparison of Flooding and Thought Stopping in the Treatment of Obsessional Neurosis. Behav Res Ther 13: 263–269, 1975
20. Hall CS, Gardner L: Theories of Personality, 2d ed. New York, John Wiley & Sons, 1970
21. Hauser MJ: Cognition Commands Change. J Psychiatr Nurs Ment Health Serv 19 (February): 19–26, 1981
22. Jacobson E: Progressive Relaxation. Chicago, University of Chicago Press, 1938
23. Jones MC: A Laboratory Study of Fear: The Case of Peter. Pedagogical Seminary and Journal of Genetic Psychology 31: 308–315, 1924
24. Kazdin AE: Effects of Covert Modeling and Coding of Modeled Stimuli on Assertive Behavior. Behav Res Ther 17: 53–61, 1979
25. Kovacs M: The Efficacy of Cognitive and Behavior Therapies for Depression. Am J Psychiatr 137 (December): 1495–1501, 1980
26. Krech D, Crutchfield RS, Livson N (with the collaboration of Wilson WA): Elements of Psychology, 3d ed. New York, Alfred A. Knopf, 1974
27. Krumbaltz JD: Behavioral Goals of Counseling. J Counseling Psychology 13 (Summer): 153–159, 1966
28. Lamaze F: Painless Childbirth: Psychoprophylactic Method. London, Burk Publishing Company, 1958
29. Lazarus AA: Multi-Modal Behavior Therapy. Springer Series in Behavior Modification. (Franks CM, series ed) New York, Springer-Verlag, 1976
30. Lazarus AA, Abramovitz A: The Use of "Emotive Imagery" in the Treatment of Children's Phobias. J Ment Science 108 (March): 191–195, 1962
31. Lindsey OR: Characteristics of the Behavior of Chronic Psychotics as Revealed by Free-Operant Conditioning Methods. Dis Nerv Syst (Manager Supp) 21: 66–78, 1960
32. Lindsey OR: Operant Conditioning Techniques in the Measurement of Psychopharmacologic Response. The First Hahnemann Symposium on Psychosomatic Medicine, pp 373–383. Philadelphia, Lea & Febiger, 1962
33. Marks IM: Review of Behavioral Psychotherapy, I: Obsessive-Compulsive Disorders. Am J Psychiatr 138 (May): 584–592, 1981
34. McMorrow MJ, Cullinan D, Epstein MH: The Use of the Premack Principle to Motivate Patient Activity Attendance. Perspect Psychiatr Care 16 (January–February): 14–18, 1978
35. McMullen RE: Handbook of Cognitive Therapy Techniques. New York, WW Norton, 1986
36. Morrison JK: The Use of Imagery Techniques in Family Therapy. Am J Family Therapy 9: 52–56, 1981
37. Moss GR, Rick GR: Overview: Application of Operant Technology to Behavioral Disorders of Adolescents. Am J Psychiatr 138 (September): 1161–1169, 1981
38. Mowrer OH: The Present State of Behaviorism. Educational Journal 97 (Spring): 4–23, 29, 1977
39. Nigl AJ: Use of Thought Stopping and Self-Reinforcement in Treatment of Depression. Psychol Rep Part 1, 38 (June): 843–846, 1976

40. Öst L-G: Fading vs. Systematic Desensitization in the Treatment of Snake and Spider Phobia. Behav Res Ther 16: 379–389, 1978

41. Percell LP, Berwick PT, Bergel A: The Effect of Assertive Training on Self-Concept and Anxiety. Arch Gen Psychiatr 31 (October): 502–504, 1974

42. Pratt SJ, Fischer J: Behavior Modification: Changing Hyperactive Behavior in a Children's Group. Perspect Psychiatr Care 13: 37–42, 1975

43. Reakes J: Behavior Reversal Revisited; A Multi-Faceted Love for the Instructor. J Nurs Ed 18 (February): 48–51, 1979

44. Reakes J: The Effects of Two Approaches to Assertive Training on Self-Esteem, Assertiveness, Laws of Control and Life Satisfaction with Women Sixty Years of Age or Over. Unpublished doctoral dissertation, August, 1979

45. Riehl JP, Roy C Sr: Conceptual Models for Nursing Practice, 2d ed. New York, Appleton-Century-Crofts, 1980

46. Rimm DC, Masters JC: Behavior Therapy: Techniques and Empirical Findings. New York, Academic Press, 1974

47. Roberts MJ, Canfield M: Behavior Modification with a Mentally Retarded Child. Am J Nurs 80 (April): 679, 1980

48. Russel A, Winkler R: Assertive Training and Homosexual Service Groups. J Counsel Clin Psychol 45 (February): 1–13, 1977

49. Sabulsky DJ: Behaviorism and Its Application to the Profoundly Retarded. Psychiatr Nurs (September–October): 10–13, 1979

50. Salzman L, Hales FH: Obsessive Compulsive Disorders: A Review of the Literature. Am J Psychiatr 138 (March): 286–296, 1981

51. Sank LI, Shaffer CS: A Therapist's Manual for Cognitive Behavior Therapy in Groups. New York, Plenum Press, 1984

52. Sideleau BF: Irrational Beliefs and Interventions. J Psychosoc Nurs Ment Health Serv 25 (March): 18–24, 1987

53. Skinner BF: About Behaviorism. New York, Vintage Books, 1976

54. Skinner BF: Freedom and the Control of Men. American Scholar 25: 56, 1955

55. Stern R: Treatment of a Case of Obsessional Neurosis Using Thought Stopping Technique. Br J Psychiatr 117 (October): 441–442, 1970

56. Teasdale JD, Rezin V: Effect of Thought Stopping on Thoughts, Mood and Corrugator EMG in Depressed Patients. Behav Res Ther 16: 97–102, 1978

57. Watson JB, Rayner R: Conditioned Emotional Reactions. J Exp Psychol 3: 1–14, 1920

58. Wolpe J: The Practice of Behavior Therapy, 2d ed. New York, Pergamon Press, 1973

17 Psychopharmacology

Deborah Jackson Antai-Otong

There are drugs to numb experience and drugs to intensify it; drugs to put a person to sleep and drugs to awaken him; drugs to intoxicate and drugs to detoxify; drugs to energize and drugs to tranquilize; drugs to expand experience and drugs to eliminate consciousness.

Sidney M. Jourard,
The Transparent Self,
1971

Chapter Preview

The focus of this chapter is the study of psychopharmacology and its impact on psychiatric–mental health nursing. The advent of psychotropic medication has generated dramatic results in the treatment of the mentally ill. The role of the psychiatric–mental health nurse is critical in the client's understanding of the importance and usefulness of these medications. Responsibilities of the nurse include recognizing the desired actions and adverse reactions of the drugs and normal therapeutic dosages, documenting medication administration, and keeping abreast of current literature on the psychotropic drugs. Another nursing responsibility involves teaching the client and family members about the client's medication.

This chapter discusses the psychoactive drugs according to their major classifications, desired effects, adverse effects, side effects, normal dosage ranges, and nursing implications. Drug interactions and contraindications are also discussed to facilitate safe administration of the psychoactive drugs.

Learning Objectives

On completion of the chapter, you should be able to accomplish the following:

1. discuss the historical development of psychopharmacology
2. identify the nursing responsibilities in administering psychoactive drugs
3. formulate a teaching plan for a client who is taking psychotropic medication
4. identify nursing actions to promote clients' compliance with medication regimes
5. discuss nursing responsibilities in administering research drugs
6. identify the actions, therapeutic dosages, uses, side effects, toxic effects, routes of administration, contraindications, and nursing implications of the following:
   antipsychotic agents
   antidepressant agents
   anxiolytic (antianxiety) agents
   antimanic agents
7. plan nursing actions to prevent or alleviate the side effects of psychoactive drugs

Historical Review of Psychopharmacology

Man's search for relief from the miseries, anxieties, and worries of everyday life has probably existed since the beginning of time. In each age, man has sought to find a means of decreasing his anxiety and elevating his moods.[36] He has experimented with some brews or natural derivatives to alter his mood, whether for medicinal, religious, or recreational purposes. He has chewed coco leaves, consumed coffee, smoked cannibus, injected opiates, and indulged in alcohol.[32]

Psychopharmacology has emerged during recent decades as a scientific discipline within the field of psychiatric–mental health care. The first accessible synthetic compounds, which appeared at the end of the 19th century, were the bromides, chloral hydrate, and morphine. World War II marked the beginning of the modern era of clinical pharmacology.[15] Barbiturates were discovered in the 20th century; the amphetamines became available initially in the 1950s.[32]

In Australia during the 1950s, Cade accidentally observed the calming effects of lithium on animals. His findings of the efficacy of lithium in the treatment of manic agitation were reported almost 10 years after his initial observations.[15] Also in the 1950s, lysergic acid diethylamide (LSD)-25 was synthesized and tested, and its effects were studied.[29]

In France during the 1950s, Laborit discovered the tranquilizing effects of chlorpromazine (Thorazine) while the drug was being initially tested as an anesthetic.[39] It was then tested on schizophrenic clients in 1952.[34] Chlorpromazine was first used in the United States in 1954 and quickly became the drug of choice in the treatment of schizophrenia. By 1970, 85% of all institutionalized psychiatric clients were receiving either this drug or other phenothiazine drugs. Because of their usefulness in managing the schizophrenic individual, the phenothiazines became known as "antipsychotic" drugs.[21]

Monoamine oxidase inhibitors were also accidentally discovered in the mid-1950s. The compound iproniazid closely resembled isoniazid, a drug used to treat tuberculosis. Early investigators observed that tuberculosis patients became less depressed and demonstrated elevations in mood during their lengthy stays in the tuberculosis sanitoria. Some patients even exhibited manic behavior in response to this antituberculosis medication. These observations and the acknowledgement that this compound produced inhibition of the enzyme monoamine oxidase (MAO) led to early speculation that a correlation existed between brain chemistry and mood.[36]

Chlordiazepoxide (Librium) was introduced in

1961. This new class of drugs, the benzodiazepines, resulted from the testing and synthesis of numerous barbiturates over a span of five decades. Toward the end of the 1950s and the beginning of the 1960s, the use of barbiturates as the sole treatment for anxiety disorders had become obsolete. Since the 1960s, benzodiazepines have dominated the market for *anxiolytic (that is, antianxiety)* drugs. Annual prescriptions written for these agents have resulted in a multimillion-dollar business.[27]

The era of the 1970s introduced diazepam (Valium) to the U.S. marketplace. This single drug accounted for approximately 53% of all hypnotic prescriptions written in the late 1970s.[49] This is useful in treating a wide range of conditions, nonpsychotic anxiety states to acute seizure disorders.[11]

Other anxiolytic agents are currently being tested. A major goal of the development of new agents is to produce a medication that decreases anxiety but is nonsedative and nonaddictive. One such agent, buspirone HCl (BuSpar), has recently been introduced. This drug seems to be less sedative and less addictive than the benzodiazepines.[17,23]

Antidepressants were initially introduced in the late 1950s under the name of imipramine (Tofranil).[37] The advent of the tricyclic antidepressants, called the TCAs, came during a time in psychiatry when the chief modalities of treatment for depression were electroconvulsive therapy (ECT), stimulants, and psychotherapy. Electroconvulsive treatment and stimulants were chiefly used for the treatment of endogenous depression; psychotherapy, on the other hand, was the major modality of treatment for reactive depression. The shortcomings of these forms of treatment alone have been documented in numerous studies.[37] The discovery of the antidepressants has brought to light the biochemical mechanisms of the brain in both normal and chemically altered emotional reactions.

Since the tricyclic antidepressants were introduced in the late 1950s and early 1960s, many clients have been able to find relief from depression. The advent of these psychotropic drugs has facilitated a shorter recovery period from depression. Despite the advantages of tricyclic antidepressants, there are some clients who have not responded to their effects. Research has continued in efforts to discover the "ideal" antidepressant. Studies have shown that about 20% to 30% of clients suffering from depression do not respond to traditional tricyclic antidepressant therapy.[44]

The 1980s have brought in a "second generation" of antidepressants, including amoxapine (Ascendin), which also has antipsychotic properties. Other pyschotropics in this group include a tetracyclic compound, maprotiline (Ludiomil), and a nontricyclic, nontetracyclic agent, trazodone (Desyrel), frequently used to manage major depression. Although all these drugs are useful in treating depression, they manifest some side effects similar to those of the tricyclic antidepressants and the antipsychotic agents—and so the search continues for the ideal antidepressant.

Over a span of several decades, the psychotropic drugs demonstrated effectiveness in controlling a broad range of mental and emotional disorders. They have revolutionized the treatment of psychiatric illness.[41] The safety of administering these medications and of monitoring their actions and side effects has similarly increased during this time. With the rapid proliferation of knowledge, the field of psychopharmacology has evolved into a group of scientific disciplines seeking to test the efficacy of various drugs and to understand their mode of action on various neuroendocrine systems.[8]

Nursing Responsibilities in Medication Administration

Ensuring Client Safety

The nurse who administers a drug is responsible for knowing the drug's action and potentialities. In addition, the nurse must know the following:

1. The prescribed dose and the maximum amount of the drug that may be safely given to the client
2. The method of administration
3. The expected action of the drug
4. The side effects
5. The adverse effects (short-term and long-term)
6. The nursing implications of the drug

In addition, the nurse is responsible for the safekeeping and storage of the drug and for the proper identification of the client, particularly the psychiatric client.[2]

The client's response to medication requires continuous monitoring of expected, adverse, and toxic effects. Nurses observe, assess, and evaluate the client's response to psychopharmacologic treatment.[12]

Documentation of these therapeutic and adverse effects of the client's medication enhances communication among mental health team members and also enhances continuity of client care (see Chart 17-1). The courts have recognized nursing's responsibility for this documentation and have held nurses accountable when appropriate communication and follow-up are not undertaken.[12]

CHART 17-1
Charting Medication Reactions

A client who was discharged 5 days ago is now in the lobby of the outpatient Crisis Unit and requests to see the physician because "something is wrong" with him. The receptionist calls the nurse to come and see the client. He was discharged on Navane, 20 mg daily.

S—"My neck is stiff, I can't move it! What's wrong with me? I can't talk right. Help me!"

O—Client is standing in the lobby of the Crisis Unit with his head in a fixed position to the right side, his tongue protruding from his mouth, with some increased salivation; speech slurred

A—Patient is experiencing a dystonic reaction from psychotropic medication, Navane

P—1. Give (ordered) prn dose of Cogentin, 2 mg IM now
2. Evaluate client's response to Cogentin
3. Reassure client that he will feel better in several minutes
4. Contact physician and arrange follow-up with client today
5. Reinforce teaching about taking oral Cogentin if symptoms recur

Signed by D. Antai-Otong, R.N.

Teaching the Client about Medication

Client teaching has always been a responsibility of the nurse; this responsibility is particularly a priority with the psychiatric–mental health client.[3] Teaching facilitates and promotes understanding of the medication that is prescribed for the client and encourages medication compliance. Compliance with his medication regime is especially important when the client is discharged from a treatment facility.

The nurse generates the client's teaching plan after assessing his individual needs, problems, diagnoses, support systems, and level of understanding (see Chart 17-2, "Medication Teaching Plan"). To compile a thorough history and assessment, the nurse interacts with the client and his family or friends. The data gathered from the client and his significant others facilitate the development of an individualized treatment plan and provide information about his past responses to medications and past compliance or noncompliance with prescribed medication regimes.

The following is an example of nursing plans to address the client's and family's teaching needs concerning the client's prescribed medication:

1. Establish family contact, preferably on the client's admission to the psychiatric treatment setting
   a. Provide information
   b. Provide support and empathy
2. Involve family members
   a. Focus on family needs
3. Structure the setting
   a. Negotiate time
   b. Arrange the environment
4. Instruct the client regarding the following:
   a. Mental disorder
   b. Medications
      Drug name
      Dose prescribed
      Time of administration
      Desired action
      Self-care
      Side effects to report to doctor or clinic
   c. Importance of follow-up, including follow-up laboratory work for clients on lithium or medications that produce blood dyscrasias or other dangerous effects

Promoting Compliance with Medication Regimen

A major problem in psychiatric–mental health care involves the client's failure to adhere to a prescribed medical regimen. Most people who are physically or mentally ill and hospitalized express a sense of loss of control over their lives. They may become dependent on the medical and nursing care providers and may feel left out of the decision-making processes regarding their daily care.

Noncompliance is influenced by the client and his family and friends (see Chart 17-3, "Therapeutic Dialogue"). For example, when a psychiatric client is hospitalized with symptoms of mental illness such as psychosis, the family may have requested that the client be "fixed." The client may exhibit impaired judgment, insight, and understanding of the disorder.[4] When these symptoms abate, the family may believe that the client is "cured." This information is conveyed by the family to the client, who has little reason to doubt that this is true because, indeed, he "feels better"—even "cured." When the discharge order is written, usually when the individual is no longer a threat to the family, both client and family members believe that the disappearance of symptoms

CHART 17-2
Medication Teaching Plan

A 21-year-old man has been discharged from an inpatient psychiatric facility on thiothixene (Navane), 20 mg at bedtime. A prn medication, benztropine (Cogentin) 2 mg, has also been ordered if extrapyramidal symptoms develop. He has been given a month's supply of medications and a follow-up appointment for the outpatient day center activities program. His medication teaching plan follows.

These are directions that will assist you in taking your medications: Take Navane, 20 mg, 2 tablets (10 mg each), at bedtime by mouth.

1. Your medication should not make you sleepy or drowsy during the day, but if your doctor increases your medication, you may be sleepy for 2 to 4 days, so give your body time to adjust to the medicine by being careful when driving or using heavy machinery during this time.

2. Your medication should not cause you to have stiffness in your back, neck, tongue, or eye muscles. If these symptoms occur, you need to take your side effect medicine, which is Cogentin, 2 mg, by mouth.

3. It is expected that your mouth may become dry; drink plenty of water. Constipation might be a problem, but do not rely on laxatives; increase the roughage in your diet or ask your physician to prescribe a stool softener.

4. Anxiety (nervousness) is a normal human emotion, but if it should get out of hand or excessive, you need to report this to your doctor as soon as possible.

5. For Navane to be effective, you must take it every night as prescribed. For example, do not wait to take it when you feel the need; if you miss a dose, make it up as soon as you remember.

6. Navane is not addictive. It is not habit-forming. You will not get "hooked" on it.

7. If you develop any of the following symptoms, you need to report them immediately to your doctor.

> Muscular twitching
> Weakness
> Dizziness
> Difficulty swallowing
> Disturbances or changes in your walking

equates "cure" and that medications are therefore no longer important.

Another misconception about psychotropic medication involves the client's and family's fear that he will become "addicted" to the drug. It is the nurse's responsibility to initiate a teaching plan for the client and family to provide them with accurate information about the psychoactive medications and the importance of following the prescribed medication regimen.[34]

The majority of psychiatric clients who do not take their medication as prescribed are those with a diagnosis of schizophrenia.[31] Several variables are responsible for this noncompliance, including the following:

1. The need for maintenance medication over a lengthy period of time

2. The experience of uncomfortable side effects from the medications

3. The nature of the schizophrenic disorder, in which the client who stops taking his medication may "feel better" or, at least, no worse[10]

C H A R T   17-3
Therapeutic Dialogue

Assessment of Compliance with Medication Regimen

Nurse: (seated at desk, facing client and his wife) What has brought you to the clinic today, Mr. A.?

Client: (avoiding eye contact, looking at wife) My wife told me I needed to come in.

Nurse: Your wife told you to come in? Do you know why your wife wanted you to come in?

Client: I don't know. Ask her! (pointing to his wife)

Client's Wife: He has been doing things that do not make sense. He's done this before and he needs medicine.

Nurse: (turning to client again) Will you tell me what your wife is talking about?

Client: I don't know, ask her! (voice becoming louder, fidgeting in his chair)

Client's Wife: He has been getting up at night and going outside in his underwear. All he needs is his medicine.

Nurse: More medicine? When is the last time you took your medication, Mr. A.?

Client's Wife: He ran out of medicine 3 months ago and at the time he was feeling good.

Discussion

One of the major problems in treating the psychiatric client is medication compliance. It is valuable to have a family member present during these discussions to substantiate what the client is or is not saying about his medications and about his behavior when he takes and does not take his medicine. The nurse assesses his behavior and ascertains how he has responded to medication in the past and how he is responding to it presently. It is also necessary to assess the family members' knowledge and understanding of the client's need for medications, particularly long-term medications for the treatment of schizophrenia and bipolar disorders.

The health professional may inaccurately assume that the schizophrenic client is taking his medication when, in fact, he is not. On the other hand, if the client's disturbed behavior does not change after the medication is prescribed, mental health care providers may incorrectly assume that he is not taking his medication.[22]

One study that involved the use of two groups of outpatients diagnosed with schizophrenia examined the effects of compliance with medication regimens. One group of clients was treated with parenteral fluphenazine decanoate; the other group was given the oral form of the same medication, with questionable compliance. The results of the study revealed equal rates of relapse between the two groups. This picture suggests that there are other factors to be examined when one concludes that a client is compliant or noncompliant with his prescribed medication.[45]

Self-medication helps to promote a sense of being in control of oneself. The capabilities of individual clients and the availability of their support systems influence who will be able to administer their own medications. Taking control over one's life and one's medication facilitates the development of confidence and self-respect and minimizes the pervasive pathologic dependence that often surfaces in the psychiatric–mental health client. Care providers need to encourage this control and sense of confidence.

Another factor influencing compliance is the fact that people want to feel as good as they possibly can. Many clients will stop taking their antipsychotic medication when they begin to feel worse. Part of this discontinuation of medication is related to the client's poor judgment inherent in the psychotic process, but there are other factors.[22] Akathisia and other side effects may be more distressing to the client than the medical and nursing staff realize. Sometimes, psychiatric–mental health caregivers tend not to listen to what the client is saying about the medication's side effects, especially if the client is not exhibiting common physical aberrations.[34] It is essential that each of the client's complaints be attended to, assessed, and documented to alleviate these side effects.[42]

The final area to examine in relation to compliance with medication regimens is, "What meaning does the client attach to taking medications?" The symbolism of taking medication is another reminder to psychiatric clients that they are mentally ill or disturbed.[21] This issue may be neglected by many mental health professionals who interact with clients; however, if this issue and other issues of concern to the client and family are examined and explored, nurses can provide factual, useful information about psychotropic medications and can alleviate the client's fears about taking medication over a prolonged period of time.

Working with Research Drugs

During the last three decades, the introduction of new psychotropic drugs has transformed the treatment of psychiatric–mental health clients. Present research is examining the effects of psychoactive drugs on the nervous system. Research findings have demonstrated that some drugs have specific effects on psychological processes, and these findings have generated a need for further research into the nature of mental illness. Examples of such effects are the chemical changes that take place in depressive and manic states characteristic of bipolar disorders.[4]

Drug treatment is based on scientific research, more so than other somatic therapies.[2] Nursing professionals contribute to the success of the research findings through the provision of continuous, 24-hour-per-day monitoring. Medication regimens are prescribed primarily by means of the documented observations of the nursing staff.[12]

Initially, the effects of a new drug are researched with the use of laboratory animals. When the drug is considered safe for the use of humans, drug trials are instituted to determine the effects of the drug on human subjects. The subjects selected have a common set of target symptoms that are expected to benefit from the drug. These clients must have access to explicit reports regarding their disorders, severity of the symptoms, and degree of incapacity. Nursing responsibilities include careful documentation of all therapeutic effects observed and the clients' reactions to them. Usually, the study involves a control group, and it is the responsibility of the nurse to administer the drug to one group and withhold it from the other group, utilizing other forms of treatment as ordered.[2]

In addition to monitoring the psychological responses of clients who are involved in psychopharmacologic research, the nurse is also responsible for monitoring and documenting the physiological responses. Physiological monitoring includes assessment of the vital signs, particularly the blood pressure, prior to and after administration of the drug. Changes in the heart rate and rhythm, palpitations, and any signs indicative of blood dyscrasias should be reported and documented carefully.[2]

Nurses involved in research of psychotropic drugs must be aware of negative feelings that may be generated by the research itself. The nurse needs to acknowledge honestly the client's participation in research that is not willingly undertaken. Ambivalence may interfere with the client's progress as well as with the benefits of the study.[2]

Finally, it is imperative that nurses who are involved in research are familiar with proper research guidelines peculiar to the health care institution.[38] These guidelines include the signed informed consent of each participant in the research study (see Chart 17-4, "Consent to Act as a Subject for Research and Investigation").

Psychotropic Medication

Table 17-1 lists names, classifications, and dosages of the psychotropic medications.

Antipsychotic Agents

Approximately 20% of the prescriptions currently written in the United States are targeted toward altering mental processes. That translates to hundreds of thousands of individuals who presently take these medications.

Antipsychotic (or neuroleptic) agents comprise a group of widely used drugs in the field of psychiatry (see Chart 17-5). They are used primarily to treat severe psychiatric disorders (*i.e.*, psychoses).[6]

The antipsychotic drugs change or alter the moods and thoughts of individuals who recognize and respond to reality with difficulty, such as clients with hallucinations, delusions, disordered thinking, and emotional withdrawal. The drugs are not selective for schizophrenia, but have other forms of clinical use-

CHART 17-4
Consent to Act as a Subject
for Research and Investigation

I hereby agree to participate voluntarily in a study of the following experimental procedure or treatment:

_____
(Name of procedure or treatment)

conducted by:

_____
(Name of person(s) or institution conducting investigation)

After careful explanation, I agree to,

1. Voluntarily participate in this study and I may withdraw at any time without interference with my treatment at _____
(Health care institution)
2. My individual results will not be identified or reported; my name will not be associated with the findings.
3. The information from these tests may help the investigators learn the best method of treatment for this participant and other patients with similar difficulties in the future.
4. According to the investigators, every effort will be made to prevent physical injury or reaction that could result from the administration of this procedure or treatment.
5. The investigators are prepared to advise in the event that medical treatment is needed due to adverse reactions. I agree to report these adverse effects.

I have received a verbal description of this study, including a fair explanation of the procedures and their purpose, any associated discomfort or risks, and a description of the possible benefits. An offer has been made to me to answer all questions about the study after its completion. I further understand that no medical service or compensation is provided to subjects by this institution as a result of injury from participation in this research.

_____   _____
(Signature of patient or person authorized to   (Date)
consent for patient)

_____   _____
(Signature of witness)   (Date)

fulness, including their antiemetic properties, their antihistaminic effects, their ability to potentiate analgesics, and their ability to treat hiccoughs.

Clients taking antipsychotic agents must be closely monitored for adverse side effects, including extrapyramidal reactions and tardive dyskinesia. There is a wide margin of safety between the doses of antipsychotic agents necessary to produce therapeutic effects and those that can cause fatal overdose. Although they are capable of producing toxic effects, neuroleptic agents have a low incidence of lethality.[43]

Nurses are responsible for observing the client for adverse as well as therapeutic effects and for reporting and documenting these effects. Client and

Table 17-1. **Psychotropic Medications**

CLASSIFICATION	CHEMICAL GROUP	GENERIC NAME	TRADE NAME	DAILY DOSAGE
Antipsychotic/ neuroleptics	Phenothiazines	Chlorpromazine	Thorazine	100–2000 mg
		Trifluoperazine	Stelazine	5–60 mg
		Thioridazine	Mellaril	100–800 mg
		Fluphenazine	Prolixin	5–20 mg
		Fluphenazine decanoate	Prolixin decanoate	12.5–50 mg q2–4 wks (IM)
		Mesoridazine	Serentil	100–400 mg
		Perphenazine	Trilafon	6–64 mg
	Dihydroindolones	Molindone	Moban	50–225 mg
	Dibenzoxazepines	Loxapine	Loxitane	20–250 mg
	Thioxanthenes	Thiothixene	Navane	10–60 mg
	Butyrophenones	Haloperidol	Haldol	1–30 mg
		Haloperidol decanoate	Haldol decanoate	50–500 mg/month (IM)
Antidepressant agents	Tricyclics	Imipramine	Tofranil	50–300 mg
		Desipramine	Norpramine	50–300 mg
		Amitriptyline	Elavil	50–300 mg
		Doxepin	Sinequan, Adapin	50–150 mg
		Nortryptyline	Aventyl, Pamelor	25–100 mg
	Triazolopyridine	Trazodone	Desyrel	150–400 mg
	Tetracyclic	Maprotiline	Ludiomil	75–225 mg
	Dibenzoxapine (metabolite of loxapine)	Amoxapine	Ascendin	200–300 mg
	Other	Fluoxetine hydrochloride	Prozac	20–80 mg
	Monoamine oxidase inhibitors	Phenelzine sulfate	Nardil	15–90 mg
		Tranylcypromine sulfate	Parnate	10–60 mg
		Isocarboxazid	Marplan	10–60 mg
Anxiolytics/ antianxiety agents	Benzodiazepines	Alprazolam	Xanax	0.5–5.0 mg
		Diazepam	Valium	4–40 mg
		Lorazepam	Activan	2–6 mg
		Chlordiazepoxide (HCl)	Librium	15–100 mg
		Clorazepate	Tranxene	15–60 mg
	Azaspirodecanedione	Buspirone HCl	BuSpar	20–30 mg
	Propanediols	Meprobamate	Equanil/Miltown	1200–1600 mg
Antimanic agents	Lithium carbonate	Lithium carbonate	Lithium	900–1200 mg (divided doses)
			Eskalith (slow-release)	900–1200 mg (divided doses) (Serum levels range: 0.5–1.5 mEq/L)
	Carbamazepine	Carbamazepine	Tegretol	400–1600 mg (dose ranges and serum levels should be maintained between 8–12 μg/ml)

family teaching is essential to promote medication compliance and to minimize the incidence of exacerbation. Support is necessary for the client experiencing adverse effects, particularly if there is any impairment in sexual functioning.

Movement Disorders

The central nervous system's potential responses to antipsychotic drugs are great. Because of the high incidence of extrapyramidal side effects of antipsychotic agents, it is imperative to discuss this subject with the client and his family. These side effects, predicted to develop in 5% to 15% of all clients who are taking antipsychotic drugs, are usually frightening, embarrassing, and uncomfortable to the client.[5, 26]

Extrapyramidal side effects of antipsychotic agents are difficult to prevent, but can be alleviated if they are diagnosed early and accurately. The allevia-

CHART 17-5
Antipsychotic/Neuroleptic Agents

Classification: Antipsychotics, Neuroleptics

Formerly called "major tranquilizers"
Improve the mood and behavior of psychotic clients without excessive sedation and without causing addiction

Actions

Block the uptake of dopamine at receptor sites
Sites of action: both nervous system (limbic, reticular activating system, extrapyramidal) and peripheral
Anticholinergic effects
Antihistamine, antipruritic
Sedation, antipsychotic effects without clouding of consciousness

Side Effects

Central nervous system: extrapyramidal with motor restlessness (akathisia), parkinsonism, seizures, dystonias, neuroleptic malignant syndrome, that is, tardive dyskinesia
Autonomic nervous system: dry mouth, mydriasis, nasal congestion, constipation, urinary retention

Cardiovascular: reversible arrhythmias, orthostatic hypotension, tachycardia
Gastrointestinal: anorexia, constipation, diarrhea, hypersalivation, nausea and vomiting, obstructive jaundice
Hematopoietic: agranulocytosis (especially with chlorpromazine), leukopenia, leukocytosis
Endocrine: amenorrhea, changes in libido, lactation, gynecomastia, impotence
Allergic: dermatitis, photosensitization
Special senses: retinopathy, visual impairment

Drug Interactions/Contraindications

Central nervous system depressants (alcohol, narcotics, barbiturates) are potentiated
Anticonvulsives—seizure threshold is lowered
Antiemetics—effects are potentiated
Tricyclics—anticholinergic effects are potentiated
Levodopa—inhibits antiparkinsonism effects
General anesthesia—effects are potentiated
Lithium—can cause encephalopathic syndrome (*i.e.,* weakness, fatigue, irreversible brain damage)
Anticoagulants—effects inhibited
Monoamine oxidase inhibitors—effects inhibited

---

tion of these symptoms decreases the client's distress and, therefore, contributes to his willingness to adhere to a medication regimen. A study involving 85 long-term schizophrenic clients demonstrated that there was a significant association between clients' taking their medications and the occurrence of extrapyramidal side effects, particularly akathisia, regardless of the severity of the symptoms.[41]

The antipsychotic agents that are associated with the highest incidence of precipitating extrapyramidal symptoms are the low-dose phenothiazine drugs (such as fluphenazine [Prolixin]) and haloperidol. The four groups of major toxic effects associated with the development of extrapyramidal symptoms are as follows:

1. Pseudoparkinsonism
2. Akathisia
3. Dystonia/dyskinesia
4. Tardive dyskinesia[5]

Pseudoparkinsonism symptoms, those symptoms that mimic Parkinson's disease, are characterized by akinesia, rigidity, and tremors. These symptoms, accounting for about 40% of all extrapyramidal side effects, may be caused by the blockage of dopamine receptors in the basal ganglia and substantia nigra.

Akathisia is characterized by a syndrome involving motor restlessness. These symptoms account for about 50% of all extrapyramidal side effects.[5]

Dystonia and *dyskinesia* are characterized by involuntary, jerking, uncoordinated body movements. *Tardive dyskinesia* normally occurs as a late symptom and is associated with the long-term use of high-dose phenothiazine drugs. Symptoms characteristic of tardive dyskinesia are mainly buccolingual movements, such as "fly catcher" tongue movements, pursing of the lips, and jaw movements. There can also be involvement of the limbs and trunks that sometimes mimics Huntington's chorea. Unfortunately, there is no treatment for tardive dyskinesia.[5]

Clients who are taking antipsychotic (or neuroleptic) drugs should be examined for the development of neurologic symptoms at least every 3 months. "Drug holidays," brief periods of time during which the client is taken off his medication, are recommended at least two times per year in order to decrease

Nursing Care Plan 17-1

The Client Taking Phenothiazines

Nursing diagnosis: Knowledge deficit regarding side effects of phenothiazines
Goal: To minimize side effects of phenothiazines and promote safety

Side Effect/Problem	Intervention	Rationale
Drowsiness	1. Administer medication at bedtime 2. Report to the physician if drowsiness persists longer than several weeks 3. Advise the client not to operate hazardous machinery or drive a vehicle while taking phenothiazine	1. To maximize sedation 2. This is usually a temporary condition; continued sedation may indicate a need to decrease or change medication 3. To prevent injury to self or others
Orthostatic hypotension	1. Encourage the client to progress slowly from a supine or sitting to a standing position (over one minute) 2. Record the blood pressure with client in lying, sitting, and standing positions; call the physician if blood pressure drops 20 to 30 mm Hg 3. Teach the client to keep head up while ambulating 4. Apply elastic hose as ordered 5. Reassure the client that this is a temporary occurrence and should disappear in several weeks	1. To enable automatic nervous system to equalize blood throughout body and decrease venous pooling in lower extremities 2. To monitor changes in blood pressure 3. To minimize dizziness 4. To promote venous return 5. To alleviate anxiety
Weight gain	1. Monitor weight daily 2. Teach the client how to plan well-balanced meals and avoid salt	1. To determine weight fluctuations 2. To provide nutritious, low-calorie, and low-salt foods that are acceptable to client
Melanosis	1. Teach the client to apply sunscreen when exposed to sunlight and to wear protective clothing and sunglasses	1. To protect the skin from sunlight and prevent pigmentation
Impaired vision (Mellaril retinopathy)	1. Teach the client symptoms of Mellaril retinopathy: blurred vision or brown-colored vision, night blindness; instruct client to report these symptoms immediately to physician	1. To minimize incidence of pigmentary retinopathy and decrease permanent damage to retina

the risk of tardive dyskinesia. This respite from medication allows symptoms that have been masked to surface.[19] (Nursing Care Plan 17-1 further illustrates precautions and interventions needed for clients on phenothiazines.)

Prevention of tardive dyskinesia is a crucial aspect of administering psychotropic drugs. Psychiatric nurses participate in this preventive effort by providing information to the client and family members; this information assists them in detecting the early signs and symptoms of these side effects and helps them recognize the importance of reporting them immedi-

Table 17-2.   **Movement Disorders**

REACTION	ETIOLOGY	SYMPTOMS	ONSET	INTERVENTION
1. Acute dystonias/ dyskinesias	1. Inhibited dopamine transmission induced by neuroleptics (antipsychotic agents)	1. Muscle tightness in throat, neck, tongue, mouth, eyes, neck, back	1. Hours to 5 days; long-acting decanoates within 72 hours	1. IM or IV Benadryl or Cogentin
2. Parkinsonism (pseudo-parkinsonism)	2. Dopamine blockage induced by neuroleptic agents	2. Rigidity, mask-like faces, shuffling gait, drooling, action tremors	2. 5 to 90 days	2. IM or IV Benadryl or Cogentin
3. Akathesias	3. Dopamine blockage	3. Motion restlessness, inability to sit still, agitation, excitement	3. 4 to 72 days	3. Decrease dosage or change neuroleptic (Inderal may be helpful)[40]
4. Tardive dyskinesia	4. Possible prolonged use of neuroleptics which increases sensitivity to dopamine in basal ganglia[51] Increased incidence: Elderly clients Females Clients with histories of affective disorders[54]	4. Insidious process *Early signs:* Tongue movement, increased blinking *Late signs:* Tongue protrusion, vermiform movement of tongue, sucking, smacking lip movements, chewing jaw movements[50]	4. Months to years	4. Prevention essential; reevaluate neuroleptic after 6 months; maintain lowest effective dose Informed consent

ately. Client and family teaching also diminishes the distress and embarrassment associated with the symptoms. Nursingcare providers must also be aware of the times of maximal risk for the development of the extrapyramidal side effects of antipsychotic agents (see Table 17-2).

Antiparkinsonism Medication

Antiparkinsonism drugs are used to treat the side effects and toxic effects precipitated by antipsychotic medications, with the exception of tardive dyskinesia. The controversy continues regarding the prophylactic use of these drugs when antipsychotic medication is initiated. Several factors feed this concern over the use of antiparkinsonism drugs.

There is a low incidence of extrapyramidal symptoms in clients who take antipsychotic medication.

Antiparkinsonism drugs produce additional anticholinergic side effects.

Antiparkinsonism drugs add additional cost of treatment for the client and family.

There is some evidence that antiparkinsonism drugs become unnecessary after 1 to 3 months of treatment and should be discontinued.[5] The antiparkinsonism drugs should not be administered until there are overt signs and symptoms of extrapyramidal side effects that respond favorably to this type of intervention (see Tables 17-3 and 17-4).[6]

Neuroleptic Malignant Syndrome

Neuroleptic malignant syndrome (NMS) is a rare, idiosyncratic reaction to neuroleptic agents. The disorder was first identified in Europe in the 1960s and in the United States in the early 1980s. Neuroleptic malignant syndrome is characterized by severe muscle rigidity, hyperthermia, and stupor.[18]

The etiology of neuroleptic malignant syndrome is not clearly understood. Studies suggest that NMS is caused by blockage of dopamine in the basal ganglia, which may be precipitated by rapid, massive overloading of neuroleptic agents over a period of time.[1,46]

Neuroleptic malignant syndrome occurs in 0.5% to 1.0% of persons taking neuroleptic drugs. The risk of NMS is increased when the individual is taking one of the high potency neuroleptics, such as the piperazine phenothiazines and long-acting, parenteral forms of the medications. Frequently the symptoms appear abruptly within several days or weeks after therapy with the neuroleptic agents.

Table 17-3.　**Antiparkinsonism Medications**

CLASSIFICATION	GENERIC NAME	TRADE NAME	DOSE (MG/DAY)	ROUTE
Anticholinergic	Benztropine	Cogentin	0.5–6.0	PO, IM, IV
	Biperiden HCl	Akineton	2.0–8.0	PO
	and Biperiden lactate		6.0–10.0	
	Trihexyphenidyl HCl	Artane	6.0–10.0	PO
Antihistamine	Diphenhydramine	Benadryl	75–150	PO, IM, IV
Other	Amantadine	Symmetrel	100–200	PO

These symptoms include extrapyramidal manifestations such as muscle rigidity, tremors, dystonias, carpopedal spasm, stupor and mutism, and autonomic disturbances such as hyperthermia, diaphoresis, tachycardia, blood pressure fluctuations, and urinary retention. The disorder may eventually progress to renal failure and respiratory failure. A 20% to 25% mortality rate secondary to cardiovascular collapse, pulmonary emboli, or acute renal failure has been reported.[16]

Treatment of NMS is generally supportive. The prescribed neuroleptics are immediately discontinued, and renal, cardiac, and respiratory functions are supported. Hypothermic measures and treatment of concurrent infections are instituted. Monitoring and treatment of the client with NMS usually requires 1 to 3 weeks.[47] (See Chart 17-10)

Antidepressant Agents

Affective disorders, or mood disturbances, include depression and mania. *Depression* is characterized by dysphoric mood, changes in appetite, changes in sleep patterns, and slowing of mental processes. Proper treatment of depression necessitates accurate diagnosis.[4] Physical problems underlying the depression are explored and treated before the antidepressant drug treatment is initiated.

Depression may be treated with tricyclic antidepressant agents, second-generation antidepressants, and monoamine oxidase inhibitors (MAO inhibitors). Tricyclic antidepressants and related compounds are the most widely used agents for the treatment of depression (see Chart 17-6); their efficacy in the alleviation of depression has been established by numerous research studies.[37]

Antidepressant medications are particularly effective in the treatment of endogenous depression, which is marked by vegetative symptoms, such as regression and decreased productivity. The therapeutic value of these agents depends on the client receiving adequate doses of the drug for a sufficient period of time. The onset of drug action for most antidepressant agents occurs in approximately 2 to 3 weeks and the optimal response takes place in 1 month. Some sedation is often desirable during early treatment with antidepressants and is noted during the administration of both amitriptyline and doxepin.[6,37]

The nurse is responsible for client teaching, emotional support, and assessing the client for suicidal potential during treatment with antidepressant agents (see Nursing Care Plan 17-2). The client needs

(Text continues on p. 284)

Table 17-4.　**Side Effects of Antiparkinsonism Drugs**

SYSTEM AFFECTED	SYMPTOMS	TREATMENT RECOMMENDATIONS
Central nervous	Drowsiness	Administer at bedtime; decrease dose of drug
Autonomic	Dry mouth, blurred vision, urinary retention	Sugar-free candy or gum; avoid activities requiring visual acuity
Cardiovascular	Orthostatic hypotension	Antiembolism hose; assist client to sit or stand slowly
Gastrointestinal	Jaundice	Stop medication; bedrest
Endocrine	Weight gain	Weight reduction diet; physical exercise
Allergic	Transient skin rashes, photosensitivity	Antihistaminic drugs; avoid sunlight

CHART 17-6
Antidepressant Agents

Classification: Antidepressants

Used in the treatment of clients with regressed and agitated depressive states

Actions

Possibly inhibits the membrane pump mechanism responsible for the uptake of norepinephrine and serotonin in adrenergic and serotonergic neurons

Reverses psychomotor retardation in depressed individuals

Improves insomnia by increasing state-4 slow wave and decreasing rapid eye movement (REM) sleep

Potent anticholinergic

Monoamine oxidase inhibitors—increase concentration of epinephrine, norepinephrine, and storage sites thoughout the central nervous system that increases the concentration of monoamines in brainstem

Side Effects

Central nervous system: drowsiness, sedation, muscle tremors, paresthesias, delusions, hallucinations, extrapyramidal symptoms, tardive dyskinesia with amoxapine

Autonomic nervous system: dry mouth, urinary retention, constipation, mydriasis, priapism with trazodone

Cardiovascular: postural hypotension, sinus tachycardia, cardiac arrhythmias, pedal edema, electrocardiogram (ECG) changes (ST-segment depression, T wave flat, prolonged QRS)

Gastrointestinal: nausea and vomiting, anorexia, obstructive jaundice

Hematopoietic: agranulocytosis

Endocrine: gynecomastia, galactorrhea, hyperglycemia, and hypoglycemia

Allergic: allergic rash

Withdrawal symptoms: abrupt cessation leads to nausea, headache, malaise (not indicative of addiction)

Drug Interactions

Antihypertensives—action/effects may be blocked

Thyroid medications—effects are potentiated

Central nervous system depressants—effects are potentiated

Monoamine oxidase inhibitors—causes hypertensive crisis, severe convulsions, and death

Antipsychotics—potentiate anticholinergic effects

Atropine—potentiates anticholinergic effects

Contraindications

Caution in clients with cardiovascular disorders (causes arrhythmias)

Increases or exacerbates psychosis in schizophrenics

Increases or exacerbates mania in manic-depressives

Increases hazards in clients receiving electroconvulsive therapy (ECT)

Caution in clients with impaired liver disorders

Caution in clients who are suicidal or who have a history of suicidal attempts (dialysis is of little value in overdoses because of decreased plasma levels)

Monoamine Oxidase Inhibitors

Drug Interactions

Tricyclics and tyramine-containing foods—cause serious hypertensive crises

Antihistamines—increase the accumulation of norepinephrine in nerve endings

Central nervous system depressants—decrease metabolic breakdown by liver

Levodopa—potentiates the action

Antihypertensives/diuretics—decrease the action

Amphetamines—potentiate the action

Dibenzypines—cause hypertensive crisis and severe convulsions

Contraindications

Foods that are high in tyramine—aged cheeses, beer, pickled herring, sherry, sour cream, chocolate, raisins, and many others

Clients with cerebrovascular defects or cardiovascular disorders

Presence of pheochromocytoma

Persons with liver impairment

Clients older than 60

The Client Taking Antidepressants

Nursing diagnosis: Knowledge deficit regarding side effects of antidepressants
Goal: To minimize side effects of antidepressants and promote client comfort and safety

Side Effect/Problem	Intervention	Rationale
Dry mouth	1. Teach the client to drink frequent sips of water or lemonade and chew sugarless gum and candy 2. Reassure the client that dryness of his mouth is a temporary reaction	1. To moisten mucous membranes 2. To decrease anxiety and increase his compliance with medication regime
Constipation	1. Teach the client to include in his diet foods that are high in bulk and fiber, (*i.e.,* brans, fresh fruits, and vegetables) 2. Encourage drinking adequate amounts of fluids 3. Encourage ambulation 4. Administer stool softeners as ordered	1. To increase bulk in stools and promote peristalsis 2. To soften stools and prevent constipation 3. To promote peristalsis 4. To lower surface tension, permitting water to penetrate and soften stool
Sedation	1. Encourage the client to take medication at bedtime 2. Teach him the importance of avoiding alcohol and other sedatives and depressants 3. Advise the client to avoid driving and using hazardous equipment	1. To promote sleep and rest 2. The antidepressants potentiate sedative effects of CNS depressants 3. To prevent accidents and injury
Urinary retention	1. Monitor intake and output 2. Check the abdomen for distention 3. Catheterize prn 4. Assess for the history of prostatic hypertrophy 5. If urinary retention persists, report to the physician	1. To assess if the client is adequately emptying bladder 2. To assess bladder distention 3. To empty bladder and decrease the risk of bladder infection 4. This condition will further increase the risk of urinary retention 5. This may be a temporary effect of the medication; therefore, persistent retention should be investigated further
Hypertensive crisis (due to monoamine oxidase inhibitors)	1. Monitor the client's blood pressure in lying, sitting, and standing positions 2. Assess neurological signs, including complaints of headache and blurred vision 3. Teach the client to avoid foods that contain tyramine, such as aged	1. To provide baseline blood pressure and to assess cardiovascular changes in response to position changes 2. Headache may be an initial sign of hypertensive crisis 3. These foods will precipitate hypertensive crisis 4. These drugs have adrenergic properties and increase the

Side Effect/Problem	Intervention	Rationale
	cheese, wine, beer, chicken livers, and so forth	potential of developing hypertensive crisis
	4. Warn the client to avoid over-the-counter cold and sinus medications and amphetamines	
Risk of suicide	1. Monitor the client's swallowing of medications	1. To prevent the client from hoarding lethal dose of medications
	2. Inform the client and his family of the time required for the drug's therapeutic effects to occur	2. To encourage and reassure the client that depressions are usually time-limited
	3. Assess the suicide potential; that is, previous attempts, family history, possession of a weapon, lethality of the plan, and so on	3. These drugs are potentially lethal and may be included in the client's suicide plan
	4. Instruct the client not to take antidepressants with central nervous system depressants	4. To minimize central nervous system depression resulting from potentiation
	5. Assist the client to explore alternatives in dealing with feelings of hopelessness and despair	5. To provide options and increase availability of support systems
Nausea/Vomiting (Desyrel)	1. Take medication with meals or light snack	1. To minimize nausea and vomiting and decrease gastric irritation
Dizziness, lightheadedness (orthostatic hypotension)	1. Encourage client to rise slowly in morning and sit for short periods before standing	1. These measures will allow client's body to adjust to changes in position from recumbent to standing, and allow for venous return
Blood dyscrasias (Desyrel)	1. Monitor WBC, CBC with differential, neutrophil count	1. These will allow monitoring of neutropenia
	2. Teach client/significant other to report sore throat, fever that persists	2., 3. These symptoms may indicate agranulocytosis; lab work will also provide baseline data regarding this disorder
	3. Report these symptoms to physician immediately	
Prolonged/inappropriate erections (Desyrel)	1. Teach client to report these symptoms immediately and stop the medication	1., 2., 3. This drug has been associated with the incidence of priapism in 1/3 of cases reported; this side effect can cause permanent impairment of erectile function or impotence; client must report these symptoms immediately
	2. Inform physician immediately	
	3. Caution the use of Desyrel in those men with histories of sexual dysfunction	
Potential for exacerbation of mania in bipolar disorders	1. Teach client/significant others symptoms of recurrent mania, *i.e.*, pressured speech, sleeplessness, restlessness, and so forth	1. This medication may cause exacerbation of mania within 5–14 days; therefore, the client and family members need to be aware of the possibility and monitor for occurrence

to be informed of the length of time necessary for optimal response to his medication. Some clients may become discouraged and possibly even more depressed if they are not told about this delayed therapeutic response.[35]

Tricyclic Antidepressants

Tricyclic antidepressant agents are potentially lethal if they are taken in amounts that are 10 to 30 times the daily recommended dose. A nursing implication is therefore to monitor the ingestion of the tricyclic antidepressants to prevent the client from hoarding the medications for a future suicide attempt. Individuals who overdose on these medications do not respond to treatment by dialysis or forced diuresis. Rather, the treatment for tricyclic antidepressant overdosage includes supportive measures and the administration of physostigmine to manage atropine overdose effects.[5]

There exists a high relapse rate with antidepressant medication treatment during the first year after recovery from acute, severe, depressive illness. The client is therefore usually treated with antidepressants for a period of at least several months.[30,31] The nurse provides further support to the client by sharing with him information that reinforces his positive response to the medication.

Monoamine Oxidase Inhibitors

The MAO inhibitors are generally considered not as effective as other forms of treatment for acute depression. The severe side effects of these drugs and their complex interactions with other drugs and foods limit their usefulness. Although MAO inhibitors are not used as often as other antidepressant drugs, they may also provide selective benefits for conditions other than depression, such as those disorders characterized by phobias and anxiety.[6]

The nursing implications of administration of MAO inhibitors include observing the client for untoward side effects, particularly hypertensive crises resulting from interaction with specific drugs and foods. It is essential for the nurse to educate the client and family about certain foods and drugs that the client must avoid while taking these medications. These foods and drugs that contain tyramine and produce a synergistic effect with the MAO inhibitors include aged cheese, wine, beer, yogurt, chocolates, pickled herring, and bananas.

Anxiolytic Agents

Anxiety is both a normal aspect of universal human behavior and a cardinal symptom of many psychiatric disorders. Anxiety is also associated with fear and serves psychobiological adaptive purposes.

Anxiolytic, or *antianxiety agents,* among the most widely prescribed drugs, are usually the drugs of choice to treat overt anxiety and somatic complaints. They are also useful in the treatment of convulsions and muscle spasms. (See Chart 17-7.)

The benzodiazepines constitute the most useful group of antianxiety agents. The conditions that respond most favorably to the benzodiazepines are those involving acute anxiety reactions of medical and psychiatric clients. It is imperative that medical causes contributing to the client's anxiety are ruled out before this medication is begun.

The nursing implications of administering antianxiety agents include recognizing the potential for both physical and psychological dependence and abuse of these agents. Abuse of these drugs may be attributed, in part, to the development of tolerance to them after approximately 3 to 4 weeks. During this time, the client may increase the dosage that was orig-

---

C H A R T   17-7
Anxiolytic Agents

Classification: Anxiolytic Agents

Formerly called "minor tranquilizers"
Reduce anxiety, tension, and agitation
Sedative effects

Actions

Possibly act on limbic system, thalamus, and hypothalamus
Produce calming effect

Side Effects

Central nervous system: drowsiness, ataxia, confusion, depression, blurred vision
Cardiovascular: hypotension, palpitations, syncope, transient ECG changes
Gastrointestinal: nausea, vomiting, diarrhea
Hematopoietic: neutropenia, aplastic anemia, agranulocytosis
Endocrine: changes in libido
Allergic: skin rash
Physical/psychological dependence: withdrawal can cause convulsions, tremors, and abdominal and muscle cramps

Drug Interactions

Central nervous system depressants—actions are potentiated

Contraindications

Clients with renal or liver impairments

Nursing Care Plan 17-3

The Client Taking Anxiolytic (Antianxiety) Agents

Nursing diagnosis: Knowledge deficit regarding side effects of anxiolytics
Goal: To minimize side effects of anxiolytics and promote client safety

Side Effect/Problem	Intervention	Rationale
Sedation	1. Teach the client to administer medication at bedtime 2. Caution the client about the use of hazardous equipment and driving a vehicle	1. To maximize the sedative effects and promote sleep 2. To prevent or minimize the possibility of accidents and injury
Physical and mental dependency	1. Assist the client to view his problems realistically 2. Assist the client to examine other alternatives in dealing with anxiety, such as physical exercise, gardening, and relaxation techniques 3. Teach the client the signs of dependency, such as the need to increase dose to obtain same effect, nervousness, and abdominal cramping 4. Instruct the client not to stop medications suddenly without consulting the physician	1. To resolve conflicts and underlying anxieties 2. To promote tension release, goal-setting, and relaxation 3. To minimize physical and psychological dependency on medications and to encourage the client to assume responsibility and control over the use of drugs 4. Abrupt withdrawal can precipitate seizures and, possibly, death

inally ordered in order to regain the initial euphoric effect.[4] The client needs to be informed that these drugs are not a "cure" for his anxiety and that the identification of the source of his anxiety may help reduce its effects. The nurse also assists the client in exploring methods of dealing with his feelings (see Nursing Care Plan 17-3).

Antimanic Agents

The primary indications for the use of lithium carbonate are treatment for acute mania and long-term prophylactic treatment of bipolar disorder, formerly termed manic-depressive illness (see Chart 17-8). Lithium is particularly efficacious in the prevention of recurrent manic episodes.

Lithium is ideally used to treat clients with normal sodium intake and normal cardiac and renal functioning. Before lithium administration is initiated, the individual must undergo an adequate medical evaluation consisting of electrolyte studies, thyroid function tests, complete blood count, blood urea nitrogen, urinalysis, and electrocardiogram.

Lithium, a salt, is not metabolized by the body. It is easily absorbed via the oral route and exists in body fluids. During the process of renal excretion of lithium, it competes with sodium for reabsorption in the proximal tubules of the kidneys.[5]

Most clients demonstrating severely manic behavior are initially treated with large doses of antipsychotic drugs (see Table 17-5). When the client evidences less disturbed behavior, in approximately 5 to 10 days, lithium is gradually introduced.

There is a low therapeutic index for lithium salts. Lithium is a potentially toxic drug that can produce degenerative changes primarily in the kidneys.[20] Despite its toxic effects, lithium may be safely administered through careful monitoring of the client's serum level of lithium. The therapeutic serum lithium range for the treatment of acute mania is 0.9 to 1.4 mEq/liter; long-term maintenance level of lithium is 0.6 to 1.2 mEq/liter. Serum lithium levels should be

C H A R T   17-8
Antimanic Agent: Lithium

Classification: Antimanic Agent

Used to treat mania and recurrent manic
episodes

Actions

Alters sodium transport in nerve and muscle
cells and effects a shift toward intra-
neuronal metabolism of catecholamines;
however, specific biochemical mechanism
of action on mania is unknown

Side Effects

Central nervous system: tremors, muscle hyper-
irritability, tinnitus, confusion, slurred
speech, clonic movements
Autonomic nervous system: blurred vision
Cardiovascular: cardiac arrhythmias, hypotension, bradycardia
Gastrointestinal: anorexia, nausea, vomiting,
diarrhea, excessive salivation
Endocrine: euthyroid goiter, hypothyroidism
(myxedema)
Urinary: albuminuria, oliguria, polyuria,
decreased creatinine clearance
Allergic: drying and thinning of hair, alopecia,
itching

Note: Plasma lithium levels require close monitoring. Therapeutic level is 0.5–1.5 mEq/
liter; the therapeutic and toxic levels are
very close in reading. Lithium levels more
than 1.5 mEq/liter produce signs of toxicity; 20% to 30% of clients with bipolar
disorders do not respond to lithium

Drug Interactions

Diuretics—increase risks of lithium toxicity
Antipsychotics—can cause encephalopathic syndrome (*i.e.*, weakness, fatigue, irreversible
brain damage)
Neuromuscular blocking agent—prolong their
effects
Nonsteroidal/anti-inflammatory agents—
increase the plasma levels of lithium

Contraindications

Clients with renal impairment
Cardiovascular disease
Clients taking diuretics
The presence of severe debilitation or dehydra-
tion, sodium depletion
Pregnant women (causes fetal anomalies)
Clients with hypothyroidism require close
monitoring

measured about 10 to 14 hours after the last dose of
the drug. Once a maintenance level of serum lithium
has been reached, blood levels should be measured
about every 3 months. It normally takes 2 to 3 weeks
of lithium administration to produce a therapeutic
level of the drug.[5]

An important nursing responsibility is client and
family education, aimed at preventing toxicity and
manic-depressive recurrences. The necessity of taking
the medication as prescribed should be stressed. Clients and family members should be instructed to notify their physician if the client experiences increased
sweating, takes diuretics, or decreases his salt intake.
These conditions lower the body's sodium levels and
increase the risk of overdose. The client needs to be
(Text continues on p. 291)

Table 17-5.   Antimanic Agents

CLASSIFICATION	CHEMICAL GROUP	GENERIC NAME	TRADE NAME	DAILY DOSAGE
Antimanic Agents	Lithium carbonate	Lithium carbonate	Lithium	900–1200 mg (divided doses)
			Eskalith (slow-release)	900–1200 mg (divided doses) (Serum levels range: (0.5–1.5 mEq/L)
	Carbamazepine	Carbamazepine	Tegretol	400–1600 mg (dose ranges and serum levels should be maintained between 8–12 mg/ml)

Nursing Care Plan 17-4

The Client Taking Lithium

Nursing diagnosis: Knowledge deficit regarding side effects of lithium
Goal: To minimize side effects of lithium and promote safety

Side Effect/Problem	Intervention	Rationale
Toxicity	1. Monitor the client for early toxic signs, such as diarrhea, nausea, and vomiting 2. Teach signs and symptoms of toxicity to the client and his family members	1., 2. There is a small index between the therapeutic level and toxicity; noting these early symptoms assists in preventing toxic effects.
	3. Obtain baseline levels of renal and cardiovascular functioning prior to beginning medications (*i.e.*, BUN, ECG, and so on) 4. Monitor laboratory results associated with renal functioning	3., 4. Lithium is excreted by the kidneys; ineffective functioning of the kidneys may result in cumulative toxicity.
	5. Monitor lithium serum levels and teach the client and his family the importance of follow-up; client needs to have lithium level drawn 12 hours after last dose, *i.e.*, HS dose at 8 P.M., lithium level approximately 8 A.M. the following day; skip A.M. dose until lab work drawn	5. To provide objective data about serum levels of lithium
	6. Teach the client how to maintain adequate sodium intake and the necessity of calling the physician if there is an increase in sodium loss via diaphoresis, vomiting, or diarrhea	6. Sodium competes with lithium in the kidneys for reabsorption; a decrease in sodium due to these conditions contributes to an increased risk of lithium toxicity
Recurrence of manic behavior	1. Teach the client and his family the signs and symptoms of recurring mania, such as talkativeness, increased motor activity, racing thoughts, inability to rest, decreased attention span, and so forth	1. To alert the client and his family that psychiatric attention is required
Recurrence of depression	1. Teach the client and his family the symptoms of recurring depression, such as crying, feelings of hopelessness, lack of attention to personal hygiene, lack of energy, and so on	1. To alert the client and his family that psychiatric attention is required

Discussing the Pros and Cons of Lithium

Mr. Carson, a 37-year-old man recently discharged from an acute psychiatric unit, has been diagnosed with bipolar disorder, manic-type, and stabilized on lithium carbonate 300 mg qid. He has been referred to a local community mental health center for follow-up of his medication regimen.

Nurse O has been scheduled to interview Mr. Carson and his wife today.

Mr. Carson: Can you tell me why I have to take this medication?

Mrs. Carson: He is not sick anymore; I also want to know why he needs medication.

Nurse O: Yes, Mr. Carson, you have a history of manic depression, or bipolar disorder, and lithium will reduce your chances of having these problems again.

Mr. Carson: But I feel great! I'm sleeping well and I plan to return to my job next week.

Nurse O: Yes I can see that you are doing well. The lithium you are taking is helping you to feel the way you are feeling right now. Lithium has made it possible for you to sleep and think more clearly. You need to take it as long as your doctor prescribes in order to reduce your chances of having a relapse.

Mr. Carson: I do not want to get dependent on any drugs. I do not want drugs to control my life.

Nurse O: I understand your feelings, Mr. Carson, but taking lithium can be compared to taking insulin to control diabetes or anti-hypertensive medications for high blood pressure. You have a chemical imbalance that makes it necessary for you to take lithium in order for you to function. I can assure that it is not addictive. When you take this medication, lithium, you have control over your life. If you do not take lithium, you will begin to have troubles like before and lose control over your life.

Mrs. Carson: Do you mean that if he stops taking lithium, he will become confused again and start doing weird things?

Nurse O: Yes, he will become disturbed again and may have to be hospitalized. I understand how difficult it must be for you to take this medication, Mr. Carson, but taking lithium will reduce your chances of hospitalization.

Mr. Carson: But I do not feel bad when I get sick. I feel I can do "anything."

Nurse O: But, Mr. Carson, what happened as a result of your "good feelings"?

Mr. Carson: I ran up all my credit cards and charged more than $15,000 for my trips to Las Vegas.

Nurse O: That doesn't sound like having control over your life to me. What do you think?

Mrs. Carson: You are right! He lost complete control and now we are knee deep in debt.

Nurse O: Mr. Carson, taking lithium may be a change in your life but the advantages far outweigh the disadvantages of not taking it.

Mr. Carson: You may be right.

Nurse O continues the interview by using a teaching plan for Lithium.

CHART 17-10
Neuroleptic Malignant Syndrome

Neuroleptic malignant syndrome (NMS) has been defined as a rare, idiosyncratic reaction to neuroleptic agents. This disorder was originally identified in Europe in the 1960s. The first recognized case in the United States was confirmed in the early 1980s. NMS is characterized by severe muscle rigidity, hyperthermia, and stupor.[18]

Etiology

The cause of NMS is not clearly understood. Theories and studies suggest that it is caused by dopamine blockage in the basal ganglia. These changes may be precipitated by rapid, massive loading of neuroleptic agents over a given period of time.[1,46]

Incidence

1. NMS occurs in 0.5% to 1.0% of clients taking neuroleptics
2. High-potency neuroleptics, usually the piperazine phenothiazines, long-acting, parenteral forms (*i.e.*, Haldol or Prolixin decanoate) increase risk
3. Frequently symptoms appear abruptly within several days or weeks after therapy with neuroleptics; occasionally symptoms occur with increased doses of neuroleptic agents after the client has been on the drug over a longer period of time
4. Rare occurrences with Mellaril (thioridazine)
5. 80% of clients are less than 40 years of age (ages range from 6 to 61)
6. Men develop NMS twice as often as females
7. Clients with parkinsonism and Huntington's chorea are at greater risk for developing NMS[13,14]
8. Sudden withdrawal of dopamine agonist (antiparkinsonian drugs)[48,52]

Signs and Symptoms

Extrapyramidal Symptoms

Widespread muscle rigidity, diffuse tremors, dystonic reactions in face, extremities, chest, neck, trismus (tightening of jaw muscles)
Hands/feet become fixed in carpopedal spasm
Hypertonicity in oropharyngeal areas
Increased salivation (sialorrhea)
Painful joints (dysarthria)
Difficulty swallowing (dysphagia)
Mutism

Stupor

Difficult to assess, but characterized by stupor and coma
Client unable to communicate because of mutism
Mental status extremely difficult to assess

Autonomic Disturbances

Hyperthermia (malignant hyperexia)
Diaphoresis
Tachycardia
Fluctuation in B/P
Urinary retention
Severe cases may be complicated by dehydration → renal failure
Myoglobinuria 2° to rhabdomyolysis
Late stage may develop dyspnea, tachypnea → respiratory failure, which may be due to pulmonary emboli or pneumonia

Conditions That Predispose Clients to NMS

1. Physical agitation
2. Physical exhaustion
3. Dehydration

Differential Diagnosis/Assessment

History-taking is essential in assisting the physician in making an accurate diagnosis of NMS and differentiating it from other febrile conditions.

1. Febrile conditions of the central nervous system, such as encephalitis, meningitis, or tetany, must be ruled out
2. History of neuroleptics (antipsychotic drugs)—name, dose, route, frequency, and length of time on the medication; ask if medication has been recently increased in dose
3. History of these symptoms in past
4. History of parkinsonism or Huntington's chorea (familial history)
5. History of extrapyramidal symptoms
6. History of heat stroke

Diagnosis

General Appearance (see chart of signs/symptoms)

1. Widespread muscle rigidity, diffuse tremors, severe extrapyramidal symptoms and dystonias
2. Temperature elevation (up to 40.7°C [107°F] rectally)
3. Hypertension (fluctuation in B/P)

(Continues on p. 290)

Labs

1. WBC/CBC reveal leukocytosis ($\uparrow$ white blood cells)
2. In CPK (creatinine phosphokinase)
   $\uparrow$ in CPK demonstrates in muscle enzymes
   $\uparrow$ in CPK and K$^+$ (potassium) indicates skeletal muscle necrosis (rhabdomyolysis)
3. $\uparrow$ liver enzymes

Treatment/Goals (generally supportive)

1. Prompt discontinuation of neuroleptics
2. Intensive care unit (ICU) for cardio-pulmonary support
3. Maintain renal function
4. Concurrent infections must be treated
5. Hypothermic measures

Note: There is controversy at the present time over the effectiveness of anticholinergic agents in the treatment of NMS. Dialysis is not effective in decreasing circulating neuroleptics because they are protein- and lipid-bound.[16]

Drugs Frequently Used in Treating NMS

Dantrolene (Dantrium) is a peripheral skeletal muscle relaxant that decreases body temperature; this drug may reverse muscle rigidity and rhabdomyolysis[24]

Bromocriptine (Parlodel) is a central acting dopamine receptor agonist that may reverse EPS and autonomic symptoms and stupor[24]

Course of NMS

Treatment and careful monitoring usually require 1–3 weeks. Neuroleptic malignant syndrome (NMS) subsides in 5–10 days if client was taking oral neuroleptics and 10–21 days for long-acting phenothiazines[47]

Mortality Rate

NMS has a 20% to 25% mortality rate, usually secondary to respiratory failure that results from pulmonary emboli, cardiovascular collapse, or acute renal failure.[16]

C H A R T   17-11
Drug Interactions with Tegretol (Carbamazepine)

Increase Serum Levels of Tegretol (CBZ)

Valproic acid
Propoxyphene (Darvon)
Isoniazid (INH)

Decrease Serum Levels of Tegretol (CBZ)

Phenytoin (Dilantin)
Phenobarbital
Primidone
Erythromycin
Haldol
Coumadin

Tegretol (CBZ) Increases Metabolism

Theophyllin
Warfarin

Increases Risk of Neurotoxicity

Lithium

C H A R T   17-12
Contraindications for Tegretol (Carbamazepine)

1. History of bone marrow depression
2. Pregnancy (increases incidence of fetal anomalies)
3. Should be used cautiously in clients with histories of latent schizophrenia (increases incidence of recurrent psychosis)
4. Should be used cautiously in elderly patients (may increase agitation and/or confusion)
5. Should be used cautiously when operating motor vehicle or undertaking dangerous tasks

Tegretol has not been approved by FDA for the treatment of bipolar disorders. INFORMED CONSENT and CLEAR DOCUMENTATION are needed.

CHART 17-13

Tegretol (Carbamazepine) Nursing Implications

Action

Exerts anti-kindling effect, specifically in the limbic system and temporal lobe region[7,9]

Uses

Temporal lobe epilepsy (TLE), trigeminal neuralgia

Psychiatry

1. Useful in treating clients with rapid-cycling bipolar disorders (four or more episodes/year)[33]
2. Alternative to lithium in preventing relapses in clients with rapid-cycling bipolar disorders who are resistant to lithium prophylaxis
3. Useful in treating clients who are sensitive to lithium

Therapeutic Levels

8–12 µg/ml

Therapeutic Dose

400–1600 mg/day

Side Effects

Hemopoietic: Aplastic anemia, leukopenia, agranulocytosis, thrombocytopenia
Neurological: Dizziness, ataxia, headaches, blurred vision, paresthesias, agitation, tinnitus, lethargy
Gastrointestinal: Nausea and vomiting, dry mouth, diarrhea, anorexia
Integumentary: Pruritus, exfoliative dermatitis, Stevens–Johnson syndrome, alopecia
Genitourinary: Urinary retention, ↑ BUN, glycosuria, albuminuria
Hepatic: Liver function test abnormalities, jaundice
Cardiovascular: Congestive heart failure, syncope, edema, hypertension, hypotension

---

able to recognize the possible side effects of lithium, such as diarrhea, tremors, and nausea, and needs to report them to his physician immediately. The client and family must also be informed of the need for regular monitoring of serum lithium levels (see Nursing Care Plan 17-4 and Chart 17-9).

Nurses provide psychological support to clients and their families in dealing with their feelings about this bipolar disorder. Parents or grandparents, for example, may experience guilt associated with feeling responsible for the client's emotional disorder. Stressing the importance of preventing recurrences by taking the medication as prescribed may encourage hopefulness for the client and family.

Summary

This chapter has focused on several areas that are significant for the safe and therapeutic use of psychotropic medication. The historical perspective presented information about the revolution of psychotropic drugs and their influence on the field of psychiatric–mental health care. Some of the other major points of the chapter have included the following:

1. The introduction of psychotropic agents has revolutionized the treatment of institutionalized psychiatric clients and has facilitated their return to community life.

Case Study 17-1

The Client Who Is Noncompliant with Medication Regimen

Mr. Irving is a 20-year-old man who has been brought to a local community crisis center by his father. His father reports that the client has been restless and agitated, pacing the floor at night, that sometimes his son talks to himself, and that he does not socialize with family members. Inquiry reveals that Mr. Irving stopped taking his medication, Navane, several weeks ago.

Mr. Irving reports that he stopped taking his medication because it made him "feel like a robot." He also explained that when he took his medication, his mouth was "dry all the time" and he suffered from constipation.

History obtained from both client and his father revealed that he was diagnosed with schizophrenia, paranoid type, 6 months ago. He was hospitalized at that time when his father found him wandering around the neighborhood half-dressed, confused, and complaining of people following him. His course in the hospital was uneventful, except he was tried on several neuroleptic agents. Navane was selected as the drug of choice and he was discharged from the psychiatric facility on 30 mg of Navane at bedtime.

Mr. Irving has always lived with his parents. He has few friends and is not close to family members at present. He is the third child of five but he always has been a "loner." His father reports that when his son takes his medication, he is less agitated and suspicious. The client concurs that he sleeps better when he takes Navane. Although his family is supportive of

Mr. Irving's treatment, his father expresses concern that his son will not take his medication if he continues to have these side effects.

Mr. Irving's present appearance is disheveled. He is agitated, suspicious, guarded, and reluctant to answer certain questions. He does not have a history of alcohol or illicit drug abuse. He has no major medical problems at present. He denies suicidal or homicidal ideations at this time and has made no suicidal or homicidal gestures or attempts in the past. He is alert and oriented in all three spheres and has no evidence of auditory or visual hallucinations at present. There is evidence of paranoia and flat affect. The client's father has been a significant informant during this interview.

The client and his father have been seen by the staff psychiatrist. Mr. Irving's prescription is refilled and he was also prescribed Cogentin 2 mg bid. In three weeks he is scheduled for a followup appointment. He and his father have been instructed to call the nurse if other problems related to side effects of the medication arise.

Poor medication compliance, a major problem in psychiatry, has been related to the occurrence of uncomfortable side effects of the psychoactive drugs. Some of these side effects can be reduced with anticholinergic agents such as Cogentin. Nurses are in key positions to provide client teaching to all individuals on psychotropic medications and to their families and instrumental in creating effective, individualized teaching plans.

Nursing Diagnosis	Goal	Interventions	Evaluation
Noncompliance related to neuroleptic side effects	Increase medication compliance	1. Teach measures that will minimize the side effects of neuroleptics 2. Develop teaching plan that lists side effects and ways to minimize them 3. Encourage client and significant others to verbalize feelings about side effects 4. Describe measures that will decrease side effects, *e.g.*, high roughage diet for constipation, sugarless candy for dry mouth	1. Within 1–2 weeks, client will take Navane under supervision of family member/significant other 2. By the end of 3–4 weeks, the client will take medication with minimum supervision of family member/significant other 3. By the end of 6–8 weeks, client will take medication as prescribed without close

Nursing Diagnosis	Goal	Interventions	Evaluation
		5. Point out that some side effects are temporary and decrease after several months 6. Encourage client to take Cogentin as prescribed 7. Encourage client to call clinic if side effects persist or worsen, *e.g.,* restlessness, agitation	supervision of family member/significant other

2. One of the more important theories of the action of psychotropics is based on the biochemical activities of the neurotransmitters, specifically norepinephrine and dopamine.

3. The psychotropic medications are classified into the antipsychotic or neuroleptic, antidepressant, antianxiety, and antimanic agents.

4. Nurses play a significant role in the development of new information from research studies of psychotropic drugs.

5. Noncompliance with medication regimens is a major problem in the field of psychiatric–mental health care.

6. One of the variables that may reduce this noncompliance with regimens and may prevent recurrences of emotional disorder is client and family teaching, an integral part of the psychiatric treatment plan.

7. The revolution that heralded the advent of psychopharmacology several decades ago has developed into continuous research processes that lead to the important drug discoveries of today and tomorrow.

References

1. Abbot RJ, Loizou LA: Neuroleptic Malignant Syndrome. Br J Psychiatry 148: 47–51, 1986
2. Altshul AT: Psychiatric Nursing, 4th ed. pp 256–261. Baltimore, Williams & Wilkins, 1973
3. American Nurses' Association: Standards of Psychiatric and Mental Health Nursing Practice. Kansas City, American Nurses' Association, 1982
4. American Psychiatric Association: Diagnostic and Statistical Manual of Mental Disorders, 3d ed, rev, Washington, American Psychiatric Association, 1980
5. Appleton WS: Fourth Psychoactive Drug Usage Guide. J Clin Psychiatry 43: 12–27, 1982
6. Baldessarini RJ: Drugs and the Treatment of Psychiatric Disorders. In Gilman AG, Goodman LS, Gilman A (eds): The Pharmacological Basis of Therapeutics, 6th ed, pp 391–442. New York, Macmillan, 1980
7. Ballenger JC, Post RM: Carbamazepine in Manic-Depression: A New Treatment. Amer J Psychiatry 137: 782–790, 1980
8. Berstein JG: Handbook of Drug Therapy in Psychiatry. Boston, John Wright & Sons, 1983
9. Birkhimer LT, Curtis JL, Jann MW: Use of Carbamazepine in Psychiatric Disorders. Clin Pharmacol 4: 425–434, 1985
10. Blackwell B: Drug Therapy: Patient Compliance. N Engl J Med 289: 249–252, 1973
11. Bloom FE: Neural Mechanisms of Benzodiazepines Actions. Am J Psychiatry 134: 669–672, 1977
12. Brands AJ, Brands AB: Responsibility. Fam Community Health 6: 63–71, 1983
13. Burke RE, Fahn S, Mayeux R et al: Neuroleptic Malignant Syndrome Caused by Dopamine-Depleting Drugs in a Patient with Huntington's Disease. Neurology 31: 1022–1026, 1980
14. Burke RE, Fahn S, Jankovic J et al: Tardive Dystonia: Late-Onset, Caused by Antipsychotic Drugs. Neurology 32 (December): 1335–1346, 1982
15. Cade JJ: Lithium Salts in the Treatment of Psychotic Excitement. Medical Journal of Australia 2: 349–352, 1949
16. Caroff SN: The Neuroleptic Malignant Syndrome. J Clin Psychiatry 41: 79–83, 1980
17. Cole JO, Orzack MH, Benke B et al: Assessment of the Abuse Liability of Buspirone in Recreational Sedative Users. J Clin Psychiatry 43: 67–74, 1982
18. Cope RV, Gregg EM: Neuroleptic Malignant Syndrome. Br Med J 286: 1938, 1983
19. Crane GE: Prevention and Management of Tardive Dyskinesia. Am J Psychiatry 129: 466–467, 1972
20. Davis JM: Overview: Maintenance Therapy in Psychiatry: Affective Disorders. Am J Psychiatry 133: 1–13, 1976
21. Davison G, Neale JM: Abnormal Psychology: An Experimental Clinical Approach. New York, John Wiley & Sons, 1978

22. Diamond RJ: Enhancing Medication Use in Schizophrenic Patients. J Clin Psychiatry 44: 7–14, 1983

23. Gershon S, Eison AS: The Ideal Anxiolytic. Psychiatr Ann 17: 156–157, 1987

24. Granada JE, Stern BJ, Ringel A et al: Neuroleptic Malignant Syndrome: Successful Treatment with Dantrolene and Bromocriptine. Ann Neurol 14: 89–90, 1983

25. Hamilton JD: Thioridazine Retinopathy with Upper Dosage Limit. Psychosomatics 26: 823–824, 1985

26. Harris E: Extrapyramidal Side Effects to Antipsychotic Medications. Am J Nurs 18: 1324–1328, 1981

27. Harvey SC: Hypnotics and Sedatives. In Gilman AG, Goodman LS, Gilman AG (eds): Pharmacological Basis of Therapeutics, 6th ed, pp 339–375. New York, Macmillan, 1980

28. Henderson VW, Wooten GF: Neuroleptic Malignant Syndrome: A Pathogenic Role for Dopamine Receptor Blockade? Neurology 31: 132–137, 1981

29. Hofmann A: The Discovery of LSD and Subsequent Investigations on Naturally Occurring Hallucinogens. In Ayd FJ, Blackwell B (eds): Discoveries in Biological Psychiatry, pp 91–106. Philadelphia, JB Lippincott, 1970

30. Hollister LE: Current Antidepressant Drugs: Their Clinical Use. Drugs 22: 129–152, 1981

31. Hollister LE: Tricyclic Antidepressants. N Engl J Med 299: 1106–1109, 1168–1172, 1978

32. Jaffe JH: Drug Addiction and Drug Abuse. In Gilman AG, Goodman LS, Gilman A (eds): The Pharmacological Basis of Therapeutics, 6th ed, pp 535–584. New York, Macmillan, 1980

33. Janicak PG, Boshes RA: Advances in the Treatment of Mania and Other Acute Psychotic Disorders. Psychiatr Ann 17 (March): 145–149, 1987

34. Kane JM: Problems of Compliance in the Outpatient Treatment of Schizophrenia. J Clin Psychiatry 44: 3–6, 1983

35. Klein DF, Davis JM: Diagnosis and Drug Treatment of Psychiatric Disorders. Baltimore, Williams & Wilkins, 1969

36. Klein DF, Gittelman R, Quitkin F et al: Drug Treatment of Psychiatric Disorders of Adults and Children, 2d ed. Baltimore, Williams & Wilkins, 1980

37. Kuhn R: The Treatment of Depressive States with G22355 (Imipramine Hydrochloride). Am J Psychiatry 115: 459–464, 1958

38. Laben JK, Mclean CP: Legal Issues and Guidelines for Nurses Who Care for the Mentally Ill. New York, Slack Inc, 1984

39. Laborit H: Note: Complimentaire concernant l'utilisation des antihistaminiques des synthese en anesthesie. Acta Chir Belg 49: 390–391, 1950

40. Lipinski JF, Zubenko GS, Cohen BM et al: Propranolol in the Treatment of Neuroleptic-induced Akathesia. Am J Psychiatry 141: 412–415, 1984

41. Newton M, Godbey KL, Newton DW et al: How You Can Improve the Effectiveness of Psychotropic Drug Therapy. Nursing '78 8: 46–55, 1978

42. Rifkin A, Quitkin F, Kane JM et al: Are Prophylactic Antiparkinson's Drugs Necessary? A Controlled Study of Procyclide Withdrawal. Arch Gen Psychiatry 35: 483–489, 1978

43. Rodman MJ, Smith DW: Pharmacology and Drug Therapy in Nursing, 3d ed. Philadelphia, JB Lippincott, 1985

44. Rudorfer MV, Golden RN, Potter WZ: Second-Generation Antidepressants. Psychiatr Clin North Am 7: 519–534, 1984

45. Schooler NR, Levine J, Severe J et al: Prevention of Relapse in Schizophrenia: An Evaluation of Fluphenazine Decanoate. Arch Gen Psychiatry 37: 16–24, 1980

46. Shalev A, Hermesch H, Munitz H: The Role of Loading Rate in Neuroleptic Malignant Syndrome. Am J Psychiatry 143: 8, 1986

47. Smego RA, Durack DT: The Neuroleptic Malignant Syndrome. Arch Intern Med 142: 1183–1185, 1982

48. Simpson DM, Davis G: Case Report of Neuroleptic Malignant Syndrome Associated with Withdrawal from Amantadine. Am J Psychiatry 141: 796–797, 1984

49. Tallman JF: Receptors for the Age of Anxiety: Pharmacology of Benzodiazepines. Science 207: 274–281, 1980

50. Tarsy D: Movement Disorders with Neuroleptic Drug Treatment. Psychiatr Clin North Am 7: 453–471, 1984

51. Task Force on Late Neurological Effects of Antipsychotic Drugs. Tardive Dyskinesia: Summary of the Task Force Reports of the American Psychiatric Association 137: 1163–1172, 1980

52. Toru N, Matsuda O, Makiguch K et al: Neuroleptic Malignant-Like State Following Withdrawal of Antiparkinsonian Drugs. J Nerv Dis 169: 324–327, 1981

53. Van Patten T: Why Do Schizophrenic Patients Refuse to Take Their Drugs? Arch Gen Psychiatry 31: 67–72, 1974

54. Wojcik JD, Gelenberg AJ et al: Prevalence of Tardive Dyskinesia in an Outpatient Population. Compr Psychiatry 21: 370–379, 1980

PART 4

Developmental Issues in Psychiatric–Mental Health Nursing

18 Development of the Person

Sylvia M. Anderson Whiting
Deborah Jackson Antai-Otong

To venture causes anxiety, but not to venture is to lose oneself.
Søren Aabye Kierkegaard

Chapter Preview

Development is the result of a combination of factors and forces that impel the individual toward a characteristic style. The nature–nurture controversy has created diverse and sometimes conflicting schools of thought. It is generally agreed, however, that development proceeds along certain specific lines called developmental phases or stages.

Although most adults can identify significant life events that they believe have affected the present, the debate continues about how these influences come about, about their effects upon the emerging personality, and about the resolution of problems. The student of psychiatric–mental health nursing needs to understand the factors influencing human development and needs to formulate a conceptual framework of mental health problems and treatment approaches.

Newborn infants subjected to identical stimuli display a wide variety of responses. These differing reaction patterns of newborns are termed constitutional baselines or complexes. For example, one infant may remain placid whereas another may react intensely to stimuli. Feeding and crying behaviors also differ widely from infant to infant. These infant behaviors require adaptive responses from the mothering or parenting figure. The resulting maternal–child or parental–child interactions are responsible for multiple adaptive or maladaptive responses affecting maturation and development. The unfolding of development has been thought to occur over a period of 2 decades to form the functioning personality.[5] Current theory asserts, however, that development is a continuous process occurring throughout the lifespan and is not limited to a few years in early life.

The reader may sometimes hear references to normal or abnormal development. These terms, it must be remembered, are relative and dependent upon many factors, such as averages or statistical norms, social norms, individual response patterns, and the presence or absence of psychopathology.[5]

This chapter will introduce the reader to theories about human development from intrapsychic, interpersonal, social learning, cognitive, and behavioristic viewpoints.

Learning Objectives

On completion of this chapter, you should be able to accomplish the following:

1. discuss the phases of psychosexual development according to Freud's intrapsychic theory

2. describe the development of self-concept according to Sullivan's interpersonal theory

3. explain the developmental tasks of the eight stages of development described in Erikson's social learning theory

4. describe the thinking of children during each of the four periods of cognitive development according to Piaget's theory

5. discuss the effects of reinforcement on learning according to behavioristic theory

6. apply developmental criteria to the assessment of clients evidencing physical and emotional health problems

7. apply the nursing process to clients who have experienced difficulty meeting developmental tasks

Theories of Development

Intrapsychic Theory

Sigmund Freud, credited with being the father of psychiatry, was a Viennese physician whose work continued until his death in 1939. Freud utilized hypnosis in the treatment of psychiatric patients and, in this way, became interested in the processes of the unconscious. The art and science of psychoanalysis developed from his description of the unconscious, which is thought to contain the repressed memories of all experiences from the first 6 years of life. An extension of this concept states that, although memories may be repressed, they continue to influence or drive all behavior. (Chapter 2 also provides information about the development of psychoanalytic and other theories and their application to the treatment of mental disorders.)

Libidinal or instinctual drives influence behavior and are related to a person's attempt to gain pleasure or satisfaction through the mouth, anus, or genitalia. The three periods during which the infant and young child focus on these orifices are known correspondingly as the oral, anal, and phallic (or oedipal) phases of development.

The psychoanalytic theorist relates psychological (often referred to as psychosexual) problems to the child's experiences during these three phases of development. Individuals with severe disturbances of the mind are believed to have experienced maladaptive maternal–child relationships during the early infantile period, the oral phase. Those with less severe mental disturbances are thought to have encountered difficulties during the later periods of early childhood; that is, during the anal phase (approximately from 18 months to 3 years) or during the phallic phase (approximately from 3 to 6 years).

Oral Phase

Encountering difficulties in any of these three phases results from anxiety of the mother or mothering person. The development of the infant's ego strength depends on the mother's security in herself and in her mothering role. During the oral phase, the infant experiences whatever the mother feels; that is, he introjects the person of closest attachment and takes on the anxiety or serenity of that person.[15] When the anxiety of the mothering person is all-pervasive, the infant is particularly vulnerable and begins life with a deficit in adaptive abilities.

Anal Phase

The mothering person may encounter no particular difficulty during the period of infancy but may cope ineffectively with the young child as a mobile toddler. The anal phase challenges the mother's coping ability because she must allow him to move away—in effect, to seek freedom or a greater sense of self. Toilet training of the toddler and other issues of the anal phase often arouse psychological problems, particularly related to the rules of custom and culture.

While the toddler strives for mastery over certain aspects of his life, he may not be ready to comply with the social expectations of his parents or other significant adults. The child's striving in two directions, compliance and noncompliance, is termed *ambivalence*. He may comply through proper elimination, thereby introjecting the values of his parents, or he may not comply through retention or inappropriate discharge of feces, which then brings retribution and further anxiety. This "holding on" and "letting go" leads to various behaviors that psychoanalytic clinicians refer to as *anal characteristics*.

Phallic Phase

As the child moves into the phallic (or oedipal) phase of development, the foundation has usually been well established for what occurs during this stage. When anxiety has been present throughout the parent–child relationship, it is likely that it will continue to manifest itself in the ongoing relationship.

In addition, a problem of a different nature may evidence during the phallic phase, when the child begins to develop an awareness of gender. The child recognizes his or her own gender and manifests an interest in the sexuality of others. He or she may also engage in sexual exploratory play, which may cause parents considerable anxiety.

The term *oedipal* refers to the Greek myth about Oedipus Rex, who was separated from his mother in childhood, was reunited with her in adulthood, and, not knowing that she was his mother, fell in love with her. Freud postulated that, during the years from 3 to 6, the child is unconsciously driven toward the parent of the opposite sex and, in effect, desires to possess that parent for himself or herself. For the male child, the issue is less complex than it is for a female child because the mother is the primary love object; for the female, however, it means competing with mother, the young girl's primary love object. The child often resolves the oedipal complex by becoming like, or identifying with, the same-sex parent.

Latent and Genital Phases

Freud called the next two stages of development the latent and genital phases. His use of the term *latent* refers to his belief that sexuality in the child from 6 to 10 or 12 years does not disappear but becomes hidden. At this age, the child engages in the larger world and is absorbed by its challenges to such an extent that his or her libidinal drive seems to assume less importance and attention.

Then, during the adolescent period, the oedipal strivings reawaken and stir a need for the adolescent child to rework and settle his or her libidinal drive toward the parent of the opposite sex. One way in which this is accomplished is by the adolescent rechanneling his or her energies toward peers of the opposite sex.

An individual's responses during the infantile or early childhood periods, which are carried into adulthood, may cause maladaptation and serious adjustment problems. When a person senses himself to be in constant jeopardy, he is unable to turn his energy away from the self and toward more productive activity. In this way, a person may become self-absorbed and defensive in the protection of the self or ego. Defensive maneuvers arising from these early phases of development include repression, introjection, projection, denial, isolation, ambivalence, regression, and sublimation.

Interpersonal Theory

The work of Harry Stack Sullivan, one of psychiatry's most influential thinkers, began in the 1920s and continued to evolve until his death in 1949.

Departing from Freudian concepts, Sullivan used the term *integrating tendencies* to describe behavior by which one moves toward others.[17] These behaviors include smiling, eye contact, verbal communication, offering an object, and so on. This interpersonal relating of one individual to another takes place, according to Sullivan, to convert us "into human beings instead of merely members of the species by assimilating and becoming part of a vast amount of culture."[17]

Security and Self-Concept

The integrating tendencies are related to the pursuit or maintenance of security or the avoidance of insecurity, so that the individual does not experience anxiety. The self comes into being through the young child's experiences. When the child experiences satisfactory fulfillment of his needs, he senses a "good mother" who relaxes the tension of his recurrent needs; this "good mother" becomes introjected as the "good me." When the child receives inadequate mothering and his needs are not satisfactorily met, he senses the "bad or evil mother" associated with the experience of anxiety, which he then introjects as the "bad me."[18] If the maternal–child relationship is, in effect, nonexistent, the child faces a more serious situation, from which there develops no sense of self or "not me." According to Sullivan's interpersonal theory, self-concept and anxiety are closely related to an individual's early-life experiences and continue their influence throughout the lifespan.

Social Learning Theory

Psychologist Erik Erikson has contributed a theory of development that has gained prominence during the past 2 decades. Erikson's theory is formulated according to three principles of organization—the somatic process, the ego process, and the societal process.

In the infantile period, the individual is influenced by somatic processes through exposure to pain, such as colic, earaches, and hunger pains, and by ego processes through exposure to anxiety, such as anxiety that is introjected from the mothering figure. Through societal processes, such as the experience of a family crisis, the infant may be exposed to panic, which affects him through the method and quality of care administered by his caretaker.

Erikson describes the psychoanalyst as a kind of historian and the history of childhood as the basis for understanding human anxiety. According to this theory, anxiety is the outcome of the ongoing interaction of somatic, ego, and societal processes.

Developmental Tasks

The eight stages of developmental tasks or ego qualities devised by Erikson are as follows (also see Chart 18-1):

1. Trust versus mistrust—infancy
2. Autonomy versus shame and doubt—toddlerhood
3. Initiative versus guilt—preschool years
4. Industry versus inferiority—school age
5. Identity versus role confusion—adolescence
6. Intimacy versus isolation—young adulthood
7. Generativity versus stagnation—middle adulthood
8. Integrity versus despair—older adulthood

Through satisfactory completion of the developmental task of each stage, the individual becomes ready to move on to each succeeding stage feeling strong and able to meet the requirements for that stage. If the individual experiences failure in any stage, he is likely to have greater difficulty achieving success in future stages of development. Each stage is also significant in its own right and results in satisfaction and need fulfillment to the individual who meets the challenges of that stage.

A further distinction of Erikson's social learning theory is his concept linking the developmental stages of individuals to certain social institutions or values. Success in living is described by Erikson in this way: "Healthy children will not fear life if their elders have integrity enough not to fear death."[8]

Cognitive Theory

Jean Piaget's theory of cognitive development states that motor activity involving concrete objects results in the development of mental functioning. For example, as an infant discovers his hand that is holding a rattle, he begins to recognize a sound that occurs every time he moves his hand with the rattle in it. Therefore, reflex activity drops out as repetition produces a result that the infant observes; his activity begins to take on purpose. Eventually, the infant identifies the shaking rattle as a producer of sound. Later, he will realize that he is able to create the sound.

Piaget's four periods of cognitive development are as follows:

1. Sensorimotor (0–2 years), during which time development proceeds from reflex activity to representation and sensorimotor learning
2. Preoperational (2–7 years), during which time development proceeds from sensorimotor representation to prelogical thought
3. Concrete operational (7–11 years), during which time development proceeds from prelogical thought to logical, concrete thought
4. Formal operational (11–15 years), during which time development proceeds from logical, concrete thought to logical solutions to all kinds or categories of problems

Tenets of Piaget's Theory

The basic tenets of Piaget's theory of cognitive development are as follows:

CHART 18-1

Erikson's Stages of Development with Adaptive or Maladaptive Characteristics Within Each Stage

Infant

Trust	Versus	Mistrust	Societal Institution
Ease in feeding Depth of sleep Relaxation of bowels The first social achievement allows mother out of sight without undue anxiety or rage		Withdrawal into schizoid and depressive states	Religious affiliation

Toddler

Autonomy	Versus	Shame and Doubt	Societal Institution
Self-control without loss of self-esteem Good will and pride Rightful dignity Lawful independence Sense of justice		Low self-esteem Secretiveness Feelings of persecution	Economic ethos

Preschooler

Initiative	Versus	Guilt	Societal Institution
Loving Relaxed Bright in judgment Energetic Task-oriented		Hysterical denial Paralysis, inhibition, or impotence Overcompensatory showing off Psychosomatic disease Self-righteousness Moralistic surveillance	Law and order

School-aged

Industry	Versus	Inferiority	Societal Institution
Productivity Task completion Steady attention Perseverance Manipulation of tools		Sense of inadequacy Mediocrity Self-restriction Constricted horizons Conformity	Technologic ethos

Adolescent

Identity	Versus	Role Confusion	Societal Institution
Idealistic Integration of identifications with libidinal vicissitudes Integration of aptitudes with opportunity Confidence		Delinquency Psychotic episodes Doubt and sexual identity Overidentification with heroes, cliques, and crowds	Ideology and aristocracy

(Continues on p. 302)

Young Adult

Intimacy	Versus	Isolation	Societal Institution
Commitment		Self-absorption	Ethical sense
Sacrifice		Distancing behaviors	
Compromise		Character problems	
True genitality			
Work productivity			
Satisfactory sex relations			

Middle-aged Adult

Generativity	Versus	Stagnation	Societal Institution
Establishing and guiding the next generation		Regression to an obsessive need for pseudo intimacy	Ethos of generative succession
Productivity		Personal impoverishment	
Creativity		Early invalidism	
		Self-love	
		Lack of faith	

Older Adult

Integrity	Versus	Despair	Societal Institution
Assurance of order and meaning		Fear of death	Charity
Experience conveying world order and spiritual sense		Sense time as too short	
New and different love of one's parents		Disgust	
Defends the dignity of own life-style against threat			
Emotional integration			
Fellowship with others			
Acceptance of leadership			

(From Erikson EH: Childhood and Society. New York, WW Norton, 1968)

Every child passes through each stage and substage of cognitive development in the same sequence, although not according to a given timetable.

Every child develops strategies for interacting with the environment and knowing its properties.

There is a gradual progression from one period of cognitive development to another, with the acquisition of each new operation building on already existing ones.

The process of development is one in which increasing differentiation and complexity is matched by increasing integration and coordination of schemata.[6]

Early Learning

Maximal learning, said Piaget, takes place through the process of contemplative recognition, which precedes intentionality. During the period from 4 to 8 months of age, the infant evidences interest in the results of his own behaviors on the environment, and he invents procedures to make interesting sights last. These reactions of the infant are forerunners of contemplative recognition.

Contemplative recognition is the function of recognizing and remembering that what has disappeared will reappear. In other words, the infant sees mother appear, disappear, and reappear frequently enough to anticipate a recurrence of the experience. This ability to recognize when an object has reappeared extends to many other objects. From approximately 6 to 11 months of age, the infant demonstrates this cognitive process when he repeatedly throws an object and waits expectantly for someone to pick it up. The game of peek-a-boo also reinforces this process.

Representational intelligence refers to the manipulation of mental representations of things and actions, the anticipation of events and consequences of actions, and the ability to evoke an image of an absent object rather than simply recognizing it when it appears. The development of representational intelligence leads to the preoperational stage, wherein objects are classified and categorized. Rudimentary cognitive function precedes language development.[6]

Piaget emphasized the maturation of the nervous system in his theory of cognitive development. The abilities developed within each stage evolve according to the individual's unique timetable of maturation.

Behavioristic Theory

According to behavioristic theory, development is influenced by the stimulus–response interaction; behavior is shaped through the consistency of responding. Researchers have conducted studies to determine the effects of reinforcement of newborns' sucking behaviors, older infants' smiling behaviors, and other developmental skills, such as toilet training, sharing, helping, and cooperating.[11]

Reinforcement of Learning

The neonate is able to learn much more than is usually recognized by parents and professionals. Neonate learning occurs through reinforcement that coincides with need satisfaction.[20] Perceptual discrimination and active learning are possible for the newborn. Therefore, when a mothering person consistently appears along with a need-fulfilling stimulus (*e.g.,* the breast or bottle), the neonate relates the two and prefers that person over all others.

Differentiation between two faces and voices has been demonstrated during the first 2 weeks of the neonate's life. Furthermore, this recognition seems to be related to the infant's development of social communication skills by means of bodily movements and, within a short period of time, by means of the smile. These forms of social communication occur through mutual interaction of mother and neonate, which is reciprocally rewarding and reinforcing.

Current Developmental Theory

The newest model of development, a biopsychosocial model, discounts the idea that the optimal period for certain developmental behaviors is always in early childhood. It asserts, rather, that the human organism possesses a complexity that defies easy or simple classifications or comparisons.

Two attributes of the human brain, flexibility and plasticity, are developmentally significant and allow for a variety of adaptive sequences.[19] Therefore, although early life influences are considered very important, they are no longer thought to produce irreversible effects on the personality.

Consonance Versus Dissonance

An interactionist model of development focuses on the concept of "goodness of fit" and the related ideas of consonance and dissonance. This model demonstrates that development in a progressive direction occurs when consonance (or goodness of fit) exists and that dissonance (or poorness of fit) involves discrepancies between the individual and the environment. Such discrepancies result in distorted development and maladaptive functioning.[19] The goodness-of-fit concept implies that environmental demands and expectations are in accord with the individual's capacity to respond. This results in consonance or a sense of comfort, which makes progressive, optimal development possible.

Consider the following application of this concept: Mary is a shy, introverted individual who has just completed college with a bachelor's degree in biology. She restricts relationships to one or two people. She has two job opportunities from which to choose, one as a research assistant in a laboratory and the other as a public relations coordinator. They pay equitable and similar salaries. Using the goodness-of-fit concept, it is likely that Mary would be more comfortable and more adaptive as a research assistant than as a public relations coordinator and that her development would continue more smoothly.[20,21]

Developmental Issues in Nursing

Nurses are frequently called upon to assess developmental processes and progression in the course of implementing the nursing process. They frequently refer to any of these theories, or a combination of them, to determine probable causes of behavior and interventions that will facilitate effective behavior change. Psychiatric–mental health nurses are necessarily interested in developmental issues, because physical and emotional health are, in large part, determined by adaptive or maladaptive responses along the developmental continuum.

One useful framework considers the presence of

Table 18-1.   **Progression from Dependence to Interdependence**

INFANCY (0–1)	CHILDHOOD (1–12)		ADOLESCENCE			ADULTHOOD
		Early	*Middle*	*Late*		
Dependency	Decreasing dependency	Conflict in dependency	Struggle toward independence	Independence		Interdependency

dependency, independency, or interdependency in progressive stages on a continuum (see Table 18-1). This framework establishes that in healthy, adaptive states, there is progressive movement away from total dependency at birth to the ultimate adult position of interdependency.

The great struggle for independence takes place during the adolescent period and is responsible for creating marked equilibrium. Ego crystallization, the crucial issue during adolescence, occurs through the process of achieving independence. When this process is incompletely experienced, often observed in adolescent rebellion, it is usually worked out during later periods of life at a time when other processes should be occurring, thereby hindering the development of those phases.

Dependency is closely related to anxiety and an emotionally restricted self. Interdependency, on the other hand, is found in persons who are relatively free of anxiety and able to view themselves as capable individuals interacting with other capable individuals.

The overall goals of human development include social competence and mastery. Many believe that the first year of life is the most important; some would even propose that the first day of life may well be the most significant one.

It is clear that the study and understanding of development is complex and multifaceted, even before the added influence of cultural differences. The development of a child in America and another in Samoa will demonstrate obvious differences in the manner in which tasks are mastered, the time when they occur, and the utilization of skills. Nevertheless, there will be consistent sequential development in numerous areas of functioning across cultures; the children within a given culture will evidence linear progression toward mastery of certain tasks expected within the cultural group.

To understand development, the nurse must consider genetic transmission, cultural transmission, temperament, motivation, physical endowment, stimulus provision, and interaction with others. The fact that these forces contribute to development lends credence to the notion that developmental outcomes are not the responsibility of one person. In the past,

mothers were viewed as totally responsible for the healthiness of a child's development. Fathers, siblings, extended family, and even the child himself were seen as mere bystanders in the scenario. Furthermore, it was held that the child's development was essentially completed in 6 years and that, from the age of 6 on, only modification of the personality took place. Little attention focused on adult development, particularly on the mid-age and late-age periods.

Current developmental theories give rise to the hope that there is continuity in the process of development, and that self-actualization may occur even in the late-age period. Many examples of persons who achieved their greatest potential only after reaching elderly status are available. Some adults appear to progress, regress, and progress according to life circumstances or crises. Late-age development was a less prominent issue in the years when life expectancy did not exceed the mid-age period for most, but survival past the age of 100 years is not uncommon anymore. The 1970 United States census revealed that there were more than 10,600 Americans past the age of 100 years.[19]

Generally, development in the elderly is not as much a matter of achieving a higher level of functioning as it is a transformation, qualitative in nature, that is concerned with maintaining adaptive behavior governed by weakened physiological structure and increased egocentricity.[18] Adaptation requires considerable compensation for the individual whose sensory apparatus, from the 4th decade on, begins to limit function. As the 7th decade begins, the person's sensory and perceptual processes become slower, requiring a longer period of time to arrive at accuracy in problem-solving. Research findings suggest that the major change in intellectual functioning from midlife to early old age is related to reaction time. An understanding of this concept is important if nurses are to avoid infantalizing the aged individual who may respond to the label if he is regarded as incapable.[13] Often, people conclude that because the elderly person does not function as well physically as the young person, he is also less capable intellectually. Nurses are in a position to reinforce the elderly individual as

(Text continues on p. 310)

CHART 18-2
Unresolved Developmental Issues and Conflicts

The developmental tasks and issues that are faced throughout a person's lifetime normally occur without significant turmoil or trauma. Although the transitional phases between the stages of development usually increase tension and stress to some degree, the person moves from one stage to another without major incident, achieving higher levels of growth.

Some individuals, however, do not make smooth transitions through these stages of development and are, therefore, more vulnerable to develop psychiatric disorders in the future than those who make healthy, adaptive transitions. Several researchers have asserted that there are variables—including biological predisposition and psychosocial and psychological stressors, as well as transitional issues—that increase susceptibility to affective disorders.[2] Other researchers attribute some psychiatric disorders to early, unresolved issues.[3,4] Individuals at risk usually have difficulty dealing with social developmental issues. They are at risk for crises and psychological turmoil with each transitional stage of development. This turmoil is often manifested by an affective disorder.

The following case histories are examples of individuals who have experienced developmental turmoil.

Diane: Role Confusion versus Identity

Diane is a 15-year-old girl who has recently been admitted to the adolescent unit with a diagnosis of suicide attempt, overdose of Valium. During her initial interview she reveals that she recently broke up with her boyfriend, whom she had dated for about 6 months before she found out he was also dating her best friend. Her discovery of this situation led to an argument with the boyfriend and girlfriend at school. Shortly after arriving home from school, she drank several cans of beer and took her father's tranquilizers.

Diane's mother found her unconscious in her bedroom and called the paramedics, who transported her to the local emergency room. Her stomach was pumped and she was transferred to the Intensive Care Unit for two days of observation.

At the present time Diane is appropriately dressed and groomed. She has poor eye contact with the interviewer and expresses regret at not having succeeded with her suicide attempt. She says she is angry at her girlfriend for dating her boyfriend and that she wants their relationship (hers and her boyfriend's) to be like Jill's and Victor's on her favorite soap opera.

Diane's history reveals that she began drinking several years ago and "smokes pot" several times a week. Her parents are professionals and she spends many evenings alone or with neighbors. She makes poor grades in school and has frequently skipped classes in the past 6–8 months. Her parents have tried to talk with her about these problems, but they said that they felt she was "too much to handle" and would eventually "grow out of her problems."

Nursing Care Plan: Diane

Nursing Diagnoses	Outcome Criteria	Intervention	Rationale	Evaluation

1. Hopelessness and high risk for suicide, related to recent attempt and inadequate support system	1. Client will not act on suicidal impulse	1. Suicide precautions/assessment must be carried out
		  Safe Climate
		  Assign one
		   nurse for
		   1-to-1 until
			1. Clients who attempt are at risk to try again within 24 to 72 hours after initial attempt; these	Client will no longer express thoughts of suicide, helplessness, or hopelessness ideation
				
				(Continues on p. 306)

Nursing Diagnoses	Outcome Criteria	Intervention	Rationale	Evaluation
		she is no longer suicidal	measures provide a safe and accepting environment	
		Establish trusting relationship		
		Remove dangerous objects from the client's room, *e.g.,* sharp cutting objects, belts		
		Assess suicidal ideations/ thoughts		This must be ongoing process during hospitalization
		Use hospital guidelines for the suicidal client		
2. Disturbance in self-concept/self-esteem, related to poor limit-setting by parents and lack of positive reinforcement	2. Client will verbalize more positive feelings about herself; parents will improve limit-setting/structure in family system and increase communication within family	2. Establish regular times to meet with client after progress from one-to-one observation	2. This will promote and establish trusting relationship ↑ positive feelings and ↓ feelings of worthlessness	2. Client will be able to demonstrate, verbally and nonverbally, positive feelings about herself; family will report greater satisfaction in interacting
		Provide activities in which she will be successful; praise when appropriate or when task completed		
		Avoid negative/angry feedback (provide constructive criticism)		
		Set limits and be consistent		
		Encourage client to ventilate feelings about recent suicide attempt, *e.g.,* how she feels about not succeeding		

Mrs. Jones: Integrity versus Despair

Mrs. Jones is a 68-year-old divorced woman who is admitted to the acute psychiatric unit with a diagnosis of major depression. She divorced several decades ago, has dated infrequently, and lived with her 90-year-old mother until her mother's death 10 months ago. She has few friends and has spent most of the past 5 years caring for her mother.

Mrs. Jones complains of difficulty sleeping, manifested by early morning awakening. She has lost about 20 pounds over the past 2 to 3 months and attributes this to a "poor appetite." She says she's having "trouble concentrating and forgetfulness." She was referred for admission by her family doctor, who felt she could no longer take care of herself.

Mrs. Jones does not have a history of previous psychiatric problems. She does not smoke or drink. She has been treated for adult onset diabetes for the past 2 years with an oral hypoglycemic agent.

Her psychosocial assessment reveals a depressed, 68-year-old woman who cries frequently and has poor eye contact with the interviewer. Her general appearance is unkempt and she mumbles often about missing her mother. She expresses feelings of hopelessness—and states that she will never recover from her mother's death. She has few friends and limited community resources.

Toward the end of the interview, Mrs. Jones expresses disgust with her life and with the fact that she is old and that no one cares about her. She says she is afraid of dying alone.

Nursing Care Plan for Mrs. Jones

Nursing Diagnoses	Outcome Criteria	Intervention	Rationale	Evaluation
1. Dysfunctional grieving, related to maladaptive coping skills	1. Client will resolve grief issues and improve coping skills	1. Encourage ventilation of feelings related to death of mother; use cognitive techniques; involve in unit activities that foster working through grief process	1. Gain insight into feelings about mother's death; these will increase her awareness and assist her in separating emotions from intellect in dealing with death of mother	1. Client will be able to verbalize to nursing staff
2. Social isolation, related to lack of meaningful relationships	2. Client will increase social interactions and improve social skills	2. Encourage involvement in group therapy activities; assign ward activities allowing her a choice of what she wants to do; prior to discharge, refer to community groups	2. Activities will decrease self-absorption in grieving and will distract her from having constant negative thoughts; involving her in groups will increase her	2. Ongoing process of noting her involvement; initially 1-to-1 with nurses; later, with a larger group *(Continues on p. 308)*

Nursing Diagnoses	Outcome Criteria	Intervention	Rationale	Evaluation
			social skills and assist her in gaining insight into her behavior/feelings	
3. Disturbance in self-concept/self-esteem, related to lack of positive reinforcement	3. Client will verbalize thoughts and feelings evidencing positive self-image and self-actualization	3. Encourage participation into activities in which she will be successful and offer praise as appropriate; avoid negative feedback and provide constructive criticism in positive manner	3. This will increase and improve her self-confidence, will decrease her negative reinforcement/self-depreciation	3. Client's ability to verbalize how she feels about herself; her general appearance, makeup, dress, etc.
4. Hopelessness and potential for suicide, related to inadequate support system and maladaptive coping skills	4. Client will not act on suicidal impulse	4. Maintain suicide precautions, close observation of client (see Nursing Care Plan for Diane)	4. Suicide precautions will provide the needed environment for client's return to safety	4. Ongoing process

Ms. Moore: Trust versus Mistrust

Jody Moore is a 30-year-old woman who requests psychiatric treatment in a crisis unit for situational depression. She was terminated from her job several months ago after working as a medical records clerk for 6 years. She complains that her supervisor was against her and was responsible for her recent job loss.

Jody complains of sleeplessness and poor appetite, which has led to a weight loss of about 12 pounds over this period of time. She also complains of irritability and difficulty getting along with her mother. She had to move back into the mother's home recently because of her financial situation, and she expresses feelings of failure because of her present living situation.

Further history-taking reveals a chronic history of relationship problems with her mother since childhood. She also reports that she "has never been able to get along with people" and feels no one likes her.

During the interview, Jody is tearful and has a depressed mood and poor eye contact. She frequently criticizes herself for her recent job loss. She expresses feelings of being a failure and reminisces about her mother "telling her all the time she wishes she were a boy instead of a girl."

Jody is dressed appropriately and wears little makeup. She expresses regret for seeking psychiatric treatment because she does not think anyone can help her.

Nursing Care Plan for Ms. Moore

Nursing Diagnoses	Outcome Criteria	Intervention	Rationale	Evaluation
1. Ineffective individual coping and mistrust, related to lack of positive, meaningful relationships	1. Client will be able to form trusting relationships	1. Set up time to meet with client Be on time Follow through with agreed meeting times Allow client to have input into meeting time, place, and date Be consistent Set limits when appropriate Encourage client to join community groups and activities when appropriate Encourage ventilation/expression of feelings	1. These activities promote trust and feelings of safety for the client This will increase her social skills and decrease social isolation Ventilation promotes insight into feelings about present stressful situation	1. Client will verbalize feeling comfortable; she will discuss feelings easily with nurse and mental health team members Client will demonstrate willingness to join and participate in groups
2. Disturbance in self-concept related to lack of positive reinforcement and recent crisis of job loss	2. Client will develop a positive self image and express feelings of self-worth	2. Encourage client to identify strengths Praise when appropriate Be genuine when giving feedback Avoid negative statements Provide opportunity for participation in activities she will succeed in Encourage her to examine reasons behind failures	2. This allows client to look into positive aspects of herself Positive feedback will increase positive feelings about herself Looking at failures will assist her in developing the ability to deal with them realistically	2. Client will be able to focus on positive aspects of herself and verbalize some understanding about failures, without seeing *herself* as a failure

a person who has wisdom, responsibility, and prestige.[13]

Summary

This chapter has presented an overview of five different developmental theories—intrapsychic, interpersonal, social learning, cognitive, and behavioristic. The integration of these theories has evolved into a body of knowledge permitting further study of developmental issues. Some of the major points of the chapter are as follows:

1. Human development is a complex and multifaceted process involving a variety of forces that effect unique personalities.
2. Development is currently considered to be a continuous process, unfolding throughout the lifespan, rather than being limited to a few years in early life.
3. No longer is the responsibility for development placed on the mothering person alone, but on the complex and interacting influences on the individual.
4. The developmental period of old age is a focus of current attention. Evidence supports the idea that a qualitative level of development continues in the increasing numbers of elderly persons in our population.
5. Healthy, adaptive adult functioning occurs at a level of interdependency.

References

1. Addario D: Developmental Considerations in the Concept of Affective Illness. Clin Psychiatry 46 (Oct): 46–53, 1985
2. Akiskal HA, Mckinney WT Jr: Overview of Recent Research in Depression: Integration of Conceptual Models into a Comprehensive Clinical Framework. Arch Gen Psychiatry, 32 (Mar): 285–305, 1975
3. Bowlby J: Attachment and Loss, Vol 2, Separation, Anxiety and Anger. London, Hogarth Press and Institute of Psychoanalysis, 1972
4. Brown GW, Prudo R: Psychiatric Disorder in a Rural and an Urban Population; Aetiology of Depression. Psychol Med 11 (August): 581–599, 1981
5. Call JD: Normal Development. In Noshpitz JD (ed): Basic Handbook of Child Psychiatry, Vol I, pp 1–10. New York, Basic Books, 1979
6. Drucker J: Development from One to Two Years: Ego Development. In Noshpitz JD (ed): Basic Handbook of Child Psychiatry, Vol I, pp 157–164. New York, Basic Books, 1979
7. Emde R, Robinson J: The First Two Months: Recent Research in Developmental Psychobiology and the Changing View of the Newborn. In Noshpitz JD (ed): Basic Handbook of Child Psychiatry, Vol I, pp 72–105. New York, Basic Books, 1979
8. Erikson EH: Childhood and Society, 2d ed. New York, WW Norton, 1963
9. Mausch I: Old Age in the U.S.: A Time to Wait. Geriatr Nurs 1 (May/June): 42–43, 1980
10. May R: The Meaning of Anxiety. New York, The Ronald Press, 1950
11. O'Leary KD, Wilson GT: Behavior Therapy: Application and Outcome. Englewood Cliffs, N.J., Prentice-Hall, 1975
12. Pierce P: Intelligence and Learning in the Aged. J Gerontol Nurs 6 (May): 268–270, 1980
13. Plawecki H, Plawecki J: Act Your Age. Geriatr Nurs 1 (September/October): 179–181, 1980
14. Robson KS: Development of the Human Infant from Two to Six Months. In Noshpitz JD (ed): Basic Handbook of Child Psychiatry, pp 106–112. New York, Basic Books, 1979
15. Roiphe H: A Theoretical Overview of Preoedipal Development During the First Four Years of Life. In Noshpitz JD (ed): Basic Handbook of Child Psychiatry, pp 118–127. New York, Basic Books, 1979
16. Rosen H: Pathway To Piaget. Cherry Hill, New Jersey, Postgraduate International Inc, 1977
17. Sullivan HS: Clinical Studies in Psychiatry. New York, WW Norton, 1956
18. Sullivan HS: The Fusion of Psychiatry and Social Science. New York, WW Norton, 1964
19. Schaie KW: Psychological Changes From Midlife to Early Old Age: Implications for the Maintenance of Mental Health. Am J Orthopsychiatry 51 (April): 199–218, 1981
20. Thomas A: Current Trends in Developmental Theory. Am J Orthopsychiatry 51 (October): 580–609, 1981
21. Thomas A, Chess S: The Dynamics of Psychological Development. New York, Brunner/Mazel, 1980

19

Sexuality and Sexual Concerns

Sharon Byers

I am a sexual being. So is she. Together, we produce an experience that is exquisite for both of us. She invites me to know her sexually, and I invite her to know me sexually. We share our erotic possibilities in delight and ecstasy. If she want me and I don't want her, I cannot lie. My body speaks only truth. And I cannot take her unless she gives herself. Her body cannot lie.

Sidney M. Jourard,
The Transparent Self, 1971

Chapter Preview

Sexuality is an integral part of the personality, a significant aspect of the functioning of the identity during varied states of wellness. Sexual activity is a form of communication, a method of self-affirmation, a pleasurable form of play, and a reflection of the individual's value system.

This chapter explores the development of sexuality throughout the life span. A humanistic perspective emphasizes the importance of identifying the client's sexual norms and needs and facilitating adaptation accordingly. The chapter describes the stages of the human sexual response cycle, traditional lifestyles and nontraditional methods of sexual expression, and sexual dysfunctions and their treatment approaches. The nurse's role and intervention with clients manifesting sexual problems or concerns are also discussed.

Learning Objectives

On completion of the chapter, you should be able to accomplish the following:

1. define sexuality, sensuality, sex role, and gender identity
2. differentiate between sex derivative, adjunctive, and arbitrary differences
3. discuss the genetic, hormonal, and psychological influences on sexual development
4. describe the stages of human sexual response
5. compare traditional and alternative sexual lifestyles
6. discuss the client's sexual needs during specific physical or emotional disorders
7. describe the common sexual problems of men and women clients who seek sex therapy
8. apply the nursing process to the care of a client manifesting a sexual problem

The Meaning of Sexuality

Sexuality is the expression and experience of the self as a sexual being. It is, therefore, a state of both the body and mind and a crucial part of the personality. Sexuality is not limited to overt sexual activity, such as sexual intercourse, but includes solitary activities like studying, walking, and relaxing. Sexuality is a part of every relationship, whether it is primarily a sexual relationship or not; it is the rapport that is established between the self and the other.[21]

An important aspect of sexuality is *sensuality*, which is the expression and experience of self as a sensual being. Sensuality means the ability to experience enjoyment through the senses, such as touching a pleasing fabric, listening to good music, or touching the skin of a loved one. Sensuality is a necessary component of fulfilled sexuality. Sensual attraction, however, does not necessarily lead to a wish for sexual activity; it refers merely to pleasure in the company of the other.

One key to unlocking one's enjoyment of sexuality and sensuality is through body awareness and acceptance. *Sex roles* are culturally determined patterns associated with male and female social behavior and may be accepted or rejected by the individual. *Gender identity,* or how one chooses to view oneself as a male or female in interaction with others, is an individual and unique expression.

Body appearance holds some limitations for self-direction. The *transsexual,* for example, is a person who is able to reject clearly his or her physical sexual appearance and prefers to undergo surgery, psychotherapy, and hormone treatments to make a complete "sex change." More common are the problems of men's and women's inabilities to accept their bodies to the fullest extent to enable sexual fulfillment. To ease the acceptance of their bodies, men and women may perceive a need to change their bodies through dieting or exercise. Nevertheless, body acceptance ultimately depends on one's ability to relax with one's body and to allow physical sensations to be accepted and experienced as they are, without defensively screening out unwanted sensations or perceptually twisting sensations.

People view sexual activity through a structure made up of religious values and stereotypical myths. Reality is shaped by choice, our assigned sets of meanings, and even by anxiety, fear, and lack of knowledge.[11] Religious beliefs and other sets of personal values usually result in our classification of sexual activity into one of three categories.

1. Procreational sex refers to sexual activity for the purpose of conceiving children.
2. Relational sex refers to sexual activity for the purpose of strengthening or fulfilling commitments of a relationship.
3. Recreational sex refers to sexual activity for the purpose of play and personal enjoyment.[16]

Sexual Differences

Sex Derivative Differences

The body holds the only inevitabilities of sexuality. These inevitable differences are that men normally impregnate women and women are normally able to lactate, gestate, and menstruate. Nothing else, including aggressivity, strength, or sex role has been found to be strictly related to either male or female.[16] The other differences are relatively arbitrary, some appearing as predispositions created by anatomic differences, such as baldness and the position one must take to urinate. These are called *sex derivative* differences and they are not absolutes. These differences vary from individual to individual according to familial tendencies, physical makeup, and personality preferences.

Sex Adjunctive Differences

Sex adjunctive differences are those seen fairly consistently from culture to culture but are even less related to real physical differences than are the sex derivative differences. Examples of sex adjunctive differences are the choice of male or female to earn money for the household and the traditional role of the woman in childrearing. These differences are based on some physical differences, such as muscle mass and the ability to lactate, but were more important determinants of male and female preferred roles in the past. These roles tend to persist due to historic precedence, but are now being questioned and challenged frequently by modern "house husbands" and career women.[7] These sex adjunctive differences are of great political importance today in the liberation of men and women; stereotypical roles have become chains to people who prefer to use choice rather than history to determine their daily activities.

These sex adjunctive differences may have been linked to hormonal or genetic programming during the days of our early primate ancestors. For example, one male hormone, androgen, does increase physical activity in the individual; however, the expression of this activity as physical aggression or dominance is not related to hormonal factors but rather to individual choice and learning—that is, androgen may influence one to be more aggressive, but ultimately the personality structure and choices of modern men and women determine behavior.

Sex Arbitrary Differences

Sex arbitrary differences are purely determined by culture and therefore vary from culture to culture. Such differences include face painting and genital mutilation. In the Anglo-Saxon cultures, it is acceptable for the female to wear colors on her face, called makeup. In other cultures men wear face paints. In Judeo-Christian cultures, it is common for men to be circumcised as infants. In other cultures, the young female undergoes similar procedures, such as removing or cutting away a part of the clitoris or the hood of the clitoris. In most of these situations of genital mutila-

tion of infants, the procedure is believed to be painless, despite the infants' cries to the contrary, and is undergone without anesthetic. The procedure is also usually explained as required by hygienic, as well as religious, needs.[16]

It is sometimes difficult to understand how basically arbitrary distinctions can be viewed as unquestionable and inevitable differences between the sexes. The explanation for this view lies in the fact that our world is shaped by a basic he-schema and she-schema. Our expectations, habits, traditions, mores, customs, norms, and the wielding of power throughout history form the basis for these schema.[20] The interpretations of difference between the sexes are evident from the first days of life, when baby boys and baby girls are handled and talked to in measurably different ways.[16] The infant's behavior is also interpreted differently according to sex-related expectations and perceptions. Choices of gifts, colors, and activities are determined according to the child's sex and perceptions of how a child of that sex should behave.

There are also age-related distinctions regarding sexual differences. For example, in our culture, children are not generally considered to be sexual. Therefore, we observe the panic of a mother finding her toddler son fondling his penis, or the horror of parents discovering their 13-year-old daughter's birth control pills. The infant's first erection and lubrication occurs soon after birth, indicating the pervasive nature of sexuality. Elderly people are also thought of as asexual by many in the American culture. Two hundred years ago, few individuals lived long enough to become elderly; we have no precedence on which to form our view of sexuality in the elderly. Our cultural perspective on the sexual needs of the elderly has not progressed as rapidly as the average life span has grown.

Nurses' Knowledge of Sexual Differences

The task of the nurse regarding sexuality is fourfold.

1. To be knowledgeable about sexuality and the "norms" of society
2. To use this knowledge to understand others' behaviors and attitudes that differ in cultural and individual perspectives from one's own
3. To use this understanding to facilitate the client's adaptation and optimal health
4. To be aware of, and comfortable with, one's own sexuality

Adaptation does not mean conforming to others' expectations or norms, but rather responding to the world without losing one's unique qualities. Through adaptation, a person maintains his choices and values while accepting those of differing choices and values.[21] The nurse's awareness of her own and others' feelings and attitudes about sexual behavior and differing choices enables her to respond to an encounter based on a sincere understanding of the needs of the client, rather than on emotional taboos or her own stereotypical beliefs.

Sexual Development

Sexual development occurs in the embryo and continues throughout the life span. A variety of influences (genetic, hormonal, and psychological) have an impact on this development.

Genetic Influences

Chromosomes initiate sexual development. Chromosomes, found in every cell of the body, are the carriers of genetic programming information. Within the ovum and sperm are the chromosomal offerings of the two parents, which determine the genetic makeup of the child. The male's sperm cell determines the sex of the embryo at conception by adding either an X chromosome or a Y chromosome to the X chromosome contained within the ovum. Two X chromosomes result in a female fetus; an X and a Y chromosome result in a male fetus.

Sometimes, these groupings of chromosomes occur differently, resulting in such variations as XXY, or *Klinefelter's syndrome*. This extra X chromosome produces a male who appears normal until adolescence, when decreased production of the male hormone (testosterone) results in small testes, infertility, and a predisposition for a low libido (or sexual interest). Behavioral differences may be associated with Klinefelter's syndrome due to genetic predisposition. These include generalized passivity, lack of ambition, and a predisposition to sudden outbursts of aggression. These behavioral and libido differences are reversed with treatments of testosterone, even when undertaken as late as in adulthood.[11] Apparently, hormonal therapy affects the libido to enable a broader range of behavioral choices.

Turner's syndrome occurs when the second sex chromosome is missing, producing the pattern XO. This syndrome results in short females without functioning gonads. Until puberty, no problems are noted; however, at the normal age of puberty, the breasts do not develop and there are no menses. The psychological problem associated with this chromosomal variation involves the effect of stigma caused by the differences between this person and the female norm. The absence of hormones during fetal devel-

opment results in possible deficits in motor coordination, range of affect, and directional sense. The patient with Turner's syndrome may seem more complacent and seem to have less initiative than other girls or women of similar age.[8] Although it is uncertain why these traits are found in women with Turner's syndrome, an answer offered by research seems to be that genetic patterning creates a predisposition that is fostered by cultural influences. Hormone therapy results in normal breast development and menses in the female with Turner's syndrome, but the short stature does not change, resulting in a woman no taller than 4½ to 5 feet tall.

The XYY chromosomal pattern produces a male with few physical differences from an XY male, except for a slightly taller stature, low sperm count, and some abnormalities of the seminiferous tubules.[18] As children, these boys appear less socially mature, more impulsive, and less successful in interpersonal relationships than their peers. As adults, these men are often found in penal institutions, perhaps due to some intellectual deficit making them more prone to break the law. These men tend to commit crimes, but not necessarily crimes of an aggressive nature.[11]

Nursing implications of the diagnosis of one of these chromosomal abnormalities include counseling with parents and child regarding the effect of the diagnosis on the developing self-image of the child. The nurse educates parents and child about the typical behavioral predispositions and appearance differences associated with the syndrome. The nurse explains that, although hormone therapy is a useful means of reducing the difference between the child and the normal male or female, it is not a "cure" for the syndrome. In all cases, hormone therapy can only change superficial differences. Counseling is recommended for intervention in, or prevention of, a crisis in response to the diagnosis as the client and family experience the loss of a "normal" identity. Counseling may also help family members learn to reinforce adaptive behaviors and shape behaviors away from predispositions that may result in maladaptive behaviors.

Hormonal Influences

During the first 6 weeks of development, male and female fetuses are anatomically alike. At 6 weeks, primitive gonads are beginning to develop but are not yet differentiated as male or female. Following this time, hormones have the greatest effect on the sexual differentiation of the fetus. At 8 weeks, if testosterone is present in sufficient levels, testes develop from the indistinct gonads. If no testosterone or a less-than-normal amount of testosterone for a male of this age is secreted by the 12th gestational week, ovaries are formed. Even if the genotype is XY, the absence of testosterone at this partricular time of fetal development causes female differentiation to occur. This would result in an anatomic female who is capable of procreation but who bears a XY genotype.

These sexual differentiations occur in the external genitalia, the internal sex structures, and the delicate nervous pathways and other portions of the brain to create the pattern for further development. The ambiguous gonadal structures develop into uterus, fallopian tube, and vagina in the absence of testosterone. With testosterone and androgen secretion at sufficiently high levels, the same structures become the vas deferens, seminal vesicles, and ejaculatory ducts.

Externally, androgen stimulation results in the urogenital folds joining to form a penis. Without androgen, this fold becomes the labia minora. The hypothalamic-pituitary-gonadal system in the brain responds to the presence of androgen by becoming noncyclic. Without androgen, female hormones result in female structures and a cyclic system, with fluctuating hormonal levels producing menses and fertility (see Fig. 19-1).[11]

A variety of hormonal imbalances may affect the development of the fetus, so that a genetic female develops male genitalia or, more likely, ambiguous genitalia with a hypertrophied clitoris. A genetic male could develop internal or atrophied testes, ambiguous genitalia (such as a penis and a small vaginal opening), or an atrophied penis. Such variations differ from those seen in chromosomal abnormalities in that the original structures determined by the genotype are sex-appropriate, but an improper balance of male and female hormones results in an ambiguous stage of sexual development of the fetus.

Diagnosis and treatment with hormone therapy assists the child with ambiguous genitalia to have a normal life and reproduce. Many times, the fetal development is so different from the genetic structure that the best decision is to raise the child as a child of the sex of the genitalia rather than the genotype. The learned element of sexuality is apparently the most important influence after birth, because these children rarely have problems developing gender identity if they are treated consistently as the sex assigned early in life. Surgery, hormone therapy, and counseling with the parents are critical elements in a healthy pattern of development. During such procedures, the child is less confused and traumatized if the situation is described as a "hormone imbalance" rather than referring to "male" or "female" characteristics. Parents will adapt more readily to the birth of a child with ambiguous genitalia if the delivery room staff do not refer to the child as either sex, until careful study results in the assignment of sex of greatest likelihood of development.[11]

Development of Gender Identity

Infants are treated differently according to their sex. Undoubtedly, differences of parental behavior result in differences of behavior of the child. According to Freudian or psychodynamic theory, the first 3 years of life are crucial in the development of gender identity because, during this time, the child identifies with the parent of the same sex and develops a complementary relationship with the parent of the opposite sex. Biochemically, these first 3 years are possibly crucial in the development of neural pathways that further result in certain predispositions of behavior according to sex. According to learning theory, the responses of others teach the child to develop a gender identity of male or female early in life. Another theory considers sexual development to occur as imprinting, so that genetic as well as environmental influences result in the development of a stable gender identity of male or female at a set age of 2 to 3 months.[19]

Many theorists, although accepting the importance of early experience, development, and learning, reject the idea of a fixed identity at such a young, and seemingly arbitrary, age. These theorists believe that a variety of influences develop predispositions (that may or may not be realized) in response to lifelong experience, development, and learning. These theorists believe that maleness and femaleness are not fixed points but exist on a continuum that is open to interpretation and expression according to cultural pressures and preferences. The choices of the individual ultimately become decisive in developing the gender identity in response to the experiences of life. The normally developed male and female human share most of the same "male" and "female" hormones, but in differing proportions according to the genetic and hormonal development of the individual. Although they are normally differentiated, the male and female are much more like one another than they are like less differentiated individuals having genotypes other than XX or XY, or than they are like individuals who developed without the influence of both types of sex hormones.

The first step of gender-identity development occurs as the child becomes aware of the differences of the sexes and perceives that he or she is male or female, as compared to others. This basic recognition of one's sex (whether anatomically clear or assigned due to anatomic ambiguity) is called *sexual identity*.[10] Sexual identity allows the child to clearly interpret the behaviors of others as behavior appropriate for a male

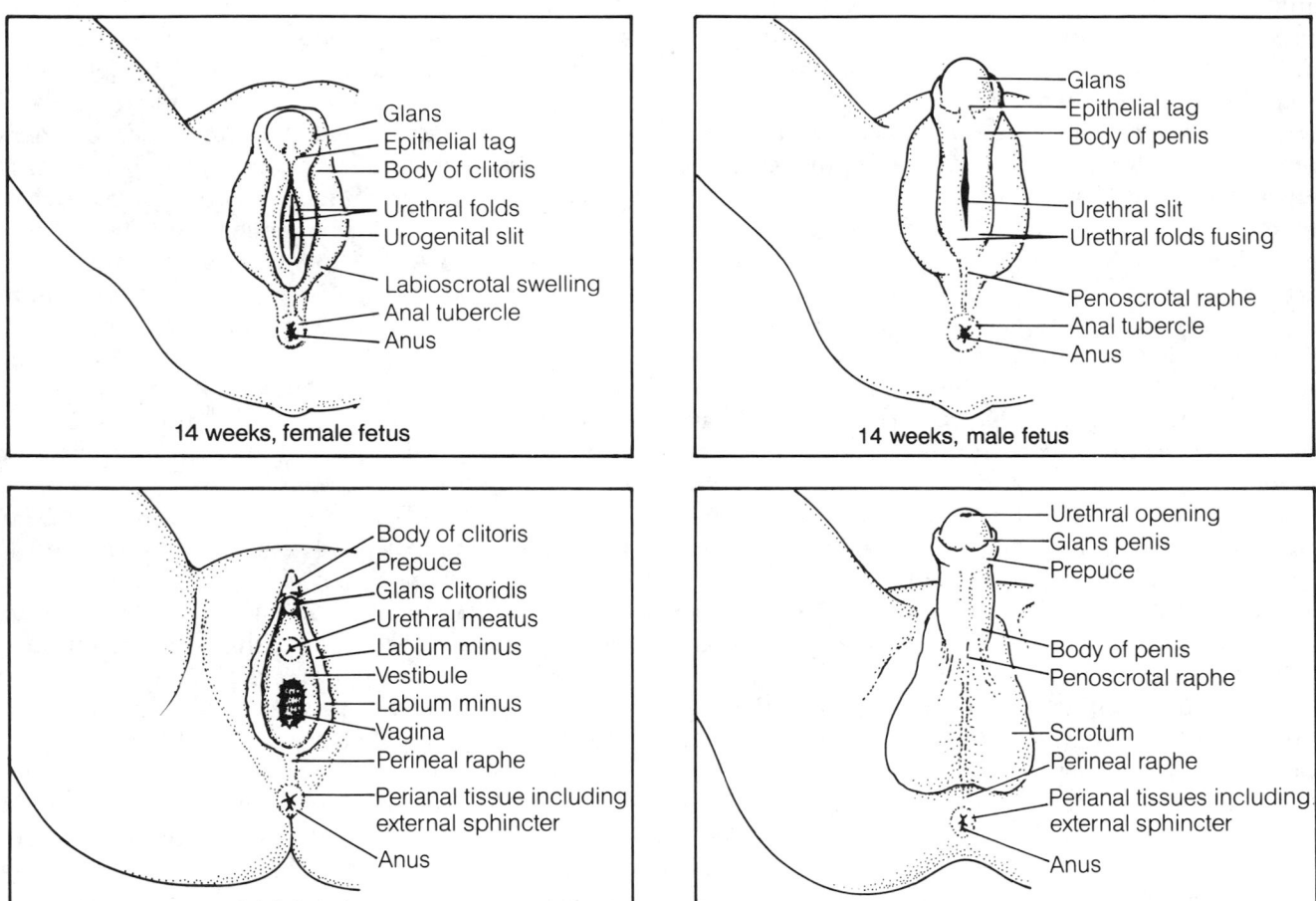

Figure 19-1. *Sexual differentiation.*

or female, and as different or the same as the sex of the child.[6]

During early childhood, the child forms bonds between himself and male and female significant people. How these bonds are formed affects how the child will prefer to develop his or her sexual identity. Par-

ents and other important adults serve as role models and teachers about how men and women act and relate with each other.

Gender identity refers to how the child feels about his or her sexual identity; that is, how the child decides to interpret his or her sexual identity for himself or herself. The development of *gender role* refers to how the child's gender identity will be expressed socially, in behavior with others of the same and opposite sex.

Children tend to prejudge themselves and others regarding sexual orientation and identity based on information and attitudes mimicked from parental behavior, because they have little real experience on which to base their own behaviors. Often, this results in very rigid distinctions of gender roles. On the other hand, if children are told about sexuality, about differences and similarities between the sexes, and about sexual behavior between the sexes before puberty, they develop a more matter-of-fact approach to sex. Later on, they are able to make important decisions about their own behavior based on information, rather than on emotions, stereotypes, or expectations of others.[16]

During early childhood, fantasies also play an important role in the child's developing gender identity. These fantasies include images of ultimate self-satisfaction and feelings of self-fulfillment. Children's fantasies do not tend to be as structured or realistic as those of adults. These fantasy associations are formed according to feelings of pleasure, and are instrumental in the development of the child's system of symbols pertaining to self. These symbols are uncensored by the expectations of society and loved ones, and are therefore truly creative events of the child. This system of symbols and fantasies takes on an erotic quality when the child reaches puberty.[16]

These fantasies guide the *choice of sexual object*; that is, the individual's choice of an object for sexual expression. For most people, symbols and fantasies are abstractions during childhood, but in adolescence they develop into an image of the ideal man or woman. For others, the system of abstractions persists, and the adult's sexual interest is invested in objects, events, or particular types of people; this is termed *paraphilias*. The fantasies of the child before puberty probably correlate with later choices of sexual expression when he becomes sexually active.[14]

The preadolescent years are an important period in the development of gender identity because, during these years, the child experiences his first bond of an adult nature. The preadolescent usually forms this intense bond or friendship with a peer of the same sex, although he may have a strong case of "hero worship" of an older person. This sensitive preadolescent period enables the child to begin to shed childhood values and interests and replace them with those of the adult world. The intense preadolescent relationship is not unlike a love relationship. It is usually not one-sided like the "crushes" of earlier childhood but may be just as fantasy-oriented and

romantically obsessive, whether the romantic element is covert or overt. These intense relationships sometimes become sexual, resulting in an early homosexual or heterosexual experience. This does not, however, indicate the life-long sexual object choice of the preadolescent. Nevertheless, the resolution and success of this bond creates early perceptions about roles in a sexual relationship.

During the adolescent phase of development, the adolescent expresses his perceptions of roles through sexual interest in another. Although sexual object choice is usually determined during adolescence, this choice can, and frequently does, change in adult years. The way in which early romantic relationships develop and satisfy the adolescent's needs and desires greatly affects his future behavior in relationships.

Life experience and opportunities and increasing self-awareness influence gender identity, gender role, and sexual object choice throughout the adult years. The early and middle adult years focus on sexually solidifying a long-term relationship and procreating. In middle age and later maturity, the focus turns again to the self and to personal fulfillment. In older age, sexual activity becomes symbolic of the continuation of social abilities and the reaffirmation of the self.

Sexual Expression

Sexual object choice determines sexual expression. This choice is formed by an internal fantasy image of the "ideal other." Dating behaviors are attempts to find this perfect other and develop a relationship rich in personal satisfaction. The success or failure of early adolescent relationships depends greatly on how well the fantasy actually fits the person. As people mature, their fantasies change. The "ideal-person" image is usually altered by learning more about the needs, desires, and behaviors of others. A more mature person may be successful in falling in love because the fantasy may be more realized.[16] If the individual's fantasy is of an object, as in the paraphilias, he may still develop feelings of concern, affection, and erotic interest in another person in response to experience.

The state of "being in love" means total involvement with, and devotion to, another person. In this state, sexual activity is undertaken according to perceived mutual needs and desires, which are expressed nonverbally during acts of lovemaking. The ability to send and receive these nonverbal cues accurately is necessary in sexual relationships. Also, people usually engage in sexual activity in a state of *abandonment*, in which each partner abandons his or her body to the pleasure of the other, and becomes totally immersed in delighting the body of the other.[16]

"Being in love" is obviously not the sole motivation for sexual activity. Sometimes, people are unable to integrate their images of an ideal relationship partner and an ideal sexual partner. They then find themselves in a relationship with one person, with whom they are "in love," but deeply sexually attracted to another person. Some people do not like the man or woman with whom they enjoy the most intense sexual pleasure. Some men and women, perhaps due to conflicting feelings about sexual activity, believe that they can only experience sexual abandonment with someone they do not like or respect. It is probably true that relationships endure when they contain the potential for both sexual and personal pleasure for both parties.

Human Sexual Response

The research of Masters and Johnson developed physiological information about the human sexual response cycle. They identified four phases of the cycle and labeled them excitement, plateau, orgasm, and resolution. Kaplan's work suggested renaming these desire, excitement, and orgasm for better understanding of the physiological process.[10] More subjectively experiential or psychological approaches suggest a pre-excitement or transitional phase during which the partners are psychologically receptive to erotic stimuli.[8] The following discussions are based on Kaplan's system. The phases are discussed as specific and consistent. In fact, individuals may experience these phases in variations of these descriptions, according to individual differences and a variety of relationship, health, and environmental influences.

Desire

This phase involves the activation of areas of the brain to produce sexual appetite or drive; it does not include actual changes in the genital organs. It is experienced as a desire to engage in a sexual encounter. This may include genital sensations, or may be experienced as a feeling of restlessness, "sexiness," or just interest and openness to sex. The exact way in which the neural system of the brain creates these sensations is not clearly understood. It is assumed that these neural pathways are connected with both pleasure and pain centers of the brain. This would explain the pleasurable, euphoric feeling people have when engaging in sex, as well as the absence of sexual desire when a person is in pain. The desire phase seems to be controlled by the individual's perception of the environment, by personal preferences and attractions to other people, and by the absence of inhibitory influences. Sexual desire will exist and build only in the absence of inhibitory forces such as fear, anxiety, discomfort, mental preoccupation (*e.g.*, worry), a higher-level need (*e.g.*, hunger), or an intense emotion (*e.g.*, anger). However, forces that are inhibitory in some people, such as pain or anger, may create a higher base level of excitement and actually increase sexual arousal in people who do not perceive these sensations as frightening or aversive. Although we do not understand this mechanism, it is another example of the highly individualistic nature of the sexual experience.

Excitement

The next phase, excitement, is brought on by the psychological stimulation of the desire phase, such as fantasy or romantic communication. Physiological stimulation, such as touching, kissing, fondling, licking, or biting erotic parts of the body, produces the genital changes of the excitement phase. The areas on the body that are particularly sensitive to erotic stimulation are called *erogenous zones*. These zones differ among individuals, but generally include the neck, mouth, breasts, inner thighs, and genital areas. The anus and navel are also erogenous areas for some people.

The petting and fondling activities engaged in during the excitement phase of the sexual response cycle are called *foreplay*. For many people, foreplay is the most important part of sexual activity. The caring, nurturing, and attentive behaviors between the sexual partners communicate concern and appreciation for the needs, desires, and sexual nature of the other. Young men and women of various ages sometimes reach orgasm (or climax) in response to intense foreplay alone. Nevertheless, this phase of sexual activity is the one most frequently omitted, especially if the couple perceives sex as relational or procreational, rather than recreational.

This phase in the female begins with lubrication, expansion of the clitoris, and nipple erection. There is a generalized tensing of muscles throughout the body, and increased heart rate, respirations, blood pressure, and motor restlessness. A fine rash or "sex flush" also appears over the abdomen and chest of many women.

In males, this phase begins with erection of the penis, elevation of the testes, nipple erection, and sometimes a sex flush. Heart rate, respiratory rate, blood pressure, and motor restlessness increase in men as in women.

In the female, vaginal vasocongestion results in a reduction of the opening of the vagina, and the development of a swollen and tensing area called the *orgasmic platform* in the lower third of the vagina and the labia minora. The clitoris retracts from the normal position. Breasts enlarge through areolar engorgement. The sex flush, generalized muscle tension, rising heart rate, blood pressure, and respiratory rate continue.

In men, there is an increase in size of the coronal area of the glans penis. The testes continue to increase in size and elevate. The sex flush and motor restlessness increase. Heart rate, blood pressure, and respiratory rate rise.

Orgasm

The next phase of sexual response is called *orgasm*. In females, orgasm consists of three to fifteen strong, rhythmic contractions of the orgasmic platform of the vagina. These may be followed by spastic contractions. During this phase the vagina remains enlarged, and the uterus contracts irregularly. There is generalized muscle spasm and loss of voluntary muscle control throughout the body. Hyperventilation, blood pressure, heart rate, and sex flush reach a peak. The rectal sphincter may contract and the urinary meatus may dilate.

In males, the orgasm phase consists of emission and ejaculation and is characterized by ejaculatory contractions along the entire length of the penis, three or four expulsive contractions, then several contractions of less intensity. Response patterns of muscles, rectal sphincter, heart rate, blood pressure, and respiratory rate are the same as those seen in women during this phase.

In the Masters and Johnson model, there is no desire phase, and the excitement and plateau stages of their model are comparable to the excitement phase of the Kaplan model discussed in this chapter. Kaplan's model corresponds to more discrete physiological as well as psychological changes. The Kaplan model does not include the stage of resolution that is included in the Masters and Johnson model, because resolution is not actually a part of sexual response. However, it is helpful to examine this return of the body to a normal state following orgasm.

In the female, this stage is marked by the return of the orgasmic platform to its normal size and position. The clitoris returns to normal size and position in 5 to 30 minutes. Breasts return to their normal size. Sex flush and muscle tension disappear as heart rate, blood pressure, and respiratory rate return to normal. In many women, lubrication recurs during the resolution phase, indicating an ability to reach orgasm again if stimulated.

In the male, the resolution phase is a similar return of the genitalia to their normal sizes and positions, but it also includes a *refractory period,* during which time ejaculation cannot occur. This refractory period varies widely in length among individuals, and it changes throughout the life span. During the resolution phase, the penis reduces in size about 50% almost immediately after orgasm. The remaining enlargement of the penis disappears more slowly, sometimes over 2 hours. Similarly, vasocongestion of the scrotum and testes reduces by 50% rapidly, then continues to resolve over a longer period of time. Sex flush, nipple erection, muscle tension, heart rate, blood pressure, and respiratory rate all normalize fairly quickly during this phase.

These phases have many variations according to the individual's health state, energy level, and environment. For example, decreased lubrication or erection may have nothing to do with decreased desire. Orgasm may not be reached, yet both partners may have experienced a fulfilling sexual encounter. The subjective experience often does not match the physiological event, especially in women. Women frequently have long or slowly increasing plateau phases. Some women may even lose excitement during this phase, yet feel fulfilled. All of these variations are normal, and it is important that clients understand them as normal. For example, some people experience orgasm as a release, but not as the intensely pleasurable or euphoric experience that other people do. Neither orgasm is "better," nor do the differences reflect any significant physiological or psychological differences. An individual's sexual response is based on more than just physiological factors and is affected greatly by attitudes about sexual activity and the relationship, as well as by many other less obvious factors.[9]

Methods of Experiencing Orgasm

Orgasm may be reached through a variety of techniques. *Masturbation* refers to the self-stimulation of erogenous areas to the point of orgasm. In men, masturbation is usually performed by gripping the shaft of the penis and moving the hand up and down. Vibrators are also commonly used in masturbation, by rubbing the moving area of the machine over and around the penis. Women masturbate by either directly or indirectly stimulating the clitoris, by rubbing over or around the clitoris, or by inserting an object into the vagina to simulate the action of the penis in intercourse.

Cunnilingus is oral-genital stimulation performed on a woman. *Fellatio* is oral-genital stimulation performed on a man. Many men and women prefer this method of reaching orgasm over other methods. Lips, tongue, and teeth are used to stimulate the clitoris and vagina in cunnilingus and the penis in fellatio. Sucking, licking, nibbling, and blowing activities are used in this method of sexual stimulation.

Anal intercourse is common among male homosexuals and also occurs in heterosexuals. A lubricant is necessary because the anus does not have the natural lubrication of the vagina. Anal intercourse is very stimulating to the penis because the anal opening is tight. The penis inserted into the anus stimulates the clitoris or penis of the receiving partner indirectly and is psychologically erotic for many people. For others, anal intercourse does not produce erotic sensations and may result in pain. Some women and men are excited by their partner stimulating the anus with a finger during intercourse. The finger or penis inserted into the anus should be washed before insertion into the vagina to avoid infecting the vagina with the normal bacteria of the rectum.

Sexual intercourse, or *coitus,* is penetration of the vagina by the penis. Coitus is performed in a variety of positions. Face-to-face–woman-above and face-to-face–side-lying positions allow more control by the woman and usually result in less depth of vaginal penetration than many other positions for intercourse. The face-to-face–man above position facilitates deeper penetration, especially if the woman has her legs over the shoulders of the man. This position does not facilitate as much ejaculatory control by the man. The rear-entry position allows deeper penetration and manual clitoral stimulation. Seated and standing positions offer varying degrees of control for either partner, depending on the position of each partner, and they tend to decrease the depth of penetration.[11]

Other activities for reaching orgasm include penetrating the vagina or anus with the hand, vibrator, or other object, simulating actions of the penis. The hand and fingers create widely different sensations than does the penis or other penis-shaped objects, and offer variations for heterosexual, homosexual, and lesbian couples. In addition, the penis, scrotum, clitoris, and vagina may be stimulated by the hand or other body part of the partner to result in orgasm.

Traditional Lifestyles of Sexual Expression

In the current, dominant society of this country, some sexual activity occurs in most men and in many women before marriage. Although this is counter to the teachings of most American religions, this practice does allow the adolescent to survey sexual attractions and erotic relationships before making a lifetime choice of marriage.[16] In addition, masturbation is common among adolescents and may help the adolescent and young adult develop his or her sexual re-

sponsiveness and range of sexual preference.[10] Dating extends through the high-school years, and the time of marriage generally depends on career choices. Many men and women choose to establish themselves in a profession or other career before marriage; however, subcultural as well as individual values, goals, and norms help determine the time of marriage.[16] Committed relationships are now commonly formed as partnerships, in the true sense of the word, with marriage contracts defining the shared responsibilities and the obligations of both partners.

With the current increase in sexually transmitted disease, sexual activity is generally initiated with a great deal of thought and consideration. *Safe sex* includes limiting numbers of sexual partners and talking in depth with potential partners before agreeing to sexual activity. If a sexual partner has not been monogamous for at least three months or has not tested negative to a sexually transmitted disease such as AIDS, condoms are used. Condoms are now being made much stronger for greater reliability, but are still not foolproof. "Safe sex" includes avoidance of oral sex with an unscreened partner and use of a glove or finger cot when exploring anal or vaginal areas and touching the penis. Kissing and hugging are generally safe, though french kissing may pose a hazard in some individuals. The general rule is to avoid contact with blood, feces, vaginal secretions, or semen.

Cultural Differences in Sexual Behavior

Sexuality in the individual is the product of psychological, biological, social, and cultural influences. The individual, of course, has choice, but this choice is greatly affected by many influences. Sexual behavior has been said to have no meaning outside a sociocultural context.[2] This becomes increasingly complex in today's mobile world. Cultures that were homogenous and "pure" in beliefs and values 15 years ago are much more diverse today, due to political and economic changes resulting in the influx of other cultural norms. Some general indications, however, can help the nurse know what to expect regarding clients' cultural values.

In the case of immigrants to the United States, the most likely predictors of "Americanized" sexual attitudes seem to be the length of time the client has been in this culture, the education of the client, and the client's parents' education level.[1] Between blacks and whites in this country, gender is a more significant variable than race in predicting sexual attitudes.[17] Similarly, a study of Indian and American men and women revealed that males of both countries had more in common regarding sexual attitudes than either group had in common with females of either country.[18] In one study of Mexican-American, Japanese-American, Black, and Caucasian groups, Mexican-Americans expressed the most discomfort with sex education, but suggested the earliest age to discuss sex education with their children. Caucasian parents, on the other hand, seemed most likely to proceed with sex education despite discomforts.[1]

Religious attitudes have a strong influence on sexual attitudes and sexual behavior in some cultures. For example, premarital sexual behavior among black women has been shown to be related to religious involvement.[3]

Sex role attitudes seem to predict attitudes about sexual behavior as well. Cultures that value equality between the sexes also reflect more liberal notions about sexual freedom and tend to be more open to discussing sexuality. In cultures that value a strictly patriarchal household, such as the Lao Hmong people and Iranians before the Islamic revolution, there is a clear double standard, with men accepted as sexually promiscuous and inclined toward extramarital sexual relationships, while women are expected to be virgins before marriage and to remain monogamous throughout marriage.[14] Such beliefs, however, sometimes are changed when these people move to a more sexually permissive country or are educated in that country.

The nurse must develop trust with the client and then interview the client to uncover his or her sexual norms and values. Nursing intervention must be based on an understanding of the client's cultural context for sexual values, norms, and behaviors.

Alternative Sexual Lifestyles

Homosexuality, Lesbianism, and Bisexuality

For about 10% of the population, the sexual object choice is a member of the same sex. For another 20% to 40%, the sexual object choice could be either male or female. Preferring a member of the same sex as a sexual partner is referred to as *homosexuality* among men and *lesbianism* among women. *Bisexuality* refers to an equal, or almost equal, preference for either sex. In addition, many bisexuals do not feel fulfilled with a solitary (or monogamous) relationship with a member of either sex, but prefer to be involved in equally intense and meaningful relationships with a man and a woman. Other people may refer to themselves as bisexual if they have had an intense sexual relationship with a person of the same sex, even if they generally prefer and are engaged in a heterosexual relationship.

The development of the homosexual, bisexual, and lesbian is probably not very different from that of the heterosexual. The homosexual who identifies himself as such is open to nonconformity and is able to tolerate risk. The imagery and early bonds of homosexuals may have been related to developing an appreciation of people of the same sex or, in the case of the bisexual, an equal appreciation of both sexes. There may be biochemical differences present in people who choose alternative sexual lifestyles, but these probably represent potentialities rather than inevitabilities, and are probably also present in many people who choose heterosexual lifestyles.

These choices of alternative sexual lifestyles are made not only due to preferences for sexual activities, but also due to a perceived ability to share emotional intimacy with either a man or a woman, and with that particular man or woman chosen for a sexual relationship. Some people believe that everyone is bisexual to one extent or another and that situations create the lifestyle choice.

Homosexuals, lesbians, and bisexuals are sometimes referred to collectively as "gays." There is, in some areas of the country, a united force of gay people working through political means for greater sexual freedom and less stigmatization in society. Aside from this aggregate created primarily for political purposes, there exists very little similarity among homosexual men, lesbians, and bisexuals. Each represents a distinct subculture with differing values, norms, and mores. There is really no such thing as a typical "gay person," just as a typical heterosexual person exists only statistically. The mannerisms and preferences of dress that are seen as associated with gay people are many times subcultural artifacts, like any fashion trend, and are sometimes exaggerated in response to stigmatization from the heterosexual world.

The sexual behavior of gay people varies as much as the sexual behavior of heterosexuals. Sexual dysfunction, bizarre sexual practices, child molestation, or sadomasochistic sexual activity are no more prevalent among homosexuals, lesbians, and bisexuals than among heterosexual groups. Neither is promiscuity more common among homosexuals than heterosexuals. Gay people do tend to enter a greater number of sexual relationships, perhaps because there are no societal supports of long-term relationships among gay people. Nevertheless, their relationships tend to last for 2 to 3 years, and they tend to be monogamous. For many homosexual people, the "gay bar" provides an opportunity, and one of the few places where it is acceptable, to meet with and talk to other homosexuals; the heterosexual, or "straight" world, on the other hand, has a variety of places within which heterosexuals can display affection for each other and be considered socially acceptable.

Transsexuality

The *transsexual,* in most cases, presents an entirely different lifestyle choice than the homosexual. Many transsexuals do not desire a homosexual relationship and are, perhaps, in successful heterosexual relationships. The transsexual believes he or she is psychologically of the sex opposite his or her anatomic gender. Surgery, hormone treatment, and psychotherapy are sought as a "sex change" process by the transsexual. The impetus for this change process is rarely a sexual relationship but is a need to ensure the integrity of his or her identity.

Paraphilias

Other variations in sexual preferences and lifestyles are termed *paraphilias* (*i.e.,* sexual or erotic attraction to objects, events, or superficial aspects of certain types of people). Although these variations are manifested by people who also have very normal sexual habits and vocational interests, the paraphilic activities may occur more often during times of stress or difficulty in heterosexual relationships. The common factor of these variations is erotic pleasure received from the inanimate and unreciprocated sexual activity. One example of the paraphilias is *transvestitism,* or a sexual desire to dress in the clothing, or adopt the mannerisms, of the opposite sex. *Voyeurism* refers to a desire to watch others in sexually vulnerable or erotic positions, such as those who are engaged in sexual activity with another or those who are undressing alone. *Exhibitionism* is an erotic desire to expose one's genital or erogenous areas to others. Voyeurism and exhibitionism sometimes involve anger toward the victim (the unsuspecting person who is observed or is the recipient of the exhibitionism) or anger toward something the victim represents. An exhibitionist, for example, may be angry with all women and may believe he hates them; he then expresses his anger through the victim's response of shock. In most cases, however, the impetus for the behavior involves no attempt at psychological violence.

The paraphilias include a sexual preference for children (*pedophilia*), a preference for sexual activity with animals (*bestiality* or *zoophilia*), and a sexual attraction to the smell and sight of death (*necrophilia*). *Sadism* is a paraphilia in which the man's or woman's preferred sexual object choice is not a type of person but is the act of inflicting pain on someone else. A *masochist* is a person whose sexual object choice is the experience of pain. In sadistic and masochistic relationships, erotic fulfillment is not achieved without either psychic or physical pain.

The paraphilias are not easily "treated," just as the sexual object choice of a heterosexual or a homosexual is not easily changed. Desensitization has been effective in dissociating the erotic experiences from the image of the paraphilia when the person is fully motivated to change.[16]

Variations in Sexual Expression Due to Physical or Mental Conditions

The Client's Sexual Needs

Illness, disability, hospitalization, and surgery are frequent factors in the disruption of the self-concept, including the sexual identity and gender identity. The client may demonstrate these disruptions as withdrawal from the family, anger toward the hospital or clinic staff, and deterioration of normal practices of hygiene and dress. Sometimes, hospitalized clients respond to crises by making obscene or sexually suggestive remarks or gestures toward nursing personnel. Although this behavior cannot be reinforced by the nurse, the response should not be one of anger. The nurse first clarifies the nature of the nurse-client relationship, and then clearly states that the nurse is interested in maintaining this therapeutic, nonsocial relationship. If the client is persistent, the nurse repeats the limits of the relationship and that she will not tolerate violation of these limits. Often, the client accepts the more clearly defined relationship and, perhaps, indicates a need for a closer relationship with staff on a therapeutic level. Illness and hospitalization weaken most normal coping mechanisms of clients and remove them from significant relationships, thereby creating a need for intimacy on some level with staff members. This need is met by an understanding nursing staff responding with emotional warmth and support within a professional relationship.

Many nurses are bothered by the client who masturbates. Perhaps one reason for this lack of tolerance and empathy is a mistaken belief that seriously ill people do not have sexual needs and desires. The nurse should provide for, and respect the privacy of, the client by knocking on the door before entering, by keeping the curtain drawn around the client's bed unless requested otherwise, and so forth. If the nurse finds a client masturbating, she should apologize for the invasion and provide the necessary privacy. It is important to convey respect and appreciation for the needs and individual values of the client. Similarly, a client may need sexual activity with his or her sexual partner while hospitalized. The nurse should be sensitive to cues of these needs and should respond by providing needed privacy. When the sexual relationship of the client is not a marital one, or is not heterosexual, the nurse may be less understanding of his needs. This is an example of the nurse's own value system being forced on the client and represents a nontherapeutic act of stigmatization.

Changes in Sexual Abilities

Certain physical and mental conditions affect one's ability to perform sexually and create a threatening crisis for the client's self-esteem. The nurse needs to be aware of such conditions and needs to encourage the client to verbalize feelings and frustrations. Many times, if the usual mode of sexual expression is not possible, an alternative method could be successful in meeting the client's sexual and relationship needs. For example, the quadriplegic client can participate in sexual intercourse if she or he is comfortable taking on a new role, perhaps a more passive one. A man who has lost the ability to achieve and maintain an erection may undergo a relatively simple procedure to have a penile implant placed surgically that enables erection, although not ejaculation. Many times, the client will feel satisfied with the ability to please his or her partner sexually, even if orgasm, as formerly experienced, is impossible.

Many surgical treatments and disease result in impotence in the male or decreased sexual excitement in women. These include perineal prostatectomies, sometimes ileostomies and colostomies, and, in some cases, diabetes. These problems may be caused by either psychological or physiological changes. The client may require referral for more tests or therapy to discern the nature of the problem. If a man has physiologically caused erectile dysfunction, he might be encouraged to try activities other than intercourse for sexual fulfillment. A penile implant might be preferred by some men. Male or female clients might be assisted to find greater sexual pleasure by trying longer foreplay periods, patience on the part of both the client and partner, and improved communication about thoughts and feelings in response to sexual activity.

Some women experience a loss of libido following bilateral oophorectomies and difficulty reaching orgasm following abdominal surgeries to create a colostomy or ileostomy. It is important that both partners understand the physiological causes of these reactions and openly communicate their responses. These are also good suggestions for clients who may have sexual changes due to diabetes mellitus. This disease may cause orgasmic dysfunction in women and retrograde ejaculation in men (which would prevent conception).[13] Some women experience *dyspareunia,* or pain with sexual intercourse, following hysterectomies and radiation treatments for uterine or cervical cancer. Coital positions providing the woman with more control in directing the penis and preventing deep penetration may restore sexual satisfaction in the relationship.

The aged person experiences changes in sexual abilities that are sometimes perceived by the elderly as an inability to engage in any sexual activity. The elderly person should be counseled regarding the normalcy of changes, such as a longer refractory period in the male, less firmness of the male erection, a longer time period required to achieve erection and reach orgasm, and occasional incidents of inability to achieve erection. Many men adapt to such changes by trying alternative sexual activities, such as having the partner stimulate the penis manually before attempting coitus, and oral sex if erection cannot be achieved fully enough to engage in coitus. Women tend to experience a loss of lubrication and some dyspareunia with the normal physical changes of aging. Sexual activities other than coitus and new coital positions allow the elderly woman to enjoy a full sex life.[11]

The Effects of Drugs

Some drugs affect libido and sexual abilities. When possible, the drug should be discontinued and a drug without this side effect should be administered. If this is not possible, the nurse explains to the client the cause of the problem and encourages him to alter his or her sexual activity as necessary. One such alteration might be the adoption of new coital positions or longer periods of foreplay before attempting coitus. Again, it is necessary that the client's sexual partner know the reason for the client's changing sexual abilities. Alcohol affects sexual interest and abilities in many men and women, but these changes are reversed when the alcohol use is curbed or stopped. On the other hand, chronic alcohol or drug use may affect the relationship to an extent that it interferes with normal sexual activity. Couples therapy or counseling may be needed to help restore open communication between the partners.

Sexual Behavior During Psychoses

The schizophrenic client may evidence bizarre sexual habits during psychotic episodes. These are usually part of the client's delusional system and probably do not represent his covert sexual desires. The client with manic behavior often exhibits increased sexual interest along with the loss of his usual inhibitions. This results in a period of sexual promiscuity and flirtatious behavior. The depressed client may experience a loss of sexual interest and ability during the acutely depressive period. It is important that family members, friends, and sexual partners of these clients be informed of the causes of erratic behavior and understand that the behavior may never recur during healthier periods for the client. The client should be protected by limit-setting of the staff; punishment or chastisement will not change his inappropriate behavior.

Post-Traumatic Syndromes

Many women and some men have unfortunately been victims of rape, incest, or other forms of sexual assault. Some researchers have gathered evidence that verifies that many people in this society condone rape.[7] Rape is a crime not of passion or sex but of power and mastery. Likewise, incest is a crime of dysfunctional family systems, not one of dysfunctional sexuality. The result of these traumatic events is often lifelong emotional trauma. Many victims of sexual abuse and assault develop psychological problems that prevent them from being vulnerable and thus accepting love, or from being strong with another and thus creating equal relationships.

Victims of sexual abuse or assault may have distorted body images or unusual anxiety and fear about sexual behavior or sexual touch. All of the common sexual problems listed in this chapter could potentially have been caused by traumatic sexual events in some period of the client's life. The nurse must ask clients if they have experienced such trauma and help them explore thoughts and feelings about this if they are willing and able to do so. Psychotherapy may be advisable for clients who have experienced sexual trauma.

Nursing Interventions

The attitudes held by health care providers can make the occurrences of sexual problems more difficult or less difficult for the client and family to cope with and overcome. During the early recovery period, the nurse or other staff member who works with the client who underwent injury or surgery resulting in a change in body image must convey an attitude of acceptance of the ostomy, the amputation stump, or the paralyzed limbs. Nurses must be sensitive to the client's cues that a concern exists and support his attempts to discuss the problem or fear. The nurse must be aware of the sexual needs of the hospitalized client, the elderly client, and the clients' sexual partners. It is also important for the nurse to facilitate the family's understanding of the client's condition. This may be done by suggesting a family meeting be held, during which the nurse supports the client in talking with the family or sexual partner. The nurse may wish to suggest a private meeting between the client and the sexual partner or the family. The nurse helps the client prepare for such a meeting by talking about the problems that need to be discussed and, perhaps, by role-playing a situation of talking with the family member about a sensitive topic. The nurse may also decide to talk with the family member or members about changes and needs of the client, with the client's permission, to make future discussions easier for him. Clear communication is an essential element in the relationship between client and family or sexual partner.

Nurses are frequently uncomfortable with topics of sexuality and discuss such topics with clinical detachment. This may be perceived by the client as disapproval, which may be harmful to the client who is struggling with the issue of how to continue as a sexual being while hospitalized or chronically ill. Our society tends to consider physically and mentally ill people as asexual or to attribute their sexual activities to their illness states. This is detrimental to the self-image of the client. The nurse can facilitate a change in this by being comfortable with sexual topics, open to discussing concerns and answering questions, and respectful of clients' sexual choices.[4]

Sex Therapy

Sex therapy is a particular approach to sex counseling that is practiced by master's-level clinicians with additional training in this therapy specialty. In addition, nurses of varying levels of preparation may employ sex therapy techniques as primary interventions. Sex therapy involves gathering careful assessments and histories of a couple's sexual difficulties, then clarifying each member's perceptions of the other and of sexual activities in general. The therapist facilitates communication between the two partners and their acceptance of each others' feelings and attitudes.[10] The approach of sex therapy is that sex is to be enjoyed and must not be viewed as an obligation of a relationship. The therapist may suggest certain exercises for the couple, most of which focus the couple on the sensual pleasures of touching and foreplay and de-emphasize the demand aspects of sexual activity. One such exercise is called the *sensate focus* exercise, a sense awareness activity during which the partners are not to attempt any activity to achieve orgasm but are to spend time relaxing and enjoying the physical closeness of the other. This exercise also encourages immediate involvement and discourages dissociation, or the spectator role.

The couple may also be taught new coital positions or different sexual activities that may better suit the needs of both partners. Other types of exercises assist the client to maintain more control during the sexual activity and to help him or her overcome fear or anxiety about sexual behavior. The *squeeze technique*

C H A R T   19-1

Role of the Nurse as a Sex Therapist

Ginger Manley, R.N., M.S.N.
Assistant Professor
Director, Center for Sexual Health Care
Vanderbilt University Medical Center
Nashville, Tennessee

I have been a registered nurse for more than 20 years, and for the past 11 years I have specialized in the area of sexual health. Since 1985, I have limited my practice to counseling with patients who are experiencing concerns about their sexual health and well-being. The decision to specialize was a gradual one, beginning with my willingness to inquire about my patients' sexual concerns, and progressing into my need to be accountable for intervening in problems described by the clients when I realized that few, if any, other health care providers were willing to deal with the area.

I have found that as I have become more comfortable with, and knowledgeable about, the topic of sexuality, my opportunities to help patients with their concerns have increased. Occasionally a patient just wants to ask me a question or seek information, while on another occasion the person may choose to do more in-depth work on a problem. Sometimes I am the primary therapist with the patient, while at other times I may collaborate with a physician or psychologist. Often I am asked to consult with staff about a particular problem or to provide an assessment and recommendation as part of a treatment plan. On an ongoing basis, I am a resource to medical and nursing staffs. I maintain a private practice in Vanderbilt University Medical Center, where I see patients on their own referral or at the recommendation of their health care provider. Frequently a "sexual problem" is a symptom of other underlying concerns that surface as a function of the therapeutic process.

Any illness or alteration in health care may provide the stimulus for a sexual health problem, biologically, psychosocially, or in combination. Whether working in inpatient or in ambulatory settings, nurses are often in positions to be responsive to the sexual health needs of their patients; often, though, we feel inhibited or unprepared to deal with these needs.

To respond to sexual health concerns, a nurse must first deal with her or his own sexuality through education and attitude studies. Often it is difficult to find role models for developing sexual health skills among faculty or practicing nurses. However, most nurses have excellent skills in the area of interpersonal communication, and these skills are a basis for giving patients permission to express and clarify their concerns. Often patients need information about potential, as well as actual, problems; less commonly, they may need referral for specific therapy. Although most nurses will not choose to specialize in sex therapy, it is important for all nurses to be accountable to patients' needs by directing them to appropriate resources.

---

is an exercise suggested to help a man prolong ejaculation during coitus to promote a mutually more pleasurable experience for the couple. This technique involves the woman stimulating the penis until near orgasm, then firmly squeezing the head of the penis with her thumb and two fingers, until the urge to ejaculate has subsided. This may be done during coitus also, if the woman is on top of her partner and can remove the penis from the vagina when her partner informs her of nearing orgasmic inevitability.[10]

Sex therapy has four general methods of treatment: simple counseling, couples therapy, individual therapy, and group therapy.[12] Simple counseling is an ideal format for the nurse and may be done individ-ually or with the couple or group. This includes education, specific suggestions (such as exercises or new positions), permission and reassurance, and facilitative communication. Couples therapy involves more in-depth exploration and intervention and is more often done by the master's-level sex therapist. This includes making homework assignments for exercises, then observing and responding to the couples' responses to the homework. Resentments and anxieties surface and are responded to during therapy. Obstacles to completion of assignments are observed and modified through the therapy process. Individual therapy proceeds in a similar manner but with increased focus on individual emotional blocks and

Table 19-1.   **Common Sexual Problems and Suggested "Homework"**

SEXUAL DIFFICULTY	EXERCISE OR HOMEWORK SUGGESTED	INTENDED GOAL OF HOMEWORK
Female orgasmic dysfunction	Sensate focus (first nongenital, then genital)	Reduces pressure "to perform," increases awareness of sensual pleasure, teaches partners about preferred areas and methods of nongenital and genital touch, teaches woman to avoid spectator role
	Masturbation or use of vibrators	Teaches woman how to pleasure herself, teaches her how to achieve orgasm, teaches her more about her genitals, sensitizes her to sexual stimulation
	Education and psychotherapy	Explores attitudes about self, sexuality, sexual behavior; increases partner's understanding
Male or female low sexual desire	Medical examination	Rules out hormonal imbalance
	Facilitative communication, psychotherapy, and education	Explores attitudes about self, partner, relationship, and sexuality; increases partner's understanding
Erectile dysfunction	Sensate focus	Reduces perception of pressure to perform sexually, teaches to avoid spectator role in sexual activity
	Facilitative communication and psychotherapy	Explores attitudes and feelings about self, partner, relationship, and sexual behavior; increases partner's understanding
	Medical examination	Rules out organic cause
Rapid ejaculation	Squeeze technique	Educates about level of sexual arousal
		Teaches inhibition of ejaculation, control of cycle for maximum satisfaction
Vaginismus	Relaxation exercises	Decreases anxiety about penetration and sexual intercourse
	Graduated dilators	Increases vaginal tolerance of and relaxation with insertion of penis
	Facilitative communication and/or counseling	Explores attitudes and feelings about self, partner, relationship, and sexual behavior; increases partner's understanding of situation

self-exploration homework through the use of a mirror, masturbation, and relaxation and imagery exercises. Group therapy involves discussion of problems and concerns, homework for individual or couple exploration, and group support and reassurance.

Common Sexual Problems

Erectile dysfunction, formerly termed impotence, the inability to achieve or maintain erection sufficiently to perform coitus, is a problem commonly seen in sex therapy. It is termed *primary erectile dysfunction* when the man has never been able to achieve erection, and *secondary erectile dysfunction* when the man has developed an inability to achieve or maintain erection but has successfully achieved erections in the past. *Rapid, or premature ejaculation* is the condition in which the man is unable to control ejaculation as long as he wishes to please himself or his partner. Both erectile dysfunction and rapid ejaculation may be caused by physical problems or by psychological conflict, such as stress or difficulties in the relationship. The cause of the sexual problem is ascertained before attempting treatment. The sensate focus exercise is often suggested as a treatment for impotence, and the squeeze technique is employed as a treatment for premature ejaculation.[10]

Women seeking sex therapy often present the problems of vaginismus or orgasmic dysfunction. *Vaginismus* is a spastic contraction or tightening of the vagina during or before penetration for coitus. *Primary orgasmic dysfunction* is an inability to achieve orgasm with no history of having had orgasm. *Secondary orgasmic dysfunction* refers to the development of difficulty attaining orgasm in certain situations. Physical causes for these problems, such as infection or nerve damage, are first ruled out. The therapist then ascertains that the woman wishes to be able to enjoy sexual activity with her partner. The woman and therapist discuss any conflicts about sexual activity or the relationship. Vaginismus is frequently treated by the insertion of graduated plastic dilators into the vagina for several minutes at a time, or even overnight. After the woman is able to tolerate one size, a larger dilator is inserted until she can tolerate penetration by a penis. When intercourse is attempted, the woman should assume a position that enables her to control the thrusts of the penis. Orgasmic dysfunctions are treated by suggesting the sensate focus exercise and periods of sexual activity during which the woman is not expected to "perform" or achieve orgasm. Coital positions are suggested that allow clitoral and breast stimulation by the partner or by the woman herself.[10]

Sexual Problems and the Nursing Process

Assessment

Assessment, the first step of the nursing process, includes reviewing the client's record for a clearer understanding of all aspects of the sexual problem. A sex history is obtained in which the client's earliest sexual experiences are described, along with how the client first learned about sex. The nurse compiles data that clarify the client's feelings and attitudes about sex. The assessment process also focuses on the sexual relationship. What are the sex roles and gender roles taken by each partner? How well do the partner's attitudes agree with those of the client? How does each perceive the needs of self and the other? How are sexual needs and preferences expressed in the relationship? Is there equal consideration of the needs of the other? The nurse may also wish to investigate the past relationships of the client and his or her partner. How have these prior relationships affected the client's current situation? Finally, how clearly defined is the client's gender identity, and how is this perceived by the partner? This information facilitates a clarification of the problems and assists the nurse in identifying educational deficits and other needs.

The nurse gathers the sexual history and explores sexual problem areas through the interview process. It is important for the nurse to maintain a relaxed, but respectful, matter-of-fact attitude through this interview. Data gathering should progress gradually from easier, more comfortable, material to more difficult material by means of focused and open-ended questions. When introducing potentially uncomfortable material, the nurse should first make an accepting statement that assumes the client has had a full range of experience in this area. An example is "When did you start masturbating?" rather than "Do you masturbate?" or "Men sometimes are unable to have an erection even when they really want to have intercourse—what is that like for you?" rather than "Do you have difficulty achieving an erection sometimes?" Also be sure to use words familiar and comfortable to the client. For example, if the client uses the word "lovemaking" instead of intercourse, the nurse uses this word also.[15]

The interview includes questions about when and how the client learned about sex, current atti-

tudes about sex, how the current health problem influences his or her sexual attitudes or behavior, and questions about current sexual habits and functioning. The interview should also gather information about self-image, body image, and sexual image. These refer to the client's feelings and thoughts about his or her body, the self in general, gender identity, sexual object choice, and sexual behavior and attitudes. Other areas to explore include history of sexual trauma, rape, or sexual abuse or harassment. It is also helpful to understand how the client's family of origin dealt with sexuality and nonsexual touching and affection. Is the client comfortable with nonsexual touch and friendly hugs? Especially important in the assessment is information about the client's current sexual relationship. How needs are communicated, how satisfied the client is with the frequency and quality of the sexual relationship, and what the client assumes his or her partner's answers to these questions would be are important areas for exploration.[8]

It is important for the nurse to include cultural data in the assessment process. The religious and ethnic influences on the client's perceptions of sexuality assist the nurse in understanding the client's responses and determining realistic treatment approaches. If the client has rejected his or her culture of origin and adopted another lifestyle or subculture, the culture of origin may still have a covert influence on his behavior and responses. If the client has chosen a lifestyle that is nontraditional, the nurse may be helpful in suggesting ways the client can respond to stigmatization, either in controlling exposure in society, or in establishing a support group and alternative system of approval. (See Charts 19-2 and 19-3.)

Nursing Diagnosis

After gathering the assessment data most pertinent to the client's sexual problem or concern, the nurse formulates a nursing diagnosis. This second step of the nursing process, diagnosis, involves the synthesis of information about the client's sexual health, needs, problems, knowledge level, and satisfaction. The nursing diagnosis of the client's sexual concern leads the nurse to a more precise plan of care. Possible nursing diagnoses include the following:

Impaired verbal communication, related to interpersonal (marital/couple) discord, evidenced by lack of discussion about sexual needs and preferences with sexual partner
Alteration in comfort, acute pain, related to intercourse, evidenced by facial mask of pain and distraction behavior
Sexual dysfunction, related to rapid ejaculation
Sexual dysfunction, related to female orgasmic dys-

CHART 19-2
Therapeutic Dialogue

Talking with the Client About Sexual Concerns

Nurse: What is the part about your relationship you dislike most?

Client: Our sex life.

Nurse: Your sex life doesn't suit you. In what ways is it unsatisfactory for you?

Client: I don't know. It's good for him, I guess. I guess that's how it always is?

Nurse: That's how what always is?

Client: It's always what suits him. I just think something ought to go my way too.

Nurse: How does sex not go your way?

Client: Well, it's when he wants it and how he wants it and you know—I never have time.

Nurse: Does your husband rush sexual activity a little too fast for you?

Client: Too much, too fast.

Nurse: It sounds like you feel your husband doesn't take enough time to get you ready for intercourse. And that maybe he doesn't ask what you like. Is that right?

Client: Yeah. And he always wants to do it.

Nurse: If he were trying things that you liked more, and taking it a little slower, would you like to have sex more often than you do now?

Client: Well, yeah, maybe. But he won't change anything.

Nurse: How much do you talk about sex, and what each of you likes and dislikes?

Client: Never.

Nurse: Have you ever told him how you feel about your sexual pattern together?

Client: He knows. I've never told him, but he has to know.

Nurse: I don't really think he can know unless you tell him. Have you ever told him what you like and don't like in sexual activity?

Client: Well, no, but I thought he was supposed to know that.

Nurse: Actually, it sounds like both of you could benefit by learning to talk about this openly.

Discussion

The client in this dialogue has been married to her sexual partner for 18 months. The couple has not as yet established satisfactory communication patterns. Difficulty expressing and discussing needs and wants is frequently manifested as a sexual problem.

---

function, low sexual desire (male or female), erectile dysfunction, vaginismus

Altered sexual patterns, related to homosexuality, transsexuality, lesbianism, bisexuality, paraphilia

Knowledge deficit, related to sexual response, need, health

Disturbance in self-concept, low self-esteem, related to prior sexual victimization, evidenced by inability to enjoy sexual activity

Planning

Treatment approaches are planned following the data-gathering and analysis processes. These approaches may be suggested by the nurse or other health care professional, based on an understanding of the cultural and religious preferences that influence one's sexuality and sexual activity. The nurse ascertains the client's acceptance of the suggested in-terventions and explains the processes involved. In most situations, it is necessary that both sexual partners accept and understand the therapy program. It is the couple, not one or the other partner, who is the client in sex therapy. The client (*i.e.,* the couple) works with the nurse through the planning process.

Intervention

The nurse's role in the intervention process is frequently one of clarification of communication. The nurse encourages expression of feelings by both partners, eliciting feedback, separating thoughts and feelings, and helping the clients learn other means of clear, open communication. The nurse often suggests activities for the couple to try to encourage the development of new sexual patterns. Many times, the nurse acts as a teacher, clarifying vague information for the client and giving him new information about sex positions or habits. The nurse might help the client ex-

C H A R T 19-3
Nursing Analysis and Diagnosis of Sexual Problems

The following are nursing diagnoses of sexual problems and assessment data supporting each diagnosis.

Assessment and Analysis of Data	Nursing Diagnosis
Thirty-year-old woman, three pregnancies, three abortions	Sexual dysfunction, related to vaginismus, fear of pregnancy
Anxiety experienced during entry of penis during intercourse and during fantasy of intercourse	
No anxiety during foreplay or masturbation or cunnilingus	
Discomfort during entry of finger into vagina and pain during intercourse	
Complaints began 3 months earlier, 2 months after last abortion	
Reported similar but milder problems following each abortion, but of brief duration (4–6 weeks)	
No signs of vaginal infection or tissue damage of any kind	
Stated fear of pregnancy but no recognition of this as cause of problem	
Observed adequate communication between partners and an apparently supportive and "healthy" relationship	
Twenty-eight-year-old woman, states she is a lesbian, complaining of boredom in sexual relationship of 2 years	Sexual dysfunction, related to presence of stress and unresolved anger in relationship, evidenced by lack of sexual enjoyment
Client denies any problem with her lesbianism; is open about this at work and with peers	
Client denies any other problems in the relationship; states she has never had this problem in previous long-term relationships	
Client describes her partner as an "unusually good lover," despite complaints of "boredom" and disinterest	
Client's partner appears to be a controlling person, insists on managing many aspects of the client's life	
Client has admitted difficulty expressing anger in the relationship	

(Continues on p. 330)

Thirty-four-year-old male, married and divorced twice; states that he cannot enjoy sex and other aspects of intimacy in these relationships	Sexual dysfunction, related to possible transsexualism, evidenced by lack of sexual enjoyment
Reports successful sexual performance but denies comfort or pleasure in the role	
Three homosexual relationships of short duration; reportedly unsatisfactory	
Reports sexual fantasies usually include self as female	
Has long felt he is more "like a woman in a man's body"	
Twenty-four-year-old male, single, complains of frequently being unable to reach orgasm or ejaculation, except when masturbating	Sexual dysfunction, related to retarded ejaculation, discomfort in relationships with women
Reports satisfactory erections during all sexual encounters	
Reports normal ejaculation when alone and occasionally when with a "casual sexual partner—somebody I just met"	
Reports this problem persists even when highly sexually aroused and sufficiently stimulated by partner	
Reports no long-term sexual relationships or close friendships with women; states he feels "too shy with women"	
Fantasies include successful sexual encounters with women—denies any homosexual fantasies or experiences	

Discussion

The nurse compiles and examines assessment data to place historical and descriptive information in the appropriate context. By considering as many aspects of the problem as can be explored, the nurse strives to understand it from the perspective that is most helpful to the client. This approach to analysis of sexual concerns is particularly important, because the problem may be related to a multiplicity of factors, including self-image, physiologic conditions, genetic tendencies, communication abilities, sensitivity to nonverbal cues, and erotic-fantasy images.

Analysis of assessment data results in a nursing diagnosis that describes briefly the problem and identifies the immediate etiology or etiologic factors. Formulation of a nursing diagnosis enables the nurse to understand the client's sexual problem in greater depth and to develop a precise, helpful care plan or initiate a timely referral to another mental health professional.

Case Study 19-1: Sarah C.

Sarah C. is a 26-year-old woman who is hospitalized for depression. During the general assessment, Sarah reveals she has concerns about her relationship of 2 years, for 18 months of which she has been married. Sarah feels her partner does not understand her and doubts that he loves her. These feelings are based on Sarah's observation that "We don't talk as much as we used to, we have more fights, and our sexual relationship is not as good."

The nurse interviews Sarah (see excerpts in Chart 19-2). The interview reveals that Sarah has probably misinterpreted her partner's behavior and does not ask sufficient questions to clarify her thoughts about his intentions or feelings. It is also learned that Sarah assumes that her husband "should just know" what she wants from him, if he "really" loves her. The nurse also interviews Sarah's husband and learns that he has similar problems in assuming that Sarah should know what he wants and that he loves

her, without his actually talking to her. During a couples session arranged by the nurse, Sarah and her husband expressed surprise at the other's thoughts, feelings, desires, and fears. Both partners agreed to talk nightly about their daily thoughts and feelings, and to try sensate focus exercises.

After two weeks, Sarah and her husband met with the nurse again. They reported that the sensate focus exercises had been very helpful. They reported having longer foreplay and feeling generally more sensitive to each other's feelings, sexual needs, and bodies in general. By this time, Sarah was stabilized on an antidepressant medication and was due for discharge in two days. The couple was given names of therapists for further counseling if needed. However, both felt they had learned useful information about their basic problem and were now ready to make necessary changes.

plore why he or she has some preference or fear, based on historical or cultural information.

The nurse is effective in interventions if she is knowledgeable and sensitive to her own, as well as the client's, sexual attitudes and concerns, and if she is comfortable with her own sexual choices and with discussing the choices of the client. Many sexual issues can be resolved through effective nursing intervention and may not require formal sex therapy.[8]

Evaluation

Nursing interventions are evaluated by follow-up sessions with the client. The nurse explores with the client whether he accepted or tried the suggested interventions. Evaluation also includes determining whether the suggested activities or positions were realistic for the client's situation. In some cases, the client may not wish to change or may not be ready to try something new. The nurse assesses the client's progress and suggests new activities, if appropriate. The nurse may decide to refer the client to someone else (perhaps someone with a perspective more consistent with the client's) or to a clinician more experienced or with greater training in sex therapy.

Summary

This chapter has discussed the development of sexuality as an integral part of the personality. Some of the major points of the chapter include the following:

1. The sexual nature of the personality affects the emotional, spiritual, and psychological natures of the self; indeed, they are not separate "natures" but parts of the personality, the self.
2. Sexual development is influenced by genetic and hormonal factors and by the development of gender identity.
3. The human sexual response cycle consists of three phases—desire, excitement, and orgasm.
4. Traditional and alternative sexual lifestyles, such as homosexuality, transsexuality, and paraphilias, are contrasted.
5. Clients who undergo injury or surgery resulting in a changed body image often suffer a blow to their sexual identity.
6. Nursing interventions with clients whose physical or mental disorders interfere with their

C H A R T   19-4
DSM-III-R: Sexual Disorders

The revised edition of the DSM-III has several diagnostic categories that are relevant to this chapter.[5]

Gender Identity Disorder of Childhood, 302.60, is a disorder in which the child experiences intense distress about his or her assigned sex or insists consistently that he or she is the opposite sex. This is not a simple nonconformity to socially appropriate sex-role behavior, such as "tomboy" or "sissy" behavior. There is more preoccupation with being or becoming or behaving as the opposite sex, and there is generally rejection of male or female anatomical characteristics. This disorder is said to begin to develop by the fourth birthday. Although this could result in the child later developing a homosexual or transsexual orientation, most do not. Gender identity disorder of childhood is not said to be related to abnormalities of sex organs, and it is assumed to be the result of inconsistent or inadequate reinforcement of normative gender-role behavior. This diagnosis is not made after puberty.

Transsexualism, 302.50, is a similar condition in a person who has reached puberty. There is a persistent preoccupation (for at least 2 years) with wanting to get rid of the primary and secondary sex characteristics, to take on the sex characteristics of the opposite sex, and to live as a member of the opposite sex. Dress, behavior, even social habits are more likely to be consistent with those of the opposite sex. The person's sexual object choice may be that of the same sex or the opposite sex, or the person may deny having strong sexual feelings.

Gender Identity Disorder of Adolescence or Adulthood, Nontranssexual Type, 302.85, is characterized again by a persistent or recurring sense of inappropriateness and discomfort with the assigned sex. There is cross-dressing, in either fantasy or actuality, but this is not for the purpose of sexual excitement as in Transvestic Fetishism. There is not a consistent preoccupation with getting rid of one's own sex characteristics and taking on those of the opposite sex. Again, the person has reached puberty and may be asexual, homosexual, or heterosexual in sexual orientation.

Gender Identity Disorder Not Otherwise Specified, 302.85, is a label for conditions that fit some but not all of the criteria for other classifications, such as brief periods of transsexualism or cross-dressing or anxiety and depression about sexual orientation.

The Paraphilias are distinguished according to severity, with "mild" being a condition in which the person has strong urges but does not act on them, "moderate" as occasionally acting on these urges, and "severe" as consistently acting on the urges.

Exhibitionism, 302.40, is a disorder in which the person has intense and recurrent sexual urges to expose the genitals to unsuspecting strangers, in association with sexually arousing fantasies, and this has persisted for at least 6 months. The person has acted on these urges or is quite distressed by them.

Fetishism, 302.81, is a condition of recurrent sexual urges and sexually arousing fantasies involving the use of nonliving objects by themselves, either for use alone or with a sexual partner. These cannot be limited to articles of clothing used in cross-dressing or devices for tactile genital stimulation. These urges are acted on or the person is markedly distressed by the urges, and the condition has persisted for 6 months or more.

Frotteurism, 302.89, is a disorder of recurrent intense sexual urges and sexually arousing fantasies regarding rubbing against or touching a nonconsenting person, and the actual touch, rather than a coercive element of the behavior, is the sexually exciting focus. The person has acted on these urges or is distressed by them, and the condition has persisted for 6 months or more.

Pedophilia, 302.20, involves recurrent and intense sexual urges and fantasies of sexual activity with prepubescent children. The person has acted on these urges or is markedly distressed by them, and must be at least 16 years old and at least 5 years older than the children of focus. This would not include a late adolescent in an ongoing relationship with a child of 12 or 13. The person may be attracted only to children or may be nonexclusive; the urges may or may not be limited to incest; and the urges may be toward same sex, the opposite sex, or both sexes.

Sexual Masochism, 302.83, involves persistent, intense sexual urges and fantasies involving real acts of being humiliated, beaten, bound, or otherwise made to suffer. These have persisted for 6 months or more. The person has acted on the urges or is distressed by them.

Sexual Sadism, 302.84, involves a 6-month or longer condition of recurring sexual fantasies and urges of performing real acts of inflicting suffering, psychological or physical, on a victim; these acts become sexually exciting. Either the urges are acted on or are distressing to the person.

Transvestic Fetishism, 302.30, must be differentiated from the gender identity disorders listed earlier. The condition has persisted for 6 months or more and involves a heterosexual male with recurrent sexual urges and fantasies of cross-dressing. The urges are acted on or are distressing to the person.

Voyeurism, 302.82, is a recurring sexual urge with fantasies involving observing an unsuspecting person naked, disrobing, or involved in sexual activity. The person has acted on the urges or is distressed by them.

Paraphilia Not Otherwise Specified, 302.90, includes disorders that are not seen commonly and that do not fit the criteria of other classifications. Examples are *urophilia* (urine), *klismaphilia* (enemas), *partialism* (exclusive focus on one body part), *necrophilia* (corpses), or *telephone scatologia* (lewdness).

Disorders of sexual dysfunction are also included in the DSM-III-R. All of these include a criterion that the disorder is not present exclusively during another major health disruption, such as depression or a serious physical illness.

Hypoactive Sexual Desire Disorder, 302.71, is a persistent or recurrent deficiency or absence of sexual fantasies or of the desire for sexual activity within the context of the person's life.

Sexual Aversion Disorder, 302.79, involves a persistent and recurrent avoidance of all or almost all genital contact with a sexual partner.

Female Sexual Arousal Disorder, 302.72, is *either* a subjective sense of a lack of sexual excitement and pleasure in female sexual activity *or* a partial or complete failure to maintain or attain a lubrication-swelling response of sexual excitement through completion of sexual activity.

Male Erectile Disorder, 302.72, is *either* a total or partial failure in a male to attain or maintain erection through completion of activity *or* a subjective sense of a lack of sexual excitement and pleasure during male sexual activity.

Inhibited Female Orgasm, 302.73, is a persistent delay in or absence of orgasm following normal sexual excitement and sexual activity of adequate focus, intensity, and duration. Some women cannot have an orgasm during intercourse unless otherwise manually stimulated. Whether this represents a normal variation of sexual response or a psychological inhibition depends on the overall situation and may be impossible to differentiate without a trial of treatment.

Inhibited Male Orgasm, 302.74, is a recurrent delay in or absence of male orgasm following normal sexual excitement and sufficiently focused, intense, and lengthy sexual activity, within the person's norm and context. This pertains not only to being unable to reach orgasm in the vagina but also to reach orgasm by other means such as masturbation.

Premature Ejaculation, 302.74, refers to persistent ejaculation with minimal stimulation or before, upon, or shortly after penetration and before the person wishes it. Again, context must be considered in assigning this diagnosis.

Dyspareunia, 302.76, is recurrent genital male or female pain before, during or after sexual intercourse. This is not assigned if the condition is due to lack of lubrication.

Vaginismus, 306.51, is recurrent and involuntary spasm of musculature of the outer third of the vagina that prevents or interferes with coitus.

Sexual Dysfunction Not Otherwise Specified, 302.70, includes disorders that do not meet criteria for other conditions, such as absence of erotic sensation despite physiological orgasm, genital pain during masturbation, or the female analogue to premature ejaculation.

---

sexual abilities include client and family teaching, support, and counseling.

7. Sex therapy may be the treatment of choice for certain common sexual problems—erectile dysfunction, rapid ejaculation, vaginismus, and orgasmic dysfunction.

8. The steps of the nursing process are applied to clients with sexual problems.

References

1. Abramson PK: Parental Attitudes about Sexual Education—Cross Cultural Differences and Covariate Controls. Arch Sex Behav 12, 5, 381–397, 1983
2. Abramson PK: The Sexual System: A Theory of Sexual Behavior. New York, Academic Press, 1984

3. Brown SV: Premarital Sexual Permissiveness Among Black Adolescent Females. Soc Psychol Q 48, 4 (Dec) 381–387, 1985

4. Campsey J: The Sexual Dimension of Patient Care. Nurs Forum 22, 2, 69–71, 1985

5. Diagnostic and Statistical Manual of Mental Disorders, 3d ed, rev. Washington, American Psychiatric Association, 1987

6. Fast I: Gender Identity: A Differentiation Model. Hillsdale, NJ, Analytic Press, 1984

7. Fingler L: Teenagers in Survey Condone Forced Sex, Ms. 9(8), 23, 1981

8. Higgins L, Hawkins J: Human Sexuality Across the Life Span: Implications for Nursing Practice. Monterey, CA, Wadsworth Health Sciences Division, 1984

9. Jayne C: A Two-Dimensional Model of Female Sexual Response. J Sex Marital Ther 7, 1 (Spring) 1981, pp. 32–36.

10. Kaplan HS: Disorders of Sexual Desire and Other New Concepts and Techniques in Sex Therapy. New York, Simon & Schuster, 1979

11. Kolodny RC, Masters WH, Johnson VE, Biggs MA: Textbook of Human Sexuality for Nurses. Boston, Little, Brown, & Co, 1979

12. Lion E: Human Sexuality in Nursing Process. New York, John Wiley & Sons, 1982

13. Manley G: Diabetes and Sexual Health. The Diabetes Educator 12, 4, 366–369, 1982

14. Meredith W, Rowe G: Changes in Lao Hmong Mental Attitudes After Immigrating to the United States. Journal of Comparative Family Studies 17, 1 (Spring) 117–125, 1986

15. Mims F, Swenson M: Sexuality: A Nursing Perspective. New York, McGraw-Hill, 1980

16. Money J: Love and Love Sickness. Baltimore, Johns Hopkins Press, 1979

17. Roo VVP, Roo VN: Sex Role Attitudes: A Comparison of Sex Race Groups. Sex Roles 12:9–10 (May) 939–953, 1985

18. Roo VVP, Roo VN: Sex Role Attitudes Across Two Cultures: United States and India. Sex Roles 13:11–12 (Dec) 607–624, 1985

19. Steiner B (ed): Gender Dysphoria: Development, Research, Management. New York, Plenum Press, 1985

20. Weinberg JS: Sexuality: Human Needs and Nursing Practice. Philadelphia, WB Saunders, 1982

21. Woods NF: Human Sexuality in Health and Illness, 2d ed. St. Louis, CV Mosby, 1984

20 Mental Health of the Aging

Patriciann Furnari Brady

An Old Lady Has the Last Word

What do you see, nurse, what do you see?
What do you think when you're looking at me?
A crabby old woman, not very wise,
Uncertain of habit, with faraway eyes,
Who dribbles her food and makes no reply
When you say in a loud voice, "I do wish you'd try."
Who seems not to notice the things that you do,
And forever is losing a stocking and shoe
Who resisting or not, must do as you will
Is that what you're thinking; is that what you see?

Then open your eyes, nurse, you're not looking at me.
I'll tell you who I am as I sit here so still,
As I do your bidding, as I eat at your will,
I'm a small child of ten with a father and mother.
Brother and sister who love one another;
A young girl of sixteen with wings on her feet,
Dreaming that soon now a lover she'll meet;
A bride soon of twenty—my heart gives a leap,
Remembering the vows that I promised to keep.
At 25, now I have young of my own who
Need me to build a secure, happy home.
A woman of 30, my young growing fast,
Bound to each other with ties that should last;

At 40, my sons have grown and are gone.
But my man is beside me to see I don't mourn;
At 50, once more babies play around my knees;
Again we know children, my loved one and me.

Dark days are upon me, my husband is dead.
I look to the future, I shudder with dread.
For my young are all rearing children of their own,
And I think of the years and the love I've known.

I'm an old woman and nature is cruel.
'Tis her jest to make old age look like a fool.
The body it crumbles; grace and vigor depart.
There is now just a stone where I once had a heart.

But inside this old carcass a young girl still dwells.
And now and again my battered heart swells.
I remember the joys, I remember the pain.
And I'm loving and living life all over again.
I think of the years, all too few, gone too fast,
And accept the stark fact that nothing can last.
So open your eyes, nurse. Open and see.
Not a crabby old woman; look closer—
        See Me.
        Author Unknown

Chapter Preview

In 1900, there were slightly more than three million elderly persons in the United States.[5] In 1976, the number of persons aged 65 and older was 22 million or approximately 10.5% of the total population.[28] Statistical projections estimate that by the turn of the century there will be 45 to 48 million elderly living in the United States.[21]

Elderly persons constitute a significant portion of our society. Recognition of the needs of the elderly and an understanding of their physical and psychosocial changes are essential for all practitioners of nursing. The focus of this chapter is to help nurses recognize their own attitudes about the elderly, to identify the physical and psychosocial changes that occur in the aging process, and to apply the nursing process to the care of the elderly.

Learning Objectives

On completion of the chapter, you should be able to accomplish the following:

1. identify those individuals in our society who are identified as the elderly
2. discuss nurses' attitudes toward the elderly and how these attitudes have an effect on health care
3. define the process of aging
4. describe the normal physiological and psychosocial changes occurring during the aging process
5. identify means for promotion of health and positive adaptation to aging, including the following:
   - preparing for retirement
   - deciding about residential placement
   - dealing with depression

The Elderly and the Nurse

Identifying the Population

Individuals who have reached the age of 65 are considered elderly in our society. Terms such as *aged, senile old woman,* and *dirty old man* are all part of the systematic stereotyping of, and discrimination against, people because they are old.[6] Nurses must recognize that each individual is unique and that the aging process is also unique for the individual.

Old age is a period of continued developmental growth. The developmental tasks of aging include conservation of strength and resources, when necessary, and adaptation to those changes and losses that occur as part of the aging experience. The ability of the elderly person to adapt and thrive is contingent on his physical health, personality, early life experiences, and the societal supports he receives, such as adequate finances, shelter, medical care, social roles, and recreation.[6]

When one thinks of the elderly, the picture that may come to mind is that of an old person sitting restrained in a wheelchair in a nursing home; however, most elderly individuals live in single family-owned homes. The largest proportion of the elderly live in independent households and the majority of these people live with a spouse or other relatives. According to the 1970 census, fewer than 5% of the elderly live in institutions.[28]

The Nurse's Attitudes

Nursing of the elderly does not command the same level of prestige as nursing in many medical–surgical nursing areas. Unfortunately, geriatric nurses and, particularly, those staff employed in nursing homes often feel and are treated like second-class nurses.[5] They may be thought of as unable to perform in "real" hospital settings; their pay is often below that of nurses who practice in hospitals. Some people believe that it does not take much skill or expertise to take care of old people and that the elderly need custodial care more than anything else.[5] In June, 1966, geriatric nursing was recognized, for the first time, as a vital specialty in nursing by the American Nurses' Association. Standards for Geriatric Nursing Practice were established in 1970 (see Chart 20-1, "The American Nurses' Association's Standards of Geriatric Nursing Practice").

Although the nurse could function as the primary guardian of the aged person's mental health and human dignity, most institutions reward nurses for their medical and technical skills. Psychological and social interventions undertaken by the nurse are deemed worthy and laudable, but more or less voluntary.[22]

Stereotyped attitudes of nurses concerning old people often interfere with treatment by preventing the nurse from seeing the individual as he really is (see Chart 20-2, "Stereotyped Attitudes About the Elderly"). If nurses and other health care providers isolate stereotyped attitudes and behaviors directed toward the elderly, they may better understand their reactions to the elderly and become better prepared to care for their aged patients.[7] It has been shown, for example, that the abnormal behavior of patients is

CHART 20-1
The American Nurses' Association's
Standards of Gerontological Nursing Practice

Standard I: Organization of Gerontological Nursing Services

All gerontological nursing services are planned, organized, and directed by a nurse executive. The nurse executive has baccalaureate or master's preparation and has experience in gerontological nursing and administration of long-term care services or acute care services for older clients.

Standard II: Theory

The nurse participates in the generation and testing of theory as a basis for clinical decisions. The nurse uses theoretical concepts to guide the effective practice of gerontological nursing.

Standard III: Data Collection

The health status of the older person is regularly assessed in a comprehensive, accurate, and systematic manner. The information obtained during the health assessment is accessible to and shared with appropriate members of the interdisciplinary health care team, including the older person and the family.

Standard IV: Nursing Diagnosis

The nurse uses health assessment data to determine nursing diagnoses.

Standard V: Planning and Continuity of Care

The nurse develops the plan of care in conjunction with the older person and appropriate others. Mutual goals, priorities, nursing approaches, and measures in the care plan address the therapeutic, preventive, restorative, and rehabilitative needs of the older person. The care plan helps the older person attain and maintain the highest level of health, well-being, and quality of life achievable, as well as a peaceful death. The plan of care facilitates continuity of care over time as the client moves to various care settings, and is revised as necessary.

Standard VI: Intervention

The nurse, guided by the plan of care, intervenes to provide care to restore the older person's functional capabilities and to prevent complications and excess disability. Nursing interventions are derived from nursing diagnoses and are based on gerontological nursing theory.

Standard VII: Evaluation

The nurse continually evaluates the client's and family's responses to interventions in order to determine progress toward goal attainment and to revise the data base, nursing diagnoses, and plan of care.

Standard VIII: Interdisciplinary Collaboration

The nurse collaborates with other members of the health care team in the various settings in which care is given to the older person. The team meets regularly to evaluate the effectiveness of the care plan for the client and family and to adjust the plan of care to accommodate changing needs.

(Continues on p. 338)

Standard IX: Research

The nurse participates in research designed to generate an organized body of gerontological nursing knowledge, disseminates research findings, and uses them in practice.

Standard X: Ethics

The nurse uses the code for nurses established by the American Nurses' Association as a guide for ethical decision making in practice.

Standard XI: Professional Development

The nurse assumes responsibility for professional development and contributes to the professional growth of interdisciplinary team members. The nurse participates in peer review and other means of evaluation to assure the quality of nursing practice.

C H A R T 20-2
Stereotyped Attitudes About the Elderly

1. Discussing sad and traumatic events of the past makes elderly patients depressed.
2. Rearranging a patient's room provides a more stimulating environment for the elderly.
3. Elderly people prefer to be with people their own age.
4. Elderly patients are not willing to discuss their emotional problems.
5. Elderly people tend to become grouchy and stubborn.
6. As you grow older, you must expect to depend on other people.
7. Most elderly patients are confused at some time during the day.
8. Elderly patients should be encouraged to perform self-care as much as possible.
9. It is bad for the elderly to talk about death and sickness.
10. The elderly tend to be childish and are more secure if treated as a kind adult treats a child.
11. Aged persons do not have sexual feelings or interest in the opposite sex.
12. Old age is a form of sickness requiring medical care and nursing.
13. Elderly patients generally have poor memories.
14. Old people often like to meddle in other people's business.
15. Older people cannot expect to lead completely full or satisfying lives.

often rewarded; hence, a decrease in normal behavior occurs.[44] Recognition of these attitudes is the first step toward improving health care and quality of life for the aging.

The Process of Aging

Each individual, including the elderly individual, develops at his own rate. The age of 65 has been chosen to signify the elderly because of the great number of psychosocial changes heralded by this age. These social changes act as a point of comparison to the younger adult.

As children begin to walk at different ages, the physiological aging process likewise occurs at different rates for each individual. The following discussion is presented as a guideline to the aging process.

Physiological Changes

The aging process begins at birth. The body does not change obviously, but a variety of cyclic aging changes, on a lesser level, are constantly occurring.[40]

The rapidity of aging depends on a person's heredity, the amount and regularity of exercise, any past illnesses, the presence of one or more chronic illnesses, and the stresses experienced throughout life.[16] Changes attributed to aging are as follows:

1. A decrease in rate of cell dimension in specialized cells that regenerate (*e.g.*, epithelial tissue)
2. A deterioration of more specialized non-dividing cells, particularly neurons and skeletal muscle cells, leading to a decreased functional capacity
3. Changes in connective tissue leading to in-

creased rigidity and loss of elasticity, producing changes in organ systems

4. A general loss of reserve functional capacity in all organ systems[16]

Respiratory System

There is generally decreased functional reserve capacity of the respiratory system in the elderly.[17] The decreased lung elasticity and changes in the thoracic bones affect the ventilation of the lungs. These are common respiratory system changes that take place with aging; unless illness occurs, elderly people adapt to these changes without difficulty.

Pneumonia and other respiratory illnesses increase in frequency in the elderly due to the inability of the lungs to handle proper ventilation. The reserve capacity of the lungs is increased, however, if the person has continued to exercise regularly.

Cardiovascular System

The heart tends to maintain its size with age; however, in some individuals, it becomes smaller.[28] Reduced cardiac muscle strength and cardiac output frequently occur; however, the anatomic and physiological changes that take place in the aged heart allow it to function adequately, unless the elderly person has coronary artery system disease.[28] Because of the decreased metabolic needs of the aged, the heart functions adequately to meet the needs of the healthy aged individual.

The older American typically shows some degree of atherosclerosis affecting the aorta, coronary arteries, and carotid arteries. Atherosclerotic changes reduce the distensibility and elasticity of the large arteries and limit the ability of the blood vessels to increase the amount of blood available to vital organs.[16] Therefore, any illness that increases the need for blood, such as fever, may produce angina or syncope.

Gastrointestinal System

The bony structures of the mouth begin to shrink with age. Aged people tend to have missing teeth that have been replaced with dentures. As the bony structure of the face changes, the person's dentures may not fit properly and may result in difficulty in chewing food properly. Meals become less pleasurable for the individual and he tends to avoid nutritious foods such as meats, vegetables, and fruit. Decreased peristalsis of the gastrointestinal tract causes a feeling of fullness, which, in turn, causes the individual to ingest less food. A slight decrease in the amount of pancreatic enzymes in the aged individual further diminishes the individual's digestion and absorption of nutrients.

Most elderly individuals have daily bowel movements despite reduced peristalsis, reduced muscular activity, and inadequate exercise.[16] Many elderly persons use a variety of medications to avoid constipation. It is the nurse's responsibility to assist the elderly with diet teaching, thereby assuring maximum nutritional benefits from food and adequate bulk to avoid gastrointestinal problems.

Genitourinary System

During the aging process, the ureters and bladder tend to lose muscle tone. The bladder may lose enough muscle tone to result in incomplete emptying, which increases the risk of urine retention and cystitis. The kidneys concentrate urine inadequately, causing frequent urination and nocturia.

Because of the relaxation of their pelvic muscles, multiparous elderly women frequently experience urinary incontinence. Older men, because of hypertrophy of the prostate and decreased bladder capacity, experience frequency of urination. These conditions frequently affect the lifestyle of the elderly, but appropriate health care intervention helps the elderly adjust to these changes. Although many elderly individuals decrease their fluid intake to alleviate frequency and incontinence, the nurse should explain the hazards of dehydration and should encourage the aged person to take in at least 2000 ml of fluids every 24-hour period, unless contraindicated.[16]

Endocrine System

Estrogen and testosterone are the hormones that generally decrease with age; growth hormones continue to be secreted in the elderly. Some hormones, such as insulin, appear to be secreted at a lower level in the elderly than in younger people.[16]

A decrease of estrogen during menopause causes many of the physiological changes of the female body. Changes in breast tissue result in less glandular tissue, reduced elasticity, and more connective tissue and fat. The uterus becomes smaller and the external genitalia shrink with age and loss of subcutaneous fat.[16]

A decline of testosterone in the aged male occurs, but does not result in an abrupt decline in spermatogenesis.[16] Benign prostatic hypertrophy is a common occurrence in elderly males.

Ears, Nose, and Throat

Visual accommodation is altered in adults around the age of 30 years and progresses throughout all of old age. This visual change is due to the inability of the lens of the eye to adapt to near vision. By the age of 40, most people need corrective lenses for near vision. With age, the pupillary sphincter causes the pupil size to decrease; therefore, bright light becomes necessary for reading. This decreased pupil size also presents an added risk of accidents when the aged person walks in poorly lit areas. Handrails may be necessary to avoid accidents. The lacrimal glands of the older individual produce fewer tears; dry and irritated corneas may result from decreased tearing.[16]

Neurologic System

Neurologic changes of the elderly may be due to physiological or psychological causes. It has been established that, in very aged people, there is a decrease in the size and weight of the brain, with some decrease in the number and functioning of neurons;[16] however, there has been no evidence to support a relation of brain size to neurologic functioning.

Recent studies have shown that those most prone to deficits in mental functioning are individuals with high blood pressure or other deteriorative vascular changes.[5] One study showed that there was minimal evidence of brain impairment in the memory and intelligence performance of men with normal blood pressure, whereas those with high blood pressure manifested marked decline.[48] Of particular relevance is the finding that the individual's intellectual functioning is related more directly to psychological adjustment than to chronological age.[14] Nurses must treat older people as intelligent adults capable of comprehending events unless they have a pathologic condition superimposed on the aging process.[16]

Sleep requirements of the elderly differ from the younger adult in amount and pattern of sleep. The elderly tend to need less sleep and the stages of rapid eye movement (REM) sleep are altered. Assisting the elderly to relax and prepare for sleep and discouraging naps during the day assure more restful sleep patterns for the aged (see Case Study 20-1).

Integumentary System

Changes of the skin, hair, and nails are common manifestations of the aging process. Decreased elasticity and dryness are the causes of wrinkled skin. The exposure to sun over a period of years contributes to the aging of the skin. Liver spots (lentigo senilis) and keratosis frequently develop due to sun exposure. The skin becomes dry, inelastic, pallid, and grayish in color due to deficiencies of protein and caloric intake.[43] Frequent baths should be avoided by the elderly because soap causes dryness. Lotion may be used to increase skin moisture. With the thinning of the epidermis, the skin is easily injured and healing is slowed by a decreased blood supply to the dermis.[21]

The toenails and fingernails of the elderly tend to become thick and to split easily. Teaching proper nail care is important to avoid injury to the fingers and toes. For example, the nurse recommends that nails be soaked prior to cutting them.

Graying of the hair begins in the middle years and progresses to the snow-white hair of old age. The hair may thin and become fine due to atrophy of the hair roots.

Musculoskeletal System

Joint, muscular, and bone changes are common conditions manifested in the elderly individual. The ability to ambulate and move our extremities is often taken for granted. In the elderly, joint changes and diminished bone and muscle mass give way to increased incidence of fractures and falls, stooped posture and shortened stature, loss of muscle power, misshapen joints, pain, stiffness, and limited mobility.[28]

Fractures in the elderly generally heal as quickly as in the young. Due to decreased activity and nutrition, the elderly may experience increased muscle atrophy and stiffness. Proper health teaching should emphasize the intake of foods high in protein, vitamins, and minerals, which can decrease these health problems. Encouragement of daily exercise, especially walking, may result in decreased muscle atrophy and stiffness.

A common manifestation of bone changes in the elderly is osteoporosis. This condition is found more frequently in older women than men due to the effect that decreased estrogen production has on the bones.

Adaptation to Physiological Change

The nurse working with the elderly focuses on assisting them to do the following three things:

1. To understand the normal aging process
2. To maintain the body through diet, rest and sleep, and exercise
3. To cope with physiological changes through adaptation

The nurse's understanding of the normal aging process facilitates the elderly patient's adaptive skills. Planning and implementing nursing care to provide for these needs is the nurse's ultimate goal.

Psychosocial Considerations of Aging

Myths of Aging

There are many myths associated with aging. These are identified as follows:

1. Physiological aging
2. Unproductivity
3. Disengagement
4. Inflexibility
5. Senility
6. Serenity[6]

Case Study 20-1: Mrs. W.

Mrs. W., a 78-year-old widowed female, was admitted to the medical floor due to complaints of weakness and dizziness. Mrs. W. lives in her own apartment in a senior citizens apartment complex. She had been functioning well at home until approximately 4 days prior to admission. Her daughter, who is married and lives in the same town as Mrs. W., stated that Mrs. W. complained of an inability to sleep at night and of falling asleep during the day. Her daughter feared Mrs. W. was sleeping through meal times. She stated that Mrs. W. formerly was an active person; for example, she knitted many presents for others.

After all medical tests were completed, no physiological cause of the problem was identified. Mrs. W.'s pattern of sleeping during the day continued. Attempts to place Mrs. W. in a wheelchair at the nurses' station during the day did not decrease this behavior. Mrs. W. remained awake from 12:30 A.M. until 5:30 A.M. and continually attempted to get out of bed.

Following a conference of the nursing staff, the following care plan was implemented to intervene in Mrs. W.'s behavior:

Nursing Diagnosis	Intervention
Sleep pattern disturbance	Discuss with client her perception of the problem and plans to change her bedtime patterns. Assist Mrs. W. with bedtime routine at 7:00 P.M. Offer 8 oz of warm milk at bedtime. Back rub at bedtime. Night light left on in the room. When awake at 12:30 A.M., permit her to sit at nursing station with knitting for a while. Then return her to bed. Back rub for relaxation.
Alteration in nutrition: less than body requirements, related to difficulty awakening for meals	Wake client at 7:30 A.M. Assist her with A.M. bath. Determine preference for certain foods. Ambulate in hall following meals. Encourage family to visit, particularly during mealtimes. Provide her with knitting supplies and provide reinforcement for knitting completed. Encourage her to participate in planning daily activity.

The nursing staff implemented this new routine for 4 days. Following day 2, Mrs. W.'s periods of wakefulness during the day increased. Mrs. W. ate all her meals and began to become interested in knitting. She did not exhibit confusion, weakness, or dizziness. Mrs. W. stated she felt like "her old self." Plans were being made for discharge, and Mrs. W. stated she intended to follow this routine at home.

(Continues on p. 342)

Questions for Discussion

1. What are the sleep requirements of an elderly person?
2. Identify the nursing interventions that assist an individual to relax and to sleep.
3. What factors contributed to Mrs. W.'s weakness and dizziness?
4. Discuss why activity was encouraged during the periods Mrs. W. was awake.
5. Why was it important for the nurses to ask Mrs. W. her perception of her problem and to encourage her to participate in planning her daily activity?

To facilitate understanding the process of aging, an attempt is made to explore these myths.

Physiological Changes. Physiological changes are part of a continuous process begun at birth. The nurse recognizes these changes in the elderly and helps them adapt to changes. Physiological changes require adaptation skills. Most physiological changes of aging bring with them psychological components that cannot be negated, such as threats to self-image, self-esteem, personal identity, and role performance. These aspects of the elderly person's psychological well-being must be addressed by the nurse and the elderly client.

Unproductivity. Current research supports a broader view of the cognitive process of aging.[5, 6, 21, 28] The variety of life experiences of the elderly contribute to cognitive adjustments to aging. Mental and intellectual functioning of the elderly do not necessarily decline during the aging process, and only at death are there apparent changes in intelligence. The changes prior to death, however, may be due to depression rather than physical causes.[22]

The necessity for learning may decrease as one ages. The elderly person's attitude toward learning or his attempts to solve problems on the basis of previous experiences may bring about this change in behavior.[28] The elderly individual tends to respond slowly to directions and this is often mislabeled as a decrease in intellectual functioning. The manner in which the elderly person perceives outside stimuli is related to his visual and auditory abilities. Due to delayed auditory perception, the aged individual's reaction time may be increased; likewise, as the amount of information associated with decision-making is increased, the time required to reach a decision is increased.[42] It has also been noted that elderly people may be more reflective in making decisions due to consideration of their previous experiences.[6] Nurses should provide the elderly with sufficient time to process information

and with the opportunity to be involved in planning their care.

Disengagement and Inflexibility. Personality development of the elderly is often described as inflexible and disengaged. Nevertheless, patterns of personality development of the aged are not dormant. The elderly person attempts to complete the final stage of personality development, which ultimately leads to a preparation for death.

Erikson has identified this final developmental task as Ego Integrity versus Ego Despair.[13] This stage involves a developmental integration of one's life, during which the individual reviews his life experiences and evaluates the successful completion of his life goals. The individual who accepts his life and the achievement of his goals achieves a new sense of ego integrity. He sees life as having meaning and does not despair for what might have been. He views life as another phase of development that one must accomplish; achieving a positive sense of self becomes his ultimate goal.[36]

Senility and Serenity. The majority of behavioral changes of the elderly are responses to poor adaptation of physiological, psychological, or environmental factors. Mild forms of behavioral changes may be caused by adverse environmental influences, such as social deprivation.[27] For example, sensory-deprived patients are reported to exhibit a loss of mental function, personality disintegration, and psychotic symptoms.[34]

Societal forces place the elderly into dependent roles. Mandatory retirement, financial limitations, highly mobile extended families, government priorities in budget allocations, incidence of chronic disease, and differential mortality rates for men and women cause dependent role positions, which may precipitate dependence in other areas.[12] In planning and providing care for the healthy elderly, the nurse needs a working knowledge of psychosocial develop-

CHART 20-3
Physical and Psychological Changes of the Aging: Diagnosis and Intervention

Nursing Diagnosis	**Interventions**
Respiratory System	
Breathing patterns, ineffective	1. Protection from respiratory infection 2. Planned exercise program, preferably walking 3. Periods of rest, if exercising and experiencing shortness of breath
Cardiovascular	
Cardiac output, alteration in, decreased	1. Periodic monitoring of blood pressure 2. Supervision and instruction in diet as directed; for example, a low salt diet 3. Exercise to maintain cardiac output; for example, walking
Gastrointestinal	
Bowel elimination, alteration in, constipation	1. Instruction to increase foods high in bulk 2. Adequate fluid intake 3. Teach proper use of laxatives
Nutrition, alteration in, less than body requirements	1. Check for properly fitting dentures 2. Encouragement of dental exam 3. Nutrition instruction related to caloric intake 4. Nutritional guidance with food planning 5. Assess elderly client's ability to prepare own food
Genitourinary	
Urinary elimination, alteration in patterns	1. Fluid intake of approximately 2000 ml/day 2. Decreased fluid intake prior to sleep 3. Bladder training, if necessary 4. Health teaching of proper cleaning technique following voiding to avoid infection 5. Physical examination of male elderly for prostate changes
Eyes, Ears, Nose, Throat	
Injury potential, alteration in eyesight	1. Provide glasses and eye examination, as necessary 2. Remove excess furniture, clear cluttered environment 3. Provide properly lighted area for ambulation 4. Handrails to assist with ambulation

(Continues on p. 344)

Nursing Diagnosis	Interventions
Eyes, Ears, Nose, Throat	
	5. Night light in bathroom and bedroom at night
Sensory peceptual alteration, auditory	1. Provide access to hearing aid, if necessary
	2. Face client when communicating
	3. Speak slowly and enunciate clearly
	4. Exclude extraneous background noises when communicating with client
	5. Use visual aids as necessary
Neurological System	
Sleep pattern disturbance	1. Discourage naps during the day
	2. Provide fresh air and exercise during the day
	3. Provide relaxing environment prior to sleep
Thought process alteration, slowing of response	1. Provide adequate time to understand communication
	2. Allow adequate time for responses
	3. Use visual aids for reality orientation
	4. Treat as intelligent adults, able to comprehend events
Integumentary	
Skin integrity, impairment, actual and potential	1. Avoid frequent baths with soap
	2. Use lotion to increase moisture to skin
	3. Teach proper nail care
	4. Safety needs to avoid injury to skin

ment of the aging individual and, in turn, she must support his independence and positive adaptation.[12]

The elderly are frequently labeled confused as a result of behavior that is disturbing to nurses and the family. Each client deserves a careful medical and social evaluation before any diagnostic label is attached. The registered nurse with physical assessment skills and mental status examination skills can determine the causes of confusion and plan appropriate nursing intervention.[4] Interactional factors and physiological status must be determined on an individual basis, and the nurse must guide and monitor adequate nursing intervention for each client. In general, the nursing activities determined to be most helpful in preventing or ameliorating confusion states are as follows:

1. Measures to prevent diminished oxygenation of the brain
2. Measures to maintain hydration
3. Measures to avoid extremes in sensory input
4. Provision of a safe, ordered, and orienting environment with familiar objects
5. Making certain that circumstances are clear and uncomplicated, communication heard and understood
6. Judicious administration of drugs[49]

Promotion of Health and Adaptation to Aging

Health care of the elderly individual requires the acceptance and implementation of a treatment model that is concerned with the psychosocial functioning of the elderly.[1,6] The long-term effects of physical health, longevity of family and social relationships, satisfying and purposeful activities, and successful resolution of psychosocial conflict are difficult to measure, but these factors appear to be instrumental in determining the quality of life for the elderly.[37]

Preventive and Therapeutic Measures

Nursing care of the elderly focuses on those preventive and therapeutic measures that assist the individual to adapt to the changes of growing older. Life review therapy and life-cycle group therapy are two forms of psychotherapy that assist older people in this manner.

Through an extensive autobiography of the individual, life review therapy helps him develop an improved self-image and helps the nurse gain a deeper understanding of him (see Chart 20-4). The consequences of a life review include expiation of guilt, exorcism of problematic childhood identifications, the resolution of intrapsychic conflicts, the reconciliation of family relationships, the transmission of knowledge and values to those who follow, and the renewal of the idea of citizenship.[6]

Life-cycle group therapy is oriented toward persons experiencing a crisis in their lives. The members of the group are concerned not only with intrinsic emotional problems, but also with preventive and remedial measures as they pass through the life cycle.[6]

Unfortunately, health care deliverers and institutions tend to be organized around the medical model concept of illness. When the behavior of the aged fits neatly into categories that are defined as appropriate illness behavior, then we can discuss, diagnose, and dispose of cases with very little difficulty.[19] Although such illnesses may be present in some elderly patients, opportunities can be provided, even for patients who are slowly deteriorating, to maximize and maintain their essential human dignities through a physical and psychosocial milieu that minimizes the patients' losses.[22]

A variety of treatment techniques, modalities, and therapies exist that assist older persons who exhibit cognitive and emotional impairment, including the following:

1. Reality orientation focuses on repetition and learning of basic information, such as the client's name, location, and time of day.
2. Resocialization groups increase the elderly client's contact with others and expand his ability to recognize available choices of living for himself.
3. Remotivation therapy encourages the moderately confused elderly client to take a renewed interest in his surroundings by focusing attention on everyday life not related to his emotional situation.
4. Attitude therapy reinforces the client's desirable behavior and eliminates undesirable behavior.
5. Reinforcement therapy proposes that a person learns to behave in a way that allows him to experience pleasant and rewarding situations.
6. Milieu therapy uses all facets of life of the older individual in the social milieu as opportunities for living-learning experiences.
7. The *prevlab* program (prevention of loneliness, anxiety, and boredom) is based on the concept that sensory input can be altered in a positive direction for most subacute or chronically ill individuals by introducing high-interest items into their immediate environment and by altering or modifying the design and decor of their environment.
8. Self-image therapy is based on the rationale that as a person grows older, he experiences feelings and reactions that affect the self.
9. Reality therapy attempts to lead clients away from denying external reality and helps them to recognize not only that reality exists, but that they can fulfill their needs within its bounds.[1]

Adaptation to Change

Besides the physiological and psychological changes of the elderly, there are also lifestyle changes that confront the elderly. These are discussed below.

Retirement

For many individuals, work is a great part of life. Many people view retirement as a crisis. If work is a focal point of one's life, retirement may threaten feelings of identity, integrity, and self-esteem. With retirement may come loss of income, influence, status, creativity, activity, social relationships, and control over the environment.[18]

To plan for retirement, adults need to develop leisure activities that will support their self-esteem. Involvement in groups, such as senior citizen or retirement groups, may provide new areas for experiences in creativity, activity, and social relationships.

Family roles may change during this period. The individual and spouse should plan together and take into consideration their needs and the effect of the changes on their financial situation. Establishing new roles and relationships takes time and requires that others support the client's and family's growth. Our mobile society has altered the extended family; now, the retiree has an opportunity to expend energy on reestablishing and nurturing relationships.

C H A R T   20-4
Therapeutic Dialogue

Life Review Therapy

Mr. J., an 84-year-old widower, has been a resident of a nursing home for 2 years. In the last 3 weeks, he frequently mentioned to the nurses that he had a son who died at 9 months of age. The nurses were aware that Mr. J. had two daughters who lived in another town, but were unaware of any children who had died. The nurses feared that Mr. J. was becoming confused; however, he participated in the home's activities and demonstrated no other behavioral changes.

The head nurse, Mrs. Brown, decided to visit Mr. J.'s room, sit with him, and participate in an activity with him to provide an opportunity for him to discuss his son. Mr. J. enjoyed doing puzzles, and she asked him to put one together with her. After 15 minutes of working on the puzzle and discussing activities at the nursing home, the following interaction took place.

Mr. J.: Do you know that I had a son die at 9 months?

Nurse: You had a son who died at 9 months?

Mr. J.: Did you ever hear of the bad flu that went around a long time ago?

Nurse: Did your son die of the flu?

Mr. J.: We were never sure. I couldn't get the doctor there in time. He had a high fever.

Nurse: The doctor didn't arrive in time?

Mr. J.: (tears in his eyes) It was snowing outside, and I had to travel 5 miles to get a doctor. It took me almost 1 hour to get to the doctor and 1 hour to return home. When we got home, I found my wife crying, and I knew he was dead.

Nurse: That must have been a difficult time for you and your wife.

Mr. J.: She cried for 3 days until the funeral. Then she never would talk about Peter. She said it was something we must forget, but I never forgot Peter.

Nurse: You would have liked to talk about Peter?

Mr. J.: He was our only son, and then we had the two girls. I love our girls, but I felt it was my fault he died, and my wife didn't want to talk about it, ever.

Nurse: You felt he died because you couldn't get the doctor there?

Mr. J.: I needed to say I was sorry. It feels good to tell someone that I did the best I could. I'm glad I could tell you.

Mr. J. returned to talking about the puzzle and did not discuss his son in the subsequent weeks. When his daughter came to visit, she confirmed that Mr. J. had a son who died at nine months of age.

Questions for Discussion

Mr. J.'s discussion with the nurse was a type of life review.

1. Discuss the benefits of a life review for the elderly individual.
2. What are the expected results of life review therapy?

Loneliness

Adjustment to recurrent loss is a prevailing theme in the lives of the elderly.[26] At one time, most of the elderly person's existence involved family life and work. It is ironic that, with the passage of time, these sources of meaning may render meaningless the later, role-deprived lives of those they once enhanced.[38] Loneliness is a constant stressor for the elderly. In a recent review of the literature related to loneliness in the elderly, Ryan and Patterson have found that elderly women complain of loneliness more than men, and that loneliness is linked to poor self-evaluation of health and a pattern of increased suicide rates among the elderly.[41]

Loneliness has been linked to alcohol use in the elderly. These may be a high-risk subgroup of elderly who might become late-life alcohol abusers.[41] It is often difficult to assess the drinking problem of the elderly. In fact, the different ways that alcohol-related problems may present are endless, with all body systems potentially affected. Elderly people also frequently take medication for various health problems; these medications may interact in a potentially lethal manner with alcohol.

C H A R T   20-5
Psychosocial Assessment Guide

Sondra George Flemming, M.S., R.N.
Associate Dean, Health Occupations
El Centro College
Dallas, TX

Date _____

Name _____   Person supplying information
Age _____   (if other than client) _____
Birthdate _____   _____
Present address _____   Relationship _____

Client Profile:
  Birthplace:
  Where have you resided most of your life?
  Occupation:
    Pre-retirement
      Occupation
      How long were you at this job?
      Occupational stresses and hazards
    Post-retirement
      Did you work after retirement?
      Where?
      How many hours per week?
      Occupational hazards
      Employed or self-employed?
      Are you now employed?
    Retirement
      Date of retirement
      Was it voluntary?
      Was it compulsory?
      Was it because of illness?
      Did you have pre-retirement preparation? (Seminars, counseling,
      etc.)
      Did you have post-retirement counseling?
  Education:
    Grammar   College
    High School   Graduate or professional school
    Later courses, other education, self-education
  Religion:
    Original family affiliation
    Present affiliation
    Are you an active member?
  Ethnic, racial, or cultural background:
    Are you an immigrant?   Year of immigration:
    Where did you immigrate from?
  Marital status:
    Present status
      Single _____ Separated _____ Widowed _____
      Married _____ Divorced _____
    Marriage most current:
      Name of spouse
      Date of marriage
      Closest anniversary attained
      Date of separation, divorce, or widowhood (specify which)

(Continues on p. 348)

Marriage, previous:
  Number of previous marriages
  Dates of previous marriages
  Closest anniversary attained
  Dates of separation, divorce or widowhood (specify which)
Describe your relationship in the present marriage
Economic status:
  Indicate sources of income:
    Employment   Insurance payments
    Social security   Annuities
    Veteran's benefits   Investments
    Railroad retirement   Savings
    Private pension plan   Assistance from family
    Public assistance   Others
  Do you have financial problems?
  Do you have health care coverage?
Home situation:
  Where do you live?
  Who lives with you?
  Any problems with living situation?
  How do you feel about the amount of space you have?
  Do you have:
    Many stairs to climb
    Toilet facilities
    Running water
    Bathing facilities
    Cooking facilities
    Heating and lighting
  Are there any problems with your neighborhood (crime, accessibility)?
  Do you live near areas with loud noises, fumes, and chemicals?
  Are you able to care for yourself in your home environment?
  Care of home:
    Who cares for the home?
    Who watches the house when you are gone?
Transportation and mobility:
  Do you drive a car?   Own one?   Have access to one?
  Do you wear seat belts?   How do you usually get around?
  Is public transportation available? Do you use it?
  Do you have any physical disabilities that affect your mobility?
  Do you feel safe going out during the day?
  Do you feel safe going out during the night?
  Do you have a telephone?
Availability of family or significant others:
  Relatives
  Friends
Hobbies and special interests:
  Hobbies
  Sports and exercise
  Commercial recreation (movies)
  Music
  Language
  Travel
  Vacation habits (frequency, what do you do during vacations)
  Gardening
  Collecting
  Pets

Use of community centers
Community involvement (memberships, clubs)
Energy levels
    Psychological
    Social
    Sexual
How do you spend an average day?
Dietary history:
    How many meals do you eat a day?   Glasses of water per day?
    How many hot meals a day?
    How do you get your meals?
    Are you on a special diet?
    Do you take vitamins?   What kind?
    Who does the shopping for the food?
    Are shopping areas accessible?
    Who does the cooking?
    How do you pay for the food?
Habits (coffee, alcohol, tobacco, soft drinks)
Personal habits (bite nails, tug hair)
Rituals (hot water in morning)
Neurological:
    Alertness
Ability to communicate and understand
Behavior during assessment
Comments:

In assessing the potential for alcohol abuse, the nurse should assess support systems at the time of loss, confusing symptoms of physical illness, and a previous drinking history.[45,46] Through proper assessment, the nurse can institute appropriate interventions and referrals.

Residential Placement

An individual's need for security and sense of identity may be threatened when it becomes necessary for him to change his lifestyle. Entrance into a residential care facility may threaten the elderly person and subject him to possible psychological stress or anxiety.[2] Significant proportions of the aged are clearly mismatched with respect to their placement in institutional settings and this results in unmet needs, serious health problems, and sometimes death.[31]

Entrance into a residential home may be regarded as a "crisis rite" for the aged—as an official acknowledgement of their inability to care for themselves, their dependence on others, or their withdrawal into the "sick role." Entrance into an institution also represents the general public's perception of old people, signifying the end of one phase of life (normal society or the outside world) and the beginning of another (institutional care or the "inside").[35] The adaptation of the elderly to such a facility is de-

pendent on pre-admission planning, pre-admission counseling, and matching the individual's needs to the proper facility.

Dealing with Depression

As some elderly individuals attempt to cope with the changes of aging, normal adaptation skills may not suffice. Failure of adaptation skills may lead to depression and depression may lead to suicide.[32]

Suicide in the elderly tends to be a response to situational problems related to the client's aging, rather than an inability to cope.[15] Elderly people make fewer suicide attempts, communicate intentions of suicide less frequently, use more lethal methods of suicide, and are more successful than younger suicidal people.[32] Single, widowed, separated, and divorced people comprise the highest suicidal groups in the elderly population.[29] Crucial factors in determining who among the elderly will attempt suicide appear to be the individual's coping abilities and the strength of his "will to live."[32] In an era when suicide among the elderly is increasing, caregivers need to understand ways in which to address intent and to follow through on statements that are serious in nature.[47]

There are eight major causative patterns of suicide in the elderly. Each pattern of suicide is actually a means of reacting to one or more of the changes brought about by the aging process. Suicide among the elderly may be a result of a reaction to the following:

1. Severe illness
2. Mental illness
3. The threat of extreme dependency or institutionalization
4. The death of a spouse
5. Retirement
6. A pathological personal relationship
7. Alcoholism or drug addiction
8. Multiple factors[32]

Precise information is unavailable regarding the number of suicides among the elderly population. Many factors, including family denial and fear of loss of insurance benefits, contribute to this lack of information.[30]

Suicide attempts by the elderly may also be life-threatening behavior, but are not always recognized as such by those caring for them. Life-threatening maneuvers are identified by three characteristics.

1. They can hasten death singly or in combination.
2. They are usually not aggressive behaviors but passive behaviors.
3. They are observed, but unrecognized, by caregivers.[30]

Life-threatening maneuvers by the elderly that are often not recognized as passive suicide attempts include the following:

1. Refusing medication
2. Not following the physician's orders and recommendations
3. Smoking and drinking against medical advice
4. Refusal to eat, or ingesting food but retaining little of it
5. Placing the self in a hazardous environment (near drafty doorway, walking on an icy sidewalk)

When the nurse recognizes these behaviors, she begins to develop a relationship with the elderly person to help him adapt to change and learn new adaptation skills. This may be accomplished by encouraging continuity of care, discouraging relocation, fostering interpersonal mutuality, and reinforcing comfort-giving behavior.[30] (See Chap. 37, "Suicide.")

The finality of suicide should make us aware of the importance of assessing the actual suicidal intent of the elderly. While interviewing the aged person, the nurse should clarify suicidal intent by inquiring about it and determine the existence and lethality of a suicide plan. Nursing intevention involves staying with the person, lending support and strength, thereby preventing the institution of the plan, and bringing in assistance and support.[47] It becomes an essential role of the nurse to assess the intent of suicide in the elderly. The persistence of symptoms of depression in the elderly over months and years may "numb" the family to the severity of the symptomology.[3]

Planning nursing intervention to respond to change brought about by the aging process can further enhance the life of an elderly individual. Purposeful nursing intervention based on a theoretical framework has been found to be more effective in decreasing dysphoria and increasing life satisfaction.[23] One case missed is a tragedy, given the level of suffering inherent with depression and the potential for a shortened life expectancy through suicide.[3]

Summary

This chapter presents three major areas of information—the elderly and the nurse, the process of aging, and the promotion of health and adaptation to aging. Some of the major concepts of the chapter include the following:

1. Aging is a process of continuous physiological change from birth to death and a continuous developmental growth process.
2. Through an understanding of the normal aging process, the nurse is better able to assist the elderly to comprehend the inherent physiological and psychological changes and to cope with these changes through adaptation.
3. The nurse is urged to recognize the myths or stereotyped attitudes about aging and to become aware of her own attitudes toward, or beliefs about, the aged.
4. Nursing provides the elderly person with the opportunity to continue to grow throughout the process of aging and to meet death at peace with himself.
5. Loneliness, the threat of retirement and residential placement, and depression and the possibility of suicide are powerful stressors to the elderly.
6. Treatment of the cognitively and emotionally impaired elderly includes reality orientation, remotivation, resocialization, reinforcement, and milieu, attitude, self-image, and reality therapies.

References

1. Barns EK, Sack A, Shore H: Guidelines to Treatment Approaches. The Gerontologist 13:513–527, 1973
2. Beland IL: Clinical Nursing: Pathophysiological–

Psychological Approaches. New York, Macmillan, 1970

3. Blazer D et al: Major Depression with Melancholia: A Comparison of Middle-Aged and Elderly Adults. J Am Geriatr Soc 35:*10*, 928–932, 1987

4. Brady PF: Labeling Confusion in the Elderly. J Gerontologic Nurs 13 (June): 29–32, 1987

5. Burnside IM: Nursing and the Aged. New York, McGraw-Hill, 1976

6. Butler RN: Successful Aging and the Role of Life Review. J Am Geriatr Soc 22 (December): 529–535, 1974

7. Campbell ME: Study of the Attitudes of Nursing Personnel Toward Geriatric Patients. Nurs Res 20:147–151, 1971

8. Combs KL: Preventive Care in the Elderly. Am J Nurs 78 (August): 1339–1341, 1978

9. Craven RF: Primary Health Care Practice in a Nursing Home. Am J Nurs 76 (December): 1958–1960, 1976

10. Davis RW: Psychological Aspects of Geriatric Nursing. Am J Nurs 68 (April): 802–804, 1968

11. Dickelmann N: Pre-Retirement Counseling. Am J Nurs 78 (August): 1337–1338, 1978

12. Dresen SE: Autonomy: A Continuing Developmental Task. Am J Nurs 78 (August): 1344–1346, 1978

13. Erikson E: Childhood and Society, 2d ed. New York, WW Norton, 1964

14. Fischer J: Competence, Effectiveness, Intellectual Functioning and Aging. The Gerontologist 13:62–68, 1973

15. Furukawa C, Somaker D: Community Health Service for the Elderly. Rockville, MD, Aspen Publishing, 1981

16. Graves M: Physiological Changes and Major Diseases in the Older Adult. In Hagstel MO (ed): Nursing Care of the Older Adult: In the Hospital, Nursing Home and Community. New York, John Wiley & Sons, 1981

17. Gray PL: Gerontological Nurse Specialist: Luxury or Necessity. Am J Nurs 82 (January): 82–85, 1982

18. Haber J, Leach A, Schudy S, Sideleau BL: Comprehensive Psychiatric Nursing. New York, McGraw-Hill, 1982

19. Hacker SL: Patients' Effect on Mental Health Professionals. The Gerontologist 12:54–57, 1973

20. Hagstel MO: How Do Elderly View Their World? Am J Nurs 78 (August): 1335–1338, 1978

21. Hagstel MO (ed): Nursing Care of the Older Adult: In the Hospital, Nursing Home and Community. New York, John Wiley & Sons, 1981

22. Herr JJ: Psychology of Aging: An Overview. In Burnside I (ed): Nursing and the Aged. New York, McGraw-Hill, 1976

23. Hirschfeld MJ: The Cognitive Impaired Older Adult. Am J Nurs 76 (December): 1981–1984, 1976

24. Hoch C: Assessing Delivery of Nursing Care. J Gerontologic Nurs 13:*1*, 10–17, 1987

25. Hoff LA: People in Crisis. Menlo Park, CA, Addison-Wesley, 1978

26. Janosik EH, Davis JL: Psychiatric Mental Health Nursing. Boston/Monterey, Jones & Bartlett, 1986

27. Kabrynski B: Innovation in Programs of Care for the Elderly. The Gerontologist 13:50–53, 1973

28. Kart CS, Metress ES, Metress JF: Aging and Health: Biologic and Social Perspectives. Menlo Park, CA, Addison-Wesley, 1978

29. Kastenbaum R, Aisenberg R: The Psychology of Death. New York, Springer-Verlag, 1976

30. Kastenbaum R, Mishara Braue L: Premature Death and Self-Injurious Behavior in Old Age. In Kastenbaum R (ed): Old Age on the New Scene. New York, Springer-Verlag, 1981

31. Leberman M: Institutionalization of the Aged: Effects on Behavior. J Gerontol 24:330–340, 1969

32. Miller M: Suicide After Sixty: The Final Alternative. New York, Springer-Verlag, 1979

33. Murray RB, Zentner JP: Nursing Concepts for Health Promotion. Englewood Cliffs, NJ, Prentice-Hall, 1979

34. Oberleder M: Psychotherapy with the Aging: An Art of the Possible. Psychotherapy 3:139–142, 1966

35. Pasner J: Notes on the Negative Implications of Being Competent in a Home for the Aged. Int J Aging Hum Dev 5:357–362, 1974

36. Pasquali EA, Alesi EG, Arnold HM, Debasio N: Mental Health Nursing: A Bio-Psycho-Cultural Approach. St Louis, CV Mosby, 1981

37. Peterson BH: The Age of Aging. Aust NZ J Psychiatry 7:9–16, 1973

38. Putnam PA: Coping in Later Years: The Reconciliation of Opposites. Image: J Nurs Scholarship (Summer): 67–69, 1987

39. Robinson L: Psychiatric Nursing as a Human Experience, 3d ed. Philadelphia, WB Saunders, 1983

40. Rossman I: Human Aging Changes. In Burnside IM (ed): Nursing and the Aged. New York, McGraw-Hill, 1976

41. Ryan MC, Patterson J: Loneliness in the Elderly. J Gerontologic Nurs 13:*5*, 6–11, 1987

42. Stone V: Give the Older People Time. Am J Nurs 69 (October): 2124–2127, 1969

43. Ubler DM: Common Skin Changes in the Elderly. Am J Nurs 78 (August): 1342–1344, 1978

44. Ullman LP, Krasner LA: A Psychological Approach to Abnormal Behavior. Englewood Cliffs, NJ, Prentice-Hall, 1969

45. Valanis B, Yeaworth RC, Mullis MR: Alcohol Use Among Bereaved and Non-Bereaved Older Persons. J Gerontologic Nurs 13:*5*, 26–32, 1987

46. Wellenberg ML et al: Alcoholism Screening in the Elderly. J Am Geriatr Soc 35:*9*, 864–869, 1987

47. Whall A: Assessing Suicidal Intent. J Gerontologic Nurs 13:*8*, 36–37, 1987

48. Wilkie F, Eisdorfer C: Intelligence and Blood Pressure in the Aged. Science 172:959–962, 1971

49. Williams MA, Holloway JR, Winn MC et al: Nursing Activities in Acute Confusional States in Elderly Hip Fractured Patients. Nurs Res 28:*1*, 25–35, 1979

PART 5

Application of the Nursing Process to Disturbed Behaviors

21　Anxiety and Anxiety Disorders

Judith A. Greene

Grief has limits, whereas apprehension has none. For we grieve only for what we know has happened, but we fear all that may possibly happen.

Pliny the Younger,
Letters

Figure 21-1. *Mental health–illness continuum.*

Chapter Preview

The phenomenon of anxiety is not new. People in every historical age and in every culture have experienced the emotion of anxiety. To feel anxious occasionally for brief time periods is considered a part of normal human life. When the experience of anxiety, however, persists, cannot be dismissed, and begins to interfere with daily existence, then an anxiety disorder is present.

Although anxiety is a clinical feature of almost every psychiatric syndrome, it is the primary symptom of the anxiety disorders. With respect to the health-illness continuum, anxiety disorders follow adaptive mental health and precede the personality disorders and psychoses (see Fig. 21-1). This schematic classification illustrates the severity of these disorders in relation to adaptive mental health and the more severe psychiatric disorders. Although anxiety disorders are considered less pathological than the personality disorders and psychoses, they can become disabling.

Learning Objectives

Upon completion of the chapter, you should be able to accomplish the following:

1. define the concept of anxiety
2. discuss the concept of anxiety and its physiologic, perceptual, cognitive, and behavioral effects
3. define anxiety disorder
4. identify the ways in which anxiety manifests itself in the five anxiety disorders
5. discuss the five anxiety disorders in terms of their major signs and symptoms
6. apply the nursing process—assessment, formulation of nursing diagnoses, planning, intervention, and evaluation—to clients with anxiety disorders

Anxiety Defined

According to Hildegard Peplau, *anxiety* is defined as the initial response to psychic threat.[13,14] In other words, anxiety occurs as the initial response to psychic stressors. Because anxiety is a form of energy, it is not accessible to direct observation. The presence of anxiety, however, may be ascertained through the individual's self-report. For example, anxious individuals may describe the subjective experience of anxiety as vague discomfort, uncertainty, self-doubt, diffuse apprehension, dread, restlessness, or feeling jumpy, jittery, helpless, powerless, or irrational.[13] On a more objective basis, the effects of anxiety may be inferred from the individual's verbal or nonverbal behaviors and physiological responses. These behaviors and responses indicating the presence of anxiety occur along a continuum ranging from mild, moderate, and severe degrees of anxiety to panic (see Fig. 21-2).[13,14]

Physiological Effects of Anxiety

Anxiety causes certain physiological responses within the individual. Initially, epinephrine and norepinephrine are released from the adrenal medulla, and cortisone is secreted by the adrenal cortex. The secretion of these hormones produces an increased heart rate, elevated blood pressure, and an increase in the rate and depth of respiration. Other physiological effects accompanying anxiety include: systemic and localized changes in body temperature; urinary frequency and urgency; dryness of the oral mucosa; anorexia; excessive perspiration of the palmar surfaces of the hands and feet; increased muscle tension; changes in the woman's menstrual cycle; sexual dysfunction of both men and women; decrease in the blood's clotting time; and release of glycogen by the liver. The extent to which these physiological effects occur depends largely upon the degree and duration of anxiety. Generally, mild and moderate anxiety enhance these effects while severe anxiety and panic tax the individual's capacity to emit these physiological responses.[13]

Perceptual Effects of Anxiety

Anxiety also affects the ways in which an individual perceives and processes sensory input. In *mild anxiety*, the human organism is capable of grasping increased sensory input. The five sensory channels—sight, hearing, taste, smell, touch—are more open to sensations. Mild anxiety thus heightens the individual's sensory awareness. *Moderate anxiety*, on the other hand, dulls perception; that is, the individual's sen-

Figure 21-2. *Anxiety continuum.*

sory channels are less open to sensory input. If, however, the individual is directed to do so, he can attend to greater sensory input.[13]

With the occurrence of *severe anxiety,* perception becomes increasingly distorted and sensory input is reduced. The processing of sensory stimuli occurs in a scattered, disorganized manner. In *panic level* anxiety, perception becomes grossly distorted.[13] At this point, the individual is incapable of differentiating real from unreal stimuli.

Effects of Anxiety on Cognition

Cognition—the ability to concentrate, learn, and solve problems—is influenced by anxiety. Mild and moderate anxiety levels are more conducive to concentration, learning, and problem-solving. The normally intelligent individual who is mildly to moderately anxious discerns relationships between and among concepts with relative ease. His concentration and problem-solving occur without undue difficulty.

In contrast, severe anxiety seriously hinders cognitive function. The severely anxious individual has difficulty concentrating and often fails to discern even obvious relationships between and among concepts. The panic-stricken individual suffers even greater cognitive impairment. Concentration, learning, and problem-solving are virtually impossible during panic episodes.[13]

Effects of Anxiety on Verbal and Nonverbal Behavior

Mild Anxiety

The speech content and form of the mildly anxious individual reflect heightened sensory awareness and cognitive function. Thoughts are logically verbalized; speech rate and volume are appropriate to content and communication context. Nonverbally, the mildly anxious person appears alert, confident, and relatively secure.

Moderate Anxiety

Verbal behavior of the moderately anxious individual is often characterized by frequent changes of topic, repetitive questioning, joking, and wordiness. Blocking, or loss of train of thought, may also occur. Speech rate often accelerates and speech volume often increases.

Nonverbally, the moderately anxious individual may change body positions frequently, use excessive hand gestures, and assume aggressive body postures towards others. Furthermore, because moderately anxious individuals do not perceive and process sensory input as efficiently as mildly anxious individuals, they tend to hesitate and procrastinate in meeting routine social and vocational expectations. Such be-

haviors often present an overall picture of restlessness and discontent that may provoke others' feelings of irritation toward the moderately anxious individual.

Severe Anxiety

The severely anxious individual displays verbal behavior indicative of highly distorted perceptual and cognitive function. Severely anxious individuals often verbalize their emotional pain by making such assertions as "I can't stand this," "I can't think," or by vociferously demanding help and relief.

Nonverbal behavior usually reveals both fine and gross motor tremors, facial grimaces, as well as other forms of purposeless activity, such as pacing and hand-wringing.[13] Severely anxious individuals present an overall picture of extreme emotional discomfort and behavioral disorganization.

Panic

Panic-level anxiety results in even greater emotional pain and behavioral disorganization to the individual. Both verbal and nonverbal behaviors suggest a psychoticlike state in which panic-stricken individuals are virtually helpless to defend themselves and to negotiate simple life demands. These individuals may scream and run about wildly, or may cling tenaciously to something or someone accurately or inaccurately perceived as a source of safety and security. Protective and calmative measures must be initiated promptly because prolonged panic states are incompatible with life.[13, 14]

Anxiety Disorders

Anxiety Disorder Defined

The term *anxiety disorder* refers to a psychiatric condition characterized by the emotion of intense terror.[9, 16, 19] This emotional state is accompanied by thoughts of impending catastrophe and continues during substantial periods of time. Individuals so afflicted rigidly cling to maladaptive perceptual and behavioral styles as they futilely attempt to reduce or eliminate their painful state.[2] Failure to achieve the desired relief usually serves to increase the severity of the individual's symptoms.

Common Characteristics of Anxiety Disorders

There are five types of anxiety disorders: phobic disorder, panic disorder, generalized anxiety disorder, obsessive-compulsive disorder, and posttraumatic stress disorder. The effect of anxiety on perception, cognition, affect, and behavior differs in each of these

CHART 21-1
Behavioral Patterns Employed to Cope with Anxiety

Individuals attempt to cope with anxiety by employing the following major behavioral patterns:

1. **Withdrawal**
   The behavioral and/or psychological retreat from anxiety-provoking experiences
2. **Acting out**
   The discharge of anxiety through aggressive behavior
3. **Psychosomatization**
   The visceral or physiologic expression of anxiety
4. **Avoidance**
   The management of anxiety-laden experiences through evasive behaviors

5. **Problem-solving**
   The use of anxiety in the service of learning adaptive behavior[13,14]

With the exception of the last item, these behavior patterns are maladaptive because they replace feelings of anxiety with feelings of pleasure and comfort at the expense of accurate perception of reality and growth toward maturity. Therefore, the primary goal for treating clients with anxiety disorders, as well as other psychiatric syndromes, is to help them use anxiety as a means to increase their commitment to reality and growth toward maturity.

---

disorders. Despite these differences, the following common features are shared by all of the anxiety disorders:

1. The individual is distressed by a single symptom or group of symptoms
2. The individual perceives the symptom or symptoms as unacceptable to the self (ego-dystonic)
3. Reality-testing, the ability to perceive reality accurately, is grossly intact
4. The individual's behavior does not violate the prevailing culture's social norms
5. The disorder endures or recurs without treatment
6. The disorder cannot be attributed to an organic factor or cause[9]

Additionally, anxiety-disordered individuals may receive both primary and secondary gains because of their symptoms. The primary gain received because of symptom(s) is defense against and/or reduction of the emotional pain associated with anxiety. Secondary gains may include relief from responsibility and receipt of extra attention or monetary rewards. Receiving both primary and secondary gains tends to reinforce symptoms and maladaptive behavioral styles associated with anxiety disorders.[18]

Etiology of Anxiety Disorders

A variety of possible predisposing factors is connected with the development of anxiety disorders. These factors include hereditary predisposition; persistent neurochemical abnormalities, such as hyperthyroid-ism; physical diseases producing continual fears of death, as in the case of mitral valve prolapse; developmental traumas producing special vulnerabilities; inadequate social or interpersonal experiences necessary for acquiring mature coping mechanisms; counterproductive cognitive patterns in the form of unrealistic goals, values, or belief sets; and exposure to extreme psychological stressors.[2,7,12]

Additional factors thought to contribute to the onset of anxiety disorders are chronic physical illness; continuous, unavoidable exposure to toxic substances; repeated exposure to physical or psychological danger; chronic, insidious exposure to subtle criticism, threats, and disapproval; and specific external stressors impinging on specific emotional vulnerabilities, as in the case of an autonomous individual being forced to conform to the strict norms of a rigid, regimented group.[2] Any of the preceding factors alone or in interactive combination with others could be considered the cause of anxiety disorders.

Incidence and Prevalence

Statistics concerning the incidence and prevalence of anxiety disorders vary considerably.[2] According to Horowitz, 10% to 15% of people in the general population have at some time experienced what might be classified as an anxiety disorder.[7] Pasnau, on the other hand, estimates that only 2% to 4% of the population has had at some time a disorder which could qualify clinically as an anxiety disorder.[12] Still other experts speculate that 5% of the population is currently suffering from an acute or chronic anxiety disorder.[9]

Based on available information, women outnumber men two to one in the occurrence of anxiety disorders. Also, current information suggests that anxiety disorders tend to run in families. While significant numbers of individuals have succumbed to anxiety disorders, there is currently no reliable information indicating that their incidence has increased.[9]

Application of the Nursing Process to Anxiety Disorders

Assessment

Phobic Disorder

A *phobia* is a persistent, irrational fear attached to an object or situation that objectively does not pose a significant danger.[2,7] As a result, the individual experiences a compelling desire to avoid the dreaded object or situation. The phobic individual usually recognizes that the fear is unreasonable or excessive in proportion to the actual threat presented.[12] Three forms of phobic disorders commonly seen in clinical practice are agoraphobia, social phobia, and simple phobia.

Agoraphobia. *Agoraphobia* is a marked fear of being alone or in a public place from which escape would be difficult and/or help unavailable in the event of suddenly becoming disabled. It is the most severe and pervasive form of the phobic disorders.[7] It can begin abruptly after severe stress or in some cases for no apparent reason. Agoraphobia can also develop slowly in association with chronic severe anxiety. The agoraphobic individual is usually excessively dependent on others and may become symptomatic for the first time when faced with the loss of a significant relationship.[4]

Agoraphobia is most intense when the individual enters enclosed spaces such as stores, airplanes, vehicles, restaurants, theaters, subways, churches, or other situations in which he or she is surrounded by crowds. The agoraphobic individual *perceives* such situations as dreadfully frightening. *Cognitively,* the individual is preoccupied with avoiding the situation, or, when in the situation, with finding an escape route or exit. In addition to experiencing severe anxiety, the agoraphobic individual also feels embarrassment and humiliation about being unable to bear a situation that is usually well tolerated, if not enjoyed, by others.[11]

The agoraphobic individual may engage in a variety of behaviors to avoid confronting the anxiety-causing situation. These may include rituals designed to check on things, such as turning off the faucet, locking the door, or turning off the coffee pot. Even-

tually, the limitations imposed by agoraphobia may cause the individual to become depressed.[12]

Agoraphobia also affects the individual's interpersonal behaviors. Often the agoraphobic individual is conspicuously dependent on a spouse or close family member. This dependency is closely bound with the agoraphobic individual's sense of security, especially if he or she must leave home to face the dreaded situation. Eventually, the agoraphobic individual may even become housebound and insist on the constant companionship of this significant other.[7] In such a case, normal life activities are greatly constricted for both the agoraphobic individual and his or her companion.

The level of adaptation achieved by agoraphobic individuals is usually seriously impaired unless they receive treatment. Prolonged remissions are rare and spontaneous cures almost never occur. Complications such as chemical dependence and major depression are common.[7]

Social Phobia. A *social phobia* exists when an individual has a persistent irrational fear of, and a compelling desire to avoid, situations in which he or she may be exposed to the scrutiny of others. Additionally, the individual harbors the fear of behaving in a manner that will be humiliating or embarrassing to the self. Marked anticipatory anxiety occurs if the individual is confronted with such a situation, and attempts will be made to avoid it.[12]

Usually symptoms of social phobias occur in personal rather than impersonal situations.[4] In such a situation, the individual may perceive others as threatening sources of criticism and the self as small and insignificant in comparison. The individual's thought patterns may become disturbed or blocked as evidenced by his or her garbled speech or inability to speak or write. Besides feeling severe anxiety, the individual may shake, tremble, blush, vomit, or experience vertigo. As these symptoms increase in severity, the individual usually resorts to behaviors designed to avoid friendships or other close associations. Consequently, the individual with a social phobia becomes socially isolated. This social isolation may extend beyond recreational pursuits to the individual's employment as well.[4] Examples of social phobias include fear of speaking in public, writing in the presence of others, or using public restrooms.[12]

Levels of adaptation achieved by individuals with social phobias are severely restricted. This condition is a chronic illness and may coexist with agoraphobia or generalized anxiety disorder. While spontaneous remissions may occur, treatment with psychotherapy and psychochemotherapy is almost always indicated.[7]

Simple Phobia.   A *simple phobia* is a persistent irrational fear of, and a compelling desire to avoid, exposure to a circumstance or class of thing other than those specific to agoraphobia or social phobia.[7] Common simple phobias include acrophobia, or fear of heights; claustrophobia, or fear of closed spaces; blood phobia, or fear of the sight of blood or injury. Other simple phobias are fear of birds, cats, furry animals, housedust, microbes, snakes, or insects.[7,12]

Upon exposure to the dreaded circumstance or thing, the individual may experience anxiety that reaches the panic level. Before probable confrontation with the dreaded object or circumstance, persons with simple phobia may behave like individuals in crisis situations. For example, they may seek a great deal of information before committing themselves to action, or become hypervigilant, or in some cases they may experience disbelief and psychic numbing.[7]

The nature of the simple phobia determines to a great extent the level of adaptation achieved by affected individuals. To illustrate, impairment may be minimal or almost nonexistent if the dreaded object or circumstance is rare in the environment and can be easily avoided. For example, snakes may be feared but can be avoided in a large city. On the other hand, a fear of riding elevators can be disabling in a large city. Usually, adults who have had a simple phobia since childhood or who have since acquired one require treatment to reach their optimal adaptation level.

Panic Disorder

The term *panic disorder* refers to an anxiety disorder characterized by recurrent, unpredictable anxiety attacks of panic proportions.[12] Although panic attacks are unpredictable in onset, they frequently occur in certain situations such as driving a car. While these attacks may be associated with a given situation, they do not necessarily occur every time the individual confronts the situation. Moreover, panic attacks may occur in other places. This feature is helpful in distinguishing panic attacks from phobias.[7]

Panic attacks are usually manifested by a sudden onset of intense apprehension or terror and are often associated with feelings of doom.[7] The clinical picture during a panic attack closely approximates the alarm reaction described in Selye's General Adaptation Syndrome, in which there is a psychologic and physiologic over-response to stressors. For example, the individual experiencing a panic attack incorrectly perceives his or her circumstances as life-threatening. Consequently, the individual experiences the following physiological reactions: dyspnea, chest pain or discomfort, palpitations, choking or smothering sensations, dizziness, vertigo, parathesias, hot and cold flashes, sweating, and fainting. Additionally, the person may report feelings of depersonalization, derealization, and fears of dying, going crazy, or behaving in an uncontrolled manner during the attack.[12] These attacks usually last for several minutes but rarely last hours.[7]

During panic attacks, the individual may make extreme efforts to escape from what is perceived to be causing the panic. Consequently, social and/or work relations may be disrupted by the individual's supposedly strange behavior.[7] Between panic attacks, the individual often remains moderately to severely anxious.[12] Thus, the individual's level of adaptation may be seriously thwarted unless treatment is sought.

Generalized Anxiety Disorder

Generalized anxiety disorder is usually characterized by chronic anxiety that is so uncomfortable that it interferes with daily life. Seldom do individuals suffering from this disorder experience eruptions of acute anxiety.[9] Rather, these individuals persistently manifest signs of severe anxiety, including motor tension, autonomic hyperactivity, and apprehensive expectation.[12] In some instances, people affected by this disorder also have chronic hypervigilance, as evidenced by their continuously scanning the environment for potential threats. Behavioral displays of impatience and irritability, as well as complaints of always feeling on edge, are common.[7]

Due to this tense hyperarousal, individuals may be unable to concentrate, may suffer chronic fatigue, and may experience sleep pattern disturbances. Additionally, they may exhibit tenseness and distractibility in social situations. For these reasons, individuals with this disorder may eventually become depressed.[7] Because of their symptoms, these people usually seek treatment to improve their adaptation level.

Obsessive-Compulsive Disorder

Obsessive-compulsive disorder is a psychiatric condition in which the individual experiences recurrent obsessions and/or compulsions.[12] The term *obsession* as used in this diagnosis refers to recurrent, persistent ideas, thoughts, images, or impulses. The individual with this disorder does not voluntarily produce obsessions. Rather, the individual feels invaded by the obsessive material and often finds the material repugnant or meaningless. Despite efforts to ignore or dismiss obsessive material, the individual remains preoccupied with unbidden ideations.[7,12]

Compulsions, on the other hand, are ritualistic behaviors that the individual feels compelled to perform either in accord with a specific set of rules or in a routinized manner. Performing the compulsive ritual is designed to prevent or reduce anxiety associated with some future event the individual wishes to prevent or produce.[12] At the same time, the person invests the obsessive act with symbolic significance by unrealistically believing that the act magically solves problems or atones for past misdeeds.[7] If the affected individual or others intervene to stop the compulsive act, anxiety results.[7, 10, 12]

The obsessive-compulsive individual may experience mild to severe symptoms. If symptoms are mild and conducive to occupational productivity, the individual may not feel the need to seek treatment. Severe symptoms that interfere with the quality of life, however, almost always result in the individual seeking help. If treatment is not sought or is unsuccessful, these individuals may become so uncomfortable that they become depressed and even suicidal.[4] Because of these factors, the adaptation level achieved by obsessive-compulsive individuals is variable.

Posttraumatic Stress Disorder

Posttraumatic stress disorder is a new diagnostic category. It is defined as the development of characteristic symptoms after exposure to a tramatic life experience capable of psychologically harming most people.[1] Unlike other psychiatric conditions, which are causally linked to the individual's psychosocial and biological makeup, posttraumatic stress disorder occurs only in response to a traumatic life experience.[12]

Traumatic events capable of causing posttraumatic stress disorder fall into three categories:

1. Natural disasters, such as earthquakes, floods, hurricanes, tornadoes
2. Accidental human-made disasters, such as nuclear plant accidents, auto crashes, industrial accidents, airplane crashes
3. Intentional human-made disasters, such as prolonged military combat, rape, muggings, armed robbery, assault, physical and/or psychological abuse (ranging from death camp experience, to public ridicule and hazing, to frightening or painful health care experiences)[8]

These traumatic events vary in *duration* and *severity*. Both factors, however, must be carefully considered in evaluating whether the stressor is capable of producing posttraumatic stress disorder. For example, short episodes of military combat, harassment, hazing, and public ridicule are not usually considered sufficiently severe to cause this disorder. They are, however, capable of producing this disorder if they persist over time.[1]

Other stressors such as rape, robbery, or assault are severe enough to cause posttraumatic stress disorder after only one exposure. Events of this nature are intentional human-made disasters that occur suddenly and are almost totally unexpected. The person is caught off guard and usually feels trapped, with no opportunity to flee or fight.[1] Because stressors such as these are not only sudden, unexpected, and inescapable but also motivated by intentional human cruelty, they cause greater psychological trauma than accidental human-made or natural disasters.

Characteristic symptoms of posttraumatic stress disorder include the following:

Reexperience of the traumatic event by way of intrusive recollections, dreams, and/or suddenly feeling and acting as if the event is recurring[12]

Psychic numbing and denial

Perceptual distortions, including illusions, intrusive images, and pseudohallucinations

Feelings of being pressured, confused, or disorganized when thinking about the event

Memory impairment

Overgeneralization of other sensory inputs so that they seem related in some way to the event

Preoccupation with the event to the extent that concentration on other topics is impossible

Hypervigilance and exaggerated startle reactions

Somatic symptoms such as fatigue, headache, and muscular pain

Alterations in activity pattern, including compulsively repeating actions associated with the event, frantic overactivity, withdrawal, and indecision about how to respond to the consequences of the event

Alterations in social role due to loss of a reality-based relatedness with the ongoing world

Paranormal experiences such as deja vu, precognition, telepathic dreams, transpersonal experiences, as well as other altered states of consciousness[8]

A latency period of months or even years may intervene between exposure to the traumatic stressor and the onset of symptoms associated with posttraumatic stress disorder. When symptoms appear within six months of the trauma, an *acute posttraumatic stress disorder* exists. If symptoms begin more than six months after the traumatic event, the condition is referred to as a *delayed posttraumatic stress disorder*.[1]

With both acute and delayed posttraumatic stress disorder, the individual's adaptation level can be positively or adversely affected. With effective treatment, the individual may recover from the disorder and also gain increased psychological resilience and coping capacity. In other instances, the disorder may increase the individual's vulnerability to development of other anxiety disorders, chemical abuse and dependence, and depression.[8] Prompt, effective treatment, however, seems to be the key to restoring the individual to his or her optimal adaptation level.

Formulation of Nursing Diagnoses

Formulating nursing diagnoses for clients who manifest symptoms of anxiety disorders is a challenging nursing responsibility. Unlike psychiatric medical diagnoses, which provide descriptive classifications for symptom sets, nursing diagnoses describe behavioral alterations and coping deficits and suggest prescriptive intervention. As such, nursing diagnoses apply not just to one psychiatric diagnosis but to several.

Nursing diagnoses applicable to clients with anxiety disorders include the following:

Sensory-perceptual alteration associated with severe anxiety

Disturbed cognitive functioning associated with severe anxiety

Disturbed cognitive functioning related to decisional conflict

Alteration of breathing pattern related to hyperventilation associated with severe anxiety

Short-term memory deficit related to exposure to a traumatic stressor

Diversional activity deficit related to preoccupation with repetitive, ritualistic activity

Self-care deficit related to preoccupation with repetitive, ritualistic activity

Disturbed cognitive functioning related to repetitive, intrusive thoughts

Exaggerated fear of being alone in assigned room

Anticipatory anxiety of severe proportion associated with preparing for shopping trip to mall

Ineffective individual coping related to chronic moderate anxiety

Ineffective individual coping related to exaggerated fear of conversing with other people

Impaired verbal communication related to severe anxiety

Decreased social sensitivity related to psychic numbing

Alteration in consciousness associated with re-experiencing a traumatic event

Sleep pattern disturbance associated with recurrent dreams and nightmares

Dysfunctional marital relationship related to decreased sexual desire associated with chronic severe anxiety

Dysfunctional group membership behavior related to chronic severe anxiety[3]

This is a fairly small sample of nursing diagnoses applicable to individuals with anxiety disorders.

Planning

Despite the differences among the anxiety disorders, the major goals for nursing care have applicability to each of them. These goals are concerned primarily with the client learning about anxiety and how to cope with it. They are as follows:

To accept the experience of anxiety as inevitable and normal

To increase self-awareness with regard to fluctuations in anxiety level

To reduce shame about exhibiting signs of anxiety

To learn and apply self-help techniques designed to reduce anxiety

To increase problem-solving and coping skills

Clients who meet these goals not only develop an increased tolerance of anxiety but also an increased awareness of their strengths and limitations.

Intervention

To help the client reach the planned goals, the nurse needs to establish a supportive relationship with the client. This relationship is characterized by trust, respect, and empathy on the part of the nurse. Displaying these attributes to the client on a consistent basis will lay the groundwork for therapy to begin.

Clarifying the Issues

To defuse the client's emotionally charged state, the nurse needs to remain calm, because anxiety is transmitted easily through interpersonal contact.[17] Conversely, calmness can also be transmitted to the client by the nurse. Because the client's perceptual and cognitive processes may be disturbed due to high anxiety levels, the nurse needs to position herself in the center of the client's visual field. Additionally, the nurse needs to speak clearly, using a voice low in volume and tone. Doing so will help the client perceive accurately what the nurse is saying. For the same reason, the nurse needs to use short, uninvolved sentences to facilitate the client's articulation of the specific issues associated with his symptoms of anxiety. Once the issues surrounding the anxious state are revealed and clarified, the nurse can then begin to intervene to help the client understand the connections between identified issues and the experience of anxiety.

For example, a client who suddenly appeared in the emergency room manifesting an almost panic-level anxiety and complaining of having been terrified of driving for the past month was admitted to the mental health unit. Shortly after her admission, she revealed that her adult son had moved back home about 2 months ago with his wife and infant, creating an upheaval in her household. The client later confided that she would just like to run away from home. Of course, as the client had become terrified of driving, she had few choices except to stay in her home or to seek refuge in the hospital. After assisting the client to clarify the issues associated with the onset of her anxious state, the nurse was able to help the client

Nursing Care Plan 21-1

The Obsessive-Compulsive Client

Nursing Diagnosis	Goal	Intervention
Self-care deficit due to preoccupation with repetitive, ritualistic behavior	Promotion of self-care activities, *i.e.*, grooming, eating, recreation	Do not overtly stop the client's performance of the ritual
		Initiate conversation with client as he performs ritual
		Assess for behavioral clues indicating an increase in anxiety
		If the client's anxiety level remains unchanged, then negotiate with the client a schedule for performing the ritual that will allow time for performance of self-care activities
		Assess client for attending to stimuli that distract him from performing the ritual
		Assess the client's anxiety level when exposed to the distracting stimulus
		If his anxiety level does not increase, then present the distracting stimulus at gradually shorter time intervals until the ritualistic behavior is extinguished

learn how to cope and solve problems more effectively.

Accepting the Inevitability of Experiencing Anxiety

The nurse needs to explain the concept of anxiety to the client in simple terms and emphasize that all people feel anxious from time to time. In doing so, the nurse reduces the client's anxiety about being anxious by "normalizing" this experience to a degree.[2] Also, this nursing intervention assuages to some extent the shame that clients may feel about losing control of their emotions.

Increasing Self-Awareness

In the case previously mentioned, the client may have viewed the change in her household situation as merely coincidental with the development of panic episodes associated with driving a car. To help the client recognize on a conscious level the highly prob-

able connection between the two issues, the nurse engaged the client in self-awareness activities. Three of these activities are as follows:

1. Ask the client to maintain a diary in which she will record when she feels anxious, what she is doing at the time, what she is thinking, and who she is with. The client—either alone or with the assistance of the nurse—may begin to recognize her "anxiety triggers."
2. Ask the client to maintain a graph, with anxiety levels on one axis and time measured in 30-minute intervals on the other axis (see Fig. 21-3) for a 24-hour period. This activity, used in combination with the diary, may help the client develop awareness not only of when, but of under what circumstances, her anxiety is mild, moderate, severe, or of panic proportions. Discussing and analyzing the findings with the client are crucial in this process.[2]

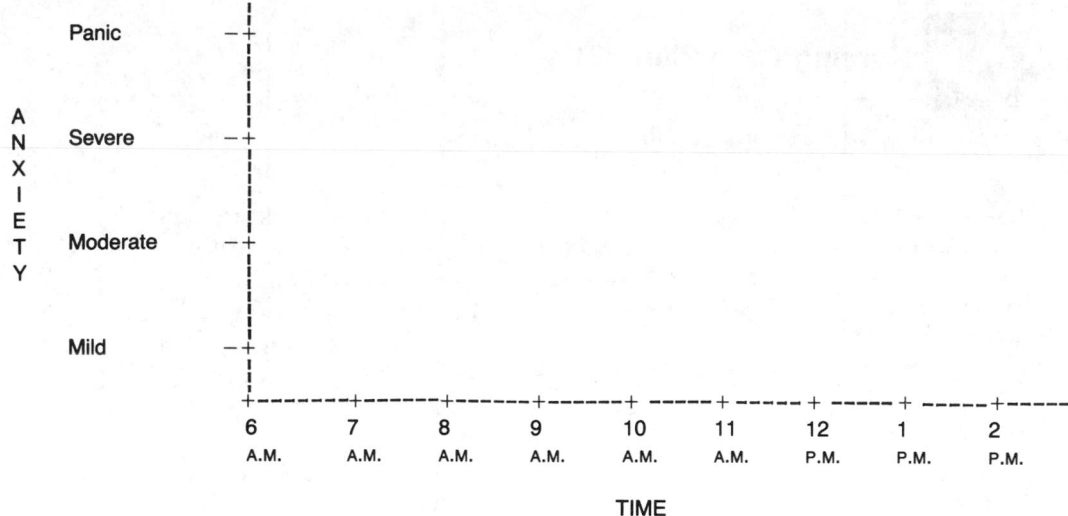

Figure 21-3. *Graph of anxiety levels.*

3. Ask the client to participate in a family conference in which family members or significant others enter the conference group one at a time. As each person enters the room, ask the client to rate her anxiety level and to record the findings on a small piece of paper. The results can be discussed in the family conference and in subsequent individual interactions with the client. Both the client and the family need careful preparation for this exercise. The purpose must be explained as helping the client and the family to identify how they affect each other.

Learning Self-Help Skills

Once the client has identified those factors associated with uncomfortable symptoms of anxiety, the nurse needs to help the client identify ways of reducing anxiety to a tolerable level. In the case previously mentioned, the client connected the onset of symptoms with the upheaval created by her son and his family moving into her home. Additionally, she was able to articulate her anger about her son's refusal to contribute money to pay for household expenses and his inattention to his wife and child. The anger the client felt was frightening to her because it meant that she had failed in her role as the "good mother." So, rather than express her anger directly to her son, she repressed and suppressed her feelings. When these defense mechanisms failed to shore in her emotions, the emotions appeared in the form of severe to panic-level anxiety. Because the client unconsciously wished to escape from her anxiety-producing situation yet realized that she could not do so for fear of appearing irresponsible, she began to experience anxiety attacks, especially when she attempted to drive her car.

To assist the client to express her feelings openly and honestly without losing control, the nurse encouraged the client to learn *assertiveness skills.* The client attended an assertiveness training class daily for 5 days. In role-play exercises with other clients, she practiced expressing her feelings—both positive and negative—to her son. Additionally, the client practiced making *behavior change requests* of her son during these role-play sessions. At the end of the 5 days, the client was able to use assertiveness skills effectively with her son and other family members in a family therapy session led by the nurse.

While the client had gained a great deal of knowledge and insight into her condition and had become more assertive with her family and associates, she still expressed doubt about her ability to drive a car without becoming overly anxious. To help prepare the client for resuming this activity, the nurse taught her how to use *positive coping statements* to allay her self-doubt and anxiety about driving. To use positive coping statements, the nurse asked the client to compose reassuring statements that she could say aloud or silently to herself whenever she felt anxiety or self-doubt about driving. The client was then asked to repeat these statements continuously until she experienced relief.

Additionally, the client was asked to close her eyes while in a sitting position and to imagine herself in her car. The nurse then asked her to imagine herself driving, feeling alert and calm, and being successful. The client was then asked to repeat this exercise, known as *covert rehearsal,* at least three times each day.

Nursing Care Plan 21-2

The Client with Posttraumatic Stress Disorder

Nursing Diagnosis	Goal	Intervention
Alteration in consciousness associated with reexperiencing the traumatic event by way of unbidden images, illusions, pseudohallucinations, and nightmares	Restoration and maintenance of normal stream of consciousness	Reassure client that these experiences are common occurrences after a traumatic event
		Reassure client that these experiences are not serious portents of psychosis, *i.e.,* "going crazy"
		Stay with the client until these experiences subside
		Encourage ventilation of feelings
		Offer reassurance and empathy as often as needed

Relaxation therapy was also used to assist the client to learn how to control her anxiety. The client learned to do progressive muscular relaxation and deep breathing exercises to decrease her anxiety. Using this form of therapy by way of audiotapes each morning and evening helped her to control her anxiety.

The nurse also suggested that the client read self-help books and pamphlets written by individuals who had successfully overcome anxiety disorders similar to her own.[5,6] This form of treatment is referred to as *bibliotherapy*. The client also attended a daily self-help group known as Emotions Anonymous. Through these experiences, the client developed an understanding of herself and her anxiety disorder and an acceptance of her tendency to feel anxious occasionally.

Increasing Problem-Solving and Coping Skills

Besides involvement in learning self-help skills, clients with anxiety disorders also benefit from individual and group therapies designed to assist them in identifying their emotions and automatic behaviors used to relieve uncomfortable feelings. When they are able to identify these, then clients can engage in problem-solving with regard to the following issues:

The extent to which their appraisals of stressors as dangerous are correct

Whether their emotional response exceeds the degree of anxiety expected in view of the actual dangerousness of the stressor

The effectiveness and appropriateness of the relief behavior

Alternative ways of perceiving and appraising stressors

Alternative coping mechanisms for allaying and discharging anxious feelings

Clients can then test out alternative coping mechanisms in therapy to enhance their generalizability to life situations.

Administering Antianxiety Agents

Usually, antianxiety agents are prescribed for anxiety-disordered clients during the initial phase of treatment. Because many anxiety-disordered individuals are at risk for development of chemical abuse or dependence, antianxiety agents—which are, for the most part, addictive—are administered sparingly and on a short-term basis. Antianxiety agents do not cure anxiety disorders, but they do calm clients sufficiently for them to engage in and benefit from therapies that may be beneficial, if not curative.[15]

Evaluation

The extent to which nursing care for clients with anxiety disorders is effective is based on the client's subjective report of his feeling state as well as changes in the client's behavior. Behavior changes indicating improvement, such as decreased muscular tension and tremors, increased appetite, normal physiologic in-

Case Study 21-1

Caring for the Client Who Has a Posttraumatic Stress Disorder

Ms. S. was brought to the hospital emergency room by a friend. Ms. S. was in a stunned, dazed state, had difficulty attending to questions or statements addressed to her, and was disoriented as to time and place. She was, however, oriented to her own identity and that of her friend. Ms. S. also seemed unable to appreciate the significance of her having been brought to the emergency room for examination and possible treatment. Her general appearance was within normal limits; she appeared well-nourished, neat, clean, and appropriately dressed.

Her friend reported that Ms. S. answered her door reluctantly when she made an impromptu visit earlier and that, when she was finally allowed to enter, Ms. S.'s home was in disarray. The friend further reported that she realized Ms. S.'s home had been forcibly entered and that she had called the police for assistance. Blood-stained clothes had been discovered in Ms. S.'s bathroom by the police, and the friend expressed the fear that Ms. S. had been raped.

When a male physician approached Ms. S. in the examination room, she displayed an exaggerated startle response and muscular stiffening. Additionally, Ms. S. recoiled and began to mumble nonsensical statements as she struggled to distance herself from the male physician.

A nurse clinical specialist with expertise in rape crisis counseling was then called to help Ms. S. The nurse was able to defuse Ms. S.'s extreme state of anxiety by acknowledging that she must have been terribly hurt by someone and that it was normal to be upset about being hurt. As Ms. S. began to attend to the nurse, she was able to admit finally that a man had hurt her. Gently, the nurse asked her if she had been raped. Although Ms. S. cried out loudly and at first was incoherent, she eventually acknowledged that she had been raped. After crying and vividly recounting details of the incident and her attempt to make herself forget by taking several baths, Ms. S. was able to undergo the necessary examination and procedures needed by rape victims.

Ms. S. was discharged from the emergency room and referred to the local mental health center for intensive rape crisis counseling. During 6 months, Ms. S. received both individual and group therapy. The primary focus of the treatment was aimed at helping her view herself as an effective survivor rather than a helpless victim.

Within 6 months, Ms. S. was completely recovered. She was able to serve an an effective witness in the identification and prosecution of the perpetrator of the crime committed against her.

---

dices, and increased attention span and concentration, may be the first signs that the client has begun to improve. Additionally, the reduction of cardinal symptoms associated with anxiety disorders and their replacement with adaptive behavior signify improvement.

The development of increased self-awareness and ability to cope with anxiety producing situations, as evidenced by the client's self-disclosures and behavioral patterns, also indicates significant improvement. More important, the client's acceptance of anxiety as an inevitable part of human existence, and his commitment to live effectively in spite of this, stand as the major advances toward recovery of adaptive mental health.

Summary

This chapter has provided an overview of anxiety as a part of normal human existence. It has discussed the occurrence of more severe levels of anxiety that persist, cannot be dismissed, and interfere with the individual's life—that is, the anxiety disorders. Specifically, this chapter has made the following points:

1. Anxiety is a clinical feature of almost every psychiatric syndrome.
2. Anxiety occurs as the initial response to psychic stressors and is ascertained through self-report, such as feelings of dread, appre-

C H A R T   21-2
Panic
Karen R. Perkins, M.S.N., R.N.
Clinical Nurse Specialist/
Clinic Manager, Psychiatric Outpatient Services
Parkland Memorial Hospital
Dallas, Texas

The following diagram is an algorithm, or decision tree, which serves as a guideline for action. Although a nursing algorithm guides nursing intervention with a client exhibiting certain kinds of behavior, the nurse recognizes that each client situation is different and individualizes care accordingly. The following is an algorithm for a client with manifestations of severe anxiety or panic.

(Continues on p. 368)

(A) Nurse Reaction

Clients experiencing severe anxiety or panic may be found in any health care setting. However, the majority of these clients are commonly encountered in an emergency department or psychiatric service. Often, it is the nurse who first initiates care for such clients. It is readily apparent that a client experiencing severe anxiety or a panic attack is in great distress. The person dramatically displays physiological, emotional, and cognitive signs and symptoms of extreme anxiety. Physiologic symptoms reflect sympathetic discharge, e.g., tachycardia, paresthesia, etc.; emotionally, a sense of unexplained/unrealistic dread or terror usually dominates the client's mood. Cognitive symptoms range from an inability to attend to all but the most simple of directions to delusional, even frankly psychotic, thinking. The client may or may not be hallucinating. He may present as desperate and clinging or dash about as if frantic to escape. He may cry, scream, and shake or simply freeze and stare as if in great fear and confusion. Such behavior can be confusing and disquieting to even the most seasoned nurse. Acute anxiety or panic is a notably contagious state of being. An awareness of this phenomenon, coupled with a planned and structured approach to panic management, can greatly decrease not only the client's, but the managing nurse's, own rising anxiety level.

(B) History

Because acute anxiety is often a manifestation of a serious medical illness, concurrent psychiatric condition, or an ongoing intrapsychic condition, a thorough medical and psychiatric history is essential in establishing a working diagnosis and initial approach to treatment. The history should include the development of symptoms (including time factors), interrelationships of symptoms, and factors that help to decrease symptoms. Psychiatric history includes any past or current treatment, medication regimen, including duration and dosage, and any problems associated with treatment. History concerning drug and alcohol use/abuse, any family psychiatric history, and any recent increase in psychosocial stressors is also important. The history may have to be obtained from a family member or close friend if the client is initially unable to cooperate; as the client begins to calm down, additional history is collected in an ongoing manner.

(C) Nursing Assessment and Goals

The nursing assessment is directed toward screening for patterns of behavior that indicate the etiology of the particular attack, i.e., drug abuse, response to psychosocial stressors, disease states, psychiatric disorders. Depending upon the client's ability to cooperate, basic nursing assessment includes information about chief complaint, complete vital signs, and an evaluation of dangerousness to self and others. Occasionally a client may become overly aggressive if he misperceives staff or the environment as being hostile or harmful. A client complaining primarily of physical symptoms requires an immediate medical evaluation. Regardless of precipitating cause, primary nursing goals include decreasing/relieving the client's immediate distress and maintenance of client and staff safety. Subsequent goals include helping the client to identify and better cope with the underlying sources of anxiety which have contributed to the particular attack.

(D) Behaviors Indicating Medical Illness

Because many serious medical illnesses produce signs and symptoms identical to those often associated with anxiety disorders, the diagnostic process must be systematic and thorough. Be prepared to assist in obtaining specimens for laboratory tests. Usually a client's panic will decrease as he is assured that others are in control and that he is being promptly and correctly evaluated and treated. Some common medical conditions in which anxiety may be a prominent symptom are: hypoxia, angina pectoris, caffeinism, pulmonary embolus, thyrotoxicosis, myocardial infarction, hypoglycemia, metabolic acidosis, pneumothorax, hyperthyroidism, and a host of infectious diseases.

(E) Behavior Indicates Psychiatric Disorder

Clients with a thought disorder, i.e., schizophrenia, may respond to the internal stimuli of delusional or hallucinatory material with increased levels of anxiety. Command hallucinations frequently lead clients to the point of panic when fears of acting on suicidal or homicidal commands overwhelm defenses. Whereas a nonpsychotic client may be reassured by appropriate physical contact, a psychotically anxious client should not be touched or approached too closely unless his condition requires physical restraint. Clients with a primary anxiety disorder usually respond to reassurance that they have a condition that is treatable with either medication or a combination of medication and psychotherapy. If a client is hyperventillating, simply having him breathe into a small paper bag while calmly reassuring him can produce a marked decrease in symptoms. The definitive treatment for generalized anxiety disorder is antidepressant therapy, but because these drugs are potentially lethal, have many side-effects, and often take a month or more to reach therapeutic levels, they are not usually started in an ER setting. The client should be referred for appropriate inpatient or outpatient treatment as indicated. True panic disorder is best treated with a regimen of anxiolytic medication and psychotherapy.

(G) Behavior Indicates Medication Side-Effects

Drug-induced akathisia is a common extrapyramidal reaction associated with many antipsychotic drugs. The restlessness and intense compulsion to move about may appear to be symptoms of an anxiety disorder—only a thorough medication and drug history, along with careful observation and questioning, can help distinguish anxiety states from drug-induced akathisia. IM or IV antiparkinson/anticholinergic agents or antihistamines may be helpful in relieving these very uncomfortable sensations. However, akathisia can be difficult to treat; it does not respond as dramatically to anticholinergic therapy as do dystonic reactions. Clients have been known to attempt suicide in an effort to escape the distress of protracted and extreme akathisia. Clients may require hospitalization until a suitable medication regimen can be established. If the client can be managed as an outpatient, careful teaching and a referral to a program that will provide comprehensive services are a primary nursing responsibility. Anticholinergic toxicity secondary to Artane and Cogentin abuse may also mimic

anxiety and is becoming more of a problem and source of abuse.

(F) Behavior Indicates Substance Abuse/Withdrawal

Panic states and high levels of anxiety are commonly associated symptoms of substance abuse and withdrawal. Such clients are seen very frequently in ER settings. Depending upon the agent abused, treatment and general approach to client management will vary. A client experiencing a "bad trip" secondary to LSD usually responds to the reassurance that he will regain control of his mind and that staff will help him through this phase. He should be removed to a quiet room with soft lighting and someone should remain with him at all times. Usually the client responds to quiet reassurance and can be "talked down." Inexperienced users of marijuana sometimes have an acute panic reaction; they too usually respond to quiet reassurance and decreased stimuli. Phencyclidine (PCP) abusers can be unpredictable and should be considered potentially dangerous to self and others. Clients are best treated by being placed in isolation in a quiet room under observation. If the client is combative or self-destructive, he should be restrained and medicated. Trying to "talk down" such a client usually serves only to further agitate him and make matters worse. Nurses should be familiar with signs and symptoms of substance withdrawal and respond according to unit protocol and procedure.

References

1. Rund D. and Hutzler J. *Emergency Psychiatry.* St. Louis, CV Mosby, 1983
2. Soreff S. and McNeil G. *Handbook of Psychiatric Differential Diagnosis.* Littleton, MA, PSG Publishing Co. Inc., 1987
3. Mancini M.E., *Decision Making in Emergency Nursing.* Toronto, BC Decker Inc., 1987

hension, restlessness, and "jitteriness," and through physiological signs, such as increased heart rate and blood pressure, excessive perspiration, sexual dysfunction, and increased rate and depth of respiration.

3. Levels of anxiety range from mild to moderate, severe, and panic.

4. An anxiety disorder is a psychiatric condition characterized by the emotion of intense terror and thoughts of impending catastrophe that persist over substantial periods of time.

5. Phobic disorders commonly seen in clinical practice include agoraphobia, social phobia, and simple phobia.

6. A panic disorder is an anxiety disorder characterized by recurrent anxiety attacks of panic proportions that occur unpredictably.

7. Generalized anxiety disorder is usually characterized by a level of chronic anxiety that is so uncomfortable that it interferes with daily life.

8. In obsessive-compulsive disorder, the individual experiences recurrent obsessions, or per-

sistent thoughts, ideas, images, or impulses, and compulsions, or ritualistic behaviors that he feels compelled to perform in a routinized manner.

9. Posttraumatic stress disorder is the development of certain characteristic symptoms after exposure to a traumatic life experience capable of psychologically harming most persons.

10. Planning and implementing nursing care for clients with anxiety disorders centers on helping the client accept the experience of anxiety as normal and inevitable, increase self-awareness regarding variations in anxiety levels, reduce shame about exhibiting signs of anxiety, learn and apply self-help techniques to reduce anxiety, and increase problem-solving and coping skills.

References

1. Andreasen NC: Posttraumatic Stress Disorder. In Kaplan HI, Sadock BJ (eds): Comprehensive Textbook of Psychiatry IV. Baltimore, Williams & Wilkins, 1985
2. Beck AT, Emery G, Greensberg RL: Anxiety Disorders and Phobias. New York, Basic Books, 1986
3. Gordon M: Manual of Nursing Diagnosis. New York, McGraw-Hill, 1984
4. Gray M: Neuroses. New York, Von Nostrand Reinhold, 1978
5. Green MD: Living Fear Free. New York, Warner Books, 1985
6. Handley R, Neff P: Anxiety and Panic Attacks. New York, Fawcett Crest, 1985
7. Horowitz MJ: In Goldman HH (ed): Review of General Psychiatry, pp. 362–375. Los Altos, CA, Lange Medical Publications, 1984
8. Horowitz MJ: A Review of Posttraumatic and Adjustment Disorders. Hosp Community Psychiatry (March) 241–249, 1986
9. Nemiah JC: Neurotic Disorders. In Kaplan HI, Sadock BJ (eds): Comprehensive Textbook of Psychiatry IV. Baltimore, Williams & Wilkins, 1985
10. Nemiah JC: Obsessive-Compulsive Disorders. In Kaplan HI, Sadock BJ (eds): Comprehensive Textbook of Psychiatry IV. Baltimore, Williams & Wilkins, 1985
11. Nemiah JC: Phobic Disorders. In Kaplan HI, Sadock BJ (eds): Comprehensive Textbook of Psychiatry IV. Baltimore, Williams & Wilkins, 1985
12. Pasnau RO: Diagnosis and Treatment of Anxiety Disorders. Washington, D.C., American Psychiatric Press, 1984
13. Peplau HE: A Working Definition of Anxiety. In Burd SF, Marshall MA (eds): Some Clinical Approaches to Psychiatric Nursing. New York, Macmillan, 1963
14. Peplau HE: Interpersonal Relations in Nursing. New York, GP Putnam's Sons, 1952
15. Roy-Byrne PP, Katon W: An Update on Treatment of the Anxiety Disorders. Hospital and Community Psychiatry 38 (August) 835–843, 1987
16. Reusch J: Disturbed Communication. New York, WW Norton, 1972
17. Reusch J: Therapeutic Communication. New York, WW Norton, 1973
18. Smith SF, Karasik DA, Meyer BJ: Review of Psychiatric and Psychosocial Nursing. Los Altos, CA, National Nursing Review, 1984
19. Stern VF, Stern EM: Keeping Faith with the Terrorized Patient: A Dialogue. The Psychotherapy Patient 1, 4 (Summer) 3–10, 1985

22 Maladaptation: The Personality Disorders

Judith A. Greene

Judge not, that ye be not judged.
For with what judgment ye judge, ye shall be judged: and with what measure ye mete, it shall be measured to you again.
And why beholdest thou the mote that is in thy brother's eye, but considerest not the beam that is in thine own eye?
Or how wilt thou say to thy brother, Let me pull out the mote out of thine eye; and, behold, a beam is in thine own eye?
Thou hypocrite, first cast out the beam out of thine own eye; and then shalt thou see clearly to cast out the mote out of thy brother's eye.

Matt. 7:1–5,
Holy Bible,
King James Version

Chapter Preview

The current period of history is rapidly becoming known as the age of narcissism.[5, 6] *Narcissism,* a love for the self, stands as a counterpoint to love for humanity. Given that many of today's most popular life philosophies advocate individual growth, individual rights, and self-improvement to the exclusion of concern for others, narcissism is an appropriate metaphor for the recent state of the human condition.[5, 6]

With this change in how individuals view themselves in relation to others, the incidence and prevalence of psychiatric syndromes have also changed. More specifically, unlike the *age of anxiety,* when people succumbed to a variety of neuroses (now referred to as anxiety states), the *age of narcissism* is resulting in the increased incidence and prevalence of personality disorders.[5] Although typologies and diagnostic criteria for personality disorders have undergone many changes that render it virtually impossible to obtain valid statistics regarding their incidence and prevalence, experts agree that personality disorders constitute a significant psychiatric–mental health problem.[5, 19, 20]

Learning Objectives

Upon completion of the chapter, you should be able to accomplish the following:

1. Define personality and personality disorder
2. Identify common characteristics of personality disorders
3. Describe the position of the personality disorders on the mental health continuum
4. Discuss selected personality disorders in terms of their perceptive, cognitive, affective, and behavioral disturbances, adaptation levels, and mental health care-seeking behaviors
5. Apply the nursing process—assessment, diagnosis, planning, intervention, and evaluation—to clients with personality disorders

Personality and Personality Disorder Defined

The *personality* may be defined as "a consistent and stable pattern of behavior shown by a person in meeting a variety of challenges and opportunities, consistent over long periods of his life and recognized as special to each person."[17] The individual's personality is an indispensable aspect of his identity in that it is ego-syntonic with his self-definition. Personality patterns or styles may be adaptive or maladaptive. When the personality of an individual is maladaptive, the designation *personality disorder* is appropriately applied.

Common Characteristics of Personality Disorders

Although several distinct types of personality disorders exist, the following characteristics are commonly found in all of the disorders:

1. A deeply ingrained, inflexible, maladaptive response to anxiety
2. Maladaptation that is most apparent within an interpersonal or social context
3. The capacity to induce others to feel extreme irritation and annoyance
4. A self-centered, inflexible approach to work and interpersonal relationships[19]

Adjectives or descriptive phrases applicable to many persons with personality disorders include narcissistic, unempathetic, inordinate sense of entitlement, dependent, lack of self-insight while giving evidence of pseudoself-knowledge, unable to self-evaluate, cynical, pessimistic, depressed, lack of objectivity, lack of self-control, egocentric, selfish, lonely, immature, manipulative, aggressive, impulsive, hostile, and suspicious.[1, 5, 19] While these terms concretize, to some extent, the four characteristics associated with all personality disorders, they also indicate the severity of these disorders.

Personality Disorders in Relation to the Health–Illness Continuum

The health–illness continuum may be used to classify personality disorders in terms of severity, with adaptive mental health at one extreme and psychoses at the other extreme. Neuroses or anxiety states follow adaptive mental health on the continuum. The personality disorders then fall between anxiety states and psychoses. (See Fig. 22-1.) This schematic classification thus illustrates that the personality disorders constitute one of the most severe groups of psychiatric syndromes.

Figure 22-1. *Mental health–illness continuum.*

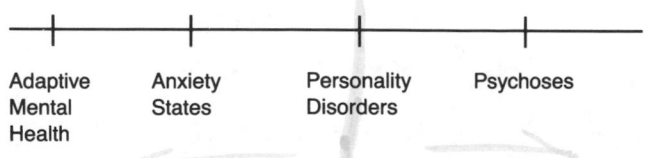

Etiology of Personality Disorders

Because typologies and diagnostic criteria for personality disorders have changed frequently, exact sources of etiology remain unverified through clinical research. It is commonly believed, however, that genetic, constitutional, maturational, and environmental factors may play a role in their emergence.[19] The social fabric of today's world, with its emphasis on indulgences of all kinds, is also thought to play a major role in the development of some personality disorders.[5,6]

Course and Prognosis

Because little information is available about the prevalence of personality disorders as they are currently defined, the study of their prognoses is difficult.[20] Based on reported clinical observations, however, the following outcomes are likely to occur:

1. Personality disorders may become permanent and may worsen over time.
2. Some persons with personality disorders may mature out of their maladaptive coping styles.
3. Still others may drop out of treatment, thus preventing further follow-up and treatment outcome evaluation.
4. Many other individuals with personality disorders may never submit to mental health care and therefore remain a totally unknown variable in the study of these disorders.[20]

Application of the Nursing Process to Personality Disorders

Compulsive Personality Disorder

Assessment and Analysis

Perception. Perceptual, cognitive, affective, and behavioral disturbances accompany compulsive personality disorder. *Perceptual* disturbances associated with this disorder include inattention to new facts or different viewpoints, sharp focus on selected details, and the inability to focus on casual or peripheral details.

Cognition. This narrow perceptual focus leads to a variety of *cognitive* disturbances. Intellectual rigidity, or the inability to voluntarily shift attention and concentration to another topic, is prominent in the compulsive personality.[16] The cognitive content associated with this tenacious cognitive form usually centers around rules, standards, or codes of a moralistic or legalistic nature.[8] Consequently, the compulsive personality is often described as dogmatic.

Affect. The compulsive personality's narrow, yet tenaciously sharp, perceptual focus also reflects an underlying *affective disturbance*. Anxiety and ambivalence lie at the heart of this disturbance. Specifically, the individual with a compulsive personality experiences anxiety concerning the ability to control a variety of desirable, but forbidden, emotions and impulses. Moralistic or legalistic injunctions serve to defend the compulsive personality against those feelings and impulses.[8] Thus the individual with a compulsive personality avoids experiencing anxiety by tenaciously clinging to a set of fixed beliefs or injunctions.

Emotional constriction evidenced by a lack of mirth, affection, lust, or frivolity occurs as an outgrowth of this concentrated focus on rules and regulations and represents another feature of the compulsive individual's affective disturbance. Furthermore, whimsical, frivolous behavior demonstrated by others often precipitates feelings of resentment and contempt in the person with a compulsive personality.[16]

Behavioral Disturbance. *Behavioral disturbances* exhibited by individuals with compulsive personalities include inflexible stubbornness, blind conformity and obedience, excessive prudence, neatness, and cleanliness, and undue preoccupation with work, efficiency, and productivity.[8] In interpersonal relationships, compulsive personalities show little ability to "give and take." Instead, these individuals insist on doing things the right way—that is, their way.[19] Issues of control and dominance thus take precedence over issues of human care and concern. For this reason, it is not surprising that the person with a compulsive personality is often perceived as cold, self-centered, and demanding. Since individuals with compulsive personalities often display verbal and nonverbal disapproval of persons whose behavior departs from their standards, these perceptions have some grounding in reality.[16]

Additionally, persons with compulsive personalities engage in a variety of behaviors designed to convince others to behave in accordance with their own rules and regulations. This need to control others stems from the compulsive individual's unconscious battle to control the self.[16] In other words, the person with a compulsive personality seeks to control the self through the control of others.

Level of Adaptation

Despite the limitations to the compulsive personality's perceptual, cognitive, affective, and behavioral functions, this disorder is adaptive and even rewarded in some occupational settings. Therefore, individuals affected by this disorder are rarely viewed as "mentally ill."[8] At worst, they are considered obstinate and boring; at best, the "ideal, efficient worker."

Moreover, individuals with compulsive personalities are not drawn to seek therapy, which would necessitate change. Because change is threatening, therapy is usually sought only if and when these individuals experience unanticipated stress that overtaxes their coping mechanisms.[8]

When some persons with compulsive personalities do appear for treatment, they commonly present with psychophysiologic discomforts, anxiety attacks, sexual problems, exhaustion, or depression.[8,16,19] Treatment therefore centers around amelioration of these presenting symptoms rather than the compulsive personality disorder itself.

Passive-Aggressive Personality

Assessment and Analysis

Perception. Individuals with passive-aggressive personalities tend to perceive the world, other persons, life in general, and themselves through a "negative lens." For example, these persons search for faults, flaws, injustices, and mistakes in almost any situation or environment in which they find themselves.[8] This *pessimistic perceptual filter* not only influences the kind of sensory input received with passive-aggressive personalities, but also influences their cognition, affect, and behavior.

Cognition. *Cognition* in the passive-aggressive personality reflects a negative mindset filled with negative thoughts about the future and criticisms of self and others. Indecisiveness about how, when, and under what circumstances to act also stands as a major characteristic of the passive-aggressive personality's cognitive set. Deficient regulatory control of impulsive, fleeting thoughts accounts for the passive-aggressive personality's indecisiveness.[8]

Affect. Underlying the passive-aggressive personality's indecisiveness is an *ambivalent* effect.[8] That is, these persons are characteristically torn between enthusiasm and pessimism, hope and hopelessness, compliance and noncompliance, love and hate, respect and envy, independence and dependence, and action and inaction. Understandably, such ambivalence leads to irritable moodiness, discontent, dissatisfaction, and contrariness. Low self-confidence and resentment toward authority figures on whom the passive-aggressive individual depends and whom he views as superior to himself are also associated with this ambivalent affect. Consequently, jealousy, hostility, and aggressive strivings occur to a significant degree in this disorder.

Behavior Patterns. The *verbal behavior* of passive-aggressive personalities reflects their characteristic manner of perceiving, thinking, and feeling. The passive-aggressive individual verbally displays negativism through incessant complaining, grumbling, and fault-finding. The content of his verbalization usually centers around themes of feeling unappreciated, unloved, overworked, and overburdened and of being unfairly treated, misused, and abused.[8]

Nonverbal behavior patterns stemming from the passive-aggressive individual's indecisiveness and ambivalence include procrastination, delay tactics, dawdling, inefficiency, obstructionism, and errors of omission.[19] These behaviors serve to vent hostile, envious feelings and aggressive strivings while simultaneously permitting the passive-aggressive personality to appear ingratiating, friendly, and even submissive. Furthermore, these covertly aggressive tactics manipulate, maneuver, or induce others to behave in a manner that will increase the passive-aggressive person's feelings of safety and security. These passive attack techniques thereby enable individuals with this personality type to avoid experiencing anxiety.

If these passive attack techniques fail and anxiety and frustration continue to mount, the individual with passive-aggressive personality may resort to angry, emotional outbursts. The content of these angry outbursts usually centers around issues of exploitation, unfair treatment, and unappreciation. The underlying intent of these outbursts is to elicit sympathy and thus to manipulate others to decrease their demands and expectations.[8] In this way the passive-aggressive person can also escape experiencing anxiety.

Level of Adaptation

Individuals with passive-aggressive personalities are usually articulate in reporting their subjective distress. Rarely, however, do they exhibit insight regarding the origins of their distress.[8] Therefore, the inner conflicts and ambivalences underlying their distress remain unrecognized.

Although these individuals complain about their discomfort and express a desire to rid themselves of it, they nevertheless avoid seeking adaptive solutions through learning and problem-solving. Consequently, it is not surprising that passive-aggressive personalities often develop anxiety and depressive episodes as well as suicidal crises. In such cases, treatment is aimed at crisis resolution and reinforcement of a more consistent and adaptive approach to life. To fulfill these treatment goals, behavior modification, family and group therapies, and crisis intervention techniques are often employed. In more severe cases, extensive, long-term psychoanalytic therapy may be indicated.[8]

Antisocial Personality Disorder

Assessment and Analysis

The term *antisocial personality* refers to an aggressive behavioral pattern. This aggressive personality type is described as "the acting out kind of person, the adventurer, the explorer, the athlete, the soldier, and the pioneer," as well as the delinquent and criminal.[14] While individuals with antisocial personalities use action as a primary form of expression, they also possess characteristic ways of perceiving, thinking, and feeling.

Perception. Antisocial personalities *perceive* other people and the world as hostile, harmful, and out to undermine their independence. Consequently, these individuals expect to experience malice, humiliation, and betrayal at every turn.[8] Viewing the world and other people from such a "hostile lens" results in antisocial persons' experiencing continual threat.

Individuals with antisocial personalities view others as sources of threat to their independence because they perceive themselves as "super-independent" individuals capable of negotiating life demands alone.[8] More specifically, these persons see themselves as assertive, self-sufficient, tough-minded, competitive, powerful, and superior. Valuing these characteristics highly, individuals with these personality types reject attributes associated with warmth, caring, or tenderheartedness in both themselves and others.

Cognition. This hostile perceptual style influences what persons with antisocial personalities *think* and *believe* about themselves and others in rather drastic ways. To illustrate, the slogans "might makes right" and "beat the other guy to the punch" could very well serve as life mottos for antisocial personalities. To state more simply, antisocial persons believe that human beings are basically evil; therefore, they believe that they are entitled to take a highly antagonistic stance toward other people and society in general. Holding these beliefs, individuals with antisocial personalities use their cognitive capacities, for the most part, to design schemes, tactics, or strategies to outwit and punish their perceived adversaries. The terms rigid, dogmatic, and cunning describe the cognitive style of these personality types.[8]

Affect. Affectively, antisocial individuals are hostile, punitive, and vengeful. Because these persons project their own malevolent attributes onto others, they mistrust people. Individuals with antisocial personalities are especially mistrustful of people who display warm, caring, or tender behaviors, because they fear that such persons are insincere, deceitful, and out to undermine their independence.[8]

Antisocial personalities also experience feelings of anxiety; they feel anxious when they cannot become independent of individuals or situations perceived as threatening.[8] To reduce their anxiety and to increase their feelings of powerfulness and independence, those with antisocial personalities *act out* in a variety of ways.

Behavior Patterns. *Behavioral manifestations* characteristic of antisocial personality disorder reflect the perceptual, cognitive, and affective patterns described above. *Nonverbally*, antisocial persons appear cold, callous, and insensitive to the feelings and values of others. While they may periodically display gracious, cheerful, and socially clever behaviors, they express neither warmth nor compassion towards others.[8]

Because individuals with antisocial personality disorder become easily bored, restless, and frustrated when faced with the tedium of day-to-day routines and responsibilities, they often impulsively seek thrills and dangers to buffer these feelings. Examples of such acting-out behaviors include aggressive sexual behavior, vandalism, fighting, dangerous sports, outbursts of explosive anger, chemical abuse, and violent abuse and exploitation of other persons.[19]

Verbal behaviors reflecting the antisocial personality style include derogating, humiliating, brusque, and belligerent verbalizations directed to or about persons perceived as threatening; vicious argument and insults; and other forms of violent, verbal abuse. Such verbal behaviors betray the tendency of antisocial personalities to become furious and vindictive when faced with threats to their independence and control over others. That is, the first inclination of these persons is to attack the perceived threat by resorting to demeaning, violent, or controlling behaviors.[8,11,20]

Despite the fact that most antisocial individuals manifest abrasive, crude, and callous behaviors, some are capable of sensitively discerning the subtleties of human interaction.[8] More specifically, these persons are not only keenly aware of the moods and feelings of other persons, they are also capable of using these perceived weaknesses to manipulate, exploit, and control others. In short, individuals with antisocial personalities use both verbal and nonverbal behaviors to accrue power and independence and to cope with anxiety.

Level of Adaptation

At one time the term antisocial personality suggested criminal and delinquent behaviors.[11] More recently, however, clinicians have come to believe that only a very small proportion of antisocial personalities actually come into conflict with the law.

Currently, it is thought that many individuals with antisocial personalities receive societal reinforcements and rewards for their tough, realistic, competitive approaches to life. In fact, most persons with these personality types find socially valued positions in business, politics, or the military. Still others find their place in society as harsh, punitive parents or spouses, "fire and brimstone" evangelists, vengeful, controlling bosses, or as irritable, punitive teachers.[8]

In any case, aggressive, action-oriented, antisocial personalities seldom seek mental health services. If and when such services are sought, antisocial individuals are unlikely to make significant progress in the direction of adaptive mental health.

Paranoid Personality

Assessment and Analysis

The term *paranoid personality* applies to individuals who display pervasive and long-standing suspiciousness. This suspicious pattern affects the perceptual, cognitive, affective, and behavioral functions of paranoid persons in some specific ways. Alterations in these functions reflect the great effort individuals with paranoid personalities must make to counter the anxiety they experience in everyday life.

Perception. The *perception* of individuals with paranoid personalities is extremely acute, intense, and narrowly focused in search of "clues" or the "real" meaning behind the behavior of other persons or life events in general. To a great extent, paranoid persons perceive the world as being composed of clues to hidden or special meanings; hence, they disregard or even disdain manifest reality. Moreover, paranoid personalities perceive unexpected or unpredictable events and behaviors as highly threatening.[16]

Paranoid individuals generally perceive other persons as dishonest, full of trickery, and out to undo them. Their extreme distrust of others stems largely from their distorted perception of self. These individuals usually view themselves as self-sufficient, objective, rational, emotionally balanced, and very important.[8]

Cognition. The great degree of perceptual distortion present in persons with paranoid personality disorder significantly influences their *cognitive function*. Cognitive disturbances may range from tran-sient ideas of reference, in which they believe that others are giving them special attention or gossiping about them, to delusional systems, in which they grossly misinterpret trivial events or achievements to fit their grandiose self-perceptions. These delusional systems may also be of a persecutory nature, in which paranoid individuals believe that others are being unduly critical or are being purposefully deceptive or malicious toward them.[8]

Paranoid persons are hypercritical of others and are prone to collect real and imagined injustices. Often they seek retribution for such injustices through the legal system. While these persons criticize others freely, they regard criticisms directed at themselves as signs of betrayal, jealousy, envy, or persecution.[8] Their cognitive function thus deals primarily with making the imagined real and the real invalid.

Affect. The paranoid individual's *affective* domain reflects a lack of basic trust. Extreme suspiciousness, vigilant mistrust, guardedness, and hostility characterize this lack of trust. Other affective attributes of paranoid personalities include abrasive irritability, defensiveness, envy, jealousy, serious-mindedness, and emotional coldness. Typically, paranoid persons assume a callous, unsympathetic approach to others in an effort to purge themselves of any tendencies to experience humor or affectionate and tender feelings. Moreover, when others express affection or tenderness toward a paranoid individual, that expression of warm feelings is likely to arouse in him fears of entrapment, deceit, and domination.[8] When confronted with humorous situations, persons with paranoid personalities often react with anger, hostility, and extreme suspiciousness.

Paranoid individuals experience profound emotional constriction in that they are virtually unable to reach out or connect with other persons in an emotional sense. Consequently, they experience little, if any, interpersonal or sensual pleasure. Furthermore, they must resort to fault-finding and projection of their own shortcomings onto others to preserve their own sense of self-esteem.[16] Through projection and psychological and social withdrawal, individuals with paranoid personalities maintain control of their fears and anxieties. Their behavioral patterns reflect these maladaptive approaches to anxiety control.

Behavioral Manifestations. *Nonverbally*, paranoid personalities present as hypervigilant, mobilized, prepared individuals who are ready for attack. Rarely do they appear relaxed or unguarded. For the most part, they remain coldly reserved and on the periphery of events, and seldom do they mix smoothly with people in social situations. Rather, these individuals remain withdrawn, distant, and secretive in social situations. Because they lack the capacity for spontaneity and abandonment, their nonverbal behaviors appear very deliberate, tense, and, at times, even rehearsed.[8,16]

Paranoid persons often engage in a variety of *verbal* interchanges designed to test the honesty of their associates. Because of the nature and lengthiness of these interchanges, their associates may become quite exasperated and angry with them. Besides testing the trustworthiness of others, persons with paranoid personalities may also display argumentative, contentious, intimidating, and cajoling verbal behaviors.[8] The content of their verbalization usually reflects themes of blame, deceit, control, persecution, and self-aggrandisement.

Level of Adaptation

Most individuals with paranoid personalities experience lifelong effects of the disorder. In some, this disorder may precede the development of schizophrenia. In still others, paranoid personality disorder may remit with maturity and the reduction of life stressors.[19]

Few individuals with paranoid personalities, however, voluntarily seek mental health services. When these persons appear for treatment, it is usually at the insistence of family members or associates.[8] Individual, rather than group, psychotherapy is indicated for persons with paranoid personalities.[19] At the outset of therapy, trust formation must take place before other therapeutic techniques are employed.[8] Genuineness, respect, courtesy, and a formal, instead of an overly warm approach facilitates the process of trust development.[19] After trust is established between client and therapist, cognitive restructuring or psychoanalytic techniques may prove beneficial.[8] Behavioristic techniques, however, are usually contraindicated because of their intrusive nature.[19] In any event, such therapeutic interventions serve to palliate, rather than reverse, the paranoid personality disorder.[8]

Schizoid Personality Disorder

Assessment and Analysis

Socially detached, shy, and introverted persons may be described as having schizoid personality disorders. This classification refers to individuals who exhibit perceptual, cognitive, affective, and behavioral patterns that fall within the healthier end of the schizophrenic spectrum.[19] This personality disorder differs from the schizotypal personality disorder in that the latter's symptomatology more closely resembles schizophrenia. Schizoid personalities, in contrast to both schizotypals and schizophrenics, do not demonstrate odd or eccentric perceptual, cognitive, and behavioral patterns.[19]

Perception. The *perception* of individuals with schizoid personalities, however, does reflect a distorted pattern. This pattern is characterized by a reduced ability to attend, select, differentiate, and discriminate adequately between and among interpersonal and social sensory inputs. Consequently, the person with schizoid personality tends to blur or mix up such inputs, resulting in disorganized perceptual function. This perceptual dysfunction appears largely confined to interpersonal and social contexts.[8] Because illusions and hallucinations do not occur as part of this dysfunction, persons with schizoid personalities remain able to recognize reality despite their faulty interpersonal or social perception.

Cognition. The *cognitive* pattern of schizoid personality types is consistent with their perceptual style. With regard to interpersonal and social situations, schizoid individuals demonstrate vague, impoverished thought processes; that is, they possess little social intelligence.[8]

Individuals with schizoid personalities are more apt to apply their cognitive abilities to mechanical problems, artistic pursuits, or metaphysical questions, and are likely to excel in these areas.[13,14,19] Inanimate objects and ideas, instead of people, become prominent topics in the schizoid's thoughts.[19]

Affect. Indifference characterizes the *affect* of the schizoid personality. This indifference manifests itself in a variety of ways. First of all, these individuals appear totally indifferent to the thoughts and feelings of other people. They appear emotionally constricted, aloof, and inappropriately serious. Some clinicians believe that fear underlies the schizoid's aloofness.[19] Even in the face of considerable provocation, however, they rarely express feelings of anxiety, anger, or depression.[8] Although they seldom become emotionally involved with people, individuals with schizoid personality disorder invest emotionally in imaginary friends and a variety of cognitive activities.[19]

Behavior Patterns. The nonverbal and verbal behaviors evident in schizoid personalities reflect a socially detached life pattern. Some prominent *nonverbal* behaviors include blank, affectless facial expression; inability to tolerate eye contact; lethargic, awkward body movements; social withdrawal and aloofness; and unfashionable dress.[19] Often, schizoid individuals appear so drab and inconspicuous that they escape the attention of other people altogether.

Verbally, persons with schizoid personalities are unproductive. While their speech is goal-directed, their verbal emissions are short and to the point. They avoid spontaneous conversation and usually remain silent.[19] Their slow, monotonous speech form reveals the use of an occasional odd metaphor or word selection.[8] Both verbal and nonverbal behaviors of these personalities can best be described as underresponsive.

Level of Adaptation

Persons with schizoid personality types live out their lives in a socially detached way; they neither desire nor enjoy social interaction. They prefer to be alone and keep other people and life experience itself at arm's length.

Very few schizoid individuals ever seek mental health services. Their social isolation and indifference reduce their motivation for doing so. When they do come for assistance, their treatment is similar to that of paranoid personalities, but, unlike paranoid personalities, they may eventually tolerate, and even profit from, group psychotherapy.[8,19]

Borderline Personality Disorder

Assessment and Analysis

The person with borderline personality disorder exhibits a cross section of almost all the perceptual, cognitive, affective, and behavioral disturbances present in the other personality disorders. In many ways, borderline personality disorder corresponds to the infantile personality described by Ruesch.[13,14] These individuals typically cannot tolerate anxiety, and, as a result, employ all the major maladaptive coping behaviors—avoidance, withdrawal, acting out, and psychosomatization—to defend themselves against anxious feelings.

Perception. An outstanding feature of the borderline personality's *perceptual* pattern is the tendency to view other people in "either-or" categories. For example, people are seen as either "all good" or "all bad." That is, the borderline personality may view other persons as either kind, rewarding, and supportive, or hateful, distant, and punitive.[7,8,19] This tendency to pigeonhole individuals into "all good" or "all bad" categories is termed *splitting.*[19]

The self-perception of those with borderline personalities is also distorted. Often they lack a clear, internal picture or image of who they are as individuals. Consequently, borderline personalities often suffer identity disturbances with regard to their self-image, sexual, social, and occupational roles.[19]

Cognition. The perceptual distortion evident in borderline personality disorder affects cognitive functioning significantly. Because these personalities tend to perceive other individuals in narrow, rigid ways, their *cognitive* function is impaired. Holding diametrically opposed and rapidly shifting beliefs about the "goodness" or "badness" of other people contributes to the borderline personality's almost constant state of cognitive confusion.[8] Lacking a clear self-perception results in a confused self-concept.

Individuals with borderline personalities also manifest cognitive dysfunction in that they fail to learn from their life experiences.[8] For this reason, they continue to repeat their mistakes over and over again. Their ability to problem-solve—that is, to cope adaptively with anxiety—is seriously impaired.

Affect. *Affective instability,* marked by shifts from normal mood to anger or depression with the return to normal mood often within only a few hours, stands as a cardinal sign of borderline personality disorder.[8] Another striking characteristic of this personality disorder is intensity of affect.[7] Anger, loneliness, depression, emptiness, impatience, self-pity, low self-esteem, and deficient self-confidence are some of the emotions experienced intensely and erratically by the person with borderline personality.[1,2] These people experience fears of loss and abandonment, intense dependency longings, and feelings of entitlement to special care or privileges. Furthermore, when authority figures do not provide immediate relief for their uncomfortable feeling states, these individuals may become rageful, hostile, and jealous.[7]

Subjectively, persons with borderline personalities report feeling scattered, unintegrated, and incapable of following self-chosen pursuits.[8] Instead, they depend on others to give their lives direction and meaning. In this sense, the borderline personality bears an exaggerated resemblance to Reisman's "other-directed person" and, as such, stands as a pitiful caricature of today's average person.[12]

Behavioral Disturbances. The behavior of those with borderline personalities dramatically reflects the perceptual, cognitive, and affective disturbances associated with this disorder. *Nonverbally,* these individuals display their highly changeable and intense affect through impulsive behaviors. Some of these behaviors are extravagant spending, sexual promiscuity, hyperingestion of food and mood-altering chemicals, and, sometimes, antisocial behaviors such as lying and stealing.[8] Furthermore, during stressful periods, they frequently exhibit self-mutilative behavior.[1,2] To a great extent, whimsical or rageful acting-out characterizes the nonverbal behavior of borderline personalities.

The individual with borderline personality disorder may display *verbal* behaviors that are self-critical, demanding, whining, threatening, manipulative, argumentative, complaining, ingratiating, and blaming.[8] Periodically, these individuals even become verbally abusive to others.[2]

The verbal and nonverbal behaviors of borderline personalities function to anger those individuals with whom they associate. Often, others feel imposed on or manipulated by the person with borderline personality disorder and, as a result, they may wish to punish him. The verbal and nonverbal expressions of intense emotions emitted by those with borderline personalities also tend to arouse feelings of fear in others. Sometimes their families, friends, and associates may actually fear for their own safety. Seldom, however, do borderline individuals become physically assaultive.[2] Nevertheless, individuals with borderline personalities are unequaled in their ability to arouse intense and contradictory emotions in their associates.

Level of Adaptation

The life histories of persons with borderline personalities reveal a series of beginnings and endings. Numerous, intense interpersonal relationships, checkered school and work records, and drastic lifestyle changes reflect the borderline personality's overall unstable pattern. Getting into and out of difficulty becomes a way of life for these persons; consequently, they seldom realize their full potential. Some may even succumb periodically to brief psychotic episodes. Their major strength, however, lies in their ability to recruit enough interpersonal or social support to make another beginning.[8]

Many individuals with borderline personality disorder seek mental health care services. Usually, they present with symptoms of depression, psychosis, or suicidal crisis. Short-term institutionalization may be needed in these instances. Treatment is aimed at reducing the presenting symptoms. Because borderline personality disorder is a deeply ingrained pattern, it is resistant to treatment. Only the most intensive and prolonged psychotherapy can effect substantial long-term behavioral changes.[2,6,8]

Behavioral Patterns Shared by the Personality Disorders

Several behavioral patterns commonly occur in individuals with personality disorders, despite their different diagnostic labels.[20] These behavioral patterns include the following:

Splitting, or the inability to evaluate and then synthesize and accept the imperfections of significant others, both past and present; instead, many individuals with personality disorders tend to divide individuals into "all good" or "all bad" categories.

Projection, or the attribution of one's own feelings and experiences onto others; additionally, personality-disordered individuals resort to excessive fault-finding, criticism, and confrontation to reduce their own feelings of inadequacy

Passive-aggression, or the tendency to turn anger against the self in a provocative manner, with the underlying motive of forcing others to comply with their wishes and needs;[20] this tendency is behaviorally expressed through such acts as wrist-cutting, nonlethal drug overdoses, and eating disorders, including obesity, anorexia nervosa, and bulimia nervosa[3]

Acting out, or the direct behavioral expression of a wish or conflict that allows the individual to avoid the conscious experience of the thoughts and emotions accompanying it

Narcissism, or the tendency to perceive the self as all-powerful and important and therefore entitled to criticize or belittle others; this individual often gives the impression of being vain and arrogant

Dependency, or the expression of incessant, unreasonable, wishes, wants, and needs in a demanding manner while strenuously denying dependent behavior

No-win relationship style, or the tendency to seek out relationships that offer a promise of something for nothing; individuals manifesting this behavior thus feel entitled to take without giving, and they usually find themselves in relationships that are difficult to end[20]

Because personality-disordered individuals display the aforementioned behavioral characteristics, they are often labeled as crocks, grumps, complainers, and manipulators. Nurses and other mental health personnel, however, must remember that personality disordered individuals suffer greatly and need careful assessments and well-executed treatment plans.

Formulating Nursing Diagnoses for Clients with Personality Disorders

Clients with personality disorders demonstrate distinct disturbances associated with their perceptual, cognitive, affective, and behavioral functioning. For this reason, nursing diagnoses targeting a particular area of dysfunction can be formulated. To illustrate, nursing diagnoses can be classified as follows:

Perceptual disturbances
Ineffective individual coping related to use of splitting
Body image disturbance related to gender confusion
Body image disturbance associated with eating disorder
Cognitive disturbances
Decisional conflict
Impaired thought processes related to overindulgence in alcohol or prescribed mood-altering drugs
Personal identity confusion
Affective disturbances
Ineffective individual coping related to labile affect
Ineffective individual coping related to depression
Ineffective individual coping related to suspiciousness
Ineffective individual coping related to ambivalence
Behavioral disturbances
Social isolation
Impaired verbal communication
Noncompliance
Potential for self-harm related to suicidal crisis

These are a small sample of nursing diagnoses that can be gleaned from the preceding assessment section.

Planning and Implementing Nursing Care for Individuals with Personality Disorders

Planning and implementing nursing care for personality-disordered clients constitutes one of the greatest challenges of psychiatric–mental health nurses. The challenge is great because these individuals inevitably trigger a negative countertransference in their therapists and other helpers. The behavioral patterns associated with these disorders are not only annoying but also difficult to change. Consequently, nurses and other mental health personnel often become irritated, frustrated, and rejecting when working therapeutically with personality disordered clients.

Self-Awareness

To plan and implement effective care for personality-disordered clients, nurses need to develop a high degree of *self-awareness*. Nurses and other mental health care providers often experience a number of emotional reactions to these individuals indicative of negative countertransference phenomena. These might include anger toward the client; defensiveness; wanting to control and dominate the client; excessive preoccupation with the client; and becoming frustrated, confused, and unable to concentrate during interactions with the client.[19] Learning to work through these phenomena requires that the nurse be able to tolerate and accept these feelings as natural reactions to personality-disordered clients, and, at the same time, to refrain from acting on these feelings. Discussing emotional reactions to these clients with a knowledgeable and trusted nurse colleague can increase the nurse's self-awareness and emotional control.

Trust Development

Because many personality-disordered clients tend to mistrust other people, the nurse needs to exercise special care to *establish trust*. A straightforward, matter-of-fact approach, as opposed to an overly warm approach, is indicated when working with these clients. Punctuality, honesty, respect, and genuineness also add significantly to trust formation.

In verbal interactions with personality-disordered individuals, the nurse should avoid interpreting the client's behavior. The reason for this is that mistrustful clients tend to view interpretations as intrusive and controlling. Instead, the nurse needs to employ open-ended questions designed to assist these clients to focus on their behavior and its consequences. Nurses must also maintain congruence between verbal and nonverbal behaviors; incongruent behavior of the nurse often results in these clients becoming more suspicious of her.[19] Some clients may attempt to use such discrepancies to manipulate the nurse and other health care providers.

Counterprojection

When working therapeutically with suspicious, personality-disordered individuals who use projection extensively, the nurse needs to avoid interjecting doubt into the client's assertions. To dispute the client will merely serve to reinforce and increase the use of projection. Instead, the nurse needs to acknowledge that the client's assertions are within the realm of possibility, if not probability. The nurse can then proceed to use empathetic techniques to help the client talk about his real feelings or motives, even though they are attributed to others rather than the self. Thus, through the use of empathy rather than confrontation, trust is promoted; this can eventually lead to the client revealing his own emotions and feared impulses.[20]

Taking Time Out

Taking time out, which involves leaving the interaction or postponing the next interaction, may be useful in working therapeutically with clients who either

CHART 22-1

Counterprojection

Mr. Barton has been hospitalized for a slight head injury due to a fall at home. From the outset of his hospitalization, he asserted that someone had tampered with his step-ladder, causing his fall. He later informed his nurse that he believed his wife's lover had secretly entered their home and tampered with his step-ladder. All diagnostic tests with regard to his mild head injury are negative. Therefore, there is no organic factor accounting for his paranoid thoughts. Moreover, his wife informs the nurse that she has no lover. She does report, however, that Mr. Barton has always been jealous of her. The wife also reports that her husband is very suspicious and has had several disputes and grievances with former employees, all of whom he had accused of undermining his authority and position. Mr. Barton has threatened his wife with physical abuse.

The psychiatric liaison nurse is asked to assess Mr. Barton for possible transfer to the psychiatric–mental health services offered by the hospital. After several sessions with Mr. Barton, the psychiatric liaison nurse decides to use the technique of counterprojection in an effort to gain Mr. Barton's trust and willingness to seek treatment.

Nurse: How do you feel when you say that your wife's lover is responsible for your falling from the ladder?

Client: (with a look of distrust) What do you mean? He is crazy and will do anything to get me out of the picture so he can be with her.

Nurse: That's a scary, frightening thought (stated with empathy). Why do you think he'd be so desperate to have your wife?

Client: He's jealous of me and wants to humiliate me. The best way to do that would be through my wife.

Nurse: You've been a successful man and have cause to take pride in your accomplishments. We need to look at some ways that we can stay on top of this situation. You and I can agree that you are a man of inner strength and it's important that you not let this situation weaken your position.

Client: Yes, I'm a strong man. But, sometimes I get worried about my marriage and my company. Sometimes I think my wife and associates might try to make a fool out of me—like if I lose control and hurt someone or destroy the business.

Nurse: I can understand how that would be of great concern to you. Let's see if there is anything we can do to help you stay in control.

Client: Well, I don't want to hurt anyone. I've got all these troublemakers at work to handle plus my wife. (When the nurse empathizes with the client and suggests their collaboration, Mr. Barton reveals his fears of losing control.)

Nurse: We can help you do that. Would you like to know about how we can do that?

Client: Yes, I would.

As a result of using counterprojection, the nurse is able to engage Mr. Barton in a therapeutic pact and to engage his cooperation in mental health treatment.

---

refuse to help themselves or who use passive-aggressive tactics to gain attention or sympathy.[20] Leaving the interaction or postponing interactions has the effect of breaking the pattern of struggle whereby the client attempts to force the nurse to do all the work during therapy. Additionally, this technique is useful to underscore the point that passive-aggressive techniques such as wrist-cutting or diet noncompliance result in less, not more, attention.[20] An extra benefit of this technique is that it allows the nurse time out to become more self-aware and emotionally controlled. (See Chart 22-2, "Time Out.")

Confrontation

Confrontation may be necessary to work effectively with some personality-disordered clients who attempt to use manipulation.[19] Pointing out a client's problematic behavior to him or her is termed *confrontation.* The purpose of confrontation is to assist the client to become more self-aware.

C H A R T   22-2
Taking Time Out

Mrs. Gabriel, a psychiatric nurse, has been having one-to-one sessions daily with her client, Ms. Simpson. Ms. Simpson is diagnosed as having a passive-aggressive personality disorder and has a past history of lashing out angrily in an attempt to devalue others.

Nurse: (using a neutral voice) I notice that you seem to have some difficulty getting to therapy today. (Miss Simpson has been late to meals, group therapy, and activities. She is also late for her session with Mrs. Gabriel.)

Client: So what's it to you? (her face reddens, her hands clench, as she speaks and glowers at Mrs. Gabriel.)

Nurse: (remains silent because further comments would possibly be interpreted as defensiveness)

Client: Sometimes I don't want to follow the schedule everyone else goes by. Is there anything wrong with that?

Nurse: Being right or wrong has nothing to do with your punctuality. The unit rules, however, which I, other staff, and clients agree to follow state that everyone will do their best to be on time for all therapies and activities.

Client: Oh yeah! Well, those rules don't apply to me because I don't agree to them. Plus, you're just being bossy and controlling. (Her voice volume is rising and her nonverbal behavior is visibly hostile.)

Nurse: From your voice tone and angry facial expression, I can see that we aren't accomplishing anything worthwhile. I'm not going to pursue this conversation any further. Perhaps when we are both less emotional, we can try again. (She calls time out to avoid further verbal abuse from the client and to allow both of them to regain their composure.)

The keys to effective confrontation include the following:

1. Pointing out the behavior as soon after its occurrence as possible
2. Being specific in describing the behavior
3. Using a nonaccusatory, nonjudgmental, matter-of-fact manner
4. Maintaining the focus on the client's actual behavior rather than the client's explanation of it

Furthermore, confrontation needs to occur in a setting in which the client feels safe and supported. The nurse must exercise sound and sensitive judgment in planning and implementing confrontations with the client. A trusting relationship between the nurse and client is a prerequisite to the use of confrontation. (See Chart 22-3.)

Limit-Setting

Manipulative, dependent, and acting-out behaviors displayed by personality-disordered clients may necessitate the nurse's use of *limit-setting*.[2] It is important to remember that limit-setting is not punitive in nature. Furthermore, limit-setting includes more than merely telling a client to stop a particular behavior. Specifically, limit-setting involves the following:

1. Identifying the behavior that the client needs to control
2. Offering an appropriate, alternative behavior for the client to pursue
3. Anticipating that the client will test the nurse to determine if she will back down
4. Remaining steadfast and consistent in the use of limit-setting

Limit-setting must be sensitively and judiciously applied to ensure effectiveness. Vacillation and backing down after setting limits with a client seriously jeopardizes the development and maintenance of a trusting nurse–client relationship.

Setting limits with clients can pose significant problems for nurses who lack maturity, self-confidence, and the ability to control their own anger and acting-out tendencies. Similarly, nurses who meet their own psychological needs by seeking the approval and affection of clients will be unable to set limits effectively. Effective limit-setting thus requires both clinical skill and personal maturity. (See Chart 22-4.)

Other Helpful Approaches and Guidelines

Working therapeutically with personality-disordered individuals can be facilitated and more effective when the nurse does the following things:

CHART 22-3
Confrontation

Mr. Samuels has been hospitalized for treatment of irritable colon. He initially presented with symptoms of abdominal cramps, diarrhea, and dehydration. Additionally, Mr. Samuels displays some behaviors associated with borderline personality disorder, such as erratic and intense moodiness, dependence, hyperingestion of foods and beverages that aggravate his irritable colon, and splitting. Despite Mr. Samuels' tendency to split staff into two groups, "the good guys and the bad guys," he has come to trust his primary nurse, Ms. Brown.

Ms. Brown has noticed that Mr. Samuels departs from his therapeutic diet frequently and that his presenting symptoms continue to persist. Mr. Samuels avoids eating his therapeutic diet by being unavailable for meals. Specifically, he is usually sleeping, feeling too ill to eat, or preoccupied with phone calls or visitors when meals are served. In place of the therapeutic diet, Mr. Samuels tells his mother and girlfriend to bring him unsuitable meals and snacks. Ms. Brown has observed these behaviors and decides to confront Mr. Samuels about his behavior.

Nurse: Have you noticed how frequently you've skipped your prescribed diet?

Client: I guess I have been too sleepy and sick to eat (whining voice tone)

Nurse: Why do you think you are either asleep or sick at mealtimes? (focusing on the meaning of the client's behavior)

Client: (changes the subject and begins talking about his desire to find a new job)

Nurse: We were discussing your not eating your prescribed diet when you started talking about something else. (refocuses client on the topic of his eating behavior)

Client: Really. I guess I didn't realize what I was doing. I'm just so tired. Anyway, what difference does it make if I don't eat what they bring me? The hospital gets paid for the food anyway. (begins to sound somewhat defensive)

Nurse: I don't know if it makes a difference or not. I do know that your irritable colon symptoms have increased. (pointing out a change in his physical condition)

Client: Yeah, so I've had a few loose stools, some stomach cramps. So what? (stated in nonemotional blasé manner)

Nurse: (Remains silent; further talk would merely be a repetition of what she's already said; Ms. Brown must be able to deal with her own feelings of anxiety during silence and to resist the client's maneuvering her into assuming the major responsibility for the interaction)

Nurse: What have you been eating in place of your prescribed diet? (uses open-ended question to gently focus client on his behavior)

Client: Well, either my mom or girlfriend brings me something to eat or drink. But I only eat a little. (sounds defensive)

Nurse: What do they usually bring you?

Client: Oh, stuff, you know. Regular food.

Nurse: This seems difficult for you to talk about. (points out client's behavior)

Client: Difficult? No, I don't think so. (facial expression looks somewhat puzzled)

Nurse: (remains silent to give Mr. Samuels time to collect his thoughts)

Client: I always eat just what I'm supposed to. (a somewhat defensive tone of voice)

Nurse: I'm sure you intend to, yet at times it's hard to stick to a diet. (gently interjects possibility of his deviating from diet without being accusatory)

Client: Maybe, uh, uh, you know, sometimes it is.

Nurse: I wonder if there are times that maybe you eat foods that you aren't supposed to? (a gentle confrontation)

Client: Once in a while. Mostly, when my mom or girlfriend brings me food.

Nurse: How do you feel physically after eating these foods?

Client: Sometimes O.K. but I guess most of the time I get sick, more diarrhea. Then, I just want to sleep.

The goal of this confrontation is to increase Mr. Samuels' self-awareness regarding the effect of his eating habits on his physical health. Toward the end of the conversation, he begins to recognize that his behavior may lead to an exacerbation of symptoms.

CHART 22-4
Limit-Setting

Ms. Musicks has been admitted to the psychiatric–mental health unit for a transient psychotic reaction associated with borderline personality disorder. By her fifth hospital day, her psychosis has remitted, and she is able to articulate clearly the stressors leading to her hospitalization. She describes being coldly and punitively rejected by her lesbian lover who reportedly ridiculed her for being overweight and lazy. Ms. Musicks has been observed gorging food at mealtimes, and between meals, by members of the mental health team. Ms. Musicks, who is 5 feet 9 inches tall, weighed 195 pounds on admission and 5 days later weighs 200 pounds. Mr. Harper, a psychiatric–mental health nurse, with the backing of the mental health team, endeavors to set limits with Ms. Musicks regarding her gorging food.

Client: (Eating a piece of cake with ice cream, and coffee in the galley of the unit)

Nurse: I notice that you spend a lot of time in here eating between meals, and that you have gained 5 pounds since your admission to the unit. What's going on that you need to do this? (points out the behavior that the client needs to control in a neutral, nonaccusatory manner)

Client: I feel rotten and eating is what I do to comfort myself.

Nurse: You feel comforted by eating. How long do you feel that way?

Client: Not long, so I keep coming back and I guess that's why I'm gaining weight.

Nurse: What else comforts you?

Client: Talking to someone who understands.

Nurse: The next time you feel the urge to eat food, other than that prescribed on your reducing diet, I would prefer that you talk to an understanding person. (offering an appropriate alternative behavior for the client to pursue)

Client: Okay. I'll do that instead of eat. (leaves the galley)

Thirty minutes later Mr. Harper unsurprisingly finds Ms. Musicks in the galley again eating ice cream and cake. Mr. Harper is unsurprised because he expected Ms. Musicks to test the limit to see if he would back down.

Nurse: We had an agreement that you would eat only your prescribed diet and no snacks in between. I expect you to hold to our agreement. (spoken in a firm, yet kind, manner)

Client: Yeh, uh, that's right. I'll go talk to Mary instead.

---

1. Requires the client to be responsible for his or her own behavior; blaming or punishing the client is seldom, if ever, effective
2. Presents the idea that behavior change is within the realm of possibility rather than demanding behavior change
3. Asks questions that help the client think through actual or intended behaviors; gaining the ability to predict behavioral consequences in advance of behavior promotes more healthful adaptation
4. Behaves as naturally as possible in order to promote trust development
5. Avoids assuming responsibility for the client's behavior; more specifically, the nurse should not attempt to rescue the client or encourage dependency
6. Encourages the client's involvement in appropriate self-help groups such as Alcoholics Anonymous, Narcotics Anonymous, Emotions Anonymous, or Overeaters Anonymous; such involvement assists the client to offer appropriate help to others who may be more needy
7. Avoids requesting or recommending the use of psychotropic medications routinely, because they cannot alter personality structure.[20]

Evaluation

Evaluating the nursing care administered to personality-disordered clients cannot be measured solely on the basis of achieved client outcomes. Despite the most effective care, these clients may not improve. Therefore, other criteria must be used to measure the quality of nursing care. For instance, the extent to which the nurse identifies her own countertransferential reactions and successfully works through these

C H A R T   22-5
Nursing Diagnoses: Personality Disorders

1. Potential noncompliance with
   Reducing diet
   Unit rules
   Medication regime
   Alcohol-free lifestyle
   Treatment plans
2. Potential cognitive impairment related to substance abuse
3. Decisional conflict related to
   Unclear life goals
   Poor problem-solving skills
   Poor self-concept
4. Anxiety related to poor stress tolerance
5. Powerlessness related to extravagant dependency needs
6. Disturbance in self-concept: self-esteem
7. Disturbance in self-concept: body image
8. Personal identity confusion
9. Unresolved independence–dependence conflict
10. Potential for violence related to
    Suicidal crisis
    Self-mutilation
11. Sexual dysfunction related to gender identity confusion
12. Ineffective individual coping
13. Spiritual distress related to value confusion

(From Gordon M: *Manual of Nursing Diagnosis*. New York, McGraw-Hill, 1984

is one important way of measuring effective clinical performance.

Additionally, the effectiveness with which the nurse sets realistic limits is another way nursing care can be evaluated. Most important of all in the evaluation process is the extent to which the nurse grows in terms of her own emotional maturity and objectivity in attempting to provide professional nursing care to difficult, and sometimes uncooperative, clients.

Summary

This chapter presents the concepts of personality and personality disorder. These concepts provide the necessary background for discussing the perceptual, cognitive, affective, and behavioral disturbances evident in the compulsive, passive-aggressive, antisocial, borderline, schizoid, and paranoid personality disorders. Some of the major points of the chapter include the following:

1. Maladaptive personality patterns or styles may be described as personality disorders.
2. The behavior of individuals with personality disorders is often narcissistic, dependent, depressed, egocentric, immature, hostile, and manipulative.
3. Compulsive personality disorder is marked by narrow perceptual focus, intellectual rigidity, anxiety and ambivalence, lack of mirth, in-

flexible stubbornness, and attempts to control others.
4. The person with a passive-aggressive personality perceives others and the world in general pessimistically, is indecisive and ambivalent, feels unappreciated and misused, and procrastinates or works inefficiently.
5. Antisocial personality disorder is characterized by hostility, antagonism, punitiveness, mistrust, callousness, and insensitivity.
6. Paranoid personalities display pervasive suspiciousness, cognitive disturbances ranging from ideas of reference to delusional systems, hypercritical attacks on others, hostility, projection, guardedness, jealousy, and emotional coldness.
7. Schizoid personality disorder is marked by social withdrawal and extremely shy behavior, impoverished thought processes, indifference, and underresponsiveness.
8. The individual with borderline personality disorder uses many maladaptive patterns to avoid anxiety; these may include splitting, avoidance, withdrawal, acting-out and psychosomatization.
9. Nursing care of personality-disordered clients requires that nurses develop a high degree of self-awareness, form trusting relationships with clients, and use counter projection, time out, confrontation, and limit-setting techniques as well as other therapeutic approaches.

References

1. Chessick RD: The Borderline Patient. In Arieti S (ed): American Handbook of Psychiatry, Vol. 3, 2d ed, pp 808–819. New York, Basic Books, 1975

2. Dubovsky SL: Psychotherapeutics in Primary Care. New York, Grune and Stratton, 1981

3. Herzog DB: Advances in Psychiatry: Focus on Eating Disorders. New York, Park Row Publishers, 1987

4. Kernberg O: Internal World and External Reality. New York, Jason Aronson, 1980

5. Lasch C: The Culture of Narcissism. New York, WW Norton, 1978

6. Marin P: The New Narcissism. Harper's (October) 45–56, 1975

7. Masterson JF: Psychotherapy of the Borderline Adult. New York, Brunner/Mazel, 1976

8. Millon T: Disorders of Personality. New York, John Wiley & Sons, 1981

9. Parsons RD, Wicks RJ (eds): Passive-Aggressiveness: Therapy and Practice. New York, Brunner/Mazel, 1983

10. Peck MS: People of the Lie. New York, Simon and Schuster, 1983

11. Rappeport JR: Antisocial Behavior. In Arieti S (ed): American Handbook of Psychiatry, Vol 3, 2d ed, pp 253–269. New York, Basic Books, 1975

12. Riesman D: The Lonely Crowd. New Haven, Yale University Press, 1961

13. Ruesch J: Disturbed Communication. New York, WW Norton & Co, 1957

14. Ruesch J: Therapeutic Communication. New York, WW Norton & Co, 1973

15. Salzman L: Other Characteristic-Personality Syndromes: Schizoid, Inadequate, Passive-Aggressive, Paranoid, Dependent. In Arieti S (ed): American Handbook of Psychiatry, Vol 3, 2d ed, pp 224–234. New York, Basic Books, 1975

16. Shapiro D: Neurotic Styles. New York, Basic Books, 1975

17. Stanton AH: Personality Disorders. In Nicholi AM Jr (ed): Harvard Guide to Modern Psychiatry, pp 283–295. Cambridge, MA, Belknap Press of Harvard University Press, 1978

18. Tupin JP, Halbrich U, Pena JJ (eds): Transient Psychosis: Diagnosis, Management, and Evaluation. New York, Brunner/Mazel, 1984

19. Vaillant GE, Perry JC: Personality Disorders. In Freeman AM, Kaplan HI, Sadock BJ (eds): Comprehensive Textbook of Psychiatry/III, Vol 2, 3d ed, pp 1562–1590. Baltimore, Williams & Wilkins, 1980

20. Vaillant GE, Perry JC: Personality Disorders. In Freeman AM, Kaplan HI, Sadock BJ (eds): Comprehensive Textbook of Psychiatry, 4th ed, pp 958–986. Baltimore, Williams & Wilkins, 1985

23 Disorders of Mood: Depressed and Manic Behavior

Susan Kah

To die: to sleep:
No more; and by a sleep to say we end
The heartache and the thousand natural shocks
That flesh is heir to, 'tis a consummation
Devoutly to be wish'd. To die, to sleep.
Hamlet

Chapter Preview

Disturbances of mood or affect illustrate, perhaps more than any other response to stress, that human feelings and behaviors exist on a continuum with no clear demarcation between "normal" and "abnormal" or between health and illness. This chapter focuses on the feelings, thoughts, and ineffective behaviors that characterize individuals who are depressed or struggling against depression. The overview of depressed and manic behavior discusses the incidence, possible causes, and types or diagnostic categories currently employed to facilitate the care and treatment of clients. A major emphasis of this chapter is the application of the steps of the nursing process—assessment, nursing diagnosis, planning, implementation, and evaluation—to individuals suffering from disturbances in mood.

Learning Objectives

Upon completion of the chapter, you should be able to accomplish the following:

1. compare the biologic and psychosocial theories regarding the etiology of mood disorders
2. contrast the incidence and symptomatic behaviors of mania and depression
3. list the types of mood disorders according to current diagnostic categorization
4. discuss primary prevention of disorders of mood
5. apply the nursing process to the care of manic and depressed clients
   assess the verbal and nonverbal behavior of clients with disorders of mood
   formulate nursing diagnoses for clients with disorders of mood
   identify nursing goals and actions designed to alleviate the problems of manic and depressed clients and their families
   formulate a comprehensive nursing care plan for a client with a mood disorder
   evaluate the effectiveness of the nursing intervention
6. recognize and discuss feelings and behaviors that may influence the therapeutic use of self

Incidence and Significance of the Problem

Unhappiness that is pathologically intense is called depression.[31] Depression has been described as the number-one mental health problem in the United States.[5,29] Perhaps 25% of the population will experience a major depressive episode over the course of a lifetime.[26] The critical nature of the problem is underscored by the fact that an estimated 15% of people with major depressions choose suicide.[26]

Manic behavior, like depression, is also a disturbance in mood. *Mania*, believed to be a defense against depression, is characterized by varying degrees of elation, hyperactivity, agitation, and accelerated thinking and speaking.

Depression occurs at all ages and does not seem to be related to the pressures produced by any particular civilization or historic age. Women are more frequently treated for depression than men. Infants are described as exhibiting *anaclitic depression* when deprived of a warm, close experience with another individual. This early form of depression in response to neglect is characterized by a lack of social responsiveness and an apathetic mood.

Contemporary mental health professionals believe that childhood depression exists and that the nature of this depression is similar to that of depression in adults.[10] Even though behaviors may be more subtle, depressed children do exhibit changes in activity level, social relationships, eating and elimination patterns, and sleep patterns; they even engage in self-destructive behavior.[12] School-age children have also been described as masking depression with aggressiveness, problematic behavior in school, and psychosomatic complaints.[1]

Adolescents develop clinical depressions with symptoms very similar to those found in adults.[26] More diffuse symptoms may include drug abuse, violence, and sexually promiscuous behavior. Suicide is now the third leading cause of death among adolescents 15 to 19 years of age in the United States.

Depressed adults are overwhelmed by feelings of helplessness, hopelessness, and sadness. These individuals have extremely low self-esteem and experience a decrease in physical and psychic energy, which results in an apathetic withdrawal from the environment. Depression is the most common psychiatric disorder in the elderly population. Late life depression is a complex phenomenon that may have multiple causes. Interpersonal and material losses, chronic illness, and frequent use of prescribed and nonprescribed medications all play a part. Somatic complaints tend to replace those of mood disturbance. Confusion due to depression, sometimes referred to as pseudodementia, may be mistaken for dementia.[35,36]

History of Depression

The history of depression includes such ancient victims as Nebuchanezzar, Saul, and Herod. Hippocrates believed depression was caused by excessive black bile or melan cholé, from which the word *melancholy* derived. Today this term is sometimes used to denote severe depression. The pains of depression have also been felt by such notables as Dostoevski, Poe, Hawthorne, Darwin, Lincoln, Churchill, and, more recently, vice-presidential candidate Thomas Eagleton and astronaut Edwin "Buzz" Aldrin. It seems that from the dawn of history, depression has been a prevalent disorder, even though an individual's specific reaction to the disturbance may have been shaped by the society in which he lived.

Etiologic Theories

As with many other mental health problems, the cause or causes of depression and mania are not definitely known. Many authorities do agree, however, that in the case of depression, either biologic or psychological factors may result in the same pathological or disturbed behavior. Consequently, theories that focus primarily on biologic or psychological causes should not be interpreted as mutually exclusive theories.

Biologic Influences

Amine Hypothesis

As a biochemical disorder, depression has been associated with a functional deficit of one or more of the brain neurotransmitter amines—serotonin, norepinephrine, and dopamine—at specific nerve cell synapses. This deficit interferes with the transmission of electrochemical impulses from one nerve cell to another. In effect, the cells are "switched off." Conversely, mania is associated with a functional excess of one or more of these amines. This amine hypothesis of the affective disorders provides a basis for understanding the pharmacologic treatment of depression. This mode of treatment of depression through medication will be described more fully later in this chapter.

Evolutionary Development

It has been hypothesized that depressive mechanisms may exist in the biochemical system because they have survival value in the evolution of the human race.[20] The dampening of emotional response may serve as a protective device when submission, passivity, and withdrawal are the most effective reactions to a particular stressful situation. Depression can, therefore, be perceived as a malfunction of an attempt to conserve energy when it would prove fruitless to do anything else.

Familial Influence

Depression seems to occur more frequently in certain families; consequently, it is believed that the predisposition for depression may be inherited. This tendency alone, however, does not necessarily result in clinical symptoms. The depressive process may be triggered by some insult to the integrity of the individual, which overwhelms the person's defenses. Scientists continue to search for the specific genetic link to depression and hope that such knowledge will help identify those who are most susceptible to the disorder. Early identification of susceptible persons should then be followed by primary preventive efforts.

Physical Influences

Depression may occur as a secondary effect of some medications, particularly hormones, sedatives, and antibacterials, and may also occur in conjunction with certain viral infections, such as mononucleosis and hepatitis. Depression that accompanies such physical states presents a much simpler mental health problem than other types of depression.

Psychosocial Influences

A frequently encountered interpersonal theory regarding the cause and dynamics of depression focuses on the importance of a real or perceived loss that the distressed individual has experienced. This sense of loss follows such events as death, divorce, physical separation, or a change in status, role, or state of health. In response to such a loss, the individual becomes profoundly depressed if resolution, the expected outcome of the adaptive grieving process, is not attained. The depressed individual responds to the loss with feelings of abandonment, frustration, and conscious or unconscious anger, much of which is turned inwardly against the self.

Psychoanalytic View

This view of depression is closely related to the Freudian or psychoanalytic belief that depression has its foundation in oral needs for love and gratification that have been frustrated, usually by a mothering figure. The resulting ambivalent feelings of love and hate produce strong feelings of guilt and a pattern of adult behavior characterized by dependency and a low frustration tolerance. The person may employ various techniques, such as submissive, manipulative, coercive, piteous, demanding, or placating behavior, to maintain this relationship that is desperately needed but that the person has essentially ambivalent feelings about.[7]

Cognitive View

A cognitive model of depression refutes the belief that depression is anger turned inward and, instead, conceptualizes depression as a negative way of thinking about one's self, one's future, and one's environment.[3]

The individual experiences sadness, loss of spontaneous motivation, loss of interest, indecisiveness, and suicidal wishes because of his idiosyncratic or peculiar views. This theory holds that the individual's cognitive disturbances precede his affective changes. The mobilization of hostility may be helpful, not because it decreases the amount of self-hate, but because it gives the individual a greater sense of control over his environment.

Believing that affect can be influenced by altering cognitions or thoughts, Beck has formulated a treatment model in which the therapist takes an active and directive position, helping the client to uncover distorted thinking and use reality-based judgments to formulate experience.[18] The cognitive approach to treating depression has implications for nursing intervention with moderately depressed clients and will be discussed later in this chapter.

Behavioral View

The behavioral view of depression is illustrated by the assertion that learned helplessness plays a central role in the development of depression. Behaviors that define "learned helplessness," such as passivity, negative expectations, and feelings of helplessness, hopelessness, and powerlessness, are also major symptoms of depression. Those persons who are susceptible to depression have encountered a lifetime of experiences that have taught them that they are ineffective and lack the ability to influence their sources of suffering and gratification.

A review of these and other etiologic theories of mental disorders leads to the conclusion that one cannot deal with the causation and symptomatology of any emotional disorder in terms of a single, discrete influence; depression is no exception. Although perceived as a primarily psychological disturbance in mood or affect, there are significant cognitive and biologic components.

Those treating and caring for the depressed client must ask several questions.

- What made the client vulnerable?
- What triggered the disturbance?
- Why did the client's defenses fail?
- What kinds of interventions will help the client to grow?

Types of Affective Disorders

The affective disorders may be categorized in a variety of ways. It may be that the various states commonly called depression are really several different disorders. It is important to remember, however, that such theoretical concerns do not necessarily interfere with offering effective help to depressed clients, especially if that help is based on specific knowledge of the individual and his environment.

If one perceives depression as existing on a continuum from health to illness, and as sometimes serving a useful function, the reaction of *grief* and the process of *mourning* would be placed at the healthy end of the continuum. Most individuals respond to losses in their lives in a fairly predictable way. Denial, usually short-lived, progresses to a developing awareness of the loss, followed by anger mixed with sadness, and then finally a resolution characterized by acceptance of the loss and, perhaps, idealization of the lost object or individual. Grief, in response to a psychic wound, such as the death of a loved one, can be compared to the pain that accompanies a physical wound. The mourning process, which may take as long as a year, can be compared to the usually more rapid healing of a physical wound. This ability to resolve losses varies greatly among individuals and is dependent upon previous interpersonal experiences, ego strength, and the support and resources that are available. Some depressions can be linked to unresolved grief.

Nonpsychotic Affective Disorders

If one moves along the continuum from health toward illness, it becomes apparent that there are some individuals who live out most of their lives in chronic states of depression, which sometimes alternate with periods of *hypomania,* an abnormality of mood ranging between normal euphoria and mania. These individuals, however, do maintain contact with reality and do not experience a personality disintegration that makes hospitalization necessary.

Cyclothymic Disorder

Those clients experiencing numerous periods of nonpsychotic depression and hypomania are described as having a *cyclothymic disorder*. Hypomania or mania is considered to be a defense or reaction formation against the painful experience of depression. Manic behavior has also been associated with an increase or surplus of neurotransmitter amines in the brain. The opposing manifestations of depression and hypomania are seen in the following pairs of symptoms: feelings of inadequacy (during depressed periods) and inflated self-esteem (during hypomanic periods); social withdrawal and uninhibited people-seeking; sleeping too much and not sleeping enough; diminished productivity at work and increased productivity.[2]

Dysthymic Disorder

Clients with *dysthymic disorders* experience periods of chronic depression or a loss of interest or pleasure in all, or almost all, usual activities and pastimes. Periods free from these depressive states may be as brief as a few days or a few weeks. The person with a dysthymic disorder does not evidence hypomanic behavior.

The chronic nature of this disorder is cause for concern because it may be accompanied by a lifelong struggle against depression, which may assume various maladaptive forms. In the attempt to escape feelings of inadequacy, emptiness, loss of energy and vigor, a pessimistic attitude toward the future, and recurrent thoughts of death or suicide, the client may intensify certain activities to generate excitement. Gambling, criminal behavior, promiscuity, and illegitimate pregnancy are examples of such "acting out" behaviors. Intensification of work, spending money, homosexual behavior, mysticism, and intensification of religious interest can also be used in the struggle against depression.

The depressed client may also turn to substance abuse (*i.e.,* the abuse of alcohol and other drugs) to dull or escape his psychic pain. The problems created by the tendency toward depression extend beyond the clinical state that is called depression.[7]

Major Affective Disorders

At the illness end of the mental health continuum, one finds the most severe disorders, which may include psychotic features. A *psychosis* implies an extreme response to stress, such as impaired reality-testing and the development of delusions, hallucinations, and affective, as well as psychomotor and physical, disturbances. The client frequently becomes unable to function either at work or as a family member, and may become a danger to himself as well as to others. This client usually requires hospitalization and responds to the structure and milieu he finds in the psychiatric facility. Psychotic episodes are also usually treated vigorously with psychotherapeutic agents. The major affective disorders can become psychotic in nature.

The major affective disorders are divided into two major categories—bipolar disorders and major depression.[2] The essential feature is disturbance involving either a manic episode or a major depressive episode. Although psychotic features may not always be present in the major affective disorders, there is extreme social and occupational impairment.

Bipolar Disorders

A *bipolar disorder* consists of one or more manic episodes, with or without subsequent or alternating major depressive episodes. These manic episodes typically begin suddenly, with a rapid escalation over a few days.

The first manic episode usually occurs before age 30, but is very rare in children and adolescents.[2,8] Most individuals who have manic episodes will eventually have a major depressive episode; however, only about 20% of the adults who experience depression have manic episodes.[8]

The bipolar disorder seems to be equally common in men and women and is frequently described as having a strong genetic or familial component. The not uncommon occurrence of bipolar disorder in the same family suggests that a biogenetic factor may be at least a contributory cause.[24]

Major Depression

Major depression is a disorder of mood wherein an individual experiences one or recurrent major depressive episodes without signs of manic or hypomanic behavior. The onset is variable in length, with symptoms usually developing over a period of days to weeks. It is estimated that at least half of those who experience a major depressive episode will have another one.[2] Major depression seems to occur more frequently in women.

Mental health professionals who work with depressed clients may encounter descriptors of mood disorders that have been used to enhance understanding of the client's situation and condition. Major depression is also referred to as a *unipolar depression*. If the major depression occurs after childbirth, it is called a *post-partum depression*. When it occurs around the 6th decade of life, it may be described as an *involutional melancholia*. If the depressed client is agitated, one says that he has an *agitated depression*; when he is almost inert, one speaks of a *retarded depression*. Depression that seems to occur without any relationship to external events is sometimes referred to as an *endogenous depression*. This is in contrast to a *reactive* or *exogenous depression*, the cause of which is evident in the client's history.

The many terms that are currently in use or have been used in the past to label depression are the result of the efforts of mental health caregivers to provide accurate descriptions of the depressive process. By formulating specific descriptions of the disorder, caregivers are better able to plan the most therapeutic nursing approaches for the depressed client.

Application of the Nursing Process to Disorders of Mood

The application of the nursing process to disorders of mood must focus on primary prevention—that is, the maintenance of mental health—as well as secondary and tertiary prevention, through the provision of care and treatment to those already identified as mentally ill. Primary prevention of the affective disorders is closely related to the etiologic theories previously presented in this chapter. Through secondary and tertiary prevention, the nurse provides needed support and resources to the client. Hopefully, mental health treatment will prevent the possible complications and long-term effects of the major disorders and will promote a higher level of functioning of the client.

Primary Prevention

Primary prevention of mental illness is specifically described as biologic, social, or psychological intervention that promotes emotional well-being or reduces the incidence and prevalence of mental illness in populations.[25] The incidence of depression as a syndrome has been described as increasing, although the presence of severe depressive illness has decreased.[3]

The rapid changes in society, with the concomitant stresses and losses of the traditional support systems such as family, church, and neighborhood, may be contributing to this increasing incidence of depression. One model of the causation of depression in the 20th century indicates that those most prone to depression seem to have the following characteristics:

To be women, the poor, young adults, the elderly, and the previously married

To have experienced a previous loss and be subjected to economic, isolating, parental, or marital stressors

To lack both employment outside the home and an intimate relationship

To have three or more children living at home

To earn feelings of love, respect, recognition, and worth in life through another person or group[19]

Primary prevention of the affective disorders, whether for the vulnerable members of society described or for others, cannot currently be achieved through biologic intervention. There are no physical means, such as a blood test, that can be used to predict depression for specific individuals. In the present absence of biologic intervention, psychological and social preventative efforts assume major importance.

Planning Primary Prevention

Two major goals in the primary prevention of the affective disorders are as follows:

1. The development of a positive self-concept, as demonstrated by self-confidence, self-respect, and even self-actualization

2. Healthy adaptation to loss

The nurse, by virtue of her professional role, finds herself in a variety of situations, such as child health care settings, in which these goals can be pursued.

The self-concept has its foundation in infancy and childhood and reflects parental perceptions and messages. The parent teaches the child overtly and covertly about his lovability, his worth as an individual, and his ability to master the environment. It is important to assess whether the child learns to initiate ideas and follow through with activity because these activities are recognized and reinforced. Instead of doing this, the child may perceive that he and his efforts are inadequate, useless, and not wanted. Rejection can be devastating to the development of a positive self-concept. Children who experience rejection sometimes conclude that they can elicit love and approval from significant others only if they assume guilt and punish themselves. Children who fail to learn to love themselves may become adults who measure their own worth solely according to the perceptions of others. These "dominant other" individuals become prime candidates for depression.

Promoting Adaptation to Loss

The nurse functions in many practice settings where children and adult clients and families are experiencing growth, development, change, and loss. Hospitalization itself results in loss of status, loss of self-determination, loss of usual family relationships, and perhaps loss of wage-earning ability. In addition, clients may be adapting to a changing body image, a changing lifestyle, and even the loss of life.

Some of these losses can be anticipated, and clients can be helped to adapt through anticipatory guidance and other supportive nursing actions that allow for verbalization, sharing of feelings, and problem solving. Some situations involving loss, such as death of a child or rape, can become crises for the individuals involved. The nurse's ability to recognize the existence of crisis and to intervene or arrange for others to do so may facilitate adaptive behaviors and may prevent depression. See Chap. 33 for more information on helping individuals deal with overwhelming stressors in their lives.

Nurses who participate in health education programs, such as prenatal and postnatal education, sexuality and family planning, genetic counseling, age-specific parenting groups, and support groups for those in transition, widows, divorcees, retirees, and so forth, are providing knowledge and exploring feelings so clients can maintain control over, and derive satisfaction from, their own lives. Nurses who practice in community health agencies, in doctors' offices, in well baby clinics, and in pediatric care settings have many opportunities to promote healthy parent–child relationships. The nurse's knowledge of growth and development can be used to help parents understand their children's behavior and, just as importantly, feel more positively about themselves.

In summarizing, the nurse, regardless of the nature of her practice, provides health education and reinforces the self-esteem of clients as integral aspects of her care. The nurse participates in the primary prevention of depression, which is certainly not limited to psychiatric treatment settings, where only a small percentage of potential and existing depression is recognized and treated.

Secondary and Tertiary Prevention

Secondary prevention seeks to reduce the prevalence of mental disorder by providing intervention that decreases the number of stressors and shortens the duration of disequilibrium. Tertiary prevention refers to measures used to reduce the level of social defects that result from mental disorder. This type of prevention often includes rehabilitation and readaptation to the environment.[25]

The nurse participates in the secondary and tertiary prevention of the affective disorders through the application of the nursing process—assessment, nursing diagnosis, planning, implementation, and evaluation—in client care settings. Although individuals with affective disorders can be found virtually anywhere, the following discussion focuses on the client in a psychiatric care setting. The nurse is reminded, however, that the application of nursing knowledge and skill is never bound by a location or setting.

Assessment

Nursing assessment and analysis of depressive and manic behaviors can be systematically accomplished through a thorough consideration of the client's affect, thought processes, intellectual processes, and physiological and psychomotor activity. The nurse identifies the client's actual or potential problems in these areas of functioning, makes nursing diagnoses, and specifies client behavior outcomes for which the nurse orders definitive interventions.

The following discussion includes observations that the nurse commonly makes when encountering clients with manic or depressive disorders. Bear in mind that no two clients present exactly the same history and behavior, and that the nurse should avoid the tendency to perceive clients with a mind set created by "textbook" descriptions.

Affective Changes

Affect in Depression. One area of assessment that provides essential data in the determination of a nursing diagnosis is the client's affect. Because depression and mania manifest themselves primarily as disturbances in mood or affect, the emotional tone of the client may be the most obvious deviation from healthy behavior. The depressed client appears sad, dejected, apathetic, and uncomfortable in his painful suffering, but does not usually exhibit bizarre behavior. He feels hopeless and, at the same time, helpless to do anything about his situation. He may verbalize feelings of guilt as well as feelings of anger or hostility. The client is unable to feel pleasure or experience joy.

These verbalized and, perhaps, unverbalized feelings are consistent with the physical appearance of the depressed client. There is frequently a disregard for grooming, cleanliness, and personal appearance. The client's stooped posture and dejected facial expression are also nonverbal messages of depression. During observation and communication with the depressed client, the nurse may begin to perceive that depression can actually be a defense against sadness and grief. Depression seems to raise the client's threshold for pain, thereby protecting the client from more pain than he is already experiencing.

Depression in Children. Because children are frequently unable to express feelings verbally, childhood depression is difficult to detect and may be reported less frequently than it actually occurs. Children tend to act out their emotional problems. Anger, aggressiveness, hyperactivity, delinquency, and school problems may be just as indicative of depression as sad, tearful faces, withdrawal from activities, and verbal expression of poor self-esteem.[1]

Affect in Mania. The manic client's mood is in direct contrast to that of the client experiencing depression. The manic client is self-satisfied, confident, and aggressive, and feels "on top of the world" and in control of his destiny. His flight into the external world, however, is also a defense against sadness and grief. The client's anger, sarcasm, and irritability become evident when the nurse attempts to set limits on his behavior or when he is frustrated by other individuals or objects in the environment.

When assessing the client's affective changes, the degree of the change is one of the most important judgments the nurse makes. Is the client mildly depressed, severely depressed, exhibiting retarded depression, or in depressive stupor? The mildly depressed client requires a less intensive approach than the severely depressed client, who sees no reason to continue living. The nurse must also observe for changes in the client's affective state, which would indicate that he is responding to other modes of therapy.

Thought Processes

Thought Processes in Depression. The thoughts of the depressed or manic client are congruent with his feelings; there is no dichotomy between thought and affect. The depressed client ruminates about his unhappy situation, discussing it repeatedly and asking the same questions, to which no one can give a satisfactory answer. Thinking may be difficult and slow; the content becomes limited to a few topics. Replies to the nurse's questions may be delayed and condensed, and the client does not reveal his private thoughts.[37]

In depression, there is frequently a heightening of awareness of inner sensations and a reduction in the awareness of external events.[31] This inability to mobilize attention to events in the outside world may lead to delusional thinking. These delusions or false beliefs, however, are consistent with the client's affective state. Delusional content is frequently characterized by self-deprecation, ideas of guilt, and remorse. There may also be a suspicious and persecutory trend to the client's ideas; that is, he may believe that he is being persecuted by others. Delusions may also be hypochondriacal in nature. The client sometimes believes he has a consuming illness that is destroying him from within, perhaps cancer.

The depressed individual thinks he is a failure and is totally pessimistic about his future. He believes that his life will not improve and he will not be convinced otherwise. The depressed client is filled with self-reproach, thinks in absolute terms, and becomes averse, rather than simply indifferent, to opportunities for change.

Suicidal Ideation. Because depression is characterized by many negative thoughts and accompanying feelings of self-hate and hostility, one of the most critical areas for the nurse to assess is the degree of the client's suicidal ideation. What thoughts does the client have about taking his own life? How great is the risk that he might try to do so? An accurate assumption for the nurse to make is that all depressed clients are potentially suicidal. The question is not "Is he?" but "To what degree is he?"

Although a data base for the assessment of suicide risk has not been scientifically established, statistics have been recorded that point toward some helpful generalizations. It has been estimated that more than 80% of the 22,000 to 25,000 suicides reported annually can be traced to a previous depressive episode.[5,13] In addition to the severity of depression being directly related to the degree of suicidal risk, there are other behaviors or symptoms that the nurse must include in the assessment of the depressed client. The presence of anxiety, hopelessness, withdrawal, disorientation, and hostility all indicate a higher risk of suicide than in depressions that are not characterized by these feelings and behaviors. Those clients who do not have social and personal resources, such as housing, transportation, money, employment, and available significant others are also at higher risk for suicide than those who do have these resources. A history of alcohol and drug abuse is a likely cause for added concern in the assessment of suicidal potential. Substance abuse behaviors are predominantly self-destructive coping strategies. Clients who have a history of multiple, high lethality suicide attempts, such as by shooting, are also greater suicide risks than those who have no such history. The client who frequently verbalizes the desire to die and describes a very specific plan is also someone who requires immediate intervention.

Depression, like suicide, is an attempt by the client to communicate a state of deprivation. If the depression does not elicit the desired responses from others, suicide may become the next course of action. Suicide can be viewed as a last desperate cry for help or love when no other avenues of communication exist for the client.

Thought Processes in Mania. Nursing assessment and diagnosis of the hypomanic or manic client's thought processes reveal different kinds of material. In all degrees of mania, there is little introspection.[24] In fact, the manic individual evades thinking and is occupied with phonetics rather than meaning in his thinking and speech. His stream of thought is characterized by a rapid association of ideas, termed *flight of ideas*, with rhyming and play upon words. Although these thoughts seem illogical, the client's remarks are very similar to free associations prompted by unconscious thoughts and feelings. The following is an example of flight of ideas.

"How do I feel? I feel with my hands. How do you feel? No, seriously, everything is wonderful; couldn't be better. Going 'from bed to worse' Benchley said. Really, honey, this is a marvelous place you've got here. Mar-vel-ous. Mar-vel-ous. Vel. I really must shampoo my hair."

In his euphoric state, the manic client is full of ambitious schemes and exaggerations that belie reality. Delusions often occur and are usually expansive, fleeting, and wish-fulfilling. The manic client may erroneously believe that he has great wealth and power. He is too busy to submit his ideas and impressions to critical examination. His desperate need to convince others of his grandiosity should alert the nurse to the very strong feelings of inadequacy that he is trying to overcome.

Intellectual Processes. Intellectual processes included in the nursing assessment of the client with a disorder of mood are perception, consciousness, and orientation. Disorders of these processes, in conjunction with the changes in affect and thinking already described, often leave the client with decreased powers of judgment and decision-making. In such instances, the nurse must determine to what extent it may be necessary to assume decision-making for the client and when this action is therapeutically warranted. Although autonomous behavior is a long-term goal for every client, there are times during acutely severe depression and mania when the nurse must make decisions for the client because he is unable to do so for himself.

Perception. The depressed client's perception may be distorted because of his intensive affective state. He perceives the world as strange and unnatural. A client with deep feelings of guilt may interpret the sound of wind in the trees as reproaching voices. This misinterpretation of a real sensory experience is called an *illusion.* The severely depressed client may less frequently experience *hallucinations,* perceptions that occur when there is no impulse created by the stimulation of a receptor. Auditory hallucinations are the most frequent form of perceptual disturbance and, if they do occur, they usually represent the projection of affective distress. An example of this projection occurs when the depressed client hears voices blaming him or telling him that he is worthless.

Hallucinations may occur in manic excitement but are not common.[24] As is the case with depression, perceptual disorders of manic clients usually take the form of illusions.

Consciousness. Among disturbances of consciousness are those imposed by disordered attention. Attention is the conscious, selective reaction by which an individual examines the external world for useful data.[24] Feeling and attitudes influence attention, and both depressed and manic clients may exhibit problems in the area of attention. The depressed client's attention may be so tenaciously directed toward his limited mental content that nothing will divert his energy elsewhere.

The severely depressed client may be so fearful of some impending disaster that he may actually become confused. Retarded depression, in which there is an inhibition of stream of thought and psychomotor activity, may result in *stupor.* In depressive stupor, there is almost complete immobility, a clouded sensorium, and intense preoccupation.

The manic client, on the other hand, is easily distracted by people, noises, and activity in the environment. Because of this inattention or distractibility,

the manic client may fail to discriminate among objects and people. The most severe form of mania, called *delirious mania,* is characterized by purposeless and continuous activity.

Orientation. Disorientation as to who one is, to where one is, and to time may occur in any mental disorder in which there is extensive impairment of the client's memory, the extent or accuracy of his perception, or his attention.[24] Because the intensely depressed or manic client may experience such impairments in orientation, the nurse assesses the client's understanding of his environment and how he locates himself in it.

A consideration of the client's intellectual processes also includes the assessment of the client's insight. *Insight,* which depends upon perceptual accuracy and consciousness, refers to the client's ability to observe and understand himself, or to the extent of self-knowledge.[24] The depressed client, acutely aware of his suffering, knows he is ill and usually demonstrates some desire to end his suffering. Unfortunately, his ambivalence and mistrust of others may interfere with an effective use of the resources available. The manic client, on the other hand, denies his many conflicts as well as the awareness that he is coping with them in a very unhealthy way.

Physiological and Psychomotor Activity. Depression and mania are physical states as well as psychological ones. An assessment of the client with an affective disorder would be incomplete without a thorough consideration of his physiological status and psychomotor activity.

Physical Effects of Depression. The depressed client has been described as an individual in whom a deficit in psychic energy is accompanied by a decrease in physical energy. All erotic, constructive, and reproductive activities come to a standstill.[31] Physiologically, depression manifests itself in a variety of ways. The client has difficulty sleeping, is anorectic, and loses weight. His muscle tone is decreased. Constipation may result from poor eating patterns and inactivity. Women may experience menstrual irregularities and amenorrhea. Sexual desire is decreased; the male client may be impotent. The client feels continually fatigued and may complain of physical symptoms for which no organic basis can be found. A delusional client may refuse to eat or drink because he believes he is undeserving of sustenance.

Unless agitated by feelings of anxiety, most depressed clients are lethargic and withdrawn, and resist social contacts. The depressed client lacks interest in personal hygiene and normal grooming routines. His hair and clothes may be unkempt and his body may be in need of bathing.

Physical Effects of Mania. The manic client presents some of the same problems for care but for different reasons. Nutritional deficits may exist because the client will not take the time to eat or cannot attend to this activity for sufficient amounts of time. Dehydration may occur for the same reasons. Because the manic client's continuous activity may not result in a feeling of fatigue, exhaustion may result.

The manic client may dress in bizarre ways and may use makeup inappropriately. He does not attend to personal hygiene. Acute episodes of mania may be accompanied by singing, shouting, writing, or destruction of clothing and property. The client may intrude in the activities of others or may collect objects. Although this overactivity is purposeful, the client does not attain his objective or goal because he does not complete tasks or projects.

The overactivity of the manic client makes it difficult for the nurse to detect signs and symptoms of physical illness that may accompany his physical debilitation. Careful nursing observation may detect signs of an infection, such as pneumonia, to which the client may be too busy to attend.

Nursing assessment of the client with an affective disorder must be a continuous process. The client's mood may change quickly and the potential for suicide is great. Physical illness may complicate the client's care. The disturbances in affect, thought, intellect, and psychomotor activity described should serve as general guidelines. The changes from the normal to depressed state are summarized in Table 23-1. When the client begins to receive treatment, especially through medication or electroconvulsive therapy, his behavior may change. The nurse must remember that somatic treatment of depression, although helpful for the client, makes nursing assessment more difficult to accomplish.

Nursing Diagnosis

Assessment data about the client with mood disorders and his or her family are gathered and analyzed to form the bases for nursing diagnoses. These diagnoses will then guide the planning, implementing, and evaluating of nursing intervention.

The following nursing diagnoses may be frequently associated with clients experiencing disorders of mood:

Table 23-1.   **Changes from Normal to Depressed State**

	CHANGES	
ITEMS	*Normal State*	*Depressed State*
Stimulus		**Response**
Loved object	Affection	Loss of feeling, revulsion
Favorite activities	Pleasure	Boredom
New opportunities	Enthusiasm	Indifference
Humor	Amusement	Mirthlessness
Novel stimuli	Curiosity	Lack of interest
Abuse	Anger	Self-criticism, sadness
Goal or Drive		**Direction**
Gratification	Pleasure	Avoidance
Welfare	Self-care	Self-neglect
Self-preservation	Survival	Suicide
Achievement	Success	Withdrawal
Thinking		**Appraisal**
About self	Realistic	Self-devaluating
About future	Hopeful	Hopeless
About environment	Realistic	Overwhelming
Biologic and Physiological Activities		**Symptom**
Appetite	Spontaneous hunger	Loss of appetite
Sexuality	Spontaneous desire	Loss of desire
Sleep	Restful	Disturbed
Energy	Spontaneous	Fatigued

(From Friedman J, Katz MM (eds): The Psychology of Depression: Contemporary Theory and Research. New York, John Wiley & Sons, 1974)

Ineffective individual coping
Hopelessness
Spiritual distress
Social isolation
Impaired social interaction
Disturbance in self-concept
Alterations in thought processes
Powerlessness
Potential for self-harm
Sensory-perceptual alterations
Self-care deficits
Potential for injury
Sleep pattern disturbance
Alteration in bowel elimination: constipation
Alteration in nutrition (less than body
    requirements)
Potential for infection

Planning

The nurse can plan care for the client with an affective disorder with a legitimate feeling of optimism. Both mania and depression are time-limited conditions; in most instances, the nurse will see the client return to a healthier, functioning state. This does not mean, however, that nursing and medical care are not needed. Both can shorten the intensity and length of these affective states and can, perhaps, save the client's life.

There is no single way to approach depressed or manic clients. It is essential that the nurse perceive the client as an individual. The nurse's perceptions should be shared and compared with those of other members of the health care team. The identification of client behavior outcomes should be a combined effort of those associated with, or responsible for, the care of the client, including the client and his family when possible.

Client Behavior Outcomes for the Depressed Client.
Frequently, assessment of the depressed client will result in client behavior outcomes that are related to the following needs:

1. Physical safety and health
2. Expression of painful negative feelings
3. Love, acceptance, a feeling of belonging rather than one of isolation
4. Feelings of being useful and needed
5. Opportunities to achieve worthwhile accomplishments
6. Opportunities for autonomy and self-actualization

These client needs are quite naturally a direct consequence of the essence of depression—a lonely, loveless, and hopeless state. They are appropriate

needs for the nurse to address as they all depend upon relationships with other human beings. They are also needs that transcend the experience of hospitalization.

Client Behavior Outcomes for the Manic Client.
Assessment of the manic client will result in a somewhat different list of needs during the manic state.

1. Physical safety and health
2. Opportunities to channel physical and psychic energy
3. Accurate perception of reality

The manic client has the same underlying needs for love and autonomy that the depressed client exhibits in a more obvious manner. During the manic episode, however, the client's strong denial necessitates that the nurse postpone most interpersonal actions that may help the client meet these needs.

Discharge Planning.
Most clients with affective disorders have functioned in society as adult family members and will be able to do so again in the future. Planning, therefore, must extend beyond the time and place of hospitalization. The client's family must be incorporated into the plan of care to prevent the client from feeling abandoned and alone.

Other resources, such as church, work, and social groups, must be maintained if at all possible.

What employment opportunities will be available to the client?
What opportunities for socialization will present themselves to the client?
Whom can the client turn to when he feels stressed?

These and similar questions must be answered as the nurse and other members of the mental health team plan with the client and his family for his return to home and community.

Intervention

Nursing Intervention for the Depressed Client.
After identifying nursing diagnoses and client behavior outcomes for the client with an affective disorder, the nurse identifies nursing actions that are designed to achieve these outcomes. It is important that the nurse remember that behavior changes slowly and that the client may have periods of regression. Realistic expectations about behavior change must accompany the nurse's actions. Even minor changes in the client's behavior should be considered significant; nursing approaches should not be discarded prematurely.

Physical Safety and Health

Decreasing Suicidal Risk. The depressed client's needs for physical safety and health require that the nurse maintain a constant vigil for the possibility of suicide and other self-destructive behaviors. Once the nurse has determined that the client is suicidal, several actions are warranted. The client should be observed frequently or continuously on a one-to-one basis. Most obviously, the nurse must make sure that the environment is as free from potential danger as possible. Items such as belts, razor blades, scissors, and other sharp objects should be removed from the client's immediate environment. The nurse should also be very aware of the medications that the client is taking and the possibility of his hoarding dosages for future lethal ingestion. Pill overdosage is the most common form of successful suicide and suicidal gesture.[13] If the client leaves the unit or hospital for any reason, he and his belongings should be carefully searched upon return. Psychiatric facilities should have a detailed written description of "suicidal precautions," which are implemented when clients are identified as suicidal. The nurse should become very familiar with these and assume responsibility for their initiation, enforcement, and modification.

There is a close relationship between suicide and crisis theory. The nurse may view the suicidal state as a therapeutic opportunity. The client may be ready to learn new coping skills that he can continue to use after the crisis has subsided. If the nurse has not already established a relationship with the client, it is imperative that the nurse or some other member of the health care team do so at this time. If suicide is a cry for love, help, and attention, the client must feel that these needs are perceived by someone in the environment and that he is cared for. The risk of suicide may be so great that the nurse may determine that the client should not be left alone, even in the bathroom. Letting the client know that his stressful situation is acknowledged and communicating that he will receive support and help in controlling his impulses are important interventions. Gratifying dependency needs during this acutely stressful period may reduce the client's level of anxiety, which, in turn, decreases the risk of suicide.

The nurse, in addition to meeting dependency needs, should also use the therapeutic relationship with the depressed client in order to help him gain an understanding of the crisis, to help him become aware of and accept his feelings, which may be very hostile, and to explore coping mechanisms other than self-destruction.

The nurse bases her reactions to the suicidal client on certain beliefs. The client who talks about suicide does commit suicide, and threats and attempts must be taken seriously. The nurse must not deny the client's feelings by shying away from discussing suicidal thoughts. Such discussions will not cause the client to commit suicide or make him more suicidal; they will probably reduce some of his anxiety. Suicidal clients are ambivalent about dying, and the nurse should maximize those arguments the client accepts or offers for living. The client who commits suicide is not necessarily psychotic or even mentally ill. In fact, in many instances, the risk of suicide is greatest when the client is emerging from the depths of depression and appears to be improving. The client then has the physical and mental energy to conceive a plan and carry it out. The client may actually feel and communicate relief once he has found a final solution (*i.e.,* suicide) to his problems. For more in-depth information about suicide, see Chapter 37.

Ensuring Physical Health. The client's physical health and safety are frequently concerns when the nurse cares for the depressed client. The severely depressed client does not attend to bodily needs and may not have the energy to care for himself. The nurse should consider the following actions as long as the client cannot do these for himself:

1. Bathing the client
2. Assisting with the client's grooming, such as care of hair and nails
3. Selecting appropriate clothing
4. Ensuring the intake of nutritious food, which may mean sitting with the client as he eats
5. Clearing the environment of potential hazards, such as misplaced furniture, slippery rugs, and poorly lighted areas
6. Maintaining a record of sleeping patterns, bowel function, and menstrual function
7. Identifying the need for further nursing and medical actions

Promoting Physical Activity. The depressed client should be encouraged to engage in physical activity for several reasons: to expel energy; to produce feelings of physical well-being and control; and to produce feelings of accomplishment (see Chart 23-1, "The Brain–Body Phenomenon"). Because joy accompanies activity, it is suggested that the client participate in active behaviors that were previously reinforcing to him, such as jogging, tennis, or housekeeping chores, even if he doesn't want to do them.[22] The client progresses from solitary activity to noncompetitive activity with others to competitive activity with others.

Monitoring Side Effects of Medication. Because the depressed client is usually receiving antidepressant medication, the nurse should also be familiar with the side effects of these medications. These fre-

C H A R T   23-1
The Brain-Body Phenomenon

Walking, Running, and Dancing Your Way to Mental Health

Although it is unclear why, physical fitness enhances mental health. Walking, jogging, bicycling, swimming, and aerobic dance are popular forms of exercise that may be powerful antidotes to depression and anxiety.

Exercise produces a sense of enhanced mental energy and concentration. Joggers express feelings of heightened mental acuity and hours of clear-headedness after running.

Exercise relieves tension. Strenuous activity is all-absorbing, not allowing the participant to worry about anything else. Tension may not return until hours after exercise. Stress on one body system may help relax another.

Exercise is adult play, accompanied by joy and lightheartedness.

Exercise produces a sense of self-worth. Participants set progressive goals that are achievable and not in competition with others. It's hard to feel sorry for yourself and exercise at the same time.

Exercise produces a sense of control. It gives the participant freedom not experienced in other aspects of life. The cyclist or jogger does not depend on anyone else for exercise.

Exercise can symbolize active participation in life and serve as a socially acceptable way of asserting oneself.

Mental energy, lightheartedness, self-worth, autonomy, and assertiveness are the antitheses of depression. Movement, through physical exercise, may be a prescription of choice for disturbances in mood.

quently include constipation, dry mouth, and sedation. Other side effects are loss of visual accommodation, headache, dizziness, nausea and vomiting, increased perspiration, and weight gain. These side effects can be minimized or avoided by gradually increasing the dosage to the optimal therapeutic level.[9] The nurse should discuss possible side effects with the client and should encourage him to report them to members of the health team.

Expression of Feelings

Exploration of Anger and Sadness. The depressed client fears open communication and intimacy; nevertheless, feelings that rage inside him need some form of expression. In every phase of its development, depression includes a component of anger, whether that anger is visible or invisible, conscious or unconscious.[31] Regardless of whether the client appears angry or not, he needs someone with whom he can share his sadness and verbalize his guilt. The nurse must not be intimidated or discouraged by these interactions with the depressed client. Sometimes, nurses mistakenly assume that it is a nursing responsibility to "make things better" for the client. Even if the client professes extreme helplessness, the nurse must not approach him as though he were a helpless being.

The nurse may find it useful to explore with the client what is helping to maintain his depression. Once the client identifies his own depression-reinforcing behaviors used to elicit sympathy from others, such as crying, the client may decide to stop engaging in these behaviors. He may even decide to stop talking about his depression.

Therapeutic Communication. The nurse engages in active listening and demonstrates acceptance of whatever feelings and thoughts the client communicates (see Chart 23-2). If the nurse withdraws or more overtly rejects the client or his feelings, she reinforces his belief that it is not safe to express himself and that others don't care about him. It is very important that the nurse does not try to talk the client out of his sadness by being inappropriately cheerful and optimistic or by offering false reassurance.

Cultural Influences. The expression of feelings is greatly influenced by one's cultural heritage. Southern Europeans and Latins tend to be very expressive; Northern Europeans and Orientals do not. Some believe that to express one's feelings is a sign of weakness to be avoided at all costs. This belief is demonstrated in the subculture of sex. In many societies, it is acceptable for girls and women to express their feelings, but not for boys and men. As the nurse implements care, these cultural differences must be considered.

Positive Reinforcement. Another helpful approach in the treatment of depression is the concept of positive reinforcement. The nurse may advocate the use of an "antidepression" kit, which contains pleasuring items, memorabilia of happy times, or reminders of future activity.[23] The client creates this kit for himself and resorts to it when he feels depressed.

Effects on the Caregiver. Depression is contagious, and depressed people tend to drive others away from them. Depressed clients are repetitively negativistic and sometimes clinging and manipulative.

CHART 23-2
Therapeutic Dialogue

Encouraging the Expression of Feelings

Nurse: Sarah, you mentioned you were in the hospital because you attempted suicide; tell me more about that. (sitting on a bed next to the client, maintaining eye contact, leaning toward the client)

Client: I took an overdose of Elavil. I ended up in Intensive Care for 4 days. I just couldn't take it anymore. I had to get out of the house. (looking at the nurse, speaking calmly and deliberately)

Nurse: Then you didn't intend to kill yourself? (asked in a questioning manner, trying to make eye contact with the client)

Client: No, it was the only way I could get away from my parents. (The client, Sarah, is a 32-year-old woman with muscular dystrophy who is confined to a wheelchair.) They don't support me; they didn't even come to see me when I was in Intensive Care. (maintaining intermittent eye contact with the nurse, wiping tears off cheeks)

Nurse: You wanted them to care? (speaking softly)

Client: Yes. You know it's hard watching your body deteriorate a little bit at a time. Every day I lose something. I remember when I could dance like everybody else. (affect very sad, still maintaining intermittent eye contact) I'm depressed, but I've got a good reason to be depressed. There's no cure for me; I'm just getting worse.

Nurse: It's a heavy burden for you. (maintaining eye contact with the client)

Client: Yes. (nodding head) So I've got to use my mind. That's the only thing I have left.

Discussion

Sarah voluntarily mentioned her suicidal behavior to the nurse who did not hesitate to explore this further. Suicide is accompanied by an intense feeling state; there is a need to verbalize and share.

The nurse attempts to clarify Sarah's feelings and the meaning of her suicidal behavior. Sarah expresses ambivalent feelings toward her parents; she wants to leave them, but she wants them to care. The nurse has not yet begun to explore the origin of these feelings, nor the alternative ways to express them.

The nurse conveys a sincere interest in the meaning of, and the feelings associated with, the client's behavior. The nurse neither moralizes about the act of suicide, nor challenges the client with the possibility that she really had no intent to take her own life.

As Sarah has explained, her depression can be associated with a very real, ongoing loss. She seems to be communicating that she needs more help to cope with the feelings of anger and frustration inherent in her situation. The nurse identifies this need, which will become an important focus in Sarah's plan of care.

Nurses often feel frustrated and angry at themselves in return. Planning and sharing the client's care with other members of the health team provide the nurse with an opportunity to express and explore her own feelings and a means of group support. The client's family, who may have been likewise frustrated, may be encouraged by learning that depression is self-limiting and that they can look toward a time when the client will recover and return to a more normal level of functioning. The family members' involvement in the client's plan of treatment may help to determine the degree of adaptation and growth that the entire family is able to achieve as a result of the depressive episode.

Feelings of Acceptance and Belonging. The nurse can initiate a therapeutic relationship with the depressed client to facilitate his feelings of acceptance and belonging. The nurse may schedule regular times to meet with the client, thereby ensuring privacy and communicating that he is important as an individual. These individual appointments with the client should be arranged only as the nurse can realistically implement and follow through. The nurse's trustworthiness and consistency are paramount issues in providing care for the depressed, or any, client.

The nurse must also maintain a sensitivity to the environment and constantly question how other clients and staff influence the depressed client. Is he

Case Study 23-1

Caring for the Client Who Is Struggling Against Depression

The S. family consists of Mr. and Mrs. S. and their two sons, 15-year-old Robert and 12-year-old Andy. Robert, tall and blond, was brought to an inpatient psychiatric treatment facility by his mother who verbalized great concern about Robert's abuse of drugs and alcohol. The admitting physician diagnosed Robert as being "depressed" and "anxious."

During the admission process, the mental health care team gathered additional data from both Mrs. S. and Robert. Approximately 3 days before this admission, Robert had been treated in a hospital emergency room for a drug overdose. At that time Robert did not know what drugs he had taken and he was very angry and fearful.

Mrs. S. described Robert as being a "bright" and "good" child, although he never seemed interested in cuddling or kissing. She perceived him as being self-sufficient and hyperactive. Mrs. S. explained that Robert's behavior changed about 1 year ago. At that time, he started missing school, he failed a grade, and his abuse of drugs escalated to the point that Mrs. S. feared for Robert's life.

Family interaction, according to Mrs. S.'s description, appears chaotic and turbulent. Mrs. S. indicated that she believes in physical discipline of her children but receives very little support with them from her husband. She described Mr. S. as uninterested in the family and pointed out that she even manages the financial affairs of the family.

Upon admission, Robert stated, "I don't have a problem," but was willing to put in the necessary time so he "could get out of here." Robert described his mother as being physically abusive to both him and his brother since Robert was 5 or 6 years old. Robert related that when he was 6, he put a plastic bag over his head and said he wanted to die.

The nurse gathered Robert's history a short time after he was admitted for treatment. When the nurse and Robert talked alone, he answered questions very briefly and offered no spontaneous comments or conversation. Robert's eye contact with the nurse was minimal; his affect was moderately depressed.

The nursing history resulted in the following additional data. Robert is enrolled in a work-study program and plans to continue with school when he returns home. Robert stated that no one at school really cared whether he attended or not. He also said he would like to enlist in the Air Force after completing high school or earn an equivalency diploma and learn to fly. If he doesn't learn to fly, he said, he'd like to work around planes in some capacity, perhaps as a mechanic. Robert's vocational experience is limited; he worked as a delivery boy for 2 weeks, but quit because he wasn't earning enough money.

Robert's interests are presently limited to drugs and rock music. He stated that he has no close friends, even though he abuses drugs in the company of others (it's "no fun," he said, to do it alone). He perceives his relationship with his parents as "not too good" because they don't approve of his behavior. Robert said he doesn't have much to do with his younger brother, Andy. When asked to describe himself, Robert replied, "I'm a regular kid doing what I want to do."

This is Robert's first hospitalization for any illness. He considers himself physically healthy. When the nurse inquired about his use of drugs and alcohol, he stated matter-of-factly that he consumes about two quarts of whiskey per week and smokes marijuana daily. During the last 2 years, he has also used mescaline, LSD, oxycodone (Percodan), and methaqualone (Quaalude). Although not clearly relating it to his use of drugs, Robert also mentioned that he is currently on probation for trespassing.

During his first week of hospitalization, Robert gradually became acquainted with the staff and some of the other clients. He was perceived as being intelligent, sometimes sociable, and usually cooperative, although somewhat guarded. He frequently paced the floor. At times, he played pool or ping pong with one or two young male clients or watched television. Robert went to bed late and got up late, sleeping 10 to 12 hours a night.

Robert's treatment included occupational therapy, recreational therapy, psychotherapy, and family therapy. The latter was considered to be especially crucial to Robert's treatment. The staff also projected that Robert would need to become involved in a drug rehabilitation program following hospitalization.

The initial family therapy session was attended by Mrs. S., Andy, and Robert. Mrs. S.

(Continues on p. 402)

described herself as being at her "wits' end" and expressed a great deal of hostility toward her husband, whom she perceived as undermining everything she tried to do. During this first session, Robert was not communicative—he denied having problems and wanted to know "what all the fuss was about."

The entire family, including Mr. S., attended subsequent family therapy sessions, and Robert was gradually able to express how his feelings were related to his parents' dysfunctional relationship. His desire to modify his behavior, however, remained questionable.

The nursing care plan for Robert focused on establishing a relationship with him to facilitate expression of feelings about his family and hospitalization. Because his inability to function at home and school precipitated his admission, Robert's day was carefully structured with activities in which he was expected to participate.

After almost 3 weeks of inpatient treatment, Robert was discharged to a drug rehabilitation program. Robert's physician judged that Robert's prognosis was guarded, however, because he lacked motivation and insight.

Questions for Discussion

1. Which of Robert's behaviors are "typical" for the adolescent? Which ones are not?
2. To what possible "losses" can you relate Robert's struggle against depression?
3. How has the relationship between Robert's parents affected him?
4. Can Robert's drug abuse be related to his mother's past physical abuse of him? How are they similar or different?
5. For Robert, could drug abuse be a form of suicide? Explain why or why not.
6. What other nursing care approaches would you formulate for this client?
7. Robert's physician indicated that Robert's prognosis was guarded because he lacks motivation and insight and his behavior is ego-syntonic. Do you agree with this? Why or why not?

being included in activities? Is he relating to others and on what level? The psychiatric–mental health nurse generally has more opportunity to make such observations and manipulate the environment to the client's benefit than anyone else on the health team.

Feelings of Being Useful and Needed and Feelings of Accomplishment. Hospitalization and illness, whether for mental or physical reasons, usually imply that the client will experience a certain degree of helplessness and dependency. Consequently, it is often a difficult task to engender in the client feelings of being useful and needed. Nevertheless, the nurse should use whatever opportunities arise to promote the development and reinforcement of these feelings in the client. As soon as he is ready, the client should participate in client groups that share in decision-making for the unit or facility in which he is receiving care. The client should also be encouraged to assume some responsibility for planning and carrying out social activities and share in other unit tasks.

A severely depressed client, drawn to a state of lethargy and inactivity, may not be able to function as an effective member of a group; expecting him to do so may reinforce a negative view of himself. The nurse must assess the client carefully before communicating her expectations. Perhaps the severely depressed client would benefit from an initial one-to-one relationship that is gradually expanded to include a larger sphere of people with whom he feels comfortable.

Nursing actions intended to mobilize depressed clients into activity have been designed using Beck's cognitive framework.[40] His approach of acceptance, reactivation, and cognition is based on the assumption that the way we think about, evaluate, or predict events around us determines how we feel and behave. Behavioral techniques to counteract helpless thinking patterns are graded task assignments, activity schedules, and mastery–pleasure monitoring.

Graded task assignments consist of breaking up large tasks into small manageable steps that allow the client to experience success. These assignments may focus on client behaviors associated with grooming, eating, and socialization. Daily activity scheduling entails an hourly designation of activities for the client which is intended to counteract the inactivity associated with negative ruminations and sadness. With the mastery–pleasure technique, the client keeps a running account of and rates experiences that provide for mastery or pleasure. This provides evidence for the client that he has certain competencies and that not everything is without some degree of pleasure.[27]

Once the client is able to engage in constructive activities, cognition is increasingly emphasized.[18] Lethargy-inducing patterns of thought, such as "I have nothing important to share with anyone," are analyzed and tested by the client and nurse. Questioning assumptions and identifying errors in thinking, such as "I have to be perfect to be loved," may be enough to disprove self-defeating ideas and allow the client to perceive his strengths.

Successful experiences within the hospital may help the client believe that he can also be effective outside the hospital. Discharge planning must include a consideration of what in this client's future life will permit him to feel needed and useful.

Are there family members to whom he is important?
Is there an occupation in need of his talent?
To whom or what does he make a difference?

Opportunities for Autonomy and Self-Actualization.

Autonomy and self-actualization are frequently identified as characteristics of the mentally healthy individual.[28] Autonomy is a component of self-actualization and implies a relative independence of the physical and social environment. The autonomous individual is not dependent for his main satisfactions on the real world, including the people in it, their opinions and affections. The need for self-actualization is exhibited by the individual who must do what he, individually, is fitted for. He must be true to his own nature. Both autonomy and self-actualization are long-term goals toward which many individuals strive during most of their lifetime.

Learned helplessness and dependency, the opposites of autonomy and self-actualization, are frequent companions of depression. The severely depressed client may not be able to take care of his own bodily needs, decide how to dress in the morning, or choose what to have for breakfast. He is, therefore, even less able to make decisions about relationships, financial needs, or occupational matters. In some situations, the nurse must make such decisions for the client until his anxiety level decreases and he shows other indications of increased decision-making ability. The nurse does what must be done to mobilize the client, and this frequently requires a very directive approach. The client is not asked if he would like to have breakfast; he is told that it is time for him to have breakfast. If given a choice, most depressed clients would decline such invitations to eat. In this instance, the nurse may appear to be taking away the client's autonomy; however, this is not so. The client cannot be deprived of his autonomy when, in fact, he has surrendered it to his depression.

As the client progresses, the nurse encourages the client to listen to himself and assume more of his own decision-making. The nurse's own problem solving skills provide both support and a corrective educational process for him. What does he perceive as his problems? What are possible solutions to these problems? What are the possible outcomes of such solutions? What puts the client in control of himself and his situation? If the client can recognize his potential for self-direction and development, he is taking a step toward health and away from a mode of thinking that plays a central role in depression-helplessness.

Nursing Intervention for the Manic Client.

Nursing care of the manic client is focused primarily on maintaining the physical health of the client until his manic state subsides, usually as the result of medication. A client who is in a manic state seeks to release tension through physical activity and may not be aware of his other physical or psychological needs. The client's flight of ideas prevents significant interpersonal contact.

Physical Safety and Health. The increased mobility of the manic client ranges from mild motor excitement to incessant activity. The client's talking, singing, dancing, and teasing are frequently accompanied by weight loss, a decrease in food consumption, insomnia, and constipation. The nurse intervenes by keeping environmental stimuli to a minimum. For example, the nurse may keep the client away from areas where others are engaging in noisy physical activity. The client is extremely distractible and reacts to almost any stimulus in the environment.

Unrealistic demands by the client are also a potential problem and are best approached with partial fulfillment of the demand whenever possible. The nurse tries to avoid direct confrontations by letting the client know what he can do rather than what he can't do. A client's request to go outside at night, for example, could be answered with the information that he will have the opportunity to go out in the morning, if this is in fact so. In this manner, the client is able to focus on the positive aspects, rather than the limitations placed on his behavior.

At times, it may be necessary to use the client's distractibility to ease him out of a troublesome situation. The client's euphoric mood can change quickly to one of irritation, or even rage, when he sees that others don't respond to his enthusiasm or react in accordance with his expectations.

Promoting Physical Health. If the client's excitability is not aggravated, the nurse may find it easier to attend to his physical needs. The client cannot be expected to sit down for complete meals, but he can be given foods and liquid to carry around with him. These foods should be high-calorie and high-protein substances to meet his increased energy expenditure. The nurse should also monitor the client's sleeping and elimination patterns because these basic needs may be neglected. Nursing or medical intervention may be necessary to promote proper rest and elimination. The client should also be observed carefully for signs of illness because he may be in a debilitated state and may ignore or be unaware of developing symptoms of physical disease.

Lithium Therapy. Nursing actions to promote physical health must also include close observation of the client who is taking lithium to counteract manic behaviors. Lithium is a potentially dangerous drug that is 80% effective in the short-term management of the manic phase of a bipolar disorder.[17] The amount of drug that is therapeutic is only slightly less than the amount that produces toxicity. This difficulty in regulating the precise dosage of the drug is compounded by the fact that no two clients respond entirely the same to lithium or absorb or excrete it at exactly the same rate.[17]

Lithium therapy requires the monitoring of clients' blood levels at frequent intervals. The initial stabilization phase may be followed by a maintenance phase during which the dose is reduced. Because some clients may be maintained on lithium for an indefinite period of time, the nurse should ascertain what the client understands about his need for lithium and should help him accept the probability of continuing therapy for an extended length of time.

The nurse should also consider introducing the client to another individual who is taking lithium so they may share information and problems. The client's family also needs to be alerted to the effects and side effects of lithium, as well as to the importance of monitoring the reappearance of manic behavior. The reappearance of manic behaviors may first evidence as a sleep disturbance or an increase in alcohol consumption by the client.

Because the client must be able to eliminate lithium from his system, kidney function tests are desirable before therapy is initiated. An electrocardiogram (ECG) and electrolyte and thyroid studies should also be performed to determine if the client is a suitable and safe candidate for lithium therapy.

Clients and their families must know that lithium should not be taken with diuretics and should be advised of the signs of lithium toxicity. Fortunately, when toxicity occurs, it usually occurs in progressive fashion and is detected before harm comes to the client.[17]

If mania is severe, the client may initially be given a major tranquilizer because lithium's therapeutic effects require at least 1 week of administration to manifest themselves. During this lag phase in the treatment, the nurse should keep in mind that high doses of drugs such as chlorpromazine (Thorazine) and haloperidol (Haldol) will mask the nausea and vomiting of lithium toxicity. Close and continuous nursing observation is essential to safeguard the client during psychopharmacological therapy.

Opportunities for Channeling Physical and Psychic Energy. A creative nursing approach to the manic client is critical in the planning of his treatment. The nurse attempts to reduce the client's accelerated manner of thinking and speaking by presenting accurate feedback to him. For example, when the client moves rapidly from one topic to the next, the nurse informs him that she does not understand him and asks for clarification. When interacting with this client, the nurse may find it necessary to refocus or redirect the conversation so that only one topic is being discussed at a time. Although these nursing approaches may meet with limited success, the nurse has an obligation to provide accurate information to the client about how he is being perceived by others. It is usually best to avoid long discussions with the manic client. If he has access to paper and pen or pencil, the manic client will often write voluminously. Writing may, in fact, provide a therapeutic benefit to the individual who can use this medium to express his feelings. The nurse may involve the client in gross motor activities, such as sweeping, mopping, or other tasks, and some noncompetitive physical exercises to channel his hyperactivity. The client's attention span is short; therefore, his participation in games and sports, which require sustained interest and adherence to rules, is usually unsuccessful. Monitoring and directing of the client's activity are essential components of the nursing care designed to prevent his exhaustion.

Reinforcement of Reality. The manic client is expansive in his thinking and may be delusional. He may believe he exerts great power and control and possesses great wealth. He may identify with the influential people in the environment; for example, he may be found making rounds with doctors or nurses. The client may communicate to other clients that he can secure hospital passes for them. The nurse mirrors reality for the client by responding to him as the client he is. The nurse does not challenge the client's beliefs, but neither does she encourage his delusional thinking.

Consistency in Approach. Because of the manic client's propensity to manipulate those in his environment, it is essential that those responsible for his care communicate with one another and respond to the client in a consistent manner. The client can be argumentative and demanding; the nurse should not respond in kind. The nurse and other mental health caregivers set limits on the client's behavior consistently and with confidence, knowing that they have planned and chosen the most appropriate interventions according to the client's need.

Other Therapies. The nurse should be aware of, and may be involved in, various other forms of therapy indicated for the client with a disturbance in mood. These therapies include various forms of group therapy, chemotherapy, and electroconvulsive therapy.

Group Therapy. Depending on his level of wellness and his ability to interact with others, the depressed client may benefit from involvement in remotivation therapy, a structured form of group therapy which focuses on reality-orientation and building self-esteem. Group therapy and family therapy may also be beneficial. A group comprised entirely of depressed clients is usually avoided, because the nature and extent of the interaction within the group would be limited. The manic client is usually disruptive to others in a structured group situation and may not benefit from this therapeutic approach.

Chemotherapy. Chemotherapy plays a significant part in the treatment of both depression and mania. Antidepressant and antimanic drugs are employed to alleviate the client's symptoms but do not resolve the psychosocial issues that may have precipitated the client's disorder. Because these drugs help make the client more amenable to other types of intervention, those responsible for the client's care must take advantage of this effect. Chemotherapy should never be the sole form of treatment for the client.

A major depressive disorder is the primary indication for the use of antidepressants that achieve their therapeutic effect by altering neurotransmitter imbalances. Antidepressant medications are expected to increase the client's level of activity, increase his appetite, and improve his sleep patterns. They are also expected to elevate mood and decrease self-accusatory or delusional thoughts.

Antidepressants are frequently divided into the following three categories:

1. The standard tricyclic antidepressants, including imipramine (Tofranil), desipramine (Norpramin), amitriptyline (Elavil), doxepin (Sinequan), protriptyline (Vivactil) and trimipramine (Surmontil)
2. The "second generation" antidepressants, including amoxapine (Asendin), maprotiline (Ludiomil), and trazodone (Desyrel)
3. The monamine oxidase inhibitors (MAOIs), including isocarboxazid (Marplan), phenelzine (Nardil), and tranylcypromine (Parnate)

Sixty to eighty percent of clients with major depressive disorders respond positively to these approved antidepressants.[4] However, all of these drugs do have side-effects and it is the side-effect profile which frequently determines the drug of choice for a particular client.

As mentioned earlier in this chapter, the standard tricyclic antidepressants and the "second generation" antidepressants, in addition to their intended therapeutic effects, may cause temporary side-effects. These include dry mouth, sedation, blurred vision, nasal congestion, and orthostatic hypotension. Additional troublesome side-effects are constipation, urinary hesitance, tremor, slowing of intracardiac conduction, and lowered seizure threshold. Antidepressants may be particularly hazardous for the elderly whose slowed metabolism places them at greater risk for these side effects.

The MAO inhibitors are usually reserved for those clients who do not respond to other antidepressant drugs. This is because of their potential to exacerbate the actions of other medications and to cause serious hypertensive crises when taken with certain foods which contain tyramine. Some of the items which clients must avoid are cheese, beer, wine, yeast, yogurt, chicken livers, and pickled herring. Other side effects are insomnia, orthostatic hypotension, dry mouth, weight gain, headache, constipation, and blurred vision.

The nurse can expect the client to show definite improvement within the 2 to 4 weeks following the initiation of antidepressant therapy, and perhaps sooner. If improvement does not occur, a change to another drug may be warranted. Medication is usually continued for 6 to 12 months after the client clinically recovers, and it is withdrawn gradually.

The nurse who administers antidepressant and antimanic drugs to clients must be familiar with the intended therapeutic effects, the signs of toxicity, the contraindications, the usual dose and route of administration, and the side-effects and related nursing management. For example, constipation can be alleviated by increasing the client's fluid and fiber intake. Fall prevention precautions are indicated for orthostatic hypotension. Seizure precautions should be initiated for clients with preexisting seizure disorders. The nurse must observe the client carefully to verify that he is taking his medication. Both manic and depressed clients may have perceptions that convince them that drugs are not necessary or that drugs are even harmful to them.

Lithium, the drug usually prescribed to treat mania, effectively decreases the client's excessive elation, hyperactivity, and accelerated thinking and speaking. Lithium may also be the drug of choice for bipolar depression. It appears to have antidepressant effects in treating acute episodes of depression and in reducing the frequency of relapse.

The potential toxicity associated with lithium therapy has been described earlier in this chapter. Additional side-effects include major impairment of urinary concentrating ability, which results in polyuria and polydipsia; intention tremor; and gastrointestinal irritability. The sustained release preparation of lithium and lithium citrate solution may be used because they are less irritating to the gastrointestinal tract.

A complete review of the medications indicated for disorders of mood is included in Chapter 17.

Convulsive Therapies

Insulin Therapy. Before the advent of chemotherapy in the treatment of psychiatric disorders, various types of shock therapy were administered to the client in the hope that behavior change would result. The use of shock therapies dates from 1933, when large doses of insulin were injected into the schizophrenic client to produce a deep hypoglycemic state as a form of treatment for schizophrenia.

Electroconvulsive Therapy. Electroconvulsive therapy (ECT), first used in 1938, is the application of a small dose of electricity to one or both sides of the brain. Both insulin and electroconvulsive therapy are in use today. There is still no satisfactory explanation for the therapeutic action that results from either type of shock therapy.

The primary indication for electroconvulsive therapy is depression. Acutely manic clients who are threatened by exhaustion may also benefit from this type of treatment. Because chemotherapy has proved to be effective in the treatment of mood disturbances, electroconvulsive therapy may be less often indicated or may be considered only when the client does not respond satisfactorily to medication.

Electroconvulsive therapy, a relatively safe procedure, sounds more ominous than it actually is. Nevertheless, the nurse should keep in mind that strong feelings of fear and anxiety may be elicited when one mentions this type of treatment to clients and families. The client may envision electrocution or death or may anticipate permanent intellectual changes. Both the physician and nurse must carefully explain what the treatment is like and prepare the client for the aftereffects. The nurse can be supportive of the client to the extent that she has knowledge about, and has resolved her own feelings about, the use of ECT. The client's fear of ECT should never be used against the client in the form of a threat or coercion.

The client is prepared for ECT in a manner similar to preparation for surgery. The nurse assures that he has no food or drink the morning of the treatment, voids just prior to the procedure, removes dentures, and wears a hospital gown or loose clothing.

The client must give his informed consent and the appropriate form must be signed. A complete physical examination of the client is required, including a spinal x-ray. Vital signs are monitored before and after the treatment.

The ECT treatment is usually administered in a room that is designated for this purpose and that adjoins a recovery area. The client is placed on a stretcher or firm bed. A rubber mouthpiece is inserted in the client's mouth to maintain an airway. In some instances, the client is given intravenously a short-acting anesthetic, such as methohexital (Brevital), and a muscle relaxant, frequently succinylcholine (Anectine), just before the electric shock is administered. Electrodes are applied unilaterally or bilaterally to the client's temples, the shock is administered, and the client experiences a typical grand mal seizure with tonic and clonic phases. The nurse and others in attendance should not attempt to restrain the client's body but should guide the extremities so that they do not become injured during the seizure activity.

When the seizure ends, oxygen may be given as a safety measure because apnea may occur physiologically in any general convulsive seizure. Consequently, airways and equipment for oxygenating the client should be readily available in the treatment area.

Once the client is transferred to the recovery area, he will regain consciousness quickly. While he is awakening, he should be positioned on his side to prevent aspiration of oral secretions. The nurse monitors the client's vital signs during the recovery period. It is usual for the client to be confused. The client must be observed carefully to insure his safety and must be reoriented to his surroundings. The client should be permitted to rest after the treatment and should then be helped to get his breakfast.

The client may or may not be hospitalized for ECT treatments. Such treatments are usually given three times a week; the number of treatments the client receives depends upon the results obtained. The physician may originally plan six treatments, but may continue to 25 or 30 treatments according to the client's response. The nurse's observations of the client during this time are important in the decision-making regarding the number of future treatments.

A frequent aftereffect of ECT is memory impairment that may range from a mild tendency to forget details to severe confusion. This memory impairment may persist for weeks or months following the last ECT treatment. The nurse prepares the patient for this confusion and assures him that it is expected and that full return of his memory will eventually occur. Evidence that unilateral treatment (ad-

(Text continues on p. 410)

Nursing Care Plan   23-1

The Depressed Client

Nursing Diagnosis	Client Behavior Outcome	Intervention
Potential for self-harm	Will not harm self	Establish a nurse–client relationship to meet client's dependency needs, reduce his anxiety, monitor risk of suicide, and help client identify alternatives to self-destructive behavior
	Will identify effective coping mechanisms to handle stress	Carefully monitor ingestion of medication
		Control the client's access to objects in the environment that can be used for self-destructive purposes, such as pointed objects, belts, light bulbs, and mirrors
		Maintain constant observation by nurse and other members of the health care team
		Engage the client in diversional activities; avoid constant focus on suicidal preoccupations
		Follow "suicide precautions" established by treatment facility, if warranted by client's behavior or ordered by client's therapist
		Encourage the client to take responsibility for his own behavior whenever this behavior is a therapeutic possibility
Self-care deficit: feeding, bathing, dressing	Demonstrate increased interest and desire to eat	Expect the client to eat regular meals; do not give him a choice about whether or not to eat
		Remain with the client during meals to determine his eating patterns; maintain intake and output records if necessary
		Allow as much time as client may need for eating; client may need to be fed
		Encourage the client to eat with whom he feels comfortable
	Relate feelings of comfort and satisfaction with body cleanliness	Bathe client daily, if necessary, and supervise related activities, such as mouth and skin care

(Continues on p. 408)

Nursing Diagnosis	Client Behavior Outcome	Intervention
	Demonstrate increased ability to dress self	Shampoo and comb hair if client cannot do it for himself
		Assist the client with other aspects of grooming, such as the use of deodorant, makeup, and nail care
		Select appropriate clothes for the client and assist with upkeep as necessary
		Recognize the client's efforts to maintain his own appearance; do not become impatient if his self-care is slow
		Reinforce what the client can do for himself rather than focus on what must be done for him
Sleep pattern disturbance	Demonstrate an optimal balance between rest and activity	Establish regular hours for sleeping and wakefulness
		Consider prohibiting daytime sleeping if the client has difficulty sleeping at night
		Expect the client to participate in physical exercise on a daily basis; try to incorporate activities the client previously enjoyed
		Gradually encourage the inclusion of others in physical activities, as they become more enjoyable for the client
		Prevent accidents; maintain a safe environment for the client
Ineffective individual coping	Verbalize feelings related to emotional state	Initiate interaction with the client on a regular basis
		Be direct and honest with your own feelings
	Identify coping patterns and the consequences of the behavior that results	Allow for verbalization of feelings, as in "You look very annoyed this morning"
		Encourage physical expression of feelings, such as striking pillows or a punching bag and hammering appropriate objects
		Avoid impulses to cheer up the client or to try to talk him out of his depression
		Explore with the client what is helping to maintain his feeling of depression (What are the secondary gains?)

Nursing Diagnosis	Client Behavior Outcome	Intervention
		Avoid focusing on physical complaints (for which there are no organic bases); redirect the client to other topics and areas of concern
		Share the responsibility for this intervention with other members of the health care team
Disturbance in self-concept	Begin to assume role-related responsibilities, develop confidence in ability to accomplish what is desired	Schedule regular times with the client that ensure privacy and communicate his importance as an individual
		Do not overwhelm the client with attention or with too many ideas at one time
		Point out to client that self-deprecating comments block communication
		Do not allow the client to ruminate about failures in the past; redirect the client to present problems or involve the client in another type of activity
		Identify with the client achievements that would make the client feel better about himself and ask the client to focus on *one* of these
		Help the client recognize opportunities to congratulate himself, however modest his accomplishment may seem
		Include the client in group activities that provide for some degree of success
		Assign responsibilities that are important yet not too difficult for the client to assume
Powerlessness	Identify factors that can be controlled by him; make decisions regarding his care, treatment, and future when possible	Make decisions for the client during those periods when the client is unable to assume this responsibility
		Support the client's attempts at decision-making
		Encourage and role model the use of the problem-solving process in decision-making
		Insist that the client delineate the problem, propose alternate

(Continues on p. 410)

Nursing Diagnosis	Client Behavior Outcome	Intervention
		solutions, and consider the outcomes
		Allow sufficient time for the client to think and act
		Clearly communicate what is expected of the client (attendance at meals, etc.)
		Be specific about the amount of time that can be spent with the client and adhere to this limit
		Spend time with the client in group situations
		Point out to the client his insensitivity to others' needs and help him identify other ways of behaving
		Help the client formulate a written schedule of activity, first on a day-to-day basis, then for longer periods of time, to foster feelings of control

ministering electric current to only one side of the brain) produces less confusion and memory loss than bilateral treatment (administering current to both sides) is being investigated by researchers.[26]

There are many theories about why ECT is effective in depression. Some authorities believe that the confusion and impairment of memory the treatment produces permit a denial that reduces the intensity of the client's conflict and his awareness of anger and disappointment.[31] Other theories hold that the client perceives ECT as well-deserved punishment and therefore feels less guilty. Electroconvulsive therapy has also been described as a "flight into health" that the client chooses over the threat of ECT. Others maintain that physical changes occur (*e.g.,* cerebral anoxia) that cause improvement in some unknown way.

Evaluation

The nurse evaluates care of the client with a mood disorder by observing the client's behaviors and comparing them with previously formulated client behavior outcomes. The nurse also collects data relating to the client's behavior by talking with the client's family and other health team members who are involved in his care. The nursing process is cyclical in nature, and evaluation results in a reassessment of the client, the formulation of new or modified nursing diagnoses and client behavior outcomes, and the specification of additional or modified nursing actions that are intended to bring the client even closer to his optimal state of health.

As the depressed client interacts with the nurse and others during this evaluation phase, the nurse can consider the following questions: Has the client's self-concept become more positive? Does the client give any indication of suicidal ideation? Has the client's outlook become more optimistic? Has the client's dependency decreased? Is decision-making easier for the client? Does the client interact more frequently with others? Does the client sleep more and complain less of fatigue and other physical maladies? Is the client's appetite improved? Is he gaining weight? Is the client attending to personal hygiene and grooming? Positive responses to questions such as these usually indicate that the client has begun to assume control over his own life and is motivated to participate in some of the activities of daily living.

When evaluating care of the manic client, the nurse may ask the following questions: Are the client's psychomotor activity and speech becoming slower and more regulated? Is the client less distractible? Does

Nursing Care Plan 23-2

The Manic Client

Nursing Diagnosis	Client Behavior Outcome	Intervention
Sensory-perceptual alterations	Experience decreased symptoms of sensory overload	Keep environmental stimuli to a minimum
		Provide the client with sufficient room in which to move about
	Describe rationale for treatment modality	Engage the client in physical activities or tasks that channel his energy, such as writing, drawing, or sweeping
		Interrupt impulsive acting out behavior whenever possible and encourage the client to work towards self-control; respond to dangerous or destructive behavior with swift and coordinated intervention
		Try to minimize the client's activity at night
		Offer warm baths or soft music to promote sleep
		Tell the client when his conversation is not understandable; help him focus on one idea at a time
Self-care deficit: feeding, bathing, toileting	Demonstrate increased ability to feed self	Provide finger foods for the client to carry around with him; do not expect him to sit down for three meals a day
	Perform bathing activity at optimal level	Choose foods for the client that will provide needed additional calories and will also meet basic nutritional needs
	Demonstrate ability to toilet self	Provide abundant fluids
		Maintain an intake and output record, if warranted
		Remind the client to bathe, brush teeth, use toilet
		Help the client select clothing that is appropriate to the climate and situation and that is easy to take on and off

(Continues on p. 412)

Nursing Diagnosis	Client Behavior Outcome	Intervention
Alterations in thought process	Express delusional material less frequently	Do not reinforce the client's delusions through discussion or validation
		Do not challenge the client's beliefs
	Describe problems in relating with others	Reinforce reality by responding to him as the person he is; do not laugh at him
	Differentiate between reality and fantasy	Be prepared to protect the client from himself; he may give away possessions
Impaired social interactions	Identify problematic behavior that deters socialization	Set no more limits than are necessary for the client, then enforce the limits
	Substitute constructive behavior for disruptive social behavior	Provide simple explanations when denying requests; avoid argumentation whenever possible
		Use persuasion rather than force
		Partially fulfill a demand, if this is feasible, to spare the client complete frustration
		Consider postponing a decision about a client's request if more data are needed
		Maintain close communication with other members of the health care team so all are responding to the client in the same way
		Control feelings of anger toward the client to prevent loss of the situation
		Point out to the client his manipulative behavior and interrupt the pattern

the client have a more realistic perception of his influence and abilities? Is the client more introspective? Are the client's dress and use of makeup more appropriate? Is the client sleeping more and able to monitor his own physical needs?

The client's return to a healthier state is dependent upon the efforts of all members of the health care team, including family members, friends, and the client himself. When the client returns home, these resources must still be accessible as he encounters many stressors that will test his newly acquired confidence. The client may have new living arrangements to which he must adapt, a new job in which he must succeed, and altered or new relationships to establish and maintain. The client must continue to have someone with whom to share his feelings and validate his perceptions and problem-solving skills.

Summary

This chapter has focused on the characteristics of two very different but related behavioral patterns, depression and mania, and the nursing care that may be indicated for each. Both depression and mania have been presented as extreme feeling states with cognitive and physical components that differ primarily in degree, rather than in kind, from those experienced by healthier individuals. The following facts and ideas have been presented:

1. Mood disorders, described early in recorded history, are a major mental health problem in the United States.
2. The cause or causes of mood disorders have not been established with any certainty; etiologic theories include both biologic and psychosocial influences.
3. Mood disorders can be chronic as well as acutely psychotic and can be masked by various maladaptive behaviors, such as alcoholism and promiscuity.
4. Manic behavior is psychodynamically perceived as a defense against depression.
5. The nurse has a responsibility to participate in the primary prevention of mood disorders as well as in the secondary and tertiary prevention.
6. The nurse is a collaborator with other members of the health care team, including the client and his family, and assumes an influential role in determining the client's care and treatment, which have both psychosocial and biologic components.
7. Nursing assessment and intervention for the depressed client focus on the client's physical health and safety, his feelings about himself and others and the expression of these feelings, and distorted perceptions and false beliefs about the environment and himself.
8. Suicide, frequently an outcome of depression, can be prevented.
9. Nursing assessment and intervention for the manic client focus on the client's physical health, the channeling of the client's energy, environmental manipulation, and reinforcement of reality.
10. Somatic therapy, including chemotherapy and electroconvulsive therapy, is a vital component of the treatment plan for a client with a disturbance in mood.
11. Nurses and other mental health professionals need opportunities to express, explore, and resolve their feelings of anger and frustration that may develop as a result of their work with depressed and manic clients.

References

1. Albright A, Murphy CM, Rhyne MC: Depression in Children: Reasons and Risks. Pediatric Nursing 6 (July/August): 9–13, 1980
2. American Psychiatric Association, Diagnostic and Statistical Manual of Mental Disorders, 3d ed, rev. Washington DC, American Psychiatric Association, 1987
3. Beck A: The Development of Depression: A Cognitive Model. In Friedman RJ, Katz MM (eds): The Psychology of Depression: Contemporary Theory and Research, pp 3–27. New York, John Wiley & Sons, 1974
4. Bowden CL: Current Treatment of Depression. Hosp Community Psychiatry 36 (November): 1192–1200, 1985
5. Brown BS: Forward to Friedman RJ, Katz MM (eds): The Psychology of Depression: Contemporary Theory and Research. New York, John Wiley & Sons, 1974
6. Campbell L: Depression: Acute Care in the Hospital. Am J Nurs 86 (March): 289–291, 1986
7. Chadoff P: The Depressive Personality: A Critical Review. In Friedman RJ, Katz MM (eds): The Psychology of Depression: Contemporary Theory and Research, pp 55–69. New York, John Wiley & Sons, 1974
8. Chapman AH: Management of Emotional Problems of Children and Adolescents, 2d ed. Philadelphia, JB Lippincott, 1974
9. DeGennaro M, Hymen R, Crannell AM, Mansky PA: Antidepressant Drug Therapy. Am J Nurs 81 (July): 1304–1310, 1981
10. Epstein MH, Cullinan D: Depression in Children. J Sch Health 56 (January): 10–12, 1986
11. Fine M, Jenike M: Electroshock: Exploding the Myths. RN 48 (September): 58–59, 61–62, 64, 1985
12. Finn PA: Self-Destructive Behavior in School-Age Children: A Hidden Problem? Pediatric Nursing 12 (May–June): 198–199, 1986
13. Fuller E (ed): Caring for the Suicidal Patient. Patient Care 14 (November 30): 101–134, 1980
14. Glazebrook CK, Munjas BA: Sex Roles and Depression. J Psychosoc Nurs Ment Health Serv 24 (December): 9–12, 1986
15. Gordon VC: Depression in Women: The Challenge of Treatment and Prevention. J Psychosoc Nurs Ment Health Serv 23 (January): 26–34, 1985

16. Harris B: Drugs and Depression. Am J Nurs 86 (March): 292–293, 1986

17. Harris E: Lithium. Am J Nurs 81 (July): 1311–1315, 1981

18. Helm SB: Nursing Care of Depressed Patient: A Cognitive Approach. Perspect Psychiatr Care 22 (July–September): 100–107, 1984

19. Jacobson A: Melancholy in the 20th Century: Causes and Prevention. J Psychosoc Nurs Ment Health Serv 18 (July): 11–21, 1980

20. Kline N: From Sad To Glad. New York, Ballantine Books, 1974

21. Knowles RD: Coping With Lethargy. Am J Nurs 81 (August): 1465, 1981

22. Knowles RD: Handling Depression Through Activity. Am J Nurs 81 (June): 1187, 1981

23. Knowles RD: Handling Depression Through Positive Reinforcement. Am J Nurs 81 (July): 1353, 1981

24. Kolb L: Modern Clinical Psychiatry, 9th ed. Philadelphia, WB Saunders, 1977

25. Lancaster J: Community Mental Health Nursing: An Ecological Perspective. St Louis, CV Mosby, 1980

26. Lobel B, Hirschfeld RMA: Depression, What We Know. Publication No. (ADM) 85-1318. Washington, D.C., National Institute of Mental Health, U.S. Department of Health and Human Services, 1985

27. Manderino MA, Bzdek VM: Mobilizing Depressed Clients. J Psychosoc Nurs Ment Health Serv 24 (May): 23–28, 1986

28. Maslow A: Motivation and Personality, 2d ed. New York, Harper & Row, 1970

29. Maurer FA: Acute Depression: Treatment and Nursing Strategies for the Affective Disorder. Nurs Clin North Am 21 (September): 413–425, 1986

30. Minot SR: Depression: What Does It Mean? Am J Nurs 86 (March): 285–288, 1986

31. Ostow M: The Psychology of Melancholy. New York, Harper & Row, 1970

32. Rogers CA, Ulsafer-Van Lanen J (eds): Nursing Interventions in Depression. Orlando, FL, Grune & Stratton, 1985

33. Rush AJ, Altschuler KZ (eds): Depression, Basic Mechanisms, Diagnosis, and Treatment. New York, Guilford Press, 1986

34. Seligman MP: Depression and Learned Helplessness. In Friedman RJ, Katz MM (eds): The Psychology of Depression: Contemporary Theory and Research, pp 83–125. New York, John Wiley & Sons, 1974

35. Shamoian CA: Assessing Depression in Elderly Patients. Hosp Community Psychiatry 36 (April): 338–339, 345, 1985

36. St. Pierre J, Craven RF, Bruno P: Late Life Depression: A Guide for Assessment. J Gerontologic Nurs 12 (July): 4–10, 1986

37. Swanson A: Communicating With Depressed Persons. In Backer B, Dubbert P, Eisenman E (eds): Psychiatric/Mental Health Nursing: Contemporary Readings, pp 165–173. New York, Van Nostrand Reinhold, 1978

38. Todd B: Depression and Antidepressants. Geriatr Nurs 8 (July–August): 203–204, 1987

39. Wold CI, Tabachnik N: Depression as an Indicator of Lethality in Suicidal Patients. In Friedman RJ, Katz MM (eds): The Psychology of Depression: Contemporary Theory and Research, pp 187–202. New York, John Wiley & Sons, 1974

40. Wright JH, Beck A: Cognitive Therapy of Depression: Theory and Practice. Hosp Community Psychiatry 34 (October): 1119–1127, 1983

24

Retreat from Reality: The Schizophrenic Disorders

Barbara Schoen Johnson

While I was at Grace Hospital, it was my sense of hearing which was the most disturbed. But soon after I was placed in my room at home, all of my senses became perverted. I still heard the "false voices"—which were doubly false, for Truth no longer existed. The tricks played upon me by my senses of taste, touch, smell, and sight were the source of great mental anguish.

Clifford Beers,
A Mind That Found Itself: An Autobiography,
1923

Chapter Preview

This chapter focuses on the disturbances in reality orientation, thought processes, and social involvement that are known as *schizophrenia*. These serious emotional disorders cause an untold burden on human lives. The overview of schizophrenic disorders will discuss its incidence, current theories of etiology, and types or diagnostic categories of the disorder. The following sections of the chapter will apply the steps of the nursing process—assessment, nursing diagnosis, planning, intervention, and evaluation—to individuals with schizophrenia and their families and communities.

Learning Objectives

On completion of the chapter, you should be able to accomplish the following:

1. discuss biologic and psychosocial theories of the etiology of schizophrenia
2. identify the types of schizophrenia
3. describe the behaviors of schizophrenic disorders, particularly the thought, affective, and social/behavioral disturbances
4. formulate nursing diagnoses and goals for the schizophrenic client and his family
5. intervene therapeutically in the schizophrenic client's thought, affective, and behavioral disturbances
6. discuss the effects of chemotherapeutic agents in the care of schizophrenic clients
7. describe the impact of a schizophrenic member on the family, community, and society
8. intervene therapeutically with the family of an individual with schizophrenia
9. evaluate the effectiveness of nursing actions designed for clients with schizophrenic disorders
10. identify means of intervention with populations at risk for the development of schizophrenic disorders
11. discuss your own feelings and attitudes when caring for schizophrenic clients and their families

Schizophrenic Disorders

Schizophrenia is a common and unsolved mental health problem in the world today. It is estimated that 1% of the United States population is, has been, or will be affected by the disorder. Its onset usually oc-curs early in life—adolescence or young adulthood—and often becomes a progressive and disabling condition. Far-reaching economic, family, and community effects add further stress to the lives of these severely disturbed individuals and their loved ones.

The stigma of schizophrenia makes it all the more tragic, as clients and families must bear not only the disease, but the stigma as well. "Schizophrenics," says one authority, "are the lepers of the 20th century."[57] Unparalleled as a stigmatizing disease, schizophrenia reaps the societal consequences of personal shame, family burden, and inadequate support of clinical care, research, and rehabilitation.[19]

The remarkable thing about schizophrenia as a disease, says Torrey, is how little attention has been paid to it, given its prevalence and severity. Its cost in the United States has been estimated at between $10 and $20 billion annually, including the costs of hospitalization, Social Security benefits for the disabled, welfare payments, and lost wages. Demographically, it is the most expensive of any chronic disease, because the individual is well during his rearing and education, then becomes ill and dependent on society just when he would become a contributing wage earner.[57]

Although multiple etiologic theories have been proposed and studied, the definitive cause, or causes, of schizophrenia remain unknown. Current methods of prevention and treatment are often inadequate and fall into the category of "too little, too late."

Some types of schizophrenia appear to exist in all populations, regardless of culture.[47,49] There are, however, different incidence rates of schizophrenia when compared cross-culturally.

Most likely, schizophrenia is not a single disease, but a *heterogeneous disorder*; that is, a group of several distinct disorders, or a collection of disorders, with some common features.[18,23] These common features include a disturbance in thinking and an extreme preoccupation with the self and with inner fantasies.

The person who has a schizophrenic disorder may live in his own world—a world inhabited by "voices" that condemn or accuse him of vile acts, and "visions" of frightening animals, monsters, or scenes. The person may be totally withdrawn from the external environment and may invest all of his energy in an internal fantasy life. He may regress to a level wherein he does not attend to personal hygiene, activities of daily living, interpersonal contacts, or even the presence of physical illness or pain.

Etiologic Theories

There exist today many theories of the etiology of schizophrenia (see Chart 24-1, "Historical Perspectives"). The search for a cause is spurred on by the

CHART 24-1
Historical Perspectives: Views of Schizophrenia

Some important figures in medical history have conceptualized, developed, and refined what today is known as "schizophrenia."

Emil Kraepelin

At the end of the 19th century, Emil Kraepelin (1855–1926) differentiated from the rest of mental disorders a condition he called dementia praecox. This diagnosis implied a fatalistic prognosis, because dementia, Kraepelin believed, occurred precociously or early in life and followed a gradual, but continuous, downhill course leading to intellectual deterioration. Kraepelin attributed the etiology of this disorder to an endogenous factor such as organic pathology or an error of metabolism, not to societal influences.

The identified symptoms of dementia praecox included hallucinations, delusions, disorders of thought and consequently speech, poor insight and judgment, flat affect, and reduced attention to the outside world.

Eugen Bleuler

The Swiss psychiatrist Eugen Bleuler (1857–1930) renamed the syndrome "schizophrenia" to indicate the "splitting" of various mental functions. Bleuler classified the disorder's symptoms into two major categories.

1. Fundamental symptoms (also known as the "four As") that indicated the underlying process specific to schizophrenia
    Associative disturbance, or thought disturbance
    Affective disorder; that is, a flat or blunted affect or one which was inappropriate or incongruous to the thought or situation
    Autism; that is, detachment from external reality and withdrawal into fantasies
    Ambivalence, or the simultaneous existence of opposing feelings, thoughts, and desires
2. Accessory symptoms, or symptoms that were frequently present but not specific to schizophrenia nor diagnostic of it, including hallucinations, delusions, and catatonic posturing.

Sigmund Freud

Sigmund Freud (1855–1939) emphasized the importance of psychological factors in the etiology of schizophrenia. He described the process of the development of hallucinatory psychoses, which, he felt, originated from frightening and unbearable ideas. He coined the term *projection* and described it in relation to paranoid disturbances.

Adolf Meyer

Attention to the psychological factors in the development of schizophrenia was also advocated by Adolf Meyer (1866–1950), a Swiss-born and Swiss-educated psychiatrist who became a prominent medical authority in America. Meyer proposed that the longitudinal study of schizophrenic patients would offer insights into various etiological influences.

Carl Jung

Carl G. Jung (1875–1961) discussed the idea of certain individuals' "predisposition" to emotional disturbance. He saw the schizophrenic patient as an "introvert" who directs a great deal of energy into himself. Jung also considered the possibility of a psychosomatic factor in operation in schizophrenia; he proposed that an emotional disorder could cause a metabolic disturbance and, eventually, physical brain damage in psychotic patients. One of Jung's important concepts was the "collective unconscious," which stores the archetypes, or mythological images, of all people. Jung thought that the symptoms of schizophrenia were "reproductions of the archetypes deposited in our collective unconscious."

Harry Stack Sullivan

An American psychoanalyst, Harry Stack Sullivan (1892–1949), examined the impaired interpersonal relations, not the intrapsychic forces, that predominate in schizophrenia. He believed that children who were later to become schizophrenic adults had undergone disturbed interpersonal relations with their parents and significant others. Sullivan's major life work was the psychotherapy of schizophrenia in which he interacted, not as an observer, but as a participant with the patient.

(From Arieti S: Interpretation of Schizophrenia, 2d ed. New York, Basic Books, 1974; Cancro R: Individual Psychotherapy in the Treatment of Chronic Schizophrenic Patients. Am J Psychother 37 (October): 493–501, 1983; and Goldstein WN: DSM-III and the Diagnosis of Schizophrenia. Am J Psychother 37 (April): 168–181, 1983) hope that discovery of the cause, or causes, of schizophrenia will result in the determination of a cure.

Currently, there are two main groups of theories regarding the etiology of schizophrenia—the biologic theories and the psychosocial theories. A biopsychosocial model of schizophrenia has been proposed to incorporate all relevant data from both the biologic and psychosocial approaches.[19] The view that schizophrenia is a collection of disorders, rather than a single disorder, implies a variety, or combination, of etiologies.[63]

Biologic Theories

According to the biologic theories, the etiology of schizophrenia is related to organic or physiological factors. These biologic theories are discussed according to genetic, biochemical, and neuroanatomic influences.

Genetic Influences. There is evidence of a genetic factor in the causation of schizophrenia.[17] A higher incidence rate of schizophrenia occurs in the relatives of schizophrenics than in the general population. It has also been demonstrated that the closer the family relationship, the higher the incidence of schizophrenia in the relatives. For example, if a man is known to have schizophrenia, the chance that his son will also develop schizophrenia is much greater than the chance that his nephew will become schizophrenic. In addition, the incidence rate of schizophrenia will be greater for both the man's son and his nephew than it would be for the general population.

Genetic influences in the development of schizophrenia have been demonstrated through the study of twins. Twin studies have shown that if one of monozygotic ("identical") twins becomes schizophrenic, the incidence rate for the other twin is significantly higher than for dyzygotic ("fraternal") twins.

Lastly, it has been shown that the rate of schizophrenia in the children of schizophrenic mothers when the child was adopted away in the first few weeks of life equals the rate that would have been expected had they been reared by their biologic mothers. The incidence rate of schizophrenia for children of nonschizophrenic mothers when the child was adopted away early in life equals that incidence seen in the general population.

More recently, the results of research studies have suggested that schizophrenia seems to occur through the interaction of a genetic susceptibility with some kind of environmental stress.[28] The presence of a major gene for susceptibility to schizophrenia has not been supported in a recent studies. Nevertheless, the genetic factors in schizophrenia have specificity, as they increase the risk of this disorder but not of other

psychotic disorders. The "new genetics" of recombinant DNA technology may offer more useful information about the genetics of schizophrenia.[3,28]

Biochemical Influences. Much recent research has focused on the biochemical influences on the development of schizophrenia. There may be biochemical differences in the nervous system of the person with schizophrenia that cause him to process sensory information in an abnormal manner. An alteration in this important mental function of information processing could result in disturbances of attention, inadequate social interaction, isolation, and hypersensitivity.[17] The attentional disorder in schizophrenia is a well-documented event and is observed especially in clients whose condition has been chronic.

Individuals with schizophrenia cannot intentionally sustain a focused attention. They attend to incidental details and accord them unusual significance. This inability to direct thought prevents full access to long-term memory. Hasty ideas are given delusional conviction when they capture the individual's attention and appear significant to him. The client, then, lacks control over his own thinking.[4]

Psychopathology research has, over the past 10 years, attempted to link schizophrenia to certain patterns of hemispheric dysfunction of the brain. Recent studies have suggested left hemisphere overactivation and consequent temporal abnormalities and delays in processing sensory information. The performance patterns of schizophrenics, however, may be a means of compensation for their generalized attentional deficits, or there may be a variety of other explanations.[59] Other pathophysiologic findings in individuals with schizophrenia include dysfunctions of eye movements; impaired modulation of stimulus input, allowing too much information to reach higher brain centers; laterality differences, in which the left hemisphere may be less efficient than the right; impaired selective attention; and directed attention in the form of vigilance.[31]

Schizophrenic disorders may be associated with a disturbance in the adrenergic systems of the brain.[37,53] An overactivity of dopamine or an insufficiency of norepinephrine at certain central synapses of the brain or an imbalance between the two substances could be among the biologic factors present in schizophrenia. Lending support to the dopamine theory of schizophrenia is the positive behavioral effect that results from the biochemical action of the antipsychotic medications, and the fact that an amphetamine-induced psychosis mimics acute paranoid schizophrenia.

It has been proposed that there may be an immunologic imbalance or, perhaps, a defect in the regulation of the immune system in some clients with schizophrenia. Nevertheless, the role of the immune system in the etiology and development of the schizophrenic syndrome is still undetermined.

Neuroanatomic Theories. Brain impairment does exist in a substantial number of schizophrenic clients.[54] Certain structural brain abnormalities in clients with chronic schizophrenia have been visualized by computed tomography (CT) scanning techniques.[60] Currently, available data suggest a complex picture of brain dysfunction in schizophrenic individuals that includes cerebral atrophy, enlargement of the ventricles of the brain, disturbances in cerebral metabolism and electrical activity, neurologic soft signs, and a variety of neuropsychological deficits.[35,54] These findings further support the belief that schizophrenia is not one disorder, but a group or collection of disorders.

Through new technologies, the brain's metabolic changes, blood flow, electrical activity, and neurochemistry can be studied with more precision than previously. Positron emission tomography (PET) produces slice images of radioisotope density. These studies have indicated relative metabolic underactivity of the frontal lobes of schizophrenics. They have also shown decreased activity in the basal ganglia that can be reversed with neuroleptic treatment.[16,38] Advances in methodologic techniques are helping neuroanatomists test their theories about schizophrenia more directly.

Psychosocial Theories

The psychosocial theories of the etiology of schizophrenia focus on the intrapsychic and interpersonal dimensions of the client's development and life experiences.

Intrapsychic Influences. An individual becomes schizophrenic, says one theorist, not because of what others did to him, but "because of what he does with what was done to him."[7] An intrapersonal approach to the etiology of schizophrenia is based on the theory that there exists a predisposition of the personality to break down under high levels of stress. Certain characteristics of the individual (*e.g.*, hypersensitivity, increased anxiety, and social detachment) may, under extensive stress, escalate into suspicion, intolerable fears, withdrawal, and isolation from others.

The child who later becomes schizophrenic may be extremely sensitized to certain negative characteristics of a parent (*e.g.*, emotional detachment or hostility) and may incorporate these feelings into his own distorted self-image.[6] His view of himself is that of a worthless, guilty, helpless individual.

Another vulnerability model proposes that schizophrenia is an episodic, and not a continuous, disorder.[64] "Triggering" life events, such as the death of a loved one, may exacerbate a crisis and emotional collapse for the person who is predisposed to schizophrenia. Some of the potential factors in the development of vulnerability include low socioeconomic status, crowding, community disorganization, lack of acculturation, social isolation, and minority status. The individual's social network, which is often diminished in schizophrenia, is an important determinant in whether he is accepted and supported or isolated and vulnerable to a schizophrenic episode.

Interpersonal Influences. An interpersonal view of schizophrenia is based on the premise that a person learns values, attitudes, and communication patterns through his family and culture. Disordered communication and interaction may, therefore, be a learned phenomenon that may also be unlearned through therapeutic intervention.

Communication within the family of a schizophrenic client may be indirect, unclear, incongruent, and growth-impeding.[51] For example, members of a family that produces a schizophrenic member often feel that they are not free to comment on whatever they observe in the family. This stifling of communication is typical of a closed family system.

Another aspect of disturbed communication is the lack of adequate feedback mechanisms. Normally, when two people communicate, one person sends a message to the other and the second person sends back a response that informs the first person of the effect of his message. Feedback and the correction of information are essential components of effective interpersonal interaction but are absent or defective in the family communication patterns of the schizophrenic.[50]

The communications of all family members are frequently discounted in the family that has a schizophrenic member. The members of the schizophrenic's family may also be forbidden to enter into any close relationships with others from outside the family.[30] The "rules" of the family of a schizophrenic often seem strange and rigid compared with the practices of other families in the community; typically, the family appears aloof and isolated.

The schizophrenic process is thought to begin early in the child's life and to destroy the emotions and personality structure of the individual as it grows. Inherent in the schizophrenic process is the fact that the parents notoriously implicate their children in their personal life.[62] Because the parents are disappointed in their mutual relationship, they may turn to their child (who later becomes schizophrenic) and expect from him all the love, acceptance, and affection they did not receive from each other.

Double-bind communication has in the past been considered to be at the core of schizophrenic maladaptation. The basic nature of the double-bind phenomenon is that the child receives two opposing messages from the parent and both of the messages must be obeyed. For example, the parent holds out his arms and says, "Come here and give me a hug, son," and then when the child runs to him, the parent pushes the child away and says, "Why would I want to touch a bad boy like you?" The child is punished if he expresses love for the parent and punished if he does not, and he can find no way out of the situation.[9]

Some families with a schizophrenic member are found to be severely *fused*, wherein the members have never adequately separated or developed into individuals with their own viewpoints, thoughts, and feelings. Rather than having separate identities, members of this family possess an *undifferentiated family ego mass*.[13] It seems that the member with the least amount of differentiation from the others is the person who often becomes psychotic in the family.

Another interpersonal influence that has received recent attention and research efforts is that of expressed emotion (EE). A negative affective climate in the home, called *high expressed emotion*, has been suggested as a particularly stressful factor in families of vulnerable individuals.[26] Expressed emotion has also been defined as a measure of relatives' expressed attitudes about the client.[46] This issue has touched off a controversy based on the misperception that expressed emotion research places blame on the families of schizophrenics.

Types of Schizophrenia

The types of diagnostic classifications of schizophrenia, according to the criteria of the Diagnostic and Statistical Manual of Mental Disorders, third edition, revised (DSM III-R), are as follows.

1. *Schizophrenia disorganized* (formerly called hebephrenic). The client is frequently incoherent and displays a flat, silly, or inappropriate affect. No delusional system is evident.
2. *Schizophrenia catatonic.* Usually, the client exhibits one or more of the symptoms of catatonic rigidity, stupor, mutism, negativism, posturing, or excitement.
3. *Schizophrenia paranoid.* The client is preoccupied with delusions of persecution, delusions of grandeur, ideas of reference, or hallucinations that involve persecutory or grandiose material.
4. *Schizophrenia undifferentiated.* The client evidences psychotic symptoms such as hallucina-

tions and delusions, but either does not meet the criteria of one of the subtypes or meets the criteria of more than one subtype.
5. *Schizophrenia residual.* The client, at one time in the past, exhibited the psychotic symptoms of schizophrenia, but is not psychotic at present. The client may still show signs of some emotional disturbance, such as withdrawal from others or flat affect.[1]

When a client is diagnosed as having a schizophrenic disorder, it is also noted whether the course of the disturbance is *chronic* (with or without an acute exacerbation of symptoms), *subchronic* (with or without an acute exacerbation of symptoms), or *in remission.*

Another approach to the classification of schizophrenia is based on prognosis.[43] *Reactive schizophrenia,* which carries the expectation of a positive treatment outcome, refers to a disorder with a rapid onset and a relatively satisfactory level of functioning before the breakdown. *Nuclear* or *process schizophrenia,* on the other hand, has a gradual onset, and is seen in persons with a socially inadequate premorbid personality. The expected treatment outcome in nuclear schizophrenia is less positive than in reactive schizophrenia.

Application of the Nursing Process to the Client with a Schizophrenic Disorder

In this section of the chapter, the steps of the nursing process—assessment, nursing diagnosis, planning, intervention, and evaluation—are applied to the client who exhibits behaviors exemplifying retreat from reality and to the client's family.

Assessment

Nursing assessment and diagnosis of the client with a schizophrenic disorder are complex processes. Chapter 7 offers general guidelines for providing the nurse with a base of information about the client. This foundation of client data, identified problems, and nursing diagnoses serves as a source of information from which treatment goals and interventions are derived. Specific nursing approaches, such as openness, honesty, cultural appreciation, and acceptance of the unique properties of the individual are essential to any comprehensive assessment.

The nursing assessment and analysis of the client who exhibits behaviors of the schizophrenic disorders are presented by addressing the following major areas:

1. Disturbances of thinking
2. Disturbances of feeling
3. Social/behavioral disturbances

Disturbances of Thinking

One of the classical signs of schizophrenia, said Eugen Bleuler, is an *associative disorder*. This disturbance in thinking has generally been considered the primary characteristic of schizophrenia. The client gives evidence of his "loose associations" or disconnectedness of thought through his verbal patterns. Because a person's speech is the only means through which one person can understand another person's thought, the nurse must be attuned to the client's communication.

Listening to the client's speech, the nurse may soon realize that his thoughts are not leading logically to the next ones. Instead, the thinking is chaotic, disorganized, and confusing. The listener feels ill at ease, unable to comprehend what is being said, and unable to take part in the conversation. At times when the client becomes more anxious, his thinking (and, likewise, his speech) becomes increasingly illogical. The uncomfortable feeling experienced by the nurse who is trying to establish communication with this client is very difficult to describe; it is, however, a readily identifiable and diagnostically important feeling once it has been experienced.

Evidence of *magical thinking* is seen in the client who believes that his thoughts or wishes can control other people or events. This form of primary process thinking can be observed as part of the normal development of the preschool child, as suggested by the familiar sight of a child skipping down the sidewalk and chanting, "Step on a crack, break your mother's back." Its presence in an adult, however, who believes that he can manipulate the actions of others through "mind control" is neither acceptable nor appropriate behavior in our society.

A schizophrenic client may have minimal or seemingly no awareness of his environment. He may wander as though he were in foreign surroundings or appear to be in a dream world. An important safety-related factor is the client's lack of regard for his own well-being. He may step in the path of oncoming traffic or perform other potentially dangerous acts, while giving the impression that he does not grasp the obvious danger.

The client may also experience feelings of *depersonalization,* wherein he feels that his body belongs to another person or that he is somehow removed from his body. He may believe that his spirit is hovering above his body and watching its movements and behavior with detachment.

The client may attempt to communicate with others through the use of *symbolism.* Again, his symbolic words and actions can be viewed as a part of his disordered thinking. Language may be private and idiosyncratic. The client may create new words, called *neologisms,* which have meaning and purpose to him alone. *Cryptic language* refers to the client speaking in an abbreviated fashion; that is, he may speak aloud only every fourth, or sixth, or tenth word of his thoughts.

Illusions may be another sign of the client's thought disorder. An *illusion* is a misinterpretation of a real sensory experience. An example of an illusion is the experience of seeing a shadow in the room when awakening in the middle of the night and immediately concluding that a robber has broken into the house. Schizophrenic clients are often disturbed and frightened by illusions.

A *delusion* is a fixed, false belief of the client's that cannot be corrected by reasoning with him. The client with paranoid schizophrenia generally has *delusions of persecution* (*i.e.,* that others are planning to harm him in some fashion, that there is a conspiracy to follow him at all times and "bug" his telephone, that creatures from other planets are controlling his mind, and so forth) or *delusions of grandeur* (*i.e.,* that he is Jesus Christ, the Virgin Mary, Napoleon, or some other important, famous, or historically significant personage [see Chart 24-2]).

These words of a client with schizophrenia are an example of a delusion of grandeur:

> I felt that I had power to determine the weather, which responded to my inner moods, and even to control the movement of the sun in relation to other astronomical bodies.[57]

To identify the presence of a delusion, the nurse must first understand the beliefs characteristic of a culture, because a delusion is a belief that is not in keeping with the beliefs accepted by a person's culture. For example, in the United States, we would term it delusional for a person to believe that semen could wander up into a man's head and cause his brain to deteriorate, and yet that belief is culturally acceptable in parts of India.[47]

A *hallucination* is a false sensory perception, (*i.e.,* without external stimulus) or a sensory perception that does not exist in reality, such as seeing "visions" or hearing "voices" (see Chart 24-3).

A client may "hear" the voice of God, the devil, or a close relative. The voice is frequently one that berates or condemns him for his past and present evils. *Auditory hallucinations* are the most common form of hallucinations; *visual hallucinations* are the second most common. Visual hallucinations are likely to be threatening, frightening monsters or scenes. Although hallucinations involving the other senses (gus-

CHART 24-2
Therapeutic Dialogue

Gathering Information About the Client's Perceptions

Nurse: (seated at table near client, looking directly at her) You were telling me, Mrs. D., about how you came to this hospital.

Client: I know why I came here. (throws her head back, stiffens her neck, and grips the arms of her chair) I have a calling.

Nurse: A calling? What kind of a calling?

Client: To help my friends. (expansive, sweeping gesture of her hand toward the others in the room)

Nurse: Who do you think called you, Mrs. D.? (questioning tone of voice, maintaining eye contact)

Client: (winks one eye and hunches forward as though sharing a secret) The Master Doctor, the Big Physician.

Nurse: Do you mean God? (straightforward, inquiring facial expression and voice)

Client: Of course, I mean God. (impatient tone of voice, frowning, stands up and shouts) Who else would I mean?

Discussion

Often the nurse wishes to gather information regarding the client's perception of the reason for, and events surrounding, admission to the psychiatric unit. At times, the client's perception is at odds with the reality-based facts of the situation.

Mrs. D. believes that she has been chosen as a special person and received this "calling" to come into the hospital to help other people.

The nurse, in interacting with Mrs. D., is asking her for clarification about this "calling," which the client believes has come from God.

The nurse neither agrees nor disagrees with Mrs. D. about the truth of her beliefs. Such agreement or attempts to disprove her beliefs usually serves to reinforce or strengthen the delusional material of the client. Instead, the nurse proceeds to gather information in a nonthreatening, supportive manner and to communicate acceptance of Mrs. D. as a valuable human being. A subsequent nursing goal will focus on the clarification of reality with the client.

tatory, tactile, olfactory) do occur, they are less common.

In American society today, there are probably only a few small religious groups that sanction hallucinations. Nevertheless, hallucinations that are not part of a psychiatric disorder may be acceptable phenomena in other societies.[47] A question that must be asked is whether the hallucination is appropriate or even expected within the cultural framework. For example, a person's role in society (*e.g.,* a medicine man or an artist) may necessitate or utilize some of the symptoms that appear to be schizophrenic in nature.

Disturbances of Feeling

The term *affect* refers to one's mood or feeling tone. Frequently, in schizophrenic disorders, there is a marked absence of affect or there is flat, blunted, or inappropriate affect. The client's apparent lack of emotional expression may cause the nurse to feel as if she is trying to communicate with a machine or inanimate object. The individual's affect may also seem inappropriate in relation to the conversation or the context of the situation (*e.g.,* the client who laughs and smiles in response to hearing some piece of sad news).

The client's apathy may increase the nurse's sense of frustration. This seeming absence of caring

Hallucinations and Delusions: How Do They Develop?

A well-known theorist and writer about schizophrenia, Silvano Arieti, has proposed that hallucinatory voices occur only in particular situations; that is, when the client expects to hear them. The client, for example, perceives hostility around him, expects to hear the neighbors talking about him, puts himself into a "listening" attitude, and then experiences the hallucination (he hears them talking about him).

Another example of this phenomenon occurs in ideas of reference. The client thinks that people are laughing at him, hears laughing and giggling, and looks at people and sees them smiling. They may not be smiling, but he may have misinterpreted their facial expressions. Or, if they are smiling, it may be for reasons that have nothing to do with the client.

The goal, says Arieti, in treating this client is to help him recognize that he sees or hears people laughing at him when he expects to. Next comes the recognition that he feels people *should* laugh at him because he is a "laughable" individual. He hears laughing, in fact, because he thinks people should laugh at him; that is, "what he thinks of himself has become the cause of his symptom."

The return to reality is slow because the client's reality is sad and worsened by his vulnerability. Therapists must be careful to promote the client's return by improving his reality. Eventually, the client moves toward mastery of his own situation, no longer the victim of external forces.

about himself or his situation may depress and anger the nurse who believes that the client must first want to improve before he will begin to make therapeutic gains. Once again, the nurse must examine the client's affective state in relation to his cultural context.

A client exhibiting inappropriate affect used these words to explain his experience:

> Half the time I am talking about one thing and thinking about half a dozen other things at the same time. It must look queer to people when I laugh about something that has got nothing to do

with what I am talking about, but they don't know what's going on inside and how much of it is running around in my head.[57]

Social/Behavioral Disturbances

The client with a schizophrenic disorder retreats from the reality of interpersonal contact. He appears aloof, uninterested in others, and content with his own inner fantasies.

His communication is either lacking or directed toward private, idiosyncratic goals. Rather than using language and nonverbal communication to establish rapport with other persons and to derive pleasure from those relationships, the schizophrenic client uses his communicative efforts as a means of self-stimulation or reinforcement of his preoccupying fantasies.

A pronounced fear of others and of himself prevents the schizophrenic client from making contact or responding to the social overtures of others. It is probable that he fears harm from other people or fears that he may not be able to control his own impulses and may, therefore, bring harm to others.

Impulsive, bizarre, or otherwise uninhibited behavior, such as masturbation in public, gesturing, or posturing, may also be signs of the behavioral disturbances of schizophrenia.

The client may show signs of extreme dependency or helplessness. This behavior is often repulsive to individuals who value independence and assertiveness and may elicit anger and frustration in even the most conscientious and self-aware mental health professionals.

The client with schizophrenia may have concerns about his sexual identity. Although little research has been conducted on this topic, a change in sexual behavior has been noted during periods of psychotic decompensation.[58] The schizophrenic client's inadequate social skills, withdrawal, and isolation contribute to his lack of sexual partners. In psychiatric hospitals, where sexual activities are generally discouraged or prohibited, chronic schizophrenic clients encounter medical, social, and cultural obstacles to their sexual expression.[58]

Assessment of the client's ability to perform his own self-care and activities of daily living, to function in his work setting, and to respond appropriately to his own physical needs are critical issues for the psychiatric–mental health nurse. At times, a client may be so removed from contact with reality that he is unaware of his body's need for food, water, and rest.

The client's role in his family and community and the availability and responsiveness of his support system are important variables in the assessment process. His eventual level of adaptation may be strongly influenced by the presence of supportive, caring significant others. The absence of a support system, on the other hand, may reinforce a lifetime of failure and rejection and may offer the client little hope for a satisfying future.

The nurse needs to assess the client's *relationships with the significant figures* in his life. From these observations and objective descriptions of family and community interactional patterns, the nurse will later formulate treatment goals and interventions for and with the client and the people who are important to him.

Positive and Negative Symptoms

There is, obviously, a broad range of symptoms of schizophrenia. To bring some coherence and usefulness out of these symptoms, investigators have begun to divide them into two major groups—positive and negative symptoms. The *positive* or *florid symptoms* tend to represent a distortion or exaggeration of normal functions; these include hallucinations, delusions, and abnormalities in language and behavior. *Negative* or *defect symptoms* represent a diminution or loss of function; these include poverty of speech and content of speech, affective blunting, and asociality-anhedonia. It has been suggested that positive symptoms may occur more frequently early in the course of the disorder and negative symptoms during the later stages of the disorder. Furthermore, once they occur, negative symptoms tend to persist. Some recent evidence suggests that negative symptoms respond less well to neuroleptic treatment than do positive symptoms.[2]

Other Unique Characteristics

In addition to these general factors that the nursing assessment of a client with a schizophrenic disorder must address, multiple variations in behaviors will also be observed by the astute and perceptive nurse. No symptom picture that is characteristic of a psychiatric disturbance is ever the same in two individual clients. Because every person is different and has unique distinguishing characteristics, he will never appear "just like all the others"—whether he is emotionally disturbed or healthy and adapting. Individualization and objectivity are key words in any nursing assessment and analysis.

Nursing Diagnosis

The formulation of nursing diagnosis is an essential component of the nursing process. The nurse analyzes the assessment data gathered during the first step of the nursing process to arrive at client/family problems and diagnoses. Many accepted nursing diagnoses are appropriate to guide the planning and implementation of nursing care of the client with schizophrenia. Some possible nursing diagnoses of the schizophrenic client and his family include the following:

Sensory-perceptual alteration: auditory/visual related to withdrawal into the self, panic level of anxiety; evidenced by poor concentration, rapid mood swings, disordered thought sequencing, and inappropriate responses.

Alteration in thought processes related to low self-esteem, repressed fears, inability to trust, possible hereditary factor, panic level of anxiety; evidenced by hypervigilance, altered attention span, distractibility, inability to concentrate, commands, obsessions, and impaired ability to make decisions, problem-solve, reason, calculate, abstract, or conceptualize

Social isolation related to weak ego development, lack of trust, regression to earlier level of development, delusional thinking; evidenced by sad, dull affect, inappropriate or immature interests and activities for developmental age or stage, preoccupation with own thoughts, repetitive and meaningless actions, isolating behavior

Potential for violence: self-directed or directed at others related to catatonic excitement, hallucinatory commands, panic level of anxiety, rage reaction; evidenced by increased pacing, overt and aggressive acts, goal-directed destruction of objects in the environment, self-destructive behavior and/or active, aggressive suicidal acts, hostile, threatening verbalizations, increased motor activity, excitement, agitation, and irritability

Impaired verbal communication related to disordered, unrealistic thinking, regression, withdrawal, panic level of anxiety; evidenced by loose association of ideas, use of slang association, word salad, neologisms, and echolalia, verbalizations reflecting concrete thinking, and poor eye contact

Self-care deficit related to perceptual or cognitive impairment, withdrawal; evidenced by impaired ability to perform hygiene tasks, dressing, grooming, maintaining appearance at satisfactory level, toileting, and eating

Alteration in family process related to presence of long-term mental illness in family member and evidenced by alteration in family's goals and plans, social activities, and daily activities according to the mentally disordered individual member[56]

Planning

Preparation of the client's treatment plans is best approached as a collaborative effort of the mental health team, which includes the client and his family. Flexibility and creativity are essential ingredients in the continuous process of planning, evaluation, and replanning of therapeutic efforts. No single treatment modality will effect the desired behavioral changes for all clients.

Although preoccupation with fantasies, poor reality contact, and symbolic forms of communication are characteristic of schizophrenia, each client exhibits specific disturbances that require individualized nursing approaches. Some psychiatric inpatient facilities may prepare standardized nursing care plans or treatment plans that offer general principles of care; these standard plans then require individualization in nursing diagnoses, specific client outcomes, and interventions for the client.

Goal-Setting

The major goals for the schizophrenic client include the following:

1. Promotion of trust
2. Establishment of a nonthreatening environment for the client
3. Encouragement of satisfactory social interaction
4. Increase of the client's self-esteem
5. Validation of the client's perceptions
6. Clarification and reinforcement of reality
7. Promotion of physical safety
8. Encouragement of independent behavior
9. Attention to the client's physical needs
10. Reduction of anxiety and psychotic symptoms through chemotherapeutic agents
11. Coordination of therapy with the client's family or significant others

Discharge Plans

Discharge planning begins at the time of the client's admission to the psychiatric inpatient unit. Many schizophrenic clients suffer not only the long-term effects of their disorder, but also "the Rip Van Winkle syndrome"; that is, they awaken from a long sleep to find a world with changed technologies, cultural values, and economics.[43] It is a frightening world for discharged clients who may cling tenaciously to the hospital environment.

An adequate discharge program needs to foster social skills, work/job skills, self-confidence in dealing with problems, and involvement in the outside community.[43] For example, before discharge from a psychiatric facility, the long-term client must learn, practice, and be tested in the basic, practical aspects of daily living, such as how to ride a bus, shop for groceries, apply for a job, cook a meal, and take his own medication. (See Chap. 40, "Community Support and Rehabilitation.")

Community involvement before discharge means that the client should be familiar with his future landlord and employer. These people, after all, are the individuals who will play a significant role in his adjustment to life outside the hospital as opposed to his readmission to a psychiatric facility. Employers and landlords must know the discharged client as a person and must realize that he needs direct and constructive feedback. He is not a fragile or helpless person and should not be treated as such. A 24-hour, 7-days-per-week, crisis telephone line to the client's former psychiatric–mental health care providers also helps smooth his discharge to his family and community.

Intervention

Certain personal characteristics are considered necessary when working therapeutically with a schizophrenic client. The mental health professional needs to be straightforward, simple, and accepting, and must hold unconditional regard for the dignity of another human being—even when that person is severely withdrawn and regressed.[6] This mandate includes, for example, demonstrating respect for the client's desire for silence, so that the nonverbal communication becomes a shared experience.

Influencing the Client's Disturbances of Thinking

Deciphering Meaning. When confronted with the client's symbolic words, actions, or other examples of his disordered thinking, the nurse remembers that, although his behavior may seem at times almost impossible to understand, it does have meaning to the client. The nurse tries to listen for the themes and search for the hidden meanings in his communication. The client's verbal and nonverbal behaviors cannot be dismissed as senseless or as gibberish.

The client's rhyming communication may also give clues to the nurse about his thoughts and feelings.

> Mary Mary dictionary
> blowing smoking
> not even caring

In these words, the client, Mary, conveys to the nurse several possible routes to explore. Is she feeling apathetic ("not even caring")? Angry ("blowing" or "smoking")? Is there a meaning to "Mary dictionary"? The nurse listens to these unusual forms of communication and attempts to decode the communication and determine, through validation, what meanings they hold for the client.

Reinforcing Reality. Much of the nurse's focus in working with the schizophrenic client will be centered on helping him to clarify reality and validate his perceptions. This is accomplished both by describing a real event or circumstance to the client and by involving the client in conversations or activities that focus on the here-and-now.

When dealing with the client with feelings of depersonalization, the nurse will need to state what she sees as a real fact (*e.g.*, that one part of his body is not dead, or that he has not become an inanimate object, and so forth) but will also need to avoid getting involved in an argument with the client. No one can argue away feelings of depersonalization or hallucinations or any other disturbances in reality-testing. Nevertheless, psychiatric–mental health professionals are responsible for stating the facts, as they see them, to the client in a manner that is simple, concise, and nonthreatening.

While she is stating these facts, the nurse also attempts to bring the client back into contact with reality by involving him in some reality-oriented activity. Perhaps the nurse could talk with the client about a picture in a magazine and attempt to interest him in this concrete topic. Perhaps involving the client in a physical activity, such as taking a walk and conversing about the objects he sees while walking, will be therapeutic for him. These are both reality-oriented activities that the nurse may employ in day-to-day contact with persons who have withdrawn from reality.

When the client is overcome with the idea that he is living in an unreal environment, he should not be left alone for long periods of time. Staying with the client is an essential step in reinforcing reality because the nurse signifies a major link with the real world for the client. Allowing the client to remain isolated only encourages him to become more involved or preoccupied with his fantasies. Again, the nurse's engagement of the client in reality-oriented activities and conversations is a helpful intervention.

Promoting Clarification. The client who has a confused sense of identity will require much clarification from the nurse. In conversations, the nurse must help the client realize what he said or did as distinct from what others said or did. When ambiguous and confusing topics arise, the nurse must stop the conversation and request clarification from the client. Because the client will often hide behind a "you know what I mean . . .," the nurse must not assume that she does know what the client means unless she has first asked for clarification. Finding out directly from the client is the only sure way to understand the message he is conveying.

The schizophrenic client's loose associations are extremely difficult to understand. Pretending to understand his line of thought only widens the gap between client and nurse. The most helpful approach to what may seem incoherent ramblings is to ask clarifying questions. Perhaps the nurse may also determine a recurrent idea or theme in the speech and further pursue its meaning for the client. The nurse and other psychiatric–mental health caregivers act as healthy role models for the client by communicating with him in a clear and concise manner.

Intervening in Hallucinations. The client who is hallucinating is one who is preoccupied and frightened; leaving him alone only deepens his preoccupation and fear. The nurse's very presence is a reassuring force that helps calm his fears. It is crucial for the nurse to remember that the hallucination is real to the client. When working with the hallucinating client, the nurse communicates to him concern that he is upset or bothered by the things he hears or sees.

At the same time, the nurse makes it clear to the client that she does not see or hear the hallucinations that he is describing. It is critical to know that the nurse never agrees with him about hearing the "voices" or any hallucinatory experience. Because it is the mental health professional's function to serve as the healthy role model for the client, the nurse cannot reinforce his retreat from reality through hallucinations or delusions. Neither is it beneficial to argue about whether or not the hallucination or delusion is real. Rather than engage in activities that strengthen the client's withdrawal, the nurse encourages the client to regain his contact with reality by gently directing him into conversation or activities focused on the here-and-now (see Chart 24-4).

It has been suggested that the "voices" appear in specific situations, when the client expects to hear them. This expectation causes him to develop a "listening attitude," especially in times of stress.[6] The nurse may help the client actively fight the hallucination, first by discovering the relation between his feelings (anxiety) and the "listening attitude," and second by disrupting the process of falling into the next stage of experiencing the "voices." The nurse administers antipsychotic medication, discussed later in this chapter, to interrupt the client's hallucinatory experience.

C H A R T   24-4
Therapeutic Dialogue

Dealing with Hallucinations

Nurse: What has been troubling you, Jeff? (sitting with the client, trying to establish eye contact)

Client: I hear voices. (looking down at the floor, shoulders hunched forward) They are punishing me and want me to repent.

Nurse: Do you want to share with me your thoughts on what you believe you heard? (leaning toward client, arms and hands open and resting on lap)

Client: (sitting very quietly, brow furrowed, staring at his hands) There were two men—one was 62 and one was 42. The 42-year-old was good. His face was in stone on the floor. When you went by, he went into your mind. It was like a strong wind. (pauses, looks at the nurse's face) You really don't want to hear this.

Nurse: (softly, maintaining eye contact) You don't think I want to hear about these "voices," Jeff?

Client: Two weeks after I was discharged from this hospital, I was walking down this road—the voices started, then the wind telling me to kill myself for my repentance. (stands up, begins to pace back and forth in front of the couch, his eyes cast downward)

Nurse: (still seated, looking up at the client as he paces) Do the wind and noises bother you a lot, Jeff?

Client: Yes, and it's always at six o'clock. (walks away from the nurse)

Discussion

Communicating verbally and nonverbally with the client who experiences hallucinations requires skilled use of therapeutic techniques.

Jeff is open in expressing the torment he is experiencing from the punishing "voices." Many clients lack the trust, reality contact, or verbal skills needed to share these hallucinatory events with psychiatric-mental health care providers.

The nurse verbalizes concern for Jeff and offers him the opportunity either to share or withhold information about "what he believes he hears." In discussing hallucinatory material, the nurse demonstrates acceptance of the client's hallucination as a "real" event to him. At the same time, the nurse neither agrees with the client nor tries to dissuade him or convince him that the "voices" are not really occurring. For the client, we must assume, the "voices" are present, and they are likely to be a source of anxiety, fear, and agitation for him.

A strong theme of guilt/repentance/punishment is evident in Jeff's conversation. The nurse has not yet begun to explore the sources of these feelings of worthlessness nor the possible ways to intervene with Jeff to reduce his unpleasant, and perhaps unbearable, feelings.

This interaction represents one aspect of the process of establishing trust and building rapport with the client.

2

Interrupting the Client's Disturbances of Feeling

Role Modeling. The nurse models appropriateness of affect by displaying a somber facial expression when discussing a serious topic or a joyful expression when engaging in a happy or pleasant topic of conversation. Using body language to convey a mood appropriate to the thought is one aspect of the nurse's repertoire of communication skills.

Developing Tolerance. Bizarre or inappropriate behavior or affect of the client must not be reinforced by nurses' smiles, nods, anger, or laughter. Although they need to demonstrate tolerance of the client's behavior, nurses and other mental health caregivers may, at times, feel disgust or amusement. It is often difficult to admit negative feelings to oneself, especially while trying hard to become therapeutic. Nevertheless, the therapeutic self is primarily a person of honesty, and any insights about one's feelings must be acknowledged openly before they can be faced. It is particularly important to deal honestly with feelings because the schizophrenic client has often learned from his family and culture to discount his own feelings. During interactions with psychiatric–mental health staff, the client may communicate that he perceives certain feelings as "dangerous." Feelings must be examined in a supportive, open environment.

3 Diminishing the Client's Social/Behavioral Disturbances

Developing Trust. The development of a trusting relationship is basic to nursing care approaches to the schizophrenic client. It is essential that nurses and other psychiatric–mental health professionals show interest in, and acceptance of, the total person who is the client. Although this goal is partly accomplished by means of the nurse's words, it is also heavily influenced by nonverbal behavior. The nurse's nonjudgmental attitude and genuineness cannot be manufactured. A genuine desire to offer assistance will be perceived accurately by the client and he will begin to view the nurse as a person who is helpful and sincere.

Through the nurse's body language, facial expression, eye contact, tone of voice, and verbalizations, the client receives messages about the nurse's trustworthiness. The client, in turn, responds to these messages. It is likely that because the schizophrenic client's past interpersonal experiences have been unsuccessful or unsatisfying, he is unwilling to take risks in his encounters with another person.

Therefore, the client's response to a nurse, even if the nurse is warm, open, and genuine, may be reticent. Establishing rapport with the client, although it is essential, will not be easy. It is hoped that gradually, as a result of continued, consistent, and pleasant interpersonal experiences, his level of trust in another person will increase. The nurse slowly breaks through his wall of isolation and assumes more and more significance for him. At this point the nurse can begin to introduce other people into his experiences. Hopefully, the client will transfer some of his trust in the nurse to another, second person, and then to a third person, and so on, until he has learned meaningful ways to interact with a larger sphere of people. If the initial interpersonal contact with the nurse is pleasant and rewarding to the client, he will be more inclined to risk opening himself to others.

On the other hand, if the nurse does not regard the client positively, fears him, or finds him repulsive or hopeless, this attitude will also be sensed by him. Sometimes, the client's perceptions are so painfully acute that he will overtly respond to whatever he senses in the other person; he will respond to the "vibes" he receives from the other person. The nurse in this situation may be saying all the correct words but will not establish a therapeutic rapport if sincerity is lacking. In fact, if one had to choose whether the actual words used by the intervener or the nonverbal behavior were the more important factor in dealing with the psychiatric client, nonverbal communication would probably be judged more influential in conveying empathy toward the client. The goal, of course, is to combine both verbal and nonverbal communication skills in order to deal effectively and therapeutically with clients.

Approaching the Client. Because the client tends to withdraw from others, the nurse needs to make the initial approach to the client. Waiting for him to make the first contact is fruitless because he often lacks the self-confidence necessary to initiate contact with another person. Remembering that the client is likely frightened of others, the nurse approaches him in a nonthreatening way. The nurse is encouraged to sit near him (but not crowding him or impinging on his personal space, because he may fear harm from close contact with others), and to speak in a soothing voice. Both of these approaches demonstrate to the client that the nurse is interested in him but willing to advance slowly and respond to his cues.

The close interpersonal relationship that develops in the therapeutic environment is, for the client, a new kind of close relationship. Other people, the client learns, can care for him, not just take care of him.[5]

Encouraging Independence. Encouraging the client's self-help skills and rewarding or reinforcing his participation in activities of daily living will help promote independent behavior. The client may need the opportunity to make simple decisions and experience small successes over a period of time. As the client is able to tolerate and accept more responsibility, he is given these opportunities in a progressive fashion.

Dealing with Hostility. The problem of dealing with the client's hostility may be of significance, because the nature of the close therapeutic relationship may engender angry outbursts from the client. It is probably the intensity of the closeness and the fear of rejection that prompt the client to reject the mental health professional. Hostility, on the other hand, may be disguised and evidenced as extreme passivity, testing behaviors, or projection.[5]

It is critical that the nurse avoid overwhelming the client with too much talk or too much closeness. Although touch is an important therapeutic technique, it must be used judiciously. Touch can be very frightening to the client if the nurse employs it indiscriminately. For example, the paranoid schizophrenic client who thinks that he can be destroyed by someone's touch will become very agitated if he is touched by psychiatric caregivers. (For a detailed explanation of interventions with the client with paranoid ideas and actions, see Chap. 25.)

4

Approaching the Client's Family

The problems faced by the family of a schizophrenic member are multiple. The schizophrenic client's failure to care for his personal needs, such as taking a bath, his inability to handle money, his social withdrawal, strange personal habits, suicide threats, interference with the family's work, school, and social schedule, and the family's fear for the safety of both the schizophrenic and other family members are all genuine and realistic concerns.[57] The family's physical and psychological resources often deteriorate to the point that the individual member's well-being and the stability and organization of the family are threatened.[45] The National Alliance for the Mentally Ill (NAMI) and other consumer advocacy groups have sprouted around the country in response to the family's need to be involved and to function collaboratively in the treatment of the mentally ill family member.[40] An example of one family's distress in helping their son with schizophrenia is found in Chart 24-5, "A Family's View of Chronic Mental Illness."[11]

Denial of the client's feelings has often been learned from, and reinforced by, the client's family. Any therapeutic work with the client who is withdrawn from reality must also be implemented with the client's family. Supportive measures must be employed to enlarge the client's and the family's social sphere, to raise their level of interpersonal functioning, and to increase their ability to become aware of feelings and learn to handle them effectively (see Case Study 24-1, at the end of this chapter). A significant degree of the success of any treatment plan depends on the mental health team's ability to effect change in the client together with his family and significant others, not as a separate entity.

Couples therapy groups for married schizophrenic clients or parents groups for the parents of young, unmarried schizophrenic clients offer problem-solving skills and provide outside contacts for the family members. Often, the discharged client will return not to his home but to a group home or some alternative living arrangement. Plans for this move to a new living situation need to be examined and worked out in detail long before the client is ready to leave the psychiatric facility.

Psychoeducation

As a result of deinstitutionalization of psychiatric clients from inpatient treatment facilities, the burden of providing community care has fallen increasingly on the shoulders of the clients' families. Current approaches to family psychoeducational intervention

may be based on a crisis intervention model, ongoing relatives' group, survival skills for relatives and ongoing family therapy, or a family behavioral model. These programs, which demonstrate effectiveness in ameliorating some symptoms of schizophrenia, incorporate the exploration of families' reactions to the mental illness of a member and provide them with information on schizophrenia.[45] In a longitudinal study, it was found that a family management approach to the schizophrenic client was superior to an individual approach of similar intensity and that the effectiveness of the approach was sustained over 2 years.[24]

An optimal approach to the client's family is to view the family not as a source of pathology but as a means of restoration to health.[7] Psychiatric–mental health professionals work with family members to help them add understanding to their personal concern, to explore the client's areas of particular vulnerability, and to learn to clarify the client's communications. The goal is to reintegrate the client into his family whenever possible.

Important Therapies

Individual Psychotherapy. The client with a schizophrenic disorder experiences difficulty relating to others and these difficulties with others are reflected in behaviors such as anxiety in interpersonal contacts, mistrust, fear, and misinterpretation of others' behavior. The therapist tries to counteract the client's anxiety, offer warmth and reassurance, and remove the fear "almost automatically aroused by interpersonal contact."[7] The client and therapist must first learn to know, trust, and not be afraid of each other.

The principles of psychotherapy of the schizophrenic client are as follows:

1. Stimulate very little or create no anxiety, and diminish the anxiety already present in the client
2. Prevent the client from returning to his premorbid (prepsychotic) state, which would promote continued vulnerability for psychosis
3. Achieve and maintain a state of "delicate balance" prior to the client's independence from treatment, because of his continued poor tolerance for frustration, discomfort, and anxiety
4. Employ a therapeutic approach by which the client moves toward gradual and progressive self-acceptance[7]

Therapists who have proved to be very successful individual psychotherapists with schizophrenic clients demonstrate certain process and personal attri-

C H A R T   24-5

A Family's View of Chronic Mental Illness

Herbert J. Barr, President
Alliance for the Mentally Ill–Los Angeles
Los Angeles, California

The nightmare started as we were preparing for the holidays. A telephone call from out-of-state said, "Come pick up your son." We had no idea what was to come or how it would affect our lives.

Our son had been off at college. He had been on the Dean's List, had 4 years of undergraduate studies, and was pursuing a degree in Pharmacology. What we found was a sick, withdrawn, almost catatonic son, who was eventually diagnosed as schizophrenic, sometimes paranoid, sometimes with depression, and at times suicidal.

At first, he required acute care in the county mental health system. He improved to the point of being warehoused in a board-and-care facility. He continued to improve and was able to get a job with an understanding large aerospace company. He lived independently in his own apartment. But this didn't last very long. He decompensated and went through several cycles: the need for acute care, stabilization, and again the need for acute care. He has recently progressed from a skilled nursing facility to a transitional living facility where he is learning to live more independently. We hope that he will progress to a satellite apartment, with the possibility that he may become capable of performing nonstressful productive vocational activities, and that he will achieve an improved quality of life.

What have we learned? Our son is ill. His illness is probably not due to any one of many stressful and traumatic childhood or growing-up experiences. The stresses he had may not have affected others, but for him, they were too much. We now know that he was probably vulnerable to the illness due to genetic/biochemical/biologic factors that are showing up in research. Stress will provoke or exacerbate the attacks, or crises. Safe, commonplace things that we take for granted—decision-making, meeting new people, dealing with problems and disappointments—are crisis-inducing experiences for those who are sensitive to stress and cannot cope in a stressful environment.

What are our frustrations? The foremost is that he may never achieve a reasonable level of happiness and the enjoyment of life that everyone strives for and that parents universally hope for for their children. Next is the frustration that there is not enough research to help the professionals learn how to diagnose, treat, cure, or prevent these chronic mental illnesses, primarily schizophrenia and the affective disorders. DSM-III-R is still a crude shotgun when aimed at understanding the subtleties of brain disorders. Next is the lack of an effective public mental illness care system. The present system's modality is governed by a shortage of tax dollars, inadequate and inhumane legal criteria for involuntary treatment, and lack of community based, low-cost housing for those who do not require expensive full-time care in state mental hospitals. And, finally, the frustration that hurts the most—because it is solvable through education and understanding of professional caregivers—stigma.

In the 1950s, theories were proposed that serious mental illnesses were caused by double-bind communication and/or bad parenting. Throughout the history of these serious illnesses, this concept had not surfaced. Witchcraft and other religious reasons had been cited, yes, but not bad parenting. Today, the originators of that theory and modern researchers have repudiated the theory, but the stigma lingers on—primarily in older texts from the 1950s and in practitioners trained in that period.

The consequence of that lingering stigma is that if you believe it, you prejudge the parents as a malevolent influence. You will not want to involve them in the treatment. They are blamed and shut out. Stigma also says that a mentally ill person is somehow "bad" and only needs to "shape up." The political and societal consequence of stigma is not wanting to fund and care for those who are seriously mentally ill. State mental hospitals were almost emptied in the 1960s, with no provisions for local community care and housing; the present homeless population, many of whom are chronically mentally ill, is an outgrowth of that stigma.

Modern teaching and education are slowly but surely correcting the problem of stigma, but treatment and long-term housing for the chronically mentally ill are dismally poor.

One of the best things that has happened to us, as a family with an ill member, is hearing about the Alliance for the Mentally Ill (AMI). It is a family support group organized to help family members understand and cope with the chronic mental illnesses and advocate for more research and better care and housing. AMI has affiliates in many communities. Families can write to the National Alliance for the Mentally Ill, 1901 No. Fort Myer Drive, Suite 500, Arlington, VA 22209-1604, for information.

It was only after we became active in AMI that we began to understand the illness and how better to help our son. At first, caregivers would not talk to us, but this situation is now improving. Many now speak at our AMI meetings, and they talk to us as caring parents. AMI also helps the caregivers through advocacy efforts and fund-raising for research. We also became appreciative of the fact that, in our family, we were being spared the heartache and grief of other families in which the mental illness was more severe, perhaps complicated with concurrent substance abuse or involvement in the criminal justice system. It is difficult enough to know that your family member has a serious mental illness, but when there is also involvement with alcohol or drugs, the problems are much more severe and there are very few, if any, provisions for concurrent treatment. This is only one hole in the care system. Likewise, it is very painful to see a mentally ill family member, in a marginally acute state and very vulnerable, thrown in jail with criminally inclined people.

As family members who care about our ill one, we are advocating more appropriate legislation that will guarantee mentally ill persons the treatment they need, rather than allowing them to remain homeless and live on the streets, with all the horrors that involves. And, finally, because too many families have been denied any and all information by many government agencies and medical practitioners regarding the location, condition, or medication of an ill family member, we are advocating that the laws of confidentiality, although reasonable for persons capable of informed consent, be modified for persons that are too ill to make judgments about their own health and welfare.

With approximately one-third of schizophrenics recovering to a normal life with or without treatment, and one-third requiring institutionalization, the remaining one-third of the population present a serious issue to the family and to the patient. Should the ill family member stay at home with the family or seek care as an independent adult? Parents receive mixed signals from professionals. We are chastised by some for not keeping our ill family member at home, but we are advised by others that it is best for the ill family member to develop his or her own coping skills as an individual and as an adult. Many families opt to keep their ill one at home, at great emotional and physical cost to both the ill person and the rest of the family. Each family has to decide for itself. Our family would dearly love to see our son stay home in a nice, warm, clean room of his own, but we have made the decision that that could lead to a great shock and upheaval when we are no longer here to take care of him. As parents, we would have failed to prepare him for the fundamental task of taking care of himself. As a result, we will advocate that the public mental health system be improved to the point that it is adequate, humane, and available for all those that are dependent on it. It has to be a public system, because the average family cannot purchase group insurance to cover a lifetime of need, and whatever financial resources the average family possesses will evaporate after a few months or a year of private care. Then what?

We would not be a caring family if we settled for less than what we are doing for our ill family member. We need to help the professionals discover better cures—and we need the support and understanding of the caregivers, because it is *our* loved one who is ill.

---

butes. These personal and process variables include the following:

Sense of self-confidence and self-worth
Honesty
Commitment to the client and his welfare
Flexibility and the ability to follow the client's lead
Persistence and hope
Ability to postpone the gratification of feeling professionally competent
Tolerance for uncertainty

Tolerance for madness without becoming frightened or rejecting
Tolerance for error[18]

The important commonalities in different effective psychotherapies may, in fact, be therapists' attitudes and attributes rather than their theoretical beliefs.

Group Therapy. Various forms of group therapy may be employed as a psychosocial form of treatment for psychotic clients in mental health facilities.

Communication with the psychotic person, in group and other kinds of therapies, may be concrete, brief, and direct, or may be psychoanalytically oriented, depending on the therapist's theoretical framework.

Behavior Therapy. In a behavioristic approach, the schizophrenic client is seen as an individual with specific and measurable problems.[42] These problems, it is believed, are treated by certain behavioral interventions, such as positive and negative reinforcement.

Although a tremendous amount has been written about various forms of psychotherapy and psychosocial treatment of clients with schizophrenia, there is very little systematic, controlled research.[36] In part, that is because this kind of research is extremely difficult to conduct. In recent years, we have seen a shift in focus from attempts to alleviate the schizophrenic disorder itself with different forms of psychotherapy to programs designed to improve the client's social adaptation, vocational functioning, and subjective well-being.[36]

Milieu Therapy. Milieu therapy is a team effort whose therapeutic effect for schizophrenic clients is related to the team's abilities to communicate and work together.[8] The psychiatric–mental health staff must feel free to talk about clients, families, events, and their own feelings to prevent a dangerous buildup of anger and frustration. The overall milieu attitude reflects the therapeutic effectiveness of the environment that has been designed for clients. Client or ward government activities may offer opportunities for clients to participate in decision-making relevant to their living situation.

Keeping in mind that the client's judgment may be impaired will alert the nurse to important safety needs. Due to his poor reality contact, the client may place himself in potentially dangerous situations both indoors and out-of-doors. Nursing responsibility dictates that the environment must be safety-oriented and that care providers must attend to the client in a conscientious manner.

If left alone, the client may neglect his basic physical needs. The nurse, therefore, assumes the responsibility for physical health when the client is unable to meet his own needs. The nurse must observe him carefully and frequently for signs of possible illness, physical deprivation, medication reaction, and so on.

Recently, however, it has been suggested that in the inpatient treatment of schizophrenia using psychosocial methods, intense and overstimulating therapies may promote or prolong regression of the client. In fact, the client's long-term adjustment may be negatively affected by this kind of treatment.[21] Schizo-

phrenia's chronicity and the schizophrenic client's vulnerability make it necessary to recommend that inpatient treatment approach him with modest, well-defined goals of therapy, gentle and supportive educational interactions, inclusion of his caregivers and support system in his care, and attention to his long-term adjustment as well as short-term symptom removal.[21]

Pharmacotherapy. The nurse is often called upon to administer psychotropic drugs to the schizophrenic client. Antipsychotic medication will act to decrease extraneous stimuli, thereby strengthening the client's contact with reality. The nurse responsible for administering this medication to the client must be aware of the drug's action, use, usual dosage, route of administration, side effects, contraindications, and nursing implications.

In the past 20 years, psychopharmacology has moved from the status of an adjunct to psychological therapies to the dominant form of treatment for psychiatric disorders. It has been found that the psychotropic drugs are useful in preventing relapse and hospital readmissions for a substantial number of, but not all, psychiatric clients.[17,52] These drugs reduce a wide range of symptoms very effectively, especially over the short term, but they do not maintain effectiveness over some of the symptoms of chronic schizophrenia, such as flattened affect.[52] They do not significantly affect the quality of the client's social or personal adjustment to life outside of the hospital.[17]

Administration of an antipsychotic medication should be a part of a comprehensive treatment program for the client with a psychotic disturbance, not the sole method of treatment. The psychoactive drugs control some of the symptoms of the schizophrenic psychoses, such as withdrawal, aggression, extreme anxiety, hallucinations, and delusions. The client who receives antipsychotic medication is, therefore, more amenable to the various forms of social, recreational, and rehabilitative therapies. The choice of any psychotropic medication depends on its effectiveness and its safety for the individual client. Most schizophrenic clients are helped by antipsychotic medications; some are unaffected and some become worse.[34]

The side effects of antipsychotic medications are distressing and harmful. The watchful nurse consistently observes the client for any of the following side effects of the antipsychotic medications: extrapyramidal effects (including tardive dyskinesia), autonomic effects, metabolic and endocrine effects, hypersensitivity reactions, and sedative effects.[23,34] More serious is the development of neuroleptic malignant syndrome (NMS). (For a thorough review of the actions, side effects, and nursing implications of the antipsychotic medications, see Chap. 17.)

To decrease the incidence of tardive dyskinesia, psychoactive medication is currently being administered in reduced amounts. This reduction in medication is accomplished either through low-dosage treatment or through intermittent or targeted medication treatment.[52] Intermittent medication administration is the episodic, rather than the continuous, use of medication for symptom reduction in some schizophrenic clients who do not need medication continuously. This method of medication administration requires the identification of prodromal symptoms, (*e.g.*, feeling "tense and nervous," or experiencing difficulty sleeping, or decreased enjoyment) and the early resumption of medication before the client becomes so disturbed that he requires hospitalization.

Although antipsychotic medications have a dramatic effect on the majority of individuals with schizophrenia, there remain a number of persons who receive little if any benefit from these drugs. At this point, the clinician may institute therapeutic trials of various combinations or dosages of medications and other treatments.[36] However, few well-controlled studies of these approaches have been conducted that suggest more than occasional benefit.

Intervening with High-Risk Populations

The children of schizophrenic women comprise a population at risk for emotional problems.[29] Often, the children's behavioral deviations are evident by the ages of 1 to 5 years. Families with a psychotic mother or father cope with their life stresses less adequately than families with nonpsychotic parents.

The children of these families are at a greater risk of educational, social, and economic deprivation. The chronic stresses facing these children include the unpredictable behavior of the psychotic parent, a chaotic household, the repeated hospitalizations of the parent, and resulting socioeconomic stress.

Suggestions for intervention with high-risk groups include the following:

1. Continuing help to the children of psychotic parents
2. Teaching the mother and father parenting skills to care for their children
3. Contraceptive information and services[29]

See Chapter 28, "The Emotionally Disturbed Child," for information on preventive programs with the children of schizophrenic parents.

Evaluation

The "success" of any treatment program is measured not only by how many clients are discharged from the program, but also by the availability of community support services and aftercare resources, and by the local community's tolerance of behavioral deviance.[43]

The schizophrenic client who is prepared for discharge needs to know that he will not be abandoned, that he will be helped to succeed in the community, and that the psychiatric–mental health staff are confident in his ability to succeed.

Evaluating the effectiveness of nursing interventions requires a reassessment process to determine what therapeutic results or gains have occurred. Has a specific nursing action had an impact on a specific disturbed behavior of the client? What is the nature of the change in affect, thinking, or social relationships? The evaluation process is a continuous one. By constantly examining changes in the client's behavior, the nurse has the opportunity to decide to strengthen or alter certain aspects of the treatment plan.

Humanistic influences that reflect on the care of the mentally disturbed today include the voiced rights of mental patients, a multidimensional understanding of behavior, respect for the basic worth and dignity of each individual, and community education that promotes acceptance and tolerance of the mentally ill.[43]

Similarly, more humanistic forms of treatment, such as open-door policies and client government, are being employed as the therapeutic modalities of choice. Evaluation of these modalities and their benefit to schizophrenic clients may encourage us to examine and critique the philosophy and practices of our own psychiatric–mental health setting.

The Nurse's Feelings and Attitudes

The nurse's own feelings are an area that deserves, but rarely receives, considerable attention. Working with the schizophrenic client, the nurse is confronted with a wide range of unusual, and sometimes threatening, client behaviors. The nurse must, in the face of "madness," remain sane and secure—essential ingredients in therapeutic effectiveness. On the other hand, it is not recommended that the nurse stay aloof or emotionally distant.

Working with a client who is in poor contact with reality is often a frustrating and frightening experience for the nurse. The delusional or hallucinatory material produced by the client is at a very primitive level and may be likened to the nightmares that each of us has experienced at one time or another. Some of our own most basic fears may be put into words or acted out by the client with a schizophrenic disorder.

It is encouraged that nurses and other mental health professionals become involved with their clients as an essential part of the therapeutic process. The client who is withdrawn from reality, however,

Nursing Care Plan 24-1

The Client Who Retreats from Reality

Nursing Diagnosis	Client Outcome	Intervention
Sensory-perceptual alteration	Client will clarify meanings	Validation of perceptions
		Detection of themes or hidden meanings
Alteration in thought processes	Client's fear and anxiety will be decreased	Remaining with client
		Calm, directive approach
	Client will verbalize reality-based thoughts	Disruption of events or circumstances leading to retreat from reality
		Orientation to nurse's name, position, and purpose in the interaction
		Acceptance of hallucinatory or delusional experience without agreement or disagreement with client
		Encouragement of reality-oriented conversation and activities
		Role-modeling of clear communication
		Consensual validation of experiences
Ineffective individual coping: incongruent, blunted, or disordered affect	Client's spontaneity and congruence of mood will be reinforced	Role-modeling appropriateness of affect
		Tolerance of bizarre behavior or affect
		Reinforcement of appropriate, socially acceptable interaction
Social isolation	Rapport will be established with client	Nonverbal communication of acceptance and trustworthiness
		Initiation of interaction
		Consistent nonthreatening approach
		Availability of support
	Client's social interaction will increase	Rewarding interpersonal experiences
		Development of trust on one-to-one basis
		Gradual increase in the social sphere
Impaired verbal communication	Communication with the client will be facilitated	Respect for silence
		Nonverbal communication through presence, consistency, and positive regard
		Acceptance of any communicative attempts

Nursing Diagnosis	Client Outcome	Intervention
Self-care deficit	Client's independent behavior will increase	• Provision of decision-making opportunities
		• Rewarding of independent behavior, such as self-care activities
		• Gradual increase in responsibility

may elicit great anxiety or similar disturbing feelings in the nurse. Seeing a person who is severely regressed, withdrawn, and apathetic is likely to be a tragic experience for any of us. Employing a repertoire of therapeutic skills with such a client may seem an overwhelming task because of the emotionally draining side effects. Although nurses need to maintain and convey hope for the client's improvement, they may find themselves distraught over the difficulties inherent in that responsibility. Feelings of guilt over "not getting through" or "not doing enough" may arise in the nurse and may further complicate the therapeutic assignment.

Understanding the facts of the client's situation and the treatment possibilities will help the nurse to set realistic goals for the client. Professional supervision sessions and involvement in a support group among colleagues in the work setting will also assist the nurse to keep a balanced view of the client's needs and gains. Nurses must cultivate close, rewarding relationships with family and friends as part of the process of personal growth and self-renewal, and to ensure their own therapeutic effectiveness.

Human involvement and caring are prerequisites to therapeutic intervention. The nurse's caring manner demonstrates to the client that he is accepted and respected as a fellow human being. In time, it will be evident to the client that he is not viewed as hopeless, but as a person of dignity and worthy of respect.

The client who is schizophrenic is likely to be very sensitive to others' feelings and to see through facades; he may arouse strong feelings of anxiety, anger, and depression in mental health professionals. The intensity of the relationship with a schizophrenic client often brings to the surface these interpersonal and emotional issues. The nurse needs to address these issues to prevent their hindering therapeutic effectiveness.

And what do the schizophrenic individuals themselves and their families say about their experiences? They eloquently recount their hopes, fears, trials, and feelings of hopelessness and of being out of control. They talk about using physical exercise and activity, work, and the support of others to maintain mental stability. They talk about being raised by a schizophrenic parent and the unpredictability and terror that accompanied them throughout childhood.[12, 15, 22, 32, 41, 48] For this important and sensitive content, see the special issue of *Schizophrenia Bulletin*, Schizophrenia: The Experiences of Patients and Families, 1987.

Summary

This chapter has presented two major areas of information—an overview of the schizophrenic disorders and the application of the nursing process to the client with a schizophrenic disorder. Some of the major foci of the chapter include the following:

1. Because it is estimated to affect 1% of the population and its onset occurs during adolescence and young adulthood, schizophrenia is considered a common and tragic emotional disturbance, or group of disturbances.
2. The biologic theories of the etiology of schizophrenia are built on data that support genetic, biochemical, immunological, or structural influences on the client and his behavior.
3. The psychosocial theories of the etiology of schizophrenia focus on the intrapersonal and interpersonal factors that lead to its development.
4. The five types of schizophrenia—disorganized, catatonic, paranoid, undifferentiated, and residual—have been explained in terms of their operational criteria.
5. Assessment and nursing diagnosis of the client are approached by examining the three major areas of disturbances of thinking, disturbances of feeling, and disturbances of behavior.
6. The foundation of an accurate assessment is a nonjudgmental attitude and careful, objective observation and description of client behaviors.
7. The psychiatric–mental health nurse is in-

Case Study 24-1

Approaching the Family System After a Member's Repeated Psychiatric Hospitalizations

The R. family, consisting of 53-year-old grandmother, Helen, a 28-year-old mother, Linda, and a 3-year-old son, Tommy, was referred to the community health nurse following Linda's third psychiatric hospitalization for a schizophrenic episode. When asked by the nurse if she knew why the follow-up visits had been recommended, Linda replied that she thought the nurse could help her with Tommy "who was still not potty-trained." This problem, perceived by Linda and her mother Helen to be the focus of concern, served as the vehicle through which the community health nurse was permitted to approach the family.

Initial contact with the R. family struck the nurse as a picture of the three family members against the world—protected in their high-rise fortress, 11 stories above street level, behind a door secured by multiple bolts and locks, and surrounded by the aged inhabitants of their apartment building. Lacking a car, a telephone, and daily newspapers, the family was fairly isolated (except for television contact or an occasional bus trip to a store) from the rest of society. Rarely would outside contacts touch the family's firmly entrenched homeostatic mechanisms. They had no relations in the southwestern United States, but Linda had a few friends and someone to date every 2 or 3 weeks. Tommy's father was not presently, nor had he ever been, involved with either his son or Linda, a fact which left her with much bitterness and distrust. Although it appeared at first that she assumed responsibility for her child, it soon became apparent that Helen fulfilled the mothering role for Tommy. Linda's relationship with her son resembled that of an older sibling, rather than a mother, to Tommy. Neither Helen nor Linda worked outside of the home; they derived their income from Social Security and Linda's disability checks.

Working with the discharged schizophrenic client means also working with the family members to promote a healthier level of functioning of the entire family system. One of the nurse's early concerns centered on Tommy and his environment. How was he to be removed from his present isolating experience and exposed to other children and adults? Research into the family backgrounds of schizophrenic clients has shown that the children at risk often require special assistance in broadening their social experiences outside their families.[14] Day care was suggested for Tommy, but until he was toilet trained, this was not possible. It seemed that neither Helen nor Linda actively attempted to toilet train Tommy because he was needed at home; without Tommy through whom to interact, the two women might have had considerably more difficulty interacting with each other.

Communication within the R. family was not the clear, direct, and congruent pattern of a healthy, adapting family. Often, Linda and Helen carried on parallel monologues and made no attempt to respond to each other's statements. Without the reaffirmation of each other's thoughts and feelings, they were both operating as isolated individuals who had no corrective mechanisms for keeping information up to date and reality-oriented. The nurse realized that neither Helen nor Linda was hearing the impact of her own or the other's messages. Focus of the intervention soon shifted from Tommy's lack of toilet training to the family's interactional patterns and payoffs.

Certain aspects of "undifferentiated family ego mass" and fusion in members' thoughts and feelings could be seen in the R. family's interaction.[13] Often, Linda would begin a sentence dealing with her emotions about a particular issue and Helen would complete the sentence. Or, Helen might speak to the nurse while Linda listened and continuously nodded her head in agreement. Rarely, especially during the initial visits, were differences of opinion expressed by the two women.

As the story of this family unfolded after several visits, it became clear to the nurse that Helen's marriage had been a source of unhappiness and frustration to her. Her husband had been a weekend drinker who, when drinking, would "lose his temper," destroy furniture, and verbally abuse her and their daughter, Linda. Helen grew increasingly alienated from him and in turn, focused a great amount of attention on Linda. The mother-child relationship became the all-important aspect of her life.

Goals of the nurse's therapeutic intervention included helping Linda and Helen develop a clearer perception of events and a greater awareness of their own and others' thoughts and feelings. Such growth in perception and awareness would permit these insecure, anxious persons to deal more effectively and less fearfully with life's problems.[14]

By helping the family members to tolerate periods of increased anxiety, the nurse hoped to demonstrate that they were not fragile, helpless people who would be harmed by their feelings. Rather, it was essential for the family to learn that anxiety is inevitable during all problem-solving situations, it is necessary for any individual's growth, and it would eventually subside. By demonstrating in face-to-face contacts that anxiety can be tolerated, the nurse hoped to show the R. family that they could live with, and learn from, anxiety. To help build the weakened self-esteem in the R. family, the nurse offered a consistently accepting and non-judgmental relationship with them.

The nursing approach to the R. family centered on support of the family leader, Linda, in making her own decisions about her future. In the past, Linda had been fearful about any ventures outside of her family. At times, she expressed ambivalence about her confining world at home and wondered aloud to the nurse if she were "smart enough to make it" on her own. Gradually, she began to make more independent choices regarding her own actions. The nurse reinforced any behavior that indicated an opening of this closed family system.

As Linda became more comfortable with her occasional social contacts (a trip shopping or ice-skating), her desire for them seemed to increase. Slowly, the nurse introduced the idea of vocational training to Linda. Again, gradually, Linda decided to investigate and, with the nurse's support and presence during the initial visit to the Vocational Rehabilitation Center, followed through with this suggestion.

A job for Linda was not without its reverberations throughout the whole family system. The job could mean loneliness and rejection to Helen, the introduction of new people and new ways of living into the family, increased self-esteem and independence for Linda, and the opening up of a wider, more reality-based world for Tommy.

Certain family "secrets" about Linda's father's drinking and abuse, Linda's repeated psychiatric hospitalizations, and Helen's feelings of guilt and responsibility for Linda's disturbance were uncovered and addressed within the family setting. It was hoped that dealing with the secret, unspoken issues openly would improve the family's abilities to interact genuinely with each other in the future. Controversial topics between Helen and Linda, such as whether they should move to another location, were not ignored but were explored with the nurse. This was done to demonstrate to them that differences of opinion do not kill either the people or the relationship involved—rather, differences offer stimulation and the opportunity for growth.

Increasing the family's interchanges with the larger community occurred most significantly through Linda's decision to enter vocational testing and training through the State Rehabilitation Commission, and through the family's decision to move to a neighborhood that offered a more open environment. The new neighborhood consisted of a younger population of residents, a peer group for Tommy, and easier access to a variety of activities for all family members. The R. family made use of, and benefited from, some planned interventions to influence their interactional patterns—both within and beyond the family.

Questions for Discussion

1. What are the potential problems facing the psychiatric client after discharge from inpatient care? How might these unique needs be met by the mental health team, the client, and his family?
2. Describe the patterns of behavior and communication that are observed in families with a schizophrenic member.
3. Discuss the therapeutic techniques that promote trust and open communication in a closed family system.
4. Create a "family nursing care plan" for the R. family.

volved in treatment planning as a collaborative effort with other members of the mental health team, which includes the client and his family or significant others.

8. Specific goals and outcomes are set for, and with, the client and his family to intervene in the present behavior and to begin preparation for discharge to the community.

9. The nurse is encouraged to be consistent and genuine in her approach to the schizophrenic client.

10. Current treatment approaches promote the

positive influence of the family on the schizophrenic member by providing information about the disorder, available treatments, and their benefits and risks.

11. The nurse's own feelings while working with the schizophrenic client must be addressed openly, as they are an important part of the therapeutic process.

12. Individual, group, and family therapy, the behavioristic approach, milieu therapy, and chemotherapy are discussed as useful modalities.

13. Interventions are proposed and advocated with high-risk populations, such as the children of psychotic parents.

14. Evaluation of nursing intervention is the continuous process of examination and assessment of the therapeutic effectiveness of each specific intervention.

References

1. American Psychiatric Association, Diagnostic and Statistical Manual of Mental Disorders, 3d ed, rev. Washington, DC, American Psychiatric Association, 1987

2. Andreasen NC: The Diagnosis of Schizophrenia. Schizophr Bull 13 (1): 9–22, 1987

3. Andrew B et al: A Study of Genetic Linkage in Schizophrenia. Psychol Med 17: 363–370, 1987

4. Anscombe R: The Disorder of Consciousness in Schizophrenia. Schizophr Bull 13 (2): 241–259, 1987

5. Arieti S: Interpretation of Schizophrenia, 2d ed. New York, Basic Books, 1974

6. Arieti S: Psychotherapy of Schizophrenia. In West LJ, Flinn DE (eds), Treatment of Schizophrenia: Progress and Prospects, pp 115–130. New York, Grune & Stratton, 1976

7. Arieti S: Psychotherapy of Schizophrenia: New or Revised Procedures. Am J Psychother 34 (October): 464–476, 1980

8. Artiss Lt Col KL, MC: Milieu Therapy in Schizophrenia. New York, Grune & Stratton, 1962

9. Bateson G et al: Toward a Theory of Schizophrenia. In Jackson DD (ed): Communication, Family, and Marriage, pp 31–54. Palo Alto, CA, Science and Behavior Books, 1968

10. Bebbington PE: Life Events in Schizophrenia: The WHO Collaborative Study. Soc Psychiatry 22: 179–180, 1987

11. Beers CW: A Mind That Found Itself: An Autobiography, New York, Doubleday & Co, 1923

12. Bockes Z: Freedom Means Knowing You Have a Choice. Schizophr Bull [Special Issue, Schizophrenia: The Experience of Patients and Families], 40–42, 1987

13. Bowen M: Family Psychotherapy, In Howells JL (ed): Theory and Practice of Family Psychiatry, pp 843–862. New York, Brunner/Mazel, 1971

14. Bruch II: Learning Psychotherapy: Rationale and Ground Rules. Cambridge, Harvard University Press, 1974

15. Brundage BE: What I Wanted to Know But Was Afraid to Ask. Schizophr Bull [Special Issue, Schizophrenia: The Experiences of Patients and Families], 32–34, 1987

16. Buschbaum MS, Haier RJ: Functional and Anatomical Brain Imaging: Impact on Schizophrenia Research. Schizophr Bull 13 (1): 115–132, 1987

17. Cancro R: The Healer and Madness. Strecker Monograph Series, No 15. The Fifteenth Institute of Pennsylvania Hospital Award Lecture, 1978

18. Cancro R: Individual Psychotherapy in the Treatment of Chronic Schizophrenic Patients. Am J Psychother 37 (October): 493–501, 1983

19. Carpenter WT: Approaches to Knowledge and Understanding of Schizophrenia. Schizophr Bull 13 (1): 1–8, 1987

20. Deutsh M, Katz I, Jensen AR (eds): Social Class, Race, and Psychological Development. New York, Holt, Rinehart, 1968

21. Drake RE, Sederer LI: Inpatient Psychosocial Treatment of Chronic Schizophrenia: Negative Effects and Current Guidelines. Hosp Community Psychiatry 37 (September): 897–900, 1986

22. DuVal M: Giving Love . . . and Schizophrenia. Schizophr Bull [Special Issue, Schizophrenia: The Experience of Patients and Families], 8–13, 1987

23. Ezrin-Waters C, Seeman MV, Seeman P: Tardive Dyskinesia in Schizophrenic Outpatients: Prevalence and Significant Variables. J Clin Psychiatr 42 (January): 16–22, 1981

24. Falloon, IR et al: Family Management in the Prevention of Morbidity of Schizophrenia: Social Outcome of a Two-Year Longitudinal Study. Psychol Med 17: 59–66, 1987

25. Fenton WS, McGlashan TH: Prognostic Scale for Chronic Schizophrenia. Schizophr Bull 13 (2): 277–286, 1987

26. Goldstein MJ: Psychosocial Issues. Schizophr Bull 13 (1): 157–171, 1987

27. Goldstein WN: DSM-III and the Diagnosis of Schizophrenia. Am J Psychother 37 (April): 168–181, 1983

28. Gottesman II, McGuffin P, Farmer AE: Clinical Genetics as Clues to the "Real" Genetics of Schizophrenia (A Decade of Modest Gains While Playing for Time). Schizophr Bull 13 (1): 23–47, 1987

29. Grunebaum H: Preventive Intervention with Psychotic Mothers: A Controlled Study. In Primary Prevention of Schizophrenia in High-Risk Groups, pp 32–37. Copenhagen, Regional Office for Europe, World Health Organization, 1977

30. Haley J: The Family of the Schizophrenic: A Model System. In Jackson DD (ed): Communication, Family, and Marriage, pp 171–199. Palo Alto, CA, Science and Behavior Books, 1968

31. Holzman PS: Recent Studies of Psychophysiology in Schizophrenia. Schizophr Bull 13 (1): 49–75, 1987

32. Houghton JF: Maintaining Mental Health in a Turbulent World. Schizophr Bull [Special Issue, Schizophrenia: The Experience of Patients and Families], 17–21, 1987

33. Jackson DD: The Question of Family Homeostasis. In Jackson DD (ed): Communication, Family, and Marriage, pp 1–11. Palo Alto, CA, Science and Behavior Books, 1968

34. Jarvik ME, Flinn DE, West LJ: Psychopharmacological Treatment of Schizophrenia. In West LJ, Flinn DE (eds): Treatment of Schizophrenia: Progress and Prospects, pp 79–98. New York, Grune & Stratton, 1976

35. Kanba S et al: Selective Enlargement of the Third Ventricle Found in Chronic Schizophrenia. Psychiatry Res 21: 49–53, 1987

36. Kane JM: Treatment of Schizophrenia. Schizophr Bull 13 (1): 133–156, 1987

37. Kety SS: Progress in the Psychobiology of Schizophrenia: Implications for Treatment. In West LJ, Flinn DE (eds): Treatment of Schizophrenia: Progress and Prospects, pp 35–43. New York, Grune & Stratton, 1976

38. Kishimoto H et al: Three Subtypes of Chronic Schizophrenia Identified Using ^{11}C-Glucose Positron Emission Tomography. Psychiatry Res 21: 285–292, 1987

39. Laing RD, Esterson A: Sanity, Madness and the Family, 2d ed. New York, Basic Books, 1971

40. Lamb HR et al: Families of Schizophrenics: A Movement in Jeopardy. Hosp Community Psychiatry 37 (April): 353–357, 1986

41. Lanquetot R: Confessions of the Daughter of a Schizophrenic. Schizophr Bull [Special Issue, Schizophrenia: The Experiences of Patients and Families], 57–61, 1987

42. Liberman RP: Behavior Therapy for Schizophrenia. In West LJ, Flinn DE (eds): Treatment of Schizophrenia: Progress and Prospects, pp 175–206. New York, Grune & Stratton, 1976

43. Ludwig AM: Treating the Treatment Failures: The Challenge of Chronic Schizophrenia. New York, Grune & Stratton, 1971

44. Merrin EL: Schizophrenia and Brain Asymmetry: An Evaluation of Evidence for Dominant Lobe Dysfunction. J Nerv Ment Dis 169 (July): 405–414, 1981

45. McGill CW, Lee E: Family Psychoeducational Intervention in the Treatment of Schizophrenia: Bull Menninger Clinic 50 (3): 269–286, 1986

46. Mintz LI et al: Expressed Emotion: A Call for Partnership Among Relatives, Patients, and Professionals. Schizophr Bull 13 (2): 227–235, 1987

47. Murphy JM, Leighton AH: Approaches to Cross-Cultural Psychiatry. Ithaca, NY, Cornell University Press, 1965

48. Piercy BP: Making the Best of It. Schizophr Bull [Special Issue, Schizophrenia: The Experiences of Patients and Families], 62–64, 1987

49. Rin H: Schizophrenia: Its Crosscultural Aspect. In Fukuda T, Mitsuda H (eds): World Issues in the Problems of Schizophrenic Psychoses, pp 90–101. Tokyo, Igaku-Shoin, 1979

50. Ruesch J: Synopsis of the Theory of Human Communication. In Howells JG (ed): Theory and Practice of Family Psychiatry, pp 227–266. New York, Brunner/Mazel, 1971

51. Satir V: Peoplemaking. Palo Alto, CA, Science and Behavior Books, 1972

52. Schooler NR, Levine J: Strategies for Enhancing Drug Therapy of Schizophrenia. Am J Psychother 37 (October): 521–532, 1983

53. Seeman P et al: Elevation of Brain Neuroleptic/Dopamine Receptors in Schizophrenia. In Baxter CF, Melnechuk T (eds): Perspectives in Schizophrenia Research, pp 195–202. New York, Raven Press, 1980

54. Seidman LJ: Schizophrenia and Brain Dysfunction: An Integration of Recent Neurodiagnostic Findings. Psychol Bull 94 (September): 195–238, 1983

55. Singh MM, Kay SR, Opler LA: Anticholinergic-Neuroleptic Antagonism in Terms of Positive and Negative Symptoms of Schizophrenia: Implications for Psychobiological Subtyping. Psychol Med 17: 39–48, 1987

56. Townsend MC: Nursing Diagnoses in Psychiatric Nursing: A Pocket Guide for Care Plan Construction. Philadelphia, FA Davis, 1988

57. Torrey EF: Surviving Schizophrenia: A Family Manual. New York, Harper & Row, 1983

58. Verhulst J, Schneidman B: Schizophrenia and Sexual Functioning. Hosp Community Psychiatr 32 (April): 259–62, 1981

59. Walker E, and McGuire M: Intra- and Inter-hemispheric Information Processing in Schizophrenia. Psychol Bull 92 (3): 701–725, 1982

60. Weinberger DR, Wyatt RJ: Structural Brain Abnormalities in Chronic Schizophrenia: Computed Tomography Findings. In Baxter CF, Melnechuk (eds): Perspectives in Schizophrenia Research, pp 29–38. New York, Raven Press, 1980

61. Wilcox JA, Nasrallah HA: Childhood Head Trauma and Psychosis. Psychiatry Res 21: 303–306, 1987

62. Wolman BB: Children Without Childhood: A Study of Childhood Schizophrenia. New York, Grune & Stratton, 1970

63. Zigler E, Glick M: Paranoid Schizophrenia: An Unorthodox View. Am J Orthopsychiatr 5 (January): 43–70, 1984

64. Zubin J: Chronic Schizophrenia from the Standpoint of Vulnerability. In Baxter CF, Melneckuk T (eds): Perspectives in Schizophrenia Research, pp 269–294. New York, Raven Press, 1980

25

Suspicious, Hostile, and Aggressive Behavior: The Delusional and Acting-Out Disorders

Mary Snyder McElvain

Growing up often means facing the anguished isolation of no longer belonging as we wander in exile through a strange world that makes no sense. Each of us must make his or her separate way through an indifferent, unfamiliar landscape in which good is not necessarily rewarded, nor evil punished. Adding to the confusion, at times we find ourselves or others graced with unearned love and happiness or burdened with "undeserved" calamity and pain.

Sheldon Kopp,
An End to Innocence:
Facing Life Without Illusions,
1978

440

Chapter Preview

Clients exhibiting delusional—that is, paranoid—and acting-out disorders experience a number of different behaviors and motivations. Nurses observe suspicious, hostile, and aggressive behavior in a variety of situations—in the behavioral pattern of a client with a diagnosed emotional disorder, and in the repertoire of responses available to any individual, in any given interaction, without that person being labeled according to a particular clinical category.

This chapter introduces the reader to the concepts of suspicion, hostility, and aggression and explores various theoretical frameworks underlying these concepts. The chapter also reviews the incidence, etiology, and dynamics of the delusional (paranoid) and acting-out disorders, and focuses on the application of the nursing process to suspicious, hostile, and aggressive behavior. It is through the creative use of personality, knowledge base, and specific techniques that the nurse, within the format of nursing process, cares for unique and individual clients.

Learning Objectives

After completing the chapter, you should be able to accomplish the following:

1. differentiate between suspicious, hostile, aggressive, and acting-out behaviors
2. discuss the incidence of delusional (paranoid) and acting-out disorders
3. discuss the psychological, biological, and sociocultural theories of the etiology of suspicious, hostile, and aggressive behaviors
4. discuss the dynamics underlying hostility and suspiciousness, impulsivity and acting-out, and anger and aggression
5. apply the nursing process to clients who demonstrate suspicious, hostile, and aggressive behavior
6. verbalize awareness of your own feelings and attitudes when interacting with a person exhibiting hostile, suspicious, or aggressive behavior

Defining Suspicious, Hostile, and Aggressive Behavior

Suspicious behavior involves hypersensitivity, alertness, and some distortion of reality.[65] The suspicious person uses selective attention to gather information that will fit his schema, confirm his beliefs, and allow rigid conclusions to be drawn.

Hostility is defined as a feeling of antagonism accompanied by a wish to hurt or humiliate others.[34,57] Because hostility is a sustained feeling, it produces responses which range from overly polite behavior to murderous rage or suicide.[35] Anger may be differentiated from hostility in that anger does not necessarily involve a wish to harm. *Anger*, rather, is a physical and emotional state in which an individual experiences a sense of power to compensate for an underlying feeling of anxiety.[57] In this way, anger may be viewed as a second-level emotion involving the wish to overpower.

Aggression is any behavior which expresses anger or its related emotions.[57] It is also a natural drive that has been classified by Freud and Lorenz as instinctive and by others as an elicited drive, described in the frustration-aggression hypothesis, or as learned social behavior.[34] Aggressive drives are greatly influenced by cultural conditioning and, therefore, may be turned toward constructive or destructive goals. Many people learn to sublimate, repress, or displace expressions of anger. The struggle for control of these expressions uses much psychic energy and is considered a crucial factor in determining the level of mental health.[27,57]

It is paradoxical that persons who find it intolerable to acknowledge their own hostility tend to perceive the world as hostile, unfriendly, and dangerous.[35] When a person fails to recognize feelings of anger in himself, he may use his anger in a destructive way and therefore may feel helpless. From this helpless and distorted perspective, the individual is constantly mistrustful of others' intentions and continually disappointed because others do not meet his needs. There becomes evident, then, a link between paranoid thinking and hostile, aggressive behavior.

Acting-out behavior consists of impulsive actions or inappropriate verbalizations to express unconscious conflicts. This pattern of behavior may be episodic or lifelong. It does not automatically include aggressive or antisocial behavior.[8] Even when a person acknowledges his acting-out behavior, he is usually unaware of what motivates the behavior or even what it may communicate to others.[27] For example, some people who chronically act-out with physical violence do not perceive themselves as having a problem with anger.[38]

Incidence of Delusional and Acting-Out Disorders

The suspicious and acting-out disorders encompass multiple behaviors and diagnostic categories, making it difficult to arrive at accurate statistical data about incidence. We could, for example, include behaviors as diverse as child abuse, vandalism, and self-mutilation in these disorders.

DSM-III-R has replaced the DSM-III diagnosis of paranoid disorder with delusional (paranoid) disorder because delusions are the primary symptom of this disorder. The type of the delusional disorder is then specified in the diagnosis and is based on one of the following delusional themes: erotomanic (one is loved by another), grandiose (one possesses greatness or a famous relationship), jealous (one's partner is unfaithful), persecutory (theme of being a victim in some way), somatic (one's body emits an odor or is infested, malfunctioning, or very unpleasant).[1]

DSM-III-R estimates the population prevalence for delusional disorder at about 0.03%. In most studies the average age of onset has been found to be between 40 and 55 years. The estimate of the prevalence of antisocial personality disorder for American males is about 3%; for American females, less than 1%. To receive this diagnosis, a person must be at least 18 years of age and have a history of conduct disorder before age 15.[1]

Persons with socially deviant behavior do not usually seek mental health services voluntarily. The incidence of socially deviant behavior traditionally has been two to three times higher among males than among females.[34] As females move into many formerly male-dominated arenas, will these statistics change, or do the statistics reflect a more basic biologic or sociological difference between the sexes to account for the difference in socially deviant behavior?

Etiologic Theories

Like so many of the behaviors studied in pychiatric–mental health nursing, suspicious, hostile, and aggressive behaviors are multi-determined. In this chapter, the antecedents of these behaviors will be discussed by means of psychological, biologic, and sociocultural theories.

Psychological Theories

Intrapsychic Approaches

Freud believed that aggression stems from redirecting the death instinct away from the self toward others.[34] Antisocial behavior, he said, involves a defective ego that is combined with a weak or immature superego, resulting in a person who is unable to control or regulate his behavior but who feels little or no guilt because of the inability.[48] Freud also portrayed paranoid processes as unconscious homosexual tendencies from which the individual defends himself through the use of denial and projection.[34]

Other intrapsychic theorists view hostile and aggressive behavior as a result of anxiety and inner conflict, or as energy that is directed into specific character orientations in relating to the world.[31] Fromm describes an "exploitative orientation," wherein the source of good and bad lies outside the self. With this orientation, a person values other people and things only for their usefulness.[22]

Another psychological factor in the development of paranoid or antisocial behavior may include "malevolent transformation," in which an individual turns rejection and hatred from the self toward others. Or the person may use "desensitization," wherein his defense mechanisms operate to deaden feelings toward others.

Other research has supported the *stimulation-seeking hypothesis,* that is, the hypothesis that psychopathic individuals engage in more stimulus-seeking than do neurotic persons.[5,13] Such findings imply that during intervention with psychopathic individuals, diverse stimuli may be needed to cue and to reinforce behavior, and a particular stimulus may work for only a brief period of time.

A *cognitive model* explains how appraisals, expectancies, and private speech mediate between aversive stimuli and aggressive reactions. Results of one study show that as aggressive behavior becomes more marked, subjects are biased to infer hostility in interpersonal relationships. The threshold for aggressive acts seems to be related to an expectation of hostility from others.[46] A further application of the cognitive model was a study of three groups to measure the joint influence of outcome expectations and beliefs in personal efficacy.[53] The data suggest that low personal efficacy may be a distinguishing characteristic of all psychiatric patients, whereas outcome expectancies may determine the specific nature of the psychiatric disorder. The depressive group in the study expected outcomes to be controlled by chance, whereas the paranoid group expected outcomes to be controlled by powerful others.[53] As research tests concepts such as these, our understanding of behavioral pathologies will increase.

Interpersonal Approaches

Antisocial behavior is often thought to stem from childhood. If, for example, parents alternately infantilize their children and then expect perfection, the child cannot internalize conflicts due to superego defects.[39] Another theory proposes that there is an interactional pattern to antisocial behavior because the behavior is unconsciously encouraged by a parent who obtains vicarious satisfaction of his or her own antisocial impulses.[60] Bowlby feels that lack of attachment to a mother figure during the first 3 years, whether by absence, changes, or deprivation, leads to acting-out behavior later in life.[6]

Considering the importance of the second stage of growth and development, *autonomy versus shame,* in learning controls, it is understandable that parental neglect or inconsistency during this period might have undesirable consequences. This is not to say that a direct cause-and-effect relationship exists between early parental deprivation and later development of an impulsive lifestyle. There is, however, some evidence that relates lack of close emotional ties early in life to affectionless lifestyles.[66]

The third stage of growth and development, *initiative versus guilt,* has also been cited as a crucial time in the formation of social or antisocial traits. If the child lacks a warm, trustworthy role model during this period, he may fail to introject societal values adequately.

Biologic Theories

Biochemical Theories

Biochemical theories of suspicious, hostile, and aggressive behavior focus on the fact that changes in blood chemistry may sensitize or desensitize neural systems for aggression. Underlying those theories is the premise that particular stimuli activate certain neural systems in the brain, resulting in a tendency for the organism to behave destructively toward those stimuli complexes. Another stimulus change thereby turns off aggression.

Alcoholism and aggressive behavior are certainly linked phenomena, as police and emergency room staffs could verify. Researchers have found that variations in the level of intoxication result in different levels of aggression.[49]

Blood chemistry variables always interact with social, environmental, and learning factors. However, other things being equal, increased androgen levels are associated with increased hostile behavior of some

kind. If the progesterone–estrogen ratio is altered, feelings of irritability accompanying premenstrual tension syndrome can be decreased. Exact endocrine–brain chemistry interactions and their causal relationship to aggressive behavior remain to be discovered.[44] Allergic aggressive reactions have been reported, but their physiology is unclear.

Biochemical theories of paranoid behavior point to the fact that increased dopaminergic activity in the brain leads to both euphoria and paranoia. An extremely small study of four cocaine abusers with histories of stimulant-induced paranoid psychoses reported a selective decrease in paranoia, but not in euphoria, when the subjects were treated with dopamine blockers (chlorpromazine and haloperidol). The author concluded that this finding implied different neurophysiological substrates for these two states.[24] Further research that might discriminate this presumed dopaminergic activation in both states will be important.

Physiological Theories

Physiological theories have examined the functional integrity of relevant neural systems. The neural system for aggression is found in much of the limbic system. For example, limbic tumors result in personality changes, with irritability as a predominant symptom. It is postulated that tumors irritate neurological mechanisms for aggression or destroy inhibitory mechanisms to aggression. Certain types of brain trauma, rabies, and encephalitis, which damage particular portions of the limbic system, are associated with a loss of impulse control. Temporal lobe epilepsy may also activate the neural system for aggression. Specific brain lesions can likewise reduce or eliminate excessive hostile behavior.

Genetic Theories

Certain chromosomal abnormalities such as Klinefelter syndrome and XYY syndrome may result in a lack of impulse control. The occurrence of these disorders points to the existence of a genetic theory. Nonetheless, more evidence is needed to support genetic theories of hostile and aggressive behavior.

Sociocultural Theories

When a person perceives society's norms as ambiguous, weak, or conflicting, he may develop socially deviant behavior.[48] This "social strain theory" proposes that misunderstanding of or rebellion against values leads to criminal acts. Certainly, the crises of everyday life among the poor are a social strain. Because different social classes hold different norms for behavior,

behavior that is tolerated or promoted in one class becomes deviant when judged by members of another social class.

Social learning theories lead researchers to look at patterns of family interaction to see how these patterns may be learned and transmitted from parents to children. A study of boys from a lower-class urban environment found three major elements affecting levels of aggression.[41] (It is interesting to speculate that these same elements could readily occur in other populations than the one studied, *e.g.,* middle-class, rural, suburban.)

First, when parents frequently used physically punitive discipline, threats, or parental rejection, such as unfavorable comments on the boys' worth, their sons were likely to behave in a highly aggressive manner. Second, high demands, overcontrolled or undercontrolled supervision, and inconsistent discipline tended to increase the level of the boys' aggressive behavior. Third, there was higher aggression in families where one parent undermined or attacked the other; that is, where parental conflict and antagonism were pervasive.[41]

Another study looked specifically at violent behavior of high school students toward their parents. This study found that youths who are violent toward parents are more likely to live in families with a low level of family integration or functioning, to have witnessed a good deal of violent, aggressive behavior within the family, and to have been the victim of such behavior.[37]

Exposure to aggressive models, especially television violence, has also been studied as a social determinant of aggressive behavior. Researchers have shown that subjects who viewed aggressive human and cartoon models on film showed almost twice as much aggression, when later frustrated, than did a control group. One can conclude that filmed aggression facilitates the expression of aggression and shapes the form of subjects' aggressive behavior.[4]

Why is television violence important? After all, it does not control instigators to aggression, nor does it provide reinforcement for aggression in real life. It does, however, teach us how to aggress. It also portrays for us the functional value of coercive behavior in achieving material rewards, social recognition, increased self-esteem, or successful retaliation against enemies.[3]

Other research found a strong positive relationship between the violence ratings of favorite programs and aggressive behavior of boys, although there was no corresponding relationship for girls.[17] The single best predictor of how aggressive a young man would be at age 19 was the violence of TV pro-

grams he preferred at age 8. This seems to be a critical developmental period when the child is very susceptible to violence on TV. Girls may have a differential ability to use TV as a fantasy experience rather than a realistic one, so that the modeling effect is decreased.[16]

Environmental determinants of aggressive behavior include noise, crowding, and heat. These extrapersonal stressors and situational determinants, such as heightened arousal and drugs, have shown inconclusive results as determinants of human aggression.[34] Recently, however, an interesting 18-year study has drawn a profile of 66 aggressive individuals from adolescence into adulthood. A few of the characteristics of children with the most extensive continuing antisocial activity are as follows:

They are mostly boys
They have the longest pre-admission history of childhood problems
Their antisocial and behavioral disturbances are the chief complaints, rather than their psychiatric symptoms
Their families have more antisocial backgrounds and there are more single-parent homes
There are more minority children from deprived and disadvantaged areas[20]

Dynamics of the Delusional and Acting-Out Disorders

Our curiosity as psychiatric nurses leads us to ask many "why" and "how" questions about human behavior and the situations, predicaments, and crises in which people find themselves. In studying patterns of behavior, the student needs to consider dynamics; that is, what forces within the individual explain particular symptoms or psychiatric syndromes. This chapter considers the dynamics of hostility and suspiciousness, impulsivity and acting-out, and anger and aggression.

Hostility and Suspiciousness

In delusional (paranoid) disorders, delusions are dominant behavioral symptoms. These delusions may be well systematized and developed logically, or they may be bizarre and changeable. In either case, suspiciousness, which results in delusions, is a defense against disintegration of the ego.

Paranoid styles of behavior usually involve projection of attitudes about the self, especially feelings of rejection, inadequacy, and inferiority. As the client becomes increasingly anxious in response to intrapersonal, interpersonal, or extrapersonal stressors, his uncomfortable inner feelings are projected and therefore perceived as a growing danger or threat from without. The client finds a focus for his projected feelings, resulting in delusions about the FBI, the Mafia, extraterrestrial beings, and so on. The client's projection may result in over-aggressiveness. Or the client may use other ego defense mechanisms, such as reaction formation against aggression, dependency needs, and feelings of affection, or denial of certain painful realities.[34]

Lack of trust, the hallmark of suspicious behavior, is probably the result of early parenting in what the child perceives as a hostile environment within an authoritarian or critical family atmosphere. The child becomes hypersensitive to imagined slights.[34] At the same time, the environment may place on the child high expectations for performance. An insecure child may use fantasy to increase his self-esteem or may develop overdetermined goals. Social failure later in life may result from rigid or unrealistic goals.

As paranoid ideation progresses, a "pseudocommunity" may develop, wherein the paranoid person ascribes malevolent motivations to real and imagined people.[34] This pseudocommunity can be thought of as the significant others of the paranoid person. The person uses considerable energy in watching for and defending against these negatively significant others.

An old term, *folie à deux,* or shared paranoid disorder, has been replaced in DSM-III-R by the diagnosis of induced psychotic disorder, which is felt to be a more accurate description of a very rare occurrence. In this disorder, a delusional system develops in a second person as a result of a close relationship with another person who already has a psychotic disorder with prominent delusions. The same delusions, often within the realm of possibility and based on common experiences, are at least partly shared by both persons. These people usually have lived together for a long time and are isolated from contact with other people.[1]

Focusing on disrupted communication rather than intrapersonal stressors constitutes an interactionist approach to suspicious behavior. This approach explains that, by exclusion and mutually perceived mistrust, delusions develop over time. In fact, by examining the social environment of the identified client, one may find that the client's significant others use many pretexts, or misstatements, to influence him or gain his cooperation.[66] This pattern of altered communication continually feeds into and fuels his mistrust of others.

Impulsivity and Acting-Out

As with suspicious behavior, impulsive and acting-out behavior has the common dynamic element of mistrust. The impulsive client demonstrates a low frustration tolerance and an inability to postpone gratification. His behavior seems to say, "If I can't have it now, I don't trust either you or me to be able to get it for me later." The client's excessive dependency, combined with a low frustration tolerance, may lead the nurse to feel conflicted and to want to withdraw from him.

Impulsive and acting-out behavior styles are generally characterized as disorders of the superego. Due to faulty identification and learning, the client does not see himself from the perspective of inner ethical principles (conscience), nor from outer standards of authority (morality). He tends to blame all of his difficulties on others; that is, he projects, which usually comes across as a "victim posture" or the attitude that "the world has the problem and must change—not me."

Although the person exhibiting impulsive or acting-out behavior does not have a thought disorder in the sense of the psychotic person's break with reality, he is deficient in the ability to predict effects of actions or to problem-solve in terms of long-range consequences. He appears egocentric and without a sense of direction, so whim becomes all important in his thinking.[66] He views the world as inconsistent, rather than as hostile.

The impulsive or acting-out person denies responsibility for the results of his behavior. He lacks the controls which refine the thinking process; he has not, however, lost control of his aggressive feelings.[28] Although he engages in a great deal of manipulation of the social environment, he feels no guilt about his exploitations.[48]

A child may develop mistrust and faulty superego functioning when parents delay in meeting his needs or act indifferently or rejecting toward him. The child who later exhibits impulsive behavior may have had no role models or models who were deceitful, superficial, or narcissistic.[28]

A newer method of studying and formulating impulsive, acting-out behavior is based on the rational-emotive therapy of Albert Ellis. Impulsive behavior, says Ellis, results from philosophic distortions or irrational beliefs. For the impulsive person, "wants" become "needs," and once a person "needs" something, he is no longer responsible for the behavior it takes to meet that need. This is an example of "the end justifies the means" philosophy. Rational-emotive therapy, however, is descriptive and does not address the question of why a person confuses his wants and his needs in the first place. Nevertheless, it does offer a framework for intervention with persons with ego-centric belief systems that will be discussed in this chapter.

Anger and Aggression

Anger is a universal human emotion. Some people deny their anger at the expense of considerable psychic energy. Anger is expressed through a wide range of behaviors which are learned and shaped through the socialization process. By identification with role models, by subtle nonverbal cues, and by the consequences of aggressive actions during childhood, individuals learn both healthy and harmful ways to deal with angry feelings.

Anger is also a cover-up. It "veils the original threat which gave rise to anxiety."[30] Anger is a means of neutralizing or avoiding anxiety that arises in response to an interpersonal threat. Chart 25-1 shows a model of the development and release of anger.

Anger and aggression may be channeled externally or internally.[11,57] The direct outward expression of anger and aggression may take place through verbal or physical means; it may either overpower others or consider the rights of others. There are degrees of direct outward expression of aggression. For example, a person may calmly state, "I am feeling angry enough to hit you," or may shout, "Get out of here or I'll kill you!" A person may break a cigarette, hit a wall, turn over a chair, break a window, or break someone's nose. These behaviors occur on a continuum from less severe to more severe and, as a consequence, may result in different kinds of responses to the aggressor.

The indirect, outward expression of anger and aggression may occur through ego defense mechanisms or passive-aggressive behavior. A person may use several defense mechanisms to deal with angry feelings. Through rationalization, he tries to justify angry behavior by giving motives other than the real ones—for example, "When I get tired, I get grouchy." A person may use reaction formation to disown angry feelings; while actually seething inside, he may show undue concern or an oversolicitous attitude toward others. By using fantasy, a person may belittle the object of anger so that it becomes less threatening. Sarcasm or ironic remarks are examples of the magical attack which fantasy entails. Through somatization, he focuses on bodily aches and pains rather than on the anger which festers inside his body. Displacement is used to direct anger toward a safer target. For example, family members are often the recipients of displaced angry feelings from the work setting, or vice versa.

A person exhibiting passive-aggressive behavior uses passivity or submissiveness to express hostility or destructive feelings. This resistive form of behavior is often seen as procrastination, dawdling, stubbornness, intentional inefficiency, or forgetfulness. Parent-child interactions which lead to passive-aggressive behaviors probably involve some inhibition of the child's assertiveness, with only partial and grudging satisfaction of his dependency needs. The child therefore develops a behavior pattern through which he learns to attract attention and, at the same time, cause discomfort to authority figures. His dependency needs insure that he seldom, if ever, expresses anger directly.

Psychoanalytic theory proposes that the inward expression of angry feelings is depression or self-destructive acts. Another view, however, states that hostility is a defense against depression, rather than a cause of it.[35]

A therapist who works within a psychoanalytic framework supports the client in expressing his repressed angry feelings in order to relieve the depression. When angry feelings are viewed as a defensive mechanism, however, the therapist may only be strengthening the client's defenses through attention to angry feelings rather than focusing on depressive ones.

C H A R T 25-1
A Model of Anger

Perceived threat (frustration, unmet
    expectations, loss of self-esteem)

↓

Anxiety is felt

↓

Anxiety is transformed to anger (anger
    gives a sense of power, which results
    in increased self-esteem, which is a
    stimulus for action)

↓

Feel relief (however, if the expression of
    anger has been forbidden, ignored, or
    ineffective in the past, the individual
    will likely experience guilt or lowered
    self-esteem)

Application of the Nursing Process to Suspicious, Hostile, and Aggressive Behavior

Assessment

The astute nurse assesses clients for cues indicating suspicious, hostile, and aggressive behavior. The nurse then uses the nursing process to defuse volatile situations or to channel the expression of these emotions as constructively as possible.

Therapeutic assessment begins with asking questions. It never assumes that the nurse knows the meaning behind a given behavior or that a certain client will respond in a particular fashion in a particular situation. To describe and explain behaviors, it is useful and helpful to ask, "Which are the problematic behaviors, for whom, and why?"

Environmental Factors

Environmental influences are important factors in assessing suspicious, hostile, and aggressive behavior. New and unfamiliar surroundings may increase the client's mistrust or frighten him to such an extent that he feels the need to protect himself. The amount of stimulation in the environment—that is, the noise, lighting, temperature, clutter, or crowding—may also cue suspicion and hostility. In locked psychiatric units, the locked door may symbolize entrapment or punishment against which a client feels powerless and, eventually, angry. Uniforms, whether worn by professionals from the emergency room, security guards, or police, may trigger feelings of rebellion against authority in a client with poor impulse control or poor reality-testing. Nurses are often able to regulate environmental stressors that negatively affect clients.

Indicators of Dangerous Behavior

The unpredictability of suspicious, hostile, and aggressive behavior bothers many beginning practitioners in psychiatric–mental health nursing. Watching for *behavioral cues* and listening carefully for the *feeling tone or latent communication* of a client enables the nurse to prevent hostile feelings from escalating into dangerous actions. Some indicators of suspicious or dangerous behavior include:

Thinking and perception. Hallucinations or delusions that threaten the client with harm or command the client to harm (for example, a new father hears voices telling him to take his baby to another town to save him from murderers)

Motor activity. Increased psychomotor agitation, which is often a signal that the client cannot tolerate physical closeness (for example, a client begins to pace the hall rapidly)

Mood or affect. Increased intensity of affect or verbalizations, or a noticeable change in the manner in which a client expresses wants and needs (for example, a client's voice quivers and she pleads with psychiatric staff to let her out of the hospital before she loses control)

Physical state. Organic states in which the client may be unable to communicate a warning, such as beginnings of seizures, delirium, brain lesions, or withdrawal states

Context. History of violent outbursts against self or others, which may include repeated criminal behavior or multiple suicide attempts (for example, a client is known to have engaged in physical fights with other clients and staff on previous admissions); and use of alcohol, other addictive drugs, or hallucinogenic drugs that remove controls on behavior (for example, a client is admitted with known PCP ingestion)[2, 27, 48, 54]

These predictors indicate that the impulse control of an adult or adolescent is disturbed in some way. There is a "childhood triad" of behaviors which is used to ascertain the seriousness of impulse control disturbance in children. These three behaviors are firesetting, bedwetting, and cruelty to animals. The consistency of this particular combination of behaviors has been found to correlate with some degree of socially aberrant behavior in children.[55]

Assessing Potential for Violence. One aspect of every mental status assessment is assessing the client's potential for violence. During initial interviews, or whenever the nurse suspects the *possibility of suicidal or homicidal behavior,* the nurse should ask, "Do you feel like hurting yourself or anyone else?" The nurse will not introduce ideas of violence into the client's head. Rather, by asking the question directly, the nurse promotes a healthy role model of verbalization in place of acting-out behavior. If the client is a poor historian or is unable to respond, the nurse may need to interview people who accompany the client to the clinic or hospital regarding the client's impulse control. The nurse asks those accompanying the client how he has managed aggressive feelings in the past.[34] At this time, the nurse may also offer information about how the hospital will help the client control his behavior.

Degrees of Suspicion, Hostility, and Aggression

Just as there are four stages of anxiety, there are several degrees of suspicious, hostile, and aggressive behavior. Some of the terms used to describe these various degrees are vigilant, sensitive, hypersensitive, paranoid, underlying hostility, thinly veiled hostility, overt hostility, belligerent, aggressive, and assaultive. The aim of nursing, of course, is not to eradicate the client's feelings, but to teach the constructive expression of these feelings and to provide a safe environment for staff and clients.

Assessing the Client's Control and Knowledge

Suspicious, hostile, and aggressive feelings and behaviors may be assessed on a continuum from less severe to more severe, or they may be assessed in relation to two ego functions, control and knowledge. By considering the correlation of *control of behavior* and *knowledge of feelings* the nurse gains direction in planning nursing interventions. In Table 25-1, possible nursing interventions are suggested for different levels of client ego functioning, different degrees of control and knowledge.

The nurse uses assessment skills to decide if a given client is in control and knows what he is feeling and doing. Judging whether someone is in control of his behavior is easier than deciding whether someone understands his feelings. Many times nurses confuse these two ego functions, control and knowledge, and insist that a client "should control" his behavior whenever he exhibits self-awareness. However, any of us may have habits of behavior that have harmful effects and yet not be "in control" or able to stop these habits at will.

Table 25-1. **Control and Knowledge of Suspicious, Hostile, and Aggressive Feelings and Behavior: Possible Nursing Interventions**

	CONTROL OF BEHAVIOR	NO CONTROL OF BEHAVIOR
KNOWLEDGE OF FEELING	No intervention needed	Behavior modification Psychotherapy Medication
NO KNOWLEDGE OF FEELING	Confrontation Role-playing Insight therapy Education	Medication Physical restraint Isolation from others

(From communication and collaboration with Marvin A. Glovinsky, PhD, Las Vegas, NV, Fall, 1981)

Nursing Diagnosis

Diagnosing the Suspicious Client

The nurse selects, from among a list of standardized nursing diagnoses, those which are relevant to a particular client. The data gathered about an individual client form the basis for the determination of the final nursing diagnosis or diagnoses. The nurse considers the following probable and possible nursing diagnoses when working with a client who is suspicious. The supporting data are given below each diagnosis.

Probable Nursing Diagnosis

1. *Anxiety*
   Client perceives threat to self-concept and lacks trust in new environment and strangers
2. *Impaired verbal communication*
   Client withdraws and refuses to speak or becomes argumentative over the precise meanings of words; either pattern of communication disrupts usual flow of conversation
3. *Coping, ineffective individual*
   Client demonstrates distortion or confusion of roles, difficulty making decisions, destructive behavior, and inappropriate use of defense mechanisms
4. *Powerlessness*
   Issues of control are manifest in client's interactions; client has heightened awareness of need to control
5. *Self-concept, disturbance in*
   Client's negative view of self is often displayed as attack on, or withdrawal from, others; client may inappropriately attempt to direct own treatment
6. *Social isolation*
   Client withdraws from others due to mistrust
7. *Thought processes, alterations in*
   Client has difficulty evaluating reality and problem-solving, has poor judgment, and may have hallucinations or delusions

Possible Nursing Diagnosis

8. *Activity intolerance*
   Client does not tolerate an increase in activity, lacks incentive to participate, and lacks trust in the person asking him to participate
9. *Ineffective family coping*
   Client's history shows evidence of ineffective or abusive relationship with parents, spouse, children
10. *Diversional activity deficit*
    Hospitalized client feels trapped in inpatient unit with nothing he wishes to do
11. *Health maintenance, alterations in*
    Client does not perceive threat to health (*e.g.,*

"There's nothing wrong with me"), resulting in refusal of medications or other therapies

12. *Home maintenance management, impaired because of mental status*
Client exhibits delusional thinking; he doesn't assume usual responsibilities around the home, or he takes control inappropriately

13. *Potential for injury related to perceptual deficit*
Hallucinations may direct or command the client to harm self or others; poor judgment may lead client to put self in dangerous situations

14. *Knowledge deficit*
Client denies his situation or inaccurately perceives his health status; client's anger may interfere with adherence to prescribed health behavior

15. *Mobility, impaired physical*
Client who is physically restrained has impaired mobility

16. *Noncompliance*
Client does not comply with therapeutic regimen due to prior negative experiences with psychiatric personnel, general lack of trust, nontherapeutic environment, unsatisfactory relationship with caregiver, expensive therapy, health beliefs that are different from professional advice, poor self-esteem, or negative side effects from psychotropic medication

17. *Nutrition, alterations in: less than body requirements*
Client believes that food is poisoned, or that staff has slipped unwanted medication into food or drink, and stops eating due to mistrust; if nutritional status changes, client may suffer from alterations in bowel elimination or fluid volume deficit

18. *Parenting, alterations in*
Stress of entire family unit is increased when one member has psychiatric problems

19. *Self-care deficit*
Client is unwilling to eat, bathe, or groom self satisfactorily

20. *Sensory-perceptual alterations*
Psychotropic medications may slow reactions to environment; client undergoes physical isolation if he is in restraints or otherwise secluded from others

21. *Sexual dysfunction*
Client experiences decreased libido or impotence as side effects of some of the psychotropic medications; lack of trust limits selection of sexual partner or hinders sexual performance; hospitalization results in separation from partner

22. *Sleep pattern disturbance*
Hospital environment or anxiety decreases ability to sleep; tranquilizing medication increases sleep or drowsiness

23. *Violence, potential for*
Perceived threat to self-esteem, misperceived messages from others, dysfunctional verbal communication patterns to relieve stress, and hostility lead to violent behaviors; client has history of lack of control or acting-out behavior

Planning

Setting Client Behavior Outcomes

How the nurse assesses the multiple factors involved in the client's expression of suspicious, hostile, and aggressive feelings will determine how she plans appropriate interventions. The client behavior outcomes anticipated for paranoid or acting-out clients are consistent with the stages of growth and development that have been negatively resolved. These client behavior outcomes include the following:

Trust in interpersonal relationships and trust in self, manifested in such ways as following through on commitments or sharing personal information about self in close relationships

Control over the expression of feelings and resultant behavior, manifested in such ways as using assertive statements rather than degrading, hostile comments in difficult interpersonal situations or choosing some form of exercise to dispel energy that has accumulated through frustration or disappointment

Social awareness, manifested in such ways as the ability to describe what co-workers are doing or verbalizing the major events reported in the news

Development of values and conscience, manifested in such ways as discussing a jury verdict from various viewpoints or paying bills on time

In addition to establishing client behavior outcomes to work toward, the nurse plans *secondary prevention activities* designed to intervene with the client's dependency needs, level of anxiety, self-esteem, low frustration tolerance, and physical needs. Planning also takes into account the greater potential for manipulation in relationships with these clients.

Discharge Planning

Discharge planning for paranoid and acting-out clients may involve coordination with social agencies other than mental health facilities; for example, public health agencies, probation departments, and welfare services. New support systems must be developed if a client has exhausted or "worn out" his former supports. Families may be frightened of a returning client if incidents of hostile and aggressive behavior were traumatic and family members have not worked through their feelings.

Paranoid and acting-out clients are likely to have many resistive defenses. They do not feel that their behavior or attitude requires any modification; they demand instead that others change their behavior. Some clients have been through their communities' legal, mental health, and various assistance programs to the extent that workers and officials offering these services are "worn out" by the client. The inclination of some mental health professionals may be to discharge them "to the streets" without referral or follow-up treatment. Other clients may be discharged on the condition that they "get out of town" and cause no further trouble in a particular community. A change of scenery for the client does not, however, alleviate stressors, nor is it a way to decrease impulsive, antisocial behavior. An exception to this is the situation where a person may be removed from a particular community for the purpose of changing friends who trigger certain undesirable behaviors.

Intervention

Nurses are challenged when intervening with clients who demonstrate paranoid and acting-out behavior because these clients frequently also exhibit hostility and resistance. The clients are usually not asking for help from mental health professionals; in fact, they may say directly, "Go away." The nurse who understands the client's sense of inadequacy and inferiority will decode his verbal and nonverbal communications as "go away closer," and therefore she will not be put off by the client's often involuntary status, resistance, and noncompliance.

Primary Prevention

Suspicious, hostile, and aggressive behavior is other-directed, social behavior. Intervention must therefore take into account the social context in which it occurs. *Primary prevention* must be addressed if mental health professionals do not wish to perpetrate conditions which foster this behavior. Our communities are often breeding grounds for continued rage and violence.[9, 28] The insanity of hunger, poverty, unemployment, and overcrowding cannot be accepted as "givens" in society. Strengthening family systems, identifying and treating maternal depression, and preventing and treating child abuse and neglect are specific areas for primary prevention efforts by mental health professionals.[48]

Intervening Before the Outbreak of Aggression

Do studies dealing with decreasing aggression among children have any bearing on reducing the frequency of aggressive behavior in adults? One study showed that aggressive behavior in children could be reduced through decreasing exposure to aggressive models.[18] Similarly, on psychiatric units, could not criticism, bickering, and dissension among staff members be reduced and greater nurturing of clients be provided as a corrective emotional experience? Modeling includes gentle but firm attitudes on the part of staff members and the selection of nonviolent television programming on units.

"An ounce of prevention" is worth more than a pound of cure when it applies to the *prevention of violence* in a psychiatric–mental health facility. Loss of control accompanied by violence always damages self-esteem and interpersonal relationships. Skill in detecting the client's wish for control and the ability to set limits without being punitive are professional hallmarks toward which nurses strive. It greatly reassures clients to know that they will not be allowed to be destructive.

A first step in intervening before the outbreak of aggression is to remember that hostility is a second-level emotion. The nurse constantly assesses the client's feeling tone and then deals with signs of his anxiety or fear that could escalate into angry feelings and behaviors. *Genuineness* and *empathy* are attitudes to be cultivated when working with hostile clients. These attitudes elicit responses which are incompatible with anger or violent acts and may deter such behavior. The nurse also keeps her verbal tone light and matter-of-fact, rather than intense and authoritarian, to avoid challenging or provoking the client who has poor impulse control.

Humor that does not demean the client may be used in some situations to elicit feelings of amusement. Humor is not useful, however, with paranoid clients because it is too likely to be misinterpreted.

The use of humor is demonstrated in the following exchanges:

Client: "Who do you think you are, telling me I seem angry this morning?"

Nurse: "You're saying that, if I were an umpire in a baseball game, that would have been a bad call?"

Client: "If that lady doesn't shut up, I'll punch her lights out."

Nurse: "That would be great on a movie set in some violent scene, but here in the hospital, control is the name of the game."

Case Study 25-1

Inpatient Treatment for an Impulsive and Aggressive Young Adult

Johnny M. was admitted to the psychiatric inpatient unit at the local general hospital for the fifth time in 2 years. Johnny is 23 years old, from a minority ethnic background. He quit school at age 15, supposedly to start working, but he drank and caroused so extensively that he was unable to hold even menial jobs. He spent several short periods of time in the county jail before he was 21 years old. It was during his time in jail that he was first referred for psychiatric observation because he had many physical fights with other inmates; however, when placed in a cell by himself, he was self-destructive. Now, when police pick him up for fighting or destroying property, they bring him to the psychiatric unit rather than booking him into jail. He is often drunk or high on street drugs when he comes to the attention of authorities.

Johnny has an older brother with whom he lives from time to time. When they have a disagreement, one of them throws the other one out. Johnny supports himself on disability checks he gets for a back injury sustained at age 19, when he worked at a construction job for 3 months. He still portrays a "macho" image and has some skill at finding women with whom to live and who are willing to support him for awhile. He was married for 6 months at age 17 and still talks about the girl because "she messed up my head." He stabbed himself when she divorced him.

When the nurse admitting Johnny asked him to comment on his frequent admissions to the psychiatric unit over the past 2 years, he said, "Hey, my friends have split and nobody wants to help me out. Everybody's interested in locking me up and throwing away the key. Only the nurses know there's nothing wrong with me. I think the cops get their kicks out of hassling me." The nurse also noted Johnny's lack of insight, his loneliness, and his use of projection. She decided to ask the treatment team to discuss Johnny's plan of care to try to break the discouraging cycle of admissions.

When the team met the next day, they decided that treatment must include attention to Johnny's psychological needs, his diminishing relationships with family and friends, and his social environment, including the drug culture and lack of job training.

Johnny is an example of the "fuzzy distinction between criminal justice and the mental health systems."[37] Because he bounces from legal system to mental health system to social or disability payment systems, his care has been fragmented, repetitive, and ineffective. Some professionals in each system have been only too glad to pass him to another system because working with him is frustrating.

At this point, the treatment team acknowledged accountability for Johnny's care. They invited Johnny to the team meeting and obtained his permission to contact family members and agency workers. They explained to Johnny that "help" involves working together to move forward, not "passing the buck" and moving in circles. Johnny's loneliness is an emotion from which he cannot escape as he has done in the past. He has finally experienced enough pain to agree to start a new treatment plan. The treatment team has no illusions that Johnny's progress will be rapid or easy to effect. His impulsiveness and hostile-aggressive feelings are habitual and, in response to stress, he is likely to regress to those styles of behaving and feeling.

Questions for Discussion

1. What is the connection between the legal system and the mental health system? What does "accountability" in those systems mean?
2. How are issues of authority, responsibility, trust, and control manifest with the young adult client who displays impulsive and aggressive behavior?
3. Discuss the therapeutic techniques that are useful and those that are noneffective in an initial interview with a client who is toxic on alcohol or street drugs.
4. Describe the new, young, chronic population of psychiatric clients.
5. Formulate a nursing care plan for Johnny M. based on needs and problems identified by the treatment team.

People want to be listened to and understood. When a client is angry, the nurse can reduce his feelings of being threatened and *minimize defensiveness* by restating the feeling and content of what he has communicated.[33] For example, the client says, "I've been in this _____ hospital for 4 days and no one will go to my apartment and get my clothes. I'm being held against my will and I'm going to sue everyone involved on this ward." The nurse might respond, "I hear how frustrated you are to be here and not to believe anyone is doing anything for you."

The initial interview is an important time to try to *defuse anger* and convey the attitude that psychiatric–mental health professionals are willing and able to work with the client. The client may stare angrily at the nurse without speaking. To meet that gaze directly communicates that the nurse is trustworthy. Instead of trying to convince the client of the nurse's friendliness, the nurse portrays professional understanding by commenting on the client's anger and mistrust. Feelings which are brought out into the open can be discussed. If the client tries to control the interview with a myriad of complaints, the nurse refocuses his attention by asking him how the nurse can be of help.[34]

Dealing with Manipulation.

When a client is struggling with the issue of control, the probability increases that he will use manipulation. *Manipulation* is the process of influencing another to meet or comply with one's own needs and wishes, regardless of the needs and wishes of the other.[27] When manipulation exists, the goals of the nurse and the client conflict. If the nurse is manipulated into believing an untrue story about the client or meeting his dependency needs, such as dressing him when he is able to dress himself, the nurse may be ridiculed by peers or counseled to "be more firm" with clients. In this situation the nurse often feels powerless and "used." As a consequence of having been manipulated, many nurses refuse to meet any dependency needs of clients and overreact to clients' need to control interactions. If nurses respond to clients with defensiveness and anger, this cycle continues and sets up barriers to effective communication.

The key to avoiding manipulation is to be as clear as possible about each other's goals; that is, to verbalize conflicts rather than operating from "hidden agendas." The nurse's own annoyance at meeting a client's request or demand is an early clue that manipulation may be occurring. The nurse then asks what is happening in the nurse–client relationship and how she feels about it. Restating what each person wants from the other may correct misperceptions of roles and expectations.

Preventing Loss of Control.

Whenever the nurse feels as though she must be very careful not to upset the client, the nurse may be detecting subtle cues of the client's impending loss of control. In this event, the astute nurse will intervene in one of the following ways:

- Environmental manipulation, by decreasing frightening stimuli or by giving the client more space
- A calm, self-assured, and helpful attitude toward the client, by identifying herself and giving succinct explanations of what is happening or what is expected of the client; allowing the client to "save face" by suggesting alternatives, such as "Let's walk off some of that energy," is more helpful than issuing commands, such as "Stop what you're doing or you'll go into the seclusion room"
- Offering medication, usually the major tranquilizers, which decreases anxiety, agitation, and delusions.[28, 66]

Indications for Medication.

The use of antipsychotics/neuroleptics to help clients control their agitation or rage is a well-established practice, especially on most psychiatric inpatient units, the notable exception being research units conducting drug-free studies. Examples of major tranquilizers used for this purpose are chlorpromazine, trifluoperazine, thioridazine, and haloperidol. Readers are encouraged to review current literature on the pharmacology associated with aggressive behavior. Now being published is information about trials of drugs other than the standard antipsychotics—such as propranolol, carbamazepine, and tryptophan—for use with aggressive patients.[42]

Patients who experience increasing levels of agitation while hospitalized may have prn orders written for them to receive additional doses of antipsychotic medication. Collaboration between physician, nurse, and patient is necessary so that target behaviors are well assessed and documented. Underuse or overuse of prn medications in these cases is a disservice to the patient and impedes the patient in regaining personal behavioral control.

Whenever a nurse gives antipsychotic medication, she should be alert to the potentially fatal complication known as neuroleptic malignant syndrome (NMS) which has symptoms of severe muscle rigidity, hyperpyrexia, and autonomic dysfunctions. Treatment for this syndrome has been the conventional antiparkinsonian agents and dantralene. Bromocriptine has also been used.[62]

It should be noted that paradoxical rage has

been observed in a few individuals receiving benzo-diazepines.[6] Chlordiazepoxide may tend to increase aggressiveness; therefore, it is useful with clients who are inhibited and could benefit from expressing aggression. On the other hand, oxazepam seems to have no effect on aggression and may be a better medication for clients with poor impulse control.[6,23] Initial studies also indicate that lithium may have a reasonably specific antihostility action, but further investigation is needed to confirm that finding.[56,61]

Validating and Expressing Feelings. If the nurse has previously established a therapeutic relationship with the client, she may intervene to prevent the outbreak of aggression by talking with him, usually on a one-to-one basis, to validate assumptions about his feelings. The nurse encourages the client to describe and clarify the present experience to *increase his awareness of feelings* and what triggers them. The nurse then helps the client choose to *express his feelings* in a socially acceptable manner. The nurse may direct the client to sublimate the energy generated by his feelings in a number of activities, or the nurse may role-play with the client the direct expression of feelings in hypothetical situations.[35,48] In these instances the nurse uses the positive aspects of her relationship with the client to neutralize his aggressive drives.[20] (See Chart 25-2.)

Removing Sensory Reinforcement. There are research data to suggest that sensory reinforcement maintains some instances of aggression.[29] The treatment implications of this finding indicate that undesirable behavior may be suppressed by *removing sensory consequences*—for example, by not yelling or acting startled if someone bangs a fist on the table. Or aggressive acts may be replaced with more socially acceptable behavior that still has sensory consequences, as in hitting a pillow or a punching bag, rather than a human.

Decreasing the Client's Suspicious Behavior

The suspicious client is one who uses avoidance, resistance, testing, and manipulation to protect a fragile self. The client will respond more readily to one or two mental health care providers working with him consistently than to a number of different staff members. Gradually he will form relationships with a few significant others. The nurse makes *undemanding, brief contacts* with the client at first, knowing that he needs distance to preserve his sense of self. The client may perceive the approaches of others as attacks.

Maintaining honesty, adhering to a schedule, and following through on commitments made to the suspicious client are important ways for the nurse to increase her credibility. A matter-of-fact, rather than a warm, approach allows the client to set the pace for closeness.[48]

In clients with mixed symptomatology, interventions may not always be clear-cut. For instance, one study found that among later-life (55 years or greater) psychiatric inpatients, there was an interrelationship between symptoms of depression, anxiety, hypochondriasis, and paranoia.[32] Because trust is at the core of the nurse–client relationship, it makes sense that decreasing suspiciousness would be one of the nurse's first goals, so that the patient would become more approachable for working to decrease other symptoms. (See Case Study 25-2, "When Behavior Is Out of Control.")

Counteracting Misperceptions. The nurse does not touch a client who exhibits suspicious behavior. Again, touch may be perceived as an attack, even as a sexual advance or threat, by a delusional client. Likewise, the nurse is careful to do nothing which may be construed as secretive in front of the suspicious client. The nurse is honest in answering questions about medication, which, for example, may be mixed with fruit juice, or any other questions about various treatment approaches. Simple, *straightforward explanations* are best because they provide the client with less material for distortion. The nurse neither whispers in front of the client nor discusses other clients within his hearing range.

Decreasing the Client's Hostile Behavior

The nurse assists the hostile client to move from reliance on external controls to his own internal controls. Nevertheless, the nurse does not hesitate to apply external controls when necessary for safety. If the client's hostility escalates to the level of assaultiveness, psychiatric nursing staff should initiate quick, decisive teamwork. The guiding principle in applying external controls is to assemble and use sufficient staff members to deal with the situation safely. Often, a "show of force" alone will subdue a client who is out of control.

Applying External Controls. On units where there is an increased possibility of physical assaultiveness, such as emergency rooms, intensive care units, and psychiatric inpatient units, all staff should be aware of a general *plan of action* and familiar with their responsibilities should an incident occur. Training staff in defensive and restraining techniques increases staff confidence and decreases staff and patient injuries.[42] There should be a clear, written policy and procedure for seclusion and restraint in every work setting where seclusion and restraint is used as an intervention.

Anxiety is communicated interpersonally; it is

C H A R T   25-2
Therapeutic Dialogue

De-escalating Angry Feelings

The client is sitting alone in the day room of an inpatient unit where several other clients are talking quietly or involved in activities.

Nurse: (approaches client) You've been sitting here for some time by yourself, Mike. I'd like to sit with you now. (sits down)

Client: Ah, get out of here. Just go.

Nurse: You're very firm in that command, Mike. I'm concerned about your feelings being bottled up.

Client: (sarcastic tone of voice) Oh sure, everyone is so concerned about me. (voice becomes louder) Then why did they drag me in here so I'll lose my job?

Nurse: That's a lot to sort out. (continuing in matter-of-fact tone) You don't want to be here, you're upset with someone, and you're afraid you'll lose your job.

Client: If you can solve all that, sister (snicker), you're a better man than I am.

Nurse: Which part of it do you want to tackle first?

Client: I just want you to get out of here and leave me alone before I blow my stack.

Nurse: You haven't blown your stack yet, which shows good control of your behavior. One way to stay in control here is to talk things out a little at a time. For now, how would you like some coffee or juice?

Discussion

When a client "looks" angry, it may be difficult for the nurse to approach him because of the nurse's fear of rejection. In many cases, however, the nurse must assume responsibility for initiating the interaction or the client will remain withdrawn. In this situation, the nurse tells Mike she will sit with him rather than asking his permission to sit; he still has a choice of whether or not he wants to talk. The nurse's metacommunication says, "You are worth my time."

Mike's initial attitude suggests that he may be testing others' concern for him because of prior negative experiences. When the nurse encounters a defensive, angry client, data must be collected regarding his skill in relating to others in the past. The nurse looks for patterns of behavior which indicate that the client is developing a beginning level of trust. During this interaction, Mike continues to "push away"; therefore, the nurse proceeds slowly.

Initially, the nurse informs Mike that she hears his wish to be left alone. The nurse then continues to verbalize her interest in him. Mike's response shows a defensive, victim posture ("they dragged me in here"), which tells the nurse his anxiety level is rising. Again, the nurse uses the communication technique of paraphrasing to list the various ideas Mike has expressed both overtly and covertly. The nurse tries to help Mike focus his thoughts and feelings rather than making global statements.

In the midst of this interaction, the nurse detects Mike's feelings of low self-esteem and of being overwhelmed. Instead of assuming the client's sense of powerlessness, the nurse conveys the idea that he can approach his problems bit by bit. By asking Mike what *he* wants, the nurse conveys to him that, with the nurse's help, he is responsible for setting goals in his treatment.

Mike's response to the nurse's attempt at goal-setting is to push the nurse away again. His response indicates a low level of frustration tolerance to demands placed on him. The nurse recognizes his rising anxiety level for the second time and his need to distance people. The nurse compliments Mike on his control, although it may be tenuous, and makes the covert issue of control overt. It is also necessary for the nurse to educate the client about the unit's expectations for maintaining control. The stated expectations offer the client the alternative of ventilating at his own pace rather than acting-out.

Finally, the nurse gives the client another alternative to his angry posture in her suggestion to use a socially approved means of relaxing. The nurse may use the client's reaction to her offer of coffee or juice for further assessment of whether an alliance is forming.

This interaction shows that nursing interventions do not have to be "heavy" to be therapeutic. In this brief encounter, the nurse was constantly aware of the client's varying anxiety level and his need for increased self-esteem. Nursing interventions, therefore, were directed to those two areas of need while attempting to build rapport and help the client focus on goals.

C H A R T   25-3
Therapeutic Dialogue

Interacting with a Paranoid Client

Nurse: (approaching client on an inpatient unit) Mr. W., It is time to attend group therapy.

Client: Is it recorded?

Nurse: No, Mr. W., there are no tape recorders in the room.

Client: But everything we say right now is being heard through those vents. (points to air conditioning vents near ceiling)

Nurse: Mr. W., those are air conditioning vents to keep the temperature comfortable. You are safe here in the hospital.

Client: They would love to know what I'm saying.

Nurse: Who is "they"?

Client: You'll probably run tell them.

Nurse: Mr. W., I'm Jack, the nurse working with you today at the hospital. You sound anxious. Please tell me how we might work together so that you can feel safe and able to attend activities.

Discussion

The client with whom the nurse is interacting is severely paranoid, as evidenced by his delusional thinking. Many people approach novel situations with caution, but for clients who mistrust, making a choice involving some interpersonal risk is especially frightening.

The nurse approaches the client with a clear, direct statement regarding an activity. Throughout the interaction he clarifies misperceptions in a straightforward but nonargumentative manner. The nurse reaffirms his own identity and assures the client of his safety as necessary. Emphasis is placed on reality-orientation to person and place because the client's delusional thinking may confuse this experience with future fantasies or past memories.

Finally, the nurse externalizes the feeling (in this case, anxiety) that may have precipitated the suspicious sequence. If the client can begin to connect his feeling state with his thought processes, he may begin to understand and to control some of the faulty conclusions he draws.

The nurse does not pursue the global pronoun "they" at this time, because the client's guardedness serves a defensive function and the nurse is working to establish trust. It would be appropriate to do so in another context. Too many questions, especially with no comments or statements interspersed with the questions, are likely to be perceived as attack by the paranoid client.

By focusing on process, or what is happening in the relationship, rather than on content, the nurse avoids the trap of trying to talk a client out of delusional thinking. Instead, he gives feedback and allows the relationship to develop at the client's pace.

---

contagious. During an incident of aggressive behavior, everyone's adrenalin seems to flow. It is the nurse's responsibility to manage anxiety levels and especially to keep herself in a mild to moderate range of anxiety. At all times staff members strive to *maintain the client's self-esteem*. The nurse's attitude of being authoritative rather than authoritarian, and of setting limits rather than punishing, is the medium through which the client's self-esteem is maintained.

When the client returns to a moderate level of anxiety, the nurse clarifies with him what occurred, what feelings were involved, and what might be learned from the situation. The nurse uses this problem-solving approach with all clients who are capable of learning from their behavior. The nurse conveys the message: "Your behavior was or is unacceptable, but you are acceptable."[48]

Use of Restraints and Seclusion. Several treatment alternatives exist for intervention in assaultive behavior. Medications, physical restraints, and seclusion rooms may be used separately or in combination, according to protocols in given treatment settings. The 1982 Supreme Court decision in *Youngberg v. Romeo* held that the professional decision to seclude or restrain a patient is presumptively valid and that liability for secluding or restraining a patient may be imposed only when the professional's decision is a substantial departure from accepted professional judgment, practice, or standards.[58]

Case Study 25-2

When Behavior Is Out of Control

Joe K. was admitted for the first time to the psychiatric inpatient unit at a local general hospital. He was a freshman at the community college, living at home, when his parents noticed increasingly bizarre behavior. The incident precipitating hospitalization occurred at the dinner table when Joe rambled on and on praying before the evening meal. When his 14-year-old sister made a sarcastic remark interrupting him, he attempted to choke her, saying that she was "possessed by Satan." Attempts by his parents to calm him after physically pulling him away from his sister were futile. Joe began threatening them also, and the police were called.

Joe's father accompanied Joe and the police to the emergency room and finally to the hospital unit for inpatient treatment. Joe was given antipsychotic medication in the E.R. and was quietly mumbling to himself when he arrived on the unit 1 hour later. Joe was shown to his room by a nurse and introduced to a roommate. The nurse said she would leave and return in a few minutes with a unit handbook and would do Joe's admission interview at that time.

When the nurse returned with the admission packet she witnessed Joe being held by his father to prevent him from leaving the room. Joe began yelling threats, the nurse called for assistance, three more staff responded, and Joe was carried to the seclusion room. Joe's father remained in the room, crying. The nurse ob-

tained an order for seclusion and for antipsychotic medication. As she gave Joe the medication she explained that she knew Joe was frightened and needed to regain control of his behavior. She further explained that Joe was now in a hospital and could not leave at present.

Questions for Discussion

1. What needs does Joe's family have at this time and how might they best be met?
2. What factors influence a decision to place a patient in a particular room upon admission? How might the presence of a roommate have affected Joe's response?
3. What indicators of dangerous behavior did Joe exhibit? (Consider thinking and perception, motor activity, mood or affect, physical state and context.)
4. What could the nurse have done differently initially?
5. What is legally involved whenever a patient is placed in seclusion?
6. Formulate a nursing care plan for Joe including short-term and long-term behavior outcomes, Joe's strengths, and the nursing interventions useful in using Joe's strengths to help him reach the desired outcomes.
7. Suggest possible staff and patient reactions to Joe based on his behavior on admission.

The reported incidence of restraint or seclusion ranges from 3.6% to 51% and seems to vary most based on the composition of the patient population and the treatment philosophy of the unit. Short-term crisis intervention units generally have higher seclusion rates than private units accepting only voluntary patients.[58] One study found that during evening and night shifts, staff use seclusion rooms more frequently than do staff on day shifts. Also, shifts which are staffed primarily with female employees use seclusion more often than shifts staffed primarily with male employees. Seclusion is, in effect, an "intensive care environment" in which the client requires additional monitoring and staff involvement.[12,52]

The purposes of seclusion and restraint are containment of injurious actions, isolation to reduce difficult interpersonal relationships, and decreased

sensory input to relieve sensory overload.[67] When a patient's behavior is so unsafe or out of control that seclusion and restraint must be used, one staff member acts as the team leader and directs the actions of everyone else according to established and practiced routines. The leader will tell the patient what is occurring and why, keeping verbalizations concise and matter-of-fact in tone. Other members of the team will be assigned limbs to safely hold and transport the patient to the seclusion room or to apply restraints. Restrictive therapies must have clear guidelines and a physician's order for continued use.

Terminating the use of seclusion rooms or restraints must depend on objective criteria, rather than on the arbitrary feeling states of the nursing staff. Criteria for release from restraint or seclusion may be grouped in the following categories:

Psychomotor agitation, assessed by means of decreased restlessness, lowered blood pressure, and pulse rate

Stabilization of mood, assessed by means of absence of physical threats, lowered anxiety level, consistency of verbal and nonverbal behavior, and feelings of trust in staff

Cognitive processes, assessed by means of insight and ability to look at precipitating incident in objective manner, increased ability to concentrate, and improved reality-testing[67]

Nursing intervention with a client who is hostile but not assaultive may require "waiting him out." Karen Horney conceptualized all behavior as motivated by the desire to move toward, move away from, or move against someone else. When we assess the angry client as moving against us in a self-defensive maneuver, we can show a willingness to listen and demonstrate respect and caring for the individual.[45] When we assure the client that he is safe with us, his defensive, hostile behavior often subsides.

Exploring and Controlling Angry Behavior.
The nurse may observe various types of hostile behavior exhibited by psychiatric–mental health clients. A *grandiose* client may state, "When I get out of here, I'll buy a decent hospital for anyone who wants to be admitted," implying that the present treatment is inadequate. The client with *hyperreligiosity* may become angered when others challenge his claims to be a deity or disagree with his interpretation of theology. Likewise, the client who is a *champion of causes* arouses hostility when followers are not forthcoming. Lastly, the client, seen especially in involuntary settings, with a *propensity for litigation* can be verbally threatening to psychiatric staff members who, in turn, often react in a defensive, sarcastic, or placating manner. A guiding principle of intervention with each of these hostile clients is to avoid power struggles and, instead, to focus on establishing a therapeutic alliance in which trust and learning occur.

Although the nurse may assess a client as angry or hostile, the client may not be aware of those emotions or may deny them. In trying to validate her perceptions, the nurse uses terms such as "You seem upset (or irritated, or frustrated)," rather than "You seem angry (or mad)," because the latter terms are emotionally loaded words which provoke an even more intense reaction.[57] Helping clients *explore their anger* is often a lengthy process and involves a great deal of reteaching, redirecting, and resetting of priorities.

Research on cognitive techniques to control anger has found that it is important to *remain task-oriented* when faced with a provocation.[47] Less anger is aroused if one defines a situation as a problem that calls for a solution, rather than as a threat that calls for an attack. Early recognition of arousal is also an important principle of anger control. The further a person has progressed into the provocation sequence, the less likely he is to initiate effective self-control.[47]

Behavior therapists may help a client become more aware of angry feelings by asking him to count the number of times each day that he experiences the feeling of irritation or anger, no matter how slight the feeling. To understand better what triggers the feelings, the therapist then asks the client to describe the situations surrounding these incidents. *Imagery* and *role-playing* are other techniques by which an individual may become more aware of his feelings and may practice his responses in given situations.[38]

Frequently the nurse is the recipient of the client's hostility. If the nurse's actions have led to the client's angry response, it is helpful to let him ventilate those emotions directly. Often, however, the nurse is a victim of displaced anger, and the nurse can point out to the client that she is not the correct target by saying, "I seem to be getting intense feelings from you that may belong somewhere else." At times the client reacts with hostility to the nurse because the nurse symbolizes the rules and regulations of the therapeutic regimen. The nurse should then recognize the importance of the issue of control and provide the client with *opportunities to exercise choice*—for example, on daily menus, in requesting passes from inpatient units, or in voluntary participation in selected activities.

Decreasing Antisocial Behavior

Interventions with impulsive, acting-out behavior often call for the application of *external controls* prior to initiating the problem-solving aspect of the therapeutic process. The nurse's aim is not to help the client resolve unconscious conflicts, but to support his basic needs regarding dependency and fear of intimacy. Due to developmental deficits in the character of the person with impulsive behavior, therapy with this individual is likely to be a long-term process incorporating education about mature ways of handling stressors.

Because the impulsive person is often oblivious to anxiety as a warning that something is amiss in interpersonal relationships, the nurse must *give feedback* to the impulsive client about the consequences of his behavior, any self-destructive results, and the social reality in which the behavior took place.[10] *Offering alternatives,* rather than telling him to stop a certain behavior, helps the impulsive client retain a sense of freedom and choice, which is essential in helping him take control of and responsibility for his actions.

Modeling Communication. Communication skills of clients with impulsive behavior are notoriously poor. Why else would these individuals act-out, rather than talk out, conflicts? Indeed, the nurse intervenes by *modeling the expression of feelings,* especially those feelings regarding the effect a client's behavior has on the nurse and others.[66]

Needs versus Wants. One interesting approach to clients with impulsive behavior is to demonstrate to them that their impulsive actions are often the result of thoughts that confuse "need" and "want" statements. "I need something and therefore I should have it" is often substituted for "I want something and will be frustrated not to have it." When wants become needs, the person may feel that he is no longer responsible for behavior necessary to fulfill those needs. On the other hand, wants are preferences one can choose to act upon or not. Such patterns are pointed out in rational–emotive therapy, a form of cognitive therapy.[64,65] *Challenging need/want confusion* may help a client redefine a situation, thereby eliciting new or different emotions. It is one way to help a client learn to tolerate anxiety.

Group therapy is often a more desirable treatment modality than one-to-one therapy with clients who use antisocial behaviors, because their manipulative style, which is often very draining on one therapist, can be diluted or exposed in group settings. Peer pressure for socially acceptable behavior is an effective method of treatment.[8]

Whenever acting-out behavior occurs, the nurse should examine her own behavior in relation to the client. Inadvertently, the nurse may encourage or reinforce acting-out behavior by being very angry or very pleased with the client's behavior. The nurse asks herself how provocative she is being with the client.[8] New rules and limits may be needed.

Evaluation

Evaluation of nursing interventions with clients demonstrating suspicious, hostile, and aggressive behavior takes into account the following factors:

Was the behavior controlled although feelings may have been intense?
Was everyone's safety maintained?
Did symptoms of paranoia and acting-out decrease?
Did the client and nurse learn any problem-solving techniques for handling these behaviors in the future?
Was the client's self-esteem maintained?

The nurse's effectiveness in evaluating what occurs in nurse–client relationships involving anger, suspicion, and impulsivity often depends on the nurse's self-awareness or recognition of these emotions in herself. While evaluating nursing interventions, the nurse is also reassessing client behavior and beginning the nursing process again.

Nurses working in outpatient settings may evaluate their interventions in supervisory conferences. Informal chats with colleagues or formal staff conferences on inpatient units should be used to discuss the effectiveness of various forms of intervention. By answering questions like the five listed above, nurses can analyze techniques and feelings and propose alternative behaviors to improve the outcomes in future situations. For example, during a mental health team conference, the staff members may discuss the fact that, when a client was restrained in leather restraints, his safety was assured and dangerous behavior was stopped but his suspicious symptoms increased. Therefore, the staff might decide that fear was an important motivator of the client's acting-out behavior. Closer observation of the client and assurances to him of his safety are needed to prevent his further acting-out.

Nurse's Feelings and Attitudes

The qualities most useful in working with paranoid and aggressive clients are nondefensiveness, realism, acceptance, consistency, and kind firmness.[48] However, when a client is noncompliant and defiant, the nurse is likely to react with uncomfortable, if not negative, feelings. It is frustrating not to have clients welcome our good intentions to help. If nurses remember, however, that the client is in the treatment setting because of such defensive behavior, they are less likely to insist that he relinquish his defensiveness as a condition of treatment.[28]

The nurse should neither ignore defensive symptoms nor run from them. The client who says in an angry tone, "Go on and talk to some other poor fellow who really needs help," challenges the nurse to pass him by. Instead of leaving him, the nurse may suggest, "Let's get to know each other without focusing on problems." In this way, the nurse offers an interaction wherein the client can feel comfortable.

Some nurses have great difficulty saying "no" to clients. Their own need to be liked by others overrides their ability to be firm. If the nurse vacillates and conciliates aggressive clients, the client gains control. If the nurse reacts kindly and with submissive reassurance, the client may become passively dependent.[7] For example, the client who tests the nurse with requests or demands for special privileges often reacts to fulfillment of each one by asking another favor. The nurse readily feels manipulated in these situ-

Nursing Care Plan 25-1

The Client Who Is Hostile and Suspicious

Nursing Diagnosis	Client Behavior Outcome	Intervention
Alterations in motor behavior, restlessness, or unpredictable behavior	Maintain self-control, *e.g.*, the client will sit in activities for minimum of 1/2 hour, or the client will discuss precedents to anxiety, or the client will choose one form of exercise and complete same for 20 min. each A.M. and P.M.	Reduce environmental stimulation Encourage verbalization of feelings Suggest diversional activities that channel energy constructively Approach in a calm manner Offer medication to decrease agitation
Alterations in conduct/impulse control	Maintain safety of self and others, *e.g.*, the client will distinguish verbally his thoughts from the need to act on all thoughts, or the client will seek out staff and request time away from others in order to de-escalate violent feelings, or the client will comply with medication regimen as prescribed	Ensure adequate numbers of staff to contain behavior Reduce environmental stimulation Provide chemical or mechanical restraints Establish one-to-one interaction with staff members involved in the client's violent episode, after behavior is controlled, to review incident for learning
Alterations in communication, not verbalizing feelings, manipulating others	Be direct in communication, *e.g.*, the client will state his feelings in a given situation, or the client will directly ask for what he wants or needs	Clearly define the nurse–client relationship Discuss behavioral expectations and consequences Encourage discussion of feelings by role-modeling Acknowledge and reward open communication
Impaired family role, dependence excess	Make decisions and accept responsibility for actions, *e.g.*, the client will set goals for therapy and write his own progress note at specified times, or the client will respond in helpful manner to others in group therapy, or the client will ask for help from others no more than one time per hour	Initiate frequent interactions, especially during initial phase of relationship Recognize "pseudo-independence" or distancing in relationship as reaction formation to unmet needs
Compulsive behavior, drug abuse	Abstain from drug use, *e.g.*, the client will comply with detoxification routine, or the client will inform significant others of	Follow medical detoxification regimen Encourage satisfying interpersonal relationships Initiate referral to rehabilitation

(Continues on p. 460)

Nursing Diagnosis	Client Behavior Outcome	Intervention
	need to abstain from all nonprescription drugs, or the client will attend AA or NA meetings	program and follow-up with referral
Alterations in perception, delusions and hallucinations	Maintain reality orientation, *e.g.,* the client will ask for medication as "voices" become more intense, the client will be oriented to person, place, time and situation, or the client will write a structured plan for activity and rest to follow daily	Use calm, directive, nonthreatening approach Follow through consistently on commitments to client Make undemanding, frequent, brief contacts with client Present nurse's reality in matter-of-fact tone and manner Comment on client's safety but recognize presence of his fear Orient client to person, place, time, and situation Connect feeling to situation at the onset of the feeling Encourage reality-oriented conversation and activities
Impaired emotional experience: excess of dominant emotions	Maintain a tolerable range of feeling, *e.g.,* the client will discuss feelings for maximum of 15 min. with staff each shift, or the client will engage in prearranged activity when feelings start to become strong, or the client will list thoughts he has when experiencing an intense feeling and discuss those thoughts with therapist	Approach in calm, nonthreatening manner Role-model appropriate verbalization of feeling Tolerate deviant expressions of affect in place of acting-out behavior Instruct client that feelings do not have to lead to bizarre or destructive behaviors Provide opportunities for alternative activities to release energizing force of feelings
Alterations in self-concept; impaired self-esteem	Maintain positive self-esteem, *e.g.,* the client will accept positive feedback from others, saying only "thank you," or the client will reward self daily for some action or thought, or the client will list those things that enhance his self-esteem, or the client will practice a specified new behavior, use the new behavior with others, and evaluate results with staff	Avoid mutual withdrawal between nurse and client Encourage and accept expression of thoughts and feelings Provide opportunities to problem-solve instead of acting impulsively Practice new behaviors in role-rehearsal or role-playing situations Give merited praise and recognition Discuss behaviors in their perspective Provide opportunities for client to experience success
Age-inappropriate behavior, pseudomature behavior as seen by low frustration tolerance	Be able to delay gratification, *e.g.,* the client will notify staff when feeling impulsive so alternative behaviors can be realized,	Provide supportive relationship Gradually increase responsibility at client's pace Promote awareness of feeling states that are warning signals of im-

Nursing Diagnosis	Client Behavior Outcome	Intervention
	or the client will develop a written plan of things to do when feeling impulsive, or the client will identify situations that usually lead to feelings of frustration and discuss ways to avoid these situations or learn to cope differently with them	pulsive or explosive behaviors Discuss alternative behaviors when warning signals occur

(From Loomis M et al: Classification of Individual Human Responses of Concern for Psychiatric/Mental Health Nursing Practice, Working Draft, American Nurses' Association, 1986)

ations. The nurse may avoid feelings of powerlessness by meeting the client's dependency needs while voicing the expectation that, gradually, he will assume more and more responsibility for meeting his own needs.

If the nurse assesses that a power struggle exists, she next identifies anxiety levels and needs.[51] Is the client asking for more limits? Is the client testing to see what controls are present? In what ways can the nurse help the client maintain control? It is best to make the covert issue overt. The nurse may tell the client that she is not interested in power struggles. She may state that she would like to see the client remain in control. She can also compliment the client on whatever degree of control he can maintain, however tenuous that control.

Psychiatry and psychiatric–mental health nursing rely on verbal rather than physical abilities. Because nursing is still primarily a female profession and women are not sanctioned to be physically aggressive in our society, many nurses have highly emotional reactions when they need to restrain a client using touching and holding. Anticipatory guidance, or talking through possible feelings, is one way to help nurses deal with this experience of restraining clients.

In the face of aggressive or assaultive behavior the universal response of all of us is fear. Feeling the fear and understanding what it signals can direct a nurse to action. Possible outcomes of this experience of fear include the following:

Countertransference reactions, due to angry feelings, leading to limit-setting without talking-through behavior, as in authoritarian relationships
Manifest anxiety reactions, due to helpless feelings, leading to flight from the situation
A therapeutic reaction or vigilance for the oppor-

tunity to teach and learn about thoughts, feelings, and behaviors.[10, 28]

Obviously, the third outcome is the most desirable.

When afraid, the nurse may "come down hard" on the client in an attacking manner, avoid any confrontation, or approach the feared stimulus in a problem-solving manner. The choices open to us when faced with stressors are the same as those of our clients. Our professional expertise and use of the nursing process help us achieve favorable outcomes even in difficult situations.

Summary

This chapter has discussed the wide range, the intensity of feelings, and the minor to severe ramifications of suspicious, hostile, and aggressive behaviors. The twofold orientation of the chapter focuses first on the development and maintenance of these feelings and behaviors and secondly on the application of the nursing process to the care of clients exhibiting paranoid and acting-out disorders. This chapter includes the following points:

1. Etiological theories from diverse frameworks are advanced to explain the origins of suspicious, hostile, and aggressive behavior and to guide intervention strategies.
2. The dynamics of hostility and suspiciousness, impulsivity and acting-out, and anger and aggression explain the "how" and "why" of these behaviors.
3. The nurse assessing the client with paranoid or acting-out disorders gathers information about altered cognitive or perceptual states, increased psychomotor activity, altered mood

or affect, environmental factors causing increased anxiety levels, and history of poor impulse control or drug abuse.

4. The nurse determines the client's ability to remain in control of his behavior.

5. In planning treatment, the nurse and client choose desired client behavior outcomes based on the needs for trusting relationships, social responsibility, and increased self-esteem.

6. Defusing and de-escalating rising feeling states and supporting the client who attempts to control his behavior in socially sanctioned ways are preferable to reactionary handling of aggressive incidents.

7. When control is an issue, manipulation is a possibility.

8. A blending of the nurse's theoretical orientation with the client's needs leads to interpersonal, behavioral, or cognitive interventions.

9. As a member of the multidisciplinary mental health team, the nurse communicates her observations and interventions to other team members toward the goal of maintaining a consistent, holistic approach to the client.

10. Working with suspicious, hostile, and aggressive clients taps surface and deep emotions in the nurse and other mental health care providers.

11. Evaluation entails a close examination of both client and nurse to determine whether client behavior outcomes were met and to decide what nursing skills and attitudes might be more effective in helping delusional and acting-out clients reach their desired outcomes.

References

1. American Psychiatric Association: Diagnostic and Statistical Manual of Mental Disorders, 3d ed, rev. Washington, DC, 1987

2. Bacy-y-Rita G et al: Episodic Control: A Study of 130 Violent Patients. Am J Psychiatry 127, 1473–1478, 1971

3. Bandura A: Aggression, A Social Learning Analysis. Englewood Cliffs, NJ, Prentice-Hall, 1973

4. Bandura A, Ross D, Ross SA: Imitation of Film-Mediated Aggressive Models. J Abnorm Soc Psychol 66, 3–11, 1963

5. Barrett JE, DiMascio A: Comparative Effects on Anxiety of the 'Minor Tranquilizers' in 'High' and 'Low' Anxious Student Volunteers. Diseases of the Nervous System 27, 483–486, 1966

6. Bowlby J: Attachment and Loss: Attachment, Vol I. New York, Basic Books, 1969

7. Carney FL: Outpatient Treatment for the Aggressive Offender. Am J Psychotherapy 31 (April): 265–274, 1977

8. Carter FM: Psychosocial Nursing, 3d ed. New York, Macmillan, 1981

9. Chwast J: Psychotherapy of Disadvantaged Acting-Out Adolescents. Am J Psychotherapy 31 (April): 216–226, 1977

10. Clack J: Nursing Intervention into the Aggressive Behavior of Patients. In Burd SF, Marshall MA (eds): Some Clinical Approaches to Psychiatric Nursing, pp 199–205. New York, Macmillan, 1963

11. Clancy J et al: The Hostile-Dependent Personality. Post-Grad Med 55, 109, 1974

12. Convertino K, Pinto RP, Fiester AR: Use of Inpatient Seclusion at a Community Mental Health Center. Hosp Community Psychiatry 31 (December): 848–850, 1980

13. DeMeyer-Gapin S, Scott TJ: Effect of Stimulus Novelty on Stimulation Seeking in Antisocial and Neurotic Children. J Abnorm Psychol 86 (January): 96–98, 1977

14. DiFabio S: Nurses' Reactions to Restraining Patients. Am J Nurs 81 (May): 973–975, 1981

15. Durkheim E: The Rules of the Sociological Method. New York, Free Press, 1938

16. Eron, LD: Prescription for Reduction of Aggression. Am Psychol 35 (March): 244–252, 1980

17. Eron LD: Relationship of TV Viewing Habits and Aggressive Behavior in Children. J Abnorm Soc Psychol 67, 193–196, 1963

18. Eron LD, Walder LO, Lefkowitz MM: Learning of Aggression in Children. Boston, Little, Brown, 1971

19. Fagan TJ, Lira FT: The Primary and Secondary Sociopathic Personality: Differences in Frequency and Severity of Antisocial Behaviors. J Abnorm Psychol 89, 493–496, 1980

20. Fareta G: A Profile of Aggression from Adolescence to Adulthood: An 18-Year Follow-Up of Psychiatrically Disturbed and Violent Adolescents. Am J Orthopsychiatry 51 (July): 439–453, 1980

21. Freud S: Collected Papers of Sigmund Freud, E Jones (ed). New York, Basic Books, 1959

22. Fromm E: Man for Himself. New York, Holt, Rinehart and Winston, 1947

23. Gardos G et al: Differential Actions of Chlordiazepoxide and Oxazepam on Hostility. Arch Gen Psychiatry 18, 757–760, 1968

24. Gawin FH: Neuroleptic Reduction of Cocaine-Induced Paranoia But Not Euphoria? Psychopharmacology 90(1): 142–143, 1986

25. Gerta B: Training for Prevention of Assaultive Behavior in a Psychiatric Setting. Hosp Community Psychiatry 31 (Sept.): 628–630, 1980

26. Gluck M: Learning a Therapeutic Verbal Response to Anger. J Psychiatric Nurs Ment Health Serv 19 (March): 9–12, 1981

27. Grace HK, Camilleri D: Mental Health Nursing, A Socio-Psychological Approach, 2d ed. Dubuque, IA, WC Brown, 1981

28. Haber J et al: Comprehensive Psychiatric Nursing. New York, McGraw-Hill, 1978

29. Hayes SC, Rincover A, Valosin D: Variables Influencing the Acquisition and Maintenance of Aggressive Behavior: Modeling Versus Sensory Reinforcement. J Abnorm Psychol 89, 254–262, 1980

30. Hays DA: Anger: A Clinical Problem. In Burd SF, Marshall MA (eds): Some Clinical Approaches to Psychiatric Nursing, pp 110–115. New York, Macmillan, 1963

31. Horney K: The Neurotic Personality of Our Time. New York, WW Norton, 1937

32. Hyer L et al: Depression, Anxiety, Paranoid Reactions, Hypochondriasis, and Cognitive Decline of Later-Life Inpatients. J Gerontol 42(1): 92–94, 1987

33. Johnson DW: Effects of Warmth of Interaction, Accuracy of Understanding and the Proposal of Compromises on Listener's Behavior. J Counseling Psychology 18 (March): 207–216, 1971

34. Kaplan HI, Sadock BJ: Modern Synopsis of Comprehensive Textbook of Psychiatry/III, 3d ed. Baltimore, Williams & Wilkins, 1981

35. Kiening Sister M: Hostility. In Carlson C, Blackwell B (eds): Behavioral Concepts and Nursing Intervention 2d ed, pp 128–140. Philadelphia, JB Lippincott, 1978

36. Kopp S: An End to Innocence: Facing Life Without Illusions. New York, Macmillan, 1978

37. Kratcoski PC: Youth Violence Directed Toward Significant Others. J Adolescence 8(2): 145–157, 1985

38. Lanyon RI, Lanyon BP: Behavior Therapy: A Clinical Introduction. Reading, MA, Addison-Wesley, 1978

39. Lidz T: A Developmental Approach to Problems of Acting-Out, E Rexford (ed), pp 6–17. New York, International Universities Press, 1966

40. Luckey JW, Berman JJ: Effects of New Commitment Laws on the Mental Health System. Am J Orthopsychiatry 51 (July): 479–483, 1981

41. McCord W, McCord J, Howard A: Familial Correlates of Aggression in Non-Delinquent Male Children. J Abnorm Soc Psychol 62, 79–93, 1961

42. Maier GJ et al: A Model for Understanding and Managing Cycles of Aggression Among Psychiatric Inpatients. Hosp Community Psychiatry, 38(5): 520–524, 1987

43. Mark VH, Neville R: Brain Surgery in Aggressive Behavior. JAMA 226, 765–772, 1973

44. Moyer KE: The Psychobiology of Aggression. New York, Harper and Row, 1976

45. Murray R: What to Do with Crying, Clinging Demanding, Seductive, Abusive and Withdrawn Patients. Nursing Life (September/October): 32–39, 1981

46. Nashby W, Hayden B, DePaulo BM: Attributional Bias Among Aggressive Boys to Interpret Unambiguous Social Stimuli as Displays of Hostility. J Abnorm Psychol 89, 459–468, 1980

47. Novaco RW: Anger Control: The Development and Evaluation of an Experimental Treatment. Lexington, MA, D.C. Heath, 1975

48. Pasquali EA et al: Mental Health Nursing: A Bio-Psycho-Cultural Approach. St. Louis, CV Mosby, 1981

49. Pihl RO et al: Attribution and Alcohol-Mediated Aggression. J Abnorm Psychol 90, 468–475, 1980

50. Quay HC: Psychopathic Personality as Pathological Stimulation-Seeking. Am J Psychiatry 122, 180–183, 1965

51. Richter JM: Power Struggle in the Clinical Setting. In Kneisel CR, Wilson HS (eds): Current Perspectives in Psychiatric Nursing: Issues and Trends, pp 115–122. St. Louis, CV Mosby, 1978

52. Rosen H, DiGiacomo JN: The Role of Physical Restraint in the Treatment of Psychiatric Illness. J Clin Psychiatry 39 (March): 228–232, 1978

53. Rosenbaum M, Hadari D: Personal Efficacy, External Locus of Control, and Perceived Contingency of Parental Reinforcement Among Depressed, Paranoid, and Normal Subjects. J Perso Soc Psychol 49(2): 539–47, 1985

54. Roth M: Human Violence as Viewed from the Psychiatric Clinic. Am J Psychiatry 128, 397–407, 1972

55. Rubin B: Prediction of Dangerousness in Mentally Ill Criminals. Arch Gen Psychiatry 17, 397–407, 1972

56. Sheard MH: Effect of Lithium on Human Aggression. Nature 230, 113–114, 1971

57. Smitherman C: Nursing Actions for Health Promotion. Philadelphia, FA Davis, 1981

58. Soloff PH, Gutheil TG, Wexler DB: Seclusion and Restraint in 1985: A Review and Update. Hosp Community Psychiatry 36(6): 652–657, 1985

59. Speck RV, Attneave CL: Family Networks. New York, Pantheon Books, 1973

60. Szurek S: Childhood Origins of Psychopathic Personality Trends. In Berlin IN, Szurek SA (eds): The Antisocial Child: His Family and His Community, pp 2–12. Palo Alto, CA, Science and Behavior Books, 1969

61. Tupin JP et al: The Long-Term Use of Lithium in Aggressive Prisoners. Compr Psychiatry 14, 311–317, 1973

62. Verhoeven WM, Elderson A, Westenberg HG: Neuroleptic Malignant Syndrome: Successful Treatment with Bromocriptine. Biol Psychiatry 20(6): 680–684, 1985

63. Walters RH, Willows DC: Imitative Behavior of Disturbed and Non-Disturbed Children Following Exposure to Aggressive and Non-Aggressive Models. Child Dev 39, 79–89, 1968

64. Watkins JT: The Rational-Emotive Dynamics of Impulsive Disorders. In Ellis A, Greiger R (eds): Handbook of Rational-Emotive Therapy, pp 135–152. New York, Springer, 1977

65. Whaley M, Ramirez L: The Use of Seclusion Rooms and Physical Restraints in the Treatment of Psychiatric Patients. J Psychiatr Nurs Ment Health Serv 18 (January): 13–16, 1980

66. Wilson HS, Kneisl CR: Psychiatric Nursing. Menlo Park, CA, Addison-Wesley, 1979

26 Substance Abuse: The Drug Dependencies

Barbara A. Thurston

O God that men should put an enemy in their mouths to steal away their brains: that we should with joy, pleasance, revel and applause, transform ourselves into beasts.

Othello

Chapter Preview

This chapter deals with the topic of substance abuse and dependency. It discusses the use of substances that affect the central nervous system and the physical and behavioral changes that occur in individuals who abuse and become dependent on them.

These substances are classified as drugs. The generic meaning of the term drug, which includes the substance ethyl alcohol (ethanol), is used in this chapter. Because of the socially acceptable status of alcohol, this substance frequently does not elicit as forceful a relationship to drug classification as the image produced by the mention of an illegal drug, such as heroin, or even prescription drugs, such as barbiturates or amphetamines. Nevertheless, the substance alcohol, by its properties and actions, is a drug and needs to be treated as such.

There are factors that all drugs of abuse and dependency have in common, as well as factors that are specific to each drug. This chapter addresses both those commonalities of substance abuse and dependency and the specific factors particular to each drug classification. Wherever possible, however, the emphasis is on the common concepts. This generic concept embraces the idea that the problem of abuse/dependency of a substance and manifestations resulting from the abuse may differ. For example, the manifestations of dependence on heroin differ from those of dependence on alcohol, but the core problem remains the same; that is, the fact that there is abuse of, or dependence on, a substance.

Individuals who abuse or become dependent on substances are impaired physically, socially, and psychologically at some time in the course of their disorder. The behavior manifested by persons abusing drugs is not tolerated or accepted in most cultures. Prolonged abuse of, or dependency on, drugs and the concomitant adverse behavioral changes that affect the individual's life and well-being usually culminate in a self-destructive course unless the substance use is discontinued or the individual's lifestyle is altered. Ultimately, drug-dependent individuals must learn to adapt to the stresses of life with means other than the abuse of drugs.

This chapter examines systems of classification of substance abuse and dependency and various concepts related to the etiology and dynamics of substance abuse and dependency. A focus of the chapter is the application of the nursing process to individuals who abuse or are dependent on drugs.

Learning Objectives

After completion of the chapter, you should be able to accomplish the following:

1. Discuss the application of Selye's theory of stress and adaptation to the problems of substance abuse and dependency
2. Define substance abuse and dependency and explain current diagnostic categorization
3. Differentiate among various types of substance abuse/dependency disorders
4. Discuss the common etiologic concepts related to substance abuse and dependency
5. Discuss the incidence and significance of substance abuse and dependency
6. Describe the dynamics, physical effects, behavioral changes, medical consequences, social and family problems, and specific group characteristics of abuse/dependency on alcohol, sedatives, hypnotics, anxiolytics, narcotics, cocaine, amphetamine, and similarly acting sympathomimetics, hallucinogens, and cannabis
7. Apply the components of the nursing process to the client who abuses or who is dependent on substances
8. Recognize the nurse's own feelings and attitudes toward substance abuse and dependency disorders
9. Explain the importance of recognition intervention, rehabilitation, and prevention in the chemically impaired professional
10. Recognize the importance of prevention in the substance abuse dependency as a physiopsychosocial problem on the continuum of human development from the unborn child to the aged adult

Stress and Adaptation and Substance Abuse

Hans Selye's stress/adaptation syndrome may be applied to problems of substance abuse and dependency, with implications for the treatment and rehabilitation of drug-dependent individuals. (See Chap. 1 for a fuller discussion of Selye's theory of stress and adaptation.)

Stress/Adaptation Syndrome

Stress, says Selye, is "the nonspecific response of the body to any demand made upon it."[81] Clearly, the source of the stress and the pleasantness or unpleasantness of the agent or situation of stress do not matter. What does matter is the intensity of the demand for adaptation or readjustment.

Stressors, or stress-producing factors, differ in various situations and in the responses they elicit from individuals. Stressors may originate from physical, chemical, physiological, biologic, and emotional sources. They may arise from the internal or external environment of the individual.

The General Adaptation Syndrome (GAS) is composed of the following three stages:

1. *Alarm stage.* The body recognizes the internal or external stress that affects its physiological homeostasis, and then prepares to resist by means of "fight or flight."
2. *Stage of resistance.* The body uses the defense mechanisms of "fight or flight" to repair the damage it suffered and/or to adapt to the stressor. If the body is unable to adapt, it will enter the third stage; if the individual adapts to the stressor, the third stage is prevented.
3. *Stage of exhaustion.* If this stage of fatigue continues, physical or emotional diseases of adaptation (migraine headache, mental disorder) may occur. If this stage is not reversed, the body will be unable to adapt and will become exhausted, and death will ensue.[80,81]

"Fight or Flight" Mechanisms

Selye emphasizes the importance of making good use of adaptation energy to prevent the diseases of adaptation. The defense mechanisms of "fight or flight" may be applied to interpersonal relationships as well as to physiological problems. That is, a person may manage interpersonal stress by running away from or passively waiting out a situation he cannot change. The choice of the proper defense, however, needs to be tailored to each situation.

To remind himself how to use these adaptation mechanisms wisely to achieve his goals, particularly when events threaten his equanimity or cause him concern or doubt, Selye created the following jingle:

> Fight for your highest
> attainable aim.
> But never put up
> resistance in vain.[81]

The process of reflection and choice of an appropriate response for the situation and circumstances may appear simple, but is really a complex task. Selye believes that each person has to live his life as his innate freedom of choice directs.[80,81]

Drug Dependence as a Means of Coping

Applying this theory of stress and proper choice of adaptation methods to the issues of substance abuse and dependency, it is necessary to consider that drug use, abuse, and dependency serve a purpose for the chemical-dependent individual. There are legitimate reasons for the use of many drugs. Ethyl alcohol is a drug and it is also a legal substance with approved recreational and social use. Many people drink alcoholic beverages without encountering problems. Some drugs, such as narcotics and sedatives/hypnotics, are controlled substances and are used for medical purposes to alleviate physical pain and emotional suffering. When taken as prescribed under medical supervision, these drugs may be used to diminish the stress of life without the serious adverse consequences of abuse and dependency.

For the individual who abuses or is dependent on substances, however, drugs have an added function. For these people, the drugs have become a way of coping or adapting to any of life's stressors. In other words, drugs are a "way of life" for these individuals.

The individual who abuses substances, for example, may use drugs to relieve feelings of anxiety or unpleasant feelings of any kind, or to experience and increase pleasant or "high" sensations. Drugs may be used to sustain a world of daydreams or an existence beyond the bounds of reality. Drugs may be used to express feelings of joy, love, anger, or hate—or to repress these emotions. Drugs not only do things *to* people who take them, they also do things *for* people who take them. It is, therefore, important to understand what these substances do for people, in order to effect primary prevention of chemical dependence and to help individuals adapt to, or cope with, the stress of life in a more effective, healthy manner (see Chart 26-1).

Individuals who abuse or are dependent on substances come from all socioeconomic and cultural groups. The spectrum covers all ages, from youth to old age. The reasons for misuse of, abuse of, and dependence on drugs generally include an attempt to adapt to the stress of life. Ironically, the process becomes a vicious cycle, because the method of adapting to life's stressors becomes, itself, another stressor.

The use of drugs as a coping mechanism destroys or diminishes an individual's ability to master life's events. "Letting go" of substance abuse as a method of adaptation and learning healthy methods of adaptation may result in successful recovery from chemical dependence.

C H A R T   26-1
Definition of Terms

Physical Dependence (Addiction):	This is a state that is manifested by withdrawal symptoms (abstinence syndrome) when the drug is removed. This state is frequently accompanied by tolerance, or the frequent taking of a drug or drugs in increased amounts over a period of time, resulting in a biochemical change in the cells of the nervous system. These cells then need the drug for normal functioning. When the drug is removed or greatly decreased, the level of the drug in the body drops and withdrawal symptoms occur. The specific symptoms that occur depend on the drug or drugs taken.
Psychological Dependence (Habituation):	This is the expression of a severe craving or compulsion to take a drug in order to "feel good." The user has no physical compulsion to take the drug, either because the drug does not produce physical dependence or because withdrawal symptoms have been medically treated, such as when a person who has withdrawn from drugs relapses.
Tolerance:	An increased amount of the dose of a drug is necessary in order to obtain the desired effect, or there is a decrease in the desired effect with regular use of the same amount of the drug.
Cross Tolerance:	After tolerance to a drug has developed, tolerance to other drugs in the same or related classes will develop. For example, a person who is tolerant to alcohol will be tolerant to other sedative/hypnotics and minor tranquilizers.
Synergism:	This occurs when two drugs act similarly.
Antagonistic Effect:	This occurs when two drugs have opposing effects.
Additive Effect:	This occurs when two drugs acting similarly are used together and the result is a simple summation, or total, of effect.
Potentiation (Supra-additive effect):	This occurs when the effects of two synergistic, or similarly acting, drugs are greater than the sum of their doses.

(From American Psychiatric Association: Diagnostic and Statistical Manual of Mental Disorders, 3d ed., rev. Washington, DC, American Psychiatric Association, 1987. Also from Rodman MJ, Smith DW: Pharmacology and Drug Therapy in Nursing, 2d ed. Philadelphia, JB Lippincott, 1979)

CHART 26-2
DSM-III-R Criteria

DSM-III-R Criteria for Psychoactive Substance Dependence

1. At least three of the following characteristics are necessary:

    Substance taken in larger amounts or over a longer period than the person intended

    Persistent desire or one or more unsuccessful efforts to cut down or control the substance use

    A great deal of time is spent in activities necessary to get the substance, taking the substance, or recovering from its effects

    Frequent intoxication or withdrawal symptoms occur when expected to fulfill major role expectations at work, school, or home, or when substance use is physically hazardous

    Important social, occupational, or recreational activities given up or reduced because of substance use

    Continued substance use despite knowledge of having a persistent or recurrent social, psychological, or physical problem that is caused or exacerbated by the use of the substance

    Marked tolerance (need for markedly increased amounts of the substance in order to achieve intoxication or desired effect, or markedly diminished effect with continued use of the same amount)

—The following characteristics may not apply to cannabis, hallucinogens, or phencyclidine (PCP):

Characteristic withdrawal symptoms (see Table 26-1)

Substance often taken to relieve or avoid withdrawal symptoms

2. Some symptoms of the disturbance have persisted for at least 1 month or have occurred repeatedly over a period of time.
3. Dependence is defined as having degrees of severity. Guidelines for mild, moderate, and severe are provided

DSM-III-R Criteria for Psychoactive Substance Abuse

1. A maladaptive pattern of use of psychoactive substance indicated by at least one of the following:

    Continued use of the substance despite knowledge of a persistent or recurrent social, occupational, psychological, or physical problem that is caused or exacerbated by the use of the substance

    Recurrent use in situations in which use is physically hazardous

2. Some symptoms of the disturbance have lasted at least 1 month or have recurred repeatedly over a period of time.
3. Does not meet the criteria for Psychoactive Substance Dependence for this substance.

Defining Substance Abuse and Dependency

The Diagnostic and Statistical Manual of Mental Disorders, Third edition, Revised (DSM-III-R) classifies the pathological use of substances into these two categories:

1. Psychoactive Substance Use Disorders (Chart 26-2) refers to the maladaptive behavioral changes that may occur in individuals who misuse psychoactive substances that affect the central nervous system.
2. Psychoactive Substance—Induced Organic Mental Disorders refers to the physical or direct, acute, and chronic effects on the central nervous system of the misuse of the substance.

These categories, although separate for the purpose of classification, are not separate entities. Individuals with a psychoactive substance use disorder will inevitably experience a psychoactive substance-induced organic mental disorder. For example, a person who abuses or becomes dependent on alcohol will manifest certain behavioral manifestations or traits, such as the inability to cut down or stop drinking while recognizing that the amount of drinking is excessive; or the person may have serious physical problems (*i.e.,* gastritis, hepatitis, pancreatitis) because of prolonged heavy drinking and continue drinking in the same manner after understanding the substance exacerbates the physical symptoms. The individual will also experience a psychoactive substance-induced organic mental disorder such as intoxication or withdrawal (DSM-III-R).[4]

Psychoactive Substance Use Disorders

Psychoactive Substance Dependence

The symptoms of dependence are the same for all categories of psychoactive substances, although in some classes of substances the symptoms are less prominent; in a few classes, some symptoms do not occur. The main characteristic of this disorder is a group of cognitive, behavioral, and physical symptoms that indicate that the person has lost control over use of the substance and continues to use it despite adverse consequences. (See Chart 26-2.)

Psychoactive Substance Abuse

This is a residual category for defining maladaptive patterns of psychoactive substance abuse that do not meet the criteria for dependence for that class of substance. (See Chart 26-2.)

Nine classes of psychoactive substances are associated with both abuse and dependence: alcohol; sedatives, hypnotics, or anxiolytics; opioids; amphetamines or similarly acting sympathomimetics; cocaine; cannabis; hallucinogens; inhalants; phencyclidine (PCP).[4]

Substance-Induced Organic Mental Disorders

The category of psychoactive substance-induced organic mental disorders describes the specific organic brain syndrome (OBS) caused by the substance. The substance may cause more than one syndrome. Table 26-1 lists substance-induced organic mental disorders by classes of substances. The specific syndromes and the substance use disorders are described in this chapter section under "Dynamics of Substance Abuse and Dependency." Some symptoms are similar; others are different. For example, withdrawal from alcohol and withdrawal from sedative/hypnotics are similar, but symptoms of opioid withdrawal differ. The symptoms of delirium are the same for any organic mental disorders, regardless of etiology, but delirium associated with drugs has a specific cause that needs to be incorporated into the planning of care.

Etiologic Factors

There is no single theoretical concept which explains the etiology of substance abuse and dependency. It is important, rather, to reflect on the complex and varied etiologic factors.

The Drug, the Environment, and the Individual

The Drug

The first consideration is the drug itself. Each classification of drug, as well as each drug within that class, has particular chemical properties and produces effects specific to its chemical structure. The second consideration is the person taking the drug. People respond to drugs according to drug dosage, frequency of administration, the route of administration, and genetic, metabolic, physiological, and psycho-

Table 26-1. **Organic Mental Disorders Produced by Psychoactive Substances**

Substance-Induced Organic Mental Disorders	COMMON SUBSTANCES							
	Alcohol	Barbiturates and Similar Acting Sedatives/ Hypnotics	Opioids	Cocaine	Amphetamines and Similar Acting Sympathomimetics	PCP	Hallucinogens	Cannabis
Intoxication	X	X	X	X	X	X	X	X
Withdrawal	X	X	X	X	X			
Withdrawal delirium	(DTs) X	X						
Delirium				X	X	X		
Delusional disorder				X	X	X	X	X
Dementia	X							
Amnestic disorder	X	X						
Hallucinosis	X						X	
Mood disorder						X	X	

logical variables. Certain individuals are more likely to become alcoholic than others (see Chart 26-3). The third consideration is the environment from which the individual emerges, including the family, social factors (*e.g.,* extreme poverty and delinquency), and the culture or subculture.

The overview of several theoretical concepts that have been postulated to explain the nature and cause of substance abuse and dependency includes some concepts specific to the drugs of abuse (*e.g.,* the disease concept of alcoholism) and other concepts with more general application (*e.g.,* the learning theory). The etiologic concept may be reflected in the treatment and rehabilitation process. For example, those who embrace the disease concept of alcoholism will strongly advise abstinence to treat alcoholism. On the other hand, some of the proponents of learning theory may believe that an individual's behavior may be modified or changed and that social or recreational drinking may be resumed.

Social or Environmental Factors

The social or environmental concepts suggest that the social condition or environment from which an individual emerges may contribute to, or predispose an individual to, substance abuse and dependency. For example, there has been a high incidence of abuse of opioid derivatives, such as heroin, in the ghettos or poverty areas of large cities. The abuse of cocaine and hallucinogens is associated with subculture groups and those seeking "mystical" experiences. There is also a reported high incidence of cocaine abuse in the upper economic bracket and among entertainers and athletes.[4, 36, 77]

Personality Factors

A review of research studies has not substantiated that one personality type is associated with substance abuse and dependency.[11, 91] Instead, there is a wide variation in personality types, including individuals from all social, cultural, and economic backgrounds.[91] Personality disorders, however, may be intensified by abuse of, or dependence on, substances, especially in the antisocial personality.[4] It is also believed that depressed individuals and those with affective disorders may abuse substances to treat symptoms related to their disorder.[4]

Although current research does not support the concept of an "addictive personality type," there are some factors that are important to those who seek to understand, prevent, and treat substance abuse. Most of the differences between individuals who abuse alcohol and those who abuse other drugs seem to reflect age, sex, race, socioeconomic status, and the use of legal or illegal drugs, rather than intrapsychic dynamics. A common factor in all forms of substance abuse

C H A R T 26-3
At Risk for Alcoholism

Epidemiologic and social studies of alcohol abuse and dependency demonstrate that certain groups of individuals are at high risk for the development of alcoholism. Although the following criteria from the National Council on Alcoholism point to persons at risk for developing alcoholism, there is no agreement on the extent of the risk for each particular case.[18]

A family history of alcoholism, including parents, siblings, grandparents, uncles, and aunts

A history of teetotalism in the family, particularly where strong moral overtones were present and, most particularly, where the social environment of the patient has changed to associations in which drinking is encouraged or required

A history of alcoholism or teetotalism in the spouse or the family of the spouse

Coming from a broken home or home with much parental discord, particularly where the father is absent or rejecting but not punitive

Being the last child of a large family or in the last half of the sibship in a large family

Having female relatives of more than one generation who have had a high incidence of recurrent depressions

Heavy smoking (heavy drinking is often associated with heavy smoking, but the reverse need not be true)

Although some cultural groups (*e.g.,* the Irish and Scandinavians) have been recorded as having a higher incidence of alcoholism than others (*e.g.,* Jews, Chinese, and Italians), alcoholism can occur in people of any cultural derivation.

(From National Council on Alcoholism: Criteria for the Diagnosis of Alcoholism. Am J Psychiatr 129 (August): 47–48, 1972)

and dependence is a negative self-concept, marked by a sense of failure, inadequacy, guilt, shame, loneliness, and despair.[11]

Self-Destructive Phenomenon

Individuals who abuse and become dependent on substances do so in spite of severe physical, psychological, and social consequences. This lack of concern

CHART 26-4
Pharmacologic and Slang Terms for Common Substances of Abuse

Substance	Generic and Trade Name	Street/Slang Name
Barbiturates	Amobarbital (Amytal) Pentobarbital (Nembutal) Phenobarbital (Luminal) Secobarbital (Seconal)	Barbs, Blockbusters, Bluebirds, Blue Devils, Blues, Christmas Trees, Downers, Green Dragons, Mexican Reds, Nebbies, Nimbles, Pajaro Rojo, Pink Ladies, Pinks, Rainbows, Reds and Blues, Red Birds, Red Devils, Reds, Sleeping Pills, Stumblers, Yellow Jackets, Yellows
Opiates Morphine		Cube, First Line, Goma, Morf, Morfina, Morpho, Mud
Heroin	Diacetylmorphine	Big H., Boy, Brown Sugar, Caballo, Chiva, Crap, Estuffa, H., Heroina, Hombre, Horse, Junk, Mexican Mud, Scag, Smack, Stuff, Thing
Central nervous system Amphetamines	Amphetamine (Benzedrine) Methamphetamine (Desoxyn, Methedrine) Dextroamphetamine (Dexedrine)	Beans, Bennies, Black Beauties, Black Mollies, Copilots, Crank, Crossroads, Crystal, Dexies, Double Cross, Meth, Minibennies, Pep Pills, Speed, Rosas, Roses, Thrusters, Truck Drivers, Uppers, Wake-ups, Whites
Cocaine		Blow, C., Coca, Coke, Crack, Flake, Girl, Heaven, Dust, Lady, Mujer, Nose Candy, Paradise, Perico, Polvo Blanco, Rock, Snow, White
Hallucinogens LSD	Lysergic acid diethylamine	Acid, Blotter Acid, California Sunshine, Haze, Microdots, Paper Acid, Purple Haze, Sunshine Wedges, Window Panes
Cannabis Marijuana		Acapulco Gold, Cannabis, Colombian, Ganga, Grass, Griffa, Hemp, Herb, J, Jay, Joint, Mary Jane, Mota, Mutah, Panama Red, Reefer, Sativa, Smoke, Stick, Tea, Weed, Yerba
Hashish		Goma de Mota, Hash, Soles

for one's own well-being has led to the view of drug dependency as a self-destructive phenomenon.[91] It is also difficult to estimate with certainty the incidence of intentional suicide by drug overdose. The risk of suicide is high in individuals who abuse substances, both in the sober and in the intoxicated states.[4,62,83,91]

Ethnic and Cultural Factors

Substance abuse and dependency are found in all cultures and ethnic groups. There are variations, however, in the incidence and prevalence of the problem,

the drug preferred, and the aspects of treatment, prevention, and rehabilitation. For example, there is a low incidence of alcoholism but a high incidence of opiate dependency reported in the Oriental culture and population.[32,91] Researchers attribute the low incidence of alcoholism to a possible genetic intolerance to alcohol, manifested by unpleasant physical symptoms when even small amounts of alcohol are ingested.[32] There is also a low incidence of alcohol dependency in the American Jewish population,[91] but a high incidence in the American Indian and Irish

C H A R T   26-5
Fetal Alcohol Effects: A First-Person Account

Alcohol is a teratogenic drug that is, when taken during pregnancy, it can cause adverse effects in the fetus. Many alcohol-related birth defects have been associated with alcohol use during pregnancy. The most clearly defined effect on the fetus is a specific pattern of neonatal defects called fetal alcohol syndrome (or FAS). Fetal alcohol syndrome is manifested by a group of congenital birth defects which includes the following:

Prenatal and postnatal growth deficiency
A particular pattern of facial malformations including a small head circumference, flattened midface, sunken nasal bridge, and a flattened and elongated philtrum (the groove between the nose and upper lip)
Central nervous system dysfunction
Varying degrees of major organ system malfunctions (Alcohol Health and Research World 10 (1): 1985.)

This is a statement written by Maureen, who is 18 years of age and in her first semester of college. Maureen is unique, not in her aspirations, but in her survival of physical and emotional trauma. She was born addicted to drugs, and it would be inappropriate of anyone to assume that most people triumph over such afflictions. Maureen is atypical in her coping ability, as well as in her development of positive self-direction. Maureen's social awareness, in combination with her internal and external support systems, created an accepting individual with a significant tolerance for social ignorance. This is Maureen's motivation for her words:

Years ago my brother and I were born fifteen minutes apart. Not knowing what to expect, just like all other newborns, we had our first reality of life. We had to deal with withdrawal from drugs. Our biological parents were dependent upon drugs. On arrival into the world we were faced with going without the drugs which we were hooked on for nine months while inside of her womb. The painful struggle for the body was hard and long. After seeing adults who must be hospitalized for being so sick with pain, can you even imagine the pain your child and my brother and I went through? No, we don't remember, no child will because they have no knowledge, but it is extremely hard and upsetting to know that our parents put us through this by their unnecessary and selfish acts. My brother is quite healthy, but I had to have surgery right after birth to disconnect my cranial plates. I lost 50% of my hearing and am blind in one eye from hypertension. A shunt has been put in my spine to catch the overflow of spinal fluid and I still have arthritis in my hands that I was born with.

It has been a life-long struggle for me to stay away from prescription drugs, because anything I take can cause blindness in my other eye. If you have any "smarts," stay away from drugs and alcohol while you're pregnant. The choice is yours, but just remember, your irresponsible acts can cause death or permanent damage to your unborn child.

So Mommy, please let me breathe, think, and look like you when I come into that wonderful world."

Maureen

---

populations, and relatively high incidences in Scandinavian and German populations.[91] The reasons for these phenomena are related to cultural drinking habits or accepted use of alcohol.[91]

Since the 1950s, research related to alcohol abuse/dependency and culture has increased.[56] The importance of ethnic factors and cultural diversity and their effect on substance abuse dependency are now being emphasized. Knowledge acquired through study and research has special application in drug prevention and treatment programs.

Learning Theory

The learning theory concept, involving a conditioned response mechanism, has been applied to substance abuse and dependency. For example, the drug use may initially produce pleasant physical responses, desired social consequences, increased feelings of self-confidence, or relief from tension or anxiety. The conditioned response is always positive in the beginning of the process; however, even after severe negative consequences occur, the repetitive or learned behavior continues, although the initial reasons for the repetitive or learned behavior are no longer in operation.[49,91]

Biologic Theory

There is a high incidence of alcohol abuse and dependency (alcoholism) in children and family members of alcoholics. Several research studies have suggested a possible inherited predisposition to alcoholism.[17,31,32]

Studies of twins with a family history of alcoholism have yielded interesting results. Monozygotic twins (those who share the same genetic material) were more concordant—that is, both twins having the same condition for alcoholism—than dyzogotic twins (those who have the same genetic material as siblings) for alcoholism. The adoptive studies, which involve examination of data of children born of alcoholic parents but separated after birth from their natural parents and raised by nonalcoholic foster parents, indicate that these children are particularly susceptible to becoming alcoholic.[17,31,32,89]

Researchers are making an effort to determine what genetic characteristics may make a person a risk for the development of alcoholism. One study is related to a hypothesis involving tetrahydroisoquinolines (TIQs or THIQs). Tetrahydroisoquinolines are potent morphinelike neurochemicals formed by the chemical combination of acetaldehyde (a major product of alcohol metabolism) and neurotransmitters. The structural similarity of some TIQs to morphine and its derivatives has led to the hypothesis that opiate addiction and alcoholism may show a common addictive mechanism involving specific receptors in the brain that bind both opiates and TIQs.[64]

Findings from other research studies have led to the hypothesis that excessive drinking could be caused by metabolic abnormalities that result in excessive production of TIQs. If this hypothesis is correct, it is possible that an inherited tendency to become alcoholic may also be due to genes that cause an overproduction of TIQs.[64] In addition, brain wave studies have revealed peculiar and apparently genetically based electrical phenomena in the brains of people at risk for alcoholism.[64]

A family history of alcoholism does not necessarily indicate that the cause of alcoholism is genetic in origin. Consider the fact that the majority of all children are raised by their biologic parents and the profound influence of social, cultural, and psychological factors within the family environment on the behavior of children. The question becomes, Does the familial aspect of alcoholism come from a learned pattern of behavior, rather than a genetic predisposition to alcoholism?[31,32] There may be, in fact, an unfamilial, as well as a familial, type of alcoholism.

At this time, no research studies have offered direct evidence that narcotic addiction is genetically transmitted.[35] Nevertheless, researchers are conducting psychobiologic studies in an attempt to identify a common link or aspect of drug addiction. Presently, there is an increase in polydrug users; that is, people who take a variety of substances, including alcohol, with no specific drug of choice.[13]

Disease Concept of Alcoholism

Viewing alcoholism as a disease rather than a moral problem originated with the work of E. M. Jellinek. A pioneer in the study of alcoholism, Jellinek classified alcoholics into five categories. The disease concept he proposed was based on the statistical analysis of a survey of 2000 male alcoholics. The classes or types of alcoholics that he identified, however, were not meant to reflect theories as to cause or nature of alcoholism.[46,47] The concept of alcoholism as a disease has had a great effect on the acceptance of alcoholism as an illness or process outside the control of the afflicted individual.

Jellinek's disease concept, labeled by some as the "traditional" model of alcoholism, has been challenged by a more recent concept of alcohol dependence as a behavioral disorder with adverse consequences on the health of individuals. This latter "new" concept has been called the multivariant concept of alcoholism.[67] Most authorities in the field of alcohol abuse continue to view the disease concept of alcoholism as the more valid approach to treatment and eventual recovery.

Incidence and Significance of Substance Abuse and Dependency

The drug of abuse is a main consideration in examining the incidence and significance of substance abuse and dependency. For example, of the many people who use the substance alcohol, a legal substance with social approval for recreational use, about 1 in 10 experience abuse or dependency. On the other hand, among the users of heroin, an illegal substance, there is a higher incidence of users becoming dependent. Also, abuse or dependency occurs more quickly for narcotics than for alcohol.[4,91]

The culture or social status from which the drug user comes also has an impact on the incidence of substance abuse. The teenage group culture may experiment with a variety of drugs, including heroin, cocaine, stimulants, alcohol, sedative/hypnotics, PCP, or almost any substance available.[77] During the Vietnam era, servicemen used and abused heroin and cannabis in large quantities with a resulting high incidence of abuse and dependency. Upon returning to the United States, some were able to stop using heroin completely or changed the class of drug of abuse.[4,72]

The type of drug used in a ghetto may be different than that used by suburban middle-class men or women who, because of class distinctions and social variables, may choose a prescription or legal drug, such as alcohol. Frequently, entertainment or sports celebrities and people of high economic status are associated with abuse of, or dependence on, cocaine.[77]

The age, sex, culture, and social setting from which the individual emerges are factors affecting the incidence and significance of drug abuse. Other considerations include the availability of the drug, the cost of the drug, peer pressure, and the drug-oriented American culture, which extols the use of alcohol and prescription drugs for relief of tension and pain. To counteract this prevalence of substance abuse, health professionals in all fields are uniting to combat abuse and dependency problems in psychological, biologic, and social areas and through treatment, research, and prevention.[77]

Dynamics of Substance Abuse and Dependency

This section on the dynamics of substance abuse and dependency will describe the chemical substance, or drug, the specific diagnostic criteria, and the particular physical, behavioral, and familial consequences.

Alcohol Abuse and Dependency

Alcohol abuse and dependency is one of the most serious public health problems in our nation. The incidence of alcohol-related accidents resulting in fatalities or in permanent disabilities is enormous. The social impact of the disorder on family members, especially on children, is devastating. Many American adolescents are affected by destructive drinking patterns or suffer alcoholism themselves; many children are born with abnormalities or suffer from fetal alcohol syndrome. (See Chart 26-6, "The Impact of Alcoholism.")

Nature of Alcohol
The chemical substance commonly referred to as alcohol is ethyl alcohol (C_2H_5OH), also known chemically as ethanol and sometimes abbreviated as ETOH.[75] It is a legal chemical substance or drug; that is, the sale and commercial distribution of alcohol-containing beverages differ from the regulation and sale of other classes of drugs.

Ethyl alcohol has pharmacologic properties that produce mind-altering and mood-altering effects on individuals. It is a central nervous system depressant similar to barbiturates and ether.[75] Chloral hydrate and paraldehyde are sedative/hypnotic drugs derived from ethyl alcohol.[75] Chloral hydrate is used to induce sleep; paraldehyde was used in the medical management of alcohol withdrawal symptoms before the introduction of modern tranquilizers.

Most of the drugs that affect the central nervous system have a use in medicine, but ethyl alcohol is not commonly used as a drug in medical treatment. In addition, although other drugs that cause physical and psychological dependence produce their effects in small quantities, alcohol usually requires large quantities over a period of time to cause physical dependence.[18]

There are several types of alcohol-containing beverages. The most common types are beer, wine, and distilled spirits, each containing the same amount of alcohol content. For example, 12 ounces of beer, 4 ounces of dry wine, or 1 ¼ ounces of whiskey have the same alcohol content.

The alcohol content of distilled spirits is expressed as proof; that is, the concentration of ethyl alcohol in the substance. In the United States, proof is twice the ethanol concentration. One hundred proof is 50% (ethyl) alcohol; 80% proof is 40% (ethyl) alcohol.

Ethyl alcohol is a central nervous system depressant, as are the sedative/hypnotics, antianxiety drugs, and general anesthetics. These drugs cause the following pattern of effects as the dose of the drug is increased—sedation, impairment in mental and motor functioning, deepening stupor with a decrease in stimulation response (including painful stimulus response), coma, and eventually death from respiratory and circulatory collapse.[73]

Alcohol is often erroneously thought to be a stimulant. The reason for this misconception is that after drinking alcoholic beverages, some individuals may become more talkative or hyperactive, display a euphoric mood, have increased self-confidence, or become aggressive. This behavior has been attributed to the disinhibiting effect produced by a low dose of the drug.[73]

Alcohol Concentration in the Body. The physical and behavioral manifestations of the effects of alcohol on the central nervous system are related to the level of alcohol in the blood and the concentration of alcohol in the brain, as well as to other contributing factors. The blood level of alcohol is expressed in the number of milligrams of alcohol per milliliter of blood, that is, mg/ml.[73]

The blood alcohol level is a laboratory blood test to determine the degree of alcohol (ethanol) intoxica-

C H A R T   26-6
The Impact of Alcoholism

Alcoholism and alcohol-related problems have considerable significance in the United States.

Variation and Prevalence of Drinking Problems

Considering all measures of drinking problems and available recent survey data, approximately 10% of adult American drinkers are likely to experience either alcoholism or problem drinking at some point in their lives.

In general, results from these recent surveys indicate that a substantial number of adult American drinkers experience serious drinking problems. Males continue to outnumber females by a fairly wide margin on most indicators of drinking problems.

Level of consumption is related substantially to both alcohol dependence and adverse effects. The higher the level of consumption, the greater the probability that a person will experience dependence symptoms and adverse physical and social consequences. Regular heavy drinking leads to adverse consequences and dependence. Intermittent heavy drinking may also result in adverse consequences.

Biomedical Consequences

Although alcohol-related mortality appears to have remained relatively constant, mortality rates for alcoholics continue to be higher than expected. One recent study reported a mortality rate for alcoholics 2.5 times greater than expected in a group of alcoholics followed over time.

Social Implications

In the United States, traffic accidents are the major causes of violent death. Between 35% and 64% of the drivers in fatal accidents had been drinking prior to the accident. Between 45% and 60% of all fatal crashes involving young drivers are alcohol-related.

Approximately one half of adult fire deaths involve alcohol. Alcoholics are 10 times more likely to die in fires compared with the general population.

Alcoholics are at particularly high risk of committing suicide. Between 15% and 65% of persons who attempt suicide and up to 80% of those who committed suicides had been drinking at the time of the event. The risk of suicide for alcoholics is as much as 30 times greater than the risk of suicide for the general population.

Prevention

The Surgeon General's Report, a World Health Organization Conference, and the Department of Health and Human Services' prevention objectives for the year 1990 indicate increased interest in the prevention of alcohol-related problems.

Intervention

Current prevention programs are aimed at minimizing the occurrences of alcohol-related problems through means other than treatment and rehabilitation. Projects for youth in education and service organizations, projects for public information utilizing mass media and communications, projects replicating earlier successful prevention strategies, and projects involving voluntary organizations and community movements have been undertaken.

Treatment and Rehabilitation

The number of persons receiving treatment for alcoholism and problem drinking has continued to increase. Nevertheless, approximately 85% of the population of alcoholics and problem drinkers are not receiving formal treatment services.

(From selected Highlights of the Fourth Special Report to the U.S. Congress on Alcohol and Health, United States Department of Health and Human Services. Washington, DC, January, 1981)

tion. It may be used in medicolegal procedures to rule out intoxication in a person who is comatose. The degree of intoxication of an individual may also be measured by breathalyzers.

The alcohol concentration in the blood depends on the rate of absorption, transportation to the central nervous system, redistribution to the other parts of the body, metabolism, and elimination. Alcohol is absorbed through the mouth, stomach, and small intestine. It is absorbed unchanged into the blood and circulates throughout the body, including the brain; it

(Text continues on p. 478)

C H A R T   26-7
Impaired Professionals
Sue Stanton, R.N., C., C.A.C.
Coordinator, Committee for Physician's Health
Syracuse Regional Office
Medical Society for the State of New York
Syracuse, New York

Treatment of chemical dependence and mental illness in the professional, in particular in physicians and nurses, is a critical issue in health care today, because of the potential harm to patients if these diseases go untreated. Substance abuse and the ensuing mental illness that result in the loss of personal well-being of the practitioner seriously compromise the delivery of safe, quality health care to the public. Alcoholism and other drug addictions, as well as some forms of mental illness, are amenable to treatment; those affected should have the opportunity to obtain treatment and rehabilitation prior to action on Licensure by the State Health Department. Because these diseases are progressive and lead to physical and mental deterioration, early detection and treatment are the primary goal of the American Medical Society (AMA) and the American Nurses' Association (ANA).

Impairment as defined by the AMA occurs when the physician is unable to practice medicine with reasonable skill and safety because of mental illness or excessive use or abuse of drugs, including alcohol. According to the ANA, nursing practice is impaired when the individual is unable to meet the requirements of the professional code of ethics and standards of practice because cognitive, interpersonal, or psychomotor skills are affected by conditions of the individual in interaction with the environment. These factors include psychiatric illness, excessive alcohol or drug use, or addiction. The Medical Society of New York State distinguishes between troubled and impaired. Within this context, physicians are described as *troubled* when their chemical dependence or mental illness has produced personal, family or other interpersonal distress but has not yet affected their medical practice. It is important to intervene on the practitioner's impairment before a patient is injured.

How many physicians are impaired? The most conservative statement is that "no ones knows." Reliable data are presently not available; however, medical societies are collecting data via computers and soon there will be more valid statistics available concerning those who are in treatment. Until the medical community becomes sophisticated enough and trusting enough of the programs in place for treatment and makes referrals to these programs, many physicians will go untreated. However, a plausible estimate is that 3% of all physicians at some time in their career are impaired as a result of drugs or alcohol abuse but others estimate this at 5%. Others feel that the figure might be as high as 18%. In the general population the figure is 10% and there is no reason to think that this figure is lower in medical practitioners and, in fact, there is some rationale to think it might be higher due to the vulnerability of this group and the easy access to drugs in the workplace. Of the cases seen in treatment, approximately 80% are treated for alcohol/drug abuse, 10% for senility, and the others are treated for mental illness.

The degree of impairment in nurses is also unclear. Again, this is due to a lack of research data on the prevalence of chemical dependence and psychiatric illness in professional groups. Psychiatric illness is even more difficult to trace because it is rare for nurses to lose licenses because of mental illness. Most action by state boards of nursing on Licensure is taken for violations of the Nurse Practice Act involving substance abuse. Of these Licensure actions, approximately 68% are due to substance abuse. The prevalence of problems of chemical dependency and psychiatric illnesses within society parallels in nursing according to most estimates. These estimates place drug at 2 to 3%, alcoholism at 8 to 10%, and psychiatric illness at 3% for psychoses and 5 to 8% for depression. If we apply the increasing knowledge that is being gathered concerning Adult Children of Alcoholics, we may consider that these percentages might be higher, i.e., that the oldest child in these alcoholic families very often chooses a helping profession as a career. This would apply to physicians, nurses, clergy, and social workers. The real answer to prevalency, therefore, lies in future research.

Physicians and nurses are at high risk to develop the disease of chemical dependency. The genetic factor cannot be emphasized enough. Many come from alcoholic families and this predisposes them to the disease and makes them at risk if they decide to use. Those who have a history of drug abuse, especially as teenagers, may continue that pattern of use in adulthood. Because the mechanics of work in medicine and nursing are often stressful and demanding and often lacking in recognition of effect and accomplishment, relief usage may be sought and seen as temporarily effective. Any group which has easy access to drugs is at risk for developing chemical dependency and certainly nurses and physicians are no exception and fall into the category of having easy accessibility.

In 1981, the American Nurses' Association resolved to address health problems of nurses. The ANA was particularly concerned with the practice by nurses whose judgment was impaired by drugs, alcohol, or psychological dysfunction. A resolution was made for action on alcohol and drug abuse and psychological dysfunction in relation to the ANA Code for Nurses. This was an effort to show responsibility to society, to self-regulate the practice of its members, and to assure quality in professional performance. This issue was emphasized heavily at the ANA convention in 1984. At the district and state levels nurses have planned and put into place programs for peer assistance for impaired nurses. Treatment is tailored to meet individual needs of the impaired nurse-client. It may include inpatient, outpatient, detoxification, rehabilitation, psychiatric treatment, and/or participation in self-help groups. The maintenance of confidentiality is critical to the program.

If the nurse-client does not cooperate with treatment recommendations, and it felt that her practice places patients in jeopardy, the nurse may be referred to the Board of Regents or State Board of Nurse Examiners for further investigation.

We believe that chemical dependency is a complex, progressive, but treatable, illness which has been largely ignored or denied in the female population as a whole and, more specifically, in the predominately female profession of nursing. To prevent the progression of these diseases, we need to recognize early symptoms, gently confront the nurse in the presence of another nurse, and offer assistance into treatment. The nurses doing the confrontation must be firm, supportive, and prepared for denial and hostility and have a plan for rejection. Early symptoms may be any combination of the following:

1. Absent or late for work, especially following several days off. Note, however, that drug-addicted nurses may never be absent and may "hang around" when not on duty because the hospital is their source of supply.
2. Odor of alcohol on the breath. Any nurse who would report for duty after drinking is assuming a terrible risk and in doing so is evidencing her loss of control and need for the drug.
3. Odor of mouthwash and breath mints. These may be used to mask the odor of alcohol.
4. Fine tremors of the hands. This symptom occurs with withdrawal from the drug. The alcoholic nurse will sometimes begin to use tranquilizers to mask signs of withdrawal and thus may develop cross dependency.
5. Emotional lability. The nurse may change from being irritable and tense to being mellow and calm. There may be inappropriate anger or crying.
6. Returns late from lunch break.
7. May be sleepy or may doze off while on duty.
8. Shuns interaction with others and tends to withdraw.
9. Makes frequent trips to the bathroom. The female alcoholic will carry her handbag with her.
10. Deterioration in personal appearance.
11. Frequent bruises or cigarette burns. These injuries are the result of crashing into furniture or falling while intoxicated or dozing off with a lighted cigarette.
12. Job performance will be affected, with sloppy or illegible handwriting, errors in charting (e.g., charting on the wrong chart), and errors in patient care.
13. Lapses in memory or confusion. There may be euphoric recall of events.
14. Shunning of job assignment or job shrinkage. The nurse is apt to drop out of professional activities.

The nurse who is stealing drugs from the unit

1. Always volunteers to give medications.
2. Medicates another nurse's patient.
3. Always uses the maximum PRN dosage when other nurses use less, or the maximum PRN dosage may always be used on one shift but not on another. (The PRN

(Continues on p. 478)

medications afford the greatest opportunity for the nurse to supply her habit)
4. Has responsibility for patients who complain that medication given on one shift is not as effective as on others, or that they did not receive medication when the record shows they did.
5. Has frequent wastage, such as spillage of drugs or drawing blood into the syringe.
6. Is working on a unit where drugs are disappearing or seals have been tampered with.

With treatment, physicians and nurses emerge with improved practice. They now are able to recognize early symptoms of chemical dependence and mental illness in their patients and able to more accurately diagnose and treat. They are able to look beyond the presenting symptom for further evidence of alcoholism or other drug dependencies. Physicians begin to look at their prescribing practices and refrain from so freely prescribing benzodiazepines, and begin to recognize the need to refer their patients for treatment of chemical dependency. So, to salvage a career for these professionals means getting improved treatment for many others.

also crosses the placenta into the fetal circulation. Intoxication occurs when the circulating alcohol interferes with the normal functioning of the nerve cells of the brain.[73]

The rate of absorption into the blood varies with the following factors:

1. Substances in the beverage, such as the carbonation (CO_2) in champagne, increase absorption.
2. The rate of ingestion of alcohol can affect the rate of absorption. Drinking alcoholic beverages slowly over a period of time may slow absorption and allow for metabolism of alcohol by the liver. Because the body metabolizes alcohol at a steady rate, when an individual drinks faster than the body can metabolize the alcohol, it accumulates in the blood.
3. The rate of drinking may vary, but alcohol leaves the body at a fixed rate.[73]

Ninety percent of the alcohol absorbed by the body is eliminated by oxidation, which takes place mainly in the liver. The other 10% of the alcohol is eliminated unchanged, through breath, sweat, urine, and other body fluids. The liver of the normal adult metabolizes approximately one drink, or 1 ounce of distilled spirits, per hour; the excess alcohol that the liver cannot metabolize continues to circulate in the blood. Food in the stomach, especially fatty food, slows absorption, whereas an empty stomach increases absorption. The emotional state of the drinker may also affect absorption of alcohol. For example, stress, fear, anger, and fatigue may increase or decrease absorption. The body size of the drinker affects the concentration of alcohol in the blood. The same amount of alcohol taken by a lightweight person (100 pounds) and a heavyweight person (200 pounds) will result in greater blood alcohol concentration in the lighter person, because there is more blood volume in the heavyweight person in which the alcohol can be diluted. An individual's body chemistry and cultural influences may also alter the behavioral effects of alcohol.[14]

Tolerance. Prolonged heavy drinking results in physical and behavioral tolerance. Physical tolerance, or tissue adaptation, means that changes occur in the cells of the nervous system, so that more of the drug is required to achieve the desired effect. When physical tolerance develops, the individual may experience withdrawal or abstinence syndrome after cessation or a decrease in consumption of alcohol. Physical tolerance to alcohol never reaches the high dose tolerance of the opiates. Cross tolerance to sedative/hypnotics and other central nervous system depressants also occurs.[73]

Behavioral tolerance to alcohol and other drugs is manifested by the ability to mask the behavioral effects; for example, the acquired ability not to slur words, to walk straight, and to function in ways that would not be possible in a nondependent person. The drinking history of alcoholics frequently reveals the ability to increase tolerance and maintain this increase for a long period of time, perhaps over several years. Frequently, this increase in tolerance is followed by an irreversible drop in tolerance; the individual becomes intoxicated with a smaller amount of alcohol.[13,14,75]

Blackout. Persistent heavy drinking frequently results in the chemically induced alcoholic blackout. This is not the same as "passing out," which is defined as a loss of consciousness. During a blackout, the individual appears to function normally while drinking, but he is later unable to remember what occurred. The blackout may be a few hours or several hours. The individual may come out of the blackout period and wonder, "Where did I leave my car last night?" or wake up in a strange city not remembering leaving his home and wonder, "How did I get here?" or "Was I with someone?" These blackouts may be a symptom of alcohol abuse and dependency.[49,77,87]

Alcohol-Induced Organic Mental Disorders

Intoxication. Intoxication occurs after drinking alcohol and is evidenced in behavior such as fighting, impaired judgment, interference with social or occupational functioning, or other maladaptive behavior. Physiologic signs such as slurred speech, incoordination, unsteady gait, nystagmus, and flushed face may accompany intoxication. Psychological signs also may be observed, as in mood changes, irritability, talkativeness, or impaired attention.

Alcohol Withdrawal. Alcohol withdrawal, or abstinence syndrome, occurs after reduction in, or cessation of, prolonged heavy drinking. A coarse tremor of hand, tongue, and eyelids may occur, as well as nausea and vomiting, general malaise or weakness, autonomic nervous system hyperactivity (*e.g.,* increased blood pressure and pulse), anxiety, a depressed or irritable mood, and orthostatic hypotension. Sleep disturbances, insomnia, and nightmares may also occur during withdrawal.

Alcohol Withdrawal Delirium. Alcohol withdrawal delirium, referred to as DTs or delirium tremens, is the most serious form of the withdrawal syndrome. It also occurs after cessation of, or reduction in, prolonged heavy drinking and can occur as long as a week after cessation of drinking. The symptoms of delirium include clouding of consciousness (unawareness of environment); inability to shift, focus, and sustain attention to stimuli in the environment; misinterpretations, illusions, or hallucinations that are usually visual and vivid; incoherent speech; insomnia or daytime drowsiness; increased or decreased psychomotor activity; frequent agitation; and increased blood pressure, sweating, and temperature. Seizures may also occur as a result of alcohol withdrawal (sometimes called "rumfits"). If untreated, this syndrome can cause serious medical complications, such as fluid and electrolyte imbalance, pneumonia, and dehydration.

Alcoholic Hallucinosis. Alcoholic hallucinosis usually occurs within 48 hours after cessation of, or reduction in, drinking. Vivid, and perhaps threatening, auditory hallucinations may develop, but clouding of the consciousness does not occur. The individual's response to the hallucinations is appropriate to its content; that is, he responds with anxiety or fear. Auditory hallucinations are usually experienced as voices, but may be experienced as hissing or buzzing sounds.

Alcoholic Amnestic Disorder. The alcoholic amnestic disorder results from heavy prolonged drinking and is thought to be related to poor nutritional intake. If the disorder is related to thiamine deficiency, it is known as Korsakoff's syndrome. Amnesia consists of impairment in the ability to learn new information (short-term memory) and to recall remote information (long-term memory). Other neurologic signs such as neuropathy, unsteady gait, or myopathy may be present.

Alcoholic Dementia. Alcoholic dementia is associated with prolonged, chronic alcohol dependence. Signs of dementia include loss of intellectual ability that is severe enough to interfere with social or occupational functioning and impairment in memory, abstract thinking, and judgment. The degree of impairment may range from mild to severe and may include permanent brain damage.

Medical Consequences

The heavy consumption of alcohol can adversely affect almost every body system. Various medical conditions may alert the nurse to the early recognition of alcohol abuse problems.

Gastrointestinal problems occur as a result of the irritating effects of alcohol on the gastrointestinal tract, resulting in gastritis or gastric ulcers. Acute or chronic pancreatitis, or inflammation of the pancreas, may occur. Esophagitis may result from the direct toxic effects of alcohol on the esophageal mucosa, from increased acid production in the stomach, or from frequent vomiting. Alcohol cardiomyopathy occurs because of both the direct toxic effects of the substance and malnutrition.[14,25]

The liver is highly susceptible to the damaging effects of alcohol because it is the primary organ that metabolizes alcohol. Alcohol has been found to be toxic to the liver regardless of the nutritional status of the individual.[6,14] Alcohol liver disease has been divided into three major types. In fatty liver, deposits of fats (triglycerides) build up in the normal liver cells. This condition is reversible.[6,14] Alcoholic hepatitis is a more serious condition, involving inflammation and necrosis of the liver cells. This condition is also frequently reversible.[6,14] Cirrhosis of the liver is the most serious condition and is irreversible. In cirrhosis, the liver cells are destroyed and replaced by scar tissue. About 90% of deaths from cirrhosis of the liver are associated with chronic alcoholism.[6] A high risk of cancer, especially of the mouth, pharynx, larynx, esophagus, pancreas, cardia of the stomach, and colon, is also associated with alcoholism.[6,53]

Recent research studies indicate that the consumption of alcoholic beverages in women may be an increased risk factor in the development of breast cancer.[68]

Major and Minor Criteria for the Diagnosis of Alcoholism

The criteria for the diagnosis of alcoholism compiled by the National Council on Alcoholism establish guidelines for the early detection of alcoholism, provide uniform terminology, and help prevent overdiagnosis. The criteria also allow for the differentiation between early, middle, and late stages of alcoholism. This staging identifies progression (*i.e.*, worsening over time) of the disease. The criteria for diagnosis of alcoholism are divided into major and minor criteria (see Tables 26-2 and 26-3). The criteria are further grouped into the following three diagnostic levels:

Diagnostic Level 1. Classical, definite, obligatory; a person meeting this criteria is diagnosed as being alcoholic

Diagnostic Level 2. Probable, frequent, indicative; a person who meets this criteria is under strong suspicion of alcoholism

Diagnostic Level 3. Potential, possible, incidental; these manifestations are common but do not by themselves give a strong indication of alcoholism; more significant evidence is needed before a diagnosis is made

The diagnosis of alcoholism may be made if one or more of the major criteria in either track are present, or if several of the minor criteria in both tracks are present.

Abuse of Controlled Substances

Drugs other than alcohol are not as easily attainable and have illegal status. These classes of drugs are regulated by the Controlled Substance Act (Title II, Comprehensive Drug Abuse Prevention and Control Act of 1970, Public Law 91-513). These federal control standards are used to decrease the illegal use and abuse of drugs in the United States.

Barbiturates and Similar Sedative/Hypnotic Drugs

Effects. The barbiturates and other central nervous system depressants are called sedative/hypnotics and anxiolytics. The main difference between a sedative drug and a hypnotic drug is the degree of sedation, or sleepiness, produced in comparison to the antianxiety-producing effects.[90] The barbiturates are the most common drugs of abuse after alcohol, which is the number-one drug of abuse in the United States. The barbiturates and similarly acting drugs are capable of producing intoxication and withdrawal.

Barbiturates are capable of producing physical and psychological dependence and tolerance. The route of administration may be oral or parenteral (*i.e.*, intravenous or intramuscular). Basically, the organs with greater blood flow absorb the drug first.[90] The majority of commonly used barbiturates are metabolized by the liver. Some barbiturates (*e.g.*, phenobarbital) are not metabolized and are excreted unchanged by the kidneys.[90]

Because barbiturates cross the placental barrier, there is potential for the fetus of a drug-dependent mother to experience physical dependence. The physical withdrawal symptoms may occur in the infant up to 7 days after delivery. The physical symptoms of the drug-dependent infant may include a high-pitched cry, tremors, restlessness, disturbed sleep, increased reflex action, hyperphagia, diarrhea, vomiting, and major motor seizures.[90]

Barbiturates and alcohol produce cross tolerance and, when taken together, will increase absorption and produce additive depression of the central nervous system. Because of this, people have taken overdoses of barbiturates while intoxicated with alcohol, perhaps unaware of the additive effects of alcohol and the sedative/hypnotics.

Patterns of Abuse. The barbiturates are frequently used by individuals who abuse or who are dependent on drugs to relieve or counteract the effects of other drugs. For example, barbiturates may be used to relieve symptoms of heroin withdrawal. The individual may be unaware that cross tolerance does not occur between opiates and barbiturates and may think that, because his tolerance to heroin is high, his tolerance to barbiturates will be high also; therefore, he may unintentionally overdose on barbiturates. Heroin addicts may substitute barbiturates for heroin when heroin is unattainable and, because there is no cross tolerance, may develop physical dependence on both classes of drugs.[90] Barbiturates may also be taken to relieve the anxiety related to flashbacks from LSD abuse or to counteract the symptoms of anxiety, paranoia, and depression due to excessive use of amphetamines.[90]

Individuals may abuse barbiturates and sedative/hypnotics or anxiolytics for the many reasons people abuse alcohol, including the relief of anxiety and dis-

(Text continues on p. 484)

Table 26-2. **Major Criteria for the Diagnosis of Alcoholism**

CRITERION	DIAGNOSTIC LEVEL

Track I. Physiological and Clinical
A. Physiological dependency
   1. Physiological dependence as manifested by evidence of a withdrawal syndrome when the intake of alcohol is interrupted or decreased without substitution of other sedation. It must be remembered that overuse of other sedative drugs can produce a similar withdrawal state, which should be differentiated from withdrawal from alcohol.

a. Gross tremor (differentiated from other causes of tremor)	1
b. Hallucinosis (differentiated from schizophrenic hallucinations or other psychoses)	1
c. Withdrawal seizures (differentiated from epilepsy and other seizure disorders)	1
d. Delirium tremens, which usually starts between the 1st and 3d day after withdrawal and minimally includes tremors, disorientation, and hallucinations	1

   2. Evidence of tolerance to the effects of alcohol (there may be a decrease in previously high levels of tolerance late in the course). Although the degree of tolerance to alcohol in no way matches the degree of tolerance to other drugs, the behavioral effects of a given amount of alcohol vary greatly between alcoholic and nonalcoholic subjects.

a. A blood alcohol level of more than 150 mg without gross evidence of intoxication	1
b. The consumption of ⅕ of a gallon of whiskey or an equivalent amount of wine or beer daily, for more than one day, by a 180-lb individual	1
3. Alcoholic "blackout" periods (differential diagnosis from purely psychological fugue states and psychomotor seizures)	2

B. Clinical: major alcohol-associated illnesses
   1. Alcoholism can be assumed to exist if major alcohol-associated illnesses develop in a person who drinks regularly. In such individuals, evidence of physiological and psychological dependence should be searched for.

a. Fatty degeneration in absence of other known cause	2
b. Alcoholic hepatitis	1
c. Laennec's cirrhosis	2
d. Pancreatitis in the absence of cholelithiasis	2
e. Chronic gastritis	3
f. Hematologic disorders	
Anemia: hypochromic, normocytic, macrocytic, hemolytic with stomatocytosis, low folic acid	3
Clotting disorders: prothrombin elevation, thrombocytopenia	3
g. Wernicke–Korsakoff syndrome	2
h. Alcoholic cerebellar degeneration	1
i. Cerebral degeneration in absence of Alzheimer's disease or arteriosclerosis	2
j. Central pontine myelinolysis diagnosis only possible postmortem	2
k. Marchiafava-Bignami's disease	2
l. Peripheral neuropathy (see also beriberi)	2
m. Toxic amblyopia	3
n. Alcohol myopathy	2
o. Alcoholic cardiomyopathy	2
p. Beriberi	3
q. Pellagra	3

Track II. Behavioral, Psychological, and Attitudinal
All chronic conditions of psychological dependence occur in dynamic equilibrium with intrapsychic and interpersonal consequences. In alcoholism, similarly, there are varied effects on character and family. Like other chronic relapsing diseases, alcoholism produces vocational, social, and physical impairments. Therefore, the implications of these disruptions must be evaluated and related to the individual and his pattern of alcoholism. The following behavior patterns show psychological dependence on alcohol in alcoholism.

1. Drinking despite strong medical contraindication known to patient	1
2. Drinking despite strong, identified, social contraindication (job loss for intoxication, marriage disruption because of drinking, arrest for intoxication, driving while intoxicated)	1
3. Patient's subjective complaint of loss of control of alcohol consumption	2

(From Criteria Committee, National Council on Alcoholism. Am J Psychiatry 129 (August):47–48, 1972)

Table 26-3.   **Minor Criteria for the Diagnosis of Alcoholism**

CRITERION	DIAGNOSTIC LEVEL
Track I. Physiological and Clinical	
A. Direct effects (ascertained by examination)	
1. Early	
a. Odor of alcohol on breath at time of medical appointment	2
2. Middle	
a. Alcoholic facies	2
b. Vascular engorgement of face	2
c. Toxic amblyopia	3
d. Increased incidence of infections	3
e. Cardiac arrhythmias	3
f. Peripheral neuropathy (see also Major Criteria, Track I, B)	2
3. Late (see Major Criteria, Track I, B)	
B. Indirect effects	
1. Early	
a. Tachycardia	3
b. Flushed face	3
c. Nocturnal diaphoresis	3
2. Middle	
a. Ecchymoses on lower extremities, arms, or chest	3
b. Cigarette or other burns on hands or chest	3
c. Hyperreflexia, or, if drinking heavily, hyporeflexia (permanent hyporeflexia may be a residuum of alcoholic polyneuritis)	3
3. Late	
a. Decreased tolerance	3
C. Laboratory tests	
1. Major—direct	
a. Blood alcohol level at any time of more than 300 mg/100 ml	1
b. Level of more than 100 mg/100 ml in routine examination	1
2. Major—indirect	
a. Serum osmolality (reflects blood alcohol levels) every 22.4 increase over 200 mOsm/liter reflects 50 mg/100 ml alcohol	2
3. Minor—indirect	
a. Results of alcohol ingestion	
b. Hypoglycemia	3
c. Hypochloremic alkalosis	3
d. Low magnesium level	2
e. Lactic acid elevation	3
f. Transient uric acid elevation	3
g. Potassium depletion	3
h. Indications of liver abnormality	
i. SGPT elevation	2
j. SGOT elevation	3
k. BSP elevation	2
l. Bilirubin elevation	2
m. Urinary urobilinogen elevation	2
n. Serum A/G ratio reversal	2
o. Blood and blood clotting	
p. Anemia hypochromic, normocytic, macrocytic, hemolytic with stomatocytosis, low fluid acid	3
q. Clotting disorders: prothrombin elevation, thrombocytopenia	3
r. ECG abnormalities	
s. Cardiac arrhythmias: tachycardia, T waves dimpled, cloven, or spinous, atrial fibrillation, ventricular premature contractions, abnormal P waves	2
t. EEG abnormalities	
u. Decreased or increased REM sleep, depending on phase	3
v. Loss of delta sleep	3
w. Other reported findings	3
x. Decreased immune response	3
y. Decreased response to Synacthen test	3
z. Chromosomal damage from alcoholism	3

CRITERION	DIAGNOSTIC LEVEL
Track II. Behavioral, Psychological, and Attitudinal	
A. Behavioral	
1. Direct effects	
Early:	
a. Gulping drinks	3
b. Surreptitious drinking	2
c. Morning drinking (assess nature of peer group behavior)	2
Middle:	
a. Repeated conscious attempts at abstinence	2
Late:	
Blatant indiscriminate use of alcohol	1
Skid Row or equivalent social level	2
2. Indirect effects	
Early:	
a. Medical excuses from work for variety of reasons	2
b. Shifting from one alcoholic beverage to another	2
c. Preference for drinking companions, bars, and taverns	2
d. Loss of interest in activities not directly associated with drinking	2
Late:	
a. Chooses employment that facilitates drinking	3
b. Frequent automobile accidents	3
c. History of family members undergoing psychiatric treatment: school and behavioral problems in children	3
d. Frequent changes of residence for poorly defined reasons	3
e. Anxiety-relieving mechanisms, such as telephone calls inappropriate in time, distance, person, or motive (telephonitis)	2
f. Outbursts of rage and suicidal gestures while drinking	2
B. Psychological and attitudinal	
1. Direct effects	
Early:	
a. When talking freely, makes frequent reference to drinking alcohol, people being "bombed," "stoned," or admits drinking more than peer group	2
Middle:	
a. Drinking to relieve anger, insomnia, fatigue, depression, social discomfort	2
Late:	
a. Psychological symptoms consistent with permanent organic brain syndrome (see also Major Criteria, Track I, B)	2
2. Indirect effects	
Early:	
a. Unexplained changes in family, social, and business relationships; complaints about wife, job, and friends	3
b. Spouse makes complaints about drinking behavior, reported by patient or spouse	2
c. Major family disruptions: separation, divorce, threats of divorce	3
d. Job loss (due to increasing interpersonal difficulties), frequent job changes, financial difficulties	3
Late:	
a. Overt expression of more regressive defense mechanisms: denial, projection, and so on	3
b. Resentment, jealousy, paranoid attitudes	3
c. Symptoms of depression: isolation, crying, suicidal preoccupation	3
d. Feelings that he is "loosing his mind"	2

(From Criteria Committee, National Council on Alcoholism. Am J Psychiatr 129 (August): 47–48, 1972) inhibiting effects. Some may believe the barbiturates are less detectable than alcohol or find alcohol unpleasant to taste. Many individuals combine or alternate alcohol with the barbiturates or similarly acting sedative/hypnotics.[90] The behavioral differences that may occur in intoxication are usually due to the individual personality of the user or the social setting in which intoxication occurs; for example, violence or aggressive behavior may be more readily exhibited in social settings where alcohol is consumed.[4, 90]

The following are two general patterns of abuse/dependency in this class of drugs:

Individuals who obtain the drug through legal means, such as prescription for medical problems, find the drug useful to relieve anxiety; they increase dosage and frequency of consumption. This pattern is often found in individuals from a middle-class background and in females between the ages of 30 and 60 years.

Individuals whose pattern is one of illegal possession of the drug are frequently in their late teens or early twenties and use the drugs to get "high" or get relief from the stimulant effects of the amphetamines.[4]

Sedative-, Hypnotic-, or Anxiolytic-Induced Organic Mental Disorders

Intoxication. Intoxication occurs after a recent ingestion of sedative/hypnotics or anxiolytics. Signs and symptoms of this class of substance are similar to those of alcohol intoxication.

Withdrawal. Withdrawal occurs hours to several days after decrease in, or cessation of, prolonged heavy use of the barbiturate or similarly acting sedative/hypnotic agent. Signs and symptoms of withdrawal are the same as those of alcohol withdrawal. The signs and symptoms do not necessarily follow a specific sequence of occurrence, and the severity of the symptoms depends on individual differences, doses, and the duration of use. Abrupt withdrawal from these drugs is not recommended; detoxification should take place in a medical setting.

Withdrawal Delirium. Withdrawal signs and symptoms from the barbiturates are the same as those of alcoholic withdrawal delirium or DTs and usually occur within 1 week after cessation or reduction of the drug. Some individuals experience delirium without seizures, some experience seizures only, and some exhibit both.[90] This condition is a medical emergency requiring hospitalization and medical intervention.

Amnestic Disorder. Amnestic disorder occurs after prolonged heavy use of barbiturates or similarly acting sedative/hypnotics. Predominant signs and symptoms of the disorder are impairment in short-term memory (inability to learn new information) and long-term memory (inability to remember past learned information). Full recovery from this disorder is possible.

Medical Consequences. Severe complications may result from intravenous barbiturate use. If the drug is inadvertently injected into subcutaneous tissue, *cellulitis,* in which subcutaneous tissues become swollen, inflamed, and painful, may result. *Vascular complications* occur if the drug is accidentally injected into an artery; these may result in loss of a hand or fingers.[90] The intravenous user may also suffer other medical complications from self-injections, particularly *serum hepatitis, endocarditis, pneumonia, tetanus,* and other *bacterial infections.* Also, *syphilis* or *malaria* may result, as well as allergic reactions to substances that may have been added to the drug.[90]

Barbiturates are frequently used in suicides. There are more than 15,000 deaths secondary to barbiturate poisoning reported yearly.[90] The extent to which these deaths are attributable to accidental or intentional suicide, however, is difficult to ascertain.

Individuals rarely use only one sedative/hypnotic drug; most use a variety of these drugs as well as alcohol. It is critical in the detoxification process to assess whether an individual used alcohol, other drugs concurrently with alcohol, or other drugs without alcohol.

The Opiates

Effects. The opiates are narcotics or drugs that produce depressant effects on the central nervous system. Included in this definition are opium and derivatives of opium such as morphine, codeine, and heroin, as well as synthetically produced drugs such as meperidine and methadone.[36]

The pharmacologically active ingredients of opium are the alkaloids, the most common of which are morphine and codeine. The opiates may be taken orally or rectally or they may be smoked; however, they are usually injected intramuscularly or intravenously.

Essentially central nervous system depressants, the opiates produce analgesia, mood changes, and sedation; depress respirations; and inhibit coughing. They are very effective pain relief medications. The physiologic actions of heroin are similar to morphine except that studies indicate that heroin is four or five times more potent than morphine.[36]

The body metabolizes heroin and morphine in similar ways. Heroin is converted by the body into morphine, metabolized primarily in the liver, with end products secreted through urine and bile.[78] Tolerance to the opiates develops rapidly and physical dependence occurs after a brief period of use.

Patterns of Abuse. Opiate abusers may be separated into two classes—those who are street abusers and those who abuse the opiate analgesics obtained from medical sources. The latter, in general, are an older, middle-class, well-established group, in comparison with the street abusers who obtain opiates from illegal sources.[7,91]

The average "street" abuser tends to be male, young, and frequently from a minority group. The individual begins using opiates occasionally but progresses to daily use and quickly develops dependence and tolerance. Frequently, there is a history of delinquent or antisocial behavior. The illegal status of the drug brings involvement in legal problems. There is a high incidence of death in this group due to suicide, homicide, accidents, and diseases such as infections and tuberculosis. The mortality rate is about 5 to 10 per 1000 for opiate users.[78]

Medical abusers tend to be women from a middle-class environment or those with pain syndromes who misuse their prescribed drugs and often misuse other drugs as well. Two high-risk groups for this type of abuse are those individuals with pain syndromes and health care workers, especially physicians and nurses.[78] Opioid abuse and dependency is usually preceded by a period of polydrug use, which continues after opioid use is acquired.[4]

Opioid-Induced Organic Mental Disorders

Intoxication. Opiate intoxication is marked by the recent use of opioids, pupillary constriction, drowsiness, slurred speech, impairment in attention or memory, euphoria, dysphoria, apathy, and psychomotor retardation. Problems in social or occupational functioning and impaired judgment may result in maladaptive behavior.

Opioid Withdrawal. Following the prolonged, heavy use of opioids and after cessation or reduction of opioid use, withdrawal symptoms may include tearing, runny nose, dilated pupils, "gooseflesh" (piloerection), sweating, diarrhea, yawning, mild hypertension, tachycardia, fever, and insomnia. Accompanying symptoms may be irritability, depression, restlessness, tremor, weakness, nausea, vomiting, and muscle and joint pains. All of these symptoms may resemble "flu" symptoms.

Duration of the withdrawal period depends on the specific drug. Withdrawal symptoms may elicit a great deal of discomfort but are usually not life-threatening unless the client has a concurrent, serious medical problem, such as cardiac disease.

Medical Consequences. The prolonged use of opiates often results in decreased motivation to quality life experiences; personal and social deterioration that usually involves problems with police and law enforcement agencies; and family and interpersonal problems.[78]

Serious medical problems may result from drug overdose, from the additives in the street drugs, from poor nutrition and health, and from infections due to unsterile needles and equipment used in self-injection. Some of the common problems encountered are *abscesses* and *infections* of skin and muscle, *tetanus, malaria, liver disease, hepatitis, gastric ulcers, endocarditis, heart arrhythmias, anemia, infections* of bones and joints, *pneumonia, tuberculosis, lung abscesses,* and *kidney failure* caused by infections of additives in street drug mixtures. Sexual functioning problems may occur secondary to low testosterone levels during chronic opiate use. In addition, serious emotional problems, such as depression, may result from opioid abuse.[78]

Amphetamines and Cocaine: Central Nervous System Stimulants

Stimulants are drugs that act directly on the central nervous system. The individual taking stimulants becomes more talkative and active and has an increased sense of well-being, self-confidence, and alertness. Stimulants are frequently used to decrease appetite, reduce fatigue, and combat mild depression. A common stimulant is caffeine, an ingredient in coffee, tea, and soft drinks.

Amphetamine is the prototype for this class of drug and other chemically related drugs with similar pharmacologic properties.[4,36] Cocaine, also a stimulant, is classified as a narcotic and falls under the Controlled Substance Act.

Effects of Amphetamines and Similarly Acting Sympathomimetics. This category includes all substituted phenylethylamine structures such as amphetamine and methamphetamine ("speed"), substances with different chemical structures but amphetamine-like actions, and some substances used as "diet pills." These substances may be taken orally or intravenously.[4] Tolerance develops within hours to days, and there is cross-tolerance to most stimulants. It is not known whether this tolerance is related to cocaine.[78]

Patterns of Abuse. As with other substances, abusers of amphetamine can be generally classified into medical abusers and street abusers.[36,78] Medical abusers may obtain these drugs to aid in weight loss or to treat fatigue. Students may use them to help stay awake when studying for exams; truck drivers may use them to stay awake during long distance driving. After the medication is discontinued, fatigue results and need for sleep leads to an increase of dose, eventually leading to chronic use.

Street abusers use amphetamine or similar drugs to get "high" or achieve an altered state of consciousness. The drug may be used alone or with depressant drugs. Another pattern is using the substance in "runs"; that is, taking the drug around the clock for 2 or even 4 days, usually by the intravenous route.[36,78]

Amphetamine- and Similar Sympathomimetic-Induced Organic Mental Disorders

Intoxication. Physical symptoms of amphetamine intoxication include increased heart rate, dilated pupils, increased blood pressure, perspiration, chills, nausea, and vomiting. The psychological symptoms of intoxication of this drug are psychomotor agitation, elation, grandiosity, talkativeness, loquacity, and hypervigilance. Individuals who are intoxicated with amphetamine display maladaptive behavior, such as fighting, interference in social and occupational functioning, and impaired judgment.

Delirium. The symptoms of amphetamine delirium usually occur within 1 hour of oral intake or immediately after the intravenous injection and subside within 6 hours. Symptoms of amphetamine delirium include hallucinations (visual, tactile, and olfactory), labile affect, and violent, aggressive behavior.

Delusional Disorder. Prolonged, chronic use of moderate to high doses of amphetamine may result in a delusional disorder. Symptoms of the disorder include persecutory delusions, ideas of reference, aggressiveness, hostility, anxiety, and psychomotor agitation. The delusional individual may experience distortion of body image or tactile hallucinations, such as feeling bugs crawling under the skin, and he may scratch intensely to relieve the sensation. The delusional disorder may last for a week or longer, even for as long as a year.

Withdrawal. Amphetamine withdrawal follows prolonged use with abrupt cessation or reduction in the use of the drug. Symptoms of withdrawal include dysphoric mood (*e.g.*, depression, irritability, anxiety), fatigue, disturbed sleep, and increased dreaming. Dysphoric mood is the main feature of this disorder; if it is severe, agitation or suicidal ideation may occur. The sleep disturbance is related to an increase in REM sleep and may be present for weeks. The withdrawal syndrome occurs within 3 days of cessation or reduction in the use of the substance and peaks in 2 or 4 days. The symptoms of depression and irritability, however, may continue for months.

Medical Consequences. The medical consequences of abuse of amphetamine and similar drugs are those associated with overdose. Problems such as *tetanus, hepatitis, abscesses,* and *infections* may also result from the complications of self-injection. The signs of *cerebral vascular accident* may appear as a result of the strong contractions of blood vessels caused by stimu-

lants; the increase in blood pressure may cause *intracranial hemorrhage*.[78]

Effects of Cocaine. Cocaine is an akaloid obtained from the plant coca bush (Erythroxylum Coca), which grows in South America. It is a white, odorless, fluffy powder that looks like snow, giving the substance one of its street names. It may be taken by sniffing through the nose ("snorting"), where it is absorbed through the nasal mucous membranes. (Cocaine can be absorbed from all mucous surfaces, including the gums or mucous lining of the mouth, rectal and vaginal mucosa, and abrasions of the skin surface. All of these routes have been utilized.) Cocaine may be injected intravenously ("mainlining"), mixed in the same syringe with heroin (called a "speedball"), or ("free basing"). Because cocaine hydrochloride decomposes at high temperature, cocaine "free base" is the term used when the cocaine alkaloid is freed from the hydrochloride salt. Users have kits to perform this process. In the United States, cocaine free base for smoking is sold in "crack" or "rock" form. The cocaine hydrochloride is processed into solid form and can be broken into "rocks" or cracks for smoking with no further preparation. Crack houses are places where crack cocaine is sold and smoked. Crack appears to be the most addictive form of cocaine.[4,20,30]

Smoking of cocaine is an efficient way of delivering the drug in a concentrated form to the brain. The alveoli of the lung offer a large area for absorption of the chemical substance. The appeal of smoking to users is the rapid circulation time from the lungs to the brain—about 6 to 8 seconds—while injection from arm to the brain takes about 16 seconds. Cocaine is metabolized by plasma enzymes and the liver and excreted in the urine.[4,20,30]

Cocaine-Induced Organic Mental Disorders

Intoxication. Cocaine intoxication is marked by recent use of cocaine, maladaptive behavioral effects such as fighting and impaired judgment, and problems in occupational or social functioning. The following physical and psychological symptoms occur within minutes to 1 hour of taking the drug. The psychological symptoms include an increased sense of well-being and confidence, increased awareness of sensory input, psychomotor agitation, elation, talkativeness, pacing, and pressured speech. Physical symptoms are increased heart rate, dilated pupils, increased blood pressure, sweating, chills, nausea, and vomiting.

Cocaine use, especially by intravenous injection, causes a characteristic "rush" or feeling of increased self-confidence and well-being. If severely intoxicated, the individual may experience confusion, incoherent speech, anxiety, paranoid thoughts, headache, and palpitations. Following the physical effects, the user is likely to feel anxious, tremulous, irritable, depressed, and fatigued. This state is known as "crashing," and the user craves more cocaine for relief of these unpleasant symptoms. Recovery from intoxication occurs in 24 hours.

Delirium. The symptoms of cocaine delirium usually occur within 1 hour of use of the substance (immediately when the substance is taken by intravenous injection) and subside within 6 hours. Symptoms of cocaine delirium include labile affect, violent aggressive behavior, and tactile and olfactory hallucinations.

Delusional Disorder. An organic delusional syndrome occurs soon after use of the drug. Symptoms include rapid development of persecutory delusions, distortion of body image, and misperception of faces. Persecutory delusions may lead to aggressive or violent behavior; tactile hallucinations, such as the feeling of insects crawling on the skin (formication), occur.

Cocaine Withdrawal. Cocaine withdrawal follows abrupt cessation or reduction in prolonged (several days or longer) heavy use of the drug. Symptoms of withdrawal include a disphoric mood (*e.g.*, depression, irritability, anxiety) along with symptoms of fatigue, psychomotor agitation, and sleep disturbance manifested by insomnia or hypersomnia. Paranoid and suicidal thoughts may occur; suicide is a major concern of withdrawal. The symptoms last for more than 24 hours after cessation of drug use.

Medical Consequences. During cocaine intoxication an individual may experience formication.[4] Severe ulcerations of the skin may result from the user's attempts to dig out these "insects." Overdose of cocaine can produce cardiac arrhythmias, convulsions, and respiratory depression.[36] Repeated heavy use by "snorting" the drug can cause tissue ulcerations in the nasal septum.[77,78] Cocaine use can produce a paranoid psychosis similar to paranoid schizophrenia disorder. This may require prolonged treatment and the use of antipsychotic medication.[20]

Hallucinogens

Effects. Hallucinogens are substances that alter mood and perception. They are also called psychomimetics. Ingestion of these drugs results in alterations in perceived time, alterations in space perception, illusions, hallucinations, and delusions. The character and intensity of these reactions depend on the drug dosage and the individual personality of the user. The results are unpredictable—a person may experience a "high" on one occasion and a "bad trip" on another.[36] Lysergic acid diethylamine (LSD) is the most potent and most common hallucinogenic drug.

Lysergic acid comes from ergot, a fungus that spoils rye grain. It was converted to LSD by a Swiss chemist in 1943. The odorless, colorless, and tasteless drug is classified as a hallucinogenic drug because it produces hallucinations.[36]

The LSD "trips" start within a half hour after taking the drug and last for varying lengths of time. It is uncertain how LSD acts on the nervous system, but it is so powerful that only small doses, 100 to 250 micrograms (one-millionth of a gram), are needed. The drug in liquid form is usually placed on a sugar cube; it has also been put on chewing gum, cookies, and blotting paper.[36]

The misuse of LSD seems to be decreasing, possibly because of the widespread knowledge that side effects such as "flashbacks" and chromosomal damage can result from LSD use. Surveys indicate that about 10% of college students have tried LSD at least once.[36]

Hallucinogen-Induced Organic Mental Disorders

Hallucinogen Hallucinosis. After recent ingestion of hallucinogens, a hallucinogen hallucinosis may result. It is evidenced by perceptual changes, dilated pupils, increased heart rate, sweating, palpitations, blurring of vision, tremors, and incoordination. Also present are maladaptive behavioral effects such as severe anxiety or depression, "fear of losing one's mind," ideas of reference, paranoid ideation, impaired judgment, and interference with social and occupational functioning. The perceptual changes, the main feature of the hallucinosis, occur in a state of wakefulness and alertness and include subjective intensification of perceptions, depersonalization, illusions, hallucinations, and synesthesias (for example, "seeing noise"). The hallucinations are often visual and colorful and contain geometric forms and patterns.

The hallucinosis syndrome begins within 1 hour after ingestion of hallucinogens and lasts for several hours. Individual variations of the experience are related to the personality of the user, the setting, and the user's expectations. Euphoria is common. The individual is usually aware that the changes in perception are due to the hallucinogen, although in some instances the individual fears loss of sanity and believes this will be a permanent state.

Hallucinogen Delusional Disorder. The use of hallucinogens may result in an organic delusional disorder that exists beyond the period of the direct effects of the hallucinogen, lasting longer than 24 hours after cessation of hallucinogen use. The perceptual changes of hallucinogen hallucinosis occur, but the individual believes that these misperceptions and thoughts are based on reality.

Hallucinogen Mood Disorder. An organic mood syndrome caused by hallucinogen ingestion may result in a disturbance in mood, often a depressed mood accompanied by feelings of guilt, fearfulness, and restlessness. The individual may be talkative and unable to sleep. The disorder may last for a brief or a prolonged period of time and may be difficult to differentiate from a mood disorder.

Medical Consequences. "Flashbacks" may occur following use of hallucinogens. Flashbacks are recurrences of hallucinations when the drug is no longer being used and may occur weeks or months after stoppage of drug use.[36] Individuals who have abused hallucinogens over a prolonged period of time are more likely to experience these recurrences of hallucinations. "Flashback" episodes cause anxiety and the fear of "going crazy." Physical dependence on hallucinogens does not develop. Tolerance develops and disappears quickly. Psychological dependence occurs in some individuals after chronic use. These individuals are known as "acid heads," implying a personality change in the individual as a result of long-term hallucinogen use. The individual becomes more passive, becomes introspective, and may lose the ability to concentrate.[36] Research has investigated the possibility of hallucinogen-induced chromosome damage that produces congenital malformations, but this has not been confirmed. Medical problems are related to self-injury during periods of impaired judgment or delusions.

Cannabis

Effects. Cannabis sativa comes from the hemp plant, which is grown in warm climates and from which marijuana and hashish are derived. Tetrahydrocannaberiol, or THC, is the active ingredient in marijuana and hashish. Marijuana is derived from dried plant leaves and is a less potent form of THC than hashish (also spelled hasheesh), which is derived from the resins of the plant flowers.[36]

The most predominant effects of the drug cannabis are euphoria and an alteration in the level of consciousness of the individual without hallucinations. The drug is usually smoked or eaten. The metabolites are excreted in feces and urine.[78] The federal government estimates that there are 16 to 20 million regular users of marijuana in the United States.[30,77] During the 1960s, the use of marijuana was popular as a means of antiestablishment protest. Presently, the use of the drug conforms to no specific social group, although many users are teenagers and young adults.[77]

Cannabis-Induced Organic Mental Disorders

Intoxication. Cannabis intoxication is marked by increased heart rate, conjunctival infection (bloodshot eyes), increased appetite (often for sweets or "junk food"), dry mouth, and the psychological symptoms of euphoria, subjective intensification of perceptions, sensation of slowed time, and apathy. Maladaptive behavioral effects of cannabis intoxication include impaired judgment and interference with social or occupational functioning, or other effects such as panic attacks, suspiciousness, paranoid ideation, and excessive anxiety.

Cannabis Delusional Disorder. This delusional syndrome may occur with persecutory delusions during an episode of intoxication or immediately following the use of cannabis. This disturbance does not usually last longer than 6 hours after cessation of the use of the drug.

Medical Consequences. Marijuana inhaled has an irritating effect on the lungs, and may result in acute or chronic bronchitis, and sinusitis in heavy smokers. Increased heart rate and a decrease in the strength of cardiac contractions invariably result from marijuana use, bringing dangerous consequences to individuals with heart conditions. Research has indicated impairment in sperm production and chromosomal damage, but results have not been conclusive. There is also research controversy concerning a causal link between marijuana use and brain damage. Another danger of marijuana use is the possibility that the use of this substance leads to abuse of more potent drugs, although this fear has not been substantiated.[78]

Application of the Nursing Process to Substance Abuse and Dependency Disorders

The discussion of the use of the nursing process with clients who evidence disorders of substance abuse and dependency focuses on general concepts applicable in all areas of practice. Although the issue of rehabilitation is addressed in relation to psychiatric inpatient settings, it is important to emphasize that nurses encounter problems of substance abuse and dependence in all areas of nursing.

Assessment

The Nurse's Attitude and Feelings

The nurse's attitude toward the individual with substance abuse or dependency is a critical component of the interview process. Individuals with substance abuse problems are often very sensitive to and perceptive of the attitudes and mannerisms of nurses and other health team members. The initial approach to interviewing the client needs to be nonjudgmental and objective. It is not unusual for the nurse to want to "rescue" the client; therefore, it is important to become aware of this possible reaction. The nurse's personal value system and personal, unpleasant contact with individuals who abuse substances may arouse judgmental feelings or attitudes toward the client. A therapeutic nurse possesses adequate knowledge about the substance abuse or dependency disorder and approaches the client with compassion and gentle firmness.

During the interview, the nurse should avoid using words or terms that may be interpreted by the client as offensive, such as "drunk," "addict," "alcoholic," and "boozer." Rather the nurse uses terms with a less negative connotation that convey the appropriate meaning, such as alcohol use, heroin use, "feeling good," and "feeling high."

The recovery process is another factor that may affect attitudes. Frequently, nurses and other health team members see more initial failures than successes. Relapse and return to drug use after treatment is not uncommon. Nevertheless, recovery does occur in many instances, and those who work in the area of substance abuse and dependence need to develop an attitude of hope. Feelings of hopelessness in the nurse or other health team workers are projected to the client; the reverse is also true.

Approaching the Client

The drug-dependent client who is being interviewed may be embarrassed about his behavior or may display uncooperative behavior. One way for the nurse to encourage cooperation is by demonstrating acceptance and a matter-of-fact manner, one that shows concern for the individual and conveys the message, "I care about your well-being" and "I know you are presently uncomfortable; I want to help you feel better."

The nurse maintains an empathetic approach during the interview and, although the client may be defensive or vague, the nurse does not respond with defensiveness or hostility. Questions should be formulated to elicit specific factual information and should be stated in such a way that they cannot be answered with evasive statements or generalities. If the client diverts the conversation, the nurse brings it back to the facts being discussed.

A format for eliciting information in major areas of assessment is provided in the Chart 26-8, "Assessment Guidelines." These guidelines are not meant to be all-encompassing. The examples of assessment data are not the only observations that may be noted; there will be others that are not listed in this assessment form.

Because of the denial frequently used by the client who abuses or is dependent on substances, some of the information obtained during the interview may be of questionable validity. A more reliable history or a clearer validation of the information obtained about the substance abuse disorder may be established by interviewing a significant other (spouse, parent, adult, child, employer, roommate) in the client's life. Although this information may also be somewhat distorted due to the emotional involvement and denial system operating in the spouse or significant other, it may nevertheless offer corroborative data about the client's substance usage and harmful consequences it has incurred. Another important reason for interviewing the significant others is to involve them in the beginning of the treatment and rehabilitation process.

Emergency Conditions

Substance intoxication, overdose, severe alcohol and sedative/hypnotic withdrawal, withdrawal delirium, withdrawal seizures, and prolonged narcotic withdrawal may be life-threatening disorders. The severity of withdrawal or abstinence syndrome depends on many factors, such as the type of drug used, the extent of the addiction, prior drug history, nutritional status, and the status of fluid and electrolyte balance.[78,91] The client may also have major medical complications, which the nurse will need to attend to in caring for him.

Intoxication. All of the drugs discussed in this chapter may cause intoxication. If the intoxication is severe, the symptoms may include lethargy and stupor, and an overdose of the drug may be a possibility. The intoxicated person may also demonstrate bizarre behavior, panic, fright, confusion, or physical problems such as vomiting or pain.[91] The treatment measures for simple intoxication may consist of careful observation of symptoms, emotional support, and protection from physical injury, until the drug has been metabolized. In most instances, intoxication resolves within a few to several hours.

Overdose. Drug overdose may be a severe medical problem and may necessitate critical care until the emergency situation is resolved. It is more frequency with alcohol, sedative/hypnotics, and narcotic drug use.[90]

Withdrawal Syndrome. Various medications are given for detoxification purposes and relief of withdrawal symptoms. The nurse is knowledgeable about the drug or drugs ingested, dose, route of administration, reactions, and possible effects and toxic effects of the drugs. Generally, the following drugs are used in treatment of withdrawal syndrome: the barbiturates are used primarily for barbiturate withdrawal and the anxiolytics, such as chlordiazepoxide (Librium) or diazepam (Valium), are used for alcohol

(Text continues on p. 492)

C H A R T   26-8
Assessment Guidelines

Demographic Data:
Name:
Age:
Sex:
Ethnic Group:
Marital Status:
Religious Affiliation:
Significant Other:

What is the reason for coming to the hospital (*e.g.*, symptoms of withdrawal, marital-family crisis, work problems, referred by legal source, wants help to "stop drinking" or using drugs, medical problems)?

What is the motivation for treatment:
General Observations:

Vital Signs:	Blood pressure (hypotensive, hypertensive)
Pulse:	Rapid, regular, irregular
Temperature:	Elevated
Respirations:	Rapid, shallow, depressed
Appearance:	
Gait:	Unsteady, normal, weaving, shuffling
Eyes:	Conjunctival infection, bloodshot, dilated, pinpoint, normal pupils, lacrimation (tearing), vacant stare, poor eye contact, good eye contact
Skin:	Perspiration, cool, clammy, dry, bruises, needle tracks, scars, abrasions, gooseflesh, excoriations, reddened palms
Nose:	Running (rhinorrhea), congested, "red"
Presence of Tremors:	Fine or coarse, slight-moderate or severe
Grooming:	Neat, unkempt, unshaven, odor (alcohol, foul)
Behavior:	
Speech:	Slurred, incoherent, loud, soft, normal, articulates clearly, monotone, hesitant, pressured, relevant, distractive
Attitude:	Quiet, calm, demanding, agitated, irritable, impatient, vague, withdrawn, suspicious, anxious, tearful, happy, silly
Dominant Mood–Affect:	Euphoric, depressed, angry, sad, appropriate, inappropriate, normal
Sensorium:	Orientation to time, person, place, changes in memory
Perception:	The presence of illusions, hallucinations, delusions, hallucinosis
Potential for Suicide:	Is the individual presently thinking about suicide? Is there a plan or a method to carry out that plan? A history of previous suicide attempts or gestures? Were attempts in intoxicated state or sober state? Is there a family history of suicide? Is there a recent loss or anniversary of a loss? (Assess need for emergency consultation and intervention.)
Potential for Violence:	Does behavior indicate potential for violence? Voice, manner, stance, verbal threats? Assess need for consultation, emergency intervention if necessary. Ask if individual has a history of violence when taking substances or during withdrawal period.
Present Drug History:	The areas that need specific assessment are the type of substance used, the amount taken, and the pattern of use.
Type:	Beer, wine, whiskey, cocaine, heroin, marijuana (cannabis), sedative/hypnotics, hallucinogens; one substance only, or a combination? This may mean combination within a class (*i.e.*,

alcohol, beer, whiskey, and wine, or alcohol and sedative/hypnotics). It may be combinations in different classes (*i.e.*, heroin and alcohol and stimulants or narcotics and sedative/hypnotics). What is the predominant substance of choice? Does the individual use "street" drugs, prescription drugs?

Amount: How much (approximate amount) does the individual drink? How many six packs, quarts, fifths? How much does he use, bags? What route (oral, intravenous, subcutaneous)? How many pills daily? Hits?

What is the pattern of use: Daily, several times a week? Increased on weekends? Only weekends? Binge or episodic drinking? Runs? Intoxicated daily? Has individual ever tried to control or cut down drinking or pattern of substance use? How?

When was last drink?
When was last drug dose? How taken?
What drugs currently taking?
Has individual developed tolerance? (explain)
When did it begin?
Has there been a change in tolerance?
Are withdrawal symptoms present?
Is there a previous history of withdrawal?
Is there a previous history of seizures?
Is there a history of hallucinations? (explain)
Is there a history of hallucinosis?
Was individual ever hospitalized? If yes, what for?
Are there are present medical problems?
Are there any chronic medical problems?
Is there a history of the following: liver disease? hepatitis? diabetes? heart disease? anemia? drug overdose?
Have there been any recent falls, injuries, accidents?
Is the individual taking any prescribed medication?
Has the individual any known allergies?
Past Drug History:
Has the individual ever stopped drinking or using drugs?
How long was the period of abstinence?
Why did the individual abstain, what was the motivation?
At what age did the individual start abusing/using substances?
At what age did the individual first begin having difficulty in life circumstances due to drug intake?
Has the individual ever been in treatment for drug abuse/dependency?
What type of treatment: detoxification, rehabilitation?
How many times in treatment for the above?
Is there a family history of alcohol abuse/dependency?
Is there a family history of other substance abuse/dependency?

Psychosocial History:

Conjugal: Married, separated, divorced, never married, widowed? What is spouse's reaction to client's abuse of substances? Does the spouse abuse substances? Is substance use causing marital conflicts?

Parenting: Are there children? How many, ages, and sex? Have children had school problems, health problems, physical, emotional sleeping problems?

(Continues on p. 492)

Intrapersonal:	What are the individual's leisure activities, hobbies? Has there been a change in participation in these activities? Has there been a change in friends or a loss of friendships? Do the social activities center on the substance use/abuse?
Occupation/Employment:	What is individual's occupation? Present employment? How long in present employment? Has the individual ever missed work from alcohol use? Drug use? Has the individual abused substances while working? Is substance use jeopardizing work or business? How long has individual been employed?
Finances and Living Conditions:	Approximate amount spent on substances? Source of income other than employment? Family suffering from less adequate housing or food due to substance abuse or purchases? What are present living conditions? Is individual living alone, in an apartment, own house, live in a room, is there no address or no permanent living arrangement?
Legal Problems:	Have there been any violations while intoxicated? Are any present legal offenses pending from substance abuse/dependency? Is present treatment court-recommended?

withdrawal. Codeine, propoxyphene (Darvon), or other opiate-type drugs are given for relief of narcotic withdrawal symptoms; if these symptoms are severe, however, drugs such as methadone or morphine may be used. Anticonvulsant drugs, particularly diphenylhydantoin (Dilantin), are given for alcohol and sedative/hypnotic withdrawal seizures. Thiamine is usually given in the alcohol withdrawal treatment phase to prevent Wernicke-Korsakoff syndrome. Multivitamins are frequently administered because of the typically poor nutritional status of the drug-dependent client.[91]

Behavioral Defenses

Defense Mechanisms. Defense mechanisms are processes within the mind (*i.e.,* intrapsychic processes) that are usually unconscious and that relieve the individual of emotional conflict and anxiety.[3]

Denial. Denial is the outstanding defense mechanism used by clients who abuse or are dependent on substances. It is especially profound in alcohol abuse and dependency.

Denial is an unconscious process used to protect against intolerable feelings, thoughts, wishes, needs, or external reality factors by blocking knowledge of these factors from conscious awareness.[3] Defense or coping mechanisms are used in normal ways to adapt to threatening situations, such as the normal grief process in terminal illness. The use of defense mechanisms becomes unhealthy when they are used inappropriately and when they interfere with healthy functioning. The individual who abuses drugs often seems unaware of the apparent adverse psychological, social, and physical consequences of the excessive drug use. Frequently, the abuse or dependency disorder develops gradually, and the use of denial and other defense mechanisms protects the individual from acknowledging the fact that the disorder is developing. This is especially true of alcoholism. Although denial can be found to some degree in all clients who abuse substances, it is most blatant in alcoholism and allows alcoholics literally to drink themselves to death.

Individuals with alcohol abuse or dependence cannot admit that alcohol is causing serious problems, and they continue drinking. One of the reasons for this denial process in alcoholism is the blackouts that occur. Blackouts are amnesia for part or all of a drinking experience, although the individual appears to others to be functioning and to know what he is doing. The guilt feelings the individual experiences as a result of his drinking, the social stigma attached to his behavior or disorder, and the possibility of rejection by others foster the development of denial.[26,49] The family and significant others also contribute by denying the drinking as a problem and by assuming caretaking or enabling roles rather than allowing the individual to experience the serious consequences of the drinking behavior.

Following are some of the defense mechanisms used by substance abuse/dependency individuals to deny or protect themselves from the acceptance of the disorder:

Projection. Projection is an unconscious mechanism whereby that which is emotionally unacceptable to the self is rejected and attributed to others.[3] The individual does not take responsibility for certain unacceptable behavior and places his behavior outside of himself, blaming persons, places, and things for his behavior.

Rationalizing. Rationalizing is an unconscious mechanisms by which the individual justifies, by seemingly believable means, feelings, behaviors, or motives that would otherwise be intolerable.[3] For example, the individual gives a reason for his excessive use of a substance other than the fact that he is dependent. The drug usage is not denied; an inaccurate, reasonable explanation is given instead.

Intellectualizing. The process of reasoning is employed to defend against dealing with unconscious conflicts and their resulting stressful emotions.[3] Rather than discussing a personal awareness of his abuse or dependence problem, the individual talks about the problem on an intellectual level, for example, analyzing the problem or giving theories related to the cause.

Minimizing. The individual admits to some drug abuse or dependence but makes it seem to be a minor problem.

Diversion. The individual uses certain tactics or techniques to change the subject to avoid the topic of abuse and dependency.

Anger. The individual expresses anger or displeasure in response to the subject of drug abuse or dependency. This reaction tends to induce the nurse or health care worker to change the subject, rather than to confront or deal with the anger the discussion produces in the client.

The nurse recognizes that the denial process is a real phenomenon; that is, the individual is not aware of the reality or extent of his substance abuse or dependency disorder. Because the initial experience with the use of the drug was pleasurable and although the pleasant aspects of the experience have diminished and unfavorable consequences have developed, the search for recapturing the pleasure remains. The psychological compulsion to continue the drug use becomes so great that it becomes the priority in a dependent person's life.[49] What begins as a stress-relief or pleasure experience becomes itself the stressor. Denial helps the drug-dependent individual maintain some sense of self-worth and remove himself from the harmful consequences of his behavior. In the process, however, he becomes progressively out of touch with the reality of the situation.[49]

Our society may well contribute to this denial process because it promotes the use of substances, especially alcohol, for relief of stress and anxiety, yet rejects the drug-dependent individual as weak-willed and amoral or as a Skid Row bum. The drug user's significant others frequently overlook situations of abuse or cover up the consequences of his behavior. In an effort to protect the individual, they enable the harmful abuse to continue; this is the meaning of the term "enablers," which is often used in the field of alcoholism.

Physical and Safety Needs

The physical needs of the client need constant assessment. The potential for infection is increased due to injuries, various medical consequences of the drugs, and factors that may result from substance-induced organic mental disorders.

The potential for physical injury is a serious problem. The safety and protection of the client from harm must be of primary consideration. The substance-induced organic mental disorders present altered states of consciousness and impaired reality-testing that will require vigilant assessment, thorough analysis, and appropriate nursing intervention.

Sleep disturbances are common, and conditions such as insomnia may result from withdrawal states, from the prolonged pattern of abuse or dependency, or from personal or family stress. Also, nightmares and increased dreaming may occur. Nursing measures to assess and alleviate sleep disturbances are undertaken because the use of sedative/hypnotics is usually discouraged owing to the abuse disorder.

Assessment and intervention methods need to be individualized to deal with the feelings of anxiety stemming from underlying conflicts and other issues related to substance abuse/dependency and cessation of use.

Depression or feelings of profound sadness due to decreased self-esteem related to substance abuse behavior or its familial, social, and legal consequences also require assessment and individualized treatment. Antidepressant medication may be used in conjunction with other supportive measures. The potential for suicide is a priority consideration and requires appropriate intervention (see Chap. 23 and Chap. 37).

Noncompliance with treatment is manifested in many ways that indicate a lack of motivation for treatment and may be due to the denial syndrome and to a lack of understanding of the disorder. The nurse needs to be alert to these manifestations and to help the client obtain insight into his behavior.

Nursing Diagnosis

Because of the wide range of physical and emotional needs of the clients with substance abuse disorders, many of the accepted nursing diagnoses are appropriate to use to guide nursing care. Some of the diagnoses applicable to the client's physical condition are: Fluid volume deficit; Alteration in nutrition: less than body requirements; Potential for injury; Potential for infection; Self-care deficit; Alteration in comfort; Ineffective airway clearance; Impairment of skin integrity; Sleep pattern disturbance; and Alteration in bowel and urinary elimination. Some of the diagnoses applicable to the client's emotional state are: Ineffective individual coping; Ineffective family coping; Hopelessness; Disturbance in self-concept: Self-esteem, role performance, personal identity; Knowledge deficit; Potential for violence; Impaired social interaction; Spiritual distress; Sensory-perceptual alteration; and Alteration in thought processes.

Planning

Developing therapeutic plans facilitates the client's participation in the treatment process and his ultimate recovery. Individualized nursing assessment and intervention help the client obtain the desired behavioral outcomes that will aid in the restoration of his emotional and physical well-being. Ultimately, the recovering individual strives for increased satisfaction in a way of life free from mood-altering and mind-altering substances.

Goal-Setting

Goal-setting for individuals who abuse or who are dependent on substances includes the following elements:

1. Provision for physical requirements
2. Maintenance of emotional stability
3. Reduction and eventual resolution of the use of pathological defense mechanisms
4. Understanding and acceptance of the substance abuse/dependency disorder
5. Identification with peers
6. Development of hope for recovery
7. Resocialization and increased interpersonal relationship skills
8. Development of increased self-worth and self-esteem
9. Establishment of alternative coping skills
10. Improvement of motivation to continued treatment and prevention of noncompliance
11. Involvement of family and significant others in the treatment and recovery process

Intervention

The Rehabilitation Process

The rehabilitation process usually focuses on the substance abuse or dependency disorder itself. The other problems that the client encounters, such as loss of job, marital conflicts, and legal problems, are often results of the drug abuse. Consequently, the individual does not benefit from the resolution of these problems if the drug dependency continues. Conversely, many problems that stem directly from the drug use, such as physical illness or family or legal problems, diminish with rehabilitation and continued abstinence. Other significant problems—physical, emotional, and social—are treated concurrently with the substance abuse/dependency disorder.

The rehabilitation process generally involves the following phases: detoxification, the restoration of physical and emotional stability, intervention methods to increase motivation to continue treatment, confrontation of the pathological defenses, intervention methods to increase self-esteem, facilitation of insight into problem areas, planning for discharge, and follow-up care.

An important aspect of the rehabilitation program is for the client to accept the responsibility for his drug abuse or dependency and to take the necessary actions toward recovery. Underlying the goal of discontinuation of the substance use and maintenance of abstinence is the necessity of a change in the individual's behavior that will lead to a new lifestyle, one of greater personal enrichment.

Breaking Through the Defenses

The breakdown of the pathologic defense mechanisms manifested in the denial system is a gradual process. The nurse is alert to recognize and understand the particular defensive maneuver being used by the client. Gradually, the nurse assists the client to come face-to-face with the objective reality that is being denied. A consistent, persistent approach is necessary. This persistent stance of the nurse and other health team members conveys the message that there is never a valid reason for the client to use the substances of abuse and dependency. When the client focuses on other problems in his life to the exclusion of the substance abuse/dependency problem, the nurse and treatment team refocus on the initial abuse or dependency problem. This approach assists the client to understand that other problems may be more effectively defined and resolved as a consequence of attacking the primary problem of substance abuse or dependence.

Understanding and Acceptance of the Disorder

The drug-dependent individual needs to attain an intellectual comprehension of the disorder. One approach is to understand that it is an illness and not a moral problem. Educational material about the manifestations of substance abuse disorder and clarification of misinformation assist in this process. An intellectual understanding helps the client accept the fact that the disorder is chronic and will not be cured. This requires acceptance of the disorder on an emotional level and recovery on a long-term, but day-by-day, basis. Most rehabilitation programs require abstinence as a prerequisite to recovery.

Identification with Peers

Peer group identification and confrontation of the abuse of or dependence on a substance is a powerful help to recovery. Individuals recognize and internalize the fact that they are not alone in their suffering, and they therefore receive emotional support and hope. The group also allows for confrontation by peers who attack pathological defense mechanisms and assist each other in the process of obtaining insight into behavior. The nurse may lead the group, encourage the client to attend the group, or discuss issues that may have surfaced after group attendance and participation.

Development of Hope

Clients enter the rehabilitation program with initial feelings of hopelessness, discouragement, and demoralization. They need to realize that escape from what may be perceived as a hopeless situation is possible. Identification with others who have the same problems and with those who have recovered or are recovering is significant in initiating a feeling of hope. The positive attitude of the nurse and other mental health team members also instills hope in clients.

Resocialization

The drug user's life becomes drug-centered and, in the process, the individual becomes self-centered. Social skills may be diminished or lacking. It is a priority to assist the client to review and rebuild the capacity for establishing interpersonal relationships that the previous self-centered attitude has eroded.

Development of Self-Worth and Self-Esteem

Generally, self-esteem and self-worth increase with the client's ability to see the substance abuse problem as an illness. In addition, the individual is helped by taking responsibility for making changes in attitudes and actions and for deriving satisfaction from achievements and relationships.

The nurse also helps the client develop self-discipline. For example, the nurse may help the client organize and adhere to a daily routine, which may be difficult for him becaue of a previously chaotic lifestyle centered around the substance of abuse. The nurse expects and conveys to the client the expectation that he take an active part in the recovery program. She encourages and supports his positive efforts to change. As the client experiences success, self-confidence, and self-esteem, hopefulness develops and he recognizes that there are alternatives to drugs. Motivation for recovery is enhanced as involvement in the program increases. Rehabilitation is a process that continues long after discharge from a treatment facility.

Other Important Therapies

Disulfiram (Antabuse) Treatment. The drug disulfiram (Antabuse) has been used in adjunct with other alcohol dependency treatment methods. The drug interferes with the metabolism to produce physical symptoms that, depending on individual variations and conditions, may be severe. The general physical symptoms experienced by the person taking disulfiram, after ingestion of even small amounts of alcohol, include flushing of the skin, pounding headache, feeling faint, weak, and dizzy, nausea and vomiting, tachycardia, chest pain, shortness of breath, hypotension, blurred vision, and confusion.[73]

The taking of the drug disulfiram does not ensure sobriety or cure alcoholism. The chemotherapeutic purpose of the drug is to assist the client to control or not act on the impulse to drink. The client understands that while the drug is being taken, these symptoms can occur after ingestion of alcohol. Therefore, the complusion to drink during that time is lessened and the client is free to concentrate on other areas in treatment. Because it takes several days for the drug to leave the body completely after the drug use has been discontinued, the client makes the decision to return to drinking on a conscious level rather than attributing it to an impulsive act. Most treatment programs offer disulfiram on a voluntary basis and a written informed consent is usually required. The client must have full understanding of the drug's action and consequences. Candidates for this form of chemotherapy must be carefully screened by the physician and baseline medical tests performed before the drug is administered.

The client must also understand that alcohol in any form (*i.e.,* in foods, cough mixtures, or other medications, as well as shaving lotions or other alcohol-containing substances applied to the skin) must be avoided because the same reaction produced with the intake of ethyl alcohol will occur. A list of these substances is given to the client, along with a medical alert card or bracelet, when he begins taking disulfiram.

Methadone Maintenance. Methadone maintenance is used in opiate dependence in conjunction with other treatment methods, although it is not a "cure." Methadone is a longer-acting narcotic that is substituted for the shorter-acting opiates, such as heroin. Methadone has similar pharmacologic properties to heroin, including addiction, sedation, and respiratory depression. It generally acts by blocking the euphoric effects of heroin and other opiates, thereby preventing the impulsive use of heroin.[91] The general purpose of a methadone maintenance program is to assist the client to develop a lifestyle free of "street drugs." This enables him to improve family and social functioning and to decrease or eliminate legal problems, traumatic injuries, and health problems associated with the obtaining and abusing "street drugs."[50,91] The drug methadone is administered in licensed clinics that have been established to control its distribution and prevent its diversion for illegal use. The clinics maintain a careful screening process for candidates and require that specific criteria for admission be met. Psychological and social rehabilitation of the client takes place concurrently.[50,91]

Drug Free Communities. Drug free communities are another approach to narcotic dependency treatment and rehabilitation. These therapeutic communities are usually long-term programs lasting up to 1 year. The client is removed from the "street culture" and given a new identity within the group community. In this program, confrontation by group members and ex-addicts helps the client gain insight into problem areas and find more successful ways of coping with life situations and stresses.[50]

Aversion Conditioning. Aversion conditioning is a behavioral approach related to the conditional response mechanism. The client may be taught not to drink by associating the sight, smell, and taste of alcohol with an unpleasant event. For example, the aversion technique may be mild electric shock to the skin.[75,91]

Other Modalities. Relaxation therapy in various modes is frequently used in programs to teach clients methods to release tension, improve self-image, and relieve insomnia without the use of drugs.

Role-playing is a technique that includes rehearsed responses to specific situations; for example, where drinking or drug-taking opportunities may be encountered—and, it is hoped, successfully refused—by the client. Social skills and responses to situations such as job interviews may be rehearsed to relieve anticipatory anxiety. Assertiveness training is another useful method to assist the client to meet dependency and interdependency needs and accept personal responsibility and satisfaction in achievements.

Self-Help Groups. The first, and perhaps the most influential, of substance abuse/dependency self-help groups is an organization called Alcoholics Anonymous or A.A. This self-help program was founded in 1935 by two men, Dr. Bob, a surgeon by profession, and Bill W., a New York stockbroker. At the time, these men were unable to obtain help for their suffering from alcoholism from the health professions. They found that, by sharing their life experiences with each other and identifying with each other in their common problem with alcohol, they were able to overcome their compulsion to drink (see Charts 26-9 and 26-10). Al-Anon is a fellowship of spouses, relatives, and friends of alcoholics that started as an outgrowth of A.A. and is now a completely separate organization. Alateen is a component of Al-Anon, and the sponsor of Alateen is usually a member of Al-Anon, although members of Alateen have separate groups and conduct their own meetings. Both groups follow the 12 steps of A.A.

Narcotics Anonymous (N.A.) is a fellowship of recovering addicts. Narcotics Anonymous follows a program adapted from Alcoholics Anonymous; that is, the 12 steps of A.A. are basis of the program of recovery.[63] Although N.A. follows the same principles of recovery as its model, the concept has been broadened to include all mood-altering substances. There is also Cocaine Anonymous (C.A.) and Adult Children of Alcoholics (ACOH) which is a component of Al-Anon, as is Alateen.

Evaluation

Evaluation is an ongoing component of the nursing process. The nurse continually assess the degree to which interventions have been successful in assisting the client resolve problems and meet short-term and long-term goals. The nurse reflects on questions related to the effectiveness of interventions. For example, if the interventions were not successful, why were they ineffective? Were there changes in the client's behavior and was the nurse able to foresee these changes? Evaluation applies to all steps of the nursing process, and modifications may be necessary because

CHART 26-9
What Is A.A.?

Alcoholics Anonymous is a program of recovery from the illness of alcoholism. It is an international fellowship of men and women who meet together to attain and maintain sobriety. It is nonprofessional, self-supporting, nondenominational, multiracial, apolitical, and almost omnipresent. There are no age or educational requirements. Membership is open to any alcoholic who wants to do something about his or her drinking problem.

What Does A.A. Do?

1. The A.A. members share their recovery experience with anyone seeking help with a drinking problem and give person-to-person service or "sponsorship" to the alcoholic coming to A.A. from a treatment or correctional facility or any other referral source.
2. The A.A. program, as set forth in the Twelve Steps to recovery, offers the alcoholic an opportunity to develop a satisfying way of life free from alcohol.
3. This program is discussed at the following A.A. group meetings:
   a. Open speaker meetings—open to alcoholics and nonalcoholics. (Attendance at an open A.A. meeting is the best way to learn what A.A. does and what it does not do.) At speaker meetings, A.A. members "tell their stories." They describe their experiences with alcohol, how they came to A.A., and how their lives have changed as a result of the A.A. experience.
   b. Open discussion meetings—one member speaks briefly about his or her experience as an alcoholic and leads a discussion on a selected subject (guilt, resentments, self-pity) or on any subjects or drinking-related problems anyone brings up.
   c. Closed discussion meetings—same format as above.
   d. Closed Step meetings—discussion of one of the Twelve Steps.

e. The A.A. members also take meetings into correctional and treatment facilities.
f. The A.A. members may, in conjunction with court personnel, conduct meetings "about A.A." as a part of A.S.A.P. (Alcohol Safety Action Programs) and D.W.I. (Driving While Intoxicated) programs. These meetings about A.A. are not to be confused with regular A.A. meetings.

What A.A. Does Not Do

A.A. does not do the following:

1. Furnish initial motivation for alcoholics to recover
2. Solicit members
3. Engage in or sponsor research
4. Join "councils" of social agencies
5. Follow up or try to control its members
6. Make medical or psychological diagnoses or prognoses
7. Provide drying-out or nursing services, hospitalization, drugs, or any medical or psychiatric treatment
8. Offer spiritual or religious services
9. Engage in education about alcohol
10. Provide housing, food, clothing, jobs, money, or any other welfare or social services
11. Provide domestic or vocational counseling
12. Accept any money for its services, or any contributions from non-A.A. sources

The primary purpose of A.A. is to carry our message of recovery to the alcoholic seeking help. The primary purpose of any alcoholism treatment modality is to help the alcoholic attain and maintain sobriety. Therefore, regardless of the road we follow, we are all heading for the same destination—the rehabilitation of the alcoholic person. Together, we can do what neither of us could accomplish alone.

(From Information on Alcoholics Anonymous, A.A. World Services, New York)

the changes reflect individual differences and responses to treatment.

Individual treatment plans are initiated together with the client, family, and members of the multidisciplinary team caring for that client. Referrals for continuing care after discharge or a return to the facility for outpatient follow-up care are frequently arranged or advocated. Referrals to halfway houses may be arranged to facilitate readjustment to community and society for clients who require resocialization in a more structured environment. Continued participation in self-help groups is strongly recommended.

CHART 26-10
The Twelve Steps of Alcoholics Anonymous

1. Admitted we were powerless over alcohol—that our lives had become unmanageable
2. Came to believe that a Power greater than ourselves could restore us to sanity
3. Made a decision to turn our will and our lives over to the care of God as we understood him
4. Made a searching and fearless moral inventory of ourselves
5. Admitted to God, to ourselves, and to another human being the exact nature of our wrongs
6. We're entirely ready to have God remove all these defects of character
7. Humbly asked Him to remove our shortcomings
8. Made a list of all persons we had harmed, and became willing to make amends to them all
9. Made direct amends to such people wherever possible except when to do so would injure them or others
10. Continue to take a personal inventory and when we were wrong promptly admit it
11. Sought through prayer and meditation to improve our conscious contact with God as we understood Him, praying only for knowledge of His will for us and the power to carry that out
12. Having had a spiritual experience as the result of these steps, we tried to carry this message to alcoholics, and to practice these principles in all our affairs

Summary

This chapter has discussed the use of substances that affect the central nervous system and the physical and behavioral changes that occur in individuals who abuse or become dependent on these substances. The focus has been on commonalities of substance abuse and dependency and the specific factors particular to each drug classification. Some of the major points of the chapter are as follows:

1. Selye's theoretical framework of the stress/ adaptation syndrome may be applied to the problem of substance abuse and dependency.
2. There is no single etiology of drug abuse and dependence; rather, theories examine multiple factors such as personality traits, genetic influences, social, cultural, ethnic, and environmental factors, and a self-destructive phenomenon.
3. Drug dependence may be viewed as a way of coping with life's stressors by individuals who abuse substances.
4. Substance use disorders are divided into the diagnosis of substance abuse and substance dependency.
5. Substance induced organic mental disorders generally include intoxication, withdrawal, and delirium.
6. Each class of substances of abuse is described in terms of its effects, patterns of abuse, diagnostic criteria, organic mental disorders, and medical consequences.
7. A nonjudgmental, objective approach is essential for establishing rapport with individuals who abuse substances.
8. Rehabilitation and eventual recovery are the focus of treatment planning and intervention with individuals who abuse, or are dependent on, drugs.
9. Problems of substance abuse and dependency are encountered in all areas of nursing practice.

References

1. Ackerman R: Children of Alcoholics. Homes Beach, FL, Learning Publications, 1978
2. Aldoory S: The Chemical Curtain: Polydrug Abuse Among Women. Alcohol Health and Research World 2 (Winter): 28–36, 1978
3. American Psychiatric Association: A Psychiatric Glossary. Subcommittee of the Joint Commission on Public Affairs (ed). Washington, DC, American Psychiatric Association, 1980
4. American Psychiatric Association: Diagnostic and Statistical Manual of Mental Disorders, 3d ed, rev. Washington, DC, American Psychiatric Association, 1987
5. Bakdash D: Essentials the Nurse Should Know About Chemical Dependency. J Psychiatr Nurs Mental Health Serv 16 (October): 33–37, 1978
6. Becker CE: Medical Consequences of Alcohol Abuse. Postgrad Med 64 (December): 88–93, 1978
7. Black C: Children of Alcoholics. Alcohol Health and Research World 3 (Fall): 23–27, 1979
8. Blume S, Dropkin D, Sokolow L: The Jewish Alcoholic: A Descriptive Study. Alcohol Health and Research World 4 (Summer): 21–26, 1980

9. Brill L, Winick C (eds): The Yearbook of Substance Use and Abuse, Vol II. New York, Human Sciences Press, 1980

10. Broadhurst PL: Drugs and the Inheritance of Behavior. New York, Plenum Press, 1978

11. Carroll JFX: Personality and Psychopathology: A Comparison of Alcohol and Drug-Dependent Persons. In Solomon J, Keeley KA, Wright J (eds): Perspectives in Alcohol and Drug Abuse: Similarities and Differences, pp 59–87. Boston, PSG, 1982

12. Cloptom JR: Alcoholism and the MMPI. J Stud Alcohol 39:1540–1553, 1978

13. Cohen S: Combined Alcohol-Drug Abuse and Human Behavior. In Solomon J, Keeley KA, Wright J (eds): Perspectives in Alcohol and Drug Abuse: Similarities and Differences, pp 89–116. Boston, PSG, 1982

14. Cohen S: The Pharmacology of Alcohol. Postgrad Med 64 (December): 97–102, 1978

15. Cornish RD, Miller MV: Attitudes of Registered Nurses Toward the Alcoholic. J Psychiatr Nurs Ment Health Serv 14 (December): 19–22, 1976

16. Cortina FM: Stroke a Slain Warrior, New York, Columbia University Press, 1970

17. Cotton NS: The Familial Incidence of Alcoholism: A Review. J Stud Alcohol 40:89–115, 1979

18. Criteria Committee, National Council on Alcoholism: Criteria for the Diagnosis of Alcoholism. Am J Psychiatr 129 (August): 127–135, 1972

19. Day S: Fetal Alcohol Syndrome. Alcoholism 1 (September/October): 35–37, 1980

20. Dougherty, DJ: Status of Cocaine Abuse 1984. Subst Abuse Treat 3. Pergamon Press, New York, 1984

21. Efinger JM: Women and Alcoholism. Topics in Clinical Nursing 5 (January): 10–19, 1983

22. Einstein S: Beyond Drugs. New York, Pergamon Press, 1975

23. Estes NJ, Heinemann EM: Alcoholism: Development, Consequences and Interventions, 2d ed. St Louis, CV Mosby, 1982

24. Ewing JA, Rouse BA: Drink: Alcohol in American Society—Issues and Current Research. Chicago, Nelson-Hall, 1978

25. Fenster FL: Alcohol Disorders of the Gastrointestinal System. In Estes NJ, Heinemann EM (eds): Alcoholism: Development, Consequences, and Interventions, 2d ed. St. Louis, CV Mosby, 1982

26. Fewell CH, Bissell LeClair: The Alcoholic Denial Syndrome: An Alcohol-Focused Approach. Social Casework 59 (January): 6–13, 1978

27. Fourth Special Report to the U.S. Congress on Alcohol and Health. DeLuca J (ed). Washington, DC, NIAAA (January), 1981

28. Fox V: Recognizing Multiple Simultaneous Drug Withdrawal Syndromes. Paper presented to NCA, AMSA Medical-Scientific Conference, Washington, DC, May, 1976

29. Gareri EA: Assertiveness Training for Alcoholics. J Psychiatr Nurs Ment Health Serv 17 (January): 31–36, 1979

30. Grabowski J (ed): Cocaine: Pharmacology Effects, and Treatment of Abuse. National Institute on Drug Abuse Research Monograph 50, 1984

31. Goodwin DW: Alcoholism and Heredity. Arch Gen Psychiatr 36 (January): 57–61, 1979

32. Goodwin DW: Is Alcoholism Hereditary? New York, Oxford University Press, 1976

33. Goodwin DW: Two Species of Alcoholic "Blackout." Am J Psychiatry 127 (June): 1665–1669, 1971

34. Goodwin DW, Powell B, Stern J: Behavioral Tolerance to Alcohol in Moderate Drinkers. Am J Psychiatry 127 (June): 1651–1653, 1971

35. Gottheil E, Evans BD, Vereby K: Research Relating to Alcohol and Opiate Dependence. In Solomon J, Keeley KA, Wright J (eds): Perspective in Alcohol and Drug Abuse: Similarities and Differences, pp 179–201. Boston, PSG, 1982

36. Green HI, Levy MH: Drug Misuses . . . Human Abuse. New York, Marcel Dekker, 1976

37. Greenblatt DJ, Shader RI: Drug Abuse and the Emergency Room Physician. Am J Psychiatry 131 (May): 559–562, 1974

38. Grinspoon L, Hedblom P: The Speed Culture. Cambridge, MA, Harvard University Press, 1975

39. Harrison J: Alcohol and the Impaired Physician. Alcohol Health and Research World 3 (Winter): 2–8, 1978

40. Haughey CW: Alcoholic Cardiomyopathy: Abstinence Makes the Heart Grow Stronger. Nursing 80 10 (September): 54–58, 1980

41. Hoffer R: Heroes and Hangovers: Pro Sports Faces Its Drinking Problem. Alcoholism 4 (November/December): 27–29, 1980

42. Huey LY: Psychiatric Problems of Alcoholics. Postgrad Med 64 (December): 123–128, 1978

43. Hughes R, Brewin R: The Tranquilizing of America. New York, Harcourt, Brace, Jovanovich, 1979

44. Inglis B: The Forbidden Game. New York, Charles Scribner's Sons, 1975

45. Jaffe J, Peterson R, Hodgson R: Addictions. New York, Harper & Row, 1980

46. Jellinek EM: Disease Concept of Alcoholism. New Haven, United Printing Service, 1960

47. Jellinek EM: Phases of Alcohol Addiction. Q J Stud Alcohol 13 (December): 673–684, 1952

48. Jones CL, Buttjes KJ (eds): Etiology of Drug Abuse: Implications for Prevention, National Institute on Drug Abuse Research Monograph 56, 1985

49. Johnson V: I'll Quit Tomorrow, rev. New York, Harper & Row, 1980

50. Jones KL, Shainberg LW, Byer CO: Drugs and Alcohol, New Yorker, Harper & Row, 1979

51. Khantzian EJ, McKenna GJ: Diagnosis and Management of Acute Drug Problems. In Brill L, Winick C (eds): The Yearbook of Substance Use and Abuse, Vol II, pp 144–169. New York, Human Sciences Press, 1980

52. Klatsky AL: Alcohol and Hypertension. Hospital Physician 16 (April): 40–43, 1979

53. Lieber CS, Garra AJ, Leo M, Warren TM: Mechanism for the Interelationships Between Alcohol

and Cancer, Alcohol Health and Research World 3 (Spring) 10–17, 1986

54. Loomis T: The Pharmacology of Alcohol. In Estes NJ, Heinemann EM (eds): Alcoholism: Development, Consequences, and Interventions, 2d ed, pp 93–101, St Louis, CV Mosby, 1982

55. Lipowski ZJ: A New Look at Organic Brain Syndromes. Am J Psychiatry 137 (June): 674–678, 1980

56. Marshall M: Alcohol and Culture: A Review, Alcohol Health and Research World 4 (Summer): 2–7, 1980

57. Martin JC: No Laughing Matter. New York, Harper & Row, 1982

58. Mendelson JH, Mello NK (eds): The Diagnosis and Treatment of Alcoholism. New York, McGraw-Hill, 1979

59. Milan JR, Kitcham K: Under the Influence: A Guide to Myths and Realities of Alcoholism. Bantam Books, 1981

60. Morin R: Sexual Dysfunction in the Alcoholic Male. Alcoholism 1 (September–October): 28–21, 1980

61. Morrissey E: Alcohol Related Problems in Adolescents and Women. Postgrad Med 64 (December): 111–119, 1978

62. Murphey GE, Armstrong JW, Jr, Hermele SL, Fischer JK, Clendenin WW: Suicide and Alcoholism. Arch Gen Psychiatry 36 (January): 65–69, 1979

63. Narcotics Anonymous. C.A.R.E.W.A. Publishing Co., 1982

64. National Institute on Alcohol Abuse and Alcoholism: Alcoholism: An Inherited Disease. U.S. Department of Health and Human Services. Maryland, 1986

65. Nightengale SL: Treatment for Drug Abusers in the United States. Addictive Diseases: An International Journal 3:11–20, 1977

66. Nir Y, Cutler R: The Unmotivated Patient Syndrome: Survey of Therapeutic Interventions. Am J Psychiatry 135 (April): 442–446, 1978

67. Pattison EM, Sobell MB, Sobell LC: Emerging Concepts of Alcohol Dependence. New York, Springer-Verlag, 1977

68. Podalsky DM: Alcohol Consumption and the Risk of Breast Cancer. Alcohol Health and Research World 3 (Spring): 40–43, 1986.

69. Reddy B, McEltresh OH: Detachment and Recovery from Alcoholism. Alcohol Health and Research World 2 (Spring): 28–33, 1978

70. Richards TM: Working with Children of an Alcoholic Mother. Alcohol Health and Research World 3 (Spring): 22–25, 1979

71. Robertson CC, Sellers EM: Alcohol Intoxication and the Alcohol Withdrawal Syndrome. Postgrad Med 64 (December): 133–138, 1978

72. Robins LN, Helzer JE, Hesselbrock M, Wish E: Vietnam Veterans Three Years After Vietnam: How Our Study Changed Our View of Heroin. In Brill L, Winick C (eds): The Yearbook of Substance Use and Abuse, Vol II, pp 213–230. New York, Human Sciences Press, 1980

73. Rodman MJ, Smith DW: Pharmacology and Drug Therapy in Nursing, 3d ed. Philadelphia, JB Lippincott, 1985

74. Rosett HL, Ouellette EM, Weiner L, Owens E: Therapy of Heavy Drinking During Pregnancy. Obstet Gynecol 51 (January): 41–46, 1978

75. Royce JE: Alcohol Problems and Alcoholism: A Comprehensive Survey. New York, Free Press, 1981

76. Santo Y: Differences in Polydrug Abuse Between Men and Women. Alcohol Health and Research World 3 (Winter): 37–39, 1978

77. Schroeder RC: The Politics of Drugs: An American Dilemma, 2d ed. Washington, DC, Congressional Quarterly Press, 1980

78. Schukit MA: Drug and Alcohol Abuse: A Clinical Guide to Diagnosis and Treatment. New York, Plenum Press, 1979

79. Schuckit MA: The Disease Alcoholism. Postgrad Med 64 (December): 78–84, 1978

80. Selye H: The Stress of Life. New York, McGraw-Hill, 1956

81. Selye H: Stress Without Distress. New York, New American Library, 1974

82. Smith DE, Wessen DR: Treating the Cocaine Abuser. Hazelton Foundation, 1985.

83. Solomon J, Arnon D: Alcohol and Other Substance Abusers. In Suicide Theory and Clinical Aspects. Boston, PSG, 1972

84. Solomon J: Perspectives in Alcohol and Drug Abuse: Similarities and Differences. Boston, PSG, 1982

85. Spotts JV, Shontz FC: Cocaine Users. New York, Free Press, 1980

86. Strug DL: The Role of Anthropology in the Treatment of Alcoholism and Substance Abuse. Alcohol Health and Research World 4 (Summer): 8–9, 1980

87. Tarter RE, Schneider DU: Blackout Relationship with Memory Capacity and Alcoholism History. Arch Gen Psychiatry 33 (December): 1492–1496. 1976

88. The Drug Abuse Council: Facts About Drug Abuse. New York, The Free Press, 1980

89. Vaillant GF: The Natural History of Alcoholism. Cambridge, MA, Harvard University Press, 1983

90. Wesson DR, Smith DE: Barbiturates: Their Use, Misuse, and Abuse. New York, Human Services Press, 1977

91. Westermeyer J: A Primer on Chemical Dependency. Baltimore, Williams & Wilkins, 1976

92. Worden M, Roselline G: Applying Nutritional Concepts in Alcohol and and Drug Counseling. Journal of Psychedelic Drugs 11 (July–September): 173–184, 1979

93. Yearwood AC, Hess SK: How Can an Alcoholic Change in 28 Days? Am J Nurs 79 (August): 1436–1438, 1979

94. Zinberg S: Principles of Alcoholism Psychotherapy. In Wallace J, Blume S (eds): Practical Approaches to Alcoholism Psychotherapy, pp 3–18. New York, Plenum Press, 1978

27

Eating Disorders: Anorexia Nervosa and Bulimia

Susan D. Decker

At age 13, I was totally immersed in self-starvation. Weighing less than 60 pounds...all the time I keep running into people who haven't seen me in a while. They all look shocked, they all say the same thing: "You're so thin! You don't look like yourself any more!" I thrive on their reactions. It's so reassuring to hear that I don't look like my supposed "self" anymore....Now, at age 30, I'm 5'5" and 120 pounds. Nicely "cured" of Anorexia Nervosa, right? I wish!

Annie Ciseaux,
1980

Mirror, mirror, on the wall. Who's the fairest of us all?
Snow White

Chapter Preview

Adolescent and young women in contemporary Western society are frequently concerned with weight and physical appearance. "Never too thin or too rich!" is a prevalent societal attitude. Two extreme manifestations of this concern with weight are anorexia nervosa and bulimia. Anorexia nervosa is a life-threatening condition characterized by an intense fear of becoming obese, emaciation, and a disturbance in body image. Many individuals with anorexia also engage in bulimia, a disorder characterized by binge eating and purging.

Why does a teenage girl determinedly starve herself, while others view her as grotesquely thin? Why can't her parents make her eat? Why does a young woman ingest enormous amounts of food and furtively vomit? The purpose of this chapter is to help the reader understand the etiology and dynamics of eating disorders and to utilize the nursing process effectively with anorexic and bulimic clients.

Eating disorders greatly challenge the nurse because of their complex psychosocial and physical problems. A sensitivity to the needs of clients with eating disorders will help the nurse to intervene constructively with clients who "resist" help and "willfully" persist in self-destructive behaviors.

Learning Objectives

On completion of this chapter, you should be able to accomplish the following:

1. define anorexia nervosa and bulimia
2. describe the incidence of eating disorders and the populations affected
3. describe the diagnostic criteria for anorexia nervosa and bulimia
4. discuss theories of the etiology of eating disorders
5. apply the nursing process to clients with eating disorders

   gather and assess the physiologic and psychosocial data of clients with eating disorders

   analyze and synthesize client data in the formulation of nursing diagnoses

   develop client behavioral outcomes

   utilize various intervention modalities with clients with eating disorders

   evaluate the effectiveness of the planned interventions for clients with eating disorders

6. recognize your own feelings and attitudes regarding the care of clients with eating disorders

Incidence of Eating Disorders and Populations Affected

Anorexia nervosa and bulimia are conditions that occur primarily among adolescent and young women. Only 5% to 10% of all cases have been identified in young men.[3] The age at onset is usually 12 to 25 years; onset after age 30 is rare.[21] However, it is erroneous to conclude that the manifestations of eating disorders necessarily disappear after young adulthood. A survey by the National Association of Anorexia Nervosa and Related Disorders indicated that among 1,400 anorexic and bulimic respondents, 5% were over age 60, 1.8% were over age 50, 2.7% were age 40 to 49, and 20.5% were age 30 to 39. The remaining respondents were below 30 years of age.[6]

Anorexia Nervosa

Anorexic clients usually come from white, well-educated, middle- and upper-class families where children are highly valued and protected. The age at onset is most commonly between 12 and 18 years of age.[13] Prior to the anorexic episode, clients are typically described as "model children" who exhibit compliance, obedience, perfectionism, and a desire to please parents and teachers. They are generally high achievers in academic and athletic endeavors. Symptoms of anorexia nervosa commonly begin following life changes such as starting high school, moving to a new city or school, or going away to camp. Although families of anorexics at first appear loving and cohesive, unresolved and denied conflicts exist among family members. Sisters of anorexics are also at risk for developing an eating disorder.[15, 32]

Although anorexia nervosa was described in the literature as early as the 17th century, health care professionals and the general public have become increasingly aware of eating disorders in recent years.[12] The prevalence of anorexia nervosa has been estimated to be as high as 1 in 200 teenage girls, with mortality rates of 10% to 15%.[20, 29] The incidence of these disorders appears to be rising, although improved diagnosis and reporting may account for some of this increase. Many anorexic and bulimic clients never seek or receive treatment. One researcher reports that approximately 40% of anorexics recover spontaneously, 20% respond to treatment, and 40% become chronic.[21] It is estimated that approximately one-half of persons with anorexia nervosa also exhibit bulimic behavior.[10, 27] Death from starvation, infection, or suicide occurs in up to 21% of cases.[26]

Bulimia

The incidence of bulimia is much higher than that of anorexia nervosa. Recent studies estimate the prevalence of bulimia among young women to be about 5%.[23, 27] It is particularly difficult to ascertain accurately the incidence of bulimia since binging and purging are generally carried out secretly and the individual's weight may be relatively normal.

The age of onset of bulimia tends to be older than that of the anorexic client. The typical bulimic is a young, college-educated woman who achieves highly at work or school. Despite her achievements, however, she tends to be passive, dependent, and unassertive. Her family may be disorganized, in conflict, and characterized by confusing sex role expectations for women.[27, 35] There is commonly a family history of affective disorders, and some researchers have proposed that eating disorders are basically a form of depressive mood disorders.[38] Bulimic clients have difficulty with direct expression of feelings, are prone to impulsive behavior, and may have problems with alcohol and other substance abuse.[34]

Definitions and Diagnostic Criteria of Eating Disorders

Definition: Anorexia Nervosa

Anorexia nervosa is a psychiatric disorder characterized by a voluntary refusal to eat. In addition to psychological symptoms, there are multiple physiologic consequences of starvation. The anorexic client has a distorted body image and, to the bewilderment of friends, views her emaciated body as "fat." While anorexics eat very little themselves, they are typically obsessed with food and cooking for others. Vigorous physical activity is often obsessively pursued to burn their "excess" calories. Physiologic changes occurring in response to the extreme weight loss of anorexia nervosa include amenorrhea, lanugo hair, hypotension, bradycardia, hypothermia, constipation, polyuria, and electrolyte imbalances.[17]

Definition: Bulimia

Bulimia is a psychiatric disorder characterized by episodic, uncontrolled, rapid ingestion of large quantities of food. Bulimia may occur alone or in conjunction with the food-restricting behavior of anorexia nervosa. The bulimic client compensates for excessive food intake by self-induced vomiting, obsessive exercise, and/or use of laxatives and diuretics. The bulimic client may consume an incredible number of calories (an average of 3,415 calories per binge episode), in a short period of time, induce vomiting, and perhaps repeat this behavior several times a day.[31] In addition to a large food bill, the bulimic client may develop dental caries as a result of frequent contact of tooth enamel with food and acidic gastric fluids.[25] Other physiologic complications may be electrocardiographic changes, parotid gland enlargement, esophagitis, gastric dilatation, menstrual irregularity, and electrolyte imbalances.[24, 25]

Diagnostic Criteria

The DSM-III-R (Diagnostic and Statistical Manual of Mental Disorders, third edition, revised, 1987) criteria for anorexia and bulimia clearly delineate the clinical features of these disorders (see Chart 27-1). An area of some controversy, however, is whether bulimia is really a separate clinical entity or more truly an extension or different expression of the same basic factors underlying anorexia nervosa. Hilde Bruch,[7] an authority on eating disorders, argues that bulimia is more accurately a symptomatic expression of anorexia nervosa. Recent research that views eating disorders as existing on a spectrum supports Bruch's point of view.[2] Many people exhibit disordered eating patterns for many years—sometimes a lifetime.[2] Such persons may fluctuate between food-restricting anorexic episodes and binge–purge episodes where weight may be low or relatively normal. Before the diagnosis of a primary eating disorder is made, other psychiatric diagnoses such as depression or schizophrenia, as well as a physiologic basis for anorexia, must be ruled out.

Etiologic Theories

Multiple theories have been used to explain the development of eating disorders. Most experts agree, however, that anorexia nervosa and bulimia develop from a complex interaction of individual, family, and sociocultural factors. Eating disorders can best be understood in terms of a multifactorial etiology. It is most likely that an eating disorder will occur when numerous risk factors occur together. A vulnerable personality, sociocultural emphasis on slimness, family functioning style, a major life change or stressor, dieting, and the onset of puberty all contribute to the development of eating disorders. Differing theories of etiology, therefore, may each add something to the understanding of eating disorders.

C H A R T 27-1
Diagnostic Criteria for Anorexia Nervosa and Bulimia

Diagnostic Criteria for Anorexia Nervosa

1. Refusal to maintain body weight over a minimal normal weight for age and height (*e.g.,* weight loss leading to maintenance of body weight 15% below that expected) or failure to make expected weight gain during period of growth, leading to body weight 15% below that expected
2. Intense fear of gaining weight or becoming fat, even though underweight
3. Disturbance in the way in which one's body weight, size, or shape is experienced (*e.g.,* the person claims to "feel fat" even when emaciated, believes that one area of the body is "too fat" even when obviously underweight)
4. In females, absence of at least three consecutive menstrual cycles when otherwise expected to occur (primary or secondary amenorrhea)[1]

Diagnostic Criteria for Bulimia Nervosa

1. Recurrent episodes of binge eating (rapid consumption of a large amount of food in a discrete period of time)
2. A feeling of lack of control over eating behavior during the eating binges
3. Regular self-induced vomiting, use of laxatives or diuretics, strict dieting or fasting, or vigorous exercise in order to prevent weight gain
4. A minimum average of two binge eating episodes a week for at least 3 months
5. Persistent overconcern with body shape and weight[1]

Psychodynamic Theory

This theoretical viewpoint proposes that the development of eating disorders stems from unresolved conflicts in early childhood. The tasks of trust, autonomy, and separation/individuation go unfulfilled and the individual remains in a dependent position. It is postulated that parents do not respond consistently to the child's cues for emotional and physical needs during infancy, resulting in feelings of ineffectiveness in the child. The child is well cared for, but everything is done in accordance with the mother's needs and feelings, not the child's demands.[7,8,28]

During toddler years, the child's assertive, autonomous behavior is unrewarded, while clinging, dependent behavior is reinforced. Instead of becoming an independent, complete self, the child develops into an overly compliant person with a strong need to please others. Self-esteem becomes dependent on receiving approval from others, rather than on an internal sense of accomplishment and effectiveness. The child eventually is unable to recognize her own impulses, feelings, and needs. A crisis occurs at adolescence, when she is unable to separate successfully from parents and engage in peer relationships.[7,8,28]

Biologic Theory

Although the biologic theory is not widely accepted, its proponents believe that eating disorders may originate from hypothalamic dysfunction. Neuroendocrine abnormalities are found in clients with eating disorders, but these are generally believed to be the result of extreme weight loss rather than the cause of the disorder. A state of malnutrition does, however, affect the client's mental status and may play a role in the self-perpetuating nature of eating disorders.[9]

Behavioral Theory

Supporters of behavioral theory argue that the client with an eating disorder may initially engage in dieting and gain approval for weight loss. As weight loss continues, this approval turns to concern. The client continues to receive attention around the issue of weight, thus reinforcing her maladaptive eating behavior.

Sociocultural Theory

Support for a sociocultural theory of eating disorders lies in the fact that anorexia nervosa is rarely found in countries with an inadequate food supply.[12] Our culture has an abundance of food and places a heavy emphasis on physical attractiveness and slimness for women.[18] This theoretical viewpoint explains an obsession with weight, but does not provide an explanation for why some individuals, and not others, go to extremes in the pursuit of thinness.

Family Systems Theory

Family systems theory is widely used to explain the etiology and dynamics of eating disorders. Issues of control are central in families of clients with eating disorders. Families often consist of a passive father, a controlling mother, and an overly dependent child. The family places a high value on achievement; the child feels she must satisfy parental standards. Minuchin identified four interaction patterns characteristic in families of anorexic children: enmeshment, overprotectiveness, rigidity, and lack of conflict resolution.[29,30]

Enmeshment

Enmeshment refers to a lack of clear boundaries between the parent and child subsystems, as well as between individual family members. Members have failed to individuate, or adequately develop their own separate identities apart from the "family identity." The enmeshed family speaks in terms of "we feel" this and "we do" that. In healthy families, the parental subsystem functions as a unit distinct from that of the children to make decisions and meet adult needs. In the enmeshed family, one frequently finds an inappropriate alliance between a child and parent. The eating disorder may be viewed as a desperate attempt by the adolescent to separate herself from the family system, particularly from an overly dependent relationship with the mother.[37]

Overprotectiveness

Hypervigilance and overprotectiveness are common in families of anorexic clients. The overinvolvement of one or both parents makes it difficult for the child to learn to think, feel, and act autonomously. Although the parents usually love the child very much, they convey a lack of trust by not allowing the child to take appropriate risks. The child does not learn to trust herself and experiences a sense of personal ineffectiveness.

Rigidity and Conflict Avoidance

The families of anorexics have a low threshold for conflict. They believe that members are "supposed" to be happy and not have problems. Children may see very little conflict or expression of strong emotions between parents, since family norms discourage this behavior. The child does, however, inevitably experience strong feelings and conflict; but as these are consistently not validated, the child learns to doubt and deny her feelings, especially those of a "negative" nature. The family's politeness and superficial pleasantness interfere with the adolescent's need for autonomous expression of self. Rather than rebelling directly, however, the adolescent becomes more obsessive and perfectionistic in a search for love, approval, recognition, and reduction in anxiety. Eventually, she does desperately try to establish her own identity by exacting tyrannical control over what she eats.

Application of the Nursing Process to Clients with Eating Disorders

Assessment

As clients with eating disorders may be secretive and unwilling to portray themselves as having problems, the nurse must be skilled in eliciting feelings and thoughts. A supportive, but firm, approach by the nurse is helpful in engaging the client in the therapeutic relationship. Knowledge of the diagnostic criteria and etiology of eating disorders guides the nurse in asking relevant questions.

Assessment of the client with an eating disorder is complex. If one examines the eleven functional health patterns, clients with eating disorders may exhibit disturbance in nearly all of the 11 functional health patterns.[19]

1. Health Perception–Health Management Pattern

The client with an eating disorder frequently has an inaccurate perception of her health status. She often does not perceive herself as ill, even though others are alarmed by changes occurring in her physical and mental health status. She frequently resists treatment and, if a minor, often receives treatment involuntarily through the actions of her parents. The nurse should explore issues with the client such as: How were you referred to treatment? Tell me in your own words why you are here for treatment.

2. Nutritional-Metabolic Pattern

Numerous disturbances exist in this pattern. The client has either a very restricted food intake (anorexia) or an excessive food intake accompanied by purging (bulimia). It is important to obtain an accurate current weight, history of previous high and low weights, and the chronology of the current weight loss episode. How fast did weight loss occur? Were there any associated circumstances such as medical illness, psychiatric illness, situational crisis, or major life change?

Since the client may be reluctant to reveal details about dieting and/or binge–purge behaviors, it is helpful to ask the client to describe food and fluid intake for a typical day. The nurse will observe for clues of preoccupation with food. Does the client cook for others? Hoard food? Talk about food constantly? Have guilt associated with eating? Physical assessment may reveal numerous symptoms related to alterations in nutritional and metabolic status: fluid volume deficit (dehydration, poor skin turgor, hypotension), impairment of skin integrity (dry skin, brittle hair and nails), hypokalemia (vomiting, using laxatives or diuretics), alteration of oral mucous membranes (dental caries, mouth sores, sore throat, esophageal inflammation), cardiac changes (arrhythmias, bradycardia), hypothermia (lowered core temperature and cold extremities), and the appearance of fine, downy, lanugo hair (state of severe emaciation).

3. Elimination Pattern

Elimination disturbances occur in both anorexic and bulimic clients. Constipation occurs as a result of restricted food intake and vomiting. Excessive use of laxatives causes diarrhea and loss of protein, fluid, and potassium in her stool. Continued use of laxatives may also lead to eventual reliance on laxatives for bowel elimination. Polyuria may be present in the client with severe weight loss.

4. Activity-Exercise Pattern

5. Sleep-Rest Pattern

Clients with eating disorders are typically very active. They compulsively exercise, are restless, and frequently suffer from insomnia. Early morning awakening is common. A lowered pulse rate often occurs in response to excessive exercise and starvation. It is amazing to others that anorexic clients are able to engage in strenuous physical activity while consuming very few calories and appearing very frail. It is helpful to ask the client to describe her activity and sleep patterns for a typical day. What kind of exercise does she engage in? Is she involved in organized sports at school? Does she have difficulty sleeping? Is she often tired or does she have a lot of energy?

6. Cognitive-Perceptual Pattern

Clients with eating disorders typically lack awareness of the connection between their eating behaviors and underlying feelings, needs, and conflicts. Presenting these clients with knowledge of eating disorders is a beginning step in helping them to acknowledge that their behavior is maladaptive. Clients with eating disorders tend to exhibit intellectualization and all-or-none reasoning. Instead of recognizing and expressing feelings, they are more comfortable with abstract concepts. The client needs to learn that strong feelings, especially those of a "negative" nature, are acceptable and that one can experience and express strong feelings without losing control. Clients with eating disorders tend to have perfectionistic personalities and to give up if something isn't done exactly right. They need to learn balance and moderation in thinking and behavior. They also tend to overgeneralize and believe that all of life's problems will be solved if enough weight is lost.

The nurse might ask questions such as: Would you describe yourself as a perfectionistic person? Do you do things over and over until you get them right? Have you ever had the experience of not being able to get something out of your mind? Of thinking about things over and over? People are often afraid of losing control over their actions. How do you feel if you lose control, such as getting very angry? Eating too much? What do you do if you feel you're losing control? Have you ever had times when you've eaten uncontrollably? If so, describe these times. What did you feel and what did you do?

7. Self-Perception/Self-Concept Patterns

Clients with eating disorders experience considerable anxiety regarding becoming obese. Anorexic clients have a distorted body image, seeing themselves as too fat even when others view them as alarmingly thin. They generally have low self-esteem even though they achieve well at school, sports, and work. They hold unrealistically rigid and high expectations for themselves and look to others for approval. Clients with eating disorders perceive a lack of control over themselves and situations. They have not developed the sense that their actions will significantly effect a desired outcome.

In order to gain knowledge of the client's perceptual accuracy regarding body image the nurse might ask questions such as: What do you like the best about your body? The least? If you could change how you look, how would you be different? To explore self-esteem the nurse might ask questions such as: What do you like the best about yourself? Least? How would you describe yourself to others? How would others (family, friends) describe you? What are your strengths and weaknesses?

8. Role-Relationship Pattern

Clients with eating disorders frequently become isolated from family and friends. They often exhibit immature interaction patterns. They remain inappropriately dependent and childlike in relationship to parents, they stop dating, and they gradually abandon good friends. If the disorder persists, deficits in social skills increase. They often remain good students and spend much time alone studying. Isolation may also result from preoccupation with weight, food, and exercise. To assess roles and relationships the nurse might ask questions such as: Tell me about your relationship with your parents. How would you describe your family to me? Tell me about your friends. Do you have a lot of friends? A best friend? What kind of things do you like to do with your friends? What is school like for you? Do you study a lot? What activities are you involved in at school? Do you feel pressure to do well in school? (Pressure from self? Parents? Teachers?)

9. Sexuality-Reproductive Pattern

As a result of excessive weight loss, reproductive hormones regress to prepubertal levels. Clients experience amenorrhea, breast atrophy, lanugo, and loss of axillary and pubic hair. Infertility accompanies amenorrhea, but once normal weight is regained and menses resume, this is generally not a lasting problem. Anorexic clients tend to be sexually inactive, while bulimic clients may exhibit impulsive sexual behaviors. The nurse might explore questions such as: How do you feel about the body changes that occur at adolescence (*e.g.,* in females, breast development, menstruation, broadening of hips)? Is dating something that you enjoy? Have you had any sexual experiences? How do you feel about the presence or lack of sexual experiences?

10. Coping-Stress Tolerance Pattern

Eating disorders are maladaptive attempts to meet life's demands, roles, and stresses. The client may exhibit the following difficulties in coping:

Inability to ask for help and nurturance
Inability to make decisions
Inability to meet role expectations of adolescence
Inability to express emotions
Perceived powerlessness

In addition to ineffective individual coping, family coping behaviors may also be compromised. Families may exhibit difficulties in expressing emotions, in dealing with conflict, and in facilitating autonomy of members. Issues of control are commonly present in families of clients with eating disorders.

In order to assess coping behaviors, the nurse might ask questions such as: Tell me how you make decisions about everyday things, like how to spend your free time: What to wear? (For example, do you usually ask someone for advice or think things out for yourself?) Is your life right now pretty much the way you want it? If not, what would you change? What can you do to make these changes? What do you do to feel better when you're sad or upset? Have you ever felt like hurting yourself when you're down? Thought about committing suicide? Have you ever used alcohol or drugs to feel better? Have you ever stolen anything (*e.g.,* food or money)? If so, how do you feel about that? Do you get along with your parents? What happens when you argue with them? What kinds of things do you argue about? What happens when you talk to them about a problem or concern you have? Tell me about your brothers and sisters. How do you get along? Can you talk to them about your feelings and problems? What about your friends? Do they help you out if you have a problem?

11. Value-Belief Pattern

Specific problems do not necessarily occur in this functional health pattern. However, because the client generally has a low degree of self-knowledge and awareness, there may be a generalized deficit in clarity of value-belief patterns among clients with eating disorders. In addition, eating disorders most frequently occur at a life stage where the individual is struggling to establish her own identity and formulate a philosophy about the meaning of one's existence. As trust develops between the nurse and client, it may be helpful for the client to explore issues such as: What is important to me? What do I care about? What is the meaning of life? Who am I? What difference do I make?

Planning

Planning involves collaborating with the client, and possibly her family, to formulate an appropriate approach to treatment. The nurse determines with the client the goals to be reached. In many settings, the nurse, physician, psychotherapist, social worker, dietician, and occupational therapist work together to formulate the treatment plan. Communication and consistency among members of the multidisciplinary

---

CHART 27-2

Quick Assessment Tool for Eating Disorders

		Yes	No
1.	Do you spend most of your time thinking about food?	☐	☐
2.	Do you panic if you gain a pound or two?	☐	☐
3.	Do you ever eat uncontrollably?	☐	☐
4.	Do you feel guilt and remorse after eating?	☐	☐
5.	Do you ever fast or restrict your diet?	☐	☐
6.	Do you vomit or use laxatives to control your weight?	☐	☐
7.	Are your periods irregular, or have you stopped menstruating?	☐	☐
8.	Do you have a strict exercise regime?	☐	☐
9.	Do you panic if you are unable to exercise as much as you'd like?	☐	☐

team are critical. The primary nurse frequently coordinates client care among team members.

Short-Term Goals

Short-term goals focus on decreasing anxiety, restoring the individual to an acceptable weight, and normalization of eating behaviors.

Client will verbalize fewer fears and exhibit decreased anxiety regarding weight gain and loss of control.

Client will have adequate dietary intake to meet body requirements and maintain weight appropriate to age and height.

Client will not engage in binge eating or purging activities.

Client will maintain an appropriate activity level.

Long-Term Goals

Long-term goals focus on helping the client and, if possible, her family resolve the psychological issues that precipitated the eating disorder and to develop more constructive coping mechanisms.

Client will recognize and verbalize her emotions and needs.

Client will exhibit a realistic thinking process and perception of her body.

Client will verbalize adequate self-esteem.

Client will perceive control over her actions.

Client will demonstrate age-appropriate autonomy.

Client will recognize maladaptive coping behaviors and demonstrate adaptive coping behaviors.

Family will demonstrate constructive communication patterns.

Family will manage conflict constructively.

Family process will assist members toward individuation.

Intervention

The treatment of clients with eating disorders is a complex process and frequently a long one. Client improvement is often gradual and characterized by two steps forward and one back. Clients may resist treatment; the nurse is challenged to establish a relationship of open communication and trust.[14] Inpatient and outpatient treatment approaches generally include one or more of the following therapies: individual psychotherapy, behavior modification, group therapy, and family therapy. Recent research suggests that treatment success is greatest with family therapy, moderate with intensive individual psychotherapy, and lowest with behavior therapy alone.[15] However, it is important to remember that different methods may be effective for different individuals and their families.

Treatment Settings

Treatment of eating disorders occurs in both outpatient and inpatient settings. Clients with anorexia nervosa are more frequently hospitalized than bulimic clients. The primary reasons for hospital admission of anorexic clients are low weight, depressed mood, low serum potassium (can cause potentially fatal arrhythmias), lack of response to outpatient treatment, and a discouraged and demoralized family. Reasons for inpatient treatment of bulimia include the client's desire for treatment, low weight, dangerously low potassium levels, or a diagnosis of maladaptive personality patterns such as an impulse disorder or borderline personality.[2]

Since many clients with eating disorders never seek treatment, nurses frequently encounter the more severely ill clients in the hospital setting. Clients with eating disorders may be admitted to general psychiatric units or to units or facilities specializing in the treatment of eating disorders. Families are frequently frustrated, angry, and scared after months of trying to get the client to eat. The temporary removal of the client from the home may relieve the family's distress and set the stage for behavior changes in both the client and her family.

Behavior Modification

Behavior modification programs are generally begun in an inpatient setting. Although programs vary, the client typically starts a program with no privileges. Privileges are gained in response to appropriate eating behaviors. A criticism sometimes aimed at behavior modification techniques is that the nurse is manipulating and controlling client behavior without dealing with underlying issues.[8] Several research studies conclude that behavior modification is useful to restore lost weight but inadequate to deal with psychological symptoms.[4,5] Behavior modification is generally used in conjunction with psychotherapy, however, and can be a very helpful approach to meeting the goals of restoring weight and nutritional status.[22] The establishment of a contract which spells out the rewards, privileges, and consequences of noncompliance is useful in eliminating power struggles with the client. If the client feels she contributes to the planning of rewards and privileges, she will perceive more control over her environment and body and be more likely to adhere to the treatment regimen. It is critical that all health team members consistently carry out the terms of the contract.[36] Even though the client may rebel against contract terms, it is reassuring to her to know that consistent limits are being maintained and she can trust the staff to help her maintain control.

The nurse communicates caring to the client

through a kind, firm, matter-of-fact approach: "When you gain 5 pounds, you will earn telephone privileges. This is your choice." The nurse avoids punitive responses, arguing over limits, bribery, cajoling, excessive vigilance, and overprotectiveness. Through her interactions, the nurse conveys to the client: "You are a worthwhile person. I care about you. I have expectations of you and you are capable of meeting these expectations."

Individual Psychotherapy

Individual psychotherapy is generally included as part of inpatient and outpatient treatment protocols. Individual therapy is particularly helpful in assisting the client to establish more realistic thinking processes, increase self-esteem, establish a healthy sense of control, and express her emotions and needs more directly.

Expression of Emotions and Needs. In working with clients with eating disorders, the nurse gives the client permission to discuss feelings. Since the client is generally fearful that strong feelings will lead to loss of control, the nurse repeatedly helps her to distinguish between feelings and behaviors. The nurse tells the client that it is okay and normal to have strong feelings that we sometimes don't like. She communicates that one can be very angry at another person without hurting him or her; even if feelings are very strong and frightening, they won't make you do anything you don't want to do. As an adjunct therapy, assertiveness training is also helpful in increasing the client's ability to express feelings directly and constructively.

Realistic Thinking Processes. Persons with eating disorders tend to have perfectionistic personalities and to think in "all-or-none" terms. This kind of thinking helps to explain the extreme fear of becoming fat that characterizes these clients. If the client eats two cookies, for example, she concludes, "I couldn't control myself. I might as well give up and eat the whole bag of cookies." The client has rigidly defined appropriate behaviors for herself in terms of "walking on a tightrope"; one must be constantly vigilant to prevent falling off such a narrow path. The client can be reassured that life is more like walking in a big meadow. One can safely move in many directions without fear of falling. The nurse encourages the client to try out new behaviors. She lets the client know that she is aware of how frightening this can be initially, but that the client will gradually learn to be more confident about her behavioral choices in all areas, including eating.

Self-Esteem. Low self-esteem in clients with eating disorders is associated with overly high self-expectations, a high need for approval and acceptance from others, and possible deficiencies in social skills. The nurse helps the client to see the association between overly high self-expectations and feelings of ineffectiveness. She helps the client identify her own positive, personal attributes and give self-approval. In addition to individual therapy, the client may improve her social skills by participating in group psychotherapy with clients with similar needs. Self-esteem can also be enhanced by successful participation with peers in activities such as recreational or occupational therapy.

Control and Autonomy. The perception of control and autonomy increases as the client learns to express her emotions and needs more directly, think in a less rigid fashion, and establish more realistic self-expectations. The nurse encourages the client to assume responsibility for choices and decisions. In order for the client to take risks and grow, it is essential that the client trust that the nurse cares about her well-being and will maintain appropriate limits. The nurse assures the client that she will learn to trust in her own ability to exert appropriate behavioral controls and act autonomously.

Family Therapy

Family therapy may occur in conjunction with inpatient treatment or entirely on an outpatient basis. Because some theories about the origin of eating disorders suggest that the family plays a major role in their development, family therapy is particularly important when the client will be returning to the home. It is important, however, not to assume that dysfunction exists in the family. Since families may already feel guilty, helpless, and frightened, the nurse should be careful to convey a supportive, nonblaming manner.

Family therapy focuses on fostering open, healthy interaction patterns among members. Some family therapists find it helpful to focus on the four dysfunctional interaction patterns identified by Minuchin: enmeshment, overprotectiveness, rigidity, and lack of conflict resolution.[29]

Enmeshment and Overprotectiveness. Members of enmeshed families have failed to establish individual identities apart from a meshed family identity. Parents are typically overprotective and intrusive toward activities of their children. In working with these families, the nurse helps all members to make "I" statements instead of "we" statements: "I feel sad" and "I am so angry!" as opposed to "We are all so

Case Study 27-1: Julie

Fifteen-year-old Julie, a sophomore in high school, 5 feet 8 inches tall and 115 pounds, was referred to the school nurse by a teacher who had heard Julie vomiting on several occasions in the bathroom. In talking with Julie, the nurse initially observed that her teeth were in very poor condition. When asked about the vomiting, Julie looked embarrassed but confided that she was worried about gaining weight and vomited when she ate too much. When asked how long she'd been vomiting, Julie reported that during the summer before her freshman year in high school, she went on a diet to lose weight. Several other girls whom she admired were on diets and Julie, although not overweight, gradually ate less and less. In a period of time between July and December her weight dropped from 114 pounds to 87 pounds. Julie stated that her parents didn't worry at first but eventually became upset about her weight loss. Julie recalls that they tried to bribe her with food and fought with each other about her refusal to eat. That whole period of time now seems somewhat unreal to her.

Right before Christmas in her freshman year, her mother took her to the family physician, who told Julie she would have to go into the hospital if she didn't eat. No other intervention occurred at this time. Julie was a "straight A" student; the idea of being hospitalized and missing school frightened her. She agreed to start eating and did so that very day. She rapidly regained the lost weight by eating everything she wanted. She couldn't remember exactly when the thought occurred to her that she could eat as much as she wanted without gaining weight if she could vomit. She soon learned that if she drank a lot of water after eating she could easily induce vomiting. With this discovery, she began eating larger amounts of food. In order that her family wouldn't be suspicious that food was disappearing so quickly, she began buying, and then stealing, candy and cookies from the grocery store and hiding them in her room. This behavior was still occurring and Julie stated that her parents did not suspect she was doing this. She said that her parents were happy when she started eating and they never talked about her weight loss again.

Julie told the school nurse that she sometimes wondered if she were crazy and that she was ashamed of her teeth. She wondered if vomiting had anything to do with dental decay, even though she brushed her teeth immediately after vomiting. The nurse provided Julie with some basic information about anorexia nervosa and bulimia. Julie didn't know that there was a name for what she was experiencing and was relieved to hear that others had the same problem. The nurse explained that there was an association between frequent eating, vomiting, and dental caries, but that Julie should not blame herself. She didn't get anorexia and bulimia on purpose and couldn't have prevented it.

With Julie's permission, the nurse called her parents in for a conference. The nurse explained what Julie was going through and that she needed assistance to cope more effectively. Without blaming the family, the nurse explained that it would help Julie if all family members would meet together with a counselor experienced in eating disorders. Julie's parents initially reacted by denying that Julie had a problem. They said that she did well in school, ate well, and that everyone in their family had poor teeth. After hearing in more detail, however, about Julie's vomiting and stealing of food they agreed to attend a family session. The family did attend family therapy for 3 months. The school nurse continued to see Julie and to provide support.

During the next year, Julie's eating patterns were normal most of the time. She reported that she occasionally binged and purged when she was experiencing anxiety. Extensive dental reconstruction had been completed, however, and Julie did not want to ruin her teeth again. Even though she had more insight into why she developed an eating disorder, she continued to feel considerable shame and guilt about her previous eating behaviors and stealing.

Questions for Discussion

1. What is the relationship between the school system and the mental health system?
2. Was the intervention by the family physician appropriate? If not, how would you have modified this approach?
3. Was the intervention by the school nurse effective? What was effective? What would you have modified?
4. What are the goals of family therapy?
5. Formulate a nursing care plan for Julie beginning at the point when the case study ended.

upset!" Members are also encouraged to speak for themselves and not for each other. Parents in enmeshed families frequently try to protect their children by speaking for them, as in "She feels happy most of the time." Members are not accustomed to identifying and expressing their own feelings and need frequent prompting from the nurse: "You look upset; what are you feeling right now?" Since enmeshed families typically have weak or inappropriate boundaries between generations, the nurse may ask siblings to sit together as a unit distinct from the parental subsystem. Such seating arrangements reinforce appropriate boundaries and help to disrupt dysfunctional alliances that may exist between a parent and child.

Conflict Avoidance and Rigidity. Families of clients with eating disorders tend to "brush conflicts under the carpet." It may be an unspoken family rule that it is not okay to feel sad or upset, or to have problems. The nurse helps family members bring existing conflicts to shared awareness. If members try to avoid or deny conflict, the nurse refocuses them on the conflictual issue. The nurse helps members to express their conflict constructively so other family members can listen and respond. For example, she teaches that it is not very effective to shout, threaten, accuse, or demand. Since the anorexic client may be accustomed to diverting parental conflict onto herself, the nurse keeps the parents talking to each other and instructs them not to involve the adolescent. For example, she may say, "Jane is not part of this conflict. This is between you and your wife. Keep talking to her and don't involve Jane in it." Family members may have difficulty listening to each other's concerns and requests. The nurse role-models appropriate communication skills and helps members repattern their communications with each other.

Group Therapy

Clients with eating disorders may also benefit from group therapy. Groups may have specific therapeutic goals such as fostering self-esteem or gaining insight into feelings and behavior. Groups may also be organized as primarily supportive or self-help groups. It is often a relief simply to know that one is not alone with a problem. Members gain self-acceptance by sharing concerns with others and receiving constructive support and feedback from peers.[16]

Evaluation

Evaluation of the care of the client with eating disorders includes examination of all phases of the nursing process. Did the nurse accurately and thoroughly assess the client's physiologic, psychological, and social status? Were nursing diagnoses accurate and comprehensive? Evaluation of the planning and implementation of care is an ongoing process. Daily evaluation of nursing care plans and client progress toward meeting goals results in modification of treatment approaches as indicated.

The nurse evaluates the client's physical and psychosocial responses to intervention. Desired physical outcomes include weight gain, normal laboratory values and vital signs, and return of secondary sexual characteristics and menstruation. Desired psychosocial outcomes include a realistic perception of body image, direct expression of feelings, improved self-esteem, a sense of control over one's self and environment, and constructive family process. As clients recover, they frequently feel guilty and ashamed of their behavior while ill. Such feelings can persist long after normal weight is attained. The nurse reassures the client that she could not have prevented herself from becoming ill. While she was ill, she behaved in ways that may now seem immature or illogical. These behaviors were ineffective attempts to cope with stressors. Now the client has increased coping skills and won't need to resort to the immature responses she used previously.

The nurse also evaluates the family's interaction patterns. Desired outcomes are that family members communicate directly with each other and deal openly with conflicts, and that parents have relinquished previous patterns of overcontrol and overprotectiveness to allow the client an appropriate degree of autonomy. Even if these goals appear to be met, most clients require follow-up treatment to reinforce behavioral changes and prevent a return of disordered eating. Followup should span at least four years because of the high rate of relapse of the eating disorders.[33]

Nursing Diagnosis

Due to the multisystem nature of eating disorders, data analysis may suggest a large number of nursing diagnoses, including the following:

1. Alteration in nutrition: less than body requirements related to refusal to ingest or retain ingested food, physical exertion in excess of caloric intake
2. Self-esteem disturbance related to unrealistic expectations from self and/or others, lack of positive feedback, striving to please others to gain acceptance
3. Ineffective individual coping related to unmet developmental tasks (trust, autonomy), dysfunctional family system
4. Alteration in family processes related to enmeshed family system, inadequate communica-

(Text continues on p. 514)

Nursing Care Plan 27-1

Clients with Eating Disorders

Nursing Diagnosis	Client Outcome	Intervention
Alteration in nutrition: less than body requirements related to reduced intake of food	Weight stabilizes within normal limits	Implement behavioral modification protocol for weight gain
	Eating patterns normalize	Monitor weight on a regular basis under the same conditions
	Exercise patterns normalize	Supervise meals to ensure adequate intake of nutrients
		Record intake and output
		Monitor vital signs on a regular basis
		Monitor activity level to prevent excessive exercise
		Supportive, firm approach in regulating eating behavior
		Focus on emotional issues versus food and eating
		Liquid diet via nasogastric tube if client is unwilling to maintain adequate oral intake
Alteration in nutrition: Less than body requirements related to binging and purging	Does not engage in binge eating and purging activities	Help client identify feelings and situations associated with binge-purge episodes
	Displays a comfortable sense of control in relationship to eating	Encourage verbalization of feelings, particularly when client feels out of control and feels the urge to binge eat or vomit
	Weight stabilizes within normal limits	Monitor client during meals and 90 minutes after to prevent binge eating or vomiting
		Record intake and output
		Monitor weight, vital signs, and electrolyte levels
Disturbance in self-concept related to perfectionism, over-dependence on appraisals and approval of others, inadequate social skills	Verbalizes a realistic perception of body	Assist client in visualizing her own and others' bodies realistically
	Verbalizes positive self-attributes	Help client identify her strengths and limitations

Nursing Diagnosis	Client Outcome	Intervention
	Exhibits age-appropriate autonomy	Help client see the relationship between overly high self-expectations and feelings of inadequacy
	Socializes effectively with peers	Encourage client to make decisions and choices for herself
		Enhance client's communication and socialization skills through promotion of information, role-playing, and participation in group activities with peers
Alteration in thought process related to all-or-none thinking, obsessions, intellectualization, over generalization, malnutrition	Exhibits behavior and verbalizations that reflect realistic thinking processes	Redirect client from obsessional thought patterns (refrain from discussing food and weight)
	Evidences age-appropriate judgment and decision-making	Help client realize that life's problems will not be solved by losing weight
	Evidences realistic body image	Facilitate a realistic body image by assisting client to compare herself with average female peers
	Sets less rigid goals and standards for self	Teach client relationship between mental status and nutrition
		Assist client in giving herself permission to try out new behaviors
Ineffective individual coping related to unmet developmental needs (trust, autonomy), dysfunctional family system	Exhibits adaptive coping mechanisms	Offer positive reinforcement for independent problem-solving and decision-making
	Distinguishes between maladaptive and adaptive coping behaviors	Role-model appropriate ways of dealing with stressors
		Explore with client ways in which she may feel control within hospital and home environments
		Help client formulate reasonable goals
Alteration in family processes related to enmeshed family system, denial of problems and conflicts, unresolved issues of control, inadequate communication patterns	Family manages conflict constructively	Encourage members to speak for themselves, to make "I" statements versus "we" statements

(Continues on p. 514)

Nursing Diagnosis	Client Outcome	Intervention
	Family encourages autonomy of members	Encourage expression of both positive and negative feelings
	Members express emotions directly	Role model direct, constructive communication patterns
		Help members identify and express conflicts constructively
		Teach assertiveness skills
		Explore with members ways to increase autonomy and decrease parental over-involvement with children

tion patterns, denial of problems and conflicts, unresolved issues of control, inability to manage conflict

5. Fluid volume deficit related to diuretic or laxative abuse, vomiting, inability to concentrate urine
6. Alterations in bowel elimination: constipation or diarrhea related to refusal to ingest or retain ingested food, chronic laxation abuse
7. Alterations in oral mucous membranes related to deficient nutritional status and frequent vomiting
8. Powerlessness related to deficiency in learning that one's actions can cause desired outcomes
9. Social isolation related to fear of rejection, impaired age-appropriate social skills, preoccupation with obsessive thoughts and compulsive behaviors
10. Altered sexuality patterns related to impaired nutritional status, social isolation, low self-esteem
11. Alteration in cardiac output: decreased, related to hypokalemia, decreased blood volume
12. Alteration in thought process related to all-or-none thinking, intellectualization, obsessions, overgeneralization, malnutrition
13. Potential for injury related to excessive exercise and deficient nutritional status

Summary

This chapter has examined two eating disorders, anorexia nervosa and bulimia, that encompass a broad range of physiologic, psychological, and social disruptions. The application of the nursing process to clients with these disorders is both complex and challenging. Some of the major points of this chapter include the following:

1. Anorexia nervosa and bulimia occur primarily among adolescent and young women.
2. Anorexia nervosa and bulimia have many etiologic factors in common and may be viewed as existing along a single spectrum of eating disorders.
3. Although multiple theories exist, most experts agree that eating disorders develop from a complex interaction of individual, family and sociocultural factors.
4. Clients with eating disorders exhibit disturbances in many or all of the functional health patterns.
5. Treatment of clients with eating disorders occurs in both inpatient and outpatient settings and is a complex, and frequently lengthy, process.
6. Treatment approaches generally include a combination of individual psychotherapy, behavior modification, group therapy, and family therapy.
7. Desired client outcomes include normalization of weight and eating patterns, improved self-esteem, development of realistic thought processes, adaptive coping mechanisms, and constructive family processes.
8. Most clients require follow-up treatment to reinforce behavioral changes and prevent a return of disordered eating.

References

1. American Psychiatric Association: Diagnostic and Statistical Manual of Mental Disorders, 3d ed, rev. Washington, DC, American Psychiatric Association, 1987
2. Andersen AE: Anorexia Nervosa and Bulimia: A Spectrum of Eating Disorders. J Adolesc Health Care 4, 15–21, 1983
3. Andersen AE, Mickahide AD: Anorexia Nervosa in the Male: An Underdiagnosed Disorder. Psychosomatics 24, 1066, 1983
4. Bemis K: Current Approaches to the Etiology and Treatment of Anorexia Nervosa. Psychol Bull 85, 3, 593–617, 1978
5. Bhanji S, Thompson J: Operant Conditioning in the Treatment of Anorexia Nervosa: A Review and Retrospective Study of 11 Cases. Br J Psychiatry 124, 166–172, 1974
6. Brozan N: Anorexia: Not Just a Disease of the Young. The New York Times, July 18, 1983
7. Bruch H: Eating Disorders: Obesity, Anorexia and the Person Within. New York, Basic Books, 1973
8. Bruch H: Perils of Behavior Modification in the Treatment of Anorexia Nervosa. JAMA 230, 1419–1422, 1974
9. Burgess A: Psychiatric Nursing in the Hospital and the Community, 4th ed. Englewood Cliffs, NJ, Prentice-Hall, 1985
10. Casper R, Eckert E, Halmi K: Bulimia: Its Incidence and Clinical Symptoms in Patients with Anorexia Nervosa. Arch Gen Psychiatry 37, 1030–1035, 1980
11. Ciseaux A: Anorexia Nervosa: A View from the Mirror. Am J Nurs 80, 8, 1468–1470, 1980
12. Crisp AH: Anorexia Nervosa: Let Me Be. London, Academic Press, 1980
13. Crisp AH, Palmer RL, Kalucy RS: How Common Is Anorexia Nervosa: A Prevalence Study. Br J Psychiatry 128, 549–554, 1976
14. Deering CG: Developing a Therapeutic Alliance with the Anorexia Nervosa Client. J Psychosoc Nurs Ment Health Serv 25, 3, 11–17, 1987
15. Doyen L: Primary Anorexia Nervosa: A Review and Critique of Selected Papers. J Psychosoc Nurs Ment Health Serv 20, 6, 12–18, 1982
16. Edmonds MS: Overcoming Eating Disorders: A Group Experience. J Psychosoc Nurs Ment Health Serv 24, 8, 19–25, 1986
17. Garfinkel PE, Garner DM: Anorexia Nervosa: A Multidimensional Perspective. New York, Brunner/Mazel, 1982
18. Garner DM, Garfinkel PE: Socio-cultural Factors in the Development of Anorexia Nervosa. Psychol Med 10, 647–656, 1980
19. Gordon M: Nursing Diagnosis: Process and Application, 2d ed. New York, McGraw-Hill, 1987
20. Halmi KA: Anorexia Nervosa: Demographic and Clinical Features in 94 Cases. Psychosom Med 36, 18–25, 1974
21. Halmi KA: Pragamatic Information on Eating Disorders. Psychiatric Clin North Am 5, 2, 371–377, 1982
22. Halmi KA, Powers P, Cunningham S: Treatment of Anorexia Nervosa with Behavior Modification. Arch Gen Psychiatry 32, 93–95, 1975
23. Hart K, Ollendick T: Prevalence of Bulimia in Working and University Women. Am J Psychiatry 142, 851–854, 1985
24. Hawkins RC: The Binge-Purge Syndrome. New York, Springer, 1984
25. Herzog DB, Copeland PM: Eating Disorders. N Engl J Med 313, 295–303, 1985
26. Kalucy RS, Crisp AH, Lacey JH, Harding B: Prevalence and Prognosis in Anorexia Nervosa. Aust NZ J Psychiatry 11, 251–257, 1977
27. Lipscomb P: Bulimia: Diagnosis and Management in the Primary Care Setting. J Fam Pract 24, 2, 187–194, 1987
28. Masterson J: The Borderline Adolescent: An Object Relations View. In Reinstein S, Giovacchini P (eds). Adolescent Psychiatry, pp 344–359. Chicago, University of Chicago Press, 1978
29. Minuchin S: Families and Family Therapy. Cambridge, MA, Howard University Press, 1974
30. Minuchin S, Baker L, Rosman B, Liebman R, Milman L, Todd T: A Conceptual Model of Psychosomatic Illness in Children: Family Organization and Family Therapy. Arch Gen Psychiatry 32, 1031–1038, 1975
31. Mitchell J, Eckert E, Pyle R: Frequency and Duration of Binge-eating Episodes in Patients with Bulimia. Am J Psychiatry 138, 835–836, 1981
32. Moore J, Cowlman M: Anorexia Nervosa: The Patient, Her Family, and Key Family Therapy Interventions. J Psychosoc Nurs Ment Health Serv 19, 5, 9–14, 1981
33. Morgen HG, Russell GF: Value of Family Background and Clinical Features as Predictors of Long-Term Outcome in Anorexia Nervosa: 4-Year Follow-up Study of 41 Patients. Psychol Med 5, 335–372, 1975
34. Pyle R, Mitchell J, Eckert E: Bulimia: A Report of 34 Cases. J Clin Psychiatry 42, 60–64, 1981
35. Rost W, Neuhaus M, Florin I: Bulimia Nervosa: Sex Role Attitudes, Sex Role Behavior, and Sex Role Related Locus of Control in Bulimarexic Women. J Psychosom Res 26, 403–408, 1982
36. Schlemmer JK, Barnett PA: Management of Manipulative Behavior of Anorexia Nervosa Patients. J Psychosoc Nurs Ment Health Serv (Nov.) 35–41, 1977
37. Sours JA: Starving to Death in a Sea of Objects. New York, Aronson, 1980
38. Swift W, Andrews D, Barklage N: The Relationship Between Affective Disorder and Eating Disorder: A Review of the Literature. Am J Psychiatry 143, 290–299, 1986

PART 6

Special Topics in Psychiatric–Mental Health Nursing

28 The Emotionally Disturbed Child

Barbara Schoen Johnson

Modern living conditions have made it much more difficult for parents to create a setting in which both their own legitimate needs and the needs of their children can be satisfied with relative ease. That is why love is not enough and must be supplemented by deliberate efforts on the part of the parent. Fortunately most parents love their children and conscientiously strive to be good parents. But more and more of them become weary of the struggle to arrange life sensibly for their children, while modern pressures create more and more insensible experiences which are added to the life of the child.

Bruno Bettelheim,
Love Is Not Enough: The
Treatment of Emotionally
Disturbed Children,
1950

The author acknowledges the assistance of Janet Pressler Devaney, RN, Charge Nurse of Child Services, Charter Hospital of Dallas, Texas.

519

Chapter Preview

There have always been children who are different from the majority of their peers. Frequently, these children exhibit behaviors that results in difficulties for them and those around them. As long ago as 1871, in the schools of New Haven, Connecticut, such children were labeled "contumacious aggressors" and segregated into their own special class.[7] More than a century later, we may continue to question our progress in the area of treating childhood disorders.

This chapter examines emotionally disturbed children, their needs, problems, and families, and urges nurses and other mental health caregivers to evaluate their own priorities, abilities, and willingness to meet those needs (see Chart 28-1). Through the nursing process—assessment, nursing diagnosis, planning, intervention, and evaluation—the nurse has an effect on the delivery of mental health care to disturbed children.

Learning Objectives

Upon completion of the chapter, you should be able to accomplish the following:

1. discuss the prevalence and causative or risk factors of emotional disorders in children

---

CHART 28-1

Working with Disturbed Children: Personal Reflections

Every field within nursing has its own unique challenges, struggles, and rewards. Working with emotionally disturbed children is no exception. During the years of providing nursing care to these children and their families, I frequently heard this question from my family and friends, "Why do you do that kind of work...how can you do it?"

Why or how does anyone choose their work? It may be because they find the work important in itself and recognize in themselves a talent, understanding, and enthusiasm for the endeavor. Child psychiatric nurses reach an awareness of the families' needs and their own abilities to help family members function more effectively and grow as a family.

The road along which child psychiatric nurses travel in their professional development, however, is frought with difficulties. Novice nurses are often bewildered by the behavior of disturbed children. "What does it mean, what could have caused it?" they ask.

At times, nurses become angry at the child's parents or guardians whose "parenting" is far from what is considered adequate by professional standards. This anger also extends to the child himself; the child's behavior may be hostile, fearful, demanding, self-defeating, aggressive, withdrawn, regressed, autistic, or destructive. The nurse is often frightened by the child's outbursts or frustrated by the seeming purposelessness of his behavior. Searching for something that will "work"—that is, something that will have an effect on the child's and family's behavior and interaction—may lead the nurse to frustration.

Sometimes, the nurse may feel hopeless and resigned to the fact that the challenge is too great. Feelings of hopelessness, helplessness, and particularly, lack of collegial support contribute to professional burnout. To prevent this occurrence, nurses can form peer support groups within which they can air their feelings and frustrations openly and receive suggestions and rewards from their colleagues.

Nurses must look to their peers in the workplace, their supervisors, their enriching personal lives, and their own strengths and resources for sources of energy, determination, and enthusiasm. The children with emotional disorders and their families cannot provide the rewards to the nurse; they are the ones in need.

2. describe the behavioral manifestations and dynamics of the emotional disorders of childhood
3. assess the family functioning and the emotional, social, educational, and cultural problems and needs of the emotionally disturbed child
4. analyze the assessment data and formulate client of family nursing diagnoses
5. identify the goals of treatment of disturbed children and their families
6. describe and compare various intervention modes for disturbed children and their families
7. discuss the child advocacy role of psychiatric–mental health nurses
8. identify measures to ameliorate the effects of multiple stressors and long-term exposure to stress on children's functioning

Emotional Disorders in Children

Prevalence

The problem of emotional disturbances in children is a monumental one. Because various researchers may employ different criteria against which to measure childhood adjustment and mental health or disorder, precise statistics regarding the prevalence of childhood disorders are difficult to determine. Other factors hampering the determination of the prevalence of childhood psychiatric disorders are difficulties with definition of the disorder, instrumentation, sampling, source of information, ages examined, and location of studies.[58]

Despite these inaccuracies, most frequently quoted estimates of emotional disorders in children assert that 10% of all children in the United States have emotional problems severe enough to disable them as adults.[46] According to the latest census reports, there are over 62 million children and youths under the age of 18 in the United States. The American Academy of Child Psychiatry estimates that 11.8% (or 7.3 million) of these children have some type of mental disorder but that only 7% of them are receiving the necessary mental health care services.[65]

Risk Factors of Disorders

Sex and Age

Certain risk factors are associated with the occurrence of emotional disorders of childhood. For example, their occurrence follows trends of sex and age. Boys generally display more disturbances than girls, in a 2 : 1 ratio, until adolescence, at which time the occurrence of girls' disorders becomes equal to, or greater than, the boys'.[10, 58] Studies show that the symptoms of emotional disorders in boys are more disturbing to parents and teachers than girls' behavioral signs; boys are referred for psychiatric treatment more often than girls.[10] For both sexes, there seems to be a slight increase in the rate of emotional disturbance between late childhood (9–12 years) and early adolescence (13–16 years).[58]

In researching the incidence of psychiatric disorders in children, Rutter and others have identified the following six familial and seemingly correlated "risk factors":

1. Severe marital distress
2. Low social status
3. Overcrowding or large family size
4. Paternal criminality
5. Maternal psychiatric disorder
6. Admissions of children into foster home placement

When examining the rates of child psychiatric disorder according to the frequency of these risk factors, an increasing progression of negative outcomes was discovered. For example, if one risk factor was present in the family, there was not much difference in incidence of disorder than if there had been no risk factors present. But, if there were two risk factors present, there was a fourfold increase in the likelihood of a psychiatric disorder; the presence of four risk factors increased the likelihood of disorder ten times.[33] This evidence certainly reinforces what we believe about the deleterious effects of multiple stressors and long-term exposure to stress on children.

Another group of children at high risk for emotional disorders is the offspring of psychiatric patients who may also be hospitalized and therefore separated from their children. A study of the indications for preventive intervention with children of hospitalized psychiatric patients built on the following premises:

1. The psychological emergency of a parent's psychiatric illness and hospitalization is compounded for the child
2. A parent's mental illness diminishes his or her parenting abilities
3. Unknowingly, mental health professionals may participate in a "silent conspiracy" with the family by overlooking the patient's children
4. The incidence of risk for psychopathology among children of psychotic parents is 40% to 50%
5. The psychiatric hospitalization of a parent may

be a turning point in preventive intervention with the child.

The study found that children do react profoundly to a parent's decompensation and hospitalization, with varying degrees of effect on their everyday functioning. While some children in the study were severely compromised by their parents' illness and hospitalization, others coped more adaptively; these "copers" had in common that they all experienced an empathetic relationship with a caring adult. That empathetic adult was usually the well parent, but for some children it was another close adult relative. An empathetic adult with whom the parental illness can be openly discussed may serve as a "buffer" for the vulnerable child.[76]

Sociocultural Factors

In addition to age and sex factors, there also appears to be a strong link between the prevalence of childhood psychiatric disorder and low socioeconomic class.[10,58] Although this correlation may be thought of as resulting from the case finders' middle-class biases, these biases may actually work in reverse. In other words, a behavior that is seen as a sign of a serious emotional problem in a middle-class child may be disregarded in a child from a low socioeconomic group.[10]

Sociocultural factors in the etiology of psychiatric disorders are probably less important in children than in adults, because most children function within a familial matrix that operates as a remarkably effective buffer to social change. Early childhood seems to be particularly immune to sociocultural influences.[10] Although children may be relatively undisturbed within the family environment when they are young, they increasingly come into contact with the larger society as they grow and develop.

Genetic and Organic Causes

Genetic and organic factors may be manifested in disorders of childhood. Some individuals may, in fact, have a genetic predisposition to handle stress poorly. (See the etiologic factors of depression, schizophrenia, and substance abuse discussed in other chapters of this text.)

Stress

Although it is generally thought that the presence of multiple stressors impacts negatively on the individual, it is possible that stress may exert the opposite effect. Stress may inoculate some children against emotional disorders by causing them and their parents to develop effective coping responses.[23]

One long-term study of children's development under stressful conditions found that children with greater assets, such as higher IQ, higher socioeconomic status, and positive family attributes of stability and cohesion appeared to be more competent; under stress, they were more socially engaged with their peers and in their classrooms. Children with fewer assets, however, appeared to be more disruptive, especially when under stress. Higher IQ and higher socioeconomic status and, for girls, more positive family attributes appeared to be protective factors against disruptive-aggressive responses to stress. Children in families with lower socioeconomic status and fewer positive qualities of stability, cohesion, and organization were both more likely to be exposed to stressful life experiences and less competent and intellectually able to deal with these experiences. The effects of these stressful events and multiple risk factors appear to be cumulative ones.[33]

Parents and Families

The role of parents and families in the child's growth and development is critical. All people bring their own concerns and anxieties to the task of childrearing. The parents' feelings of fear, guilt, depression, and anxiety, as well as love, make an impression on the child.

An important task of families is maintaining two essential family boundaries—the generational boundary and the division between the two sexes.[28] The generation boundary divides the family into the parents, who nurture, lead, and direct, and the children who are nurtured, follow, and learn. Division of the sexes results in gender awareness, identification, and security.

Disturbances in family functioning are multidimensional; a "problem" of one family member exists not in a vacuum, but as a function of family dynamics. Five areas of family task deficiencies include the following:

1. Individual pathology of a parent, such as a schizophrenic mother or alcoholic father
2. Deviant parental coalitions, such as chronic parental discord
3. Faulty nurturance, such as failure to promote the child's growth toward independence, or child abuse
4. Faulty enculturation, such as parental behavior that is dramatically atypical of the surrounding culture and leads to estrangement of the children
5. Emancipation problems, which are likely to surface in disturbance after the child has reached adulthood, married, and become a parent, thereby continuing the cycle of emo-

tional disorder from one generation to the next.[28]

Several of the family factors associated with conduct disorders of children are parental separation or divorce, marital discord, parental disorder and criminality, and a large number of siblings.[58]

Many countries, including Great Britain, France, Denmark, Holland, Canada, and the United States, have recently experienced tremendous increases in divorce rates. Two-thirds of the women who divorce in the United States are under the age of 30, and most children are younger than 7 years old at the time of their parents' separation or divorce.[50] What is not known about these and other risk factors of child psychiatric disorders is how they operate independently or interact with each other.

One of the unique features of parenting is that child development may be thought of not only as a result of parental actions, but also as an extension of the parent's self.[47] What parents, including emotionally disturbed parents, believe about the world and their place in it may be extended to their children. In one study of affectively ill mothers' beliefs about their children, it was found that unipolar depressed women were selectively satisfied with their children's development, being more concerned about the children's socioaffective development than their cognitive development. Both the unipolar and bipolar depressed mothers felt greater helplessness about their children than did the well mothers; they also were more likely to believe that their children's development was the result of uncontrollable factors or change.[47] This cognitive pattern of helplessness and chance happenings is in accordance with the way in which a depressed individual thinks and perceives his environment. The effects of this cognitive pattern on the child of a depressed mother would seem to reinforce depressive outlooks on life.

Dynamics of Childhood Disorders

Some emotional disorders are specific to childhood, such as conduct disorders and infantile autism. Others may be variations on adult disturbances. In this chapter, personality disorders will not be discussed, although you are encouraged to refer to Chapter 22. Psychophysiologic disturbances and the eating disorders of anorexia nervosa and bulimina, which often surface in late childhood or adolescence, are discussed in Chapters 27 and 32. In addition, this chapter does not discuss the problems of psychoactive substance use disorders; this is certainly not meant to ignore their substantial importance in the study and treatment of children with mental disorders. See Chapter 26 for this material.

Adjustment Disorder

The adjustment disorders of childhood are transient disorders of any severity that occur in a child who may or may not have a preexisting emotional disorder. They are acute maladaptive reactions to an overwhelming, identifiable psychosocial stressor or stressors.[3] The maladaptive reaction is seen either in an impairment in the child's functioning in school or in his usual social activities or relationships with others, or in symptoms that exceed a normal and expectable reaction to the stressor.

A common example of this type of reaction occurs when a child becomes ill, is hospitalized, and is faced with surgery. While in hospital, the child frequently exhibits regressed, fearful, and acting-out behavior. After he is discharged from the hospital and returns home, the child usually continues to show temporary increases in anxiety, hostility, fearfulness, clinging to mother, and disruptions in eating, sleep, and toilet routines. Evidences of such behavior may gradually diminish, after 3 to 6 months posthospitalization.

Attention Deficit Disorder

For the past 20 years, hyperactivity has been perhaps the most frequently diagnosed child psychiatric disorder. Formerly called *hyperkinetic reaction of childhood,* *minimal brain damage,* and *minimal brain dysfunction,* the disorder is now termed *attention deficit hyperactivity disorder* according to the Diagnostic and Statistical Manual of Mental Disorders, third edition, revised (DSM-III-R).[3, 73]

Children who are hyperactive are more often called "difficult," "aggressive," and "disruptive" than nonhyperactive children. They also engage more frequently in risk-taking behavior than other children, resulting in mishaps, scratches, scrapes, and broken bones. Hyperactive children are more likely to be academic underachievers, although they don't score significantly lower on intelligence tests, especially individually administered intelligence tests.[73]

Children with attention deficit disorder are referred for treatment for three general types of problems.

1. Problems in learning leading to school failure
2. Difficulty relating to peers
3. Difficulty complying with adult requests and commands[73]

Significant behavior of hyperactive children is their inability to sustain attention, control impulsivity, and control activity level. In fact, the four core symptoms of attention deficit disorder are distractibility, excitability, impulsivity, and excessive activity.[73] Certainly, these behaviors are inappropriate to certain contexts, such as school.

The child with attention deficit hyperactivity disorder will display, to a degree greater than that of other children the same mental age, the following behaviors:

Squirming and fidgeting
Distractibility by extraneous stimuli
Difficulty remaining seated when requested
Difficulty taking turns in games and in classroom
  settings
Blurting out answers to questions that have not
  been completed
Difficulty following through on others' instructions
Difficulty sustaining attention in tasks or play
Frequent shifting from one uncompleted activity
  to another
Excessive talking
Frequent interruptions of others
Difficulty playing quietly
Appearance of not listening to what is being said
  to him
Frequent loss of things necessary to school work or
  other activities
Engaging in physically dangerous behavior without
  considering the consequences[3]

A similar disorder, undifferentiated attention-deficit disorder, is seen when the child has many of these symptoms but not the signs of impulsiveness and hyperactivity.[3]

Conduct Disorder

A repetitive and persistent pattern of behavior in which the child violates the basic rights of others or major age-appropriate social dicta is termed a *conduct disorder*.[3] The child with a conduct disorder displays antisocial behavior in the form of physical violence against another person, theft outside the home, firesetting, assault, or callous or manipulative behavior.

Children with conduct disorders may engage in the following behaviors:

Stealing covertly ("borrowing" and not returning
  other's possessions), forgery, shoplifting, steal-
  ing with or without confrontation of a victim
Running away from home
Frequent lying
Setting fires
Frequent truancy
Breaking into someone's home, building, or car
Deliberately destroying other's property
Exhibiting physical cruelty to animals
Forcing someone into sexual activity with him
Using a weapon in more than one fight

Initiating physical fights frequently
Exhibiting physical cruelty to other people

At an older age, the physical violence may take the form of rape, assault, or rarely, homicide.[3]

One of the ways that a child may act out his feelings of rejection, isolation, and hostility is through cruelty to animals. Cruelty to animals usually occurs concomitant with certain other symptoms, such as aggressiveness to younger siblings and other small children, firesetting, interest in sex, enuresis, learning problems, hoarding, bulimia, and imperviousness to pain.[84] This behavior is seen most often in young and preadolescent boys (8 to 10 years). Although cruelty to animals and the associated symptoms may indicate a personality disturbance or mental retardation, they occur most commonly in children from chaotic homes with aggressive, violent parental models.[84]

Firesetting is a dangerous symptom that must be controlled rapidly. Children who set fires also display many other forms of acting-out, including running away, stealing, lying, truancy, and sexual acting-out. One study of 29 children, two girls and 27 boys, aged 5 to 14 years, in which a family crisis-oriented model of therapy was used, demonstrated interruption of the firesetting behavior in all but two children after the initial session.[14] The primary goal of this intervention technique with children who set fires is to bring the firesetting behavior under control by means of reinforcing the child's desire to control this behavior, developing a therapeutic alliance, and using a graphing technique, which helps the child visualize, concretize, and correlate his feelings and behavior.[14]

One study of juvenile homicide found that, counter to many case reports and theoretical contentions, very few of the adolescents who committed homicide were psychotic at the time of the offense.[20]

Oppositional Defiant Disorder

Children with oppositional defiant disorder demonstrate some of same behaviors of a child with conduct disorder, such as disobedience and opposition to authority, but do not violate the rights of others or major age-appropriate norms.[3] The child displays negativistic, hostile, and defiant behavior but does not physically assault others or destroy their property. The oppositional and defiant behavior is seen much more commonly in children with this disorder than in other children of the same mental age.

Children with oppositional defiant disorder are usually seen as argumentative with adults, angry, and resentful. They may be spiteful and vindictive. They use foul or obscene language, lose their tempers frequently, are easily annoyed by others, actively defy the requests or rules of adults, and blame others for their problems. The child himself does not usually see himself as defiant or oppositional, but justifies his behavior in light of his circumstances. Frequently these behaviors of the child are seen at home or with peers whom the child knows very well, but may not be evident at school or with strangers.[3]

Anxiety Disorders

Anxiety may be defined as a fear that is not justified by reality or an extreme reaction to a real threat. The younger the child, the more difficult it is for him to separate inner and outer reality.

Children with anxiety disorders experience repressed conflict between intense, but unacceptable, feelings and the defenses against them. The resultant behavior pattern, an anxiety disorder, is the most successful compromise the child is able to reach. The child may react as if imagined or past events are a real and continuing part of the present.[46]

Two of the most common anxiety disorders in children are phobias and sleep disturbances. A *phobia* is a morbid, irrational, and persistent fear. Childhood phobias are so common that mild, passing fears are considered part of normal development.[46] Frequently, the child may fear school, transportation (such as travel by car or plane), and animals. He may have exaggerated fears of burglars or kidnappers or concerns about dying. Many children fear dogs and become uncomfortable around them. The child with a phobia, however, is preoccupied with the prospects of meeting a dog, in a constant anticipatory anxiety state, and may not want to go to school or even out of the house to insure that he doesn't see a dog. Obviously, a phobia can be quite crippling.

Phobias may result from the following causes:

1. A real and frightening incident that conditioned the child to the fear
2. A vicarious frightening experience
3. Repression of the child's forbidden, secret wish or action leading to guilt and the substitution of another object or person to fear.[46]

School phobia is a symptom that cannot legally be ignored for long. The child may fear some aspect of the school situation, such as the teacher, classroom, trips to and from school, or lunch routine. Often, the child also has some somatic symptom that disappears when he is told that he can stay home from school. School phobia may occur at any age, but is seen more commonly in the lower elementary grades.[46] It may be described as a form of separation anxiety between the child and his parents or as a form of trouble accepting the child's increasing independence.

Sleep disturbances are also tied to separation anxiety, considering that the very young child views sleep as separation. A transitory, common experience of sleep disturbance may be seen, for example, in 2-year-olds to 3-year-olds who fear loss of control over their bodies while asleep, which results in wetting the bed. The preschool child's oedipal struggle may become translated into frightening monsters at night. The child may be afraid of sleep itself, for fear that a horrible event, even death, may befall him during his sleep. Nightmares peak during the ages from 4 to 6, and may be the cause of the child's inability to remain asleep. Children awaken from nightmares feeling helpless and afraid and in need of comforting. At the extreme, night terrors leave children feeling panicked and experiencing difficulty reorienting to reality, being comforted, and regaining self-control.[46]

The anxiety disorders include separation anxiety disorder and avoidant disorder of childhood, in which anxiety is focused on specific situations, and overanxious disorder, in which anxiety is generalized to a variety of situations.[3] A child with separation anxiety disorder exhibits excessive anxiety, to the point of panic, concerning separation from the person or persons to whom the child is attached. When separated from significant others, the child may be preoccupied with morbid fears that accidents or illness will befall the parents or himself or he may be extremely homesick, almost to the panic level. He feels distress when he travels independently away from the house, and he may refuse to visit or sleep at friends' houses, go on errands, or attend camp or school.[3] Physical complaints, such as headaches, stomach aches, nausea, and vomiting, are common. The child may cling to, or "shadow," the attachment figure.

Children with avoidant disorder of childhood exhibit excessive shrinking from social contact with unfamiliar people to the point of interfering with interpersonal functioning with peers. At the same time, the child desires increased contact with family members or peers he knows well. The child with this disorder will appear socially withdrawn, embarrassed and shy when in the company of strangers and very anxious if asked to interact, even minimally, with strangers.[3]

Overanxious disorder is marked by excessive or unrealistic anxiety or worry. The child with this disorder is extremely self-conscious and tends to worry about both future and past events, his own competence, and behaviors. The physical concomitants of anxiety, headaches, gastrointestinal distress, nausea, shortness of breath, and dizziness may also be present. The child is particularly tense and unable to relax.[3]

Mood Disorder

Childhood depression often presents as headaches, chest pains, abdominal pain, and other somatic, or bodily, complaints. Depression is often seen in children and adolescents with chronic illnesses, gastrointestinal disorders, and chronic orthopedic problems.[39]

Until recently, it was thought that children rarely, if ever, become depressed. Now, however, we know that children do experience depression. The child's behavior, which may mask his depression, may take the form of acting-out behavior or somatic complaints. The depressed child may express depressive themes in his play, fantasy, dreams, and verbalizations.[39] The various symptoms of depression are specific to the child's age or developmental level. For example, prepubertal children may evidence separation anxiety as a sign of depression; depressed adolescent males may exhibit negativistic and antisocial behavior, sulkiness, social withdrawal, and school difficulties.[16] Among psychiatric child inpatients, depressive symptoms are seen more often in physically abused than nonabused children.[43]

Some of the behaviors which we typical associate with depression in adults (see Chap. 23, "Disorders of Mood: Depressed and Manic Behavior") may or may not be seen in depressed children. For example, one recent study found that depressed children showed less facial expressiveness, smiling, and intonation, and more tearfulness, frowning, and response latency than nondepressed children, but that boys showed more, and girls less, body movement and head shaking in depression.[44] Although clinical observations and evaluation measures, such as the Depression Self-Rating Scale and the Children's Depression Inventory, are invaluable tools for discerning the presence of depression in children, optimal assessment of the depressed child involves the use of multiple measures and informants.[4]

Specific risk factors for suicidal behavior in children include the following:

1. The child's depression
2. The child's concepts about, and preoccupations with, death
3. Suicidal tendencies of the child's parents[61]

The family variables related to suicidal risk in childhood include parental separation, divorce, abuse, particularly abuse to the mother, ineffective communication patterns, crowding, family history of suicidal behaviors, and acute stressful events. Children fantasize suicide by stabbing themselves, jumping from heights, hanging themselves, and drowning themselves in a sink.[61]

Self-injury may also be seen in children who are mentally retarded. This behavior may be an attempt to reduce guilt, establish "bodily reality," or direct aggression inward, or it may be a form of autoerotic activity.[90]

One approach to the evalution of suicidal risk focuses on the assessment of *imminent danger* rather than on the intensity of his depression or hopelessness. The interviewer evaluates the youth's current suicidal plan or ideation and the presence of more than five positive responses to the following suicide-related factors:

Male sex
A past suicide attempt with a method other than
    ingestion
More than one previous attempt
A history of antisocial behavior
A close friend who committed suicide or a family
    member who attempted suicide
Frequent drug and alcohol use
Depression
Incompatibility with the social environment

The second phase of the interview is based on the youth's ability to behave in nonsuicidal ways, specifically the following:

1. The youth is able to promise in writing that he will not engage in suicidal behavior for a specific period of time, such as two weeks
2. The youth is able to compliment himself and others
3. The youth is able to differentiate and assess his own feelings by placing them in a hierarchy of intense emotional states
4. The youth is able to formulate specific plans to ward off suicidal situations

A child or adolescent who is unable to perform these tasks is considered by the evaluator in imminent danger of suicide—coping skills needed to fight off suicidal tendencies are not available to him.[72]

Autistic Disorder

Austistic disorder, or infantile autism, is a rare pervasive developmental disorder with onset in infancy or childhood that occurs three to four times more commonly in boys than in girls.[3,46] It was first described by Leo Kanner in 1943. The distinguishing characteristics of infantile autism are a lack of responsiveness to others and withdrawal from social contact, gross impairment in communication, and bizarre responses to the environment, such as peculiar interest in, or attachment to, animate or inanimate objects and insistence on routines. The onset of these behaviors is evident before 30 months of age.

The impairment in reciprocal interaction of the

child with autistic disorder may be seen by the child's marked lack of awareness of the existence or feelings of others, no (or abnormal) seeking of comfort in times of distress, no (or impaired) imitation of others, no (or abnormal) social play, and significant impairment in his ability to establish peer friendships.[3]

As infants, autistic children fail to respond to the sight or sounds of others. They give no evidence of a "social smile," or of pleasure in being with the mother or mothering figure. They do not physically reach out; they have no reaction to strangers. Because they are not demanding and don't fuss when separated from parents, these children are sometimes mistakenly called "very good babies." Social games, like peak-a-boo, do not interest autistic children.

The child with autistic disorder displays severe impairment in verbal and nonverbal communication. This may include no verbal communication; abnormal nonverbal communication (stiffens when held, does not look at the person or smile when in a social situation); no imaginative activity; abnormal speech production, such as in volume, tone, and pitch; abnormal form or content in speed, such as the use of "you" when "I" is meant; inability to initiate or sustain a conversation with others despite adequate speech.[3]

The autistic child fails to use speech for the purpose of communication. He may not talk at all, or he may talk in a mechanical, parrotlike manner. He may repeat stereotyped or nonsensical phrases, or he may echo what is said to him. If a certain word results in the child getting what he wants, he may use it over and over—not according to its meaning. The child is unable to generalize word usage. He may, in fact, be so unresponsive that deafness is suspected.[46] His response to sounds is likely to be inconsistent.

If the autistic child has speech, it is likely to be echolalic, and he will probably employ his own private language. He may use the third-person pronoun to refer to himself, indicating poor differentiation of self from others, and he may reverse other pronouns.[3,92] The child may also engage in rocking, twirling, or other self-stimulatory behavior.

The child's restricted repertoire of activities and interests may include his preoccupation with parts of objects, attachment to unusual objects, stereotyped body movements, marked distress over changes in trivial aspects of the environment such as moving an object on the table, unreasonable insistence on following routines in precise detail, an extremely restricted range of interests, and a preoccupation with one narrow interest.[3]

The autistic child is usually fascinated with objects, especially ones that spin, twirl, or reflect light and shadow. An important differentiation here is that the normal child values a toy largely because it came from a parent; an autistic child finds joy in the toy's ability to be spun, manipulated, rolled, rocked, or put together.[46]

Autism is a chronic disorder. It seems to be due to biologic factors because it occurrence is associated with maternal rubella, phenylketonuria, encephalitis and meningitis. It is unclear whether the development of autistic children follows an erratic "lag-spurt" course, a steady rate, or a stable rate within a specific area of development over time.[79]

About 40% of autistic children have an IQ below 50; about 30% have an IQ of 70 or higher.[3] Even when the child is not retarded, he may be perceived as such because autism hides whatever cognitive ability or potential the child has.[46]

Childhood Onset Pervasive Developmental Disorder

Formerly called *symbiosis psychosis, childhood schizophrenia,* and *atypical development,* childhood onset pervasive developmental disorder develops after 30 months of age and before 12 years. The DSM-III-R terms this a pervasive developmental disorder not otherwise specified.[3] It is a rare disorder, marked by a profound disturbance in interpersonal relations, such as lack of peer relationships, asocial behavior, inappropriate affect, and clinging.

This disorder is also characterized by behaviors such as sudden excessive anxiety; inappropriate or constricted affect; resistance to change; bizarre movements, such as posturing or walking on tiptoe; speech abnormalities, such as monotony of voice tone; hyposensitivity or hypersensitivity to sensory stimuli; and self-mutilation, such as head-banging or self-biting.

The child who develops a childhood onset pervasive developmental disorder may appear developmentally normal until the age of 2 to 3 years, at which time behavioral pecularities start to become evident. The child's odd postures or mannerisms are especially noticeable when one tries to play or talk with him.[46]

Some severely disturbed children cannot tolerate separation from the mother and become overwhelmed with panic when not with her; this behavior may include agitated, extreme temper tantrums. Normal children experience fears and fantasize but are able to distinguish between real and "pretend" experience. The severely disturbed child loses the distinction, particularly when he is overcome by fear or anxiety.[92]

The severely disturbed child may also show disparity among verbal, motor, social and adaptive skills appropriate for his age. This pervasive developmental disorder occurs more commonly in children with low IQs. It is a chronic and incapacitating disorder.

Psychosis in Children

Childhood psychosis is characterized by the following:

1. Severely disturbed interpersonal relationships, including lack of interest in others, unawareness of others' presence, or inability to separate from others
2. Difficulties communicating with others, including lack of meaningful speech, lack of play, or preoccupation with sensory stimuli or inanimate objects
3. Lack or impairment of contact with reality, such as insufficient distinctions of self from nonself
4. Striving for constancy
5. Uneven development of intellectual, motor, emotional, and social skills[46,77]

The psychotic child lives in a "world of his own," and that private world is unavailable to anyone but himself. He may be preoccupied with sensory stimuli (visual, auditory, or kinesthetic) that have little thought content. For example, a toy car is fun for the psychotic child not because he can pretend he is driving it, but because its wheels spin. "Psychotic children do not make believe," says one author, "they exploit their toys for their physical properties."

Psychosis in children may be thought of as a massive failure of the ego to synthesize and organize the personality.[54] These children are unable to differentiate between inner and outer reality, are often aggressive and unable to tolerate frustation, use language associatively, display stereotypic, compulsive behaviors, and perceive the world as persecuting them.[77]

Application of the Nursing Process to Emotionally Disturbed Children

When children are referred for psychological treatment, the referral may have been initiated by the child's school, parents, health care providers, or the court. A family crisis, acute or chronic physical illness, or other stressors may precipitate the seeking of therapeutic intervention for a troubled child. This section of the chapter examines the application of the steps of the nursing process to the care of emotionally disturbed child clients and their families.

Assessment

Family Functioning

In child psychiatric–mental health nursing, the treatment team assesses the disturbed child and his family and then, together, analyzes the information that has been gathered.

Assessment of the family, particularly members of extended family who may help define the family's beliefs and values about child-rearing, is best approached before the assessment of the child. This initial focus on the family, rather than on the individual child, gives a clear message to all involved that no one in the family will be exempt from looking at the "problem" and participating in problem-solving (see Case Study 28-1).

The nurse assessor or other mental health caregiver asks openended questions such as, "How are things for the family?" This form of questioning allows the family to feel free to respond with whatever information they wish to share. Usually, the parents respond first to opening questions and generally attempt to identify the problem.

Next, the nurse focuses on the child, who is typically the "identified patient" in the family. The question to the child, "How are things going?" often brings a response of "I don't know," "Fine," or "My parents (or teachers) are mad at me."

Sources of Information. Although parents and teachers are probably better informants for the assessor on the child's observable behavior, such as hyperactivity, academic problems, antisocial behavior, or difficulties with peers, the child is the best source of information about symptoms that reflect subjective experiences.[22] For example, the child should be assessed directly regarding suicidal ideation, disordered moods, feelings of guilt or low self-esteem, and hallucinations.[16]

Throughout the assessment process, the nurse seeks information from the child, parents, siblings, extended family, teachers, and health care professionals. The nurse also notes the congruencies or incongruencies among the perceptions of each of these sources of information.

Communication Patterns. During the initial assessment interview, the nurse observes the behavior of parents and children and asks, What is their body language communicating? How does the family sit? How do they arrange themselves in the room? Who speaks for whom? Who is the primary spokesperson for the family? In well-integrated, healthy family systems, each family member is free to speak—there is room for everyone's opinions and ideas. Other ways of determining the openness of the family system are exploring their extrafamilial interactions and influences, their tolerance of differences of opinion among family members, the clarity of the boundaries, and their ability to deal with current issues. (See Chap. 15, "Families and Family Therapy.")

Case Study 28-1

Assessing Eddie H. and His Family

Eddie H., a 7-year-old white male, was brought to the Child and Family Mental Health Clinic by his mother, 30-year-old Hazel W. "Eddie," said his mother, "is rebellious and destructive to school supplies and toys, tells lies to get his younger brother Ralph into trouble, throws temper tantrums, doesn't listen to his teacher, and can't understand the meaning of the word 'no.'"

Eddie is the oldest of Hazel's three children; the others are 5-year-old Ralph and 4-year-old Lucille. Hazel was married briefly to Eddie's father. Each of the children has a different father; her current husband, Mr. W., is "out of the picture," she says, and she plans to divorce him as soon as she can afford to do so. Presently living in the home are Hazel, her sons Eddie and Ralph, and sometimes Frank, Hazel's 18-year-old boyfriend. Her daughter Lucille is in foster care.

Additional information was supplied by the family's case worker from the Department of Human Resources. Eddie's behavior is disruptive in school, he spends his time drawing pictures instead of doing his school work, and he seems to block out what is going on in the classroom.

When questioned about an event that precipitated her bringing Eddie to the clinic, Hazel reported that a few days ago he took some powerful pain pills from the medicine cabinet and tried to give them to his younger brother Ralph (who refused them). During the interview Hazel also frequently referred to a car accident 2 years ago, which, she believes, brought on much of the family's troubles. The accident occurred when Hazel was driving a friend's car. She lost control of the vehicle and hit a bridge overpass. The entire family was taken to the emergency department of a local hospital. Eddie had a scalp laceration, Ralph a minor injury, Hazel a broken leg and multiple lacerations, but Lucille suffered internal injuries including a ruptured spleen and "brain damage" resulting from a skull fracture. Hazel was charged with driving while intoxicated (DWI) and Lucille was placed in foster care.

Eddie was a full-term infant, the product of an unplanned pregnancy during which Hazel felt "OK physically," but unhappy, anxious, and apprehensive that the baby might "be abnormal because of Rh." She was upset because the father of the child didn't want the child and often said that the child was not his. Hazel reported that she was in labor for 19 hours but "wouldn't dilate," that she received Demerol every 2 to 3 hours, and that Eddie was "taken with forceps." He was very sleepy when he was born as a result of the Demerol she received and he experienced difficulty starting to breathe on his own. Hazel said that she "could not afford the gamma globulin shot" after Eddie was born, but that she has had no complications with her later children.

Hazel stated that she believes that Eddie was "spoiled" as a baby and that, as his siblings arrived, he began to have more problems. He sleeps poorly and frequently wakes up screaming with nightmares. He does not talk with his mother and rarely makes eye contact with her.

Eddie's interests include riding his bike, working on art projects, fishing, and being out-of-doors. His relationships with peers are described as poor—he is "beaten up" by his peers from time to time and actively discourages the friendship of his classmates.

According to his mother, Eddie responds to the discipline of standing him in the corner or sending him to his room. Spanking or "getting after him with a switch" sometimes controls him, says Hazel, but for the past few years he "won't cry," which both puzzles and upsets his mother.

Observation in the playroom revealed that Eddie played appropriately, not destructively, with the toys. He seemed anxious and somewhat depressed, but able to interact well. He said that he "never gets mad at anybody," but sometimes worries when his mom gets upset.

When asked to draw a picture of his family doing something (a kinetic family drawing), Eddie quickly responded, "I don't have a daddy, but I'll draw one anyway." He said he drew "kids trick-or-treating at their house and having lots of fun." In fact, the only two members in the drawing were his sister Lucille "dressed up like a princess" and his brother Ralph "as a vampire."

Hazel related that 3 years ago, during a period of extreme stress, she entered a state psychiatric hospital, remained there for 57 days, and then attended outpatient therapy at a neighborhood community mental health clinic. She refused, however, to take the medications prescribed for her, because she thinks that taking medication is a sign of weakness. Presently, she

(Continues on p. 530)

cannot get to the clinic because of lack of transportation.

This family appears to live from crisis to crisis, but the mother, Hazel W., is a resourceful woman who knows how and where to find help when she needs it. She is a very anxious woman who exhibits pressured speech, a great deal of ambivalence, and dependence in her interpersonal relationships. Her current crisis was triggered by a number of factors: losing her job at a convenience store, Eddie's behavior in school and his anger at her for working away from the home, increasing debts, and her noncompliance with her prescribed medications. Eddie is anxious, mildly depressed, not overtly aggressive or destructive, but reacts to the family's stressors with his own behavioral responses of acting-out in school and against his younger brother.

The goals of treatment for Eddie, his

mother Hazel, and the other family members include the following:

1. To explore the family's previous coping skills, strengths, and supports during crises
2. To help the family reach an understanding of this crisis and its effects on the family functioning
3. To examine the family's alternate coping methods, which could result in a healthier resolution of their current crisis
4. To provide crisis intervention twice weekly for Hazel and her family for the next few weeks or until the crisis is resolved
5. To construct a long-term plan of treatment for Hazel, her son Eddie, and other family members that would teach parenting skills for Hazel and communication and coping skills for all family members

Identifying the Problem. As the child and his family define the "problem," the nurse assesses its severity, duration, and impact on family functioning, and asks, For whom is the problem most distressing? For example, conduct disorders are likely to be very upsetting to parents, siblings, teachers, and other adults, whereas school phobia may be most disturbing for the child.

The nurse also asks, How functional or dysfunctional is the problem? A child may be very manipulative with adults and, although the problem is distressing and they don't feel comfortable with him, his growth and development continue satisfactorily. Some mental health problems are dysfunctional for the child and family. When a child has anorexia nervosa, it is not uncommon for everyone in the family to try to placate the anorexic child. If a child exhibits aggressive behavior, as in a conduct disorder, the mother may interact with the child as the strict disciplinarian, while the father tries to create some positive interaction with him; this conflict may certainly lead to marital problems.

Family Relationships. The nurse assesses the family members' genuineness of concern for each other. The family members are asked to describe their relationships and roles, including the child's role in the family. In addition, the family is often requested to perform a certain task, such as planning a family vacation. This experiential task demonstrates the actual relationships, roles, degree of autonomy or enmeshment, and empathy of family members.

Is the child functioning as a family scapegoat? In other words, is he being blamed and held responsible for everything that goes wrong in the family?

Perceptions of the Child. The parents' level of knowledge about the normal processes of child development and behavior influence how realistic their role expectations for him will be. For example, is the 6-year-old male child expected to be "the little man" of the family?

The nurse asks the parents, On what level do you think your child should be functioning now? They are asked to define what is different about this child. They are asked to assess the child's disposition or temperament and his talents and strengths. The latter will be incorporated later into a plan to maximize the strengths.

Sociocultural Influences. Socioeconomic and cultural information from the family give another perspective to the nurse assessor about the family's childrearing and the aftercare planning for the child. This information includes the parents' and other family members' educations, occupations and incomes and the family's cultural beliefs and practices.

Sharing with Parents. During the assessment process, the nurse asks the family whose idea it was to seek help for the child and what intervention measures they have already tried. The nurse acknowledges the seriousness of the problem and compliments the family on their concern and love for the child, which is evident in their seeking treatment for him and the family.

The question, What do you wish your child were like now? yields information about the parents' values, expectations, culture, and attitudes and biases about parenting.

The parents are asked to describe what they hope the treatment team (therapist, caseworker, nurse, and so on) can do for them and their child. Their hopes for their child's future reveal what the parents believe about his career, standards of behavior, and relationships.

The parents need time to ask their own questions. They may fear they "did something wrong" that resulted in the child's becoming hostile, aggressive, or withdrawn. The nurse might briefly explore with them the possibility of a multiplicity of factors in the development of an emotional disorder of childhood.

The Child

History-Taking. Taking a history of factors pertinent to the child's emotional problem includes the following:

1. A history of psychiatric disorders, alcoholism and drug dependence, or organic illnesses in members of the nuclear and extended families
2. A thorough assessment of the growth and development of the child, including prenatal and perinatal factors
3. The time of onset of the problem and any significant events that occurred at or around the time the problem became manifest
4. The child's health and social history

The parents, teachers, and child are asked to describe his strengths and weaknesses and how he is functioning at home, at school, and in the neighborhood. The child's social skills, interests and hobbies, and unusual or troublesome habits are noted.

Physical and Emotional Assessment. A thorough physical examination should be conducted. The child's age, size, nutritional status, speech and hearing, and the presence of "soft" neurological signs are assessed.

A structured mental status examination of the child includes the following:

1. Appearance—dress, gestures, posture, tics
2. Mood or affect—predominant feelings, mood fluctuations, ease or constriction in displaying feelings, appropriateness
3. Manner of relating to the examiner—child's perceptions of the reasons for the interview, rapport with or distance from the examiner, use of play, activity, verbalization, or relationships
4. Modes of thinking and intellectual skills—development of child's thinking, conceptualizations of causality, body image, memory, problem-solving
5. Capacity for play and fantasy—amount and kind of involvement in play, use of play materials, themes of play, spontaneity of play, use of examiner in the play
6. Sensorimotor development—fine and gross motor activities, symmetry of movement, eye–hand coordination, and right–left discrimination[22]

(See Chart 28-2, "The Mental Status Exam for a Child.")

Because children's ability to express themselves verbally is limited, the assessment of children is conducted primarily through the medium of play. A variety of play materials, including dolls, hand puppets, art materials (paint, clay, paper), movement toys (cars, trucks, planes), age-appropriate games, punching bag, toy telephone, rubber-tipped darts, and doll house and furniture are provided as the means through which the child tells his story.[22]

Diagnosis. The word *diagnosis* is derived from the Greek and means "a thorough understanding." A diagnosis should provide the psychiatric–mental health care provider with an understanding of the cause and associated features of the disorder, age of onset, cause, incidence according to sex, diagnostic criteria, and degree of impairment. It should also lead to treatment implications.

Diagnosis of the disorders of childhood is a particularly difficult problem for the following reasons:

A child is often inconsistent and unpredictable in his behavior.

The child's relationship and degree of comfort with the examiner will definitely affect the results.

The child is an immature organism and is constantly developing.

The child is affected and being shaped by his parents.

The assessment session sets the tone for the rest of the intervention with child and family. The parents are likely to approach the mental health professionals

(Text continues on p. 536)

C H A R T   28-2
The Mental Status Exam for a Child
Nancy A. Moeller Sanchez, M.S., R.N., C.S.
Staff Development Director
Green Oaks Psychiatric Hospital
Dallas, Texas

When the nurse is conducting an assessment of a child, it is sometimes a great challenge to elicit data through the direct question-and-answer format used with adolescents or adults. It is vital that the nurse establish a sense of rapport and put the child at ease. One way to approach this is by allowing the child to explore the office and its contents—toys, games, and art supplies. While the child is examining the office, the nurse is able to make pertinent behavioral observations and ask some nonthreatening questions: "What's your name? How old are you? What grade are you in?"

As the child becomes more comfortable with the nurse, it is important to find out if the child is aware of why he is being brought in to talk to the nurse. Many children are unaware of the purpose of their visit to the nurse; parents may have made up an untrue reason for the visit to entice the child. Parents also may have told the child they'd see a "doctor" or "nurse," and this may have frightened or worried the child, especially if past experiences with nurses or doctors have been negative or frightening.

At this point, the nurse should explain that in order for her to know the child better it will be necessary for her to ask some "silly" questions and to have him use his imagination for a few minutes. Once the child indicates a willingness to respond more directly, the following questions may be helpful in evaluating the mental status of the child:

Orientation

What day/month/season is it today?
What would you like to be when you grow up?

Sexual Preference

If you had a chance to decide, would you rather be a boy or a girl? Why?

Relationships

How do you get along with your family?
Your friends?
Describe what you like to do with your friend(s).

Fantasy Life

Who would you like to take on a trip to the moon?
If you had three wishes, what would you wish for?

What animal would you like to be? Why?
What is your favorite daydream?
When you dream at night, what do you dream?
Do you ever have nightmares? [If yes] Tell me about them.
What are you most afraid of?
Do you ever see or hear things no one else can see or hear? [If yes] Please describe them.
Do you ever have strange thoughts or ideas?

Affect/Mood

I'm going to name a feeling and then you tell me when you feel that way.
  I feel *sad*   when
  I feel *mad*   when
  I feel *happy*   when
  I feel *scared*   when
What do you *do* when you feel
  Sad?
  Mad?
  Happy?
  Scared?

Art Assessment

Now I want you to draw a few pictures. [Have about 10 pieces of blank 8½″ × 11″ paper and a No. 2 pencil available.] You don't have to be a great artist, just do the best you can.

1. Draw a picture of a house. [Ask child each time about the picture when completed]
2. Draw a picture of a tree.
3. Draw a picture of a man.
4. Draw a picture of a woman.
5. Draw a picture of a family doing something together.

[After the art assessment, ask the more difficult questions that follow.]

Risk Behavior

Suicidal:	Do you ever feel like hurting yourself?
	Have you ever tried to hurt yourself?
Homicidal:	Do you ever feel like hurting others? Who?
	Have you ever tried to hurt them?
Use of chemicals:	Have you ever tried using any drugs? What? How often?

Have you ever tried drinking alcohol? How much? How often?

Abuse: Has anyone ever touched you or made you touch them in the areas covered by your bathing suit (or private zones) [or point to genital, breast area on nurse]?
Did this make you feel funny or "not right"?

At the completion of the above, the nurse should thank the child for his cooperation and allow time for him to ask questions. If risk behavior is revealed, the nurse must explain that this information will help to be sure the child is going to be protected and safe.

Attached are samples of drawings done by the following children:

Sample A

Drawn by a 6-year-old girl who has an average IQ, but whose drawings show signs of some emotional/developmental problems.

Notice absence of body parts

Notice disjointed drawing of house

Sample B

Drawn by a 7-year-old boy who has a low average intelligence, was very disturbed emotionally, and may have signs of organic impairment.

Notice the house's lack of shape or detail

(Continues on p. 534)

The drawings of people (boy and family) are disjointed, missing body parts

The kinetic family drawing shows the father whipping the child, saying, "Be quiet" to the child

Sample C: Normal Sample

Drawn by a 7-year-old girl who has an average IQ and very few problems.

Notice house and tree are fairly symmetrical

The family seems happy as they are "camping out"

In addition to the above, the mental status assessment will need to include the nurse's impressions of the following:

Appearance/dress
Motor activity
Nutritional status
Mannerisms
Tics

Attitude and General Behavior (mark what is appropriate)

Anxiety _____ Fearful _____
Suspicious _____ Compliant _____
Alert _____ Cooperative _____
Relates well _____ Relates poorly _____

Mental Activity

Spontaneous _____ Blocked _____
Relevant _____ Tangential _____
Memory _____
Evidence of thought disorder _____

Emotional Reactions

Mood _____ Affect _____

Impulse Control

At present:
    Good _____ Fair _____ Poor _____
History:
    Good _____ Fair _____ Poor _____

Orientation

Time _____ Person _____ Place _____

Client's story about why he came to the mental health agency:

Nurse's summary of assessment process:

Tentative diagnosis:

Recommended further assessment needs:

The man has all body parts

The author extends appreciation to the artist who prepared the children's art for publication—Mr. Anthony Ravagnani.

with some degree of dread; they fear what they will hear about their mistakes in parenting. They have fears that their child is "crazy" or hopeless. Dealing with and calming these fears, supporting the parents' desire to be "good parents," and teaching them new ways to interact with their child and manage his behavior are some of the nurse's foci in child psychiatric–mental health care.

Nursing Diagnosis

After gathering assessment data from the child and family, the nurse analyzes the data to formulate nursing diagnoses that will guide nursing intervention. Some of these are as follows:

1. For a child with anxiety disorder, sleep pattern disturbance related to child's anxiety and fears, evidenced by interrupted sleep, difficulty falling asleep except when in presence of parent, listlessness and lethargy during daytime activities

2. For a child with autistic disorder, impaired verbal communication related to withdrawal into the self; pathophysiologic changes occurring in response to maternal rubella, meningitis, encephalitis, phenylketonuria, evidenced by lack of speech, echolalia, or abnormal form or content of speech

3. For a child with conduct disorder, potential for violence: self-directed or directed at others related to certain neurologic disorders, retarded ego development, poor impulse control, dysfunctional family system, evidenced by aggressive body language, overt and aggressive acts, self-destructive behavior, hostile and threatening verbalizations, rage, possession of destructive means, and increased motor activity

4. For a child with adjustment disorder, ineffective individual coping related to maturational and situational crises, inadequate support systems, low self-esteem, retarded ego development, evidenced by inability to meet age-appropriate role expectations, inability to problem solve, and verbal hostility toward others

5. For a child with attention deficit disorder, impaired social interaction related to self-concept disturbance, poor attention and concentration, ready distractibility, excessive gross motor activity, evidenced by observed discomfort in social situations, observed inability to communicate a sense of belonging or shared interest, and dysfunctional interaction with peers and family

6. For any child with emotional disorder, alteration in growth and development related to existence of mental disorder, evidenced by a variety of maladaptive behaviors[86]

Planning

Planning with parents and child is a collaborative effort. It begins with the assessment and analysis of the information about the child's developmental level and his and the family's needs and problems; it also involves sharing this information with the family. Planning also takes into account the nature of the emotional disorder and the resources available to the child and family.

Determining Client Outcomes

Some of the outcomes of child and family mental health treatment are as follows:

1. The child and family will experience fewer symptoms of disorder and distress
2. The child's development will proceed along normal lines
3. The child will display increasing degrees of autonomy and self-reliance
4. The child's behavioral gains will be reinforced
5. Therapeutic changes will occur in the child's home or school environment[74]

Priority-Setting

Planning also considers the priorities of psychiatric–mental health care. A 13-year-old, for example, admitted to an inpatient treatment facility following a suicide attempt, requires a treatment plan that first attends to the physical safety of the child. Caring for the child with a decreased level of consciousness, assessing blood levels of the drug taken, and instituting antidotal therapy take precedence over psychosocial assessments of the child and family.

Intervention

The form of psychiatric–mental health treatment of children is selected according to the needs and problems of the child and family. In the past, various forms of physiotherapy were employed to treat the emotionally disturbed child. As recently as the 1950s, shock treatments for psychotic children were attained through electricity, pentylenetetrazol (Metrazol), or insulin. Other physiological measures, such as sleep therapy and psychosurgery, have not been an acceptable part of treatment of children.[29]

Prevention

The primary focus of intervention for emotional disorders of childhood is prevention. *Prevention* may be defined as any activity undertaken before individuals are identified as "clients." Approximately 3 million children and youths, therefore, are not receiving needed care. Many of these children are responding to difficult life experiences such as parental abuse or the loss of a parent through divorce, death, abandonment, or illness.[65] We know, however, that early identification of, and intervention with, children at risk *can* prevent more serious mental disturbance later in life. Unfortunately, preventive intervention has not been a priority of our mental health care system. In fact, until recently, it was thought that parenting required no special knowledge or skills; now, adolescents are often able to study parenting in school.

It has been shown that, to be effective, primary prevention programs must take into account the total sociocultural environment in which the child lives.[67] Therefore, brief exposures to interventions will not produce long-term effects in children who continue to live in a disturbed or chaotic environment.

The goals of preventive measures are as follows:

1. Reduce the incidence of new cases of the disorder
2. Reduce the incidence of disabilities in the population
3. Raise the immunity of individuals or groups to stress
4. Decrease stress in the environment
5. Improve the quality of life in a targeted population
6. Raise the general health of children[67]

Children and families at risk for emotional disturbance are the targeted populations of preventive efforts. The stress points in the life cycle that may require intervention to prevent disturbance are pregnancy, birth (particularly prematurity), crisis situations such as the maturational crises of adolescence, marriage, retirement, and dying, and the situational crises of serious illness, divorce, and rape.

Individual Therapy

Relationship Therapy. Therapy with emotionally disturbed children may focus on the individual needs and problems of the client. A therapist whose intervention effectiveness depends on the therapist–client relationship must possess a respect for the unique nature of the child.[55]

Approaching the child client may be difficult for nurses and other mental health care professionals due to what Anna Freud called "the fluidity of the child's personality."[30] The child is growing and developing—his needs are not constant.

The role of the therapist may be that of a participant–observer. The therapist hopes to become an important adult in the child's world, someone with whom the child can identify as he moves along in the growth process.[56]

Although Sullivan never treated children, his interpersonal theory has had far-reaching effects on child theory and therapy.[37] His view of maturation processes centers on communication, skills of communication, and the factors that contribute to anxiety, thereby interfering with development.

Brief Psychotherapy. Elective, brief psychotherapy with children is a form of individual psychotherapy based on ego psychology; it is not a fragment of long-term therapy nor an attempt to condense long-term therapy into a short period of time.[88]

This form of therapy is useful in the treatment of relatively healthy children; for example, those suffering from reactive disorders. The therapist or, more significantly, the child delineates a central issue that can be dealt with in the available time period.

The goals of brief therapy focus on the central issue or problem, which is openly discussed with the child and his family, and the termination date is set. The child's relationship with the therapist may become a "model for future relationships—trusting, positive, but limited relationships."[88]

Play Therapy. Nondirective play therapy offers the child an opportunity to experience growth under the most favorable conditions. Because play is the child's natural medium for self-expression, he uses the therapy time to play out his accumulated feelings of fear, tension, confusion, frustration, and aggression.

When the child plays out his feelings, he allows them to surface, faces them, and learns to control, accept, or abandon them. Through this process, the child gradually realizes that he is an individual in his own right and is capable of thinking and making decisions for himself. For a more complete description of this form of treatment, see Chart 28-3.

Family Therapy

Family therapy is based on the premise that the behavior of an individual within the family cannot be understood or changed without understanding and effecting change within the entire family system.[36] Because behavior does not occur in isolation, intervention is not directed at only one family member.

The family therapist observes the family system in action, noting patterns of interaction among family members, and questions, "What interactional patterns in this family support the child's symptoms?"[36] The therapist then intervenes to change the patterns to ones that support new behavior and personal competence and growth.[36,59]

(Text continues on p. 540)

CHART 28-3
Play Therapy: What's It All About?

Linda Agler, Ph.D.
Psychologist, Private Practice
Dallas, Texas

Many parents are reluctant to seek professional help for their emotionally troubled child, no matter how serious and long-standing the child's difficulties. Parents are likely to tell themselves they should be able to "fix" all their children's problems and to view their inability to do so as a personal failure in their roles as parents. Often parents hold themselves responsible for having caused the child's problems in the first place and fear a therapist will discover that they are to blame for the child's adjustment difficulties. When the initial resistance is overcome and parents reach the decision to seek professional help for their child, the therapist is likely to recommend play therapy. Many parents are confused about how "playing" can help their child. "What's it all about?" they ask.

To understand play therapy, it is necessary to consider how children learn. "A child's play is his work," the old saying goes. Infants first learn about objects and people in their environment by touching and exploring. Later, in creative play, children reveal their understanding of the world and their relationship to it. Children are unable to verbalize many of their thoughts, feelings, wishes, and fears. In play therapy, toys become the medium of communication between child and therapist.

A perceptive therapist will utilize the child's responses to the various objects in the playroom (including responses to the therapist) to understand the child's personality, conflicts, and defenses. For instance, the manner in which a child initially responds to the toys and the therapist in the playroom is significant. These first reactions may reveal the child's usual approach to new people and unknown situations. Is the child fearful and guarded, waiting for the therapist to make the first move and provide all the structure? If signs of anxiety and insecurity are present, is the child still able to initiate contact, cope, and make decisions? Or does the child wander from toy to toy, unable to focus thoughts and actions? Some children avoid human contact by a withdrawal into the toys and internal fantasies; others allow the therapist to participate as an equal partner; some children retain careful control over all the activities and attempt to dominate the therapist.

Similarly, the themes children develop through imaginative stories and games reveal the problems and concerns they are confronting in their lives. The child who repeatedly sets up games in which the therapist is always the loser may be demonstrating a need to be "on top" in order to maintain feelings of self-worth. The games may provide a starting point for a discussion of how the child is able to feel good in the "real" world where peers and parents forbid cheating and success is often left to chance. Or, the cheating may reflect an ambivalence toward authority, a rebellion against the many rules and regulations adults impose. Methods of expressing these rebellious feelings more productively are discussed, and possibilities for communicating displeasure with unwanted limitations in more straightforward ways are sought. Some children are not given sufficient opportunities for developing self-control in the home environment—they are overcontrolled by their parents, or no external controls are provided. A preoccupation with winning competitive games by any means may indicate that issues of domination or self-esteem are important for the child.

Determining exactly what the child is feeling based on interactions and observations in the playroom is not always easy. The therapist will suggest possibilities to the child and wait for the child to indicate the significance of the play activities by verbal response or by changes in the style of playing. Many children have little or no awareness of their true feelings. For instance, some children turn all their hurts, sadness, and fears into anger, while others internalize all of their feelings into depression or physical illnesses. Thus, some time may be required for the child and therapist to understand the feelings expressed in the play.

Goals of Play Therapy

Although therapeutic goals differ for each child, the following goals are the same for all who come to therapy:

GOAL 1: Helping the Child Better Understand Feelings, and How Feelings Relate to Behavior

Most children who come in for therapy, even those who are very verbal and able to talk about their problems, have little insight into what makes them act as they do. This goal is worked on as the therapist makes observations about the child's actions and relates those actions to internal feelings. For example, if a child begins aggressively pounding with a toy hammer after having been told he may not write on the walls, the therapist may say, "I see you are hammering very hard on those pegs; maybe it's because you are angry with me for not letting you write on the walls." Often the therapist is wrong: the sudden aggression may have appeared for a different reason of which even the child is not aware. Being wrong is not too important, though, since the underlying message is the same, "You are acting for a reason; maybe together we can discover what that reason is."

GOAL 2: Helping the Child Find More Appropriate Ways of Expressing Feelings

One child may develop play stories about monsters that attack children in their beds at night. This same child wets the bed almost every night. In therapy the child and therapist talk about how scary nighttime can be, how real those nightmares can seem, how one time he actually saw a snake under his bed. Instead of keeping the fears inside they are talked about or acted out (perhaps by playing in the therapy office with the lights turned out). Getting up in the middle of the night to go to the bathroom may seem less ominous when the child has been allowed to imagine and confront his worst fears in the playroom.

GOAL 3: Helping the Child Find Ways to Solve Personal Problems

Is a lack of assertiveness a problem for this child? In the playroom the child may use puppets to develop stories about bullies who pick on others during the bus ride to school. The stories may be enacted in various ways. One time the child sits and cries when the bullies begin their taunts. One time the child tells the bus driver, who chides him for tattling. One time he steals other children's pencils to avenge the insults. One time he stands up to them and insists they leave him alone. The possibilities are many. It is important to examine all of them until the child finds the solution that works best for him.

Phases of Play Therapy

Although each child is different, the process of play therapy is similar for most children. The following are the most common phases that children go through:

1. Introductory Phase

The first task of the therapist is to gain the child's trust. This may happen in 5 minutes or 5 months, depending on the personality and prior experiences of the child. Until trust has been firmly established and the child is able to reveal inner thoughts and feelings, it is difficult to accomplish other goals. For some children, not being able to trust that others care about them is their biggest problem. They may push everyone away, including those who might be supportive and able to offer nurture. When such children are able to trust the therapist, they are soon able to trust others, and a major goal has been accomplished.

2. Honeymoon Phase

Children, like adults in therapy, usually go through a honeymoon period when the relief from finally being able to express some of their anxieties is so great that their demeanor at home and school improves dramatically. In some children the improvement is so marked that parents wish to terminate therapy at this point. However, the relief from talking often lessens when children realize their problems are still there. Much work remains to be accomplished if enduring change is to take place.

3. Rebellious Phase

After trust has been established and the honeymoon stage has passed, the rebellious phase usually beings. At this point the child often voices strong anger about having to attend therapy sessions. Usually the child is voicing strong anger about almost everything else as well, and parents begin to wonder whether therapy is a constructive or destructive endeavor. This sudden rebellion, the constant venting of anger (of which parents often bear the brunt), is actually a positive sign. It indicates that the repressed feelings that have resulted in much anxiety and/or depression are beginning to surface. In therapy the child has been encouraged to express feelings. Now the child is, indeed, expressing them at home, at school, and in the neighborhood. Unfortunately, the child does not yet know how to do so appropriately, and temper tantrums are likely to appear. Learning to express feelings more acceptably will come with continued work in therapy sessions and help from parents at home.

4. The Working-Through Phase

Becoming aware of what one is feeling, learning more productive methods of expressing feelings, and developing healthier defenses does not happen quickly, but it does happen. There will

(Continues on p. 540)

be times when it is clear that the child is really "getting it together," only to be followed by periods in which the child returns to previous modes of responding and interacting. Occasionally the behavior may actually deteriorate or the symptoms intensify. Although such periods are relatively short, they may be very upsetting to parents and others who are involved with the child. Such regressive episodes may indicate that old defenses are weakening. For instance, the child with poor self-confidence who suppressed all his feelings until an explosive temper tantrum resulted may begin reacting to a series of trivial slights from peers. The old defenses that served to ward off the feelings of insecurity are no longer operative. While this may increase the child's distress, it provides an opportunity for an examination of the underlying feelings of worthlessness the child has harbored all along, so that healthier defenses against external threats to his self-confidence can be developed. Sometimes it seems that the child has merely substituted one set of problems for another: the child who used to bang her head when frustrated now breaks her toys instead. Although both are serious problems, the fact that the child is learning to externalize her anger is a positive sign. It is sometimes difficult for parents to see that the overly compliant, controlled child with many somatic complaints is progressing by suddenly defying even simple parental demands for civilized behavior. Yet this may be a very important first step for some children.

5. Termination Phase

Terminating therapy sessions with children is a difficult process. Memories of past separations the child has endured often surface, along with the old fears of rejection and abandonment.

The longer and more intense the sessions have been, the more difficult termination will be for the child. Parents usually find it difficult to understand both the importance of therapy sessions to the child and the depth and intimacy of the relationship that can be formed between therapist and child in just 1 hour a week. Parents may not understand that the relief they feel about ending therapy is not shared by the child. It is not uncommon for many of the child's original symptoms to reappear. This is probably due to the stress caused by the termination; it may be the child's way of convincing everyone that therapy is still needed. Other children may insist that they never want to see the therapist again when discussion of termination begins. This may be a way to avoid the sadness of saying the final farewell, or to retaliate against the therapist for the perceived rejection. Again, each child is different, but terminating the sessions and saying "goodbye" to a person with whom one has been so close and shared so much is painful for most children. If proper time is not allowed to work through all of the strong emotions generated by the separation, therapeutic gains may not be maintained.

Unfortunately there are no guarantees that the time, money, and energy a parent spends on obtaining professional help for a child will result in all of the hoped-for benefits. The therapist must help the parent be as realistic as possible in setting goals for the child. In the end, therapy is like education: the conditions for learning are provided, but it is up to the child to accept or reject the available possibilities for growth and change. The therapist is not a miracle worker, only a person whose knowledge of child development and sensitivity provides a basis for understanding and intervening to help the child.

The successful treatment of children necessitates the modification of the reinforcement patterns that are part of the child's environment. Therapeutic changes are unlikely to generalize without interventions that extend to the child's home environment. It is important to train parents to become therapeutic agents of change.[62] This training may occur in parent groups that focus on home-related problems and problem-solving.

Behavior Therapy

Behavior therapy is based on the premise that emotional disorders represent learned behavior. There-fore, principles of learning are applied to the modification of these disorders.

Behavioral approaches to therapy with emotionally disturbed children include the use of special techniques such as token economies, "time out" (from positive reinforcement), and rewards for certain behaviors.[2,18,71] This mode of treatment also employs less rigorously structured behavioral techniques. Teaching parents and teachers how to use these techniques necessitates that they be observant of child behavior, select the appropriate technique for the behavior, and apply it consistently.[91]

One example of the use of behavior therapy is

teaching the autistic child language by training him in verbal imitation, through differential reinforcement, resulting in the establishment of verbal responses in the child. After this has been accomplished, the child is taught the meaning of the verbal response.[51]

Another example of the use of behavior therapy is in parent training for the management of antisocial behavior of children. In one study, children whose parents participated in this behavior management program and who themselves attended cognitive-behavioral problem-solving skills training showed significantly less aggression and externalizing behavior at home and at school and greater prosocial behavior and overall adjustment.[42]

Educational Approaches

An emotionally disturbed child's sense of failure is heightened by his staying out of school, because attendance and accomplishment at school make up a significant aspect of the child's developmental strivings for completion. It is estimated that 42% of identified behaviorally disordered children are served in regular classrooms and 44% in special classes. Slightly more than 10% are in separate public schools and the remainder in residential or hospital settings.[29] The dilemma of the school becomes how to control or contain an unstable child and how to teach him what he needs to know.[7]

Goals of special education for the emotionally disturbed child include the following:

To decrease the child's deviant behavior
To accelerate the child's rate of learning to enable him to "catch up"
To reintegrate the child into regular classes as soon as possible[93]

Some of the techniques of working with children with emotional disorders in the classroom are to provide a high degree of structure (which lowers the child's anxiety, gives him the security of defined limits, and serves as a vehicle for expectations for his behavior) and to maximize the development of group cohesiveness and use of peer pressure.[93]

Almost all disturbed children have experienced very little success in school. In the face of repeated failure, it is extremely difficult for the child to think positively about academic learning. The teacher's task is to provide a climate that helps the child become motivated; the teacher accomplishes this task through awareness of the child's individual needs, teaching skills, and use of materials of great interest to the child, and by not defining the child as a failure.[93] It is critically important that there exist effective coordination between educational systems and the other systems of health care delivery.[29]

Milieu Therapy

Milieu therapy in a psychiatric inpatient unit or residential treatment facility focuses on the living environment of the child and the relationships between the child and the staff. The living environment of the child and his relationships with other children and the staff are the essential therapeutic features of a milieu.[8] Effective milieu therapy involves an environment organized to provide the child with corrective and restitutive experiences designed to restore his sense of trust in himself and others.[1] These experiences include opportunities for learning, group socialization, reality testing, sublimation, and positive identification with adults. Through the day-to-day living experiences of waking up, attending school, eating meals, participating in play and other activities, watching TV, preparing bedtime snacks, and so forth, the child learns new and more effective ways to relate with others, to deal with his feelings, and to manage his daily activities.

The standard repertoire of milieu therapy with children includes negotiating, avoidance of power struggles, talking a child down, slow-down periods, relaxation techniques, self-soothing skills, coping and stress-reducing strategies, and safe, gentle holding. When placing a child in a seclusion room is not an alternative for inpatient staff, they are forced to use other methods to resolve crises, prevent escalation, and manage behavior.[40]

The staff who work in a therapeutic milieu become, in actuality, family surrogates for the child—examples of supportive, respectful, cohesive adults who engage in open, healthy adult-to-adult and adult-to-child communication. The milieu staff, composed of child psychiatric–mental health professionals and paraprofessionals, constantly role-model for the children.

The milieu environment provides safety, security, structure, clear and reasonable limits, behavioral consequences, age-appropriate activities and expectations, pleasant surroundings, and the presence of mature, caring, knowledgeable, ethical staff members who are available to the child 24 hours per day. If seclusion or restraint are an aspect of the milieu, they should be used in a consistent manner and according to well-thought-out rationale.[32] Music, dance, art, and other expressive activities may be incorporated into the milieu.

Psychopharmacology

Psychopharmacology is one facet of a comprehensive therapeutic program. It must be remembered that giving a child medication is not the sole solution to his emotional problems but, combined with family or parental counseling, individual therapy, and special educational plans, medication may provide the child with much greater opportunity to improve his overall functioning. Unfortunately, it is difficult to identify the effects of certain chemotherapeutic agents on the behavior of the child, and for this reason extra caution in the administration of these agents is required. One survey of clinicians, for example, showed that drugs were being prescribed very conservatively for emotionally disturbed children, and that the drugs that were chosen and administered to children were given in neither large enough doses, nor for as long a duration of time as is considered appropriate for maximal therapeutic effect.[38]

The use of psychopharmacology with children is different from its use with adults. The emotionally disturbed child may be resentful of medication and think that the drugs and their side effects may be a punishment for his bad behavior or a way to force him to comply with adult authority.[48]

The six categories of psychoactive agents used most commonly and successfully in the treatment of disturbed children are as follows:

1. *Hypnotics and Sedatives:* The barbiturates—most widely used since the early 1900s, infrequently used with children

    Examples—phenobarbital (Luminal), amobarbital (Amytal), pentobarbital (Nembutal), and thiopental (Pentothal)

    Cellular depressants, but can produce paradoxic excitation in children and the aged

    Used to treat anxiety and produce sleep, but not safe for long-term use

2. *The Antipsychotic Agents:* The phenothiazines and related compounds—antihistamines and effective tranquilizers, their use for antipsychotic properties was begun in the early 1950s

    Examples—chlorpromazine (Thorazine), prochlorperazine (Compazine), and trifluoperazine (Stelazine)

    To sedate the acutely agitated child; decrease motor activity of hyperactive or hyperaggressive child; decrease impulsiveness, excitability, anxiety, and hyperdistractibility; and create a general calming effect

    The most important pharmacotherapeutic agents for psychotic and severely disturbed children, but prolonged use can lead to serious complications; therefore, they must be monitored carefully

    Example of piperazines—fluphenazine (Prolixin)

    Example of piperidines—thioridazine (Mellaril)

    Example of butyrophenone—haloperidol (Haldol)

    Lithium is a metal ion effective in treating bipolar disorder (manic-depressive psychosis); trade names may be Lithobid, Lithonate, Lithane, or Eskalith; effective therapeutic dose is, in many instances, near toxic level, so regular serum lithium levels should be determined in all patients taking the drug

3. *The Anxiolytic Agents:* Prescribed for anxiety, phobic states, insomnia, irritability, and hyperactivity in children, the diphenylmethane compounds

    Examples—diphenhydramine (Benadryl), hydroxyzine (Vistaril)

    Useful in treating children with behavior disorders and high anxiety levels

    The benzodiazepine compounds

    Examples—chlordiazepoxide (Librium), diazepam (Valium), lorazepam (Ativan)

    Sedative action, useful in mild to moderate anxiety states or hyperactivity, but inconclusive data available about their effectiveness

4. *The Psychostimulants:* Used in the management of hyperactive behavior in conjunction with parental counseling; in adolescents and adults, as an antidepressant; in children, to treat hyperactivity, hyperaggressivity, hyperdistractibility

    Example—methylphenidate (Ritalin), pemoline (Cylert)

    Acts by increasing alertness, concentration, motor activity, decreasing fatigue and sleepiness, suppressing appetite; also used to treat hyperactivity in children

    Paradoxical effect of Ritalin on the hyperactive child resulting in calming via unknown mechanism (perhaps by raising the child's low threshold to stimuli, helping him focus attention and increase concentration power)

5. *The Antidepressants*

    Examples—imipramine (Tofranil), amitriptyline (Elavil), nortriptylene (Aventyl), trazodone (Desyrel), doxepin (Sinequan)

    Used to treat depression, with or without anxiety, in children by elevating mood and improving sleep and appetite patterns and to treat enuresis in children

Sometimes imipramine is more effective in the treatment of children with attention deficit disorder than the CNS stimulants, particularly in the case of children with higher levels of anxiety or depression or both

6. *The Anticonvulsants*

Example—diphenylhydantoin (Dilantin), carbamazepine (Tegretol)

Used in childhood behavior disorders with or without associated convulsions, and to treat hyperactive children with organic impairment; in experimental trials, carbamazepine is being used for the treatment of other disorders of childhood[38,64,68]

Evaluation

The outcome of child psychotherapy—that is, its effectiveness—is determined by a variety of factors. These factors include the treatment, the therapist, the child and family client, the specific problem for which treatment was sought, and the treatment circumstances. Within the issue of effectiveness, two problems arise: How to define success and how to measure therapeutic change. Does success mean reducing the symptoms (maturation alone can alter those), reducing the child's anxiety, improving academic performance? Does psychopathology mean normal development gone awry, so that success in treatment means a return to an appropriate developmental course?

Research that evaluates the outcomes of child therapy must rely upon objective observations and upon information provided by significant others such as parents and teachers. The child's progress within therapy, however, does not ensure that he will make similar progress outside of therapy. Nontreatment factors, such as the child's school, may play an important role in his behavioral change and must be considered when evaluating the outcome of intervention.[63]

Evaluating psychiatric–mental health care of emotionally disturbed children and their families includes examining the behaviors of children and families following the implementation of therapeutic measures and determining, together with the client and family, whether treatment goals have been reached. "Treatment" in child psychiatry is not synonymous with individual psychotherapy.[18] A variety of therapeutic modalities is available to children and families, and often a combination of approaches provides the optimal effect for the client. Periodic reassessment of treatment techniques and their effectiveness is needed, and when indicated, the nurse and other members of the mental health team should be able to shift their approach to maximize the benefits for the child and family.[18]

Advocation for Emotionally Disturbed Children and Their Families

The child is not a "miniature adult, but a developing person" within a family system.[53] His needs are not those of an adult, but those of an individual within an emotional, and often confusing, world.

Children have legal rights, as well as physical and emotional needs. Under British law, children did not have recognized rights separate from their parents. Within the last 10 to 15 years, the courts have significantly expanded the rights of children and have affirmed that children have the same constitutional rights as adults.[15] The rights of the physically and mentally disabled are especially important in relation to children. These include the following rights:

1. To equal educational opportunity provided by the public schools
2. To freedom from involuntary sterilization
3. To equal access to quality medical care
4. To own legal counsel in any proceeding that could lead to the child's institutionalization
5. To care and treatment in the least restrictive setting[15]

Advocacy for children's rights may be formal, such as when a nurse appears in a court case on a child's behalf. Often, however, the advocacy is informal, in the form of an affirmative role of nurses to promote the respect of children's rights. Strategies that inform parents, professionals, and institutions of children's rights, attempts to overcome budget restrictions, recognition of individuals' rights, and cooperation with other advocates for children and families (case workers, attorneys, and so forth) are examples of informal advocacy for children. Child psychiatric–mental health nurses are in unique positions to advocate for the welfare of children and families; whether a nurse assumes this responsibility is an individual ethical choice.

Summary

This chapter has focused on the prevalence, causative factors, dynamics, behavioral manifestations, and treatment of children with emotional disorders and their families. Some of the emphases of the chapter are as follows.

1. The primary intervention in childhood emotional disorders is that of prevention.

Nursing Care Plan 28-1

The Child with a Psychotic Episode

Nursing Diagnosis	Client Outcome	Intervention
Sensory-perceptual alteration related to lack of awareness of surroundings and interactions	The child will be safeguarded The child's sense of reality will be reinforced	Assess the child's judgment Provide supervision to ensure safety; 1:1 supervision may be required
Alteration in thought processes related to confusion and misperceptions	The child's reality will be clarified	Use brief, simple comments to explain events, including cause and effect, to child Explain and restate as necessary the daily schedule to be followed, expectations of his behavior, and what to expect of caregivers Use specific expectations: "It's time to get up now, come with me to the bathroom…"
Impaired social interaction with other children	The child's interaction with peers will be encouraged	Keep the child present in routine activities Maintain eye contact with the child during conversations Ask the child to look at the adult or other child while talking
Social isolation evidenced by lack of eye contact, staring at wall	The child's contact with reality will be reinforced	Help the child discuss and identify feelings Teach appropriate means of expressing feelings
Impaired verbal communication evidenced by disjointed, inappropriate speech	The child will express feelings appropriately	Give specific instructions for behavior—at the table, in the classroom, and so on—and reward these behaviors
Ineffective individual coping evidenced by ritualistic behavior: rocking, tearing paper, flipping a straw, twirling, placing shoes in a certain order, rubbing the rim of a glass before taking a drink	The child's anxiety and ritualistic behavior will be decreased	Allow certain amount of time to perform these rituals, then move the child into the expected activity Do not reward rituals by smiling or laughing at the behavior

2. Emotional disorders in children constitute a serious mental health problem in the United States with estimates suggesting that at least one in ten children is in need of psychiatric–mental health services.

3. Many theories of childhood emotional disturbances postulate an interactive effect of genetic, biologic, physical, intrapsychic, familial, sociocultural, and environmental factors.

4. Assessment of emotional disorders of childhood requires an examination of both family functioning and the individual child.

Nursing Care Plan   28-2

A Child with a Conduct Disorder

Nursing Diagnosis	Client Outcome	Intervention
Ineffective individual coping related to lack of impulse control	The child will display evidence of impulse control	Teach and role model ways for the child to express needs in an acceptable manner, such as asking for an object rather than grabbing it
Ineffective individual coping related to poor frustration tolerance	The child will delay gratification of needs and effective/adaptive coping skills	Encourage the child to "take turns" during an activity Teach the child to "think before acting"; for example, by allowing a pause, which helps him to learn cause and effect Incorporate a social aspect or interaction into the child's activity Include the child in group activities with children of similar functioning levels to reduce the child's frustration
Impaired social interaction evidenced by maladaptive relationships with parents and peers	The child will exhibit acceptable social behavior	Involve the child in a "skill class" covering material such as how to introduce somebody, what to say to others during conversations, and how to compliment someone
Disturbance in self-concept: self-esteem	The child will evidence an increased self-esteem level	Build in opportunities to help the child experience success through inpatient milieu management, classroom assignment, and so forth Assign reasonable tasks that can be accomplished Reward/praise the completion of tasks
Potential for violence directed toward others	The child will evidence self-control or be appropriately restrained as needed	Allow the child to role play a situation that "makes him mad" and see how he handles his anger; tell about acceptable ways to deal with angry feelings, such as using a punching bag, pounding clay, and so on Encourage the child to express anger verbally, such as "I know that you're angry at Joey... What happened that

(Continues on p. 546)

Nursing Diagnosis	Client Outcome	Intervention
		you're angry at Joey?...Tell Joey that you're angry at him because..."
		Reinforce the child's use of verbal communication to express his feelings, such as "That was super that you used your words to tell Joey that you're angry. You did not throw a chair."
		Establish rules about not hurting self, others, or property
		Restrain the child physically when necessary
		Interrupt a physical outburst before an aggressive act occurs; if the child does commit an aggressive act, have him "undo" his behavior as much as possible; for example, if he throws a chair, allow him a period of time to calm down, then have him pick up the chair and place it in its proper position

5. Treatment planning is a collaborative activity involving the child, his family, and the mental health team.

6. Nursing intervention with the emotionally disturbed child requires maturity, thoughtfulness, and an ethical orientation to psychiatric–mental health care.

References

1. Adler J: General Concepts in Residential Treatment of Disturbed Children. Child Welfare 47 (Nov): 519–523, 1968

2. Aitchison RA, Green DR: A Token Reinforcement System for Large Wards of Institutionalized Adolescents. Behav Res Ther 12 (Sept): 181–190, 1974

3. American Psychiatric Association: Diagnostic and Statistical Manual of Mental Disorders, 3d ed, rev. Washington, DC, American Psychiatric Association, 1987

4. Asarnow JR, Carlson GA: Depression Self-Rating Scale: Utility with Child Psychiatric Inpatients. J Consult Clin Psychol 53, (4): 491–499, 1985.

5. Bailey D, Garralda ME: The Use of the Social Stress and Support Interview in Families with Deviant Children: Methodological Issues. Soc Psychiatry 22, 209–215, 1987

6. Barack RS: Hospitalization of Emotionally Disturbed Children: Who Gets Hospitalized and Why? Am J Orthopsychiatry 56 (April): 317–319, 1986

7. Bardon JI, Bennett VC: Helping Children in School. In Wolman BB (ed): Manual of Child Psychopathology, pp 1058–1087. New York, McGraw-Hill, 1972

8. Barker P, Ward PA: Milieu Therapy in a Child Psychiatry Unit. Nursing Times 68 (December 14): 1579–1581, 1972

9. Bazelon DL: The "Problem Child"—Whose Problem? J Am Acad Child Psychiatry 13 (Spring): 193–201, 1974

10. Besier M: Etiology of Mental Disorders: Sociocultural Aspects. In Wolman BB (ed): Manual of Child Psychopathology, pp 150–188. New York, McGraw-Hill, 1972

11. Bettelheim B: Love Is Not Enough: The Treatment of Emotionally Disturbed Children. New York, Free Press, 1950

12. Biederman J, Munir K, Knee D: Conduct and Oppositional Disorder in Clinically Referred Children with Attention Deficit Disorder: A Controlled Family Study. J Am Acad Child Adolesc Psychiatry 26, (5): 724–727, 1987

13. Brown AR, Avery C (eds): Modifying Children's Behavior: A Book of Readings. Springfield, IL, Charles C Thomas, 1974

14. Bumpass ER, Fagelman FD, Brix RJ: Intervention with Children Who Set Fires. Am J Psychother 37 (July): 328–345, 1983

15. Burgdorf MP: Legal Rights of Children: Implications for Nurses. Nurs Clin North Am 14 (September): 405–416, 1979

16. Cantwell DP: Childhood Depression: What Do We Know, Where Do We Go? In Guze SB, Earls FJ, Barrett JE (eds): Childhood Psychopathology and Development, pp 67–85. New York, Raven Press, 1983

17. Carr R: The Role of Medication in the Treatment of the Disturbed Child. In Steinhauer PD, Rae-Grant Q (eds): Psychological Problems of the Child in the Family, 2d ed, pp 635–663. New York, Basic Books, 1983

18. Chess S: Selectivity of Treatment Modalities. In Chess S, Thomas A (eds): Annual Progress in Child Psychiatry and Child Development, pp 448–462. New York, Brunner/Mazel, 1982

19. Chung SY, Luk SL, Lieh Mak F: Attempted Suicide in Children and Adolescents in Hong Kong. Soc Psychiatry 22, 102–106, 1987

20. Cornell DG, Benedek EP, Benedek DM: Juvenile Homicide: Prior Adjustment and a Proposed Typology. Am J Orthopsychiatry 57 (July): 383–393, 1987

21. Crewe HJ: Fears and Anxiety in Childhood. Public Health 87 (July): 165–171, 1973

22. Critchley DL: Mental Status Examinations with Children and Adolescents. Nurs Clin North Am 14 (September): 429–441, 1979

23. Earls FJ: An Epidemiological Approach to the Study of Behavior Problems in Very Young Children. In Guze SB, Earls FJ, Barrett JE (eds): Childhood Psychopathology and Development, pp 1–15. New York, Raven Press, 1983

24. Earls F, Jung KG: Temperament and Home Environment Characteristics as Causal Factors in the Early Development of Childhood Psychopathology. J Am Acad Child Adolesc Psychiatry 26, (4): 491–498, 1987

25. Eason LJ, Finch AJ, Brasted W, Saylor CF: The Assessment of Depression and Anxiety in Hospitalized Pediatric Patients. Child Psychiatry Hum Dev 16 (Fall): 57–64, 1985

26. Erikson EH: Childhood and Society, 2d ed. New York, W. W. Norton, 1963

27. Erlenmeyer-Kimling L, Cornblatt B, Golden RR: Early Indicators of Vulnerability to Schizophrenia in Children at High Genetic Risk. In Guze SB, Earls FJ, Barrett JE (eds): Child Psychopathology and Development, pp 247–264. New York, Raven Press, 1983

28. Fleck S: Some Basic Aspects of Family Pathology. In Wolman BB (ed): Manual of Child Psychopathology, pp 189–204. New York, McGraw-Hill, 1972

29. Forness SR, Sinclair E, Russell AT: Serving Children with Emotional or Behavior Disorders. Am J Orthopsychiatry 54 (January): 22–32, 1984

30. Freud A: Normality and Pathology in Childhood: Assessments of Development. New York, International Universities Press, 1965

31. Galdston R: Mind Over Matter: Observations on 50 Patients Hospitalized with Anorexia Nervosa. J Am Acad Child Psychiatry 13 (Spring): 246–263, 1974

32. Garrison WT: Aggressive Behavior, Seclusion and Physical Restraint in an Inpatient Child Population. J Am Acad Child Psychiatry 23 (July): 448–452, 1984

33. Garmezy N: Stress, Competence, and Development: Continuities in the Study of Schizophrenic Adults, Children Vulnerable to Psychopathology, and the Search for Stress-Resistant Children. Am J Orthopsychiatry 57 (April): 159–174, 1987

34. Godsey WC, Cottrell WL, Jr: Using Reality Therapy Techniques with Children and Youth. J Tenn Med Assoc 66 (October): 935–936, 1973

35. Goldman J, Stein CL, Guerry S: Psychological Methods of Child Assessment. New York, Brunner/Mazel, 1983

36. Goren S: A Systems Approach to Emotional Disorders of Children. Nurs Clin North Am 14 (September): 457–465, 1979

37. Green MR: The Interpersonal Approach to Child Therapy. In Wolman BB (ed): Handbook of Child Psychoanalysis: Research, Theory, and Practice, pp 514–566. New York, Van Nostrand Rheinhold, 1972

38. Greenberg LM, Lourie RS: Physiochemical Treatment Methods. In Wolman BB (ed): Manual of Child Psychopathology, pp 1010–1031. New York, McGraw-Hill, 1972

39. Hughes MC: Recurrent Abdominal Pain and Childhood Depression: Clinical Observations of 23 Children and Their Families. Am J Orthopsychiatry 54 (January): 146–155, 1984

40. Irwin M: Are Seclusion Rooms Needed on Child Psychiatric Units? Am J Orthopsychiatry 57 (January): 125–126, 1987

41. Kanner L: Child Psychiatry, 3d ed. Springfield, IL, Charles C Thomas, 1957

42. Kazdin AE, Esveldt-Dawson K, French NH, Unis AS: Effects of Parent Management Training and Problem-Solving Skills Training Combined in the Treatment of Antisocial Child Behavior. J Am Acad Child Adolesc Psychiatry 26, (3): 416–424, 1987

43. Kazdin AE, Moser J, Colbus D, Bell R: Depressive Symptoms Among Physically Abused and Psychiatrically Disturbed Children. J Abnorm Psychol 94, (3): 298–307, 1985

44. Kazdin AE, Sherick RB, Esveldt-Dawson K, Rancurello MD: Nonverbal Behavior and Childhood Depression. J Am Acad Child Psychiatry 24, (3): 303–309, 1985

45. Kerr MM, Hoier TS, Versi M: Methodological Issues in Childhood Depression: A Review of the

Literature. Am J Orthopsychiatry 57 (April): 193–198, 1987

46. Kessler JW: Psychopathology of Childhood. Englewood Cliffs, NJ, Prentice-Hall, 1966

47. Kochanska G, Radke-Yarrow M, Kuczynski L, Friedman SL: Normal and Affectively Ill Mothers' Beliefs About Their Children. Am J Orthopsychiatry 57 (July): 345–350, 1987

48. Koupernik C: Chemotherapy in Child Psychiatry. Br Med J 3 (August 5): 345–346, 1972

49. Lambert NM, Hartsough CS, Sassone D, Sandoval J: Persistence of Hyperactivity Symptoms from Childhood to Adolescence and Associated Outcomes. Am J Orthopsychiatry 57 (January): 22–32, 1987

50. Leahey M: Findings from Research on Divorce: Implications for Professionals' Skill Development. Am J Orthopsychiatry 54 (April): 298–317, 1984

51. Lovaas OI: The Autistic Child: Language Development Through Behavior Modification. New York, Irvington Publishers, 1977

52. Mattsson A: Emotional Problems in Asthmatic Children. Virginia Medical Monthly 100 (November): 1024–1029, 1973

53. McDermott JF, Jr, Char WF: The Undeclared War Between Child and Family Therapy. J Am Acad Child Psychiatry 13 (Summer): 422–436, 1974

54. Montanari AJ: A Community-Based Residential Program for Disturbed Children. Hosp Community Psychiatry 20 (April): 103–108, 1969

55. Moustakas CE: Psychotherapy With Children: The Living Relationship. New York, Ballantine Books, 1959

56. Niles GT: Karen Horney's Holistic Approach: A View of Cultural Influences. In Wolman BB (ed): Handbook of Child Psychoanalysis: Research, Theory, and Practice, pp 501–513. New York, Van Nostrand Rheinhold, 1972

57. Norvell N, Brophy C: The Relationship of Anxiety to Childhood Depression. J Pers Assess 49 (April): 150–153, 1985

58. Offord DR: Classification and Epidemiology in Child Psychiatry: Status and Unresolved Problems. In Stenhauer PD, Rae-Grant Q (eds): Psychological Problems of the Child in the Family, 2d ed, pp 117–129. New York, Basic Books, 1983

59. Parsons BV, Jr, Alexander JF: Short-Term Family Intervention: A Therapy Outcome Study. J Consult Clin Psychol 41 (October): 195–201, 1973

60. Pfeffer CA et al: Psychiatric Inpatient Treatment of Childhood Schizoaffective Disorder. Am J Psychother 40 (January): 125–134, 1986

61. Pfeffer CR, Zuckerman S et al: Suicidal Behavior in Normal School Children: A Comparison with Child Psychiatric Inpatients. J Am Acad Child Psychiatry 23 (July): 416–423, 1984

62. Philipp R: Conducting Parent Training Groups: Approaches and Strategies. In Shamsie J (ed): New Directions in Children's Mental Health, pp 23–30. New York, SP Medical & Scientific Books, 1979

63. Phillips RD: A Primer for Conducting Child Psychotherapy Outcome Research. Psychotherapy 24 (Summer): 178–185, 1987

64. Pliszka SR: Tricyclic Antidepressants in the Treatment of Children with Attention Deficit Disorder. J Am Acad Child Adolesc Psychiatry 26 (2): 127–132, 1987

65. Pothier PC: The Issue of Prevention in Psychiatric Nursing. Archives of Psychiatric Nursing 1 (June): 143–144, 1987

66. Proctor JT: Hysteria in Childhood. Am J Orthopsychiatry 28 (April): 394–406, 1958

67. Rae-Grant N: Prevention. In Stenhauer PD, Rae-Grant Q (eds): Psychological Problems of the Child in the Family, 2d ed, pp 591–610. New York, Basic Books, 1983

68. Rapoport JL: Stimulant Drug Treatment of Hyperactivity: An Update. In Guze SB, Earls FJ, Barrett JE (eds): Childhood Psychopathology and Development, pp 189–202. New York, Raven Press, 1983

69. Reinherz H, Walker DK et al: Clinical Assessments and Maternal Judgments: Concurrent and Predictive Relationships. Am J Orthopsychiatry 54 (April): 236–249, 1984

70. Ross AO: Behavior Therapy. In Wolman BB (ed): Manual of Child Psychopathology, pp 900–925. New York, McGraw-Hill, 1972

71. Ross AO: Child Behavior Therapy: Principles, Procedures and Empirical Basis. New York, John Wiley & Sons, 1981

72. Rotheram MJ: Evaluation of Imminent Danger for Suicide Among Youth. Am J Orthopsychiatry 57 (January): 102–110, 1987

73. Rubinstein RA, Brown RT: An evaluation of the Validity of the Category of Attention Deficit Disorder. Am J Orthopsychiatry 54 (July): 398–414, 1984

74. Rutter M: Psychological Therapies: Issues and Prospects. In Guze SB, Earls FJ, Barrett JE (eds): Childhood Psychopathology and Development, pp 139–164. New York, Raven Press, 1983

75. Schuster FP: Family-Centered Therapy of the Scapegoat Child. Southwestern Medicine 52 (November): 215–219, 1971

76. Shachnow J: Preventive Intervention with Children of Hospitalized Psychiatric Patients. Am J Orthopsychiatry 57 (January): 66–77, 1987

77. Sloate PL, Voyat G: Cognitive and Affective Features in Childhood Psychosis. Am J Psychotherapy 37 (July): 376–386, 1983

78. Sloboda SB: The Children of Alcoholics: A Neglected Problem. Hosp Community Psychiatry 25 (September): 605–606, 1974

79. Snow ME, Hertzig ME, Shapiro T: Rate of Development in Young Autistic Children. J Am Acad Child Adolesc Psychiatry 26 (6): 834–835, 1987

80. Stotsky BA, Browne T, Philbirck WA: A Study of Outcome of Special Schooling of Emotionally Disturbed Children. Child Psychiatry and Human Development 4 (Spring): 131–150, 1974

81. Sylvester CE, Hyde TS, Reichler RJ: The Diagnostic Interview for Children and Personality Inventory for Children in Studies of Children at Risk for Anxiety Disorders or Depression. J Am Acad Child Adolesc Psychiatry 26 (5): 668–675, 1987

82. Szurek SA, Berlin IN, Boatman MJ: Inpatient Care for the Psychotic Child, The Langley Porter Child Psychiatry Series, Vol 5. Palo Alto, CA, Science and Behavior Books, 1971

83. Szykula SA: Child-Focused Strategic and Behavioral Therapy Processes. Psychotherapy 24 (Summer): 202–211, 1987

84. Tapia F: Children Who Are Cruel to Animals. Child Psychiatry and Human Development 2 (Winter): 70–77, 1971

85. Thomas A, Chess S, Birch HG: Temperament and Behavior Disorders in Children. In Barten HH, Barten SS (eds): Children and Their Parents in Brief Therapy, pp 93–110. New York, Behavioral Publications, 1973

86. Townsend MC: Nursing Diagnoses in Psychiatric Nursing: A Pocket Guide for Care Plan Construction. Philadelphia, FA Davis, 1988

87. Treffert DA: Children and Adolescents: Hospital Treatment Programs, Administering a Residential Program. Hosp Community Psychiatry 19 (August): 237–240, 1968

88. Turecki S: Elective Brief Psychotherapy with Children. Am J Psychother 36 (October): 479–488, 1982

89. Wertlieb D, Weigel C, Felstein M: Measuring Children's Coping. Am J Orthopsychiatry 57 (October): 548–560, 1987

90. Williams C: Self-Injury in Children. Dev Med Child Neurol 16 (February): 88–90, 1974

91. Winberger HC, Kogan KL: A Direct Approach to Altering Mother-Child Interaction in Disturbed Children. Arch Gen Psychiatr 30 (May): 636–639, 1974

92. Wolman BB: Schizophrenia in Children. In Wolman BB (ed): Manual of Child Psychopathology, pp 446–496. New York, McGraw-Hill, 1972

93. Woodward CA, Johnson Y, Santa-Barbara J, Roberts RS, Pipe M: A Collaborative Special Education Program for Emotionally Disturbed Children: Philosophy, Design and Outcomes. In Shamsie J (ed): New Directions in Children's Mental Health, pp 41–51. New York, SP Medical & Scientific Books, 1979

29

The Emotionally Disturbed Adolescent

Mary Snyder McElvain

"Who are you?" said the caterpillar. Alice replied rather shyly, "I-I hardly know, sir, just at present—at least I know who I was when I got up this morning, but I must have changed several times since then."

Lewis Carroll,
Alice's Adventures in Wonderland

Chapter Preview

This chapter addresses an increasingly important and complex mental health problem in our society—emotional disturbance in adolescents. Accepted parameters for normal adolescent development, theories of adolescent disturbance, and the incidence and significance of this problem are presented. The chapter also discusses the dynamics of several important disorders occurring during adolescence.

The steps of the nursing process—assessment, nursing diagnosis, planning, intervention, and evaluation—are applied to adolescent disorders. There are emphases on assessment of the adolescent based on the nurse's knowledge of developmental variables, on planning with the adolescent and his or her family (including discharge planning), on principles of intervention through a variety of treatment modalities, and on evaluation of the outcomes of nursing interventions. Mental health professionals are encouraged to examine their feelings and attitudes about working with persons in this age group.

Learning Objectives

On completion of the chapter, you should be able to accomplish the following:

1. describe the components of normal physical, sexual, emotional, and mental adolescent development
2. discuss various theories of adolescent development
3. describe the incidence of various types of adolescent disturbance
4. discuss the variables of family communication, child-rearing style, personality, social pressures, and sense of alienation as they contribute to the etiology of adolescent disturbance
5. identify the dynamics of adolescent disorders
    adjustment disorders
    acting-out behavior
    substance abuse
    depression and suicide
    anxiety disorders
    eating problems
    juvenile delinquency
    psychosis
6. apply the nursing process to emotionally disturbed adolescent clients
7. discuss the nurse's own feelings when interacting with an adolescent client and his family

Adolescent Development

In the 20th century, as technology has advanced and economies have reverberated from its effect, our culture has artificially extended the period of adolescence and has made it increasingly difficult for the adolescent youth to contribute to society in a meaningful way. Nevertheless, this same society has focused increasing attention on this pivotal period in the life span. At times, adults and adolescents search together for answers as they experience novel situations such as computer literacy, AIDS awareness, and media exposure of political mistakes.

It now takes some young people until their mid-20s or beyond to assume adult roles. What is happening developmentally during all that time? Adolescent development is a mutually interactive, influential process between individual, family, and society. Adolescents help shape their environment even as their environment helps shape them.

Several myths of adolescent development may be difficult to erase. These myths include the following:

1. Adolescence is a time of universal storm and stress.
2. Rebelliousness is the typical pathway to autonomy.
3. Peer–parent conflict is inevitable during adolescence.
4. Peers replace parents as the major social influence in adolescence.[65]

For most adolescents, development proceeds in an orderly, if not rapid, sequence in which they successfully master growth tasks. "Developmental turmoil" is often, in fact, symptomatic of a disturbance requiring intervention.

Physical Development

Differences among individuals within each sex are almost as marked as the biologic differences between the sexes. Some adolescents finish maturing physically almost before others begin adolescent biologic development. Chart 29-1 shows age ranges for accelerated growth.

Endocrine glands are most involved in adolescent development. The pituitary gland, ovaries, testes, and cortex of the adrenal gland themselves undergo a growth spurt.[25] The average span of the pubertal process lasts for 5 years.[65]

Sexual Development

Physical development is largely outside the control of the individual except as nutritional, health, and safety (or plastic surgery) practices may alter one's biologic

C H A R T   29-1

Age Ranges for Accelerated Growth of Secondary Sex Characteristics and Height

Females		Males	
Ovaries	7–9 yr	Volume of testes	10–$13\frac{1}{4}$ yr
Pubic hair	8–14 yr	Penis	11–$14\frac{1}{2}$ yr
Breast buds	8–13 yr	Pubic hair	10–15 yr
Height spurt*	$9\frac{1}{4}$–$14\frac{1}{2}$ yr	Height spurt*	$10\frac{1}{2}$–16 yr
Median age menarche	12 yr 9 mo	First ejaculation of semen	11–16 yr

* Usually, the peak of height spurt in girls occurs during the year after menarche. The peak of height spurt for boys occurs most frequently after age 14, about the age of first ejaculation of semen.[22]

heritage. Sexual, emotional, and mental development takes place within certain genetic and environmental boundaries; however, learning seems to play a large role in the development of sexuality, intellect, and emotional coping.

An important question to ask in relation to adolescent sexual development is, "How does learning sex roles influence overall adjustment, ability to function as adults, and relations with peers and others?"[39]

Numerous studies of both teenage sexual activity and teenage drug use conclude that the family is a crucial factor in whether a teenager does or does not engage prematurely in either activity. Receiving sex education from a parent and having a number of sexual topics dealt with by the parents decreases the likelihood of premarital sex or of multiple partners. Teenagers in fatherless families were more likely to be sexually active, as were those who had unhappy, conflicted relationships with parents.[89]

Sexuality coexists with the adolescent's search for identity. The process of sexualization begins with dating, which provides an opportunity to practice social roles progressing from hand-holder to kisser to petter to partner in intercourse.[87,92] The adolescent defines values and standards within these social roles. Personal characteristics, such as being "sexy" or not, become part of the self-concept. Expectations for sexual behavior, sex object, and courtship style evolve out of who one thinks one is; these expectations help determine who one becomes. Sexuality is manifest in relationships with others. Does an individual confide in others of the same or opposite sex, or is the individual isolated? Finally, experimentation with sexual conflicts provides an experience for testing autonomous behavior in stressful situations.[92]

Sexual intimacy among adolescents is a concern because of the emotional ramifications and because teenage pregnancies continue to increase while the American birthrate on the whole has declined. Factors that have a significant effect on whether or not an adolescent will be sexually intimate are dating frequency, peer-group-oriented sex education, adolescent sexual experimentation, love relationships with peers, values of peers, a partner who is willing or asking to advance the level of intimacy, and the prospect of marriage.[87] Family attitudes toward sexuality do not appear to be very influential in the adolescent's sexually intimate behavior except as they affect these other variables.

The media have done much to present, and educate about, human sexuality. The average adolescent watches 2 to 3 hours of television per day, and television seems to reinforce a narrow and rigid view of sex roles.[1] In adult television programming, about 75% of the leading characters are male; in children's programming 89% to 90% of the leading roles are male. Males engage in a wider range and variety of activities than females on television.[88] The subtle message is that the male role is more interesting and appealing.

Emotional Development

Of all of the growth tasks in which the adolescent is engaged, the consolidation of his identity into an independent, fully-functioning adult is probably most challenging and crucial. Self-concept is the cognitive aspect of identity development, self-esteem the affective aspect.[36] When childhood has provided the foundation of positive social interaction and positive self-regard, adolescence is used to refine the self. If childhood, however, has provided little in the way of expectations, too few models, or inconsistent rules, then adolescence is used to define a self previously not started.[36]

The process of achieving emotional independence in adolescence involves multiple intervening factors. Assessment of the parents' readiness to let go, the adolescent's readiness to take hold, and the sense of timing is important. There must be opportunities for trying out new social and intellectual skills and a support system that will remain in place regardless of success or failure in achievement. One observer describes this interplay by explaining, "Adulthood comes about 2 years later than the adolescent claims and 2 years earlier than the parents admit."[36] The adolescent's predominant emotions as he strives for independence from parents are guilt, or "How can I leave them?" and inadequacy, or "Maybe I'm not able."

Child-rearing style provides the context in which emotional development takes place. One way to dichotomize parental discipline is between warmth–control, where parents "guide and show," and warmth–restrict, where parents "order and tell." Studies have shown that warm–restrictive parents tend to have passive, fearful, dependent, and generally well-behaved children. Warm–controlling parents tend to have children who feel responsible, assertive, self-reliant, and independent.[5,7] Needless to say, there are numerous possible child-rearing styles; however, because responsibility and independence are emotionally healthy traits, it would seem that nurses should practice, advocate, and teach parent–child interactions that foster warm–controlling traits.

The adolescent's self-consciousness is evident if one has ever watched members of this age group at an awards banquet; there is a great deal of blushing, giggling, swaggering, and so forth, all designed to maintain an image. The term for these behaviors is *adolescent egocentrism,* in which the adolescent assumes that others are as consumed with his behavior and appearance as he is. The adolescent continually constructs and reacts to an imaginary audience.[23]

Some adolescents appear to foreclose prematurely on options to develop autonomously before merging with a significant other. Many adolescents marry to escape perceived neglect or domination at home. The deck is often stacked against them. In the first 5 years of marriage, the divorce rate of both males and females who marry younger than 20 is more than twice that of those who marry at later ages, and this rate remains consistently higher than average throughout life.[17]

Emotional development proceeds within given societal boundaries. The line between psychopathology and cultural adaptation has always been thin and highly permeable, however. Alienation may now be so prevalent in our society that it can no longer be regarded as deviant or pathologic in the usual sense. One author describes an alienation syndrome which includes a basic sense of loneliness, a sense of estrangement, and a chronic sense of frustration.[61] It is logical, then, that counterculture movements would be especially attractive to adolescents who are most alienated from themselves and significant others.[15,73] Mystical and religious cults seem to recruit most successfully among college freshmen and seniors, two years during which major transitions occur. One explanation of this phenomenon is that cults promise definitive answers, give a protecting and structured environment, and provide a "father" who judges right and wrong.[36]

To emerge in adulthood with a positive self-esteem, one must navigate adolescent waters successfully. Emotional development influences and is influenced by extrapersonal circumstances, interpersonal relationships, and intrapsychic stressors.

Mental Development

Jean Piaget's theory of intellectual development describes the final period of formal operational thought, which is consolidated during adolescence. By the time adolescence is reached, the individual's system of mental operations has progressed to a high degree of equilibrium; that is, his ways of thinking, or his cognitive structures, are almost fully formed.[31] These structures may be applied to new problems with resultant new knowledge, but the structures themselves undergo little modification.

Adolescent thought is flexible and effective; an adolescent can imagine many possibilities inherent in a given situation and can deal in abstracts and hypothetical propositions. During adolescence, the individual gains an ability to form concepts, to understand time, and to generalize.[99]

Not all adolescents are capable of formal operational thought, and even those adolescents who use formal operations do not do so all of the time. Findings show that only 45% of adolescents reach formal operations by age 15 and 65% by age 30.[48] Factors such as fatigue, boredom, unstimulating environment, or inadequate education may limit an adolescent's ability to use formal operational thought. Cognitive advancement occurs as a function of the following factors:

Appropriate neurological development
Proper social environment
Experience with objects and events
Internal cognitive reorganization[31]

Adolescent Disturbance

Theoretical Frameworks

Of all the developmental theorists, Sigmund Freud spends the least amount of time on the adolescent period. According to Freud, at the time of puberty, the Oedipus complex reappears and children must again free themselves from parents as libidinal objects and discover a foreign object of love.[99] During adolescence, a relatively strong id confronts a relatively weak ego.[29] The adolescent reworks parental beliefs, values, and standards. Behavior may reflect disorganization of the superego in preparation for adult restructuring.[34]

Anna Freud states that the following ego defenses are predominant during adolescence:

Asceticism—the adolescent becomes idealistic and mistrusts enjoyment
Intellectualization—the adolescent achieves mastery through thinking imaginatively
Identification—the adolescent may isolate himself from his family and superego in order to find substitutes for abandoned parent objects; that is, he displaces his feelings to idealized adults other than his parents in order to desexualize his parents, and yet learn about adult sexuality[34]

Erik Erikson looks at adolescent development as a time of review and integration of past stages of development. He has termed the stage of adolescent development *Identity vs Self-Diffusion,* an apt name for the preoccupation with self-image that occurs during this time. In establishing identity, the adolescent looks for ideas and objects to believe in, performs independently, becomes ambitious about some felt capability, and chooses his life work.[99]

Harry Stack Sullivan's interpersonal theory of anxiety focuses on the importance of the early mother–child relationship for the development of the self-system. His theory does not center on the sexual aspects of this early relationship as did Freud's. Sullivan posed three stages of adolescent development.

Preadolescence is the stage in which the intimate "chum" relationship occurs. Intimacy here is not necessarily sexual, but is a closeness that permits validation of personal worth. The "chum" relationship is, in essence, a prototype of all future love relationships because it deals gradually with the issue of intimacy.
Early adolescence is characterized by heterophilic relationships. The genital drive and an awareness of orgasm appear, and responsibility in one's interpersonal relationships becomes an issue.
Late adolescence is the stage in which satisfactory genital activity is achieved. This activity is always accomplished within the taboos of a particular culture.[34,99]

The learning theory approach to adolescent development focuses on learning to recognize cues to the drives one feels and using those cues to direct and select behavior. The theme of reworking past experience occurs again in the learning theory approach. There is a contradiction between the teenager's previous learning and new expectations of society so that the teenager uses novel approaches to problem-solve.[56]

Within these developmental theories, one begins to observe a pattern in which separation, sexuality, and responsibility are issues. Conflict in these areas is necessary for a clarification of personal identity. Conflict in these areas is also interpersonal; therefore, it follows that emotionally absent adults in contact with adolescents are as destructive as if they were physically absent. Adolescents need adults with whom they can argue, struggle, and sort out issues. They do not have to be in turmoil and rebellion, but they must learn to be responsible for their choices.

Theories tell us that, as adolescence progresses positively, the individual matures. Maturity is measured by the capacity to be loving, to wait for emotional satisfaction, to consider the future, and to control hostile and aggressive impulses.[62] Maturity also implies the ability to function autonomously. In families in which adolescent ego autonomy is impaired, parents delineate the adolescent as subject to their control, and the adolescent has increased anxiety about his capacity to exist separately from parents. The development of autonomy may even carry a threat of alienation from parents in families of disturbed adolescents.[83]

Adolescents must never be portrayed in terms of a single image. There are vast differences between youths in Malaysia and those in Brooklyn, between those in the Ivy League colleges and those in the ghettos.[74] The nurse must apply generalized theories with caution to a given individual to avoid squeezing "square pegs into round holes."

Incidence and Significance of the Problem

Among adolescents, true psychopathology is relatively rare.[93] The difficulty arises in distinguishing normal strains of the adolescent period from serious disturbance because, if the seriously disturbed teen-ager does not receive appropriate treatment, the chances are remote that he or she will "grow out of" the problem. This viewpoint seems to be confirmed in a longitudinal study in progress at the University of California at Los Angeles.[65]

One observer has summarized data from several studies with somewhat differing definitions of psychological disorder and concludes that about 20% of adolescents experience disturbances severe enough to interfere with their functioning, 60% experience occasional episodes of anxiety or depression, but not to an extent causing major disruption in their lives, and the other 20% show no signs of psychological disorder.[95]

Some statistics demonstrate the significance of certain problems of adolescence. In one survey of adolescents who were seen in an outpatient clinic, for example, the following diagnostic categories were represented: 4% acute and chronic brain disorder; 10% mentally retarded; 6.5% schizophrenic; 11% to 18% neurotic (males had a smaller pecentage); 23% to 30% personality disorders (females had a smaller percentage); and 36% transient situational disorder.[74] It appears that the majority of adolescents seen in treatment settings fall in the "adjustment reaction" category.

Statistics on sexual attitudes and behaviors support general beliefs about adolescent sexuality. Between ages 13 and 15, boys' sexual behavior is more advanced, but by ages 16 to 17, approximately equal numbers of males and females engage in petting and premarital intercourse.[26]

Very little of what is experienced as homosexual contact during adolescence or preadolescence will develop into an adult pattern of homosexuality; only 3% to 4% of adolescents who report homosexual experience will become homosexuals as adults.[32]

The incidence of acting-out behaviors among adolescents has been researched. Census estimates are that there are approximately 1 million teenage runaways per year.[38] More than half of all serious crimes are committed by youths aged 10 to 17.[88] The issue of whether to use drugs is virtually universal in our society and can be viewed as a developmental problem faced by adolescents and their families.[67]

Statistics of drug use among adolescents vary widely. Six of every ten seniors (61%) have at least tried some illicit drug by the time they leave high school, according to one study.[42] A more encouraging fact is that, in general, there has been some appreciable reduction in drug use. The percentage of adolescents using any illicit drug declined approximately one-fourth between 1979 and 1984 (from 39% to 29%). The downturn in drug use halted in 1985, for reasons not entirely clear.[42]

Research data suggest that there is merit in physicians reducing their prescriptions of psychotherapeutic drugs for adolescents. Those adolescents who received prescriptions of minor tranquilizers, barbiturates, or amphetamines had rates of illicit drug use that exceeded those for youngsters who never were prescribed such drugs. Further studies are needed in order to establish a causal connection.[42]

Possibly as many as 5% of teens aged 14 to 18 have serious drug and drug-related problems.[8] Other data suggest that white adolescents have a higher lifetime prevalence of illicit drug use than black or hispanic youth.[8] Most compulsive, dedicated users are multiple drug users. Drug use patterns show that marijuana, alcohol, and amphetamines are most commonly used, in that order, by youths 19 years and under.[8] Daily smoking rates remained at 20% of high school seniors in 1985.[42] Minority youth tend to be much more likely than whites to use heroin and cocaine. Primary PCP abuse and inhalant abuse is more prevalent among hispanic youth.

The data from one recent study indicate that drug abuse in both sexes is highly associated with both major depressive disorder (MDD) and other psychiatric diagnoses. This study of 424 college students aged 16 to 19 years found the prevalence of MDD to be 6.8%, of alcohol abuse to be 8.2%, and of drug abuse to be 9.4%. In this sample, students were almost always subject to depressive illness first, followed by alcoholism or substance abuse. The possibility of self-medication as a factor in the development of alcohol or other substance abuse should be further investigated. Early drunkenness is an important risk factor both for substance abuse and major depressive disorder.[20]

Even studies showing that 15% to 25% of adolescents experience "problems" in development have failed to show what proportion of these individuals are true casualties of adolescence, as opposed to casualties of childhood.[65] In interpreting research about adolescent disturbance, then, one must be careful to note whether statistics are purely descriptive or whether they are inferential, and, if they are the latter, one must note what conclusions are being drawn about the adolescent period.

It is possible to make some summary statements regarding adolescent disturbance. The more behavior problems an adolescent displays, the longer these problems persist beyond an age when they might be expected, and the more they involve cognitive and behavioral difficulties instead of, or in addition to, emotional upsets, then the more likely the young person is to be psychologically disturbed.[95]

Etiologic Theories

A comprehensive, but general, etiologic theory of disturbance in adolescence states that it is caused by the interaction of a certain level of genetic or constitutional disposition (diathesis) and certain kinds of demanding experience (stress).

One theory concerns communication within the family. It states that families with "high expressed emotion" contribute to continued stress in an already disturbed teenager. Specific manifestations of "high expressed emotion" include: parents giving personal criticism of fundamental qualities of the adolescent, rather than aspects of behavior; parents intruding in the adolescent's life both behaviorally and psychologically; and high degrees of hostility, anger, and resentment.[65]

Another study suggests that children most likely to conform blindly to peer values clearly come from the most extremely authoritarian or permissive families.[65] These theoretical explanations concern childrearing style. It seems that both limits that are too confining and insufficient limit-setting drive the adolescent out of the family sphere of influence.

A disrupted family unit may predispose some adolescents to certain disturbances. The major psychological effects of divorce on adolescents appear to be the following:

A sense of rejection and fear of abandonment
Intensification of typical adolescent conflicts
Fear that own marriage will fail
A sense of confusion and disillusionment about
life[86]

It is estimated that by 1990 half of all children under 18 will experience a parental divorce or separation, spending some time in a single-parent household.[21] A study of the effect of single parenthood on adolescents found that those in mother-only households were more likely to make decisions without direct parental input and more likely to exhibit deviant behavior. Interestingly, the study also found that the presence of any other adult in a mother-only household brings control levels closer to those found in two-parent families.[21] Although the data in this study need to be updated, they point to some important considerations, such as identifying the functional equivalents in our society of two-parent families.

The factors associated with drug use illustrate the complexity of etiologic theories of adolescent disturbance. Personal, social, and familial factors are associated with how frequently adolescents use drugs and with their likelihood of using drugs at all. The inclination to use drugs is directly related to a high degree of openness to experience, tolerance of deviance, interest in independence, and a low degree of conformity, social inhibition, interest in achievement, and involvement with religion. Socially, the more an adolescent's friends use drugs, the more closely he interacts with these friends, and the more he values these friends' affection and approval, the more likely he is to use drugs.

Familial factors—including absence of a parent, lack of perceived closeness to parents, lack of closeness between parents, unconventional parents, excessively passive mothers, and drinking and drug use patterns of parents—have been positively correlated with drug use.[8] In addition to the above factors in drug use, there is emerging evidence that genetic factors contribute to the disposition to become an addictive drug user. Studies of twins and adoptees identify family patterns that cannot be accounted for by shared experience or parental modeling alone.[95]

Dynamics of Adolescent Disorders

Adjustment Disorders

Adjustment disorders are reactive or situational in nature. They are developmental lags without serious mental disorder. Stress temporarily overwhelms the capacity of the individual to problem-solve. Symptoms of adjustment disorders express a conflict over independence and arise in new life situations that call for increased independence.[45]

Acting-Out Behavior

Acting-out behaviors express conflicts through actions rather than through words. For the adolescent, acting-out behavior is a way of defending against sexual impulses and a direct means of expressing aggressive drives.[65] Acting-out behavior is often impulsive. The adolescent feels overwhelmed by affect and does not think through the consequences of his actions.[34] In this chapter, three behaviors are identified specifically as acting-out—running away, being truant, and problematic sexual activity.

Runaway behavior involves typically immature, timid adolescents who have difficulty directing their anger, or who feel unsafe or unwanted.[34] Seventy percent of runaways interviewed in one study had low achievement and little, if any, involvement with school.[4] The act of running away may involve either much fantasy about the effect the behavior will have on the person or persons left behind or feelings about the family too painful to acknowledge in thought.

Truant behavior usually occurs in youngsters who dislike school and are doing poorly academically. Although school phobia, or exaggerated fear of attending school, is probably more common than truancy, it is not necessarily seen as acting-out.

Problematic sexual behavior involves using sex to decrease feelings of loneliness and anxiety.[34] Sexual acting-out among adolescent young women is believed to reflect the breakdown of parental control, a rebellion against authority, and an acute disturbance in the parent–adolescent relationship.[30]

Adolescent pregnancy is an increasingly serious health and sociological problem. One in five births in the United States involves a teenage mother.[71] Teenage pregnancy is often unplanned and conflicts with other goals. Pregnancy interferes with the teenager becoming comfortable with her body image. The mental disequilibrium usually associated with any pregnancy can be frightening and alarming to persons whose egos are not fully integrated. Placed within the context of Erikson's psychosocial developmental tasks, the pregnant adolescent is working on generativity before she has accomplished a sense of identity or achieved the task of intimacy.[62]

Prostitution has been explained dynamically by at least two different schools of thought. The psychoanalytic theory focuses on a negative self-image of the female, due to rejection by her father, and states that prostitution is a symbolic way to degrade the self and defend against the need for love. Psychosocial theory suggests that the prostitute rejects society's values rather than rejecting the self. One study reinforces the idea that the sex act is not valued by prostitutes, but instead takes on different meanings. Almost all of the teenage prostitutes interviewed in this study stated that sex was unpleasant for them, something they did only in order to get money.[50]

Substance Abuse

Investigators have found substantial evidence of psychopathology in drug abusers, whereas drug users (*i.e.*, the experimental and social types) are much more like their non-drug-using-peers.[98] Whether heavy drug use is a cause or a result of psychosocial difficulties is difficult to determine from available research.[95]

There are several etiologic theories of drug use. First, the *peer influence theory* proposes that adolescents take drugs to be accepted by contemporaries.[44] A recent study showed that the variable that was consistently found to be the strongest correlate of adolescent cigarette smoking is whether his friends smoke. These researchers suggest using the concept of social disaffection (*i.e.*, taking issue with or not meeting conventional norms) to explain one factor that may predispose an adolescent to associate with others who smoke.[49] The peer-influence theory implies that adolescents are more likely to work for short-term social reinforcement than for long-term individual benefit.

The *parental influence theory* claims that drug-taking behavior is learned (this is especially true of drinking behavior but not strongly proven with mari-

juana use) and that a poor parent–child relationship seems to be related to the use of illicit drugs other than marijuana.[27]

The *anticipatory socialization theory* asserts that role-taking behavior, in the case of drug use behavior, is perceived as exercising personal direction or independence.[40] There is recent empirical research that suggests that alcohol-related expectancies play a significant role in the drinking behavior of adolescents.[97] Positive expectancy factors include: increased social and physical pleasure, increased power and aggression, increased social assertiveness, and decreased tension. Expectations about the negative consequences of alcohol use seem to be unrelated to drinking behavior. The clinical implications of this research would seem to indicate that the nurse should focus on positive cognitions rather than negative consequences. For example, providing relaxation training as an alternate means of tension relief, and stating that everyone does *not* drink, are ways to teach positive thinking in regard to alcohol.[97]

The *drug-prone personality theory* is based on a longitudinal study that found that drug users were nonconforming, independent, and adventure-seeking. The non-drug users were conformists, achievement-oriented, and nonimpulsive. What isn't known is whether these characteristics are cause or effect.[46]

The *deviance theory* maintains that because a deviant subculture is stigmatized and punished, its members adopt values and attitudes to survive in a hostile environment.[9,41] One 5-year longitudinal study, which supports this last theory, found that rebelliousness was the best predictor of drug use.[85]

Depression and Suicide

The normal developmental process presents teenagers with many real losses and threats to their sense of adequacy.[95] Even if development progresses seemingly smoothly, the adolescent may fear not being able to live up to the concept of self that he or she has constructed. This fear of failure may lead to a loss of self-esteem resulting in depression. Another "normal" loss in growing up is the loss of the image of parents as perfect; therefore, many adolescents are in a mourning process and feel quite alone.[70]

Depressive disorders emerge primarily in response to the experience of loss in genetically predisposed persons. Individual variation in sensitivity to loss appears to be due to developmental experiences.

A cognitive model of depression proposes that negative thoughts and attitudes are core features of depression. Loss is seen as the loss of some self-attribute necessary for happiness. According to this theory, depression-prone individuals encounter unfavorable life situations disposing them to overreact to being deprived.[64] Depriving early life experiences include parental absence, dislike of the child, or ignoring the child.[95] The child attributes a lack to himself, rather than to others, when later facing loss.

Another theory relates depression to learned helplessness, or the belief that one's actions have little impact on one's destiny.[81,82] The experience of loss that precipitates depression is a loss of control. When they were children, these individuals felt that they couldn't do anything about unhappy circumstances.

A behavioral model proposes that depression reflects an individual's inability to gain positive reinforcement.[53,54] Developmental experiences have provided insufficient opportunities to learn gratifying ways of responding to people and events.

The symptoms of depression in adolescence are often acting-out behaviors. Acting-out is seen for several reasons—the adolescent's intolerance for intense feelings, his learned behavior, or a lack of verbal skills. Remember that the adolescent is ambivalent about dependency needs versus needs for independence. If a teenager admits that he needs help, he may perceive his request for help as a regression back to childhood.[57] Suicide is acting-out in the extreme.

Of the estimated 400,000 teenagers in the United States who attempt suicide every year, 5,000 to 10,000 succeed. Verbal and behavioral clues before attempts vary widely. A helpful rule of thumb is to investigate any markedly different behavior in a teenager as a possible warning sign of a suicide attempt. The teenager may be unable to express feelings clearly; he depends on a caring, knowledgable professional to take him seriously about suicidal ideation or attempts.[91]

Eating Disorders

Two startling eating disorders of adolescence are anorexia nervosa, a starvation syndrome, and bulimia, a binge-purge syndrome. Certainly, nutrition can become problematic for any teenager, as the body requires more nutrients for growth during adolescence or as the teenager responds to dietary fads; however, this chapter examines the two pathological syndromes.

Anorexia nervosa is a self-imposed starvation whose mortality rate is 5%.[18] A fear of not being in control is the central issue in anorexia nervosa. What makes anorexia nervosa especially interesting and also difficult to treat in the clinical setting is that we are still unclear as to how much of the manifestation, both medically and psychiatrically, is a reflection of the effects of hunger and starvation per se.[11] Anorexia nervosa occurs primarily in white adolescent females from middle to upper social classes.[12]

There are three predominant areas of disturbed psychological functioning in anorexics. They are as follows:

1. Body image
2. Misinterpretation of internal and external stimuli, especially hunger
3. Overwhelming feelings of ineffectiveness

Hilde Bruch, an expert in eating disorders, describes the life of the anorexic as an ordeal of living up to family expectations. The child has, in many cases, been overvalued by parents. The child's view becomes "If you are given much, much is expected of you."[12]

Anorexics' cognitive development remains in Piaget's stage of concrete operations, characterized by egocentricity and magical thinking. The new ways of acting and thinking, which are a normal part of adolescence, are frightening to the anorexic child. She acts out the conviction that by being skinny and in need of protection, she ensures eternal love and care from her parents.[12]

The child who becomes anorexic is usually described as previously being loving, devoted, and well-behaved. The child's compliance probably concealed the fact that she was deprived of living a life of her own. Throughout childhood, her parents failed to acknowledge or confirm the developmental progress she initiated, so that her parents perceive growth and development as their accomplishment, not hers. Other characteristics of the anorexic are excessive involvement in preparing, cooking, and talking about food and being socially isolated during the year preceding the onset of the disorder.[12]

An individual's family may foster excessive concern with bodily needs. Members of the families of anorectics are overinvolved in each other's lives, with a resultant loss of individuation.[64] Transactional patterns in these families are characterized by enmeshment, overprotectiveness, rigidity, and lack of conflict resolution.[76]

Bulimia is an episodic, uncontrolled, rapid ingestion of large quantities of food over a short period of time (binge eating), resulting in feelings of physical and emotional discomfort. These episodes are typically ended by exhaustion, social interruption, or self-induced vomiting. Bulimia is commonly associated with anorexia nervosa (25% of anorexics engage in this behavior). Whereas the anorexic denies hunger, the bulimic person gives in to impulses and then controls body size through purging.[55] Definite precipitating factors are unknown, but onset often occurs during the senior year in high school, which is a transitional period. Severe weight loss does not occur in bulimia as it does in anorexia nervosa, and amenorrhea seldom occurs.[12,45]

Bulimia is a relatively common condition among

female adolescents, with a conservative prevalence of at least 1% in high-school and college settings. Most of a bulimic's life revolves around disturbed eating habits.[55]

The major medical problems associated with bulimia are consequences of self-induced vomiting, laxative abuse, and diuretic use. These include hypokalemia, alkalosis, hypochloremia, hyponatremia, dental enamel erosion, parotid and salivary gland enlargement, "lazy bowel syndrome," and malabsorption.[55]

Compared with anorexics, bulimic patients have been found to be more anxious, depressed, interpersonally sensitive, and somatically inclined. Much evidence supports a relationship between affective disorders and bulimia. A number of persons with bulimia have improved in response to antidepressants. Also, because emerging data indicate that families of bulimic persons are significantly disturbed and disturbing to live with, family therapy would seem to be an important treatment modality for this group. There is still, however, much work to do in identifying etiologic factors and effective treatments.[55]

Juvenile Delinquency

Delinquency includes a wide range of illegal acts. An individual's social class has an effect on whether or not a behavior is classified as delinquent. Some youngsters are *sociologic* delinquents, in that they have few psychological problems and are well-integrated members of a delinquent subculture. Other delinquent youngsters, whose deviant behavior results from *psychological* problems, show one of the following three patterns of disturbance:

1. *Neurotic delinquency* occurs when illegal acts are committed to communicate needs, especially needs for affection and status. Punishment for the acts may relieve guilt feelings.
2. *Characterologic delinquency* involves impulsiveness, low frustration tolerance, inadequate motivation, and a characteristic lack of guilt.
3. *Psychotic and organic delinquency* results when illegal acts are used as a defense against unrealistic fears of anxiety and annihilation.[84, 94]

Gang members are often sociologic delinquents. Youths who join gangs are different from non-gang joiners because they are more likely to have divorced parents or parents with a criminal history, they are more likely to do poorly in school and to have low IQ scores, and they enjoy violence. In fact, physical and verbal aggression are preferred coping mechanisms of gang members.[47] The gang functions as a family substitute for the adolescent whose strong dependency needs are displaced onto the peer group.[14] Sociologic delinquents usually have good family relationships during early life, but lack adequate parental supervision during elementary school and adolescence.[95]

Neurotic delinquency consists of acute, situationally determined lawbreaking, which is precipitated by current psychological distress and stops when distress is relieved. This behavior is especially likely to occur when parents inadvertently foster or reinforce antisocial behavior. For instance, parents may model minor disrespect for the law or may be inconsistent in discipline, which tacitly communicates approval of delinquent acts.[95]

Characterologic delinquency, like psychopathy, is typically associated with a childhood history of early and severe parental rejection, followed by inadequate discipline and supervision during middle childhood and adolescence. Psychopathy never develops in adulthood in the absence of a developmental history of escalating antisocial behavior.[95]

Psychotic delinquency emerges primarily in schizophrenic youngsters, or in those with minimal brain dysfunction, poor impulse control, or a form of epileptic disorder characterized by psychomotor seizures, all of which may lead to antisocial behavior.[95]

Psychosis

Most forms of schizophrenic disturbance begin during or soon after adolescence. The majority of schizophrenic adolescents initially show a mixed picture in which features of schizophrenia are secondary to, or obscured by, other difficulties, usually depression or antisocial behavior.[95]

One author has suggested that one characteristic of severely disturbed adolescents, irrespective of how a specific pathology manifests itself, is an irreconcilable, unanswerable quest to do something about their bodies.[51]

Schizophrenic youngsters withdraw from the world of reality, where they are unable to cope, and undergo profound regression to primitive thinking. In the face of overwhelming anxiety, a "retreat into psychosis" provides a degree of relief, comfort, and security.[34] There is a high price for the coping mechanism of psychosis, however protective it may be for the ego.

Application of the Nursing Process to Adolescent Disorders

Assessment

Using the theoretical knowledge bases just discussed, the nurse is prepared to assess each individual adolescent according to his developmental progress and special needs, analyze the data, and formulate nursing diagnoses (see Chart 29-2, "Nursing Diagnoses"). Assessment of adolescents is challenging because of the wide range of individual variation. It is crucial to assess the whole person and then make comparisons with normal limits of feelings, thoughts, and behaviors in an age group.

Identity Formation

The nurse assesses the adolescent's sense of identity because identity consolidation is the major developmental task of adolescence. Areas of functioning that the nurse explores to assess the adolescent's sense of ego identity include the following:

1. How distinct from others does the individual feel?
2. How is the individual aware of himself/herself? Does this awareness come from all senses? Does the individual describe experiences, memories, perceptions, and emotions?
3. Can the individual make choices from among alternatives?
4. What is the quality of the individual's interactions with others?
5. Does the individual have self-respect?
6. Are the individual's ego functioning and interests stable over time?

When assessing identity formation and maintenance, the nurse will remember that adolescence ends with a sense of ego identity. It is not until around age 17 to 22 that individuals consolidate initial adult identities.[62]

Independent Functioning

Another growth task of adolescence for the nurse to assess is psychological and financial independence or dependence in regard to parents. The 16-year-old may express a desire to "get away from parents," but the 22-year-old may have the means to carry out this theme. Our society does not define or describe the specific steps involved in the process of moving from the status of dependent child to independent adult.[62] Some steps the nurse may look for are as follows:

1. Taking responsibility for completing school work
2. Self-initiation of projects and hobbies
3. Employment that leads to, and eventually results in, self-support
4. Self-assertion in conflict situations

These steps may be attained in varying degrees; some steps may be completed while others have not been attempted. The adolescent in an inpatient unit may have many of these steps curtailed, but the nurse can still assess progress toward independent functioning.

Self-Image

Self-image is the perfect and ideal self that one imagines oneself to be, after identifying with an idealized conception of what the self should be.[100] When the adolescent says, "You don't know the real me," he is likely to be referring to self-image. *Self-concept,* on the other hand, reflects the perceived status of the self; it includes characteristics and personality traits and an evaluation of the worth or desirability of these traits.[24] The adolescent who says, "I care about others, and I'm a good student and I think that's pretty worthwhile," is reflecting self-concept.

Self-awareness is the recognition of one's own existence and characteristics and of the evaluations of others toward the self.[25] An adolescent might indicate self-awareness by a statement such as, "When I get scared of other people, I get sort of inconsiderate of them because I want to keep away and not get hurt."

Body image is a mental picture of one's body. As adolescents' bodies change, they must keep restructuring their body images. They must also come to accept a less-than-perfect body unless they are one of the lucky few to have a body that conforms almost exactly to society's current definition of perfect body type. It is hard to convince a distraught teenager that "beauty is in the eye of the beholder." Self-image, self-concept, self-awareness, and body image can be assessed by listening carefully to the adolescent's self-statements as well as by direct questioning about these issues. The disturbed adolescent will always have a disturbance in one or more of these areas.

Strengths

The adolescent is likely to overvalue or undervalue his strengths and talents. He may play down strengths without a firm sense of identity or with a negative self-concept. Conversely, the adolescent may glorify his abilities and worth, thereby showing a characteristic heightened narcissism. This narcissism comes from projecting a model of what he would like to be in an attempt to actualize the ideal image of self.[78] The nurse should assess how realistic the adolescent is in his self-evaluation of strengths, yet remember that increased narcissism is expected.

Impulsivity

Nursing assessment of an adolescent includes the degree of *impulsivity* in behavior because society expects that a person's impulsivity will decrease as he achieves adult status. As a person reaches higher levels of intellectual and moral development, he should retain spontaneity, but with minimal impulsive behavior. To assess impulsivity, the nurse watches an adolescent's reactions to situations for the cognitive component. She might ask, "Did the adolescent think of the con-

C H A R T   29-2
Nursing Diagnoses

Because the emotional problems of adolescents cover such a wide range and lead to such diverse behaviors, the appropriate nursing diagnoses will depend entirely on the data the nurse gathers for each individual. The following examples serve as guidelines to linking certain information with standardized nursing diagnoses.

Possible Nursing Diagnosis	Type of Data Supporting the Nursing Diagnosis
1. Anxiety	1. Perceived threat to self-concept; conflicts over decisions, choices
2. Coping, ineffective individual	2. Maladaptive styles
3. Ineffective family coping	3. Adolescent's problems occur within disturbed family system
4. Knowledge deficit	4. Regarding health status, economics, relationships; still in age span when formal learning is occurring
5. Nutrition, alterations in: less than body requirements	5. If anorexic or bulimic, dieting, or substance abusing; may be eating junk food rather than balanced diet
6. Noncompliance	6. May be negative toward authority figures or mistrustful of professional adults
7. Powerlessness	7. Parents, teachers, health professionals reluctant to relinquish control over decisions affecting adolescent's life; may even be rescued from experiencing consequences of own actions, such as in situations of overprotective guardians; lack of opportunity for employment or other meaningful contribution to society
8. Self-care deficit	8. May be unwilling to meet standards of self-care required in a given facility; may rebel against following rules for eating, bathing, or grooming in attempt to define identity or be accepted in peer group
9. Self-concept, disturbance in	9. Struggling to form or consolidate identity; may distort strengths and/or weaknesses
10. Sensory-perceptual alterations	10. If psychotic
11. Social isolation	11. May have difficulty finding a place in new peer group, especially if hospitalized; May feel like a misfit among peers at school
12. Thought processes, alterations	12. If psychotic
13. Violence, potential for	13. May not cope with conflicts verbally, but may instead resort to impulsive acting-out; obtain history of incidence of lack of control
14. Potential for injury	14. Suicidal adolescent or substance abuse leading to impaired reality-testing

sequences before acting in a given fashion?" To assess juvenile delinquency, the nurse examines these two factors:

1. The social context of the behavior and the life experiences of the perpetrator
2. Whether the behavior constitutes a repeated pattern or is impulsive[99]

Interpersonal Relationships

Adolescence is a time when emancipation conflicts are at a peak. The nurse assesses both the quality and quantity of peer relationships and support groups such as club membership, church affiliations, or job ties, and the nature of family interactional patterns. The diagnosis of adolescent problems is usually child-focused. In most instances, however, the adolescent's difficulties reflect the dysfunctional interaction between the youngster and the parents.[34] This statement does not place blame on parents but recognizes each party as bringing stressors to the interaction.

Sexuality

A final area of assessment is the adolescent's sexuality and sexual behavior. Body image reflects sexual identity. Internalization of body changes takes much longer than the actual physical change. The nurse assesses both physiological variables and the adolescent's cognitive internalization of bodily changes.[62]

Sorting out masculine and feminine identity and the role behavior associated with that sexual identity is a major task. The process of assuming sexual identity and role includes fantasy, role-playing, introjection, projection of self in the role, and finally, role internalization.[77] Role-taking occurs in interaction with another person; therefore, many of the areas of functioning already discussed will interface with sexuality and sexual behavior. For example, an isolated adolescent has no one available with whom to try out sexual role behaviors, so fantasy may be this adolescent's primary mechanism.

The nurse also assesses the adolescent's need for knowledge concerning sexual issues. Creating a comfortable climate for discussion about masturbation, homosexuality, sexual intercourse, contraception, pregnancy, or abortion becomes a challenge for the nurse. The cognitive level of the adolescent determines how "in-depth" the discussion may be.

In summary, no medical history of a teenager is complete without a full drug and sexual history being taken (with appropriate confidentiality assured).[89]

Nursing Diagnosis

In the second stage of the nursing process, nursing diagnosis, the nurse analyzes the data gathered from the client and his family and friends during the assessment phase. The formulation of the nursing diagnosis then becomes the basis for planning and prescribing nursing interventions for this particular client. When working with adolescent clients and their families, the nurse may formulate many different nursing diagnoses to guide their care. The following are some of the possible nursing diagnoses that may be employed:

Ineffective individual coping related to unrealistic perceptions, inadequate support systems, situational and/or maturational crises, personal vulnerability, evidenced by verbalization of low self-esteem, chronic anxiety, chronic fatigue, chronic depression, inability to meet age-appropriate role expectations, inability to problem-solve

Disturbance in self-concept: low self-esteem, related to lack of positive feedback, poor parent–child relationship, dysfunctional family system, evidenced by self-destructive behavior, lack of eye contact, inability to form positive interpersonal relationships, self-neglect, difficulty accepting positive reinforcement

Anxiety related to situational and/or maturational crises, dysfunctional family system, feelings of helplessness over own life, evidenced by increased tension, apprehension, fearfulness, poor eye contact, increased helplessness

Alteration in nutrition: less than body requirements (if anorexic or bulemic), related to excessive use of laxatives, diuretics, and/or diet pills, refusal to eat, bingeing followed by purging or self-induced vomiting, evidenced by excessive loss of hair or presence of lanugo, pale conjunctiva and mucous membranes, poor muscle tone, extreme weight loss, amenorrhea

Impaired social interaction related to self-concept disturbance, negative role models, substance abuse, dysfunctional family system, evidenced by verbalized or observed discomfort in social situations, observed use of unsuccessful social interaction behaviors, verbalized or observed inability to receive or communicate a satisfying sense of belonging, caring or interest, dysfunctional interaction with peers, family, and/or others

Potential for violence: self-directed or directed at others, related to threat to self-concept, negative role-modeling, dysfunctional family system, evidenced by body language indicating violence potential, overt and aggressive acts, self-destructive behavior and/or active aggressive suicidal acts, hostile threatening verbalizations, increased motor activity, agitation, irritability, possession of destructive means, rage, inability to verbalize feelings, provocative behavior

Planning

During the process of assessing and diagnosing the adolescent client, the nurse interacts with him. The nurse begins to establish rapport and trust in the initial contact with the client. The adolescent is particularly sensitive to being listened to, to being understood, and to being accepted. It naturally follows that the adolescent should be included in the planning of professional intervention in his life.

Client Involvement in Decision-Making

In the case of emotional and behavioral difficulties, some person other than the adolescent has probably sought out mental health professionals. It becomes imperative, therefore, that the adolescent be given the opportunity to involve himself in the decision-making. For example, even the adolescent who has been referred for psychiatric treatment by the courts can be given a choice of two or more times when he will be seen by the therapist. The metacommunication to the adolescent when professionals involve him in planning is that maturing includes being active in one's behalf or taking some degree of responsibility for the self.

Setting Behavioral Outcomes

Planning includes learning how to achieve behavioral outcomes derived from assessed needs. Two general outcomes of treatment are that the adolescent will be able to identify meanings of his behavior and that he will verbalize a problem-solving process indicating that conflicts are worked through and emotions stabilized.[99]

Planning takes into account the following questions:

1. What alternative services are appropriate to meet the client's assesssed needs?
2. What outcome can be expected from each alternative?
3. Which alternative is most cost-effective?
4. Are some alternatives less restrictive than others?
5. Do the alternatives allow the adolescent to continue his education, to be in contact with peers, and to work on the psychosocial growth tasks of adolescence?
6. How long is treatment expected to be necessary?

Family Involvement

The entire family should be incorporated into the treatment of an adolescent's problems.[2] The family system must be considered when planning care because intervention in one part of the system will impact on all other parts of the system. Most state laws require that individuals of certain ages may only be treated with parental consent. If an adolescent insists on strict confidentiality, even from parents, his insistence may be taken as symptomatic of dysfunctional family processes. The therapist points out this fact to the adolescent and tells the adolescent of pertinent legal requirements for treatment. A major decision made in the planning phase will be whether the adolescent will be treated individually, in family therapy, or some combination of both.

Some factors influencing the decision as to the most appropriate treatment modality would be whether the presenting problem is intimately related to the current family interaction pattern or whether the family's effort is needed for crisis alleviation and symptom reduction.[28]

Discharge Planning

Discharge planning involves a future orientation that concerns realistic issues of what will happen to the adolescent after treatment. It deals with how the client will manage his own health problems after therapy. In the case of inpatient care, discharge planning includes where the adolescent will live, what difficulties might be anticipated in readjusting to community life, and any available aftercare services.

Intervention

Several modalities are available to the nurse who intervenes with adolescent clients. They include specific modalities such as family therapy, group therapy, individual therapy, and behavior modification. Other general principles of intervention, such as effect of the milieu, limit-setting, and communication with adolescents, are also used.

Psychotherapy with adolescents focuses on relationship building, to help them experience engaged, trusting, mutual relationships with others, and on reality testing, to correct inaccurate perceptions of the self, environment, and consequences of action. These goals may be achieved in either family, group, or individual psychotherapy.[95]

Family Therapy

With very few exceptions, adequate treatment for disturbed adolescents requires involvement of their parents.[95] Family therapy is a formal involvement of all family members. When the adolescent or parents refuse family therapy, the chances are great that destructive reactions will continue to occur. The family system may resist improvement of the client and sabotage treatment plans in a subtle or not-so-subtle fashion. Parents may feel guilt over their child's problem and become either oversolicitous or rejecting.[95]

If family therapy is not possible, then at least some effort should be made to informally educate the parents about their adolescent's difficulties and needs. This effort is necessary to help the adolescent be reintegrated emotionally and physically into the family system upon discharge from inpatient care.

In family therapy, the therapist meets jointly with the disturbed adolescent, his or her parents, and as many as possible of the siblings and other relatives who live in the home. Although the adolescent is usually referred to as the "identified patient," the approach focuses more on problems of family interaction than on the young person's abnormal behavior.[95]

Some areas of family functioning addressed during family therapy include the following:

1. Information processing—what kind of information is sought by family members and how is it used?
2. Decision-making—how can the decision-making process be described for a given family?
3. Emotional tenor—what is the emotional atmosphere of the family?
4. Conflict management—how are individual differences handled?
5. Strengths and weaknesses[99]

Intervention strategies that a nurse uses in family therapy sessions include the following:

1. Helping family members articulate feelings and needs in ways that can be heard
2. Refocusing problems as shared difficulties, rather than one person carrying the burden for the entire family unit
3. Facilitating the reminiscence and recall of the parents' own adolescence
4. Refocusing on the marital relationship to defuse parent–child conflict
5. Helping the adolescent to modify and control responses to irritating situations
6. Modeling and facilitating the negotiation process as a way of defining and implementing limits[34]

The family is dealt with as a whole and dysfunction in any of the above areas is related to family processes rather than intrapsychic processes. It is assumed that as the family begins to relate in healthier ways, individual behavior will become more satisfying.

Group Therapy

Group therapy is particularly advantageous with adolescents because adolescents function well normally by role-taking in groups. Peer groups allow the adolescent to test behaviors by setting standards and making comparisons. For the adolescent struggling with issues of intimacy, a group setting for relationship building is less anxiety-provoking than a one-to-one relationship. For the psychotic adolescent, group therapy presents reality orientation.[95]

Two therapists of different sexes in group therapy can provide a corrective emotional experience for the adolescent who is reworking oedipal conflicts. Therapists of different sexes may also provide role models for the socially inept or withdrawn teenager. Co-leadership of adolescent groups may be necessary to manage behavioral acting-out and to reinforce limit-setting.

Adolescent group therapy may be called a "special problem group," which is a homogeneous group (all adolescents) whose purpose is to attack directly a problem of concern to all clients in the group. Homogeneous groups seem able to penetrate defenses more quickly. In homogeneous groups, members experience a greater feeling of being understood and accepted, which leads to group cohesion, rather than a sense of discrimination and isolation, which perpetuates defensiveness.[58]

Individual Therapy

Individual therapy may be the preferred mode of treatment if other modalities are not available, if the adolescent needs an intense relationship with a significant other to develop trust, or if the adolescent refuses to communicate in the presence of family members or group members. The particular focus of individual psychotherapy depends upon the assessed needs of the client and the theoretical framework and therapeutic skill of the therapist.

It is a therapeutic challenge to gain adolescents' trust and to motivate them to change. Therapists must demonstrate that symptomatic behavior is self-defeating. The majority of therapeutic approaches to adolescent psychopathology are directed toward psychic reintegration, not toward uncovering and resolving unconscious conflicts. This is a matter of emphasis, however, because often supportive or educative types of treatment also become involved with deeper layers of the personality.[45]

Psychotherapy with adolescents usually combines a dynamic focus on gaining self-understanding and a behavioral focus on symptom removal.[95] The goals of individual therapy with the adolescent include the following:

1. The development of a consistent sense of self
2. The ability to use foresight and to have fun
3. The wish to be with others and the capacity to be alone
4. Thinking that people are neither all likeable nor all unlikeable
5. Confidence in the ability to make choices, with some choices being wrong but not devastating[13]

The therapist provides the adolescent with an adult figure with rational authority and reliability. The choice of topics during therapy sessions is less important than the atmosphere in which the discussion occurs. Because the adolescent dreads to be insignificant, the therapist discusses meaningful, pertinent issues such as trust and competition, sex role satisfaction and responsibility, submissive dependence versus compulsive independence, worthlessness versus omnipotence and denial of abilities, and dedication to suffering.[13]

Behavior Modification

Because many adolescent clients with emotional disturbances are not at the intellectual stage of formal operations (*i.e.,* using logic and making abstractions) and because there is high energy and a propensity for acting-out at this age, it is often useful to plan an emphasis on behavior and observable events in therapy, rather than on inferred mental states and constructs. Studies have looked at the lasting efficacy of institutional behavior modification programs and uphold the notion of improvement in behavioral outcome measures and an increased level of independent living at 1 and 2 years post-discharge.[66]

Techniques of behavior modification that may be used with adolescents include systematic desensitization, positive reinforcement, extinction, rolemodeling, and role-playing. Many inpatient residential units for adolescents use a behavioral therapy philosophy. Tokens, or *reinforcers,* are given for certain behaviors and behaviors are tied to privileges the adolescent may earn. Expectations for positive behavior are clearly spelled out as well as consequences for maladaptive behavior. Movement through the treatment program with increasing levels of responsibility and freedom is not arbitrary, but it can be monitored and planned in relation to individual behaviors. Behavior modification programs are matter-of-fact; there is little emphasis on motivation or intent because consequences are based on well-defined behaviors and not on words or feelings. Manipulative behavior between client and staff tends to be decreased when expectations and outcomes are made known to everyone involved.

Therapeutic Milieu

Because residential care for adolescents takes them out of their usual developmental mainstream, the decision to place an adolescent in an institution is not taken lightly. When a decision is made to hospitalize an adolescent, an inpatient unit staff must pay particular attention to the effect of the milieu on a given client. Should adolescents be placed in an alladolescent unit or in a mixed adult–adolescent unit? Opinions vary, but it seems that successful treatment depends less on the mix of the patient population than on whether the unit includes staff who are particularly interested in and knowledgeable about adolescent problems.[95]

The milieu is the total context in which treatment occurs. The physical setting, the atmosphere generated by interpersonal exchanges, and the opportunities available to experience challenge and growth all become important therapeutic tools. Certain principles from milieu therapy and social learning theory explain why the milieu influences behavior.[72] These principles are as follows:

1. *The Law of Expectancy.* The frequency of a behavior depends on the expectation communicated while or before it occurs. For example, a nurse tells an agitated adolescent that she expects him to maintain control by going to his room to listen to music, rather than hitting a peer with whom he has argued.
2. *The Law of Involvement.* Acquiring or maintaining new or different behavior requires personal participation in challenges or crises. For example, the nurse guides a practice decisionmaking session with several adolescents on whether or not they will continue to live with a parent after discharge.
3. *The Law of Effect.* The frequency of behavior depends on the effects or consequences it produces. For example, visiting privileges are reduced for a patient because of sexual actingout behavior on the unit.
4. *The Law of Association by Contiguity.* Objects, actions, or environmental changes that occur simultaneously will come to be associated, function in similar ways, or mean the same thing. For example, the peer group praises an adolescent for assertive behavior, which both increases the adolescent's self-esteem and gives him a sense of belonging to the group.

When considering the effect of the milieu on adolescents, it is important to stretch out thinking to include nontraditional treatment approaches. One study specifically assessed mental health needs of adolescents and reached the conclusion that more out-reach and "off-beat" approaches are needed, such as a milieu in which alcohol abuse, employment problems, and emotional problems are treated simultaneously.[69] If combining services seems too unrealistic, then at least we might consider helping the adolescent to integrate the experience of having to deal with several different milieus. Perhaps that's what coping is all about.

Pharmacologic Treatment

Psychopharmacology in adolescents appears to be changing from a nonspecific modifier of behavior to a model of choosing medications with specific brain effects to treat specific diagnostic categories. Adolescent psychiatric disorders respond to medications in essentially the same way as those disorders in adults. Two important differences are that adolescents have a shorter mean half-life of most medications than do adults, so they may in some cases require a higher dosage than an adult, and that medication compliance may become a struggle around the issues of adolescent autonomy and independence.[79]

Studies in progress are investigating changes in adolescent body composition at puberty and the resulting effect on the volume of distribution of drugs as well as changes in organs (*e.g.*, the liver), on subsequent changes in drug metabolism, and on drug elimination. Hein has very detailed examples of pharmacologic principles for this age group.[37]

Women usually have twice as much fat per unit of body weight as men. Therefore, if a drug is distributed largely in body water, the dose for males may be higher than for females after puberty, but similar before puberty. If the drug is fat-soluble, mature females might require a higher dose than younger females or mature males. The more fat present in the body, the greater the amount of the drug distributed, particularly if the drug is highly lipid-soluble, such as anesthetics, marijuana, and imipramine.[37]

Symptomatic or asymptomatic hepatitis is a common disorder during adolescence. Regardless of etiology (drug related, viral, or toxic), hepatic dysfunction can impair drug metabolism and drug elimination. An unsuspecting teenager with hepatic dysfunction is at risk for acute behavioral changes or a change in level of consciousness if he combines illicit drugs with prescribed or over-the-counter drugs that are transformed by the liver.[37]

Tricyclics, usually imipramine, desipramine, amitriptyline, or nortriptyline, currently are often used for the treatment of adolescent major depression. For the first three antidepressants, doses range up to 5 mg/kg/day; for nortriptyline, the usual dose is 1–2 mg/kg/day in adolescents, titrated by plasma level.

A baseline EKG should always be obtained before treatment with a cyclic antidepressant, to rule out the possibility of a preexisting conduction defect. Continuing precautions with all tricyclic antidepressants are twofold: guarding against overdose and monitoring for development of cardiac conduction delays.[79]

Clinical reports indicate successful treatment of adolescent bipolar illness with lithium carbonate. Considering the dietary restrictions necessary and the possibility of use of street drugs (especially amphetamines and cocaine) that would be very dangerous in combination with MAO inhibitors, affective disorders in adolescents should be treated with means other than the monoamine oxidase (MAO) inhibitors.[79]

There are few, if any, controlled studies of the use of medications for anxiety disorders of adolescence. Initial research in this area suggests that imipramine or clomipramine may be useful for separation anxiety with school phobia and obsessive-compulsive disorder.[79]

Neuroleptics are effective medications for schizophrenia in adolescents, as with adults. Tardive dyskinesia is the most troubling of many possible adverse effects of neuroleptics because of its potential irreversibility. The nurse, along with the physician, should be alert to early manifestations of this side effect in the long-term care of adolescent-onset schizophrenia, as signs of tardive dyskinesia may occur after as little as 3 months of neuroleptic treatment.[79]

Therapeutic drug monitoring for drug concentration is useful under the following conditions:

1. It is clinically necessary for a client to remain within a therapeutic range
2. There is wide interindividual dose variation
3. There is impaired absorption or excretion
4. A medication is unexpectedly toxic or ineffective

Depending on the reason for measuring the level, a peak or trough level is obtained. Saliva levels rather than blood or plasma levels are useful with some drugs such as phenytoin.[37]

It is hoped that the number of medications with definable therapeutic ranges will increase in the coming decade, and that individual tailoring of medication regimens to teenagers will become a reality in the clinical, rather than the research, setting. Nurses will be called upon to document even more carefully each adolescent's response to medication in terms of target symptoms and side effects.[37]

Limit-Setting and Follow-Through

Too often, the term *limit-setting* brings to mind verbalizing a hard and fast rule. Instead it should mean a process of determining boundaries in a relationship. Setting limits can be understood as an indication of caring enough to bother with the other. This process becomes very important developmentally with the adolescent who is consolidating ego identity. Questions of "Where do I stand in your opinion?" and "What controls do I have?" become pivotal guides or limits to behavior in adolescence.

Limit-setting involves reaching consensus about consequences of behavior, verbalizing expectations clearly, and following through consistently with consequences. Limits to behavior must be geared to the abilities of the adolescent to perform those behaviors. For example, expecting an adolescent who is hallucinating to apologize for throwing lunch on the floor will not be as effective as removing her from the lunchroom.

Providing an opportunity to discuss limits and their implementation is another part of follow-through. Strict adherence to rules is not the prime objective in successful treatment on an inpatient unit.[99] The struggle around those rules forms the basis for problem-solving. We often call this struggle "testing." Adolescents may appear to regress and use maladaptive coping measures from past experience when they find themselves in a difficult situation. The process or struggle should be discussed with the adolescent to highlight the usefulness of conflict in forcing some kind of resolution. The nurse presents the possibility of healthier resolution of difficult conflict situations. Reviewing and analyzing how limits are set and why they are broken helps the adolescent understand more about functioning as an adult in the world.

Communication with Adolescents

"But you don't understand!" is such a common statement associated with the adolescent that one may decide adolescents are impossible to understand. Do not, however, allow the adolescent to stop communication with you by his defensive posture. A response to such a statement is, "I would like to understand." Communicating with adolescents entails first listening, then clarifying, restating, and giving nonjudgmental responses.[1]

The nurse working with the adolescent must be able to tolerate ambiguity. The adolescent may not know what to say before he says it, and then it may not "come out right." After all, the adolescent is in the process of consolidation, not closure. It is critical that mental health caregivers show the adolescent that they respect any effort at dialogue.

Both verbal and nonverbal skills are important in communication with the adolescent. For example, attentiveness, smiling, lifting the arm in a "well-done"

sign, and hugging are positive warm gestures the nurse may use with adolescents. The nurse must anticipate and understand the adolescent's unconventional language and profanity and then strike a balance between using words familiar to the adolescent and appearing phony or ridiculous by overuse of teenage slang.[91]

The nurse should also expect resistance to her efforts at communication. A young nurse may be viewed as a "sell-out to the establishment" and an older nurse may appear too parental or authoritarian. In either case, trust is difficult to establish. The adolescent's familiar role may be a negative image, so tolerating good feelings from staff or accepting kindness involves a huge and difficult change.

Any pretense of unauthentic emotion with an adolescent client is doomed to failure. The nurse should develop qualities of honesty and a sense of humor as well as the ability to say, "I am angry when...," "I am concerned when...," "I am disappointed when...," to describe the nurse's real feelings in a given situation.

Evaluation

Evaluation of the adolescent's progress toward attaining specific behavioral outcomes as a result of nursing interventions is not a difficult step in the nursing process if the outcomes were clearly stated at the start of treatment. Adolescent progress often involves movement of "one step forward and two steps back"; therefore, stating outcomes in small increments, rather than major changes, aids in evaluating the adolescent's progress.

If all outcomes have been reached, the adolescent should be discharged from treatment. If some of the behavioral outcomes have been reached, the nursing process begins again with another assessment of needs. Nurse and adolescent may decide to continue to pursue the remainder of the original behavioral outcomes, to set new behavioral outcomes, to change or alter interventions, or to lengthen or shorten the time period until the next evaluation. The adolescent's participation and cooperation in all stages of the nursing process are significant in promoting his separation from parental figures and his eventual assumption of responsibility for meeting his own health needs.

In addition to the evaluation of individual behavioral outcomes for a given client, the nurse may participate in or design treatment outcomes studies for entire programs. For example, there have been few systematic attempts to determine which treatment environments, program conditions, or treatment methods are most effective in treating adolescent

CHART 29-3
Therapeutic Dialogue

Interacting with an Adolescent

The following therapeutic dialogue is a portion of the third session between a nurse and Lara, a 14-year-old middle child.

Lara: I couldn't wait to get here today because something awful happened last week. You know how you told me to write things down that were important to me so that I could make the best use of my hour with you?...well, this one I will always remember! I debated a lot about whether I should say anything because it makes my Mom sound terrible, and I don't know whether to be mad or sad, or maybe it's no big thing.

Nurse: You've been really struggling. Let's take a look at it.

Lara: She's a liar.

Nurse: Your Mom?

Lara: Yeah.

Nurse: And that's heavy for you.

Lara: Who wants to think her mother is a big phony? (voice louder)

Nurse: Give me some of the particulars and let's see how you came to that conclusion.

Lara: I went into her drawer to borrow some nylons and found some joints under all her stuff. I mean, my own mother smokes. How can she stand there and tell us not to? Why didn't she tell me? Why couldn't she be honest? She's always wanting me to talk to her, but she never talks to me.

Nurse: Something was hidden from you and you consider that dishonest, even a lie.

Lara: I guess she couldn't come right out and say, "I like grass." I mean, I've never seen her high or anything.

Nurse: So your first reaction was to think she's a liar, but you can understand why a parent might not tell her kid everything she does.

Lara: Yeh, like I don't tell her everything I do. (smiles)

Nurse: You'd like to be close and want to talk to her, but not tell her everything. What else about the joints bothers you?

Lara: She shouldn't be doing it.

Nurse: You've said "should" and "shouldn't" a couple of times today.

Lara: Well, she shouldn't. It's against the law.

Nurse: And why might someone break the law?

Lara: They don't think they'll get caught.

Nurse: What else?

Lara: They think the law is wrong.

Nurse: What else?

Lara: I don't know.

Nurse: I don't know either. We're just speculating. Maybe they're not thinking about the law at the time. Or maybe it's fun to take a risk. People are pretty complicated. Using the words "should" and "shouldn't" can shut our minds to how complex people and relationships are.

Lara: But you're taught since you were a little kid that there are things you should and shouldn't do.

Nurse: And part of growing up is looking at those "shoulds" and "shouldn'ts" and deciding which are valid and important in your life.

Lara: Breaking the law is breaking the law.

Nurse: Yes, laws give us security by providing limits. We also get security from our parents, but now your security is shaken because you don't see Mom as quite so perfect.

Lara: I thought you would tell me to go talk to my mother about the whole thing.

Nurse: You decided what I would say before you came to see me?

Lara: Yeah. These sessions never go like I think they're going to beforehand.

Nurse: You plan to direct them more or to have more control?

Lara: I'd like to!

Nurse: That's something to learn about yourself.

Discussion

When an adolescent brings up conflicts with others, it is so easy to focus on the motives of the other or to defend or attack particular actions in the situation. This nurse never addresses whether it is right or wrong for Mother to smoke marijuana or whether in fact, Mother does! Instead, the nurse keeps the focus on the patient, her struggle as she is disappointed or surprised by others, and the issues of trust and control, which are developmental issues of adolescence. When the nurse asks the client why people might break laws, she is not focusing on others. She is asking the adolescent to reach beyond quick and simple answers in order to expand the adolescent's understanding of others.

As Lara begins this session, she repeats some things the nurse has said previously, indicating that there is some kind of positive relationship developing between nurse and client. Knowing that Lara feels support in the relationship, the nurse can prod Lara later in the interview to consider alternatives and to listen to the nurse's hypothesis regarding insecurity.

At first, Lara catastrophizes with words like "awful" and "terrible." The nurse recognizes the pain involved and invites Lara to continue in a steady, matter-of-fact way ("let's take a look"). When Lara calls her mother a liar and a phony, the nurse ignores the labels. The nurse continues to use language comfortable for the nurse, but not technical jargon or theoretical interpretations. Because the client is operating at a feeling level by calling her mother names, the nurse now gives her an opening to analyze her thinking in order to see how her thinking and feelings are connected. Making the connections won't occur in one session.

When Lara talks about the issues of trust with Mother and the unequal sharing between parent and child, the nurse knows these are parallel issues in nurse–client relationships. The nurse plans to use this example in later sessions to look at Lara's feelings for the nurse. Such interventions should be carefully planned, and will be timed differently by different therapists.

One of the growth tasks of adolescence is moving from the safety of rigid rules to judging circumstances and then choosing actions. Lara at times retreats to black-and-white simplifications; at other times, she is capable of tossing ideas back and forth with the nurse. The nurse gently coaxes Lara to expand her thinking, knowing that she will have more options available to her as an adult if she can see more possibilities in situations.

Adolescents often feel impotent in the real world. Lara opens up this issue when she talks of planning the sessions beforehand. Instead of engaging in a power struggle at this point, or becoming defensive, the nurse simply acknowledges Lara's statement and invites Lara to learn about the need she may have to control. The nurse respects Lara and does not pretend to have magic answers.

Questions

1. How might the nurse have begun if the client was less verbal, entered the session tearfully, sullen, or frightened?
2. This nurse focuses on cognitive aspects; for example, how the client decides things, how she uses "should" and "shouldn't" to guide her thinking in a rather narrow way. Where in the interview could the nurse have focused more on feelings? On behaviors?
3. As additional reading, review Alfred Adler's theory on birth order. How might Lara's middle position in her family have influenced her views on fairness and closeness?
4. What are Lara's strengths that the nurse uses in working with her?

drug abusers. Data from the few existing studies indicate that social skills training may be effective in treating institutionalized adolescent substance abusers and that, in spite of increased involvement in productive activities after treatment, adolescents continue to use alcohol and marijuana at pretreatment levels.[8]

The Nurse's Feelings

Whenever impulsiveness, emotional lability, and other issues of self-control are paramount in a treatment setting, nurses need to heighten their vigilance in regard to their own feelings. The nurse may become impatient with the adolescent who is particularly slow to complete growth tasks. Adolescent conflicts within the nurse may be tapped or reawakened. The nurse may unconsciously encourage acting-out by the adolescent because of identification with him and the vicarious satisfaction that defense brings.

Another type of identification is with the parents. The adolescent client often tries to recreate the home situation using staff in parent roles. In this case, the adolescent may expect adults to reject or abandon him and may attempt to set up a situation in which staff will fulfill his negative expectations.

The nurse may become frightened of the adolescent with tenuous self-control. The nurse who is not secure in his or her own sexual identity may pro-

Case Study 29-1

Outpatient Treatment for an 18-Year-Old Male Client

When Bob M. came home tearfully from college after only 6 weeks, he reluctantly agreed to see a nurse therapist. He felt lost, alone, and confused. His mother accompanied him to his first appointment and explained that Bob was very much like her and was a "homebody." Bob did agree to see the nurse therapist on his own for a series of appointments.

Bob's family history revealed two professional parents and one older sister who had run away from home at age 15 to marry "beneath her social class." Parents had "disowned" the older sister for 1 year and then had begun to speak to her again and to give her gifts and money. Bob idealizes his mother and believes that he is like her. He respects his father but believes that he cannot live up to the standards his father sets; he can never be "good enough" in his father's eyes.

Bob had entered a small college in another state to please his parents. A marginal student, he enjoyed sports but found that neither academics nor sports could help him over his panic at being away from home. He didn't feel he belonged in college.

Bob had one or two dates in high school with girls but was shy and uncomfortable around them. He felt quite at ease with males. He felt some pressure to be dating from his parents, who tried on a few occasions to arrange dates with daughters of their friends.

When the nurse therapist first saw Bob individually, Bob had a depressed affect. He described himself as "lazy," with his days spent watching TV or "goofing around with friends." He thought he might enroll in a local community college the next semester to overcome his guilt at "disappointing everybody." He was ambivalent about wanting to continue living at home.

The nurse therapist set the following treatment goals with Bob:

1. To separate from parents by moving to an apartment by himself or with friends
2. To become aware of his own needs as different from the needs of others by deciding on school enrollment
3. To decrease feelings of depression and guilt as reflected in an increased number of positive statements made about himself
4. To take responsibility for his own feelings and behavior through a process of rational decision-making rather than impulsive actions

During 18 months of individual therapy, Bob made progress and had setbacks. He enrolled once again in college, but did not complete the semester due to his inability to discipline himself to attend classes and study. He dated females once or twice, but continued to prefer the company of his group of male friends. He went on a trip to the beach with the group and on a ski trip, both of which he enjoyed. These trips did cause conflict with his parents, who reluctantly paid his way. His parents later insisted that he move out of the house and support himself, at which point he found a job at a carwash and moved into an apartment with a friend.

Bob terminated therapy 3 months after his parents stopped paying for his sessions because "my budget is too tight." He felt a sense of accomplishment that he had remained on his own for 6 months and he was thinking of ways he could get into a small business with a chance for advancement. Bob felt positive about his gains in thinking through conflicts rather than running away from his painful emotions. He was starting to verbalize awareness of his similarities and differences from parents and to feel more confident in his own decisions, regardless of whether or not he had parental approval for those decisions.

Questions for Discussion

1. Discuss the interaction of maturational and situational crises in Bob's life.
2. Which etiologic variables of adolescent disturbance help explain Bob's feelings and behavior?
3. How do the issues of separation, sexuality, and responsibility enter into Bob's treatment plan? Are there other important issues?
4. Would you have set the same treatment goals with Bob as the nurse therapist did? Explain your rationale.
5. Describe specific interventions that might have been used at various stages of Bob's therapy (*e.g.*, communication techniques or behavioral techniques) to accomplish treatment goals.
6. What qualities would the nurse therapist need to engage successfully Bob in a therapeutic relationship?

ject that insecurity by overreacting to situations or by not providing limits when an adolescent is testing with sexual behavior. It is hard to be on the receiving end of a barrage of hostile remarks, and the nurse may feel like retaliating against the belligerent adolescent.

The examples of many feelings destructive to therapeutic relationships with adolescents may be discouraging. There are, however, just as many instances of positive feelings.

Nurses who are considering working with this age group should carefully examine memories of their own adolescence. It might even be helpful to evaluate to what extent each of the adolescent growth tasks were completed by the nurse. The nurse's own self-awareness, by whatever means attained, is the best way to avoid being caught off guard emotionally or intellectually when interacting with adolescents. Nurses who can be honest with themselves are most likely to be honest with clients.

Positive expectations must also be emphasized in working with adolescents. Adolescents want to be accepted, loved, and understood. If the nurse clarifies which behaviors are likely to lead to satisfying relationships and increased self-esteem, the adolescent can choose whether or not to try out the new behaviors. On the other hand, the adolescent who meets only criticism may have a decided poverty of ideas regarding any other way to behave. The adolescent's message to the nurse caregiver may well be, "Do not lead, I may not follow; do not push, I may give up; walk beside and help me discover my way."

Summary

This chapter has introduced some of the parameters of normal adolescent development. Several theories providing frameworks for understanding adolescent disturbance have been presented. Some of the major foci of the chapter have included the following:

1. The adolescent undergoes marked physical change with individual differences within each sex almost as great as the differences between the sexes.
2. Sexual development proceeds by role-taking, which progresses toward sexual intimacy.
3. Emotional development includes defining or refining the self.
4. Mental development consolidates in the intellectual stage of formal operations for many adolescents.
5. The incidence of adolescent emotional disorders is difficult to identify because of varying diagnostic biases.
6. Etiologic theories of adolescent disturbance

examine the variables of family communication, child-rearing style, personality, social pressures, and the sense of isolation.
7. In the assessment phase of the nursing process, the nurse gathers data about the adolescent's sense of identity, independence/dependence, self-image, strengths and talents, impulsivity, support systems, and sexuality.
8. In the nursing diagnosis phase, the nurse analyzes and categorizes client data and formulates nursing diagnoses.
9. In the planning stage, the nurse includes the adolescent and, ideally, his family in decisions regarding outcomes of treatment based on assessed needs.
10. Various intervention strategies for working with disturbed adolescents may include family, group, individual, and milieu therapies, as well as behavior modification, psychopharmacology, limit-setting, and communication skills.
11. The result of the evaluation phase may be to decide that the adolescent is ready for discharge from treatment or to decide to restart the nursing process with a fresh assessment of needs.
12. Working with adolescents is exciting and demanding and requires a firm awareness of self and a willingness to confront issues such as identification, separation, sexuality, and self-control.

References

1. Adams JF: Understanding Adolescence: Current Developments in Adolescent Psychology, 4th ed. Boston, Allyn & Bacon, 1980
2. Admini F, Salasnek S, Burke EL: Adolescent Drug Abuse: Etiological and Treatment Considerations. Adolescence 11, 281–299, 1976
3. Baumrind D: What Research Is Teaching Us about the Differences Between Authoritative and Authoritarian Child-Rearing Styles. In Hamacheck DE (ed): Human Dynamics in Psychology and Education, 3d ed. Boston, Allyn & Bacon, 1977
4. Bayh B: Runaway Youth. Washington, DC, US Government Printing Office, 1973
5. Beck AT: Depression: Causes and Treatment. Philadelphia, University of Pennsylvania Press, 1970
6. Beck AT: The Development of Depression: A Cognitive Model. In Friedman RJ, Katz MM (eds): The Psychology of Depression. Washington, DC, Winston, 1974
7. Becker WC: Consequences of Different Kinds of Parental Discipline. In Hoffman ML, Hoffman LW (eds): Review of Child Development Research. Vol. 1. New York, Russell Sage Foundation, 1964

8. Beschner GM, Friedman AS: Treatment of Adolescent Drug Abusers. International Journal of the Addictions 20, 971–993, 1985

9. Braucht G: Psychosocial Typology of Adolescent Alcohol and Drug Users. In Proceedings of the Third Annual Alcoholism Conference of the National Institute on Alcohol Abuse & Alcoholism. Washington, DC, US Department of Health, Education, and Welfare, 1974

10. Brook JS, Lukoff IF, Whiteman MM: Peer, Family and Personality Domains as Related to Adolescents' Drug Behavior. Psychol Rep 41, 1095–1102, 1977

11. Bruch H: Psychological Antecedents of Anorexia Nervosa. In Vigersky RA (ed): Anorexia Nervosa. New York, Raven Press, 1977

12. Bruch H: The Golden Cage: The Enigma of Anorexia Nervosa. Cambridge, MA, Harvard University Press, 1978

13. Bryt A: Modifications of Psychoanalysis in the Treatment of Adolescents. In Masserman JH (ed): Adolescence, Dreams and Training, Science and Psychoanalysis, Vol IX, pp 81–88. New York, Grune & Stratton, 1966

14. Burton CA: Juvenile Street Gangs: Predators and Children. In Dacey JH (ed): Adolescents Today. Santa Monica, Goodyear Publishing, 1979

15. Carroll JW: Transcendence and Mystery in the Counter-Culture. Religion in Life 42, 361–375, 1973

16. Coche E, Thomas AT: Evaluative Research on a Therapeutic Community for Adolescents. J Youth Adolesc 4, 321–330, 1975

17. Conger JJ: Adolescence and Youth, 2d ed. New York, Harper and Row, 1977

18. Crisp AH et al: The Long-Term Progosis in Anorexia Nervosa: Some Factors Predictive of Outcome. In Vigersky RA (ed): Anorexia Nervosa. New York, Raven Press, 1977

19. Cross HJ, Kleinhesselink RR: Psychological Perspectives on Drugs and Youth. In Adams JF (ed): Understanding Adolescence: Current Developments in Adolescent Psychology, 4th ed, pp 363–382. Boston, Allyn & Bacon, 1980

20. Deykin EY, Levy JC, Wells V: Adolescent Depression: Alcohol and drug abuse. Am J Public Health 77 (2): 178–182, 1987

21. Dornbusch SM et al: Single Parents, Extended Households, and the Control of Adolescents. Child Dev 56 (2): 326–341, 1985

22. Eichorn DH: Biological Development. In Adams JF (ed): Understanding Adolescence: Current Developments in Adolescent Psychology. 4th ed, pp 56–73. Boston, Allyn & Bacon, 1980

23. Elkind D: Egocentrism in Adolescence. Child Dev 38, 1025–1034, 1967

24. Encyclopedia of Sociology. Guilford, CT, Dushkin Publishing Group, 1974

25. Fairchild HP (ed): Dictionary of Sociology. Ames, IA, Iowa State University Press, 1955

26. Finkel ML, Finkel DJ: Sexual and Contraceptive Knowledge, Attitudes, and Behavior of Male Adolescents. Fam Plan Perspect 7, 256–260, 1975

27. Forslund MA, Gustafson TJ: Influence of Peers and Parents and Sex Differences in Drinking Behavior by High School Students. Quarterly J Studies in Alcoholism 31, 868–875, 1970

28. Frances A, Clarkin JF: Considering Family versus Other Therapies after a Teenager's Suicide Attempt. Hosp Community Psychiatry 36 (10): 1041–1042, 1985

29. Freud A: The Ego and the Mechanisms of Defense, rev ed. New York, International Universities Press, 1966

30. Friedman A: Therapy with Families of Sexually Acting-Out Girls. New York, Springer Publishing, 1971

31. Ginsburg H, Opper S: Piaget's Theory of Intellectual Development, 2d ed. Englewood Cliffs, NJ, Prentice-Hall, 1979

32. Gordon S, Dickman IR: Sex Education: The Parent's Role. Public Affairs Pamphlet No. 549. New York, Public Affairs Committee, 1977

33. Green MR: The Problem of Identity Crisis. In Masserman JH (ed): Adolescence, Dreams and Training, Science and Psychoanalysis, Vol IX, pp 74–75. New York, Grune & Stratton, 1966

34. Haber J et al: Comprehensive Psychiatric Nursing, 2d ed. New York, McGraw-Hill, 1982

35. Halni K et al: Pretreatment Evaluation in Anorexia Nervosa. In Vigersky RA (ed): Anorexia Nervosa. New York, Raven Press, 1977

36. Hamachek DE: Psychology and Development of the Adolescent Self. In Adams JF (ed): Understanding Adolescence: Current Developments in Adolescent Psychology, 4th ed, pp 81–91. Boston, Allyn & Bacon, 1980

37. Hein K: The Use of Therapeutics in Adolescence. J Adol Health Care 8, 1, 8–35, 1987

38. Huba GJ, Wingard J, Bentler PM: Beginning Adolescent Drug Use and Peer and Adult Interaction Patterns. J Consult Clin Psychol 47, 265–276, 1979

39. Huston-Stein A, Welch RL: Sex Role Development and the Adolescent. In Adams JF (ed): Understanding Adolescence: Current Developments in Adolescent Psychology, 4th ed, pp 230–289. Boston: Allyn & Bacon, 1980

40. Jessor R, Jessor S: Adolescent Development and the Onset of Drinking. J Studies of Alcoholism 36, 27–51, 1975

41. Johnson BD: Marijuana Users & Drug Subcultures. New York, John Wiley & Sons, 1973

42. Johnston LD, O'Malley PM, Bachman JG: Psychotherapeutic, Licit, and Illicit Use of Drugs among Adolescents: An Epidemiological Perspective. J Adol Health Care 8, 1, 36–51, 1987

43. Jones SL: Family Therapy: A Comparison of Approaches. Bowie, MD, Robert J. Brady, 1980

44. Kandel DB, Kessler RC, Margulies RZ: Antecedents

of Adolescent Initiation into Stages of Drug Use: A Developmental Analysis. J Youth and Adolescence 7, 13–40, 1978

45. Kaplan HI, Sadock BJ: Modern Synopsis of Comprehensive Textbook of Psychiatry/III, 3d ed. Baltimore, Williams & Wilkins, 1981

46. Kay EJ et al: A Longitudinal Study of Personality Correlates of Marijuana Use. J Consult Clin Psychol 46, 470–477, 1977

47. Klein MW: Street Gangs & Street Workers. Englewood Cliffs, NJ: Prentice-Hall, 1971

48. Kohlberg L, Gilligan C: The Adolescent as a Philosopher: The Discovery of the Self in a Post-Conventional World. Daedalus 100 (Fall): 1051–1086, 1971

49. Krone MD et al: Social Disaffection, Friendship Patterns and Adolescent Cigarette Use: The Muscatine Study. J Sch Health 56, 4, 146–150, 1986

50. Kurz S: Teenage Prostitutes. Equal Times (Nov. 13):6, 1977

51. Laufer M: Adolescence and Psychosis. Int J Psychoanal 67, 3, 367–372, 1986

52. Lewinsohn PM: Clinical and Theoretical Aspects of Depression. In Calhoun KS, Adams HE, Mitchell KM (eds): Innovative Treatment Methods in Psychopathology. New York, John Wiley & Sons, 1974

53. Lewinsohn PM: A Behavioral Approach to Depression. In Friedman RJ, Katz MM (eds): The Psychology of Depression. Washington, DC, Winston, 1974

54. Lordi WM: Hospital and Residential Treatment of Adolescents. In Novello JR (ed): The Short Course in Adolescent Psychiatry. New York, Brunner/Mazel, 1979

55. Lustick MJ: Bulimia in Adolescents: A Review. Pediatrics 76, 4 (Pt 2):685–690, 1985

56. McCandless BR: Adolescents: Behavior and Development. Hinsdale, IL, Dryden Press, 1970

57. McCoy K: Coping With Teenage Depression: A Parent's Guide. New York, New American Library, 1982

58. Marram GD: The Group Approach in Nursing Practice, 2d ed. St. Louis, CV Mosby, 1978

59. Masterson JF: The Symptomatic Adolescent 5 Years Later: He Didn't Grow Out of It. Am J Psychiatry 123, 1338–1345, 1967

60. Mattheis RF: Holistic Health Concepts. In Haber J et al (eds): Comprehensive Psychiatric Nursing, 2d ed, pp 76–136. New York, McGraw-Hill, 1982

61. Meissner WW: Adolescent Paranoia: Transference and Countertransference Issues. Adolesc Psychiatry 12, 478–508, 1985

62. Mercer RT: Perspectives on Adolescent Health Care. Philadelphia, JB Lippincott, 1979

63. Miller D: Adolescence. New York, Jason Aronson, 1974

64. Minuchin S, Rosman B, Baker L: Psychosomatic Families. Cambridge, MA, Harvard University Press, 1978

65. Moore DC (ed): Adolescence and Stress. Report of NIMH Conference, US Department of Health and Human Services, PH Service, 1981

66. Moyes T et al: Long-term Follow-up Study of a Ward-based Behaviour Modification Programme for Adolescents with Acting-out and Conduct Problems. Br J Psychiatry 147, 300–305, 1985

67. Niven RG: Adolescent Drug Abuse. Hosp Community Psychiatry 37, 6, 596–607, 1986

68. Norton AH: Evaluation of a Psychiatric Service for Children, Adolescents and Adults. Am J Psychiatry 123, 1418–1424, 1967

69. Nuttall EV, Nuttall RL, Polit D, Clark K: Assessing Adolescent Mental Health Needs: The Views of Consumers, Providers, and Others. Adolescence 12 (Summer): 277–285, 1977

70. Pasquali EA et al: Mental Health Nursing: A Bio-Psycho-Cultural Approach. St. Louis, CV Mosby, 1981

71. Population Reports, Series J. Washington, DC, George Washington University Medical Center. No 14 (March), 1977

72. Rhoades LJ: Treating and Assessing the Chronically Mentally Ill: The Pioneering Research of Gordon L. Paul. NIMH Science Reports, Department of Health and Human Services (ADM): 81–1100, 1981

73. Robbins T, Anthony D, Curtis T: Youth Culture Religious Movements: Evaluating and Integrative Hypothesis. Sociol Rev 16, 48–64, 1975

74. Rogers D: Issues in Adolescent Psychology, 3d ed. Englewood Cliffs, NJ, Prentice-Hall, 1977

75. Rosen BM et al: Adolescent Patients Served in Outpatient Clinics. Am J Pub Health 55, 1563–1577, 1965

76. Rosman BL et al: A Family Approach to Anorexia Nervosa: Study, Treatment, and Outcome. In Vigersky RA (ed): Anorexia Nervosa. New York, Raven Press, 1977

77. Rubin R: Attainment of the Maternal Role. Nurs Res 16, 237–245, 1967

78. Rubins JL: The Self-Idealizing and Self-Alienating Process During Late Adolescence. Am J Psychoanal 25, 27–37, 1965

79. Ryan ND, Puig-Antich J: Pharmacological Treatment of Adolescent Psychiatric Disorders. Journal of Adolescent Psychiatric Disorders 8, 1, 137–142, 1987

80. Sedgwick RA: Family Mental Health, Theory and Practice. St. Louis, CV Mosby, 1981

81. Seligman MEP: Depression and Learned Helplessness. In Friedman RJ, Katz MM (eds): The Psychology of Depression. Washington, DC, Winston, 1974

82. Seligman MEP: Helplessness: On Depression, Development, and Death. San Francisco, WH Freeman, 1975

83. Shapiro RL: Identity and Ego Autonomy in Adolescence. In Masserman JH (ed): Adolescence, Dreams, and Training, Science and Psychoanalysis,

Vol IX, pp 18–23. New York, Grune & Stratton, 1966

84. Smiley WC: Classification and Delinquency: A Review. Behavioral Disorders 2, 184–200, 1977

85. Smith GM, Fogg CP: Teenage Drug Use: A Search for Causes and Consequences. Personality & Social Psychology Bulletin 1, 426–429, 1974

86. Sorosky AD: The Psychological Effects of Divorce on Adolescents. Adolescence 12 (Spring): 123–136, 1977

87. Spanier GB: Sexualization and Premarital Sexual Behavior. In Rogers D (ed): Issues in Adolescent Psychology, 3d ed, pp 240–241. Englewood Cliffs, NJ: Prentice-Hall, 1977

88. Stein AH, Freidrich LK: The Impact of Television on Children and Youth. In Hetherington EM, Hagen JW, Kron R, Stein AH (eds): Review of Child Development Research, Vol 5. Chicago, University of Chicago Press, 1975

89. Strasburger VC: Sex, Drugs, Rock 'n' Roll: Are Solutions Possible? A Commentary. Pediatrics 76, 4 (Pt 2): 704–712, 1985

90. Swift P: Inner City Teens. Parade (September 18): 5, 1977

91. Valente S: The Suicidal Teenager. Nursing 85, (Dec): 47–49, 1985

92. Wagner CA: Adolescent Sexuality. In Adams JF (ed): Understanding Adolescence: Current Developments in Adolescent Psychology, 4th ed, pp 267–301. Boston, Allyn & Bacon, 1980

93. Weiner IB: Psychological Disturbances in Adolescence. New York, Wiley-Interscience, 1970

94. Weiner IB: Juvenile Delinquency. Pediatr Clin North Am 22, 673–684, 1975

95. Weiner IB: Child and Adolescent Psychopathology. New York, John Wiley & Sons, 1982

96. Weiner IB, Del Gaudio AC: Psychopathology in Adolescence: An Epidemiological Study. Arch Gen Psychiatry 33, 187–193, 1976

97. Whaley AL: Cognitive Processes in Adolescent Drug Use: The Role of Positivity Bias and Implications for Prevention Policy. Int J Addict 21, (3): 393–398, 1986

98. Wieder H, Kaplan EH: Drug Use in Adolescents. Psychoanal Study Child 24, 399–431, 1969

99. Wilson HS, Kneisl CR: Psychiatric Nursing. Menlo Park, CA, Addison-Wesley Publishing Co, 1979

100. Wolman BB (ed): Dictionary of Behavioral Science. New York, Von Nostrand, 1973

30

Mental Retardation

Peggy J. Drapo

Like the surprise and wonder of finding the sky, revolution can't be planned. It happens when you least expect it. Its clerics are not bigger than life but humble and simple souls. Like the person next to you. Revolution is a Rosa Parks, who decides one day not to ride in the back of the bus. Or a navy nurse named Mrs. Nelson, who suddenly refuses to let her children be condemned to a label.

Ron Jones,
The Acorn People,
1976

Chapter Preview

This chapter focuses on the definitions, causes, and descriptions of retardation. The many causes and manifestations of mental retardation lead to misunderstanding and often to poorly planned care of the retarded.

The chapter defines mental retardation, discusses the varied aspects of daily living and its problems for the person who is retarded, and explains the application of the nursing process to the care of the retarded. It is hoped that a greater awareness of the causes of mental retardation will strengthen the nurse's interest in preventive efforts.

No one chapter in any book can teach all there is to know about mental retardation; it is a nursing specialty in its own right. Another aim of the chapter, therefore, is to stimulate nursing interest in the field so that we may become instrumental in demystifying the problems of mental retardation for the general public.

Learning Objectives

On completion of the chapter, you should be able to accomplish the following:

1. define mental retardation
2. identify levels of mental retardation as described by Stanford-Binet, Cattell, and Wechsler
3. discuss the incidence of and significant issues related to mental retardation
4. identify the leading causes of mental retardation
5. discuss the effects of the birth of a child with a mental or physical disorder on family relationships
6. apply the nursing process to the care of a child or adult who is retarded

    assess the biologic, sociologic, and psychological functioning of the retarded client

    identify nursing interventions to assist the client to achieve goals

    formulate plans to reduce the prenatal, perinatal, and postnatal risks of retardation

    design a care plan for a mentally retarded child or adult

    design a care plan for an emotionally disturbed retarded client

    evaluate the effectiveness of nursing intervention with the retarded client

7. recognize the role of the nurse advocate in the care of clients with mental retardation and related physical disabilities

Defining Mental Retardation

Mental retardation is defined by the American Association of Mental Retardation (AAMR) (formerly The American Association of Mental Deficiency [AAMD]) as a significantly subaverage general intellectual functioning existing concurrently with deficits in adaptive behavior manifesting itself during the developmental period.[22] This definition refers to an intelligence quotient, or IQ, two or more standard deviations from the mean average (100) for the population tested. Therefore, two standard deviations below the score would be an IQ of 70 or below. Two standard deviations above the score would be considered IQ ranges for the gifted.

Educators and scientists have not all agreed with the AAMR definition of subaverage intelligence because they feel the upper limit of 70 excludes from special education and other services some persons who would benefit from such programs. Many states use a cutoff score of 75.[16] The 1983 definition of the AAMR, while it continues to define significant subaverage intelligence as an IQ below 70, also emphasizes that the upper limit may be extended to 75 or beyond, depending on a variety of tests and individual characteristics, especially in school settings. The nurse should be aware that there may be some disagreements between professionals and states. This is significant because it poses a problem for families who are seeking services or who move from one state to another.

Mental retardation is actually a constellation of symptoms, rather than a disease, although it may result from a disease. Terms used in the descriptions of mental retardation are often confusing. Subaverage intellectual functioning, according to the AAMR, means that the client's performance on objective testing is below that expected for his chronological age. Adaptive behavior refers to the maturation, learning, personal independence, and social adjustment of the client. Maturation is the period of development from conception to 18 years.[3] This definition distinguishes mental retardation from other behavior disorders that may occur after the developmental period.

Classification of Mental Retardation

Labeling is a difficult and serious responsibility in the field of mental retardation. Systems of labeling vary, and the danger in attaching labels is that they may affect the care, treatment, and education of retarded persons. Parameters for classification should take into consideration the complex other factors that often surround the diagnosis of mental retardation. These include symptom severity, symptom etiology, syndrome description, adaptive behavior, educability expectations, and behavioral manifestations.[3]

The accepted classification is the use of the labels *mild, moderate, severe,* and *profound,* rather than old terms of *borderline, moron, imbecile,* and *idiot.* Depending on the test used, the symptom severity may vary slightly. The scoring accepted by the AAMD places the mildly retarded person in the IQ range of 69 to 55; the moderately or trainable person in the 54 to 40 category; the severely retarded in the IQ range of 39 to 25; and the profoundly retarded at less than 25.[9]

Controversy arises in issues related to educational placement of minority individuals who are poor achievers and disadvantaged. Here labeling takes on a negative connotation, as a disproportionate number of these children are in classes for the mildly retarded.[3]

Testing

The standard tests usually employed during childhood are the Stanford-Binet and the Wechsler Intelligence Scale for Children. During the first 3 years, the Cattell, Gesell, and Bayley tests are most often used. The latter three tests are reliable determinants of the child's developmental quotient and are rather accurate predictors of future problems with mental retardation.

According to Stanford-Binet and Cattell, levels of intellectual functioning are as follows:

Mild	68–52
Moderate	51–36
Severe	35–20
Profound	19 and below

The standard deviation for this test is 16.

The Wechsler scale has a standard deviation of 15 and the following levels of intellectual functioning:

Mild	69–55
Moderate	54–40
Severe	39–25
Profound	24 and below

Tests are set up to evaluate certain skills. The Wechsler Intelligence Scale for Children (WISC), for instance, uses subtests that cover verbal skills of general information, general comprehension, arithmetic, similarities, vocabulary, and digit span. Performance is tested by picture completion, picture arrangement, block design, object assembly, coding, and mazes. Performances on tests are compared to average abilities of persons at different chronological ages. The Stanford-Binet uses various tests to measure a wide range of abilities closely associated with various mental ages.[36]

The figures or numbers in IQ ranges do not mean a great deal unless you know that mildly retarded individuals may be able to learn academic skills up to sixth-grade level during school years and are capable of social and vocational adequacy in adulthood if given opportunities and instruction. Moderately retarded persons generally can learn the basics of self-care in childhood, functional academic skills to grade-school level during school years, and, as adults, may be able to accomplish a semiskilled occupation. The severely retarded need controlled environments in which, by adulthood, they are able to learn the skills of communication, self-protection, health habits, and sheltered workshop vocations. The profoundly retarded usually need complete care and supervision during all of their lives, but may exhibit some motor and speech development.[43]

Incidence and Significance of the Problem

The incidence of mental retardation in the United States is thought to be approximately 3% of the population or about 6½ million persons; however, these figures are theoretical and other authors suggest that the incidence and prevalence of mental retardation may change with the accumulation of data or with changing definitions. Until it is feasible to collect more data, the most quoted and accepted figure is 3% of the population.[3]

Two very distinct groups are labeled mentally retarded. The first is the relatively mildly impaired who are physically normal in appearance, who come from lower socioeconomic backgrounds, and who may have other family members that are so affected. The second is the severely impaired whose appearance is different from that of other family members. Those in the latter group are found at all socioeconomic levels with equal frequency.[3]

The problem confronting professionals who work with the mentally retarded is that mental retardation is not always a separate entity that affects the child. Most often, it is associated with other conditions. Caring for the retarded child means knowing how to care for the accompanying developmental disabilities. The nurse who chooses to work in the field of mental retardation must also be able to care for children with a spectrum of impairments. Nevertheless, all nurses should know the basics of care for individuals with mental retardation, because these people are living longer and normalization efforts are bringing them out of institutions into the mainstream of society. Increasing numbers of children are being cared for in the home with the help of outreach professionals who help the family learn how to care for their child with handicaps.

For nurses in general, the aspect of prevention of mental retardation is of greatest importance. The goals of the nurse should be, first, to promote preventive efforts and, second, to prevent problems related to mental retardation. Nevertheless, before one can prevent disorders from occurring, the nurse must first recognize the causes and manifestations of retardation.

Every outreach team and education team should include a nurse who is knowledgeable about mental retardation and the physical disabilities that are often associated with it. Every newborn nursery nurse, pediatric nurse, and public health nurse should be able to perform an assessment that will discern disabilities, should be skilled and comfortable teaching and listening to families, should recognize risk factors, and should assist families to find resources.

Legislation

Every year, more than 125,000 infants are born who will be diagnosed at some point in their developmental history as mentally retarded. One in 10 persons in America will have a mentally retarded person in his immediate family. Probably because of the growing interest in the rights of members of our society who are mentally or physically handicapped, the federal government has tried to ensure through laws what society has neglected to do by itself. Recent legislation such as Public law 94-142, the Education of All Handicapped Children Act of 1977, and the Developmentally Disabled Assistance and Bill of Rights Act of 1975 (P.L. 94-103) shows a trend toward more humane treatment of persons with disabilities.

Public Law 94-142 ensures that extensive child identification procedures will be carried out to find children who are handicapped and in need of education. The parents are assured of full service and are also assured that those programs will be maintained. Within these programs, children are to be educated in the least restrictive environment and with nondiscriminatory testing and evaluation. The provision of a free, appropriate public education at no cost to the parents or guardians is also assured.

Public Law 94-103 is a bill of similar language that details the rights of the developmentally disabled for services, treatment, and habilitation in institutions and other residential programs.[5]

These bills and others like them were long overdue but are having far-reaching implications for education and services. Currently, many programs serving the retarded are gravely concerned that funding will be reduced or that new legislation will erase the gains made because of the conservative mood of the government. The success of the legislation that has been passed requires appropriate funding, social incentives, and administrative action. Interest in legislation that affects retarded clients and their families should be a nursing concern.

Parents who are more informed about the rights of their children and advocates who are willing to lobby for the rights of a fellow human being have wrought many positive changes for mentally retarded persons in our courts of law. The AAMR in 1973 issued position papers that led to testing in courts of many clients' basic rights. Some of those rights, as stated in the position papers, are as follows:

Freedom of choice within the client's ability and within the limitations that are placed on all people in the society

The right to live in the least restrictive environment that is individually appropriate

The right to be gainfully employed with fair pay and fair working conditions

The right to be part of a family

The right to marry and have a family as appropriate for the individual's ability to be responsible

The right to have freedom of movement and not be interned without just cause and due process of law[3]

Further extensions of the basic rights also state that the client has the right to publicly supported and administered comprehensive habilitative programs and services designed to minimize handicaps. Another basic right is to have available publicly supported and administered programs of training and education, which may include, but are not restricted to, basic academic and interpersonal skills.[3]

At the present time, deinstitutionalization is a result of 15 years of discussion about mental retardation and of litigation. The realization of the legal rights of clients to the least restrictive environment and the right to habilitation has led to differing opinions among organizations and parents. Some see large state-run institutions as "warehousing" of the retarded and physically disabled individuals and press for community group homes or foster homes as the only acceptable living arrangement outside of the client's own family. Others see the institution as a secure and permanent home with decent food, medical services, and physical comforts. Many states are witnessing a backlash by families who are discontented with the movement of their children out of the institutions against their wishes. These parents and some mental retardation experts believe that there is a need for both types of living arrangements.[48] Perhaps state institutions, with all of the expertise available to the community and with sound governmental backing, should become centers of research and advocacy. Certainly colleges of nursing and medical schools should take advantage of such places to develop clinical learning experiences for students. They are a rich environment that provides valuable information and skills related to the needs of people with mental retardation and developmental disabilities. Such a relationship is, in the long run, beneficial also to the institution and to the clients.

Ethical and Moral Issues

Mental retardation and physical disability raise significant ethical and moral concerns. Nurses need to evaluate their own feelings in regard to several factors that have customarily been linked with retardation. Some of the nurse's self-directed questions are as follows:

1. How do I feel about the worth of retarded or physically disabled persons? Do I consider them of use to society?
2. Am I willing to support legislation that insures human rights of the disabled? Am I prepared to be an advocate who works to insure that these laws are carried out in more than a token fashion? Am I willing to educate the public, legislators, and the profession to bring the needs of the disabled and legislation in closer proximity?
3. What are my thoughts on institutionalization?
4. Some forms of prevention of mental and physical disability may entail issues such as abortion. What do I believe about the use of abortion as a method of prevention?
5. What are my thoughts and feelings about the use of high technology and high-cost efforts to preserve the life of premature infants?
6. Am I willing to support financially, through my taxes, programs that stress prevention?
7. How do I feel about the corrective surgery needs of disabled individuals when these surgeries may prolong their lives?

Recent legislation has also raised questions about the educational preparation of nurses. Prior to normalization efforts, the retarded and physically handicapped were placed in specialized institutions for custodial care. If nurses cared to work within this specialized area they had to receive on-the-job training. With the advent of community living, nurses in all health care settings need to be aware of the special needs of handicapped patients. Clinical care opportunities and theoretical information about mental retardation and related disabilities should be included in the basic curricula of nursing education.[28]

Etiology

The causes of mental retardation are multiple. In surveying a list of factors, one is able to envision that nearly all areas of nursing specialization are challenged. Our efforts must be directed at prevention as well as treatment. The etiology of mental retardation arises from two main sources, genetic and acquired factors.

Genetic Factors

Mental retardation is often associated with genetic aberrations. Chromosomal abnormalities, such as errors in the number of chromosomes, result in too many or too few chromosomes. The normal structure of the chromosome may also be changed because of breakage and subsequent loss, or by addition of pieces to a chromosome. Another cause of chromosomal abnormalities may be changes in genes, in which cases no karyotype differences are noticed.

To visualize the chromosomes for study, a cytogenetic lab technician photographs a cell from blood or skin samples during metaphase, enlarges it several thousand times, and then cuts and pastes these enlarged pictures of the chromosomes, matching pairs together. This procedure is called karyotyping. A karyotype is a picture of the chromosomes matched in an order based on length, position of centromere, and banding (see Fig. 30-1). In the banding process, dye is applied to the cells and the dye is absorbed by deoxyribonucleic acid (DNA). Bands of DNA material are visible in the photographs and can be matched to bands on homologous chromosomes. Each pair of chromosomes has a unique banding pattern that is characteristic for humans (see Fig. 30-2). Chromosomal aberrations can be visualized. A broken piece of chromosome without a centromere can reattach and heal, translocate, or become lost. The resulting problems are either an inheritance of too many genes, as in translocation, or the loss of the genes. The problem to the fetus depends on the quality and quantity of the genetic material. The karyotype is useful to illustrate these problems; therefore, scientists are able to visualize the abnormal chromosome(s) more readily.

A recent development by image enhancement experts (who formerly conducted research at the Johnson Space Center and at NASA's Jet Propulsion Laboratory) is the Genetiscan Digital Karyotype System. This piece of equipment, located in the Genetic Screening and Counseling Center in Denton, Texas, is one of only ten such machines in the country. It uses the latest in digital technology to help classify each of

Figure 30-1. *Photo of a normal male karyotype.*

the chromosomes and arrange them into karyotypes. After scanning and organizing the chromosomes, the system produces a high-resolution image of the karyotype that allows great accuracy in the detection of small abnormalities such as very small deletions and additions of chromosomal materials. The chromosomal image is then stored in the computer; it can be easily retrieved for further study, which may be preformed directly on the monitor screen. After completing all desired procedures, the lab technician can create a laser-printed copy of the karyotype complete with all computer enhancements. This machine takes about one-half the time needed by the previously described karyotyping method.

There are normally 46 chromosomes in a human cell. In preparing a karyotype, one begins row 1 with the 3 longest pairs of chromosomes (group A) of which pair number 1 is the longest. Group B contains pairs 4 and 5. The second row (group C) consists

of slightly smaller chromosomes which are pairs 6 through 12. The third row contains group D (13–15) and E (16–18). The fourth row is group F (19–20) and G (21–22). The other two chromosomes, known as the sex chromosomes, are the X and Y chromosomes which belong to groups C and G, respectively, located at the bottom of the karyotype. If the karyotype is a female, there are two X chromosomes (XX); for a male, there are an X and a Y.

Down syndrome is a condition in which, during the process of gametogenesis, nondisjunction occurs (see Fig. 30-3). Normally, the spindle fibers of the cell pull the chromosomes apart from each other and new cells are formed containing half (23) of the complement of chromosomes. Sometimes this process goes awry. The result is one cell lacking a chromosome and the other cell now containing two. In Down syndrome, the number 21 chromosome undergoes nondisjunction. The germ cell (ovum) now contains

Figure 30-2. *Enlarged photograph of chromosomes showing banding technique.*

many of those persons who are institutionalized have Down syndrome. The reader needs to be aware that some genetic diseases are due to mosaicism; however, this is beyond the scope of this chapter and will not be discussed.

A piece of a chromosome may break off and attach itself to another chromosome. This is called *translocation* (see Fig. 30-4). Down syndrome is sometimes transmitted by this method also. A piece of a number 21 chromosome breaks off and attaches to another chromosome, such as the number 15. If, during oogenesis, the normal number 21 chromosome and the number 15 chromosome with the translocated number 21 piece are grouped in the same ovum and fertilized, the result is two normal number 21 autosomes, one from each parent, and two number 15 autosomes, one of which contains extra number 21 material.

Turner syndrome (XO) is a situation in which one of the X chromosomes is missing due to nondisjunction, resulting in a female with 45 chromosomes (see Fig. 30-5). If the ovum containing no X chromosome is fertilized by sperm with the Y chromosome, the zygote is not viable; however, if the sperm contains an X chromosome and fertilizes an egg containing no X chromosome, the resulting individual has the physical characteristics of a female, but is usually sterile and secondary sex characteristics develop poorly at puberty. Approximately 20% of individuals with Turner syndrome are mentally retarded.

Another condition called polysomy of X (three or more X chromosomes per cell) results in individuals having female sex characteristics. This condition is commonly called "super female." The result is not accentuated femaleness, but mental retardation and behavior problems.

Klinefelter syndrome (multiple X and Y chro-

24 chromosomes instead of the normal 23. If this cell is fertilized by a sperm containing 23 chromosomes, the resulting zygote has 47 chromosomes—22 pairs of autosomes plus one extra number 21 chromosome, and two sex chromosomes. The consequences of this nondisjunction are an altered physical appearance of the infant and retardation. Down syndrome may also occur as a result of nondisjunction in the first cell division of the zygote. These two possibilities account for the high incidence of Down syndrome, and the results are children born with full trisomy 21. A great

Figure 30-3. *Graphic depicting normal cell division and nondisjunction.*

NORMAL   **NONDISJUNCTION**

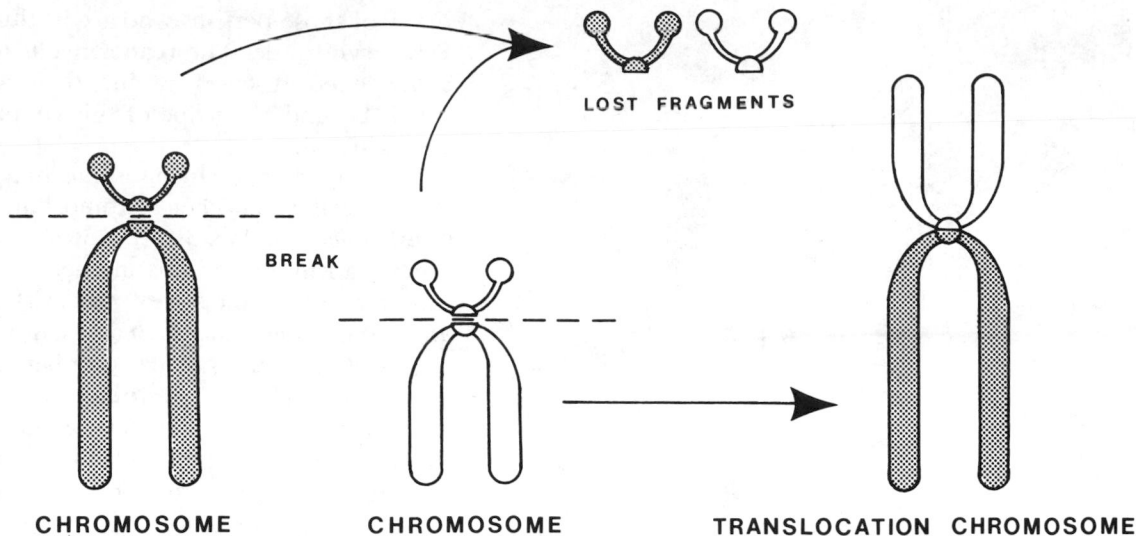

LOST FRAGMENTS

BREAK

CHROMOSOME   CHROMOSOME   TRANSLOCATION CHROMOSOME

Figure 30-4. *Graphics of translocation.*

mosomes) depicts a masculine appearance because of the presence of a Y chromosome, but the problem results from one or more extra X chromosomes (see Fig. 30-6). At puberty, female sexual characteristics develop. The male gonads are undeveloped and ster-

ile. Mental retardation and behavioral problems usually, but not always, occur. Males may also be born with an XYY anomaly. This condition may produce a dull mentality, usually in the 80 to 95 IQ range. Internal and external genitalia are often affected and the

Figure 30-5. *Photograph of karyotype of Turner syndrome.*

Figure 30-6. *Photograph of karyotype of Klinefelter syndrome.*

individual is usually quite tall. Some studies indicate that the aggressiveness attributed to these males with an XYY anomaly is related to their height acquired early in childhood, which resulted in teasing by peers. Other studies attempt to link their behavior with significant psychological differences.

There are now 3,907 disorders catalogued by McKusick that are known to be transmitted by the mendelian inheritance patterns in man.[35] Mendelian inheritance refers to rules governing the transmission of unit factors (genes) that were first described by Gregor Mendel in 1866 as a result of his experiments with garden peas. In essence, his first law states that an individual is formed as a result of the union of a sperm and an egg, each of which receives half of the genetic material found in the somatic cells of the father and mother, respectively. Genes for the traits may be either dominant or recessive.

Chromosomal differences remain the problem

but these differences are genic; that is, they are chemical or submicroscopic in nature. Some of these differences at the cellular level may affect many body systems. Some genetic disorders of metabolism involve the following:

1. Amino acids causing phenylketonuria (PKU)
2. Mucopolysaccharides leading to Hunter or Hurler disease
3. Lipids causing Tay-Sach disease
4. Carbohydrates causing galactosemia
5. Purines causing Lesch-Nyhan syndrome

There are also hereditary, degenerative diseases and endocrine disorders that may cause mental retardation. One endocrine disorder that causes mental retardation is a deficiency of the thyroid hormone leading to cretinism, a failure to develop both physically and mentally.

Some of the above conditions are transmitted in

a dominant or recessive fashion. The presence of an abnormal recessive gene, if paired with a normal dominant gene, will not be expressed. If, however, the abnormal recessive gene is paired with an abnormal recessive gene from the other parent, the trait or disorder will occur. A dominant gene will produce its effect whether its homologous allele is dominant or recessive (see Fig. 30-7).

Dominantly inherited genetic disorders are said to be milder than those which are due to recessive or X-linked genes. Mental retardation resulting from a dominantly inherited disorder is usually mild; recessive disorders are more serious (see Fig. 30-8). Phenylketonuria is such a disorder. Profound retardation often occurs with inborn errors of metabolism. These errors may appear on the X chromosome also. The Lesch-Nyhan syndrome, for instance, will cause profound retardation. There are about 150 disorders and traits resulting from altered genes on the X chromosome, but the mode of inheritance is slightly different.

Approximately 5 years ago, advanced technology enabled geneticists to visualize the cytogenetic cause of a syndrome which they had been observing in patients in the clinical area for some time. The condition is now labeled Fragile X syndrome. Through examination of chromosomes isolated from white blood cells, the defective site is now more clearly visible at the end of one of the long arms of the X chromosome. The importance of this finding is that it has identified a syndrome that accounts for a significant amount of mental retardation among newborns in the United States, second only to Down syndrome. The syndrome produces disabilities ranging from learning disabilities to mental retardation. Other anomalies are listed in the physical assessment checklist.

Since the defective site is on the X chromosome, females, who normally inherit an X from each parent, will be less affected than males. When one has two like chromosomes, both carry the same type of genetic material. The nonaffected chromosome will cover most of the effects of the defect on the other one, but the female is a carrier of this condition.

Males, however, receive an X from the mother and a Y chromosome from the father. If the X chromosome that the male has received from the mother has the defect on it, the Y chromosome, which carries different genetic material from the X chromosome, is not able to provide a backup for the faulty X chromosome. However, the condition is perplexing in that not all of the females escape the effects and about 20% of the males who inherit the gene are unaffected. Carrier females may have normal intelligence or are less retarded. Normal brothers may carry the gene and be able to transmit the condition to their offspring.[12,43]

Acquired Factors

Acquired mental retardation involves prenatal, perinatal, and postnatal factors. Prenatal factors are infections, irradiation, toxins, drugs, and unknown causes. Perinatally, one of the most common causes of mental retardation is prematurity. Other factors are anoxia, brain damage, and infection. *Postnatal* conditions include childhood diseases, accidents, infection, anoxia, poisoning, hormonal problems, and influences in the child's environment.

Birth defects such as cerebral palsy, deafness, and blindness may lead to sensory deprivation and may, therefore, result in mental retardation. Early childhood intervention is of great importance in preventing retardation resulting from these problems and will be discussed in more detail later in the chapter.

Psychiatric disorders may retard learning progress because of problematic behavioral activity. Child

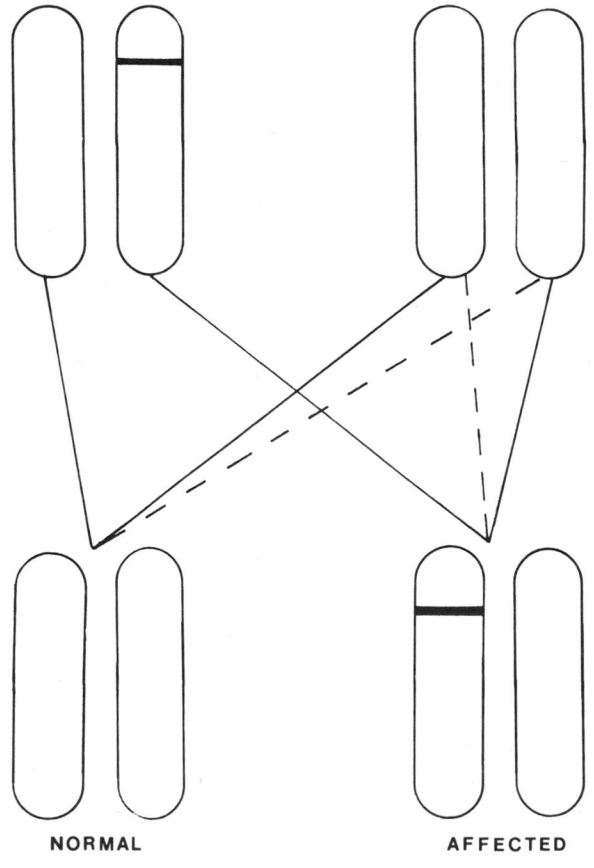

NORMAL AFFECTED

DOMINANT

Figure 30-7. *Graphic of dominant Mendelian inheritance in man.*

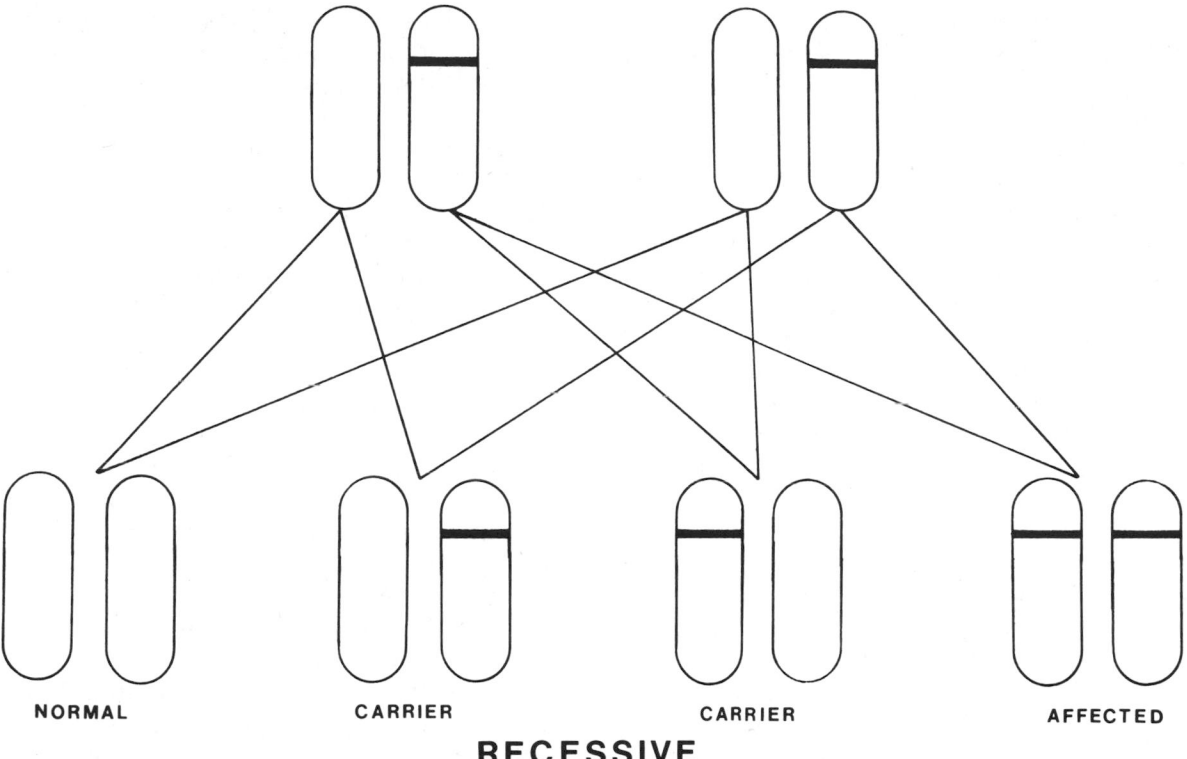

NORMAL   CARRIER   CARRIER   AFFECTED

RECESSIVE

Figure 30-8. *Graphic of recessive Mendelian inheritance in man.*

abuse may cause mental retardation through trauma or deprivation.

It is clear that prevention of mental retardation begins as early as family planning and continues throughout the developmental years. The nursing process is a tool in the preventive efforts.

Dynamics of Mental Retardation

In today's nuclear family, both parents usually pursue a career or job before the birth of a child. Many continue to work outside the home after the birth due to financial or career reasons. Inflation and high interest rates are tremendous burdens on young people trying to establish a home. The new issues related to women's rights also affect the nuclear family. Sometimes, the mother works outside the home because she wants a career and a life apart from that of housewife and motherhood. Finding adequate child care and resolving conflicts surrounding the changing lifestyle of young couples today create problems. A new child in the family may create unity toward a common goal or may result in such dramatic lifestyle changes that parents are caught up in conflict and stress.[53]

Mothers who choose to breastfeed often face difficulties arranging breastfeeding to fit with a job schedule. Guilt and anxiety may be outcomes of trying to manage a home, parenthood, and a career. Old friendships with childless couples are altered, thereby changing social outlets for the young parents. Apartments or other rental properties in which children are welcome are not easily located.

Parents are not, however, without compensation when a child is born. The birth of a beautiful baby is the outcome of prior planning and the wait during the months of pregnancy. Family and friends delight with the new parents during this happy occasion. The fun of planning showers, creating a nursery and layette, and buying baby equipment is shared by all who are close to the couple.

Future life is family-oriented. Friends begin to have families also. New friends are found with common interests. Vacations revolve around activities that can be shared by the family, such as trips to the mountains, the beach, sight-seeing, and involving the family in favorite recreation activities. As children are added to the family, the lifestyle continues to evolve.

The birth of a child with a disability is often a cataclysmic event to the family. For a young couple, already in transition, it is particularly traumatic. Every member of the extended family is affected by this event. Support, both psychological and financial, is of prime importance and often difficult to obtain. Misunderstanding about the cause of this disability and the need to place blame by well-meaning family members and friends cause additional stress to the family.

For the friend, family member, or professional who spends limited time within this situation, the viewpoint is not the same as it is for the parents who spend all of their time with the child. A once-busy social life grinds to a halt. The parent, frustrated at trying to find resources and help for the child, is often regarded as an "overanxious parent," a term used by a great many sources, many of them professional.

In order to develop a therapeutic relationship with the family, it is imperative for nurses to understand the normal sequence of stages a parent must work through before intervention can be planned that will be most useful.

Stages of Recognition and Acceptance of a Disability

Some authors believe that parents move through several stages before they are able to recognize and accept the reality of their child's disability. Before parents can begin to receive help they first must develop an awareness that a problem exists. Following this, recognition of the basic problem must occur.[40] For some parents of infants who are severely handicapped, recognition of the disorder is immediate.

The impact of the birth of a handicapped child may cause stress disorders at a time when the parent is also trying to resolve stressful situations of childbirth and maturational status. A mother must resolve several maternal tasks following birth before she feels normal and whole again.[37] These tasks are psychological processes bringing even a normal birth to a full course. They are as follows:

1. Grief work—relinquishing expectations of herself and infant and adapting to reality
2. Infant's performance—measuring the infant's ability to function compared to other infants, before she will lose fearfulness about infant's wholeness
3. Mothering skills—expending energy on developing and performing simple mothering skills
4. Redefining roles—renewing the relationship with the child's father, which is important to her emotional adjustment
5. Resuming other responsibilities—moving from the passive-dependent role to that of taking over responsibilities at home

These normal tasks for the new mother are seriously jeopardized if the child is born with mental retardation or physical disability. The postpartum nurse, through early intervention, may be the first caregiver to assist the family with these maternal tasks.

The next stage is the parent's search for a cause. Whether the cause of the child's condition is genetic in nature, the result of a maternal–environmental condition, or due to infection is important to the family. Blame-placing is an outcome at this point. No one likes to feel that the child's condition may result from a fault on his or her side of the family.

The fourth stage is the searching for a way to heal the child. Until this stage is worked through, the parent may run from one doctor to another or one therapeutic method to another. This often is frustrating to the physician who is the primary caregiver when he discovers that the parent is also putting the child through such things as polyvitamin or megavitamin therapies, patterning, consultation for surgeries, and various adaptive devices, all of which the physician has neither recommended nor planned for this child.

It is only in the final stage, that of acceptance, that the parent is able to work optimally toward goals of care for this child. Early childhood intervention is of primary importance. A dynamic infant stimulation program can "run defense" for both child and parent. Research has shown that early intervention increases children's learning capacities and social awareness.[19] Likewise, without this therapy the child can, early on, learn helplessness. A handicapped infant is more likely to experience failure and learn to be helpless because those who care for the infant are prone to do everything for the baby. Helping the family overcome this tendency and become more therapeutic is, more than anything else, the rationale for infant stimulation programs.

By understanding phases and stages that parents experience, the nurse is able to plan effective intervention to expedite the acceptance process. Denial, guilt, and grief, if not worked through successfully, may lead to pathology in the final stages of withdrawal and rejection. These stages, in the extreme, can lead to a lifetime of behaviors that will hinder acceptance of the child.

Application of the Nursing Process to the Mentally Retarded Client

The nursing process is based on assessment, nursing diagnosis, planning, intervention, evaluation, and revision of the plan. A client does not have to be ill for the nurse to use this process. The nurse easily uses the process to help prevent problems and to maintain wellness. The nursing process is simply a method of applying nursing care in any health care setting. This section of the chapter outlines some ways that nurses use the nursing process to promote optimal wellness of the retarded client.

Assessment

During infancy and early childhood, developmental screening is of primary importance in finding children at risk for mental retardation. All of the systems need to be assessed, particularly the neurologic, muscular, and skeletal systems, all of which may offer indications of problem areas.

It is not too early, during the family planning stage, to begin preventive nursing. Nurses who have the opportunity to work with families may begin the assessment of risk factors at this time. A good way to start a risk factor history is through a pedigree chart, which is a diagram in which family health or genetics is arranged in graphic form for easy visualization.

Knowledge of growth and development is necessary in screening infants and children for signs of mental retardation. Chart 30-1, "Physical Assessment: Checklist for Developmental Defects," is a beginning point for the nurse assessor. It is meant to serve as a guide to normal growth and development and to the recognition of deviations from the norm. Many children have some of these deviations and are considered normal. Genetic counseling centers urge nurses to refer clients or their families who have two or more minor anomalies for genetic counseling because several small birth anomalies may signify a more major defect elsewhere. Major anomalies, of course, must be referred. Careful follow-up of developmental lags should be accomplished as the child develops. Early intervention is very important to the child and assists the parent in his care. Assessment parameters also include social and peer interaction. Newborns are assessed in the following areas:

Response to light, sound, and pinprick
Orientation to inanimate and animate visual and
    auditory stimuli
Alertness
Muscle tone and pulling to sit
Cuddling
Defensive movements
Consolability
Excitement
Irritability
Activity
Tremulousness
Color changes of skin
Startle behavior
Self-quieting
Hand-to-mouth movements
Smiling

Assessment of an infant's behavior using tools, such as the Brazelton scale, gives clues to the child's developmental outcomes. Abnormalities are easily spotted when this tool is used to assess children at risk for retardation or disability.

Normal Developmental Tasks

Developmental tasks for infants and children are as follows:

1. Acquire motor skills
2. Acquire feeding skills
3. Develop effective communication skills
4. Develop beginning control of bowel and bladder function
5. Form simple concepts about the self and environment
6. Develop social and emotional relationships with others whom the child perceives as significant

Developmental tasks of preschool children are as follows:

1. Refine motor skills
2. Further establish communication skills
3. Accomplish toilet training
4. Develop pre-operational thought processes
5. Learn to relate to peers and adults in the outside world
6. Develop value sense
7. Develop sexual identity and modesty
8. Develop ideas of self-worth

Developmental tasks of school-aged children are as follows:

1. Develop and use logical thought
2. Define sex role and self-identity
3. Develop competencies
4. Develop a peer group
5. Expand autonomy
6. Develop internal controls for moral code
7. Develop the ability to handle stress

Developmental tasks for adolescents are as follows:

1. Utilize abstract thought
2. Establish self-identity and sexual role
3. Establish independency and develop interdependent relationships
4. Choose an occupation and prepare for it
5. Develop a personal value system[39]

When assessing any child or young person, these are the tasks that must be observed and evaluated. The person who is retarded has the same needs, and

(Text continues on p. 590)

C H A R T   30-1
Physical Assessment: Checklist for Developmental Defects

Head

Size—Normal range for male is approximately 34.5 cm at birth → 49 cm at 2 years

Normal range for female is approximately 34 cm at birth → 48 cm at 2 years

Microcephaly—limited brain size two standard deviations below norm; may have abnormality of brain tissue

Hydrocephaly—increase in amount of cerebrospinal fluid; brain size may be normal or smaller than average; head size increases due to increased fluid

The size of head is extremely important because the first 2 years of child's life is vital for brain growth. A larger than normal head, sometimes by as much as two standard deviations, is found in Fragile X syndrome.

Shape—should be normocephalic; abnormal findings may be in these areas:

Prominent forehead—as found in Hurler syndrome and in Fragile X syndrome

Premature closing of suture lines—giving rise to oxycephaly, scaphocephaly, plagiocephaly, trigonocephaly

Late closure of fontanels—most will be closed by 9 to 19 months. Late closure could indicate cretinism, Down syndrome, rickets, osteogenesis imperfecta, hydrocephalus, or syphilis; mean anterior fontanel diameter 2.1 cm two standard deviations above or below (0.6 and 3.6 cm, respectively) are important; posterior fontanels rarely exceed measurements of 0.5 cm

Face

Observe for spacing of features, symmetry, and signs of paralysis; width of a newborn face is approximately 8 cm; children with Fragile X syndrome have long thin faces and midface hypoplasia

Eyes

Eyes are same level and normally spaced

Hypertelorism—refers to wide-spaced orbits, frequently associated with some syndromes of mental retardation; mean distance between inner canthi for term infant is 2 cm; 3 cm is judged as hypertelorism

Hypotelorism—abnormally close-set eyes; may indicate lack of nasal bridge or trigonocephaly

Microphthalmia—may indicate encephalo-ophthalmic dysplasia, toxoplasmosis, or retrolental fibroplasia

Protruding supraorbital ridge—found in mucopolysaccharidosis and Marfan disease

Ptosis of lids—some neurologic problems may cause this; sometimes it is an inherited trait; family history is important

Slanting of eyes—downward slant may be indicative of Treacher Collins syndrome; upward slant may be Down syndrome

Epicanthal folds—may be present in some normal children; most will disappear by 10 years of age; may be present as a result of Down syndrome, glycogen storage disease, renal agenesis, or hypercalcemia

Eye lashes—very bushy; may indicate some syndrome disorders such as Hurler syndrome; if absent on inner two-thirds, may indicate Treacher Collins disease.

Eye brows—that grow together in center and may indicate a genetic syndrome such as the Cornelia de Lange syndrome

Color of iris—permanent color will be established in all children by 1 year; pinkish coloration may indicate albinism, light or white speckling (Brushfield spots) often found in children with Down syndrome

Lens—absent red reflex may indicate cataracts; these can be due to many problems leading to mental retardation; a dislocated lens may be the result of Marfan syndrome or homocystinuria

Ears

Normally, the upper part of the pinna should meet an imaginary line that is drawn from the lateral aspect of the eye straight backward. This will indicate if the ear is normally positioned or low set. The rotation of the ear is also important. A vertical line is drawn from the lobe of the ear straight up crossing the horizontal line. The measurement should not be more than a 10-degree angle. Abnormally shaped ears are also found in various disorders and should be reported. Look to see if both ears are at the same level. Are they flat or protruding? Are they bigger or smaller than normal? Check the size and completeness of ear lobes. Check for sinuses or tags of skin on the ear. Children with Fragile X syndrome have ears that are longer in length, often by two standard deviations, and are often posteriorly rotated. The ears are soft due to cartilage hypoplasia.

Nose

The nose should be observed to be at the middle and upper part of face. In many syndromes, the nose is shaped differently than the normal nose. In some cases, it is broad and flat, small and turned up. Notice if the nose is straight. Are the nares symmetrical? Palpate to examine bone and cartilage. Transilluminate with a flashlight on one nare and look into the other to determine if perforation of the septum exists.

Mouth

Is the mouth symmetrical? Are there clefts in the lip or palate? Drooling starts about 3 months and continues until the child learns to swallow saliva at about 9 to 12 months. Examine the palate for a gentle slope. Report a high arched palate. If a notch is noted at the junction of the soft and hard palate, report this as it may cause future speech difficulty. The lower jaw that is excessively small or large may indicate genetic problems that warrant further evaluation. Teeth that are delayed past 1 year of age may be a result of cretinism. Gums that have a black line along the margin may be a sign of metal poisoning. Do not confuse this with the normal dark pigmented coloration on the gums of black children. A prominent jaw is found in persons with Fragile X syndrome.

The tongue that seems large for the mouth may indicate Down syndrome, cretinism, or Hurler syndrome. Protrusion of the tongue is a common finding in mental retardation. Note the normal developmental sequence of feeding. The rooting reflex disappears by 3 months. Sucking-swallowing remains for 3 to 5 months. The gag reflex diminishes slightly after child begins to chew or at about 7 months. The bite reflex disappears about 3 to 5 months. Lip closure begins about 6 to 8 months.

Hair

Normally, head hair should begin high over the forehead. Some syndromes have hair growth low on the forehead, such as Hurler syndrome. Hair patterns found in Noonan and Turner syndromes allow growth of hair far down on the neck. Color is important. White hair may indicate albinism and a white patch may be related to Waardenburg syndrome. One important factor in prevention is the color changes that occur in diets that are deficient in protein. These children may have red or greyish streaks in their hair. Hair whorls are usually located on the top at the back of the head. Number and location of whorls should be noted.

Neck

The average length of the trachea is 4 cm. An extra thick or a webbed neck may indicate Noonan or Turner syndrome. Extra skin folds at the back of the neck may be indicative of Down syndrome. Check for reflexes that should have disappeared earlier (primitive reflexes). These include a symmetrical tonic neck reflex or an asymmetrical tonic neck reflex, the startle reflex, or the tonic labyrinthine reflex. These will cause future problems, particularly in feeding the child.

Chest

Any irregular shape of the chest should be reported. When the sternum protrudes from the chest wall, the child should be evaluated for syndromes such as Marfan or Morquio disease. Funnel chest is also found in Marfan disease. Spinal deformities may be a problem. A horizontal circumference of the thorax at the level of mammary glands with respiration is 34 to 35 cm.

Abdomen and Back

Note whether two arteries and one vein are present in umbilicus. Omphaloceles on the abdomen where the peritoneal contents bulge through a muscular defect are sometimes seen. It is important to know that up to one half of these children have other associated defects. Distribution of hair that is not normal should be reported. A dimpling in the spine can be associated with spina bifida and should be evaluated. The spinal column and hips should be evaluated for defects. Many are related to genetic and developmental problems.

(Continues on p. 590)

Arms, Legs, Hands, and Feet

The extremities are evaluated for deformities. Children with genetic problems often have defects of the extremities; for instance, in Fragile X syndrome the hands are often found to be at least two standard deviations greater in length than is normal. Hands are also soft, fleshy and hyperextensible in this syndrome. Specific things to look for are number of fingers and toes, nail growth, any webbing of toes and fingers, and short fingers due to missing phalanges. Enlarged toes and fingers are also significant findings. A large space between the large toe and second toe is important. Any curving inward of small fingers (clinodactyly) should be reported. Fingers that over-ride or cross over each other are sometimes seen in children with trisomy (18) syndrome. The thumb often has the appearance of another finger. Feet are rounded on the bottom and are called "rocker bottom." Dermatoglyphics of hands and toes often vary in children with syndromes. Down syndrome, in particular, has very different patterns from the normal population. An increased carrying angle of the elbows should alert the nurse to the possibility of gonadal dysgenesis in both sexes.

Genitalia

Examination of the genitalia in the developing child is important. In small children, abnormalities of the genitals may indicate problems with other developmental disabilities. In young boys, abnormal genital enlargement is often the result of neurogenic or idiopathic sexual precocity or of Fragile X syndrome, in which the testes are significantly enlarged after puberty. In older boys, small genitals can be the result of Klinefelter syndrome or an endocrine disorder. Secondary sexual characteristics may be missing in young women with Turner syndrome.

---

if normalization is to succeed, he must be helped to acquire as many skills as possible.

Eating Ability

The skill required to eat in an acceptable manner is one that must be developed if the child is to achieve autonomy. Many retarded individuals may reach adulthood spilling food, eating with their hands, stealing food from others' plates, and picking up food off of the floor and eating it. An assessment of the individual's eating ability is the forerunner of a program to upgrade the individual's skills. Chances to practice are important and, as the client learns, opportunities to eat in public are effective training methods.

Communication Skills

Language skills are crucial for all individuals. Speech is simply one form of language development. Language skills are still being learned as the retarded person grows to adulthood and becomes more independent. Information skills about the environment must also be assessed. Many young adults learn to sight read signs related to health and safety in the community. Use of a telephone is important, as are the abilities to tell time and use money. Motivation for, and mastery of, these skills must be assessed.

Some children, because of their other disabilities, do not have effective language skills. They may be able to use a communication board. Assessing the ability for using such a board can be accomplished by working with pictures and having the child point to the object named. If a child cannot use his hands or arms, but has head control, he may point with a pointer taped on a helmet. Pictures should be as similar to the child's environment as possible. For instance, a child who lives in an institution cannot relate to pictures of a bathroom or bedroom such as is found in a home situation, unless he also spends time at home. Colored pictures or black and white pictures may present problems to children with perceptual motor problems. Assessing the child's perceptual skills is essential before the nurse attempts to use visual aids in health teaching. Children may have trouble learning if there is a problem with eye-hand coordination, figure-ground discrimination, position in space, spatial relations, or form constancy. Collaboration with an occupational therapist or a speech therapist is helpful in this area. The Frostig Developmental Test of Visual Perception is a valuable tool for assessment.

The Child's Environment

Assessment of the child's environment is a valuable piece of data that will assist the nurse to plan effective interventions. All children need stimulation suitable for their physical and emotional needs. Areas that need to be assesssed are as follows:

1. Does the child have opportunities for social stimulation that promote intellectual growth? Is there a caring person in the child's environment with whom he can derive social experi-

ences? Does the child have auditory, visual, and tactile stimulation? What types of stimulation are provided and are they appropriate for the child's particular health needs?

2. Does the child have control of some things in the environment? Does he receive reinforcement for his activities that help build constructive social responses? When he is not able to succeed at a task, is he encouraged to change behavior or activities so that he will succeed?

3. Does the child possess readiness capabilities for interacting with, and benefiting from, the environment? Can he observe, pay attention to, and notice when things are different? Is he persistent in pursuing a problem? Can he imitate and anticipate? Can he see another's point of view? Does the child have the ability to explore, manipulate, or move about? Does the environment seem enriched or is it void of learning experiences?

Nursing Diagnosis

The nurse formulates nursing diagnoses to plan, implement, and evaluate nursing intervention. Several nursing diagnoses are appropriately applied to the care of the mentally retarded client and his family, including the following:

Dysfunctional grieving
Ineffective family coping: compromised or disabling
Alteration in family process
Spiritual distress
Social isolation
Disturbance in self-concept: self-esteem, role performance
Anxiety
Alteration in growth and development
Impaired swallowing
Self-care deficit: feeding, toileting, bathing/hygiene, dressing/grooming
Impaired verbal communication
Potential for infection or injury
Impaired home maintenance management
Knowledge deficit

Planning

The planning stage of the nursing process calls upon all of the communication and interpersonal skills of the nurse. The family of a mentally retarded child may be at any point from shock to acceptance at the time of the nurse's initial contact with them. Meeting the family's needs also favorably affects the retarded child. Initially, the nurse guides the family through the stages of shock, grief, anger, resentment, and, finally, acceptance. Planning revolves around the nursing assessment and analysis/diagnosis of the assessment data. Does the family need counseling at this point, the nurse asks, or are they ready to progress to the stage of securing help for the child?

During the child's infancy, the family needs to work with the nurse and other health care professionals to provide stimulation and activities that promote growth and development. Planning may include special training for parents to learn handling and special techniques to enhance the child's physical and mental condition. As the child becomes older, his needs and goals of care change. Services that meet the changing needs of the child must be identified and secured. Long-range plans should be formulated so that the parents have a time frame to help them understand what is required of them as they plan for the child's future.

Issues such as employment needs of the parents, respite care, and institutionalization should be dealt with during the planning stage. The nurse considers the needs of siblings and helps the parents work through their feelings about siblings.

Perhaps plans need to include visits to various agencies with which parents will deal at certain times in the child's development. If the nurse is not familiar with institutional life, a visit should be made to such an institution.

Legislation related to handicapped or mentally retarded persons must also be understood for informed planning with the parents and client. Moral and ethical problems must be addressed by parents, nurses, and other health care providers. A sensitive interview offers insight into how the parents feel about these issues as they pertain to their own child and his condition.

Intervention

Working with the Grieving Family

Nursing intervention is based on a careful and thorough assessment, thoughtful analysis of the client and family data, and collaborative planning. Nurses assist the grieving family to grow in a desired direction. Support of the family is critical.

We know that grief presents symptoms that are both psychological and somatic in nature and can be elicited by an experience of loss. The birth of a child with a handicapping condition triggers the grief response because the expectation or dream the parent had for a normal child is now impossible. Without supportive intervention, a sense of helplessness, hopelessness, and despair may result. Very often, both parents and the normal siblings react in this mourning process by wishing the child were dead. Some families experience additional guilt reactions because of these feelings. Grieving is a process that must take place; it assists families to solve problems and look to the future.

How does the nurse support the family? One of the first responsibilities of nursing is to guide the family through decision-making processes related to issues such as whether the parents should keep the child at home or whether they will allow corrective surgeries for some disability related to the child's diagnosis.

Within the community, there are many sources of assistance for these periods of decision-making. Nurses should be familiar with how to put the family in touch with available resources (see Chart 30-2).

It would be ideal if all families were able to keep their children who are handicapped at home—nurturing, loving, and accepting them and their disabilities. We know that this is not possible in some families. How can nurses present reality to parents?

The nurse helps the parents deal with one issue at a time, one day at a time. Resources for each need can be found. Nurses also help families think through the consequences that each major decision about the child will have for the child and the other members of the family.

Crisis Intervention

During the *crisis period* of the family, often soon after learning of the child's diagnosis, family members are likely to experience confusion, disorganization, helplessness, dependency, anguish, and anger; the client and family are in need of immediate supportive intervention. Information must be presented to the family based on the developmental expectations and capabilities of the child. Services must be secured for the child and support groups must be located to which to refer the parents. A place needs to be made for the child within the family value system.

Crisis intervention is a supportive nursing intervention for the family of a retarded child until the family is able to solve problems by means of their own strengths and abilities. During crisis periods in which families are unable to function in a healthy manner, nursing intervention may mean stepping in and giving direction to the family or simply listening to family members and helping them shape their thinking and behavior.

Meeting Developmental Needs

Problems that the retarded child will face begin in infancy and can best be appreciated by examining the normal needs of all children. If these needs are not met for some reason, the child has troubles. Retarded children are at greater risk of not being able to have their needs provided for.

The retarded child's emotional, sensory, and motor needs are the same as those of "normal" children. Meeting these needs may call upon the creativity of the nurse. The child's emotional adjustment depends on provision of security through affection, acceptance, and approval. It also calls for understanding the intrinsic behavior patterns of the child as he proceeds through growth and development. In an encouraging atmosphere, where there is acceptance of the child developmentally and optimism regarding his developmental capacity, the child is more likely to attain his fullest potential.[3]

Social development relates to the child's acceptance of the society in which he lives. His role models are his parents, siblings, and friends. The parents' culture and values influence the child. As the child progresses through the maturational process, he needs to develop autonomy and independence. Peer relationships become important and play provides opportunities to help him shape qualities and character. Sexual identification and interest in himself as a sexual person is a lifetime experience, the roots of which are in infancy.

Progressing through these normal patterns of growth and development is extremely difficult for the mentally retarded or handicapped child. Mentally retarded children need special services, which are sometimes difficult to find, to help them achieve some degree of autonomy and independence. The retarded child may grow to adulthood being regarded as the "eternal child" and never experiencing independence beyond the most basic skills of daily living. Only in the past decade has it become possible for a mentally retarded individual to be considered a peer or a functioning part of society in which he lives.

As with the general population, the population of retarded people is growing older. This is in part due to the better medical services available today. As nurses we need to make ourselves aware of the bio-psycho-social needs of this aging population as well as those of the general population.[25]

Teaching the Retarded Child

One of the most pressing needs of parents is to learn techniques to teach their retarded child. Families should be taught positive reinforcement tools, which include using food as a reward, providing feedback to the child about his performance or behavior, social approval such as verbal praise, attention, and affection, and tokens that can be redeemed for something desirable to the child as payment for good behavior.

Other methods to influence the child's behavior are punishment, restriction from a desired event, or

CHART 30-2
Learning About the Diagnosis of Down Syndrome

Two Mothers' Stories

These two women are mothers of children with Down syndrome. Phyllis B. is a woman in her mid-50s. Her son Kevin, now 20 years old, was born during a second marriage. He has three half-sisters who are school teachers. Mary J. is a young woman in her late twenties. She has a 4-year-old daughter and a 2-year-old son, Larry, who was born with Down syndrome.

The women agree that the single most devastating event for them was the way they were informed of their infants' diagnosis. Phyllis relates her story with tears and emotion as readily as if it had been yesterday. The wounds, she informs us, never heal.

She was alone in the postpartum unit on the third day after her son's birth when the obstetrician came in to inform her that her son Kevin was a mongoloid, a term that is no longer used today. She remembers:

> I did not even know what that word meant. He looked perfectly beautiful to me—with his cherub face and chubby little body. Imagine the horror I felt when told my precious child had something wrong with him! I remember the doctor telling me that it was nothing we could do anything about and it would be good if we thought about placing him in an institution and getting on with our lives. He said that such babies often die before they are 10 years old. I remember that I hysterically called my husband to leave work and come to the hospital. I will never forgive the doctor for the callous way he told me about my son's condition. I was a school teacher and I should have known about such things, but if you remember, that was before children like ours were mainstreamed into school and society. I honestly never knew what a child with Down syndrome was like, and even if I had, how could I relate that knowledge to my precious son?
>
> As a family, we have weathered a great deal, but we have remained together in spite of it all. Kevin is now living independently in a group home in our city, which is a part of the community return program provided by the state school for the mentally retarded in our area. We had him admitted at a younger age, but kept him at home until he was 18 years old. He comes home every weekend possible and he is doing very well there. It seems a most natural thing for us all.

Mary J. is a registered nurse who worked with a local physician prior to the birth of her second child. Her pain lies in remembering how even her colleagues did not seem to be able to talk to her after diagnosing the child. She tells of her anger and resentment that no one could look her in the eye or face her when they spoke. Nurses whom she knew and with whom she had attended classes avoided her room after the baby was born.

When she later took her baby to the physician's office for check-ups, he could not seem to find a single good thing to say about him. Mary says:

> The doctor would almost avoid looking at me or at the baby. I desperately wanted my friend to say one word of kindness about Larry. No one, not even family members, said, "Isn't he cute."

Mary pulls out a large picture of a darling little red-headed boy. It is obvious that he has Down syndrome, but in spite of it, he is a beautiful baby. She continues:

> I used to dress him up in new little outfits and take him places, just longing to hear someone say a good thing about him. Heck, I knew he had Down syndrome and I know he has a few problems, but he is not grotesque. He is a doll.
>
> What hurt me the most of all is that most of my friends are doctors and nurses, and their attitudes don't seem to be any different from anyone else's. They should have been the people with therapeutic methods when they confronted me—even in the name of professionalism, if not friendship.

Each woman represents a different era and demonstrates dramatically different stages of grief. Although a great deal has changed in the last 20 years, many things have not; attitudes are still much the same within our profession.

(Continues on p. 594)

Phyllis relates that services for her child were very rudimentary at the time of his diagnosis, unless one sought full institutional care. Mary, on the other hand, found services in several agencies in the community. People offered her reading material, but a great deal of it was outdated and inappropriate. She is presently involved in collecting updated material for young parents and has requested that her colleagues call her when other young couples are facing this diagnosis. She says:

> I can find something warm to say to those parents. Sure, it is a hurtful experience, but I know some of the good things about these children to tell them about and I know what help they will need.

ignoring him when he is doing something wrong (that is, not giving feedback to him).

Methods that help the client establish a right way to perform an activity include modeling the desired behavior and allowing the client a time and place to practice. Self-help skills are divided into very basic early, intermediate, and advanced skills.[2] *Basic readiness skills* are such things as looking when called and following a simple command, whereas *basic motor skills* are holding and releasing objects and finger painting. Walking is also a basic motor activity goal and drinking from a cup is a self-help goal. *Intermediate self-help skills* include threading a belt through loops or washing hands and brushing teeth. Examples of *advanced self-help skills* are tying shoes, bathing, setting a table, and so forth.

Prior to teaching parents to work with their retarded child, the nurse should discuss with the parents their expectations for the child's learning at that time. Expectations that are too high risk frustration and failure; expectations that are too low slow the child's progress. The amount of assistance given to a child should also be discussed; parents must be careful not to do everything for a child. Learning to become independent depends largely on the family's allowing the child opportunities to do some planning and carry out tasks by himself. What kind of reward system will the parent choose to increase motivation? Praise, encouragement, and attention are excellent methods.

By dividing needed skills into three categories, parents can form check-off lists of self-help skills, home-care skills, and information skills. An excellent booklet recently published to help parents assist their child become independent, complete with assessment tools, is Toward Independent Living by Bruce Baker, Alan J. Brightman, and Stephen Hirshaw. Publishers are Research Press, 2612 North Mathis Avenue, Champaign, Illinois, 61820. The manual is exceptionally helpful in pointing out ways the parent can set limits for the child's behavior and it gives examples and methods of teaching.

Providing Information

Nurses need to give information. There are many resources available that the nurse can utilize as teaching tools. If there is a university within close enough proximity, the nurse will have a ready source of information. The Association for Retarded Citizens (ARC) is an organization with chapters in every state. Its goals are broad. Experienced parents who belong to the organization strive to help new parents deal with problems. Membership includes interested professionals, community members, family members, friends of the family, and the clients themselves. The ARC educates families about services available for the child with disabilities. Advocacy, and particularly self-advocacy, is a high priority. Prevention of mental retardation is also one of the major goals of the group.

The ARC follows and explains legislation to members. Members are asked to participate fully with legislators when the law affects the needs of the retarded. The ARC endeavors to meet the needs of the retarded in the community and the nation.

The American Association of Mental Retardation (AAMR) is an organization of 9,000 interdisciplinary professionals serving persons with mental retardation and other developmental disabilities through publications, conferences, and governmental liaison. The AAMR has state, regional, national, and international chapters and groups. Active nursing divisions in each chapter recently produced standards for the clinical nurse specialist in developmental disabilities/handicapping conditions, in conjunction with the American Association of University Affiliated Programs. A copy of the standards may be ordered through the Department of Health and Human Services, Public Health Service, Health Resources and Services Administration, Rockville, MD 20857.

Outreach teams are groups of professionals who work out of specialized centers such as state schools, birth defect centers, and school districts. Their membership is made up of any combination of teachers, nurses, occupational therapists, physical therapists, speech therapists, and specially trained aides. These outreach teams travel to the home to work with family members so that parents can give appropriate intervention to their handicapped child, assisting him to develop as normally as possible or helping him progress by formal assistance. Naturally, the delay of learning during early years places the child greatly behind schedule developmentally.

Handicapped children need many special services. Most communities have speech, hearing, physical therapy, and occupational therapy services in local or state agencies. Depending on the disability, professional interventions such as dentistry, child psychology, psychiatric services, and social work may be needed. By contacting the school administration office in your school area, you can find out the name of service centers if they exist in your state. For example, the Education Service Center, Region XI, in Fort Worth, Texas, handles audiovisual materials designed for pupils and teachers and has a computer list of all resources available to handicapped children in the area. These are only a few of the services offered by this center. Schools pay $1.50 per child to participate, and the state matches that with $1.

Respite Care

Respite care is one of the services that families will need to utilize in times of family crises, vacations, or even time away from the child for shopping or various appointments when both parents need to be away from the home. Respite care is a temporary separation of the child from the family either in the child's home or outside of the home. The time may be for as little as a few hours or as much as 30 or more days in some cases. Home health aides may perform this respite service in the home, or the child may be placed in an agency.

Careful, thoughtful investigation must be made prior to placing a child in the hands of another caretaker. Some things to inquire about include the following:

1. Does the aide have special training to work with the child's disability?
2. Are personal references available?
3. What is the total cost?
4. What services can be rendered?
5. Is medical coverage available if necessary?

Agencies providing care for the retarded child should be visited at various times; be wary of an agency that does not allow a spontaneous visit. Naturally, an agency should insist that a person from the agency escort the parent around, because it would be dangerous for outsiders to be allowed free access to the facility. Nevertheless, it is reasonable to be able to drop in to the agency for a visit and ask to be escorted to the place where the child would be cared for.

Reinforcing the Family's Strengths

Working with the client and his family requires that the nurse develop a harmonious relationship with them. Through the family assessment, the nurse demonstrates to the family those factors inherent in their situation that can keep the family unit stable. This provides the family with a view of their own strengths. By allowing the family and client an opportunity to express feelings, develop problem-solving skills, and experience the nurse's support, the family begins to trust the caregivers. The nurse's caring attitude helps to validate the self-worth of the client. The family who perceives that the nurse's concern is genuine responds with greater openness.

Evaluation

Evaluation of the plan and the interventions designed for client care should be a responsibility of the total health team, which includes the client and his family. Evaluation is an ongoing activity, aiming toward the next goal the client will reach. Another form of evaluation involves examining terminal behaviors of the client at the end of a formal program. Accurate documentation enhances the evaluation process.

The nurse works with the retarded person and his family in areas related to preventive health practices such as hygiene, accident prevention, disease prevention, nutrition, and grooming. Nurses function in a school situation, in which clients are screened for vision, hearing, health problems needing regular attention related to the disability or its complications, and physical assessments. Nurses are also interested in the retarded person's need for vocational education, sex education and birth control measures, securing of resources, monitoring of ongoing health, and skills needed to live in the community, whether at home with parents or in a group home. Nurses and other health care professionals strive to help the client develop and maintain a good self-image.

Vulnerability of the Mentally Retarded Client to Emotional Disorders

Incidence

If we who are "normal" experience stress and health problems leading to emotional disorders, consider the higher degree of risk of the retarded individual. The trauma or congenital defect that led to his particular cerebral dysfunction may also cause hyperactivity. The child who is born with disability is certainly at higher risk for rejection by his significant others. If normal children sometimes are unable to adjust to the environment in which they live, imagine the problems faced by a person who has no neighborhood peers nor even a sibling with similar problems. Those personality traits that we find hard to accept in normal persons, such as tension and anxiety, prevent retarded individuals from making friendships, further increasing their adjustment difficulties.

Studies of the retarded in institutions before 1960 found a range of 16% to 40% frequency rate of emotional disturbance. More recent studies indicate that among institutionalized children with Down syndrome, 56% display emotional disturbance at the time of their admission to an institution. Among the child population, the rate is 14% to 18%; in the general adult population, it ranges to 40%. These figures indicate an increased susceptibility to emotional disturbance among the retarded.[36]

Dynamics

It is difficult to define emotional disturbances in mental retardation. Mental retardation may result from many causes and is associated with many physically handicapping conditions. Through the normal growth and developmental phases, children and their needs change continually. Mentally retarded persons are less able to relate to their family and community in general. Root causes of emotional problems in the retarded are hard to separate from those related to mental retardation. Mentally retarded children are, as a group, subject to a high incidence of behavioral and psychiatric disturbances, which are very often not recognized and go untreated.[42,49]

Some of the emotional disturbances that affect the mentally retarded are psychotic disorders, which give rise to several differential diagnosis problems because it is difficult to discern whether the primary diagnosis is a functional psychosis that resembles severe mental retardation or a functional psychosis in the retarded.[36] *Behavioral reactions* are clusters of symptoms such as hyperactivity. *Transitory situational disturbances* are reactions to stress in the environment in which clients who do not have emotional disorders are not able to deal with certain troublesome events. When the client is removed from that situation, the symptoms are no longer seen. *Psychoneurotic reactions* are symbolic behaviors that the client has found useful when dealing with anxiety, and that he continues to use thereafter for any anxiety-causing problems. *Personality disorders* may occur when the client cannot face frustration and conflicts in a socially acceptable manner. Behavior may vary from passivity to delinquency or antisocial behavior. The social isolation of retarded adults often leads to such disorders as depression or anorexia nervosa. Down syndrome clients are particularly susceptible because of their easily recognized phenotypic features and their interaction or lack of interaction with society.[50]

The Nursing Process and the Emotionally Disturbed Retarded Child

Assessment and Nursing Diagnosis

Descriptions of psychotic reactions in the mentally retarded generally include bizarre gestures or posture, communication problems, lack of discrimination between inanimate and animate objects, and deviant affective expression. The child may not make eye contact with, or relate to, the examiner. Speech may be monotonous or echolalic, or it may involve a variety of abnormal responses. Motor behavior is repetitive or preoccupied. Children may also engage in unusual motor activity such as hand flapping or tiptoeing. Psychosis is a syndrome of behaviors that cannot be separated from the cause, age of onset, the child's inheritance, and the environment in which the child exists.[36]

Personality disorders produce behaviors that involve an inability to delay gratification, impulsiveness, irresponsibility, and failure to adjust socially by learning from previous interactions with others. These personality disorders are not thought to be related to the causes of mental retardation and are not found in the mentally retarded population in greater proportions than in the normal population.

Planning and Intervention

In the past, it was considered not feasible to treat the retarded with psychotherapy because therapy required good verbal skills. More recent thinking, however, has suggested that treating the client in a humane and accepting manner in therapy is more important than the use of techniques that require the client's use of sophisticated intellectual skills.

Planning should include both the parent and the client, when possible. The treatment of emotionally disturbed retarded clients may require parent counseling, individual or group therapy, and drug therapy. Client–therapist contact may begin on a one-to-one basis and may then enlarge to include a therapy or activity group. Nurse-managed group activities may include planned activities to strengthen self-concept, such as a "This Is Your Life" party in which the client is featured. In this activity, each person in the group has a chance during one of the weekly sessions to tell about himself, hobbies, family, and friends. The nurse group leader helps the client plan his program, and the client may invite guests or family members to describe life at home; he may also bring pictures of himself, pets, and friends, examples of his hobbies, and a teacher, school counselor, or work supervisor to talk about him at school or work.

Play therapy is an intervention mode for children who are retarded and is useful even if the client has limited verbal skills. Music therapy and recreational therapy are activities that can be planned around the client's needs. Through demonstration or modeling, the client may be shown certain behaviors that need to be corrected and then shown the correct behavior. Art therapy is another useful tool incorporating many different media of expression such as clay, finger paints, and designing prints on fabric. As the client's behavior improves, he is gradually moved out of the therapy group and into a transitional group.

Evaluation

Nurses must be accountable for their nursing care through the careful recording of plans, intervention, and client progress. Plans should reflect ways in which goals and objectives are evaluated. Video tapes and progress notes describing outcomes are methods to accomplish this. Meticulous records documenting the behavior of each client and legal consents are time-consuming but worthwhile, particularly when the nurse has a large case load or long-term interaction with clients.

The Nurse's Attitude

The nurse who is an advocate for her clients invests time, energy, and skills promoting those things that she believes will help the client maintain health, prevent injury or illness, and live effectively within his environment (see Case Study 30-1). Every client is unique, with individual needs. The attitude of the nurse sets the tone for client interaction and for movement toward achieving the goals of care.

Because the mentally retarded are moving into the community in ever-increasing numbers and are consumers of health care, nurses must be prepared to care for them. Retarded individuals are more like the general population than they are different from it, but sometimes the differences spell failure in achieving independence.

Professional development is the responsibility of the nurse. Basic curricula to help those nurses meet their career needs are the responsibilities of the educational programs preparing nurses; however, few programs give nursing students the opportunity to become directly involved with the retarded in clinical areas.[28]

Now is the best time in the history of nursing to become involved as an advocate for the client. Moral and ethical issues surrounding the care of the mentally retarded or physically handicapped are churning. Budget reductions are threatening some programs of prevention and treatment. Prisons are being told to reform, and many of the prisoners in state correctional facilities are retarded. One state prison board member in Texas stated that almost one-seventh of the prison inmates are retarded.[46] If the needs of the normal prisoner are not met, how much more are the needs of the retarded inmate being neglected? Retarded prisoners are at great risk for physical and sexual abuse when mixed with nonretarded prisoners. Although many states have problems related to funding and political disunity over prison administration, one thing is clear—retarded individuals do not belong in the same prison system with nonretarded individuals, at least not without special considerations.

The enlightened nurse has a responsibility for the public's awareness of the needs and rights of the mentally retarded and the historic attitudes that have been detrimental to the handicapped. Architectural barriers must be eliminated and the need for recreational facilities must be demonstrated. The client who is mentally retarded and sometimes physically disabled is every nurse's concern. We must share information and treatment ideas with clients, parents, and each other.

Summary

This chapter has focused on a condition affecting about six and a half million persons, or about 3% of the population. There are many causes of mental retardation, but categorically, two main causes can be listed—genetic and acquired factors. The dynamics of the family into which a retarded child is born are complicated and often crisis-laden. Some of the emphases of the chapter include the following:

1. Genetic factors may be chromosomal abnormalities, such as errors in numbers of the chromosomes (nondisjunction) or errors in the structure of the chromosome due to breakage or translocation.
2. According to the laws of Mendelian inheritance, genetic disorders may be passed from generation to generation by traits found on the autosome or the sex chromosome in a dominant or recessive manner.
3. Acquired factors leading to mental retardation may occur prenatally, perinatally, or postnatally;

(Text continues on p. 600)

Case Study 30-1

A Success Story Called Mary

Her face was a wreath of wrinkles crowned by a blue stocking cap. Black men's galoshes, unbuckled at the top, flopped when she walked, letting both snow and rain inside. An old faded navy coat hung on her thin frame, and the lumps around her ankles indicated she was wearing long underwear under thick brown cotton stockings.

Mary wore that garb the first time I saw her in our nursing clinic, and, according to her case worker, she would wear it with very little variation until summer.

The psychiatric institutions in our community had begun to deinstitutionalize some long-term residents. They placed these individuals in programs throughout the city to help them become independent citizens requiring minimal supervision.

No one could explain to the professionals in our center, where Mary was placed for vocational rehabilitation, why she had been institutionalized in the first place. Mary was a passive, simple person, certainly; however, it was apparent after she attended the center for a short time that she had neither a psychiatric problem nor a serious retardation problem. Nevertheless, she had lived in a psychiatric institution most of her life. Her old admission records were buried somewhere in forgotten or long-lost boxes of files. Her case worker could not remember ever having read them.

Mary's dentures were loose and wobbled about in her mouth when she ate or talked. She needed to learn a great deal about community adjustment. The habits and neglect learned over a lifetime were not easy to slough off. Most of the clients who came to the center were younger, but Mary was given a chance to develop a skill and to live in an apartment with two other women. She had no family, as far as anyone knew, and holidays were particularly lonely for her. Her younger roommates were invited home to visit with relatives.

Christmas, though, was not lost on Mary; she was the Santa Claus of the center that first year. She was so happy to be out of the institution and meeting new people that she showered everyone with gifts. She had spent many years attending arts and crafts classes in the institution and had collected boxes full of her hand-made crafts—purses, flower vases made out of jars, paper flowers, beads of every color, and lots of old shoes covered with macaroni and sprayed with gold paint. She never had a family to whom she could give these presents, so she had saved them. After making her rounds of various offices and department Christmas parties, she returned to her apartment to spend her first Christmas alone.

The rehabilitation center assigned a team to work with Mary's many problems. Mary's transition to community living was not miraculous; it was a slow and tedious process involving several years of classes, counseling, and smoothing out of her many social, emotional, and health problems. New dentures and clothing and improved hygiene and grooming habits have contributed to a more positive self-image. She has learned to prepare nutritious food, manage her own money, shop, and travel about the city. She is more assertive and self-confident and has found a job outside the vocational center.

Mary still keeps in touch with some of us who worked with her. From time to time she sends us her picture, in which we see a woman dressed like everyone else. The old stocking cap and men's galoshes are gone; she looks quite stylish, in fact. Mary has a job in a box factory making labels for orders that are to be shipped. She has her own apartment and is no longer followed by a social worker. She pays taxes like any other wage earner.

Although she still has no family with whom to gather on holidays, she does not sit at home in a lonely apartment sipping tea and eating leftover party cookies. Now she has something useful to do during the holiday season. This year, she tells me, she has a "volunteer job," wheeling about older women in a nursing home a few blocks from her apartment. She has been invited to join them for holiday dinners. "Poor ladies," she writes, "they don't have nobody to love them. I have been going to see them since summer, and now they will not be alone. Nobody should be alone at holiday times." Who would know that better than Mary?

(Note: During the summer of 1987, I received word that Mary had died of complications of heart disease, which she had before her release from the institution.)

CHART 30-3
Nursing Process Guidelines

Preconceptual Period

Assessment and Analysis

Subjective Data:

Nutritional interview—Lack of protein may be a risk factor. Check the mother's weight and counsel her if she is below 50 kg.

History of disease or illness—Has the mother a history of diabetes mellitus, cardiac disease, or chronic renal problems?

Reproductive history—Interview for miscarriages, abortions, previous premature deliveries, a history of any previous delivery of an infant with congenital abnormalities. These are increased risks for the next pregnancy.

Family history (include genetic)—The easiest form is a pedigree chart. A history of retardation among family members, particularly males, may be indicative of Fragile X syndrome.

Age of mother—Very young mothers (younger than 16) have higher risk for translocation types of Down syndrome. Older mothers (over 35) have higher incidence of trisomy 21 (Down) syndrome.

Education of parents—Assess social and behavioral areas as well as formal education.

Objective Data:

Results of nutrition testing and metabolic workups

Evaluation of pedigree information

Results of testing of Adult Behavior Rating (test that rates adaptive behavior of an adult and examines risk factors prior to conception)

Planning and Intervention

Depending on the results of the assessment, the nurse may plan patient education and referral, which, as risk factors warrant, may include the following:

Nutrition education
Referral to appropriate agency for financial assistance
Diet therapy
Genetic counseling
Birth control information and assistance
Family life education

Evaluation

This area is very important in prevention. Follow-up is a major step in the accountability of nursing care. Areas that will enhance evaluation procedures are as follows:

Follow-up visits
Physical assessments (ongoing) for weight gain
Nutritional follow-up
Family interview

Babies are at risk if parents have one or more risk factors that are not corrected.

Prenatal Period

Assessment and Analysis

Subjective Data:

Complaints of maternal infections, rubella, toxemia
Does the mother use drugs?
Has she been exposed to radiation?
Is there a history of Rh incompatibility?
Diet history
Financial status of parents
Is there a history of psychiatric problems?
Is this child wanted?

Objective Data:

Study lab work for results of the following:

Infections—Maternal infections may cause malformations, low birth weight for baby, or prematurity.

Toxemia—It may result in poorly perfused placenta and poor fetal growth.

Polyhydramnios—It may indicate intestinal obstruction or the possibility that the fetus is unable to swallow.

Oligohydramnios—Possible urinary tract malformation

Amniocentesis—Results may indicate a genetic problem.

Sonogram—Results will provide information on placement of placenta, size of child, and developmental disability.

Maternal psychosis—A suicide threat is a potential danger for the mother. The child is also at risk for harm.

Planning and Intervention

The assessment parameters may indicate nursing care needs. At-risk individuals may need counseling, psychotherapy, and, possibly, termination of pregnancy.

(Continues on p. 600)

Perinatal Period

Assessment and Analysis

Subjective Data:

When did labor start? This is important because of trauma damage resulting from long labor.

Last meal eaten—This information is important to anesthesiologist for prevention of aspiration of stomach contents.

Any bleeding or loss of fluids—This information will alert nurse to dangers of infection or impending miscarriage.

Previous prenatal care—Lack of previous medical care may be a risk factor, because these mothers have not been evaluated for problem areas.

Objective Data:

Monitor for complications. Areas to evaluate include hemorrhage, distocia, trauma, placental damage, caesarean section, prematurity, or postmaturity.

Planning and Intervention

Monitor for fetal presentation
Evaluate maternal-infant condition
Assist with procedures for birth
Newborn Apgar score
Newborn care
Notify nursery if problems are expected
Orders for special lab work if needed

Evaluation

Look at the results of the laboratory work following birth to determine if nursing care was given correctly for each situation. What were the results of cord blood tests? What care is being given to the child as a result of a low Apgar score? Is the recovery of the mother following a normal process? If not, what nursing care is being carried out to assist her?

Postnatal—Early Childhood Period

Assessment and Analysis

Subjective Data:

Pitch and quality of the child's cry may be indicative, in some cases, of problem areas

Observe interaction of mother with infant

Objective Data:

Assessment throughout the child's developmental period must include the following factors; they should be carefully recorded by maternity, pediatric, or public health nurses for future use.

Apgar scores
Gestational age
Head size
Weight and length
Trauma
Infection
Neurologic assessment results
Physical evaluation for birth defects
Maternal depression
Signs of child neglect or abuse
Prolonged separation from child

Planning and Intervention

Report any abnormalities to physician; parents and child may be referred to genetic counseling
Support parents if defect is found
Make other referrals as needed
Sensory stimulation may be needed for delayed infant
Behavior modification for client if needed
Parent education

Evaluation

Ongoing monthly physical and developmental checks are desirable if the child is at risk. These are performed at 6 months, 1 year, 18 months, and 24 months of age. A behavior problem checklist is valuable to maintain and should be followed up in progress notes. Testing of the child's cognitive level should be done early. Language skills and achievement test reports will serve to indicate if the individual program plan is adequate.

---

these disorders may arise from trauma, disease, or infection of the mother during pregnancy or of the child following birth, or from environmental problems such as malnutrition, lead poisoning, or child abuse.

4. Usually, those conditions more readily seen at birth causing multiple physical defects are the most difficult for parents.

5. Most mental retardation is mild in nature and is usually not diagnosed until some time after birth, when the child fails to develop academic skills.

6. Feelings ranging from guilt, depression, withdrawal, or rejection to denial or anger are normal following the birth of a retarded child, and the nurse must communicate effectively with the parents to help them work through these feelings.

7. When the family has progressed past the crisis stage and is more accepting of intervention for the retarded child, referrals are made to find sources of parent teaching and infant stimulation.

8. Normalization (or social role volarization, as it is now called) is a widely accepted concept in the area of mental and physical disability that insures that the client will not be segregated from the general population and made more deviant by lack of basic skills and appropriate dress and activities for age.

9. The nurse becomes an advocate for the client and the family by directing them to every resource that meets the needs of the client at each point in his life span and by providing nursing care that accents prevention, support, guidance, and teaching.

10. An advocate is also interested in the rights of the mentally retarded as a citizen, including becoming involved in the legislative process and in ethical issues that affect the client.

11. Knowledge and experience help the nurse to dispel old wives' tales and false beliefs that many people still hold and that continue to separate the retarded from the mainstream of society.

References

1. Anastasiow J: Development and Disability. Baltimore, Paul H Brookes Publishing Co, 1986
2. Baker BL, Brightman AJ, Hinshaw SP: Toward Independent Living. Champaign, IL, Research Press, 1980
3. Baroff S: Mental Retardation: Nature, Cause and Management, 2d ed. Washington, Hemisphere Publishing Corp, 1986
4. Bates B: A Guide to Physical Examination and History Taking, 4th ed. Philadelphia, JB Lippincott, 1987
5. Braddock D: Federal Assistance for Mental Retardation and Developmental Disabilities II: The Modern Era. Ment Retard 24 (August): 209–218, 1986
6. Braddock D, Fujuira G: State Government Financial Effort in Mental Retardation. Am J Ment Retard 91 (March): 450–459, 1987
7. Braddock D, Heller T: The Closure of Mental Retardation Institutions I: Trends in the United States. Ment Retard 23 (August): 168–176, 1985
8. Braddock D, Heller T: The Closure of Mental Retardation Institutions II: Implications. Ment Retard 23 (October): 222–229, 1985
9. Capute AJ: Mental Retardation. In Haslam RZ, Vallentutti PJ (eds): Medical Problems in the Classroom, pp 217–233. Baltimore, University Park Press, 1979
10. Castellani PJ, Downey NA, Tausig MB, Bird WA: Availability and Accessibility of Family Support Services. Ment Retard 24 (April): 71–79, 1986
11. Chadsey-Rusch J, Karlan GR, Riva MT, Rusch FR: Competitive Employment: Teaching Conversational Skills to Adults Who Are Mentally Retarded. Ment Retard 22 (October): 218–225, 1984
12. De la Cruz FT: Fragile X Syndrome. Am J Ment Defic 90 (September): 119–123, 1985
13. Dickey SB: A Guide to the Nursing of Children. Baltimore, Williams and Wilkins, 1987
14. Dokecki PR, Zoner RM: Ethics of Dealing with Persons with Severe Handicaps. Baltimore, Paul H. Brookes Publishing Co, 1986
15. Downey NA, Castellani PJ, Tausig MB: The Provision of Information and Referral Services in the Community. Ment Retard 23 (February): 21–25, 1985
16. Frankenberger W: A Survey of State Guidelines for Identification of Mental Retardation. Ment Retard 22 (February): 17–20, 1984
17. Frankenberger W, Harper J: Variations in Multidisciplinary Team Composition for Identifying Children with Mental Retardation. Ment Retard 24 (August): 203–207, 1986
18. Gellin MA, Geraci D: Pediatric Case Studies: A Clinical Approach. St. Louis, CV Mosby, 1985
19. Gitter MJ: Infant Stimulation Programs for the Handicapped: Rationale. In Hernandez-Logan C (ed): Care-Giving: A Multidisciplinary Approach, pp 45–49. Palo Alto, CA, RE Research Associates, 1981
20. Goldfarb LA, Brotherson MJ, Summers JA, Turnbull AP: Meeting the Challenge of Disability or Chronic Illness: A Family Guide. Baltimore, Paul H. Brookes Publishing Co, 1986
21. Goodman RM, Gorlin RJ: The Malformed Infant and Child. New York, Oxford University Press, 1983
22. Grossman HJ (ed): Manual on Terminology and Classification in Mental Retardation. Washington, DC, American Association on Mental Deficiency, 1983
23. Harel S, Anastasiow NJ (eds): The At-Risk Infant. Baltimore, Paul H. Brookes Publishing Co, 1985
24. Halburn CS: Import of a Legal Advocacy Program on Services in a State Residential Facility. Ment Retard 20 (Dec): 254–259, 1982
25. Janicki MP, Wisniewski HM: Aging and Develop-

mental Disabilities. Baltimore, Paul H. Brookes Publishing Co, 1985

26. Johnson SH: Nursing Assessment and Strategies for the Family at Risk, 2d ed. Philadelphia, JB Lippincott, 1986

27. Jones R: The Acorn People. New York, Bantam Books, 1977

28. Judkins BL, Harrison A: Nursing Practice, Education, Mental Retardation. New York, Ways of Caring, 1981

29. Kornblatt ES, Heinrich J: Needs and Coping Abilities in Families of Children and Developmental Disabilities. Ment Retard 23 (Feb): 13–19, 1985

30. Karones SB: High-Risk Newborn Infants, 4th ed. St. Louis, CV Mosby, 1986

31. Legator MS, Harper BL, Scott MJ: The Health Detective's Handbook: A Guide to the Investigation of Environmental Health Hazards by Nonprofessionals. Baltimore, Johns Hopkins University Press, 1985

32. Lewis KD, Thompson HB: Manual of School Health. Menlo Park, CA, Addison-Wesley Publishing Co., 1986

33. Lyon J: Playing God in the Nursery. New York, WW Norton and Co, 1985

34. McDonald EP: Medical Needs of Severely Developmentally Delayed Persons Residing in the Community. Am J Ment Defic 90 (September): 171–176, 1985

35. McKusick VA: Mendelian Inheritance in Man: Catalogs of Autosomal Dominant, Autosomal Recessive, and X Linked Phenotypes, 7th ed. Baltimore, Johns Hopkins University Press, 1986

36. Menolascino FJ: Challenges in Mental Retardation: Progressive Ideology and Services. New York, Human Sciences Press, 1977

37. Mercer R: The Nurse and Maternal Tasks of Early Postpartum. MCN 6 (Sept–Oct): 341–345, 1981

38. Nelson NP, Beckel J: Nursing Care Plans for the Pediatric Patient. St. Louis, CV Mosby, 1987

39. O'Neil SM, McLaughlin BN, Knapp MB: Behavioral Approaches to Children with Developmental Delay. St. Louis, CV Mosby, 1977

40. Powel TH, Ogle PA: Brothers and Sisters: A Special Part of Exceptional Families. Baltimore, Paul H. Brookes Publishing Co, 1985

41. Pueschel SM, Tingey C, Rynders JE, Crocker AC, Crutcher DM: New Perspectives on Down Syndrome. Baltimore, Paul H. Brookes Publishing Co, 1987

42. Reiss S, Benson BA: Psychosocial Correlates of Depression in Mentally Retarded Adults I: Minimal Social Support and Stigmatation. Am J Ment Defic 89 (Jan): 331–337, 1985

43. Rogers RC, Simensen RJ: Fragile X Syndrome: A Common Etiology of Mental Retardation. Ment Retard 91 (Mar): 445–449, 1987

44. Sattler JM: Assessment of Children's Intelligence and Special Abilities, 2d ed. Boston, Allyn and Bacon, 1982

45. Schulman ED: Focus on the Retarded Adult Programs and Services. St. Louis, CV Mosby, 1980

46. Separation of Retarded Inmates Urged. Fort Worth Star Telegram, Section 1, p 13A, Dec 22, 1981

47. Smith W: Recognizable Patterns of Human Malformation. Philadelphia, WB Saunders, 1982

48. Spreat S, Telles JL, Conroy JW, Feinstein C, Colombatto JJ: Attitudes Toward Deinstitutionalization: National Survey of Families of Institutionalized Persons with Mental Retardation. Ment Retard 25 (October): 267–274, 1987

49. Szymanski LS: Prevention of Psychosocial Dysfunction in Persons with Mental Retardation. Ment Retard 25 (August): 215–218, 1987

50. Szymanski LS, Biederman J: Depression and Anorexia Nervosa with Down Syndrome. Am J Ment Defic 89 (November): 246–251, 1984

51. Tausig N: Factors in Family Decision-Making About Placement for Developmentally Disabled Individuals. Am J Ment Defic 89 (January): 352–361, 1985

52. Tesini DA: Providing Dental Services for Citizens with Handicaps: A Prototype Community Program. Ment Retard 25 (Aug): 219–222, 1987

53. Turnbull AP, Summers JA, Brotherson MJ: Family Life Cycle. In Gallagher JJ, Vietze PM (eds): Families of Handicapped Persons Research Programs, and Policy Issues, pp 45–65, Baltimore, Paul H. Brookes Publishing Co, 1986

54. Urban H, Schassar L, Rogers C, Kirkpatrick N: Meeting the Nutritional Needs of the Multiply Handicapped, p 11–12. Buffalo, United Cerebral Palsy Association of Western New York, 1981

55. Williamson GG: Children with Spina Bifida. Baltimore, Paul H. Brookes Publishing Co, 1987

31 Organic Mental Disorder

Cheryl Steudtner Detwiler

It is no easy matter to accept that one is growing old, and no one succeeds in doing it without first overcoming his spontaneous refusal. It is difficult, too, to accept the growing old of someone else, of one's nearest and dearest. That of a mother whose kindness, welcome and understanding used to seem inexhaustible, and with whom one begins to hesitate to share one's intimate confidences, because they no longer arouse in her the warm, lively echo they used to. The aging of a father whose judgment and advice always used to seem so sound, but whom one can no longer consult because he must not be worried, or because his faculties are failing. The aging of a friend to whom one no longer talks as one used to, because it would be necessary to shout out loud things that used to be said quite quietly. It is hard to accept the decay of conversation into banality, empty optimism and insignificance.

Paul Tournier,
Learn to Grow Old,
1972

Chapter Preview

This chapter presents those mental disorders that are attributed to a dysfunctioning or diseased brain. The effects of the various disorders are considered in terms of their incidence and occurrence in the general population. Etiologic factors and clinical manifestations of the organic mental disorders are discussed. Nursing interventions, as derived from the application of the nursing process, are provided, with the ultimate goal of achieving optimal care for people affected by these disorders and for their families.

Learning Objectives

On completion of this chapter, you should be able to accomplish the following:

1. define organic mental disorders
2. discuss the incidence and significance of organic mental disorders
3. compare the possible etiologies of the organic mental disorders
4. identify the behaviors associated with various organic mental disorders
5. apply the steps of the nursing process—assessment, nursing diagnosis, planning, intervention, evaluation—to clients with organic mental disorders

Defining Organic Mental Disorders

The classification *organic mental disorders* encompasses those abnormal psychological or behavioral signs and symptoms whose origins lie in an identified cerebral disease or dysfunction. This is a fairly recent classification; previously, there was no real differentiation between the psychotic behavior of a person with an intact, healthy brain and the psychotic behavior of a person with a pathophysiologically impaired brain. It has now become evident that a person with a dysfunctioning, diseased, or injured brain can manifest the same morbid psychological phenomena as the person with a functional psychiatric disorder who is believed to have a physiologically healthy brain.

The critical difference in the two similarly manifested clinical syndromes is that, in an organic mental disorder, the disturbed behavior is secondary to the brain's transient or permanent dysfunctioning or diseased state, not a primary functional problem in and of itself. The key to the diagnosis of these disorders lies in the tangible proof, obtained from the clinical history, physical examination, or laboratory findings, that there exists an organic problem affecting the brain tissue, or that by description an organic brain syndrome is present.[2] This organic factor may be a primary disease of the brain, a systemic influence originating in another body system, or an exogenous substance that is either currently affecting the brain tissue or that has left some residual, chronic deficit.

Collecting the data for a definitive diagnosis of an organic mental disorder is difficult, but the implications for treatment make it imperative. When a person with an organic disorder is treated as if he had a functional disorder, the assumption of the therapist is that the brain is an intact, healthy organ when, in fact, it is not.[37] This individual cannot respond nor can he be expected to respond to the therapy in the same manner.

In some situations an individual with an organic mental disorder who is demonstrating maladaptive behavior as a result of that malady may exhibit further psychotic behavior as an emotional reaction to the organic mental disease. In this case, the ensuing disturbed behavior is a result of two disorders, one functional and one organic. This is not an uncommon finding, but it is a complex problem that necessitates the laborious procedure of collecting and sifting data to support the diagnosis of an organic mental disorder. This differentiation must be done to initiate valid medical treatment of potentially correctable disorders.[37]

Incidence and Significance of Organic Mental Disorders

The mental health community is becoming increasingly aware of the presence of organic mental disorders, stemming from the increasing occurrence of these disorders in the mushrooming geriatric population, in the chronic-disease-survivor population, and in the population of acute-care facilities. More than one million persons, or 5% of the American population over the age of 65 years, are affected significantly enough by the dementia of organic mental disease to deter independent living. This means that 60% of the residents of nursing homes manifest organic mental disease. In addition, another 10% of the American population over 65 years of age is so affected by intellectual impairment that only semi-independent living is possible.[14] Twenty percent of the first admissions to psychiatric hospitals enter with the diagnosis of organic mental disorder, and another 40% of the chronically hospitalized have that diagnosis.

Medical intervention that has prolonged the lives of those requiring critical care and the lives of those with chronic diseases has also created a completely new entity of cerebral damage and dysfunction, which are iatrogenic realities. Systemic metabolic disturbances originating in the cardiovascular, respiratory, or renal systems may affect the homeostasis of the brain. Drug therapies, antineoplastic therapies, and post-trauma resuscitation are therapeutic modalities utilized by the increasingly sophisticated medical community, and these modalities result in a rising psychiatric morbidity.[16] Although there is now an awareness of this psychopathology in the survivors of the intensive-critical/chronic-care treatment regime, at this point, little has been done in terms of investigation to document the magnitude of the problem.[14,37]

Etiologic Factors

By definition, organic disorders must be shown to be the result of the following:

1. A primary brain disease
2. The brain's response to the influences of systemic disturbances
3. The brain tissue's unique reaction to an exogenous substance
4. The residual effects of, or withdrawal of, an exogenous substance.[2]

Table 31-1 gives examples of etiologic factors in each category of disorder.

The etiologic factor responsible for the disorder may indicate the potential for the acuteness or chronicity of the organic mental disorder. Previously, the terms *acute brain syndrome* and *chronic brain syndrome* were applied to individuals with organic mental disorders. Because the terms *acute* and *chronic* became erroneously synonymous with the prognostications of reversible and irreversible, these terms are hesitatingly applied to a client with organic mental disorder. There is value, however, in ascertaining the etiologic factor. If, for example, the factor can be eliminated from the individual's system, there is a possibility for a more favorable prognosis. In time, the symptoms may disappear altogether or, at least, their progression may halt.

It is not to be assumed that any list of plausible etiologic factors actually exhausts the possible reasons for the development of organic mental disorders. Recognition must be given to the interplay between the physical and the sociopsychological components of an individual that helps to establish, maintain, or destroy his mental homeostasis. Portnoi, working with the data obtained from Wang, has schematically diagrammed the dynamics of the interactions among the physical, psychological, and sociological spheres (see Fig. 31-1).[27,36] The discerning practitioner will consider all of these factors when determining the etiologic elements of the client's disorder.

Primary Brain Disease

This category incorporates those indigenous diseases and factors that pathologically affect the brain tissue. Table 31-1 indicates many of the known specific diseases or factors that produce an organic mental disorder.

Organic Brain Syndrome. Also included in this category are the organic brain syndromes. They are traditionally included in the category of organic disorders, although proof of their existence lies only in the description of their presence rather than in tangible proof of an organic etiology. An organic factor is assumed to be the underlying etiology of the disorder and, consequently, tangible proof is not required. (This is an exception to the qualifying definition of organic mental disease.) Should an organic etiology be proven, the organic descriptor is dropped and the etiologic factor is substituted; that is, organic delirium syndrome may become alcoholic delirium syndrome.

The organic brain syndromes are categorized into the following six groups:

1. Delirium and dementia
2. Amnestic syndrome and organic hallucinosis
3. Organic delusional syndrome and organic affective syndrome
4. Organic personality syndrome
5. Intoxication and withdrawal
6. Atypical or mixed organic brain syndrome

These may also result from other factors; for example, from a systemic metabolic disturbance affecting the whole organism.[2]

Wernicke-Korsakoff Syndrome. One example of the organic brain syndrome, or amnestic syndrome, is the Wernicke-Korsakoff syndrome. Although it is also seen in hospitalized patients with chronic intravenous therapy, in the United States this syndrome is more commonly seen in chronic alcoholics whose compulsion for ingestion of alcohol supersedes the need for nutritional intake.[19] This syndrome is usually found in the 40- to 70-year-old alcoholic with a steady and progressive intake of alcohol. In time, this individual develops a vitamin B_1 (thiamin) deficiency that directly interferes with the production of the brain's main nutrient, glucose.[18]

Table 31-1.   **Etiology of Organic Mental Disorders**

Primary brain disease	Cerebral hypoxia/vascular spasms Congenital dysfunction/birth defects Dementias: Alzheimer's, Pick's Huntington's chorea Infections: meningitis, encephalitis, German measles Intracranial tumors Irritation from blood breakdown products Neurosyphilis Normal pressure hydrocephalus Trauma: hematoma		Pituitary Electrolyte imbalance Stress: pain/fear/fever Sleep/sensory deprivation Abnormal reactions to drugs

		Exogenous substances	Heavy metals
			  Lead
			  Mercury
			  Manganese
			Tranquilizers
			  Diazepam (Valium)
			  Chlordiazepoxide (Librium)
			Anticholinergics
			  Atropine
			  Scopolamine
			Sedatives/Hypnotics
			Barbiturates
			Antihistamines
			Substance abuse
			  Marijuana
			  Phencyclidine (PCP)
			  Cocaine
			  Opium derivatives
			  Amphetamines
			  Alcohol
			Hallucinogenics
			Digoxin
			Antihypertensives
			  Aldomet
			Parkinson drugs
			  Amantadine (Symmetrel)
			  Benztropine mesylate (Cogentin)
			  Trihexphenidyl hydrochloride (Artane)
			  Leva-dopa
			Antidepressants

Systemic disturbances	Infections
	  Systemic
	  Respiratory: pneumonia, atelectasis
	  Cardiac: rheumatic fever, subacute bacterial endocarditis
	  Immunodeficiency: acquired immune deficiency syndrome
	Surgery
	  Hypoxia from anesthesia
	  Cardiac (decreased cardiac output), cerebral emboli
	  Transurethral resection
	Organ failure
	  Renal
	  Hepatic > toxin build-up
	  Cardiac: congestive heart failure
	Nutritional deficiencies
	  Vitamins-thiamin: Wernicke-Korsakoff nicotinic acid
	Metabolic imbalance
	  Thyroid
	  Pancreas
	  Parathyroid
	  Adrenal		

		Withdrawal/residual effects of exogenous substances	Potential exists for any of the drugs listed in the above category

Dementia. *Dementia* is a term describing clinical behavior that manifests itself in the insidious development of the following:

1. Memory deficit
2. Intellectual deficit
3. Disorientation
4. Decreased cognitive functioning[13]

Dementias arising in the senium (after 65 years of age) or the presenium (before 65 years of age) constitute a significant portion of the primary brain disease from the organic brain syndrome dementia, in that there is some tangible proof of their organic etiology.

Alzheimer's Disease. The most characteristic disease of the senile dementias is Alzheimer's disease, which is seen twice as frequently in women as in men. This disease has an unknown etiology, although noteworthy findings have generated several theories. Physiological studies indicating that there are degenerative changes in the cholinergic neurons and biochemical changes involving the biosynthetic enzyme for acetylcholine give credence to an etiology of a neurotransmitter deficiency.[5] Also, higher than normal amounts of aluminum deposits have been detected in the brains of Alzheimer's diseased patients. These deposits may be a cause, or a result, of the disease. Other studies have shown an abnormally high titer of antibodies present in Alzheimer's patients, giving rise to the question of whether the disease is a result of an immunological defect. A higher incidence of Alzheimer's has been associated with adult Down syndrome patients and also with close relatives of Alzheimer's patients, leading to the theory that there may be some chromosomal defect involved in the disease's etiology. Finally, serious head injury victims have a reported greater propensity to develop Alzheimer's than their counterparts, making tissue injury suspect as a predisposing factor to the disease.[33] Ninety-six percent of the individuals affected with Alzheimer's disease are over the age of 40, and 10% of the American population over the age of 65 is affected with this disease to some degree.[32] Amazingly, Alzheimer's disease accounts for 80% of the dementias of old age.[22]

The microscopic findings of senile plaques and neurofibrillary tangles present in the brains of individuals with Alzheimer's disease closely resemble the pathological changes documented in the individual whose brain exhibits "normal aging." This resemblance is so close that differentiation between the disease state of the brain in Alzheimer's disease and the state of the brain in normal aging is not always substantiated in the histological findings at autopsy. Sometimes, the disease can be substantiated only by the documented aberrant behaviors of the individual.

Pick's Disease.   Another senile degenerative dementia resembling Alzheimer's disease, although oc-

curring less frequently, is Pick's disease. This disease occurs equally in males and females who are in their early to mid-50's. The actual cause of the disease is unknown, but it is suspected that there are genetic tendencies. The general microscopic findings include atrophies of the frontal and temporal portions of the brain. Why these atrophies occur is not clearly understood but they are believed to be associated with the aberrant behaviors seen in Pick's disease.[32]

Multi-Infarct Dementia.   Another dementia seen in the senium is multi-infarct dementia. This is a primary disease of the vascular system of the brain. Although atherosclerosis may be an accompanying factor, the main pathology results from multiple infarcts occurring throughout the brain as a result of numerous occlusions within the smaller cerebral arteries. Extensive destruction of brain tissue occurs and, when the infarcts collectively produce a minimum of 50 grams of tissue destruction, the signs and symptoms of this particular dementia appear.[14] Individuals with multi-infarct dementia often have a history of either hypertension or diabetes.[30]

Huntington's Chorea.   Huntington's chorea is an example of a dementia occurring in the presenium. It is a familial disease that is passed on through the genes by an autosomal dominant trait. Huntington's chorea manifests itself in individuals between the ages of 45 and 55 years. The clinical history is the most reliable

(Text continues on p. 610)

Figure 31-1.   *Factors leading to dementia.* (From Portnoi V: Diagnostic Dilemma of the Aged. Arch Intern Med [May] 734–737, 1981)

C H A R T   31-1
Organic Mental Disorders and AIDS

Karen R. Perkins, M.S.N., R.N.
Clinical Nurse Specialist/Clinic Manager, Outpatient Psychiatry
Parkland Memorial Hospital
Dallas, Texas

AIDS (Acquired Immune Deficiency Syndrome), ARC (AIDS Related Complex), HIV (Human Immunodeficient Virus) positive; these terms do not begin to indicate the profound impact that these diagnoses generate on a personal, medical, political/legal, societal and economic level. At this time, most AIDS patients are homosexual and bisexual males and intravenous drug users. This is a population that is already greatly stigmatized. Such widespread opprobrium, coupled with the general misunderstanding and mass hysteria surrounding AIDS and related HIV positive diagnoses, greatly increases the challenge of providing adequate, much less optimal, health care for this group of patients. Even those patients viewed by society as "innocent victims," *e.g.*, hemophiliacs, blood product recipients, and infants born HIV positive, are often treated with the same irrational fears and discrimination generally reserved for the gay and IV drug user population.

Because AIDS, ARC, and HIV positive patients can develop such a wide variety of associated diseases and medical problems, all fields of medicine will encounter these patients in increasing numbers. Consequently, whether a nurse practices in surgery, general medicine, dermatology, maternal-child, emergency, psychiatry, public health, addictions nursing or any of the myriad other nursing specialties, AIDS and HIV positive patients will compromise a certain portion of a nurse's caseload. Therefore, just as diagnosed patients must come to terms with the implications of their diagnoses, so must nurses develop a universal but personalized *concept* of AIDS. A personal concept of AIDS includes working toward "coming to terms" with one's own feelings and fears concerning homosexuality, drug users, death, and the rage and sense of impotence that often accompanies working with patients who have a life-altering, and ultimately fatal, disease.

Integral to a concept of AIDS is an understanding of the prevalence of neuropsychiatric problems associated with AIDS and AIDS-spectrum disorders. So common is the presence of neuropsychiatric disease (which includes both CNS disease states and organic mental disorders) that recently the CDC's official criteria for establishing a diagnosis of AIDS has been expanded to include recognition of this fact. Prior to August 1987, AIDS was primarily diagnosed following the development of Kaposi's sarcoma or *Pneumocystis carinii* pneumonia in an HIV positive patient. Now, AIDS may be diagnosed in an HIV positive patient on the basis of "clinical findings of disabling cognitive and/or motor dysfunction interfering with occupation or activities of daily living, or loss of behavioral developmental milestones affecting a child, progressing over weeks to months in the absence of a concurrent illness or condition other than HIV infection that could explain the findings."

Neuropsychiatric symptoms may range from barely perceptible changes in a person's normal psychological presentation to profound dementia. Nurses must be familiar with and able to recognize signs of organic mental disorders (OMD) and be able to differentiate these signs from the functional reactions expected in patients who are diagnosed with a terminal and socially denigrated disease such as AIDS. Estimates concerning the percentage of AIDS patients who will develop a discernible neurological syndrome during the course of their illness range from 40% to 70%. Autopsy studies provide even greater evidence of CNS disease by time of death. In approximately 10% of all who test HIV positive a neurological syndrome may be the first manifestation that a person has been infected with HIV. Opportunistic infections in the central nervous system account for approximately 80% of all CNS disease processes in AIDS and ARC patients; CNS neoplasms account for less than 10%. A significant portion of CNS infections are treatable but require rapid, accurate diagnosis and aggressive and prolonged treatment. Even so, relapse and death, rather than recovery, are the norm. Current evidence strongly indicates that HIV is neurotropic and may itself be responsible for acute and chronic encephalitis and meningitis. It may also be the major cause of subacute encephalitis/dementia syndrome as well as myelopathy and neuropathy in AIDS-related syndrome patients.

Organic mental disorders, both acute and chronic, are overly represented in AIDS and ARC patients. Delirium is the major acute organic mental disorder and dementia is the most common chronic organic mental disorder seen in these patients. Organic affective and organic personality syndromes are not infrequently encountered. The longer a patient is sick and is plagued with opportunistic infections, the greater the probability that he/she will develop some form of organic mental disorder.

A primary nursing responsibility is to be able to recognize signs of delirium and dementia and to assure that a patient receives a prompt medical work-up for the precipitating cause. This may well include a referral to a psychiatrist who is conversant with the often difficult diagnostic dilemmas presented by these patients. Depending upon the etiology of the organic mental disorder, treatment recommendations and patient management will differ. It is always important that a baseline of mental status be established and that it be recorded for future comparison. Patients should be questioned as to difficulties with recent memory, language, and motor and integrative functions. Initial impairment may be so subtle that a patient may not be aware of problems but others close to the patient may, and they should also be interviewed. Once a baseline is established, periodic mental status assessment should be routinely accomplished, documented and checked against previous mental status documentation. Any change in status needs to be assessed by appropriate personnel, and treatment plans should be changed to reflect this new knowledge.

The health management of AIDS and AIDS-related syndrome patients should be mul-tidisciplinary in scope and practice. It is very often the nurse who coordinates the treatment team's efforts to provide comprehensive health care services to the AIDS patient and his/her significant others. Patient management programs developed for Alzheimer's patients can prove to be very helpful in developing a plan for organic mental disorder AIDS patient management from a nursing perspective. Patients with organic mental disorder are often considered difficult and time and resource intensive. Not all health professionals find working with this population to be exciting or rewarding. When AIDS confounds the picture, even fewer willingly accept the challenges of working with this population. Elizabeth Kubler-Ross closes her book, *AIDS: the ultimate challenge,* with this poignant challenge:

> *AIDS poses its own threat to mankind, but unlike war, it is a battle from within, knowing no borders or national boundaries. Are we going to choose hate and discrimination, or will we have the courage to choose love and service? Yes, I truly believe that AIDS is the ultimate challenge for all of us. Choose wisely, take the highest road you can, so that you will have no regrets at the end.*

> *Blessings to all of you who are willing to serve and to love unconditionally.*

Think about this challenge when developing a personalized concept of AIDS. If ever there was a disease that is nursing intensive and calls for the very best that nursing has to offer, AIDS is it.

References

1. Centers for Disease Control. Revision of the CDC Surveillance Case Definition for Acquired Immunodeficiency Syndrome. MMWR 1987;36(suppl no. 1S:S3-S15).
2. Durham, J., Cohen, F. *The Person with AIDS: Nursing Perspectives.* Springer Publishers, New York. 1987.
3. McKusick, L. *What To Do About AIDS: Physicians and Mental Health Professionals Discuss the Issues.* University of California Press, Berkeley. 1986.
4. Kubler-Ross, E., *AIDS: The Ultimate Challenge.* McMillan Publishing Co. 1987.

diagnostic finding, although at autopsy the brain is seen to have frontal cerebral atrophy. Research laboratory findings suggest that this disease may be the result of biochemical changes within the brain cells.[37]

Systemic Disturbances

Organic mental disorders can be a direct result of the brain's response to a systemic problem present in the individual. It is not always possible to predict the tissue's response to a systemic imbalance, especially because the individual's vulnerability may be heavily influenced by the environmental stress factors that are bombarding him. Although the causes of such systemic disturbances are almost infinite, a partial listing is found in Table 31-1.

Exogenous Substances

The inventory of those substances that may precipitate an organic mental disorder is almost limitless. The problem is compounded when more than one element is present; by itself, an exogenous substance may be innocuous, but when in the presence of, or in combination with, another substance, it may become noxious. Table 31-1 gives a partial listing of these exogenous substances.

Residual Effects and Withdrawal of Exogenous Substances

The aftermath of exogenous substances can be more devastating than their initial effect. The withdrawal of an exogenous substance may produce unique physiological responses within the neuronal structures of the brain. Accordingly, when the acute response to the substance subsides, the remaining chronic deficits may be more deleterious than the initial ones. The reaction to the absence of an exogenous substance may be seen clinically as one of the organic mental disorders.

Behaviors Associated with Organic Mental Disorders

The behavioral manifestations associated with organic mental disorders are many and varied. There are no essential features predictably present in every patient. Frequently, the most significant behavioral problems are due to the individual's emotional reactions when he becomes aware of the cognitive deficits resulting from an organic mental disorder.[2]

Behavior is the response of the individual as he adjusts to continual changes in his internal and external environment. The physiological soundness of the brain is a necessary ingredient for the successful adaptation of human behavior to these changes. When the organic integrity of the brain is interrupted or interfered with, maladaptive behavior will often follow.[37] This is the essence of what is seen in an individual with an organic mental disorder. Some of the disorders, especially the dementias, have commonalities of behavior, but this is not true of most of the acute brain disorders (see Chart 31-2).

Generally, the behavioral dysfunctions seen in organic mental disorders can be grouped into either global impairment of intellectual functions or limited impairment of intellectual functions.[22] The behavioral aberrations of organic mental disorders include deficits in the following areas:

1. Sensorium
2. Attention
3. Orientation
4. Perceptions
5. Memory capabilities[36]

Sensorium and Attention Deficits

Deficits in the sensorium stem from the individual's inability to use the information collected by his five senses to discern his environment. If this discernment does not take place, the individual experiences confusion that affects his attentiveness to the environment and, ultimately, his level of consciousness. As the level of consciousness decreases, the individual also develops an inability to concentrate on any specific event. His attention span decreases and he becomes highly distractible.

Disorientation

Disorientation occurs when an individual is hampered from successfully receiving and centrally integrating the data obtained from his internal and external environments. When the sensory inputs falls below the individual's minimum need requirements, and when the brain is affected structurally in such a way that it can no longer perceive and interpret the stimuli adequately, decreased orientation results. The disoriented individual does not know where he is, how he came to be where he is, why he is there, or how he fits into the environmental milieu.

Perceptual Disturbance

Frequently, the individual with an acute organic mental disorder will experience the perceptual abnormalities of illusions and hallucinations. (These behaviors are described in detail in Chap. 24.)

Memory Deficit

Memory disturbances are the most frequently found deficits in organic mental disorders. Recent memory

CHART 31-2
Aberrant Behaviors Associated with Organic Mental Disorders

Alzheimer's Disease

Cognitive: Global (or general) intellectual impairment of insidious onset ranging (initially) from "mistakes in judgment" to inability to comprehend to (finally) agraphia, aphasia, and ultimately unresponsiveness

Level of consciousness: No clouding until late in disease

Memory: Initially memory losses of recent vintage, gradually memory losses incorporating both recent and remote events

Appearance: Initially may not be affected, gradually poor grooming due to forgotten social behaviors and decreased coordination required to dress

Emotional: Depression and anxiety over recognized regression to (finally), loss or severe dampening of emotions; subtle loss of interest in work or family to (finally) loss of skills to do work and inability to recognize family members

Pick's Disease

Cognitive: Intellect intact; lack of insight into the disease process

Level of Consciousness: Not affected

Appearance: Slovenly

Emotional: Dramatic personality changes; socially inappropriate behavior; flip beyond reasonable propriety

Multi-Infarct Dementia

Focal signs dependent upon area involved; usually abrupt onset of symptoms resembling a stroke

Huntington's Chorea

Cognitive: Insight into the psychological deteriorative changes

Appearance: Choreiform movements; sloppy

Emotional: Moody; from apathy to aggressive behavior, inappropriate; despair over changes taking place; suicidal; decreased interest in job

Wernicke-Korsakoff Syndrome

Cognitive: Cannot learn new information because cannot retain facts

Level of Consciousness: Alert

Memory: Suspended in time; no memory prior to 2 to 3 minutes before this moment; extensive memory loss

Appearance: Unsteady gait due to peripheral neuropathies

Communication: Use of confabulation to supply information lost in recent memory gaps.

---

impairment is the most common finding in this disorder; however, remote memory may sometimes be impaired. The inability to register, retain, and retrieve accumulated information is one of the key clinical manifestations of organic mental disorders and may affect the intellectual capability of the individual.[36]

Disorientation and recent memory impairment must be present to confirm the diagnosis of *acute organic mental disorder*. These behaviors, in combination with any of the others described, often appear in a fluctuating manner, waxing and waning in severity from hour to hour or day to day. Empirically, the aberrant behaviors worsen during the hours after sunset, termed the *sundowning effect*.[29] The nurse on night shift will frequently report that the individual mistook hospital personnel for a brother or sister, hallucinated, or became frankly combative.[10]

Degenerative Impairments

Many of the organic mental disorders with a chronic dimension tend to have behavioral manifestations that are predictively associated with their degenerative nature, especially if an irreversible pathology is a known part of the disease progress. None of the organic mental disorders should be isolated and typed initially as acute, chronic, reversible, or irreversible. Any of these disorders may encompass acute, chronic, reversible, and irreversible features or evolve into them. Labeling may negatively influence attempts of the health team to help the client and family. The terminology of chronic and irreversible should be applied only in those disorders, such as Alzheimer's disease, whose known degenerative pathology is an established medical fact.

Many of the degenerative organic mental disorders are difficult to diagnose initially. The impairments that occur are global in nature and the intellectual deterioration is often artfully concealed by the well-preserved social skills of the individual.[22] Nevertheless, some of the symptoms of the diseases listed in Chart 31-2 are worth noting.

Application of the Nursing Process to Clients with Organic Mental Disorders

The nurse may participate in facilitating the recovery of, or improving the quality of life for, a client with an organic mental disorder. The nursing process of assessment, nursing diagnosis, planning, intervention, and evaluation is discussed as it is applied to the care of individuals with organic mental disorders.

The first step in determining treatment and nursing approaches for this client is a clinical screening for any treatable physical causes of the problem. This involves an extensive history-taking, physical examination, and laboratory work-up. Laboratory and diagnostic evaluation of the client often includes the tests listed in Table 31-2.

When the results of the screening tests prove to be noncontributory, the physician may look to other, more subjective factors. Is the client a victim of sleep and sensory deprivation or overload? Is the client experiencing pain? Is the client postoperative? Is he experiencing an inordinate amount of stress and anxiety from personal losses? Any or all of these elements may be the causative culprit(s) in the disorder. When the contributing factors are determined, they must be aggressively treated or, if possible, eliminated.

Assessment

The nursing assessment of a client with an organic mental disorder focuses on the present behavior of the client. The client's family is one of the most reliable resources for information about his behavior, because he may not know when the behavior began or have insight into its sequential progression. The nurse gathers and compiles behavioral reports because the client's disruptive behavior may at first be overlooked by the family or regarded as an idiosyncrasy or crankiness due to "old age."

The nurse attempts to break down the component parts of the client's behavior and assess how deficient or intact each component is. Intellectual or cognitive deficits may be assessed by the use of the short,

portable mental status questionnaire (SPMSQ) developed by Pfeiffer (see Chart 31-3). The nurse observes and documents the client's level of consciousness and his sensorium. The amount of stimulation it takes to elicit a response from the client is also to be assessed. This stimulation may range from simply calling the client's name in a normal tone of voice to vigorously shaking him and shouting his name. The attention span of an individual may be appraised by asking him to repeat six or seven digits forward, or by asking him to cross out all the "a's" he finds in a paragraph he is asked to read. Failure to perform tasks such as these indicates that the client is probably having difficulty concentrating.

Information concerning perceptual disorders may be gained by direct observation of the client's behavior and by asking him about any strange or unusual feelings or sensory experiences that he has mentioned. The family may also be able to contribute information about observing such behavior or hearing the client voluntarily express concerns about the "bugs," "roaches," and so forth that he sees.

The assessment includes an evaluation of the client's orientation to his person, environment, time, and date. Simply asking the client for this information by means of the questions "Who are you?" "Where are you?" and "What are you doing here?" will provide the needed data. The family of the client should also be questioned to ascertain if the client experiences the "sunset effect"; that is, decreased orientation with the onset of the evening hours.

Those who are living with the client or who are in daily contact with him will be able to provide much information concerning his ability to take care of himself and his personal affairs. The social interaction that takes place between the family and the client should be observed and described; it will reveal many of the client's present social assets and deficits.

The nurse spends time with the client to determine the quality of his communication efforts. Many of his social skills may remain long after the intellectual deterioration takes place. Social behavior is usually deeply ingrained by the time adulthood is reached. When talking, people give many verbal clues to one another that indicate the proper response. For example, clues such as nodding and smiling indicate a positive atmosphere in which a reciprocal nod or smile is appropriate. It is a kind of mindless, learned response. For this reason, the nurse needs to ask the client questions that solicit more than a "yes" or "no" response.

The client's memory is also evaluated during the nursing assessment. Incidents evoking remote memory are usually easy to elicit from the client. Recent

Table 31-2. **Screening Tests**

TEST	CLINICAL IMPORTANCE
1. WBC with differential	1. Infection
2. Sedimentation rate	2. Infection or vasculitis
3. Urine exam and toxicology test	
a. Sugar & acetone	a. Diabetes
b. Leukocytes	b. Infection
c. Barbiturates and other toxic substances	c. Toxicity
d. Albumin	d. Renal failure
e. Porphyria screen	e. Renal failure
4. Serum tests	
a. Blood urea nitrogen	a. Renal failure
b. Creatinine	b. Renal failure
c. Sugar	c. Diabetes, hypoglycemia
d. T_3, T_4	d. Thyroid disease
e. Electrolytes	e. Evaluation for imbalance including Na^+, K^+, Ca^{++}, Cl^-, $PO_4^=$, parathyroid-induced changes in calcium, phosphorus
f. Mg^+, Br^+	f. If available, bromides are still present in some common drugs and overuse may inadvertently lead to toxicity
g. Serum folate level Vitamin B_{12} level	g. Nutritional problems, thiamine deficiency
h. SGOT, SGPT	h. Liver failure
i. VDRL	i. Syphilis
j. Drug levels—specific search for evidence of drugs—ETOH, etc	j. Barbiturate, other drug overdose
5. X-rays, routine	
a. Chest	a. Infection, heart failure
b. Skull	b. Evidence of increased intracranial pressure, fractures, etc.
6. EEG	6. Ictal phenomenon
7. CT scan	7. Brain tumor, subdural hematoma, infection, hemorrhage
8. Spinal tap	8. Infection, hemorrhage
9. Invasive neuroradiologic procedures	9. Suspicion of tumors, vascular lesions, hydrocephalus

(From Staub R and Black F: Organic Brain Syndromes pp 109–110. Philadelphia, FA Davis, 1981)

memory, however, may be assessed by the client's response to questions that ask for the recall of the events of the previous day or week. Assessing these components of the client's behavior and then analyzing the information help the nurse lay a foundation of understanding of the client problem and a basis for nursing care planning (Chart 31-4).

Nursing Diagnosis

There are as many nursing diagnoses for the client suffering from organic mental disorders as there are possibilities of symptomatology. Although nursing diagnoses must reflect the uniqueness of each client, a plan of care might include some of the following:

CHART 31-3
Short, Portable Mental Status Questionnaire (SPMSQ)

Instructions:
   Ask questions 1 through 10 in this list and record all answers.
   Ask question 4A only if patient does not have a telephone.
   Record total number of errors based on 10 questions.

+   −   1.   What is the date today?_____
                                             Month   Day   Year

         2.   What day of the week is it?_____

         3.   What is the name of this place?_____

         4.   What is your telephone number?_____

      4A.   What is your street address?_____
                  (Ask only if patient does not have a telephone)

         5.   How old are you?_____

         6.   When were you born?_____

         7.   Who is the President of the U.S. now?_____

         8.   Who was President just before him?_____

         9.   What was your mother's maiden name?_____

        10.   Subtract 3 from 20 and keep subtracting 3 from each new
                  number you get all the way down

For white subjects with at least some high school education, but no
more than high school education, the following criteria have been established:

   0–2 errors   Intact intellectual functioning
   3–4 errors   Mild intellectual impairment
   5–7 errors   Moderate intellectual impairment
   8–10 errors   Severe intellectual impairment

(From Pfeiffer E: A Short Portable Mental Status Questionnaire for the Assessment of
Organic Brain Deficit in Elderly Patients. J Am Geriatr Soc [Oct]: 433–441, 1975)

1.   Thought processes, alteration in, related to decreased ability to interpret external stimuli

2.   Violence, potential for: self-directed related to awareness of mental deterioration

3.   Social interaction, impaired related to inability to employ effective communication

4.   Self-care deficit: dressing/grooming related to deficit in motor skills that enable hygienic tasks to be accomplished

5.   Powerlessness: related to inability to halt the debilitating progress of the disorder/disease

6.   Coping, ineffective family: disabling related to financial and spiritual bankruptcy by the relentlessness of the disease's/disorder's debilitating progress

7.   Injury, potential for related to lack of retention of any memory for personal actions maintaining personal safety

8.   Self-concept, disturbance in: role performance related to inability to maintain mental acuity defined by role in work performance and family position

Planning

When the design for care is constructed, a necessary ingredient is the involvement of members of client's family, which usually includes the spouse and the adult children of the client. If the client's prognosis is, realistically, that of continued degeneration, family

Assessment Guide

I. Subjective Data
A. Behavioral changes (often asked of the family)
1. Is there a change in the behavior? If so,
a. How does the present behavior differ from former behavior?
b. When was this change in behavior first recognized?
B. Emotional changes
1. Are any of the following present?
a. Depression
b. Anxiety
c. Paranoia
d. Agitation
e. Grandiosity
f. Confabulation
2. Does the client have insight into the fact that "things are not right"?
3. Is the client complaining of many physical ailments for which there are no bases?
4. Are certain previous personality traits becoming predominant or exaggerated?
C. Social changes
1. Is the client exhibiting embarrassingly loud and jocular behavior?
2. Is there sexual acting-out beyond the bounds of propriety?
3. Have the following developed?
a. Short-temperedness
b. Irritability
c. Aggressiveness
4. Is there an increasing inability to make social judgments?
D. Intellectual behavior
1. Has the ability to remember recent events decreased?
2. Has the ability to problem-solve decreased? (This might be especially apparent in the work or job area.)
3. Do new environments or even old environments result in the client's disorientation?
4. Is it difficult for the client to carry out complex motor skills? Do his efforts result in many errors?
5. Are any of the following language problems present:
a. Has the language changed?
b. Does the language ramble and wander from the point of the conversation?
c. Is the point of the conversation never clearly stated?
d. Is there difficulty comprehending complex material?

e. Does the client have trouble remembering names of people and objects?
f. Does the client have difficulty writing?

II. Objective Observations
A. Level of consciousness
1. Is the client confused, sleepy, withdrawn, adynamic, apathetic?
B. Appearance
1. Is there decreased personal hygiene?
C. Attention
1. Does the client have decreased ability to repeat digits after the interviewer?
2. Do other stimuli in the environment easily distract the client from the interviewer?
3. Does the client focus on only one of the stimuli in the environment and is he unable to turn attention from the one stimulus?
D. Language
1. Outflow of words decreases.
2. Patterns of repetitive, tangential, or concrete speech appear.
3. Writing skills decrease more rapidly than the spoken word.
E. Memory
Tests client's ability to remember four unrelated words and recent events. (Confabulation and anger will often be used by the client to move the interviewer away from questions related to memory.)
F. Constructional ability
The client is instructed to copy a series of line drawings; he is often unable to do this or his ability to do so will decline dramatically over a period of time.
G. Cortical function
1. The client's ability to perform arithmetic is faulty, reveals many errors
2. Proverb interpretation—usually, the client will give only a concrete interpretation of the proverb.
3. Similarities—The client will often deny similarities between two objects and give instead a concrete answer. For example, when asked, "What is the similarity between a tiger and a cat?" the client may reply, "One is small and one is large. There is no similarity."

participation becomes even more crucial as family members assume increasing responsibility for care.

The conflict and the stress brought about by the changes in the family dynamics, as well as the debilitating effects of the organic mental disorder, compel those involved in planning care to include plans that will encourage family cohesiveness and stability. Necessity demands that discharge planning be initiated early in the treatment process. It must be decided what responsibilities family members can assume and what "relief" persons, such as neighbors and friends, may be secured to prevent exhaustion of the future primary caregivers.

The general goals of care and subsequent outcomes for the person with an organic mental disorder are threefold:

Goal I. To eliminate the organic etiology if possible

Client outcome: The client will demonstrate no signs or symptoms originating from an active organic etiology and minimal residual symptomatology from a formerly active organic etiology

Goal II. To prevent the acceleration of symptomatology

Client outcome: The client will exhibit no or minimal increase in the signs and symptoms of the disease process

Goal III. To preserve the dignity of the client

Client outcome: The individual will at all times command the respect of his caretakers, family, and friends as a fellow human being

These goals are facilitated by the following supportive goals and outcomes:

1. To maintain peak physical health, with the outcome that the client will demonstrate the highest level of health on the wellness continuum that he is capable of reaching
2. To promote a structured environment, with the outcome that the client will operate in an environment that is safe for his decreasing mental and physical capabilities
3. To promote socialization, with the outcome that the client will continue to participate within the social context that his faculties allow him
4. To promote independent functioning, with the outcome that the client will actively care for himself to the extent that his mental and physical resources allow him to do so
5. To preserve the family unit, with the outcome

that the family will continue to support the active participation of the client as a member, as well as be supported in its efforts to maintain its "normality" by the cooperative efforts of the health team

Intervention

Maintaining Peak Physical Health

One of the most essential nursing actions in helping the client with an organic mental disorder is to facilitate his optimal level of functioning by maintaining his peak physical health. Realizing that exogenous substances can dramatically initiate aberrant behavior, the nurse must become very sensitive to the client's response to his drug therapy. In addition to knowing the side effects and toxicity reactions of the specific drugs that the client is receiving, the nurse pays particular attention to possible drug interactions.

The nurse also assesses the client daily to recognize any symptoms of an ensuing physical disorder. Cardiovascular and respiratory disorders have a particular effect on those persons already affected by senile dementias.[15] Prompt recognition of symptoms and appropriate intervention by the nurse prevent acceleration of the client's already existent mental deterioration.

The nurse also endeavors to minimize the client's sensory impairments. Poor vision necessitates well-fitting eye glasses that are actually worn by the client and not carelessly set aside. Diminished hearing requires a hearing aid or giving louder, slower, uncomplicated instructions while standing directly in front of the client. The client may participate in activities, but may require a slower pace or simpler instructions prior to the activity to allow him sufficient time to compute the significance of the input from his faulty sensory organs. When the nurse recognizes a sensory deficit in the client, she should initiate steps to compensate for it.

Structuring the Environment

Structuring the client's immediate environment is an important nursing intervention. The nurse may increase or decrease the client's level of the sensory input. When the client experiences sensory overload, he may be moved to a quieter area or private room where environmental stimuli are kept at a minimum and where he can rest or sleep. The nurse may place "orientation" clues in the environment; clocks, calendars, and seasonal pictures provide sensory input that is important for the client's orientation to time and place. The number of family members, friends, and hospital personnel entering the environment should be controlled to provide for optimal stimulation. The

CHART 31-5
Therapeutic Dialogue

Reality Orientation: Presenting Concrete Information

Nurse: (seated beside the client in her room, looking directly at her, with one of the nurse's hands touching the client's arm) Good morning, Mrs. S., I see that you have just finished your bath.

Client: (nodding vigorously and smiling) Yes, yes. (pats the nurse's hand)

Nurse: Mrs. S., since it is 11:00 in the morning, would you like to walk with me to the day room in this hospital to see the beautiful sunshine?

Client: Yes, oh my yes.

Nurse: Mrs. S., since you are here in St. Luke's hospital, I will walk with you. It is such a pretty day outside. I want you to enjoy the sunshine before noontime when you will eat your lunch.

Client: Yes, dear. Oh my. (Remains sitting until the nurse stands and gently pulls upward on her arm and begins to walk to the door)

Discussion

Often, the client with a senile dementia retains impressive social skills even though she has lost both cognitive capability to understand and orientation to person, time, and place.

In this dialogue, the nurse constantly reminds Mrs. S. who she is, where she is, and where she is going. The nurse also reminds the client of the time through specific facts and references to the sunshine, lunch, and so on, all of which help orient Mrs. S. to time. Note that none of this interaction took place in a manner demeaning to the client. Particularly helpful during this conversation were the "signals" given to Mrs. S., by means of touch and body language, that she should stand and walk, for without these signals, she would have understood less of the conversation.

---

people and objects within the environment should be as familiar to the client as possible. This may very well imply that the same hospital personnel need to care for the client on a consistent basis.

The perceptual difficulties of hallucinations or illusions may decrease by simply controlling the light in the environment. Light may easily eradicate the "sundown effect." Safety is an important factor that requires that any environmental hazards be eliminated. An agitated individual may become even more panic-stricken if restraints are used as a method to ensure safety. In this situation, the client might benefit from environmental structuring in which someone, either from the hospital or from the family, remains with the client to keep him from injuring himself by such acts as climbing over the bed rails, pulling out tubes, removing dressings, and so forth.

Promoting Socialization

The promotion of the client's socialization may be approached in a variety of ways. The client who is exhibiting signs of fairly severe disorientation may benefit from reality orientation therapy. Through this technique, psychiatric–mental health nurse professionals consistently bombard the client with four or five concrete facts that help to remind him of who he is, where he is, why he is here, and what is expected of him. To assist in accomplishing this goal, "reality orientation boards" are placed throughout the environment. These bulletin boards highlight for the client the date, time, place, and so forth.[23] Although this re-educative program has not been shown to significantly improve the mental status of a client, it does seem to slow the rate of decline.[15]

Another action that promotes the socialization of the individual with an organic mental disorder is that of including him in group work. The group provides a safe, empathetic atmosphere in which the individual may be motivated to utilize all of his faculties to their remaining potential. Food, touch, and music are therapeutic vehicles within the group that add to the re-establishment of self-esteem and resocialization.[15]

Promoting Independent Functioning

The nurse promotes the client's independent functioning by, first, maintaining his peak physical health and, second, helping him accomplish his activities of daily living. It is particularly helpful to make it easier

C H A R T   31-6

Alzheimer's Disease: Nurse—Client—Family

Justine Hoffman-Schmitt, M.S.N., R.N.
Nursing Instructor, Trinity Valley Community College
Formerly, Psychiatric Clinical Nurse Specialist/Coordinator,
Special Needs Units, Dallas Home for Jewish Aged
Dallas, Texas

Alzheimer's disease (AD), the most common form of dementing illness, is a progressive, debilitating, neurological disease affecting 3 million Americans today. It is the fourth leading cause of adult deaths; 150,000 people will die of Alzheimer's disease in 1987–1988. It is truly a universal disease, with 30 million victims worldwide. Alzheimer's disease is not a disease in isolation because family members are also the victims. Day by day they witness the deterioration in cognition, activities of daily living, social skills, and behavior in their loved ones afflicted with Alzheimer's disease. As a client's husband said, "There is not one thing left that reminds me of the lovely woman I married. This disease is a living death!" How can the nursing profession help?

The nurse is often the pivotal person to provide resources, call together a team of health care professionals, and coordinate treatment planning that is meaningful to the client with Alzheimer's disease and the family. Nurses join with the client and his family to help them attain some quality of life. Care of the client with Alzheimer's disease is most challenging and requires all of one's knowledge, skill, and ability. It requires, in fact, the art and science of nursing. The nurse's goal is to meet the bio-psycho-social and spiritual needs of the Alzheimer's victims by utilizing the nursing process. Maintaining physical health, developing and/or sustaining cognitive capacity, enhancing safety and security, assisting with quality of life issues, managing and interpreting behavior, correcting sensory stimulation, and helping with esteem, love, and belonging are all nursing goals. Individually and collectively every effort is made to help the client's and family's efforts toward these goals.

The multiplicity of issues and the complexity of care encourage a multidisciplinary approach to Alzheimer's disease. Treatment planning must be specific and individual. Clients can be variable, unpredictable, and dependent according to their functional disabilities and degree of brain damage. They require increasingly more of us, and this is difficult—too difficult, in fact—for one person to handle. Look around you and find others who may be helpful to you, the client, and the family. Care givers can be families, volunteers, professional and nonprofessional staff. They may be the social worker who works with the family and the grief process, the dietician who addresses the client's chronic weight loss, the volunteer who reminisces about "the good old days," the physical therapist who helps with balance, the spiritual advisor who comforts, the psychiatrist who medicates, the aide who sings "Down by the Old Mill Stream" during bath time. The health care team needs to reflect expertise, creative ability, and enthusiasm for the elderly demented resident and family. Holistic health concepts and a problem-solving approach unify the members of the team.

Care of the client with Alzheimer's disease involves good common sense, finely tuned communication skills, congruent staff behaviors, continuity of care, and the use of oneself in a careful and considerate manner. Developing a therapeutic nurse-patient-family relationship is our primary vehicle—a crucial intervention.

Empathize with what it must feel like to be terrified, out of control, lost, mute, and lonely. This is what Alzheimer's disease clients can experience. Their families express grief, guilt, loneliness, embarrassment, and frustration. People with Alzheimer's disease are not deliberately stubborn, suspicious, inappropriate, or ungrateful; their behavior is beyond their control. Nurses need to interpret this behavior and help the family understand the "whys." Nurses also model appropriate behavior and communication with both the family and client. With patience the nurse reorients, breaks tasks down into manageable steps, listens to feelings, observes moods, praises accomplishments, reinforces social skills, and maintains the client's dignity. Showing nursing's love, care, and concern is often a statement in itself.

Families are members of the multidisciplinary team. Invite them to join you in finding the best possible solutions to the dilemmas of cognitive impairment. They have a wealth of invaluable insight, family history, and personal experience. You will come to know the victim of Alzheimer's disease as he once was; in turn, the nurse can help the family accept the client as he is. We cannot cure Alzheimer's disease. We can cooperate to provide the victims with quality care, support, and professional nursing expertise.

The Alzheimer's Disease and Other Re-

lated Disorders Association (ADRDA), founded in 1980, has 300 chapters and many family support groups in the United States. Educational materials, volunteer training in respite care, information and research are privately funded. An information hotline has been established on a nationwide, 24-hour basis to link families who need assistance; the number is 1-800-621-0379.

for clients to accomplish their tasks of daily living. Making the materials for daily care available and accessible, keeping the routine of care simple and consistent, and giving the client time to complete those tasks that he is able to complete are supportive nursing actions.

Preserving the Family Unit

The nurse does not forget the importance of preserving the family unit. Discussing with the family ways in which relief may be provided by interested neighbors or by home health aides provides a respite for the family from the heavy responsibilities of full-time care of the client with an organic mental disorder. Day care for the client is one possibility that would allow family members to continue with their daily activities and responsibilities. Through day care, the spouse may be able to retain his or her job and income and have the energy to care for the client during evening and weekend hours. Family therapy may help any family who is experiencing undue stress or having difficulty coping with the situation and its demands. Planning family goals and addressing specific family problems add to the preservation of the family unit.[15] (The family's responsibilities and responses to a member with an organic mental disorder are discussed in Chart 31-6, "Alzheimer's Disease: Nurse-Client-Family".)

Evaluation

Because the client with an organic mental disorder is constantly in the dynamics of change, nursing actions must be regularly evaluated for their successful outcome and relevance. The client's physical and psychosocial changes may ineffectualize the nurse's efforts that had been previously successful. The nurse also realizes that, when dealing with the degenerative aspects of an organic mental disorder, success may be measured in terms of slowing down the process, rather than stopping or curing the problem.

The Nurse's Attitudes and Feelings

Working with clients who have organic mental disorders may be discouraging for the nurse. In certain situations, neither the institution nor the medical staff desire, or are able, to provide the supportive environment and milieu necessary for the client. For example, the client with an "acute" episode of aberrant behavior may experience attention to his physical needs only, while his psychological needs are merely tolerated. The chronically deficient individual may elicit pity from the staff, not the dynamic intervention that is reserved for the "curables." Any or all of these attitudes may pervade the environment in which the nurse works, making it difficult for her own feelings or philosophy to prevail.

Few patients have such intensive needs in both the physical and psychological realms as do those individuals with organic mental disorders. It is hoped that the nurse views this as a tremendous challenge for which she draws upon all of the resources available *in* her as well as those available *to* her.

Summary

This chapter has dealt with one of today's mushrooming problems, organic mental disorders. Appearing not only in the aging population but also in the general population as well, these disorders are becoming increasingly prominent in the critical care areas as a result of iatrogenic therapeutic modalities. Some of the major emphases of the chapter are as follows:

1. The possible etiologies of organic mental disorders include primary brain disease, systemic disturbance, influences of exogenous substances, and withdrawal and residual effects of exogenous substances.
2. Aberrant behaviors associated with these

Nursing Care Plan 31-1

The Client With Alzheimer's Disease

Nursing Diagnosis	Client Outcome	Intervention
Injury, potential for falling	Provide a safe environment	1. Maintain bed in low position 2. Keep in close visibility—room close to the nurses' station 3. Keep the bed rails up 4. Use shoes that tie (as opposed to slip-ons) when patient is walking 5. Assist patient to walk
Coping, ineffective individual	Maintain a structured, simple environment	1. Provide the same, consistent caregivers whose body language connotes friendliness and warmth 2. Monitor "excessive" stimuli; monitor traffic in and out of the room; keep radio/TV on soothing music, slower-moving programs 3. Guide through new procedures (tests, daily menu selection, etc.) allowing as much independence as possible, yet intervening to decrease overload 4. Establish a schedule of care as close to home routine as possible
Communication, impaired verbal	Promote effective communication	1. Use low-pitched, unhurried tone of voice 2. Always identify self and establish eye contact 3. Address patient by name 4. Ask only one question at a time 5. Break instructions into simple actions taken one at a time 6. Establish supportive nonverbal communication through gentle touching

disorders may include deficits in the sensorium, attention, orientation, perception, and memory.

3. Symptoms of organic mental disorders may be approached in terms of the nonpredictable findings usually associated with "acute" episodes and the more predictable findings associated with diseases that tend to be long-term in nature.

4. Gathering and analyzing assessment data regarding a client with an organic mental disorder requires participation of family members or friends who have been in close contact with the client.

5. Goal-setting for the client with an organic disorder focuses on elimination of the organic etiology, if possible, prevention of acceleration of his symptoms, and preservation of his dignity.

6. Specific nursing interventions strive to maintain the client's optimal physical health, to structure his environment, to promote socialization and independent functioning, and to preserve the family unit.

7. The nurse approaches the client with an organic mental disorder as a challenge to her professional skills.

References

1. Another Aspect of AIDS. Emergency Medicine 19, 7 (April 15): 44–45, 1987

2. American Psychiatric Association: Diagnostic and

Statistical Manual of Mental Disorders, 3d ed, rev. Washington, DC, American Psychiatric Association, 1987

3. Beam I: Helping Families Survive. Am J Nurs 84 (February): 229–232, 1984

4. Blass J: Pragmatic Pointers on Managing the Demented Patient. J Am Geriatr Soc (34) 7 (July): 548–549, 1986

5. Campbell E, Williams M, Milynarczyk S: After the Fall—Confusion. Am J Nurs 86 (February): 151–154, 1986

6. Coyle M: Organic Illness Mimicking Psychiatric Episodes. J Gerontological Nursing 13, 1, 31–34, 1987

7. Foreman M: Acute Confusional States in Hospitalized Elderly: A Research Dilemma. Nurs Res 35 (1): 34–38, 1986

8. Geriatrics Panel Discussion: Practical Considerations in Managing Alzheimer's Disease: I. Geriatrics 42 (September): 78–98, 1987

9. Geriatrics Panel Discussion: Practical Considerations in Managing Alzheimer's Disease: II. Geriatrics 42 (October): 55–65, 1987

10. Guze S: Acute Brain Syndrome. Hosp Med 13, (4): 63–69, 1977

11. Hays A, Borger F: A Test in Time. Am J Nurs 85 (October): 1107–1111, 1985

12. Jaspers K: General Psychopathology. Chicago, University of Chicago Press, 1963

13. Katzman R: Dementias. Postgrad Med 64 (August): 119–124, 1978

14. Katzman R: Early Detection of Senile Dementia. Hosp Pract 16 (June): 61–67, 1981

15. Kennie D: Management of Senile Dementia. Am Fam Physician 26, 12, 105–111, 1980

16. Lipowski ZJ: A New Look at Organic Brain Syndrome. Am J Psychiatry 137 (June): 674–677, 1980

17. Lukasiewicz-Ferland P: When Your I.C.U. Patient Can't Sleep. Nursing 87 (November): 51–53, 1987

18. Luckman J, Sorenson K: Medical Surgical Nursing: A Psychophysiological Approach. Philadelphia, WB Saunders, 1980

19. McKinney AS: Appropriate Investigations of Stroke and Dementia. Geriatrics 36 (June): 41–48, 1981

20. Mace N, Rabins P: The 36-Hour Day: A Family Guide to Caring for Persons With Alzheimer's Disease, Related Dementing Illnesses and Memory Loss in Later Life. Baltimore, Johns Hopkins University Press, 1981

21. Montgomery, Carol: What You Can Do for the Confused Elderly. Nursing 87 (April): 55–56, 1987

22. NIA Task Force: Senility Reconsidered. JAMA 244 (July): 259–263, 1980

23. Nursing Services, Tuscaloosa Veterans Administration Hospital: Guide for Reality Orientation. Tuscaloosa, AL, 1974

24. Pajk M: Alzheimer's Disease Inpatient Care. Am J Nurs 84 (Feb): 216–222, 1984

25. Pfeiffer E: A Short Portable Mental Status Questionnaire for the Assessment of Organic Brain Deficit in Elderly Patients. J Am Geriatr Soc 23(Oct):433–441, 1975

26. Pluckhan M: Alzheimer's Disease: Helping the Patient's Family. Nursing 86 (Nov): 63–64, 1986

27. Portnoi V: Diagnostic Dilemma of the Aged. Arch Intern Med 141 (May): 734–737, 1981

28. Reisberg, B: Stages of Cognitive Decline. Am J Nurs 84 (February) 225–228, 1984

29. Robins P: Management of Irreversible Dementia. Psychosomatics 22 (July): 591–597, 1981

30. Seltzer B, Sherwin I: Organic Brain Syndromes: An Empirical Study and Critical Review. Am J Psychiatry 135 (January): 13–20, 1978

31. Shapira J, Schlesinger R, Cummings J: Distinguishing Dementias. Am J Nurs 86 (June): 698–702, 1986

32. Staub R, Black F: Organic Brain Syndromes. Philadelphia, FA Davis, 1981

33. Theories and Therapies. Am J Nurs 84 (February): 223–224, 1984

34. Tomlinson BE, Blesses G, Roth M: Observations on the Brains of Demented Old People. J Neurol Sci 11 (September): 205-242, 1970

35. Verwoerdt A: Clinical Geropsychiatry. Baltimore, MD, Williams & Wilkins, 1976

36. Wang HS: Dementia in Old Age. In Walls CE (ed): Dementia, pp 15–23. Philadelphia, FA Davis, 1977

37. Wells C: Chronic Brain Disease: An Overview. Am J Psychiatry 135 (January): 1–11, 1978

38. Williams, L: Alzheimer's: The Need For Caring. J Gerontol Nurs 13, 1, 31–34, 1987

32 Psychophysiologic Disorders

M. Suzanne Doscher

We are not ourselves
When nature, being oppress'd, commands the mind
To suffer with the body

Shakespeare,
King Lear, Act II, Scene 4

Chapter Preview

Early beliefs that man was composed of a dichotomous mind and body have given way to a view of man as a system composed of interrelated parts. This chapter focuses on the interrelated parts, or systems—psychological, biologic, and family—that affect a person's choice to communicate through psychophysiologic responses. The overview of psychophysiologic disorders relates the incidence, possible causes, and examples of types of responses that traditionally have been considered psychophysiologic in nature. The latter sections of the chapter address application of the nursing process—assessment, nursing diagnosis, planning, intervention, and evaluation—to individuals who communicate psychophysiologically.

Learning Objectives

On completion of the chapter, you should be able to accomplish the following:

1. define psychophysiologic behavior
2. discuss the etiologic influences on psychophysiologic responses
3. describe the dynamics of the development of psychophysiologic disorders
4. differentiate between somatoform disorders and physical conditions that have organic bases
5. identify typical behaviors of individuals with common psychophysiologic disturbances of the gastrointestinal, respiratory, cardiovascular, and integumentary systems
6. describe physiological responses to depression, grief, loss, and change
7. apply primary prevention nursing activities to the care of individuals and families at risk for psychophysiologic disorders
8. apply the steps of the nursing process—assessment, nursing diagnosis, planning, intervention, and evaluation—to individuals who exhibit psychophysiologic behavior
9. identify and deal with your own feelings and attitudes in the care of individuals with psychophysiologic disorders

Mind-Body Interrelationship

For years, the term *psychosomatic* was used to describe individuals experiencing certain physical disease processes. Diseases such as bronchial asthma, essential hypertension, peptic ulcer, ulcerative colitis, and rheumatoid arthritis were classified under the umbrella of psychosomatic illness. It was assumed that these diseases had a primarily psychological etiology and that other diseases were primarily physical in origin. This view strongly suggested a mind-body dualism in man.

These early beliefs have rapidly given way to the current view of man as a composite of interrelated systems. Disruption or unrest in any one system affects the whole system. This view transcends the boundaries of discrete disease entities and focuses on the interrelationship between psychological and physiological factors present in every person. Strictly speaking then, there are no disease categories considered purely psychosomatic. Emotional factors influence all body processes and organic disease affects changes in the psychological state.[1]

Although clinical experience and scientific reports document the fact that psychological factors play an important role in initiating, exacerbating, or maintaining a number of physical disorders, the individual person may not be consciously aware of the psychological factors affecting organic processes, or vice versa. In two major epidemiologic surveys, 59% to 69% of the subjects did complain of symptoms with both physical and psychological components.[10, 16] It seems that the remaining subjects may have been unaware of the interrelationship of psyche and soma or the meaning of the interrelationship.

Etiology of Psychophysiologic Responses

Given similar life situations, why does one person become physically ill and another person does not? Susceptibility to physical illness depends on many factors. Few, if any, authors would support a single explanation of any disease; rather, multifactorial causation, with a delicate interaction of psychosocial, biologic, and familial factors is at the root of psychophysiologic responses.

Psychosocial Influences

Psychoanalytic View. The work of Franz Alexander in the 1940s offers the hypothesis that unresolved unconscious conflicts are central to the development of disorders that he classified as psychosomatic. Alexander emphasized that a precipitating event that is of emotional significance to the person triggers an increase in anxiety and activates his underlying conflict. Over time and depending upon the nature of the conflict, specific physiological alterations occur. For example, according to Alexander, a person who pervasively maintains a facade of independence, in an effort to cover up a need to be taken care of, experiences anxiety. The constant arousal of the independence-dependence conflict generates anxiety. The partnership of conflict and anxiety plays a key role in the development of peptic ulcer disease.[1]

Psychodynamic View. The psychodynamic approach to the relationship between psychological factors and physical disease asserts that, under stress, persons with certain personality constellations will develop physical disease. This view proposes the individual's personality type is the basis for certain physical illnesses.[5] For example, according to this theory, the person most likely to develop ulcerative colitis is meticulous, compulsive, scrupulously prompt, excessively clean, and passively angry. This idea of the significance of the basic personality has again received popularity in the description of the Type A personality who is prone to coronary heart disease.[6]

Life Experiences. Careful history-taking at the onset of physical illness frequently reveals the accumulation of many life changes in the recent past. Studies indicate that a variety of illnesses coincide with a high life-change profile.[7] Marriage, death of a loved one, retirement, trouble at work, buying a house, and financial changes are but a few of the common and often inevitable events that occur in life (see Table 32-1). The psychological impact of one or more of these events varies among individuals. For some individuals, it seems that an accumulation of these events serves as the foundation for the development of physical illness. The meaning the individual gives to the event(s), especially the issue of "not being in control" of his life, seems to be relevant in the initiation, exacerbation, and perpetuation of the illness.

Family Influences. Mechanisms used to adapt to stress are frequently learned in the family arena. Children are easily and greatly influenced by how their parental role models react and adapt to stressors such as conflict, loss or change, or disappointment. Also, at a time of stress, each child as well as each parent plays a distinct, separate role within the family system.

For some families, the prime mode of adaptation to emotional tension is through physical disorders. Generally, one child is the physical symptom bearer and, in essence, communicates the emotional pain of the entire system. Minuchin believes that the "psychosomatic family" has certain distinct characteristics that are absent from a nonpsychosomatic family.[11] These families are frequently overinvolved (enmeshed) with one another, deny the existence of conflict, have a poor ability to resolve differences, and

have a narrow, rigid, and often ineffective repertoire of responses when faced with change.

Biologic Influences

Neuroendocrine Systems. According to biologic theories, physiology rather than psychology plays a key role in the development of somatic disorders. These theories emphasize that the body, particularly the autonomic nervous system and the endocrine system, reacts in a predictable, organized manner to stress.

Cannon's studies in the 1920s led to the discovery of the adaptive function of adrenalin in assisting the body to strive for "homeostasis" when experiencing stress.[3] Later, in the 1940s, Hans Syele focused on the role of the pituitary–adrenal mechanism in the body's reaction when defending against stress.[14] Syele calls this reaction the "general adaptation syndrome." Both Cannon and Syele believed that if the body experiences a prolonged adaptive struggle to combat stress, the individual is likely to develop a "physical disease of adaptation."

Genetic Factor. It has been hypothesized that everyone has one bodily organ or system that is more vulnerable to illness than others.[12] Under stressful circumstances, underlying unconscious conflicts are activated and coping occurs via the development of a physical illness involving the weakest bodily system.

Dynamics and Manifestations of Psychophysiologic Disorders

None of us holds claim to immunity from a short-lived response to anxiety that produces temporary disruption in our physical well-being—preclinical diarrhea, predate hives, preexamination sweaty palms or pounding heart. Although we would like to control these episodes totally, the unconscious and the autonomic nervous systems seem to win out.

The response to anxiety previously described is temporary in nature, but if it were to remain or recur frequently in relation to events that the individual perceived as stressful, prolonged or chronic physical problems could ensue. All people have unique ways of relieving anxiety; however, if useful, functional "relief valves" are unsuccessful, or perhaps unknown, the individual may unconsciously choose to relieve anxiety by becoming physically ill.

Although anxiety is one feeling state that may be associated with the development and maintenance of physical illness, it certainly is not the only one. Anger that is within or outside the person's awareness and

Table 32-1.   **The Social Readjustment Rating Scale**

RANK	EVENT	VALUE	SCORE
1	Death of spouse	100	_____
2	Divorce	73	_____
3	Marital separation from mate	65	_____
4	Detention in jail or other institution	63	_____
5	Death of a close family member	63	_____
6	Major personal injury or illness	53	_____
7	Marriage	50	_____
8	Being fired at work	47	_____
9	Marital reconciliation with mate	45	_____
10	Retirement from work	45	_____
11	Major change in the health or behavior of a family member	44	_____
12	Pregnancy	40	_____
13	Sexual difficulties	39	_____
14	Gaining a new family member (*e.g.*, through birth, adoption, oldster moving in)	39	_____
15	Major business readjustment (*e.g.*, merger, reorganization, bankruptcy)	39	_____
16	Major change in financial state (*e.g.*, a lot worse off or a lot better off than usual)	38	_____
17	Death of a close friend	37	_____
18	Changing to a different line of work	36	_____
19	Major change in the number of arguments with spouse (*e.g.*, either a lot more or a lot fewer than usual regarding childrearing, personal habits)	35	_____
20	Taking out a mortgage or loan for a major purchase (*e.g.*, for a home, business)	31	_____
21	Foreclosure on a mortage or loan	30	_____
22	Major change in responsibilities at work (*e.g.*, promotion, demotion, lateral transfer)	29	_____
23	Son or daughter leaving home (*e.g.*, marriage, attending college)	29	_____
24	In-law troubles	29	_____
25	Outstanding personal achievement	28	_____
26	Wife beginning or ceasing work outside the home	26	_____
27	Beginning or ceasing formal schooling	26	_____
28	Major change in living conditions (*e.g.*, building a new home, remodeling, deterioration of home or neighborhood)	25	_____
29	Revision of personal habits (*e.g.*, dress, manners, association)	24	_____
30	Troubles with boss	23	_____
31	Major change in working hours or conditions	20	_____
32	Change in residence	20	_____
33	Changing to a new school	20	_____
34	Major change in usual type or amount of recreation	19	_____
35	Major change in church activities (*e.g.*, a lot more or a lot less than usual)	19	_____
36	Major changes in social activities (*e.g.*, clubs, dancing, movies, visiting)	18	_____
37	Taking out a mortgage or loan for a lesser purchase (*e.g.*, for a car, television, freezer)	17	_____
38	Major change in sleeping habits (a lot more or a lot less sleep, or change in part of day when asleep)	16	_____

(Continues on p. 626)

RANK	EVENT	VALUE	SCORE
39	Major change in number of family get-togethers (*e.g.*, a lot more or a lot fewer than usual)	15	_____
40	Major change in eating habits (a lot more or a lot less food intake, or very different meal hours or surroundings)	15	_____
41	Vacation	13	_____
42	Christmas	12	_____
43	Minor violations of the law (*e.g.*, traffic tickets, jaywalking, disturbing the peace)	11	_____

(From Holmes TH, Rahe RH: The Social Readjustment Rating Scale. J Psychosom Res 11:213–218, 1967)

that goes unexpressed can wreak havoc on visceral functioning. Just as mounting prolonged anxiety needs an outlet, the same is true for anger that may be "swallowed down" and allowed to mount. Unfortunately, many people do not receive permission to feel angry and express anger in childhood. Therefore, some individuals progress through life operating in the style of "turn the other cheek," "forgive and forget," and denying angry feelings. In some instances, relief is not obtained in a functional way; faulty adaptation occurs when the person's body responds by "becoming ill."

Some people feel shame or guilt about expressing or seeking functional ways of meeting their needs for affection, dependency, security, or a sense of belonging. When faced with situations that evoke these dependency longings, they experience anxiety and are apt to defend against the anxiety by blocking out, or failing to recognize, the dependency needs. Physical symptoms become the only outlet available to the person and serve to meet his dependency needs and, possibly, to punish him for needs and feelings that he deemed unacceptable.

Types of Psychophysiologic Responses

The revised third edition of the Diagnostic and Statistical Manual (DSM-III-R) no longer identifies a group of specific physical diseases that are labeled psychophysiologic. Instead, the manual delineates two categories that predominantly and inextricably interrelate the mind and body. The two categories are somatoform disorders and psychological factors affecting physical condition.[2]

In the absence of organic pathology, individuals experiencing somatoform disorders do in fact experience physical symptoms. Among the somatoform disorders is *conversion disorder*. Conversion disorder or conversion reaction is characterized by a loss or alteration in physical functioning without an underlying physiologic cause. Examples of conversion symptoms are blindness, paralysis, and aphonia. Individuals di-

agnosed with this disorder manifest little anxiety about the symptom or the attendant disruption to their lives. This absence of reaction is termed *la belle indifference*.[2]

Another somatoform disorder is *hypochondriasis*. Hypochondriacal individuals fear or believe that their bodies house serious disease. However, medical support for a physical diagnosis is nonexistent. In contrast to the absence of anxiety displayed by individuals experiencing conversion symptoms, individuals diagnosed with hypochondriasis appear anxious about their symptoms even though loss of physical function is not evident.[2]

A third somatoform disorder is identified as *somatization disorder*. This disorder or syndrome begins before the person reaches the age of 30 and is chronic in nature. The individual has multiple physical complaints that involve more than one body system.[2] Examples of possible symptoms include pain, dizziness, bowel problems, and sexual indifference.

Whereas somatoform disorders occur in the absence of organic pathology, the DSM-III-R category psychological factors affecting physical condition refers to physical conditions that have organic pathology underlying the illness. These conditions have an emotional overlay which contributes to or complicates the disease process.[2] The next section of this chapter identifies a number of physical conditions that most often exist in concert with psychological variables. Also, emotional states that elicit physiological responses are described. These examples are offered in an effort to illustrate the unquestionable holistic nature of human beings.

Gastrointestinal Disturbances

Peptic Ulcer. The typical person with peptic ulcer disease has been described as hard-working, strong, unemotional, and independent. These persons are often in executive occupational positions and, despite successes in these positions, are never quite satisfied with their performance or achievement.

Although peptic ulcer disease has no single cause, it is believed that strong dependency longings exist beneath the facade of independence. Gratification in meeting dependency needs may be blocked for external reasons or because of feelings of shame in expressing these needs. It is also thought that a genetic predisposition to gastric hypersecretion may exist in certain individuals.

Ulcerative Colitis. Experiences of intense anxiety or stress, many times associated with loss, frequently precipitate the onset or relapse of ulcerative colitis. Many people with ulcerative colitis tend to guard against becoming emotionally involved with another and are particularly sensitive to rejection, abandonment, or anger from others. When situations develop that evoke angry feelings, the person tends unconsciously to allow the values of staying in control, "being good," and remaining stoic to overshadow the need to express anger directly. Instead, the overactive colon indirectly communicates the feeling. Individuals with ulcerative colitis are frequently quite ambitious, energetic, and highly responsible, yet inwardly they feel inferior. Outwardly, these people may exhibit characteristics of compulsiveness, conscientiousness, meticulousness, indecisiveness, and a strong sense of duty and honesty.

Anorexia Nervosa. Although the cause of anorexia nervosa is unknown, individual psychological and family issues seem to play major roles in the etiology. Adolescent girls whose parents either are affluent or convey an attitude of success are most likely to be affected by this disease. These individuals are frequently described as having been "model children," the pride and joy of their parents. In effect, they have not learned to trust their own initiative or to behave in response to their own needs or wants. Rather, the needs of the parents are paramount, and the child does not learn that she has needs and wants separate from the parents', nor does she learn how to distinguish between the two sets of needs and wants.

Early issues of separation and individuation are unresolved, and in adolescence, when the struggle for identity and for a sense of independence again surges, the young person experiences intense anxiety and ineptness. One way that she discovers to establish a sense of control, identity, and independence is to starve and lose weight. In essence, the adolescent becomes a powerful master over a weakened slave, the body.

Paralleling the anorexic adolescent's childhood, which is described as trouble-free, is the family constellation described as happy, harmonious, and successful. The apparent marital harmony is, however, but a facade for underlying conflict and dysfunction. This disharmony is circumvented by parents, especially the mother, who is protective and controlling and who seeks self-satisfaction and affection from the "ideal" child. Typically, the families of anorexics are overinvolved in one another's lives and individuation is therefore lost.

Respiratory Disturbance

Asthma. A wide variety of personality types is seen among asthmatics. Some persons with asthma have an intense need to be protected and an exaggerated need to retain dependence and bonding to the mother. If the attachment to the mother figure is threatened in reality or symbolically in later life, insecure feelings and fears associated with abandonment and rejection are heightened. Some asthmatic persons are hypersensitive to other persons; others are openly aggressive or hostile.

Cardiovascular Disturbances

Cardiovascular Disease. In addition to the advent of significant medical cardiology knowledge, treatment techniques, and equipment during the past few decades, new relevance has been placed on the relationship between psychological factors and the development of cardiovascular disease (*i.e.*, coronary artery disease, congestive heart failure, and myocardial infarction).[13] Friedman and Rosenman described a "Type A" personality as being associated with high risks of developing cardiovascular disease.[6] Type A individuals are described as competitive, driven, hardworking, controlling, and aggressive. Frequently, these individuals occupy managerial or executive positions and, in a sense, their life is their work or "their work drives their life." Self-permission to enjoy life, relax, and have fun is usually at a minimum for these individuals.

Although the concept of the Type A personality certainly has relevance in all levels of cardiovascular disease prevention, it is not the only risk factor associated with the disease. Genetic factors such as predisposition to high cholesterol levels, social factors such as smoking, and factors such as obesity and lack of exercise interrelate with personality variables of individuals at risk. Nevertheless, when the person enters the health care system for treatment, the personality factors usually receive little, if any, attention. In fact, the attention may be in the form of some well-meant but superficial advice to "slow down" or "take life easy." The old concept of the mind-body dualism seems to surface and dominate. Nurses can play a significant role in preventing this hasty approach to psychophysiologic behaviors.

Essential Hypertension. As with other physical disorders, the etiologic basis of essential hypertension is related to more than one variable. The emotional component of repressed hostility, "bottled-up anger," seems to play a significant role in the lives of persons who have essential hypertension.

In encounters with people, especially within meaningful relationships where a typical or functional response may be anger, the individual with essential hypertension allows the guilt component of anger to serve as a barrier to the expression of his real feelings. In a sense, the person consciously or unconsciously chooses to "keep the lid" on his anger. Such pervasive responses of internalizing anger create mounting stress and tension. The avenue for expression of the tension related to repressed anger may be vasoconstriction of the blood vessels, which results in essential hypertension.

This method of viewing anger as an unacceptable emotion may have been learned in early life or through family experiences. The implied message from significant adults to the young person may have been, "Strong, responsible, mature people don't feel angry, or certainly don't express anger if they feel it." In addition to early learning experiences of individuals who have essential hypertension, the possibility of a genetic predisposition cannot be dismissed when considering etiologic variables. Other variables that seem to relate to the development and maintenance of essential hypertension include socioeconomic status and cultural and ethnic origin.

Skin Disturbances

Unlike other bodily systems, the skin is visible—it is not camouflaged easily. No doubt all people have experienced or observed the relationship between certain feeling states and skin responses. Physical responses to underlying emotions are readily apparent in the goose flesh of excitement or fear, the blush of the face or neck when one is embarrassed, and the sweating of palms or underarms accompanying anxiety or anger. These responses, under the control of the autonomic nervous system, are common to all and assist the body to maintain homeostasis. They generally do not represent the primary mode of communicating feelings.

Some skin disturbances, however, are not transitory in nature; they are severe and longer-lasting. Individuals suffering from these disturbances may engage in frequent itching or scratching or may complain of pain. Disfigurement of the skin in the form of excoriation or loss of pigmentation may ensue. The exact cause of skin disorders of this type is not known, even though evidence does suggest that some conditions are psychological in origin.[15] It is proposed that the individual may house an unconscious conflict between wanting and not wanting to express a feeling, and that this conflict is not generally in his awareness. During periods of stress, it is not uncommon to observe individuals with skin disturbances communicating little, if any, verbal or direct emotional unrest. Instead, they frequently suffer exacerbations of skin disorders. This expression often serves as a means of receiving concern and attention from self and others.

Physiological Response In Emotional States

Depression. As described in Chapter 23, depression is a state of being that, in a sense, exemplifies the psychophysiologic unity of human beings. Depression may be expressed through the affect, the thought processes, and the physical channels available to the individual. Thoughts and feelings of self-doubt, dejection, or worthlessness affect the availability and utilization of psychic as well as physical energy. If physical energy is depleted, bodily functions slow and the person is apt to describe himself as weak and "tired all the time."

In addition, it is not uncommon to hear people who are depressed talk about "aching all over" in the joints and muscles. The adage, "I feel like I have the world on my shoulders and I can't get it off," aptly describes both the psychic and bodily experience of many individuals who are depressed.

Another common occurrence in depression is a change in eating habits and gastrointestinal functioning. An individual who is agitatedly depressed and who manifests overt anxiety within the depression is a likely candidate to eat more than usual and to have diarrhea. In contrast, a person whose depression is more retarded in nature is apt to eat less and have constipation.

Although these physiological alterations are common symptoms in obvious depressive states, an individual's depression may be masked or may appear in the guise of physical illness. Extensive medical testing may reveal no anatomic or physiological rationale for somatic symptoms that may preoccupy the individual. The somatic illness is very real to the person and should signal the astute health care professional to intervene in ways that help the person get in touch more directly with the underlying depression. Even if there is a structural or functional basis for physical illness, it has been estimated that 70% of persons hospitalized for medical reasons are suffering from depression. This fact has significant implications for the delivery of nursing care, which attests to the belief that man is a biological-psychosocial being.

Grief, Loss, and Change. In varying degrees, loss and change are familiar experiences to everyone throughout the life cycle. Even the young infant who is weaned from the mother's breast in a sense relinquishes or loses an object that has provided pleasure and nourishment. Similarly, a young child entering school, or a late adolescent entering college, has the opportunity to experience the exciting, frightening, yet potentially satisfying aspects of growing independence while simultaneously meeting the challenge of facing the accompanying aspects of change and loss of the familiar. As individuals experience loss and change, it is not uncommon for physical problems to surface. The common cold, the "splitting" headaches, and the nagging backache are a few of the possible physical reactions to the stress of loss and change. In some instances, the physical responses may be more severe and more debilitating than these examples.

Although it is true that not all individuals experience a physical response to loss and change, studies have indicated that life changes do positively correlate with health disruptions. After analyzing 5000 case histories of patients' life situations at the onset of illness, Holmes and Rahe developed a social readjustment rating scale (see Table 32-1), which focuses on the amount of life-change events present in the subject's life at the onset of illness.[8] The scale gives a value of from 100 to 11 (referred to as Life Change Units, or LCUs) for each life event. The authors found that the higher the value of LCUs, the greater the likelihood that the individual would develop an illness. In fact, almost 80% of people with more than 300 Life Change Units in a year become sick in the near future.[8]

Loss and change are inevitable; however, having information about the potential ramifications of the life change events may assist individuals to recognize the risks and plan for ways to cope adaptively rather than becoming physically ill.

Application of the Nursing Process to Psychophysiologic Disorders

Because stress plays a significant role in the initiation, exacerbation, and maintenance of any psychophysiologic response, the nurse has a responsibility to participate in all levels of preventative care. Through primary prevention, the nurse intervenes in ways that assist people to become more aware of potential stressors and to develop or maintain functional methods of adaptation. Secondary prevention focuses on interventions that demonstrate genuine caring and support, as the nurse assists the client to improve his physical health, enhance self-knowledge, examine current methods employed to express his needs and feelings, adapt to stress, and consider alternatives for coping other than becoming physically ill. Through

tertiary prevention, the nurse supports the client as he tries out new means of expressing his needs and feelings and coping with stress.

Primary Prevention

Promoting health and striving to reduce the incidence and prevalence of disease are at the forefront of nursing care in these last years of the 20th century. Accompanying this charge to nursing is the charge to every person in Western society—to cope with a world of ever-mounting stress and challenge. For nurses the charge is dual—take care of themselves and assist others to discover ways to adapt that facilitate emotional and physical well-being.

Some individuals choose to adapt to stress or to express emotional needs by becoming physically ill. Bottling up feelings, being frightened or unsure of how to express needs, and receiving reinforcement for such responses may well be at the root of many physical illnesses.

In primary prevention, nurses must direct intervention to the family as a target of care. All people launch on the journey of growth and development in the family unit and learn patterns of behavior that are either functional or dysfunctional. High-risk families for psychophysiologic responses are those in which one or both parents express needs and feelings through psychophysiological illnesses. Regardless of the setting, a thorough nursing assessment and analysis may reveal information suggesting that the client is at risk for using psychophysiologic behavior as a means of coping. Early preventive measures may be influential in choices made as growth and development progress.

Another vulnerable group for the development of psychophysiologic illness is individuals who have experienced multiple life changes. Changes are inevitable in life, yet the nurse engaging in primary prevention can offer information that assists people to cope functionally with change and stress, rather than relinquishing control to the event or stressor.

Planning and Intervening

Goals directed at the primary prevention of psychophysiologic behavior include the following:

1. The development of family relationship patterns that do not foster the use of psychophysiologic behaviors
2. Functional adaptation to life changes

The nurse practices in many settings where she can share her knowledge and skill by role-modeling, teaching, and supporting parents and entire families in fostering functional relationships with one another. The nurse utilizes interventions that facilitate the prevention of psychophysiologic disorders and the promotion of functional family relationships by assisting families to do the following:

1. Create an atmosphere within the family that is caring, accepting, safe, and supportive
2. Develop and nourish communication patterns that are open and honest and that permit direct expression of feelings and needs
3. Accept, encourage, and respect the expression of differences in ideas and opinions
4. Negotiate and cooperate at times of conflict
5. Employ a flexible approach to problem-solving
6. Achieve a balance between belonging needs and separation needs (autonomy)
7. Establish supportive resources beyond the family matrix

Promoting functional adaptation to life changes may occur in a variety of settings. Opportunities for nursing practice in primary prevention far surpass the traditional hospital setting. Conducting speaking engagements at Parent Teachers Organization meetings, participating in health fairs, teaching prenatal and postnatal classes, and working with persons experiencing transitions in life are some of the settings in which anticipatory guidance may be practiced. Indeed, there are a myriad of life changes, and perceptions of the effect of similar events may vary from person to person. The nurse assists individuals to prepare for changes and consider options for coping when stress mounts. Active nursing involvement may help individuals cope with the stress in ways other than becoming physically ill.

Secondary Prevention

By the time the nurse meets the individual with a psychophysiologic disturbance who is in need of secondary prevention, the disturbance is already present. Through application of the nursing process—assessment, nursing diagnosisis, planning, implementation, and evaluation—the nurse helps to shorten the duration of the existing disorder, thereby reducing the prevalence of the disorder.[4]

Because most individuals in need of treatment for psychophysiologic responses do not seek psychiatric care, the nurse is apt to meet these individuals in secondary care settings, such as outpatient and inpatient nonpsychiatric care settings.

Assessment

Viewing the person as a system that is greater than the sum of its parts, or subsystems, assists the nurse in directing assessment at the whole person, rather than centering attention only on the most obvious—the physical body. Indeed, collecting and analyzing data relative to the manifested physical disorder are significant nursing activities. The nurse's knowledge of the possible multiple causes of the illness facilitates the performance of a comprehensive assessment that includes psychological, social, and family influences on the individual. Analysis of the assessment data focuses on a thorough examination of the possible interrelationships of all systems assessed. While assessing the individual, the nurse simultaneously uses the self and conveys behaviors that exemplify understanding of therapeutic relationships. (See Chap. 5.)

The nursing assessment of the individual who exhibits psychophysiologic behavior addresses the following major areas:

1. Physical examination
2. History-taking (physical and psychosocial life)
3. Emotional themes

Physical Examination. Performance of a thorough examination is a skill that nurses even 20 years ago did not practice. In most nursing curricula today, the nursing student begins to develop and master physical assessment skills. These skills linked with knowledge of the physical sciences enable the nurse to monitor continuously the individual's physiological status and to plan nursing interventions accordingly.

History-Taking. During the history-taking portion of the assessment process, the nurse aims to help the client report factual information relative to his current and past health status. In addition, the nurse meets the challenge of blending the more traditional medical history-taking format, which focuses on areas such as pertinent demographic data, present illness, past health status, and family health, with a psychosociocultural assessment model, which focuses on areas such as the client's perception of himself, his perception of changes in his lifestyle that might be associated with his current health status, his emotional responses to his health, and his relationships with others and his culture. (See textbooks of medical-surgical nursing or physical assessment.)

The client's psychosociocultural assessment includes the following significant assessment areas:

1. What are the client's attitudes toward his physical illness as well as his knowledge about the illness? How does he feel about being ill? What does he think about being ill?
2. What does the client perceive as his strengths and his limitations?
3. How does the client usually adapt to stress or tension?
4. Have significant others in the client's past

made use of behaviors similar to his when adapting to stress?

5. What events preceded or precipitated this physical illness?

6. What relationship does the client perceive between his physical illness and his emotions or behavior?

7. What tasks has the illness prevented the client from performing?

8. In what ways has the physical disorder changed the client's or his family's lifestyle?

9. What roles have changed in the client's family because of his physical illness?

10. How does the client generally get his emotional needs met?

11. What interpersonal resources are available to the client?

It is useful for the nurse to remember that assessment is not complete after the first nurse-client contact. In fact, based upon the client's physical status and the nurse's perception of his comfort and trust level, the nurse may decide that pursuit of psychosocial assessment is inappropriate during the initial contact. (See Case Study 32-1.) As the client's physical status improves, or as trust and rapport are built between the nurse and client, the nurse actively facilitates the client's thinking about, and disclosing, pertinent psychosociocultural history.

Emotional Themes. As an open, trusting nurse–client relationship develops, information becomes evident pertaining to the client's usual ways of behaving within relationships and ways in which the client expresses his needs and feelings. Because all human behavior has meaning, the nursing assessment focuses on analysis of the behavior, which includes speculation and validation of underlying emotional themes.

Through the client's interaction with the nurse, the nurse may perceive that the client has difficulty openly expressing dependency needs. For example, the client may describe himself as very self-sufficient and independent, yet the nurse notices that at least every hour, many times right after she has left his room, the client rings his call light and wants something. Similarly, assessment might indicate that the client has difficulty with openly expressing anger and, instead, seems to "swallow it down," suppress it, and remain physically ill.

Difficulties expressing dependency needs and anger are not the only emotional issues that may interfere with the client's functioning. Other emotions such as pervasive anxiety, guilt, powerlessness, loneliness, and insecurity may seem to be at the core, yet covered by the veneer of the physical illness. During the assessment and nursing diagnosis phases, as well as during the entire nursing process, it is within the nurse's role to approach the client with caring and acceptance while striving to learn about the client and assisting him to know himself in a fuller way.

Nursing Diagnosis

When formulating nursing diagnoses for clients with psychophysiologic disorders, the nurse is faced with the challenge of accurately describing the client's physiological response (*e.g.,* Alteration in comfort: pain, acute or chronic, Alteration in bowel elimination: diarrhea) and carefully describing the etiology or "related to" statement in terms of the client's emotional responses and needs. Chart 32-1, Nursing Diagnosis and Long-Term Goals, offers examples of the ways in which the client's anxiety, experience of loss, and feelings of powerlessness may contribute to his physical symptoms.

Several accepted nursing diagnoses are appropriate to use in planning the nursing care provided to a client with a physiologic disorder. For example, the client with ulcerative colitis may experience emotional responses such as anxiety, knowledge deficit, and disturbance in self-concept: body image, self-esteem, role performance, and the physical responses of alteration in comfort: pain, and alteration in bowel elimination: diarrhea.

Planning and Intervening

When planning care, the nurse must prioritize the client's needs and intervene accordingly. In some instances, the client may be acutely physically ill, and his physical condition therefore mandates that the nurse's attention be directed primarily to physical care. Even in these situations, the nurse blends knowledge and skills in the physical aspects of delivering care in a caring, compassionate, and helpful manner. The therapeutic use of self allows the nurse to minister to the physical needs of the client while simultaneously responding to his verbal and nonverbal cues that may indicate underlying emotions such as fear or anxiety. As the client's physical condition improves, the nurse is likely to find that the single most important ingredient of intervention is using herself in a manner that communicates openness, empathy, caring, and acceptance. These behaviors are likely to facilitate the client's decision to adapt in ways that are more functional and satisfying.

Because psychophysiologic behavior is communicated by means of various bodily systems, assessment and analysis may reveal that specific goals and interventions need to be directed toward the care of

Case Study 32-1

Planning Care for the Client Who Is Diagnosed with Ulcerative Colitis

Deanna, a well-dressed, pale-appearing secretary in an advertising agency, was admitted to the medical unit with a diagnosis of ulcerative colitis. During the admission interview with the nurse, Deanna reported that her physical symptoms had started approximately 1 year ago, and that she had experienced a weight loss of 20 pounds and bouts of bloody diarrhea during the past 3 months. With a flat tone of voice she stated, "I have followed the doctor's orders to a tee. Those steroid enemas and Azulfidine just haven't helped enough. I wanted so much to avoid hospitalization, but this mess seems to have gotten the best of me. My doctor says that resting here should help my colon settle down."

While caring for Deanna during her early days of hospitalization, the nurse learned that Deanna had an older and a younger brother who lived approximately 150 miles away, in the same city as her parents. She was the only daughter of a father who managed "a successful business started years ago by his grandfather." Deanna said little about her mother; however, she did state, "I told her about my being hospitalized because I knew she'd expect to know, but I hope she won't come to visit." When the nurse encouraged Deanna to elaborate on this comment regarding her mother, Deanna chose to shift the topic to talking about her work.

She described herself as a very conscientious, reliable, and dependable secretary. The advertising agency for whom she worked had undergone a change in organizational structure during the past year and Deanna's workload had increased considerably. She explained, "I never seem to be able to clear my desk completely anymore. I do the secretarial work for so many more people than when I started working there, 5 years ago. Now that I'm in the hospital with this colon problem, I guess I'll be even further behind when I get back to my job. I'm so tired of all this diarrhea." As Deanna talked about her role at work, the nurse noted that she did not verbalize directly about her feelings relative to the stress she was experiencing, but tended to focus on the fact that her hospitalization would impact negatively on her productivity at work.

Goals of nursing care established early during Deanna's hospitalization include the following.

1. Reducing the inflammation of the colon by assisting Deanna to follow the prescribed medical regime (that is, diet and medication)
2. Encouraging and providing opportunities for Deanna to experience adequate comfort and rest
3. Facilitating the development of a nurse–client relationship that would provide emotional support while reducing emotional stress

Deanna's somewhat debilitated physical condition mandated the nurse giving high priority to monitoring Deanna's response to the prescribed diet and sedative, antidiarrheal, steroids, and antibiotic drugs. While encouraging activity within the limit of Deanna's physical capabilities, the nurse geared interventions toward promoting and supporting rest. As with any nurse–client relationship, facilitating trust development and maintaining acceptance of the client were of prime importance as the nurse related to Deanna.

The nurse moved at Deanna's pace as she gradually began to talk about her relationship with her mother and Deanna's perceptions of her mother's unreasonableness in her expectations of Deanna. Deanna continued to deny the possible relationship between or among her increased responsibility at work, her reaction to the stress she experienced at work, her conflictual relationship with her mother, and her development of ulcerative colitis.

Questions for Discussion

1. Discuss your values, attitudes, and beliefs that might affect your care of Deanna.
2. What additional psychosocial assessment data would be useful in planning care for Deanna? Why?
3. Describe Deanna's primary ways of coping with stress (anxiety) at this time. How might you as the nurse intervene?
4. What possible emotional themes underlie Deanna's psychophysiologic behavior? Formulate a nursing care plan for Deanna, using one of these themes as a basis of problem identification or nursing diagnosis.

affected bodily organs—cardiovascular, gastrointestinal, or any other. Nevertheless, assessment of the total person may indicate that, in addition to goals related to physical needs, goals also need to address the following:

Recognition and ownership of feelings and needs
Provision of opportunities to express feelings and needs in an open, direct, functional manner

When intervening to help the client meet goals other than those associated with specific physical needs, the nurse recognizes that the client is frequently unaware of the relationship between physical and emotional aspects of his being. Frequently, the mental mechanisms of denial, repression, and suppression are operating; therefore, awareness of feelings and their effect on his behavior and choices are not known consciously by the client. These defenses are frequently strong and serve an important purpose for the client. Therefore, the nurse uses care and caution in approaches to help the client become more insightful (see Chart 32-2).

CHART 32-1
Nursing Diagnosis and Long-Term Goals

Clients with Psychophysiologic Disorders

Nursing diagnoses and long-term goals for clients experiencing psychophysiological disorders are offered as examples and are not meant to be conclusive. The nurse is reminded that specific nursing diagnoses are based on assessment of the individual client's behavioral manifestation of a problem and the contributing stressors. Although two clients may, in fact, have the same medical diagnosis (*e.g.,* asthma), the nursing diagnoses for these individuals may vary because of their uniqueness.

After identifying the nursing diagnosis, long-term goals designed to eradicate or modify the actual problem are identified. After identifying long-term goals, the nurse develops short-term goals that involve more specific and measurable outcomes.

Nursing Diagnosis	Long-Term Goal
Recurring headaches related to expressing anger in an indirect, passive manner	Facilitate direct, active expression of anger
Painful joints related to anxiety from perceived powerlessness and loss of control in work situation	Promote the adoption of self-control and power over reaction to stress at work
Pruritus and excoriation of the skin related to the loss of significant other	Facilitate the experience of grieving in an adaptive, functional manner
Bronchial constriction and wheezing related to anxiety from marital discord	Facilitate the utilization of problem-solving skills to cope with anxiety
Recurring bouts of diarrhea related to unrealistic self-expectations and expectations of others	Encourage realistic appraisal of strengths and weaknesses of self and others
Pseudo-independent behavior related to denial of dependency needs	Support more functional ways of fulfilling dependency longings
Adoption of sick role related to anxiety from increased role responsibilities as parent	Facilitate the utilization of problem-solving skills to cope with anxiety
Disturbed body image related to anxiety from identity confusion	Encourage realistic appraisal of self

CHART 32-2
Therapeutic Dialogue

Approaching the Client Who Has Essential Hypertension

Nurse: (seated facing client, Mrs. S., in the outpatient clinic examining room, preparing to take client's blood pressure)

Client: You know, you'd think the kind of life I live would help this blood pressure of mine go down. I couldn't be more sedentary at home. After John goes to work in the morning, it's just me, the house, and the dog. (looking at nurse, soft tone of voice)

Nurse: (placing blood pressure cuff on the table, arms and hands open and resting on lap) Tell me about a usual day for you.

Client: Well, my typical day really amounts to fixing meals for my husband and having things ready when he comes home from work. He likes his lunch at 12:00 noon and supper at 6:00 P.M. The two of us don't go out much in the evenings because John likes to be in bed by 10:00 P.M. (questioning tone of voice, maintaining eye contact)

Nurse: So, the structure you operate within revolves mostly around your husband. (pause) What about things you do for yourself?

Client: Well, let me see. (pause, thoughtful expression) I really don't know how to answer that question.

Nurse: Are you saying that your husband is your full-time job? (leaning towards client, maintaining eye contact)

Client: Well, I hadn't thought about it like that, but now that you mention it, it seems like that's so.

Nurse: (nodding) That makes sense to me.

Often, when people are busy focusing primarily on others, they tend to overlook themselves.

Client: Yeah, you know, when you take care of people and make sure that all the things that have to happen, happen, there isn't much time and energy left over. (maintaining eye contact)

Nurse: So from your perspective, the only place left to do without your time and energy is you, and what you do for you, for yourself.

The client's opening comment gives the nurse a clue that Mrs. S. is thinking about the possible relationship between her life situation and her essential hypertension. In an effort to offer support, the nurse directs her attention to Mrs. S. rather than to her illness; that is, by looking at and talking to Mrs. S., rather than taking her blood pressure. Active listening and genuine interest are demonstrated as the nurse encourages Mrs. S. to describe her thoughts.

Throughout the interaction, the nurse's approach is nonthreatening and accepting as she moves at Mrs. S's. pace. She encourages Mrs. S. to focus on herself—not on her hypertension or her husband—and to reflect on how she goes about "taking care of herself."

The nurse supports Mrs. S. as she considers the new awareness that she apparently chooses to define herself in terms of her husband. The nurse does not push Mrs. S. to explore her possible reaction to this choice; that is, essential hypertension. Although a goal in future interactions may be exploring her reaction, at this time, the nurse appropriately chooses to continue establishing trust and supporting the client in her recent insight.

A good principle of therapeutic practice is never to remove a person's defense unless or until you can offer a replacement that is more functionally sustaining. Sometimes, zealous health care providers think they know the answers to the client's problem and eagerly "lay the cards on the table." This type of zeal can, in fact, be destructive and may reinforce the client's dysfunctional modes of adaptation. Instead, attitudes and behaviors that convey a genuine willingness to help the client discover for himself options to solving his problems are potentially far more constructive and useful. This requires patience on the part of the nurse and a genuine belief in the client's capability to unfold self-understanding, meaning, and healing.

Because the emotional themes of unmet dependency needs or unexpressed anger frequently underlie the client's psychophysiologic behavior, the following nursing approaches are recommended.

Nursing Interventions for Unmet Dependency Needs

1. Be aware of your own feelings and how you allow these to affect your behavior. Because the client's need is often communicated by means of a facade of independence and demanding or manipulative behavior, the reaction of the nurse may be that of anger and resistance. Develop an awareness and understanding of this dynamic and seek supervision for dealing with your own feelings if necessary.

2. Accept the client's feelings. The client will quickly pick up on nonacceptance, which tends to reinforce his maladaptive position.

3. Begin by meeting the client's dependency needs, then gradually help him meet more of his own needs. Developmentally, the client may well be in a position like a young child who needs consistent caring and mothering. The nurse is in the position to offer the needed nurturing while recognizing the client as a responsible individual.

4. Anticipate the client's dependency needs. Remember that the client's denial of his dependency needs or his feeling that it is not acceptable to ask directly to have his needs met is likely to be strong. Expecting that he will quickly give this up is apt to lead to feelings of anger, distance, and resistance in the nurse and feelings of anger and anxiety in the client. Therefore, recognition and anticipation of needs early in the relationship are useful in meeting the client's needs and building a solid foundation of trust within the relationship. This trust becomes an especially valuable vehicle in helping the client develop greater insight, self-acceptance, and functional independence.

5. As the trusting relationship progresses, support and encourage any cues of functional independence. Assist the client, if need be, but don't usurp his responsibility and ability to think and do for himself. Of great importance is your support, caring, and willingness to follow through with your commitment to him and acceptance of him.

6. Throughout the process, use yourself in modeling and facilitating open communication. Assist the client in thinking about and talking about his thoughts and feelings. As the client becomes aware of his dependent behavior and, it is hoped, moves toward growing independence, he is likely to experience feelings of anger, shame, guilt, or anxiety. Encourage him in identifying and working through these feelings.

Nursing Interventions for Hostility

1. Be aware of your own feelings and how you allow these to affect your behavior. Considering that the client's expression of hostility is usually passive or diverted outwardly to an inappropriate source, the nurse's reaction may be frustration, avoidance, or anger. Allowing these feelings to influence your behavior negatively is likely to prevent the client from exploring his real feelings and the source of his feelings.

2. Accept the client and his feelings. Acceptance is likely to facilitate the client in gradually developing a higher level of insight and eventually adapting in a more functional manner. Consider that the client fears rejection and abandonment if he deals directly with his feelings; therefore, nonacceptance may reinforce his fears. Repressing his anger is the client's prime way of adapting. Repression is usually strong and serves as a significant protective mechanism. Patience and acceptance are important approaches as a relationship builds and develops.

3. Assist the client with recognizing his anger, identifying the source of his anger in current situations, and exploring alternative ways of dealing with his anger. This may be a very slow process because the client learned his maladaptive behavior over a long period of time. Through a trusting nurse-client relationship, the client may decide that open, direct dealing with feelings affords him a welcomed release from the anxiety and tension experienced when he "bottled up his feelings."

4. Consider that the client is apt to direct his anger towards you. This may occur by means of criticism, profanity, or in other derogatory ways. Set limits on the behavior while at the same time showing acceptance of the client and his feelings.

In addition to individual care for the client, the family must likewise be a focus of nursing care. Reminding herself that the client did not exist or develop in a vacuum when he chose psychophysiologic responses as a mode of adaptation is useful in guiding the nurse to broaden her perspective toward the family. There is therapeutic value in the nurse developing a relationship with the family and intervening as needed. The nurse also assists the family to examine ways the whole family system affects the client's physical status, as well as how the physical status of the client affects the family.

Evaluation

Evaluation is an ongoing process and overlaps with each phase of the nursing process. Because individuals who respond psychophysiologically communicate their needs through various bodily systems, evaluation of the effect of care on the client's physical status is contingent upon the bodily system involved and the degree of progression or regression of the physical malady. Regarding the effect of nursing care on the client's emotional well-being, the nurse-client relationship may be the most valuable measure of the client's status.

The nurse directs her focus to the established goals when engaging in evaluation. For example, a goal for the client might have been to identify thoughts and feelings relative to being physically ill. When evaluating whether or not this goal has been met, the nurse examines interactions with the client and cites progress, regression, or status quo. Evaluation allows the nurse to continue or adjust the plan of care and is crucial to the delivery of quality nursing care.

Tertiary Prevention

The major focus of tertiary prevention may be to support the individual who is considering whether or not he wants to make changes that could potentially reduce the likelihood of responding to stress by becoming physically ill. It is not uncommon for individuals who respond psychophysiologically to resist change in lifestyle, attitudes, and behavior. Along with change comes loss—loss of a customary, familiar way of adapting; that is, physical illness. In a sense, the physical illness has offered the person a sense of security. The idea of change is frightening, but the nurse is in a position to "be with" the person as she assesses his readiness to consider change and as he chooses whether or not to move through the problem-solving process.

Planning and Intervening

The major goal for tertiary prevention of psychophysiologic behavior is to develop functional adaptation to life stressors, without psychophysiologic behavior.

It is important for the nurse to remember, when planning interventions, that patterns of adaptation are not changed readily. Behavior changes slowly and the nurse must monitor her expectations of herself and of the client. Expecting too much of either herself or the client only serves as a major obstacle to helping the client consider more functional methods of adaptation. An important goal for the nurse may be to eradicate any expectations that she might hold. This would free the nurse to be herself and to assist the client in being realistic as he examines himself.

Interventions that focus on the change process are the major ones during tertiary prevention of psychophysiologic disorders. See literature on the change process for a thorough presentation of steps in the process. The following interventions are offered for consideration:

1. Assist the individual in examining and clarifying his values and goals.
2. Assist the individual to examine realistically how he currently copes with stress and to consider what, if any, incongruence there might be between his mode of coping and his values and goals.
3. Be honest in sharing your perceptions regarding the negative consequences of his current coping pattern.
4. Assist the person with considering alternative modes of coping. Facilitate identifying pros and cons of all alternatives and help him consider ramifications for himself and significant others.
5. Offer support as the person decides to change.
6. Positively reinforce functional change and do not abandon the person when and if he regresses to old modes of adaptation.

Evaluation

When evaluating the care offered during the tertiary phase of prevention with a person who responds psychophysiologically, the nurse directs focus to the modes of adaptation the person chooses in order to cope with stress. It may be useful for the nurse to consider the following questions:

What evidence exists to suggest that the person views stress as a growth-producing experience rather than a destructive one?
What change in lifestyle, attitude, and behavior does the person exhibit?
Has the person given up physical ills as a mode of adapting?
How is he currently adapting?
Is the person open with expressing and dealing with feelings?
Is problem-solving easier for the person?
What changes are evident in the family's style of relating?

Answers to these and similar questions may indicate whether or not the person has decided to adopt a more functional coping pattern and is striving to exercise self-control instead of allowing events and situations to control his life choices.

in the process of change is the focus of nursing practice.

Summary

This chapter has focused primarily on a view of physical illness as a mode of communicating physiological dysfunction as well as emotional unrest. Suggestions for nursing care during primary, secondary, and tertiary prevention have been offered. The following ideas have been included:

1. The human being is a composite of interrelated systems; therefore, the mind and the body cannot be divorced from one another.
2. There is no single cause for psychophysiologic responses; etiologic theories include psychosocial, biologic, and familial factors.
3. Physical illness may be a means of communicating feeling states and needs such as anxiety, anger, and dependency.
4. The integral relationship between an individual's thinking, feeling, and physical status may be evident in physiological disorders involving the gastrointestinal system, respiratory system, cardiovascular system, and integumentary system, as well as in the individual's response to depression, grief, loss, and change.
5. The nurse has a responsibility to participate in primary, secondary, and tertiary care aimed at preventing psychophysiologic disturbances.
6. During the primary prevention of psychophysiologic behavior, the nurse aims to promote functional family relationships and functional adaptation to life changes.
7. Most individuals in need of secondary prevention for psychophysiologic disorders are nonpsychiatric patients.
8. Assessment, intervention, and evaluation for the psychophysiologically disturbed person focus on physical and psychosocial life, as well as on the expressions of emotional needs and feelings.
9. The emotional themes of unmet dependency needs or unexpressed anger frequently underlie psychophysiologic behavior.
10. During the tertiary prevention of psychophysiologic behavior, the client's engagement

References

1. Alexander F: Psychosomatic Medicine: Its Principles and Applications. New York, WW Norton, 1950
2. American Psychiatric Association: Desk Reference to the Diagnostic Criteria from DSM-III-R. Washington, DC, 1987
3. Cannon WB: Bodily Changes in Pain, Hunger, Fear and Rage. New York, Appleton, 1920
4. Caplan G: Principles of Preventive Psychiatry. New York, Basic Books, 1964
5. Dunbar F: Emotions and Bodily Changes. New York, Columbia University Press, 1954
6. Friedman M, Rosenman RH: Type A Behavior and Your Health. New York, Alfred A. Knopf, 1974
7. Holmes TH: Life Situations, Emotions, and Diseases. Psychosomatics 19 (December): 747–754, 1978
8. Holmes TH, Rahe RH: The Social Readjustment Rating Scale. Journal of Psychosom Res 11:213–218, 1967
9. Leighton AH: My Name is Legion: Foundations for a Theory of Man in Relation to Culture, Vol. I: Sterling County Study of Psychiatric Disorder and Sociocultural Environment. New York, Basic Books, 1959
10. Looney JG, Lipp MR, Spitzer RL: A New Method of Classification for Psychophysiologic Disorders. Am J Psychiatry 135 (March): 304–308, 1978
11. Minuchin S, Roseman B, Baker L: Psychosomatic Families: Anorexia Nervosa in Context. Massachusetts, Harvard University Press, 1978
12. Mirsky IA: The Psychosomatic Approach to the Etiology of Clinical Disorders. Psychosom Med 19:424, 1957
13. Rosenman RH: The Impact of Anxiety on the Cardiovascular System. Psychosomatics 26, 11 (November): 6–15, 1985
14. Selye H: The Stress of Life. New York, McGraw-Hill, 1956
15. Sheppard NP, O'Loughlin S, Malone JP: Psychogenic Skin Disease: A Review of 35 Cases. Br J Psychiatry 149, 636–643, 1986
16. Srole L, Langner TS, Michael ST et al: Mental Health in The Metropolis: The Midtown Manhattan Study. New York, McGraw-Hill, 1962

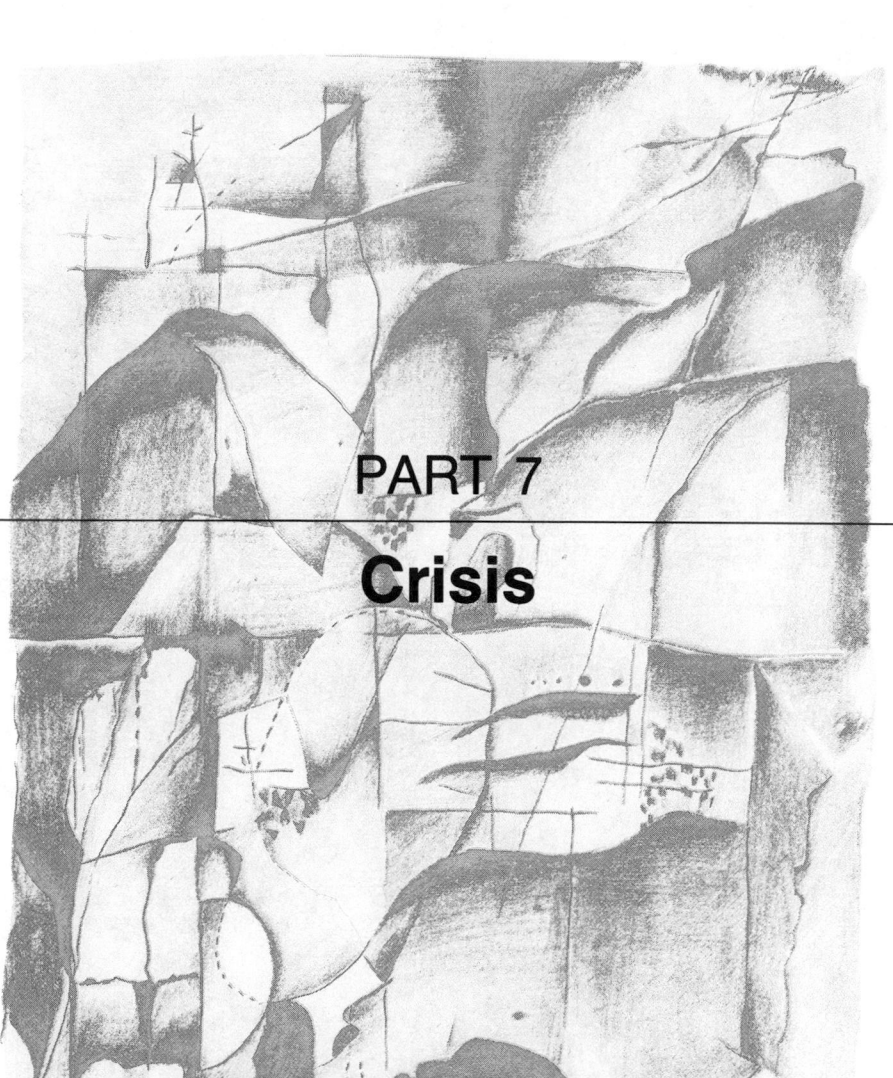

PART 7

Crisis

33 Crisis Theory and Intervention

Sandra Carter Chandler

A small trouble is like a pebble. Hold it too close to your eyes, and it fills the whole world and puts everything out of focus. Hold it at proper viewing distance, and it can be examined and properly classified. Throw it at your feet, and it can be seen in its true setting, just one more tiny bump on the pathway to eternity.

Celia Luce

Chapter Preview

In our vocabulary today, crisis and stress are common words that are often used interchangeably; however, stress and crisis are not synonymous. Many events in everyone's life are stressful—a new career, prematurely gray hair, the loss of a friend, or the acquisition of dentures. As long as the individual is able to cope with the stressful event and is not overwhelmed by it, he does not experience a crisis. On the other hand, any stressful event could precipitate a crisis for the individual, depending on his perceptions, his coping skills, and the support available to him. This chapter focuses on crisis theory and the types and development of crises. Crisis intervention is explored through the application of the nursing process to individuals in crisis.

Learning Objectives

On completion of the chapter, you should be able to accomplish the following:

1. discuss the development of crisis theory
2. describe the phases of a crisis
3. differentiate between maturational and situational crises
4. discuss the goals and methods of crisis intervention
5. contrast crisis intervention and traditional forms of therapy
6. apply the nursing process to a client or family in crisis
   - assess the perception of the precipitating event, the coping skills, and the available support system of the client in crisis
   - identify the nursing diagnoses of the client in a crisis
   - plan goals and an appropriate time frame for the resolution of a crisis
   - implement nursing actions to resolve a crisis in a healthy, adaptive manner
   - evaluate the effectiveness of the nursing actions
7. discuss the feelings and needs of the intervener in crises
8. formulate a comprehensive nursing care plan for the client in crisis

Crisis Theory

Crisis means a turning point, whether in disease or another condition. Two symbols in the Chinese language communicate crisis—they are "danger" and "opportunity."

In time of crisis, an individual is not sure what to do. His usual methods of problem-solving are not effective or are unavailable to him. As his anxiety and pain increase, the person becomes more willing to try new ways of problem-solving. In his willingness to try new methods of coping lies the opportunity for growth. Good mental health is thought to be predominantly the result of a life history of successful crisis resolutions.[5] Intervention during crisis has been found to reduce greatly the incidence and severity of mental disorders.

Development of Crisis Theory

Although people have been vulnerable to crises since the beginning of human existence, crisis has been an issue of serious study only in the past 30 years. Caplan defines crisis as a threat to homeostasis.[10] During crisis an imbalance exists between the magnitude of the problem and the immediate resources available to deal with it. This imbalance results in confusion and disorganization.[10] The active crisis state lasts a relatively short period of time—approximately 4 to 6 weeks. The individual is unable to tolerate this level of anxiety and imbalance for very long. Quick, appropriate intervention is of paramount importance in helping individuals in crisis return to an optimal state of functioning.

A number of researchers contributed to the development of crisis theory. Lindeman studied the survivors and families of the victims of the disastrous Coconut Grove nightclub fire in Boston in which many people died. Based on those observations and his study of other families who had lost a family member through death, Lindeman described the commonalities of the experience of crisis and bereavement.[26] From this classic study in 1944, some of the basic tenets of crisis theory were developed. Caplan has done the most extensive work on crisis theory and was influenced by the research and writings of Lindeman, Parad, Rapaport, Erikson, and others.[21] Crisis theory is derived from psychoanalytical theory and the work of ego psychologists. Ego psychology stresses the human ability to learn and grow throughout life.[21] The research upon which crisis theory is based involved the study of crisis in bereavement, the reactions of parents to the birth of a normal or premature child, crisis of surgery, crisis experienced by Peace Corps volunteers, responses to the ordinary upsets of early married life, and crisis as a result of war.[10]

Crisis theory emerged in an era of increased social consciousness. John F. Kennedy passionately addressed the Congress and the nation about the need for a national health program with a new approach to mental illness. He maintained that the promotion of mental health was everyone's responsibility—government at every level, private foundations, and individual citizens. Congress directed the establishment of a Joint Commission on Mental Illness and Health. As a result of the work of this commission, funds were made available for a nationwide system of community mental health centers whose emphasis was the prevention of emotional disorders. John F. Kennedy has been credited as an instrumental force in the revolution in American psychiatry.[10]

What Happens in a Crisis

According to crisis theory, an individual strives to maintain a constant state of emotional equilibrium. If he is confronted with an overwhelming threat and is unable to cope, crisis ensues.[1]

This state of disequilibrium, known as crisis, lasts approximately 4 to 6 weeks. Because the crisis state is accompanied by high anxiety, the individual will either adapt and return to his previous state of mental health, develop more constructive coping skills, or decompensate to a lower level of functioning.

The factors that influence the outcome of the crisis are as follows:

1. The individual's previous problem-solving experience
2. How the individual views the problem
3. The amount of help or hindrance from significant others in his life[21]

Maladaptive crisis resolution increases the probability that the individual will unsuccessfully resolve crises in the future.

During the crisis state of disequilibrium, the person is more open to receiving professional help and learning new ways of problem-solving. He is also more likely to make changes in attitude and behavior in a short period of time.

The focus of crisis intervention is on the problem or stressor that precipitated the crisis state rather than on personality traits. Some examples of stressors are marriage, loss of a limb, and death of a child. The person in crisis is viewed as essentially normal, capable of problem-solving, and capable of growth with a little assistance from others.[20, 21, 29, 35]

Phases of a Crisis

To better understand how a crisis develops, we will examine the phases or steps that lead to an active crisis state. The first phase of a crisis is an increase in anxiety in response to a traumatic event.[10] The person tries to use his familiar coping mechanisms to resolve the feeling of increased anxiety. If his coping mechanisms are effective, he will not be in crisis; however, if they are ineffective, he will enter the second phase of crisis, which is marked by an increase in anxiety due to the failure of his usual coping mechanisms.

In the third phase of crisis, the person's anxiety continues to rise and he usually feels forced to reach out and try to find some assistance. If the person is emotionally isolated before he experiences the traumatic event, it is usually impossible for him to avert a crisis.

The fourth phase is the active state of crisis, wherein the person's inner resources and support systems are inadequate. The precipitating event is not resolved and stress and anxiety mount to an intolerable level.

The individual in an active state of crisis demonstrates certain typical behaviors. He has a short attention span, ruminates, and looks inwardly for possible reasons for the traumatic event and how he might have changed or avoided it. This rumination is accompanied by a great deal of anguish, apprehension, and distress. The person's behavior becomes increasingly impulsive and unproductive. His relationships with others usually suffer. He becomes less aware of his environment and begins to view others in terms of their ability to help solve his problem. His searching behavior appears confused and disoriented.[6]

Due to the high level of anxiety he is experiencing, the individual may think that he is "losing his mind" or "going crazy."[21] His perceptive ability is greatly affected by high levels of anxiety, but this is not the same as psychosis. The individual in crisis often needs this explanation and the reassurance that, when he feels less anxious, he will be able to think clearly again.

Types of Crises

Maturational Crisis

There are two types of crisis—*maturational*, precipitated by the normal stress of development, and *situational*, precipitated by a sudden traumatic event. Erik Erikson identified specific periods in normal development when there is a predictable increase in anxiety or stress that could precipitate a maturational crisis.[12] Some common events that may precipitate a crisis during the various developmental stages are birth, mastering control of body functions, starting school, puberty, leaving home, marriage–parenthood, loss of physical youthfulness, and retirement.

A maturational, or developmental, crisis may occur at any of the transitional periods in normal growth and development. Because each stage of development is dependent on the previous stage, the inability to master the tasks of one stage thwarts one's growth and development in subsequent stages of life. Why are these times considered a crisis for some and not for others? One explanation is that some people are unable to make the numerous role changes necessary for the new maturational level.[18] For instance, the birth of the first child brings numerous role changes for the parents. Some parents are able to adapt and make the necessary role changes; others, due to a variety of reasons, such as emotional immaturity, marital discord, financial stress, and unmet dependency needs, may not be able to adapt readily to the new roles.

There are three main reasons why an individual may not be able to prevent a maturational crisis. First, he may not be able to visualize himself in the new role due to inadequate role models. For example, a male child reared without the love and guidance of a father or adult male may have difficulty assuming the role of a loving, guiding, involved parent. Second, the individual may lack the interpersonal resources to make the appropriate and necessary changes. For example, he may lack the flexibility to alter his life goals in order to avoid a midlife crisis, or he may lack the communication skills needed to maintain a long-term relationship. Third, other people may refuse to recognize the individual's maturational role change. Some parents fail to acknowledge their adolescent's movement toward adulthood and attempt to keep him in a child's role—precipitating a crisis for the adolescent.

In each stage of development, a person needs nurturance from others to work through the tasks of that stage and to obtain the necessary skills for the next level of development.[21] When adequate social support from family and friends is available, the individual is able to channel his increased anxiety and resultant energy into constructive growth and a feeling of accomplishment. Maturational crises are predictable and occur gradually; therefore, it is possible to prepare for these stressful transitional periods and prevent the occurrence of a crisis. Premarital counseling, preparation for parenting, and planning for retirement are examples of anticipatory guidance in crisis prevention.

Situational Crisis

A situational crisis is a response to a traumatic event that is usually sudden and unavoidable. When the stressful event threatens the physical, emotional, or social integrity of the individual, the likely result is a crisis.[1]

A situational crisis usually follows the loss of an established support. The individual's usual way of presenting himself is disrupted, and this disruption consequently threatens the way he views himself. From infancy on, each person develops an image of himself through the feedback he receives from the important people in his environment. Later in his development, the person defines himself according to the various roles he assumes. Throughout life, self-image hinges on the continuity of roles and the establishment of new role relationships. The threat or loss of a role viewed as necessary to maintain self-image will usually lead to a crisis state. The loss of a job, the loss of a spouse, the birth of a retarded child, or the diagnosis of a chronic or terminal illness will affect the way a person perceives himself.[19]

The most common response to a loss or deprivation is depression. An important point to remember in crisis intervention, however, is that if the person perceives the threat or loss as a challenge, he is more likely to move toward effective problem-solving.[32]

The difficulty in dealing with a situational crisis is compounded when it occurs while the individual is struggling with a developmental crisis.[15] Take note of this as an element in crisis intervention. A client, J. R., related that, without any prior discussion, on his 18th birthday, his father told him it was time for him to be out on his own. This occurred 2 months before Christmas and J. R. said that he was unsure of where to go or what to do. He felt hurt and abandoned. J. R. packed his suitcase and went to Europe. He spent the most miserable Christmas he could ever remember. Not long after that, his van exploded, resulting in a loss of most of his possessions. He also sustained burns on his face and hands. He remembers wandering around in a daze without being able to think clearly. The American Embassy helped him get home. Possibly, J. R. could have coped with the trauma of the fire if he had not been so vulnerable, struggling with his response to being forced to leave home.

Balancing Factors in a Stressful Event

There are certain factors that determine whether a person will enter a crisis state.[1] The balancing factors are as follows:

1. How the person perceives the event
2. What experience he has had in coping
3. His available coping mechanisms
4. The people who can be supportive to him

Aguilera and Messick devised a paradigm to assist the crisis intervener analyze and resolve a crisis situation (see Fig. 33-1).[1] It is important to remember

* Balancing factors (From Aguilera DC, Messick JM: Crisis Intervention, 5th ed. St Louis, CV Mosby, 1986)

Figure 33-1. *Paradigm: the effect of balancing factors in a stressful event.*

that the paradigm is a guide to help the intervener think clearly about the problem, not a solution to the client's problem. The person in crisis will need assistance working through some of the feelings associated with what has happened to him.

Crisis Intervention

The goal of crisis intervention is to assist the person in distress to resolve his immediate problem and regain his emotional equilibrium. This problem-solving will, it is hoped, lead to a higher level of coping ability to deal with future stressful events.

The role of the intervener is one of active participation with the individual in solving his present problem. Because the crisis state is not an illness, the helper does not take over and make decisions for the person unless he is suicidal or homicidal.[19,21,27] Crisis intervention is a partnership.[31] The underlying philosophy of crisis intervention is that, with varying degrees of assistance, people can help themselves.[21] To maximize the opportunity for growth, the person in crisis must be actively involved in resolving the problem. Crisis intervention is a thinking, problem-solving approach.[6]

The intervener helps the person in crisis analyze the stressful event, encourages him to express his feelings, and tells him that he has a right to his feelings no matter what they are. He explores methods of dealing with stress with the client and reinforces his strengths and abilities. The client is encouraged to seek support from friends, family, and other resource groups in the community. Planning designed to avert possible crises in the future is accomplished through anticipatory guidance.[1]

Crisis Intervention versus Traditional Therapies

The goal of traditional Freudian therapy is personality change. Its emphasis is on the client's past and the exploration of his subconscious. The Freudian therapist is usually nondirective and the length of therapy may be years.[1]

Briefer therapy attempts to remove the client's symptoms or prevent the development of more severe neurotic or psychotic problems. Depression and phobias are commonly diagnosed and treated by brief therapy, such as Gestalt therapy, behavior modification, or transactional analysis.[4]

Crisis intervention, on the other hand, assists a person in resolving an immediate problem that he perceives as overwhelming. Sometimes, the crisis stirs up unresolved issues from the client's past. These issues are not dealt with, however, until after the resolution of the crisis.

Crisis intervention emphasizes the healthy aspects of the personality, not pathology. There is no diagnosis of mental illness in crisis work. The individual is evaluated in terms of his ability to cope, his strengths and potentials, and his ability to problem-solve. The major focus of the therapeutic approach is the social structure of the individual, rather than the dynamics of the personality. It is assumed that the person will make appropriate decisions when given the necessary information and support. Crisis intervention requires a much more directive approach than traditional therapies.

Characteristics of the Crisis Intervener

To intervene in crises effectively, a therapist must demonstrate calmness and empathy. Because the person in crisis is often confused, the intervener must be able to identify the facts in a situation and think clearly in order to plan solutions to the problem.

The intervener should also be nonjudgmental and aware of different cultural values. There are different established patterns of response to death, illness, divorce, and pregnancy in various cultural, ethnic, and religious groups.[21] Crisis intervention is effective as long as the intervener does not impose a different lifestyle or value system on the client. A single woman, for example, overwhelmed with an unplanned pregnancy should not be subjected to chastisement or cool indifference in the "helper."

It is essential that the intervener possess cour-

age. The pain involved in a crisis is never pleasant. It is difficult to listen to the tragic things that happen to people; however, that is what the person in crisis needs—someone who will make the commitment to work with him until the problem is resolved, someone who can tolerate the uncomfortableness, the sadness, the anger.

Crisis Intervention and the Nursing Process

Assessment

Assessment of the person in crisis is the most important, and often the most difficult, step of crisis intervention. First, the nurse must determine whether the person is really in a crisis state. Tears, anger, and being upset do not automatically mean that the person is overwhelmed and in a crisis state.[3,21] If, however, the client is experiencing a great deal of anxiety, is having difficulty thinking clearly, and is unable to identify solutions to the problem, then it is helpful to encourage him to talk about the events that immediately preceded his distress.[1] This verbalization frequently calms the client and helps the nurse and client to establish rapport, the beginning of a relationship (see Chart 33-1, "The Client in Crisis"). The nurse must focus on the client's immediate problem, not his past history. Usually, when people in crisis reach out for help, the precipitating event has occurred within the previous 14 days; however, the event may have occurred within the past 24 hours.[1] The situations that can precipitate a crisis are countless—an unwanted pregnancy, the loss of hearing, the diagnosis of a terminal illness, the loss of a girlfriend, or the discovery of a spouse's extramarital affair.

The Client's Feelings

The nurse asks the client to describe the feelings he is experiencing. By accepting the client's feelings without judgment, the nurse assists him to accept his own feelings. The nurse will naturally feel some discomfort in the presence of a person in pain. The human inclination is to stop the person from crying, and to stop talking about what is horrible and upsetting to him. By avoiding the topic of his distress, the client could at least appear to be in less pain. Nevertheless, it is beneficial for the person in crisis to express his feelings and experience the pain or frustration firsthand. Therefore, the nurse must learn to tolerate these feelings of discomfort.

Usually, the nurse's increased anxiety stems from fear of saying "the wrong thing" or feeling inadequate to deal with the situation. It is important for

C H A R T 33-1
Therapeutic Dialogue

The Client in Crisis

Nurse: (walks into client's room, notices that Mr. T. is staring out the window with a sad expression on his face) Mr. T., you look sad to me. Is there something upsetting you?

Client: Oh, you don't have time to listen to me.

Nurse: Mr. T., I have 15 minutes now and I'll have more time later. Let's go for a walk and talk.

Client: (puts on his robe and continues to look at the floor as he walks down the hall)

Nurse: I want you to know that I'm available to listen to whatever is troubling you. So, just take a deep breath and get it off your chest.

Client: Well, you know I'm here because my ulcer is acting up, but what is really bothering me is I was fired from my job 2 weeks ago.

Nurse: Well, what are your feelings about that now?

Client: It's strange, it's like my life changed overnight. I've been working for this company for 10 years. I'm just stunned. I feel I'm a failure. Maybe I am a loser. Who is going to want to hire a failure? Until 2 weeks ago, I felt confident, I enjoyed socializing with the people I work with. Now, I feel like they are avoiding me.

Nurse: Do you want to see the people you work with right now?

Client: Well, yes and no. I don't know what to say to them.

Nurse: If you could get support from anyone you wanted to right now, who would it be?

Client: I'm not sure.

Nurse: Who do you trust?

Client: My father, but I'm so ashamed. I don't want to tell him.

Nurse: Let's examine your feelings of being ashamed. Mr. T., have you ever been fired before?

Client: No, never! Work has always been important to me.

Nurse: Tell me about the jobs you have had.

Client: I have worked for 25 years for three different companies. In this last one, I moved up to a mid-management position.

Nurse: Well, it sounds to me like you have had a lot of success in your career. You have worked for 25 years, right? That's a lot of years—25 years and never been fired before now. Mr. T., that doesn't sound like the work record of a failure to me.

Client: Well, my company has been having problems for a while. I just didn't think it would be me that they would let go. I thought Mr. J., my supervisor, appreciated what I have done in my department.

Nurse: How did you receive notice that you were let go?

Client: I received a letter.

Nurse: It never ceases to amaze me how poorly administrators deal with people.

Client: Yes, I always respected Mr. J. I expected more from him than that.

Nurse: Mr. T., after you are feeling better maybe you will want to go in and talk with Mr. J. about what actually happened. But right now, let's talk about your father. The news is full of companies in trouble and people losing their jobs. Don't you think your father will be hurt if you don't tell him?

Client: Yeh, he probably would be.

Nurse: How about giving him a call right now.

Client: Well, I guess I might as well get it over with. I'll call him at his office.

Nurse: I'll be back to talk with you in about an hour.

In this interview, note the distorted perception of the stressful event. Because Mr. T. was fired from his job, he felt that he was a failure. In reality, he had worked for 25 years without this occurrence. The nurse tried to encourage Mr. T. to view the situation in more realistic terms and to mobilize the social support of his father.

the nurse to understand both cognitively and emotionally that, ultimately, the client must make his own decisions. In fact, it is not expedient for the nurse to have all the answers to the client's problem. In order for the individual to grow, much of the work of problem-solving must come from him.

To help the crisis intervener focus on the problem, Aguilera and Messick devised a paradigm of the balancing factors in a stressful event.[1] It is often helpful, as a means of clarifying one's thinking, to write down and then evaluate the individual's perception of the event, his coping mechanisms, and his support systems.

Perception of the Event

The nurse who assesses the client in crisis first determines his perception of the stressful event. How threatened is the person? Is the person realistic or is he distorting the meaning of the event?[1]

Support Systems

After determining the client's perception of the event, the nurse focuses on who will be available to be supportive to the client. Questions such as "Whom do you trust?" "Who is your best friend?" and "Is there a member of your family to whom you are particularly close?" can help identify the client's support systems.

The nurse should also inquire into the religious beliefs of the individual in crisis because for many religious families, God is a source of comfort and strength. The individual's or family's religious affiliation may be an excellent resource for support.[17] It is best to have several supportive people involved with the client. Because a crisis period lasts for a brief time and the nurse will be involved only temporarily, the client needs others on whom to rely for continued support.

Coping Skills

To assess the individual's coping skills, the nurse asks him what he does when he cannot solve a problem; or the nurse may ask, "How do you deal with anxiety or depression?"[21] In any event, the nurse must encourage the client to describe his methods of coping as specifically as possible. The nurse then determines whether the client's coping mechanisms are adaptive or maladaptive. Assess the degree to which the individual is affected by the event. Is the person still functioning in his job? Is the person still attending school and fulfilling other roles, such as wife and mother? How are the significant people in the individual's life affected? Are they also upset?[1,21] The significant others may need crisis counseling as well.

Potential Self-Harm

An assessment of the person in crisis is not complete without asking him if he is having thoughts of hurting himself or "doing himself in." Most people will not volunteer this information, but when asked, will readily talk about suicidal thoughts. If the client has ever attempted suicide or has decided how, when, and where he will kill himself, the person needs protection. The suicidal client should not be left alone and needs an experienced therapist (see Chap. 37).

From the assessment data, the nurse should know the nature of the client's feelings, his perception of the precipitating event, whom he has to support and nurture him, how he copes with stress, and what his suicidal or homicidal potential is (see Chart 33-2).

Nursing Diagnosis

A crisis or precrisis state is neither a psychiatric illness nor a prolonged, disabling condition. While gathering assessment data from the client and family members, the nurse begins to conceptualize the appropriate descriptions of the client's responses to his health problems in terms of nursing diagnoses. Responses that are particularly evident in crisis are client and family ineffective coping, high level of anxiety, altered thinking and problem-solving, low self-esteem, social isolation, and impaired social interaction. In addition, the client in crisis may be experiencing powerlessness, alteration in parenting, disturbance in role performance, sleep disturbances, impaired communication, and impaired home maintenance management.

Some of the possible nursing diagnoses for the client in crisis include the following:

Anxiety related to situational and maturational crises, threat to self-concept, unmet needs, traumatic event, evidenced by restlessness, in-

---

C H A R T 33-2
Mental Note

All actions of the crisis intervener should be guided by the goal of safety for the client as well as for the intervener. In an emergency or during a crisis episode, it helps to have a ready mental cue to assist in problem-solving. Ask yourself:

What do I need to do to keep this person safe?

What do I need to do to remain safe myself as well?

somnia, verbalization of fear of going crazy and feelings of inadequacy, fearfulness, focus on self

Ineffective individual coping related to inadequate support systems, overwhelming problem, inadequate coping method, personal vulnerability, evidenced by inability to problem-solve, alteration in societal participation, inappropriate use of defense mechanisms, inability to meet role expectations, anxious mood

Alteration in thought processes related to situational and maturational crises, threat to self-concept, high anxiety level, evidenced by inability to problem-solve or make decisions, inaccurate interpretation of the environment, egocentricity, altered attention span/distractibility, inappropriate affect or thinking

Impaired social interaction related to self-concept disturbance, unmet dependency needs, evidenced by verbalized or observed discomfort in social situations, verbalized or observed inability to receive or communicate a satisfying sense of belonging and caring, dysfunctional interaction with peers, family, and others

Social isolation related to high level of anxiety and possible regression, evidenced by absence of supportive significant others (family, friends, group), uncommunicative and withdrawn behavior, preoccupation with own thoughts

Disturbance in self-concept: self-esteem, role performance, related to perception of overwhelming problem, lack of support systems, high anxiety level, evidenced by self-destructive behavior, lack of responsibility for self-care, verbalization of sense of worthlessness, inability to recognize own accomplishments, lack of role-appropriate behavior

Planning

No matter how critical the time factor, a plan is necessary.[18] Crisis intervention is a structured, objective, problem-solving approach. After collecting the data, the nurse obtains from the client a specific statement of the problem. To insure success of the plan, the client must be actively involved in planning solutions to the problem. An example of planning for a client without adequate participation of the client and family follows.

> Mrs. H. was hospitalized with a fractured hip. It was determined that, due to her cardiac condition and the rehabilitation needed for her hip, she could no longer live safely alone in her home. Her son and daughter were both married, had their own families, and were employed full-time.

> The daughter stated to the nurse, "I don't think we are going to be able to care for Mother at home." The nurse talked with Mrs. H.'s doctor and together they called the social worker to find a nursing home placement for Mrs. H.

> When Mrs. H. learned of the plan, she refused to go to the nursing home. Her family was upset and the nurse was irritated because she felt she had gone out of her way to be helpful.

> A difference in cultural values was part of this problem. In the nurse's family, moving into a nursing home when one can no longer live independently was expected and accepted. In the client's family, it was neither. For a crisis to be resolved successfully, the solutions to the problem must be in keeping with the cultural values of the client.

A universal response to crisis is a feeling of helplessness and of being out of control. The basic tenets of crisis intervention state that people can help themselves with varying degrees of assistance from others, and that crisis is an opportunity to grow and develop more constructive coping skills for future use. Therefore, it is essential that the client and significant others are actively involved in the planning stage of problem-solving.

The intervener should convey the attitudinal message that the client will be able to work through his crisis and take charge of his life again. Successful planning is dependent on thorough assessment and diagnosis of the client's level of functioning and his dependency needs. A basic rule of thumb is not to do things for people when they can do them, but always to do for people in crisis what they cannot do for themselves.[18] The more distraught and confused the client is, the more directive the intervener needs to be. Together, the nurse and client define a time frame and goals for resolution of the crisis.

Often, in planning, it is helpful for the intervener to outline the problem and available resources, using the paradigm of the balancing factors in a stressful event. In addition, by using the decision counseling approach, the intervener can clarify with the client the boundaries of the problem.

What are the agreed upon tentative solutions?
Where will the solutions be tried?
What is the time frame?
Who will do what?

Follow-up is critical and should be part of the initial plan.

Goal-Setting for the Client in Crisis

The major goal of crisis intervention is to assist the client in reestablishing his equilibrium. To reach that end, the following goals are set:

1. Establishment of a working relationship with the client
2. Identification of the specific problem
3. Reduction of the distortion of the client's perception of the event
4. Improvement of the client's self-esteem
5. Decreasing of the client's anxiety
6. Promotion of the involvement of family and friends
7. Reinforcement of healthy coping mechanisms
8. Validation of the client's ability to solve his problem

It is sometimes difficult, but is absolutely essential, for the nurse to accept that the goals of crisis intervention are different from the goals of other therapies. It is not the task of the crisis intervener to deal with all the client's problems or to orchestrate major changes in the client's life.[1,6] The aim of crisis intervention is to assist the individual in solving the immediate problem that was so overwhelming that he was unable to cope. Once he has regained his emotional equilibrium and is able again to cope, the work of crisis intervention has been accomplished.

Intervention

Realizing the Potential for Growth

Crisis intervention has been called "psychological first aid."[20] Nurturance, caring, listening, and willingness to help are powerful and saving forces for people in crisis. Within any crisis situation is the potential for the individual who is faced with an overwhelming stressor to develop a higher level of coping ability than he possessed prior to the precipitating event. Whether this possibility for growth is realized or not attained depends, in part, on the appropriateness of the crisis intervention.

The nurse and client reexamine any feelings that might block adaptive coping. When an individual has extremely negative feelings, for example, about mental illness or physical disabilities, it is particularly difficult for that person to be faced with similar circumstances. The person must deal with those feelings before he can adequately cope with his situation.

Learning to Ask for Help

In a crisis state, it is natural to feel isolated and withdrawn. Therefore, the client must be helped to communicate directly with significant others in his life. Often, the client has to be taught how to ask for help. The nurse can help demonstrate this skill to the client through role modeling. People who place a high value on their independence may need assistance in recognizing interdependence as a healthy balance.

Using Adaptive Coping

The nurse also teaches and helps the client develop healthier coping skills. During a crisis, an individual is more open and amenable to trying some new means to relieve his anxiety. The nurse encourages the client to use adaptive coping mechanisms, such as the open expression of feelings, progressive relaxation, physical exercise, and drinking warm milk or herb tea to help him relax and sleep, rather than relying on maladaptive coping through excessive alcohol or drug ingestion, social withdrawal, suicide, or homicide.[19,21]

Focusing on the Problem Resolution

As the crisis intervener, the nurse keeps the client focused on the problem and specific goals leading to its resolution. The client's high anxiety level may make it difficult for him to focus on one issue, and he may need direction to avoid fragmentation of his efforts. After the client has attempted some of the alternative solutions to his problem, he and the nurse evaluate their effectiveness and decide whether additional plans are needed. The nurse reinforces the client's abilities by reviewing the crisis event, how he has been able to cope, and any new methods of problem-solving or coping that he has acquired.

Team Approach

A crisis team approach is sometimes employed in short-term, inpatient psychiatric treatment facilities. A group of four to six clinicians of different educational preparation and experience comprise a crisis team. The team rotates leadership and may consist of a psychiatrist, a psychiatric–mental health nurse, a psychologist, a social worker, a psychiatric aide, a minister, and students in the mental health field. One clinician assumes the role of the primary person responsible for the management of a client; however, continuity of care is built into the system due to the fact that a number of people are involved with the client. The crisis team meets daily to discuss the client's progress. Decisions involving the client are made by the group. The psychiatrist outlines clinical indications for the client and the other team members implement the plan and decide on time of discharge and method and frequency of follow-up. As in any crisis intervention mode, the goals have to be kept clearly in mind, and, as soon as they are reached, the client is discharged, even if it is his day of admission.[25]

A young woman, S.L., was admitted to a crisis unit following notification that her husband was reported missing in South Korea. The client had no relatives who could be supportive to her. She had not been able to eat or sleep for the last 3 days. Her only friend brought her to the hospital for admission.

S.L. was becoming dehydrated; therefore, the physician ordered IV therapy and a mild sedative to be discontinued the following day. After the initial interview, the team met to discuss the areas in which S.L. needed assistance to facilitate coping with her distress.

In the interview, the crisis team learned that S.L. was ordinarily independent, held a responsible job, and had coped well with living alone in her husband's absence; however, S.L. was expecting her husband home in 2 weeks. It was agreed that S.L. needed more people to be supportive in order for her to deal with this crisis. The nurse made plans to introduce S.L. to other clients who would be particularly supportive, and she encouraged S.L. to contact some of her co-workers. The minister investigated what community support was available. The social worker phoned the Red Cross to see if they could assist in communications with the government. In 3 days, S.L. was eating again and able to sleep better. She had decided to move in with her friend temporarily. S.L. was discharged from the inpatient unit to outpatient status, where she was followed through four weekly appointments.

Crisis Groups

The goal of a crisis group is the same as individual crisis intervention—that the members regain their precrisis functioning ability or develop an even higher level of ability to problem-solve. For some people, a crisis group is more beneficial than one-to-one therapy, paticularly when the person has difficulty with interpersonal relationships. Others who may benefit from a crisis group are people who have difficulty accepting information from psychiatric professionals or from people they see in an authority position.

Advantages of a Crisis Group. Some advantages of a crisis group are that the individual members feel less isolated and that they often make social contact with some of the members in and outside of the group. By seeing other people express their feelings, the members realize that other people have similar feelings and problems. Often, the reticent individual can more easily express opinions and feelings after observing other people in a similar situation. Members offer each other suggestions for coping and solving problems; by helping each other within the group, the members' self-esteem is bolstered.

Disadvantages of a Crisis Group. There are some disadvantages, however, of a crisis group. It is difficult to keep each individual's crisis in focus in a group setting. Another problem in crisis groups is the destructive forms of coping or maladaptive problem-solving, which may be suggested by group members.

These problems substantiate the need for a trained crisis group leader.[1]

Format and Rules of the Group. Crisis groups are usually scheduled for 1½ to 2 hours, once a week, for 6 weeks. Five to seven members is considered ideal in a crisis group. Some crisis groups are homogeneous, with every member having a similar problem. For example, successful supportive groups have been formed for divorced people, victims of incest, parents in crisis, homosexuals, cancer patients, and many other similar groupings. Some peer groups, organized by lay people rather than by professionally trained people, have also been successful. The best known group among these is probably Alcoholics Anonymous. A heterogeneous group is one in which the members have different problems but are all in crisis. The group may be an open one, in which new members come in and others work through their problems and leave the group. This gives members an opportunity to deal with feelings about intrusion and separation. A closed group does not accept new members after it is formed and continues for a specified time.

Assessing members and clearly stating the purpose of a group are both crucial aspects of group formation.[21] The members must agree to the rules of the group, such as confidentiality, and they must be able to accept other responsibilities required of group membership. A crisis group can offer an excellent opportunity for people to develop new skills, more successful ways of interacting with others, and ways to increase self-confidence and self-esteem.

Families in Crisis

Seldom does a person live in total isolation. Usually, a crisis occurs within a family constellation and affects all those who are in close contact with the client. It is not uncommon for parents to be struggling with midlife crises at the same time their adolescent is struggling with establishing his separate identity.[14, 18] People in crises are either helped or hindered by the people in their social network.[21, 30] Anyone with whom a person routinely interacts, such as friends, family, hairdresser, doctor, teacher, or employer, is part of his social network. The issues of crisis may be viewed within a social framework; until severed social relationships are reestablished, the crisis remains unresolved.[19]

While working with families in crisis, the nurse determines which member of the family is most obviously upset in the crisis state. Different labels may be used: Who is the scapegoat? Who is the symptom bearer? Who is the identified client?[21] Next, the nurse identifies all members of the individual's social network who were involved before, or are involved now because of the crisis. Then, the social resources that would be helpful to the client in crisis resolution are determined. The nurse explains the crisis to the person in crisis and tells how others could assist him.

The intervener is very directive in bringing together the person in crisis and all members of his social system for a conference. During the conference all those involved in the crisis analyze the problem and the effect it has on each family member. Everyone is given an opportunity to verbalize comments or complaints. Available resources and possible solutions are discussed. It is important that, by the end of the conference, the participants have developed a definite plan of action. They must establish exactly who is going to do what and when. The nurse should set a follow-up meeting and help the group decide the time, place, participants, and established purpose of the meeting. The social system approach is very effective in dealing with many-faceted crisis situations, such as family crises.

Frequently, the hospital is the scene of family crises:

A 16-year-old male was admitted to the hospital with the diagnosis of leukemia—he is a juvenile diabetic with a white blood cell count of 300. Previously, he had been active in sports and suddenly he was too tired to do anything but watch television. His father had recently died due to a myocardial infarction. His mother refuses to allow her son to be informed about his illness and planned therapy.

Another admission may look like this:

A 12-year-old girl has attempted suicide by taking an overdose of butalbital (Fiorinal). She has been living with her mother and stepfather; however, she wants to live with her father and stepmother. The mother states that the child's father wants no communication or contact with the child. The mother told the student nurse, "Don't talk with my daughter about taking the pills. It just upsets her."

Evaluation

In the evaluation process, the nurse and client together evaluate whether the problem has been solved. Has the person regained his equilibrium and his usual level of functioning? It is important for the nurse to know when to "let go" of the client. Before dissolving the partnership, the nurse and client should engage in anticipatory planning so that the client's ability to avoid crisis responses in the future will be maximized.[11,34] The client may need additional information about community services or community re-

sources. After working through the crisis response, some clients are motivated to seek additional therapy to resolve old conflicts; therefore, referrals may be made.[18,21]

The Nurse's Feelings and Attitudes

Nurses often refer people in crisis to other professionals they believe are better qualified to handle the situation.[2] This is unfortunate because nurses are frequently the first health care professionals available to the client. From the standpoint of crisis intervention, the client facing an overwhelming threat needs assistance quickly. Nurses can, and must, provide effective crisis intervention.

The nurse's first experiences in crisis intervention will be neither easy nor comfortable. Often, the novice needs assistance in determining the appropriate expectations for an intervention for both client and nurse.[8] Feelings of apprehension, frustration, anger, and wanting to escape from the situation are not uncommon. Even the most experienced crisis intervener needs a colleague or supervisor who will help him discuss feelings and plan strategies, and will offer support and encouragement.

Anyone who works with people in stressful situations needs to be aware of his own vulnerability to crisis.[9] Symptoms of crisis may go unnoticed in nurses because of their caregiver roles.[16] Nurses who have learned to cope well with the inherent stress of the hospital setting have often created their own support system within the work environment. In one hospice unit, for example, the nurses met together for a few minutes at the beginning and end of each shift to share what was going on with each other. Frequently, they brought food to share as well. When a nurse was having a difficult time, the others felt comfortable offering her comfort as they would comfort a family member.[22,36] Support of this nature is advantageous, if not mandatory, in maintaining mental health.[1]

Summary

This chapter has examined how individuals and families respond when faced with an overwhelming stressor; it has also examined the therapeutic approach to help them avoid or grow from the crisis. The major points of the chapter are as follows:

1. Crisis theory evolved from the study of grief and bereavement by many researchers.
2. An individual who is faced with an overwhelming threat tries his usual coping mechanisms and, if they are unsuccessful in solving

J. L. was a 36-year-old woman, a mother of two children (7 and 9 years old), and a full-time student in nursing school. One year before completing her nursing program, J. L. learned that her husband had been having an affair with a 20-year-old woman. He informed J. L. that he was moving out and intended to live with the other woman.

J. L. came to the Community Mental Health Center for counseling because she was not maintaining a passing grade average and feared that she would not be able to remain in school. She was having difficulty coping with both the abrupt changes in her personal life and the pressures of nursing school—and she desperately wanted to finish school.

J. L. felt alienated from everyone. Her parents, particularly her father, thought it must be her fault that her husband left. J. L.'s father remembered the trauma of his parents' divorce and he did not want his grandchildren to grow up the way he did. Some of J. L.'s friends were not able to spend much time with her. J. L.'s usual method of coping was to "work hard" and "stay as busy as possible." This coping tactic had not been useful for her lately because of her inability to concentrate, frequent crying spells, and insomnia. J. L. felt she was a failure as a woman and was concerned about her attractiveness to men.

The nurse, as crisis intervener, and J. L. agreed that the immediate problems were the impending divorce and staying in school. Financial options were explored, such as loans, scholarships, and working part-time. J. L. was given permission and encouraged to get the help she needed. The nurse told her, "You have nothing to be ashamed of. You are having a difficult time as anyone would in your situation. Ask your teachers for the help you need." J. L. was encouraged to reach out to some of her classmates for support.

An important point to consider when dealing with people who are getting a divorce is that, often, the person's support system breaks down. Parents grieve the loss of their child's spouse and the family unit. Friends grieve as well; they will never interact as couples in quite the same way. Friends also experience fears and doubts about their own marriages. The person in crisis needs help in understanding the effects of the divorce on everyone. Through teaching direct communication and helping the client acknowledge with the parents and friends the natural sadness and loss, grieving is shared. It may be necessary to role-play with the client how she might handle a difficult situation. For example, J. L. might role-play her encounter with her father. "Dad, I know you are very sad and hurt. This must bring back the feelings you had when your dad and mother got a divorce. I want you to know that I love you. That hasn't changed, and I need you to love me." If communication cannot be worked out with family and friends, the nurse must supply the emotional support to the client.

Other means of support should be explored, such as groups at the college's women's center. J. L. was able to work out better communication with her family and friends, which increased her feelings of being in control and also increased her self-esteem. The children came into counseling for one session to work out communication problems within the family.

The nurse encouraged J. L. to make out a schedule for each day of the week and to include a treat every day—lunch with a friend, coffee in bed, and so forth. J. L. was frequently reminded to think highly of herself and to treat herself with respect. The nurse praised any efforts J. L. made to communicate with others and meet her own needs.

In dealing with J. L.'s feelings about being a failure as a woman because her husband left to live with another woman, J. L. was helped to realize that, for the last several years, she and her husband developed different goals that were in conflict. The reasons for the divorce, she began to understand, had nothing to do with her attractiveness as a woman.

After several weeks, J. L. was a member of a study group and was again making passing grades. She looked better and stated that she felt better. J. L. was able to juggle care of her children, school, work part-time, and socialize occasionally with the help of classmates who were in similar circumstances. J. L. related that the divorce was the most painful experience of her life, but she was stronger than she ever thought possible and felt better able to cope with her present and future life.

Questions for Discussion

1. What does divorce mean in our society today? What are the cultural variations of the meaning of divorce?
2. Discuss the effects of divorce on family members and friends. Why is divorce such a devastating experience for most people?
3. What actions of friends and family might help the client avoid a crisis situation?
4. How could health care workers assist the client and her family?
5. Discuss therapeutic techniques to use when working with a client with a distorted perception of the stressful event.

Nursing Care Plan 33-1

The Client Who Is in Crisis

Nursing Diagnosis	Outcome	Intervention
Ineffective individual coping related to inadequate support systems, overwhelming problem	Establishes a working relationship	Establish availability 1. Time you are available (*e.g.,* 9–5 M–F); emergencies call _____ 2. Emotional availability—caring attitude, willingness to help Provide measures to help the individual to feel important "I would like for you to feel comfortable. Would you like some coffee or something else to drink? Are you warm enough?" Show acceptance—both verbal and nonverbal; sit beside the person, not behind a desk
Anxiety related to situational and maturational crises, threat to self-concept, evidenced by restlessness, insomnia	Verbalizes means to deal with manifestations of anxiety; verbalizes relief of anxiety	Teach healthy coping skills Suggest walking, drinking herb tea, warm milk, eating comforting foods; give permission to accept comfort measures as if the person were physically ill Reassure that strange feelings, such as, "I'm losing my mind," are due to high anxiety
Alteration in thought processes evidenced by impaired ability to make decisions, problem-solve, reason, or conceptualize	Identifies the specific problem precipitating the crisis; verbalizes the use of coping mechanisms that worked in the past; evidences problem-solving ability	Take a directive approach "What happened that upset you enough to call? Try to be as specific as you can." Example: "Even as stressful as this has been for you, you have managed to continue working." Ask what the person does when things go wrong. Reinforce healthy coping skills. Teach possible coping methods. Diagram the problem according to Aguilera's paradigm. Ask for a commitment from the individual to participate in solving the problem. Then, both parties should agree on specific solutions to attempt (*e.g.,* nurse will call Bread Basket for emergency food; client will call best friend to help with the children for a couple of days).
Alteration in thought processes evidenced by inaccurate interpretation of the environment (the event precipitating the crisis)	Verbalizes decreased distortion in perception of precipitating event	Gently point out the facts Example: One failing grade does not make a person a failure

Nursing Diagnosis	Outcome	Intervention
Disturbance in self-concept: low self-esteem	Evidences rise in self-esteem; verbalizes own strengths	Comment on strengths; individualize approach to client; call by name
Social isolation evidenced by absence of supportive significant others (family and friends)	Verbalizes an increased involvement of family or friends	Encourage the expression of feelings and direct communication with friends and family

the problem, experiences a mounting level of anxiety.

3. A crisis occurs when an individual is unable to solve a problem that he perceives as overwhelming, when his usual coping mechanisms fail to solve the problem, when his perception of the event is distorted, and when he lacks the necessary social support.

4. People experiencing a crisis are more open to learning new coping skills to deal with their problem.

5. There exists the potential for a person in crisis to develop more adaptive coping and, therefore, healthier functioning capabilities after the crisis experience.

6. Maturational crises result from developmental changes and milestones, such as puberty, marriage, old age, and death of a loved one.

7. Situational crises result from sudden, unexpected events, such as divorce, illness, injury, and loss of a job.

8. Crisis intervention is a thinking, directive, problem-solving approach that focuses only on the client's immediate problems.

9. Nurses are often the first health care professionals in contact with the client in crisis; therefore, they are uniquely positioned to intervene in crises.

10. Any crisis intervener needs a colleague or supervisor with whom he can discuss feelings and plan approaches and from whom he can receive support and encouragement.

References

1. Aguilera DC, Messick JM: Crisis Intervention: Theory and Methodology, 5th ed. St Louis, CV Mosby, 1986

2. Ballow M, Rebich C: Crisis Intervention: A Call for Involvement for the Health Professional. J Sch Health 47 (December): 603–606, 1977

3. Baird SA: Helping the Family Through a Crisis. Nursing 87 (June): 66–67, 1987

4. Bellak L, Small L: Emergency Psychotherapy and Brief Psychotherapy, 2d ed. New York, Grune & Stratton, 1978

5. Bloom BL: Definitional Aspects of the Crisis Concept. In Porad H (ed): Crisis Intervention: Selected Readings, pp 303–311. New York, Family Service Association of America, 1973

6. Berchopp GW: Crisis Intervention: Theory, Process and Practice. In Lester D, Berchopp G (eds): Crisis Intervention and Counseling by Telephone, pp 89–104. Springfield, IL, Charles C Thomas, 1973

7. Bosse LA: A Disaster with Few Survivors. Am J Nurs (July): 918, 1987

8. Burgess AW, Baldwin BA: Crisis Intervention Theory and Practice: A Clinical Handbook. New York, Prentice-Hall, 1981

9. Caplan G: Mastery of Stress: Psychosocial Aspects. Am J Psychiatry 138 (April): 413–419, 1981

10. Caplan G: Principles of Preventive Psychiatry. New York, Basic Books, 1964

11. Caplan G, Grunebaum H: Perspectives on Primary Prevention. Arch Gen Psychiatry 17 (September): 333–345, 1967

12. Erikson EH: Childhood and Society, 2d ed. New York, WW Norton, 1963

13. Fitzpatrick JJ, Reed PG: Stress in the Crisis Experience: Nursing Interventions. Occupational Health Nursing (December): 19–21, 1980

14. Gaston SK: Death and Midlife Crisis. J Psychiatr Nurs Ment Health Serv 19, 1, 31–35, 1981

15. Golan N: Using Situational Crisis to Ease Transitions in the Life Cycle. Am J Orthopsychiatry 50 (July): 542–550, 1980

16. Grant JM: Nurse in Crisis. NZ Nurs J 71 (7): 18–21, 1978

17. Griffith JL: Employing the God-Family Relationship in Therapy with Religious Families. Family Process 25 (December): 609–618, 1986

18. Hall YE, Weaver BR: Nursing in Families in Crisis. Philadelphia, JB Lippincott, 1974

19. Hansell N: The Person in Distress. New York, Human Services Press, 1976

20. Hausman W, Rioch DM: Military Psychiatry. Arch Gen Psychiatry 16 (June): 727–739, 1967

21. Hoff LA: People in Crisis: Understanding and Helping. California, Addison-Wesley, 1978

22. Hoffman Y: Surviving A Child's Suicide. Am J Nurs (July): 955–956, 1987

23. Jacobson GF: Crisis Theory and Treatment Strategy: Some Sociocultural and Psychodynamic Considerations. J Nerv Ment Dis 141 (August): 209–218, 1965

24. Kliman AS: Crisis: Psychological First Air for Recovery and Growth. New York, Holt, Rinehart, 1978

25. Lieb J, Lipsitch I, Slaby A: The Crisis Team: A Handbook for the Mental Health Professional. New York, Harper & Row, 1973

26. Lindeman E: Symptomatology and Management of Acute Grief. Am J Psychiatry 101 (September): 141–148, 1944

27. Manglass L: Psychiatric Intervention You Can Use in an Emergency. RN (November): 38–39, 1986

28. Mitchell CE: Identifying the Hazard: The Key to Crisis Intervention. Am J Nurs (July): 1194–1196, 1977

29. Narayan SM, Joslin DJ: Crisis Theory and Intervention: A Critique of the Medical Model and Proposal of a Holistic Nursing Model. Advances in Nursing Science 2 (July): 27–39, 1980

30. Paschal JH, Schwann L: Intensive Crisis Counseling in Florida. Children Today (November/December): 12–15, 1986

31. Phelan LA: Crisis Intervention: Partnership in Problem Solving. J Psychiatr Nurs Ment Health Serv 17(9): 22–27, 1979

32. Rapoport L: The State of Crisis: Some Theoretical Considerations. Soc Serv Rev 36 (June): 211–217, 1962

33. Ruditis SE: Developing Trust in Nursing Interpersonal Relationships. J Psychiatr Nurs Ment Health Serv 17(4): 20–23, 1979

34. Schulberg HC, Sheldon A: The Probability of Crisis and Strategies for Preventive Intervention. Arch Gen Psychiatry 18 (May): 553–558, 1968

35. Taplin JR: Crisis Theory: Critique and Reformation. Community Ment Health J 1 (March): 13–23, 1971

36. Taylor PB, Gideon MD: But Who Will Minister to You? Nursing 81 11(10): 58–61, 1981

37. Wardell SC: Acute Intervention: Nursing Process Throughout the Life Span. Reston, VA, Reston Publishing Company, 1979

38. Wollersheim J: When Your Patient's Depressed You Can Make a Difference. Nursing Life 6 (March/April): 18–21, 1986

34 Rape and Sexual Assault

Sally Francis

The world breaks everyone and afterwards many are strong in the broken places.

Ernest Hemingway,
A Farewell to Arms

Chapter Preview

Rape is a crime of violence that touches everyone at some time, in some way. It is estimated that one of every ten women in the United States is a victim of rape and a rape occurs once every 6 minutes in the United States.[34] Consequently, the woman and her family, friends, co-workers, and acquaintances must acknowledge and face their own individual fears of vulnerability, loss of control, perversion, bodily harm, and death. Our hope in a crisis event that affects so many people is that all can "become strong in the broken places" and that psychiatric–mental health nurses will recognize and respond to the needs of the rape victim and her significant others during the mending and healing process.

This chapter will describe rape and sexual assault, its theoretical perspectives, the emotional effects and recovery, and intervention programs. The nursing process will be discussed during the immediate or emergency phase, the intermediate phase, and the recovery phase of the rape crisis. Through application of the nursing process—assessment, nursing diagnosis, planning, intervention, and evaluation—individuals and families affected by rape or sexual assault can be assisted to grow "strong" in their coping and adaptation.

Rape can, and does, occur with men as victims. Men raped by other men have been found to have long-term depressions, difficulties in peer relationships, and sexual dysfunction.[29] In addition, men raped by women report sexual dysfunctions and depression.[34] However, the overwhelming majority of rape victims are female. For this reason the focus of this chapter will be the female rape victim. It is reasonable to assume that the nursing process as applied to women can also benefit male victims.[29]

Learning Objectives

Upon completion of the chapter, you should be able to accomplish the following:

1. identify the typology of rape and sexual assault
2. define rape trauma syndrome and discuss the behaviors of a victim during the acute, reorganization, and recovery phases of rape trauma syndrome
3. identify and define unresolved rape trauma and silent rape trauma
4. discuss primary motivating forces of the assailant in crimes of rape and sexual assault
5. discuss primary offender treatments
6. apply the nursing process to the care of the victim of rape or sexual assault

    assess the physical and emotional status of clients who have been raped or sexually assaulted

    formulate nursing diagnoses for clients who have been raped or sexually assaulted

    plan nursing goals and actions designed to prevent or alleviate the rape victim's identified problems

    formulate a comprehensive nursing care plan for a client who has been raped or sexually assaulted

    evaluate the effectiveness of the planned intervention
7. recognize and discuss your feelings that may influence the therapeutic use of self with victims of rape and sexual assault

Theoretical Perspectives of Rape and Sexual Assault

Rape and sexual assault can be viewed from historical, legal, psychological, and sociological perspectives. It is curious that, until recent years, this overwhelming physical assault has received so little attention from research. The mythology of the ancient Greeks contains descriptions of rape which have continued through the centuries. References to rape appear in literature from each century of civilization's development. Nevertheless, it was not until the early 1970s that researchers attempted to describe the victim and rapist in terms that could lead to intervention and that could influence the psychological impact of rape.

Legal Perspective

Definition of Rape and Sexual Assault

Rape is a crime involving lack of consent, force or threat of force, and sexual penetration. Sexual assault refers to forcible sexual acts performed without the victim's consent and against his or her will. Specifically, rape is defined as a crime by the legal statutes of individual state governments. In 1982, 77,000 cases of rape were reported in the United States.

An important concept in identifying rape or sexual assault is the use of force against one's will. In this light, the crime of rape or sexual assault is one of force and violence in which sex becomes the means of expressing violence, just as, in a murder, a gun may become the means of expressing violence.

Psychological Perspective

One of the most traumatizing aspects of the crime of rape or sexual assault involves the victim's feelings about being physically forced to do something against her will. The life-threatening nature of the crime, the helplessness, the loss of control, and the experiencing of self as an object of rage all work together to result in overwhelming fear and stress for the victim. This experience has been described as the *rape trauma syndrome.*[5,6] This syndrome is viewed by some as a particular example of post-traumatic stress disorder as defined in the DSM-III-R. This classification can be made when the following four conditions are met:

1. Existence of a recognizable stressor
2. Re-experience of the trauma as evidenced by recurrent recollections of the event
3. Numbing of responsiveness or reduced involvement with the external world
4. Two additional symptoms, such as: sleep disturbances; guilt about surviving or behaviors required for survival; memory impairment; difficulty concentrating; avoidance of activities that arouse recollection of the traumatic event; intensification of symptoms by exposure to events that symbolize or resemble the event[6,19]

Regaining internal equilibrium and the ability to reorganize life into a meaningful and productive whole becomes, therefore, the goal of intervention.

Types of Sexual Assault

Burgess and Holstrom were the early researchers in the study of rape trauma syndrome.[10] Based on their study of 146 rape victims in the early 1970s, they identified four types of sexual assault: the blitz rape, the confidence rape, accessory-to-sex with inability to consent, and the sex-stress situation.

Blitz rape occurs when the woman has neither previous knowledge of, nor threat of vulnerability from, the rapist. Although blitz rape usually occurs in the woman's home, the attacker may suddenly accost the woman in a parking lot, on the street, or any place where he can strike "out of the blue."

> "I thought I was having a bad dream—that I was screaming. As I regained consciousness, I felt like I was moving up from a dark hole, screaming. It seemed like I slowly realized I wasn't dreaming. I was awake and screaming. A man was holding me down on the sofa where I had fallen asleep earlier in the evening. He had his hands on my face, pushing me down and trying to cover my mouth. He kept telling me to shut up, to stop screaming."

Confidence rape refers to a rape that involves some interaction between the assailant and victim be-

fore the rape occurs. Access to the victim is obtained by the rapist by gaining her confidence in some way. For example, the man may ring a doorbell, ask to use the phone for some assistance, gain entry into the woman's territory, and then rape her.

Accessory-to-sex describes sexual acts with an individual who is unable to consent to sex. The inability to consent results from the female's immature stage of personality or cognitive development, which prevents her from recognizing or understanding the overtures and sexual events. An example of the accessory-to-sex type of sexual assault is a mentally retarded woman who is seduced by the promise of material goods in exchange for sexual activity.

Sex-stress situation refers to events arising after initial consent to sex is given. For example, a woman may agree to a sexual experience with a date who later becomes violent and physically abusive. She then withdraws her earlier consent and he rapes her. *Date rape* is similar, in that consent to be with the individual (a date) has been given, but consent to sexual activity has not been given.

In each of these situations, sexual acts become a means for acting out distorted perceptions held by the male. The female becomes an object who experiences this objectification, powerlessness, and loss of self as a basic, consuming fear. The resultant trauma reaction of the victim, rape trauma syndrome, serves to promote self-preservation; it is a "flight" reaction when fight is not possible. Rape trauma syndrome identifies the psychological work in which the ego must engage to preserve its identity and integration.

Sociological Perspective

Myths About Rape

Although the motivation to rape arises from personality, societal attitudes influence the incidence, prevalence, and treatment of rape and sexual assault. The sociological perspective includes the myths that society holds about rape.[11] These myths and stereotypical views of rape define how a victim sees herself in relation to society, how society views the victim and the rapist, and the difficulty or ease with which a victim receives support from society. For example, the prevalent myth of rape is that it is motivated by sexual desire and that, in fact, the woman who is raped must have "asked for it." Rapists are seen as exaggerations of the "macho" male. If the victim is a person who society believes would not "ask for it," for example, a child or an elderly woman, the rapist is viewed as a very sick, disturbed, psychotic individual. A young woman hitchhiking, who is raped but not beaten by a driver who picks her up, is frequently viewed with little sympathy; however, her fears, helplessness, and loss of control can be as traumatizing as the fears experienced by a woman badly beaten in a blitz rape. Not infrequently, women who are raped, as members of the society, share the myths of the society. They experience self-blame and guilt and feel that they should have done something, or not done something, that could have prevented the assault.

> "A part of me was relieved when the police came that I looked so bad, that there was blood, that the door had been broken open, the house was torn up, and there were fingerprints. There couldn't be any doubt that something awful had happened to me."

Who Is to Blame?

Public education programs have made progress in changing society's attitudes about rape and sexual assault. Nevertheless, rape continues to be one of the most frequently underreported crimes. In an attempt to understand public attitudes, several studies have examined how various segments of society attribute blame for the crime of rape.

In one study, four predominate causal attitudes toward rape were identified—blaming the victim, blaming the offender, blaming society, or blaming the situation.[37] Another study included ineffective law enforcement and judicial procedures as potential causes of rape.[17] The multidimensional nature of societal attitudes toward rape has been demonstrated by two studies in which victim blame, offender characteristics, situational characteristics, and societal blame emerged as factors in the development of these attitudes.[16,32] Other studies have determined that there are sex differences regarding attitudes toward rape.[11,12,39] Women tend to place greater blame on society for the occurrence of rape and sexual assault. Feminist writings and popular literature have explored the socialization into sex roles and the role of violence in our society. In a society, they say, that both encourages the treatment of women as sex objects and encourages violence, women cannot avoid attack.[4,23,24] What can change is who will be attacked.

Characteristics of Rapists

Who rapes and why? Groth, a leading researcher in the area of rape offenders, concludes that rape is more than an illegal act or an extreme of cultural role behavior.[21] It is a sexual deviation wherein the offender's pathology becomes the etiology of the victim's trauma. Although similar acts may be performed, rapists are not alike. Rapists perform sexual acts in the service of nonsexual needs. It is through these needs, rather than through other behavioral characteristics, that rapists can be classified and described.

The *power rapist* attempts to place a woman in a helpless, controlled situation where she cannot resist or refuse. This situation provides the rapist with a reassuring sense of strength, mastery, security, and control, all of which compensate for his underlying feelings of inadequacy. Usually, the offender has no conscious intention to hurt his victim. His aim, rather, is to have complete control over her. Nevertheless, there may be an increase in aggression over time as the offender becomes repetitive and compulsive in his behavior and more desperate to achieve the feelings of power, control, and adequacy, all of which he lacks.

> "He had a knife but he didn't use it. Thank God he didn't cut me. He used his fists instead and he pulled me around by my hair. All the time he was verbally abusive: called me names and told me if I did what he told me to, he wouldn't kill me. He made me get down on my hands and knees and crawl while he pulled me around by my hair. There was no way out of the room; he was in complete control. When the trial started, there were nine of us who had been raped by this one guy. It was amazing how much alike our stories were. He did the same things, used the same words. The most frightening part was that the police thought there were more; one woman was murdered."

The *anger rapist* uses sexual assault as a means of expressing and discharging feelings of intense anger, frustration, and contempt. The sexual assault is an impulsive act of aggression to retaliate against a world for wrongs that he believes have been committed against him. The assault is not compulsive as is the power rape; instead, it is characterized by more brutality and physical harm due to the expression of rage. The anger rapist derives satisfaction, not from sexual gratification, but from the relief resulting from the discharge of anger and the degradation and humiliation of the victim.

The *sadistic rapist* finds pleasure in the premeditation and ritualistic acts of violence, which usually involve bondage and torture. The rapist's anger and need for control become sexualized through the intense pleasure derived from hurting, degrading, and, frequently, destroying the victim.

The *date rapist* is known to the victim, who has given consent to be with him. Frequently, rape by an acquaintance (following consent to shared company but not to sexual activity) is not reported. In a study of 71 self-disclosed college students who had raped, the significant influence came from the male's reference group (a supportive hypererotic male culture with peer-group pressure for sexual activity) and less from violence as a sexual stimulant. In date rape, the male fails to recognize or disregards female rejection and continues to the coital experience. The coital experience, manifest and anticipated benefit, and the accompanying reaffirmation of self-worth as developed through the reference group appear to be the primary motivations.[25]

Treatment of Offenders

Treatment for sex offenders has gained support, as criminal prosecution does not completely prevent the offender from posing a continued threat to society. Estimates are that many offenders are back in their communities within 6 months to 4 years after conviction.[33] Early treatment is urged as an attempt to prevent deviant sexual activity from escalating into more violent activity. In 1985, 16 states in the United States had laws dealing with the treatment of sex offenders.

Treatment can occur in both residential and community-based programs. Four basic approaches have been used. They are behavioral techniques, social skills training, psychodynamic techniques, and organic approaches.[20] An Oregon program that is obtaining positive results uses aversion therapy, confrontation with victims (not those victimized by the offender), and—to a lesser extent—drug therapy. As of 1987, only one of 20 male offenders who completed the 4-year program was known to have reoffended.[33] Effective treatment of sex offenders described by McCarthy has four components, which can be carried out individually or in groups. These are reduction in deviant arousal using aversive conditioning techniques; sex education, assertiveness training, and competency training; confrontation that causes offenders to feel increased empathy with victims, to label deviant behavior as inappropriate, and to apologize to victims; and having an appropriate adult sexual outlet.[27]

The type of rape committed has implications for the treatment of both victim and offender. Anger rape is the most frequent type of rape; however, power rapists make up the larger population of incarcerated offenders. Conviction rates may be higher when there is more physical, bodily harm to introduce as evidence in court proceedings.[27,30] Just as the physical abuse and harm is distressing to the victim of an anger rapist, the woman who was not outwardly harmed by a power rapist also has fears.[31] These fears can be complicated by the knowledge that there are fewer arrests and convictions of power rapists. The victim of a power rapist may have recurring fears if the offender was not convicted. She cannot, for example, be reassured by the knowledge that "at least, he's locked up." How women cope and adapt to these overwhelming fears is discussed as the rape trauma syndrome.

Rape Trauma Syndrome

Rape Crisis

Rape crisis is the internal and external disequilibrium experienced by the victim of rape or sexual assault. The encounter with a life-threatening situation evokes extreme feelings of fear and vulnerability. Freeing oneself from this fear, redefining one's feelings of vulnerability and helplessness, and regaining control and equilibrium in one's life is the process of adaptation known as *rape trauma syndrome*. The clustering of symptoms in response to the trauma of rape appears to be fairly consistent. It occurs during both an acute phase and a period of integration and resolution and constitutes a nursing diagnosis.[5,6,10]

Acute Phase: Disorganization

The *disorganization phase* includes the rape victim's immediate expressed or controlled reactions, her physical reactions, and her emotional reactions to a life-threatening situation. In the acute phase, the prominent feelings experienced by the woman are fright, anxiety, anger, and disbelief.[8]

These feelings can be seen in an expressive response in which the victim actively displays and discusses feelings. Second-guessing often occurs in this phase, when, for example, the victim asks herself, "Did I do everything I should have to avoid this happening to me?" The second-guessing phenomenon of self-recrimination can be a source of guilt frequently experienced by victims and, in some instances, can lead to a severe depression. Self-blame can also be an adaptive coping process that allows the victim to identify changes she can make in the environment to increase feelings of control and mastery.

A *controlled reaction* is present when the rape victim appears outwardly calm and composed. Although conventional wisdom might lead us to expect victims of rape or sexual assault to be crying, hysterical, or visibly upset in some other manner, many women do not respond in these ways. A woman who has a controlled reaction to the rape has no less internal suffering and fear, just a different way of handling herself in the acute phase.

> "I went next door to get my neighbor. I remember she said I seemed so calm while we waited for the police. Inside, I was shaking with relief to be with a safe person but I didn't want to talk much until the police came. I think a shock reaction was setting in. By the time I got to the hospital I was not so much calm as simply exhausted."

Physical reactions during the acute phase vary according to the bodily injury incurred. Often, there are feelings of soreness, which may be generalized as muscle tension eases, or localized to parts of the body that were a focus of the assault. Sleep disturbances, eating pattern disturbances, and symptoms specific to the attack occur frequently.

> "In the first days and weeks after the rape, I couldn't fall asleep until it was daylight. My scalp was sore for days and then just sometimes it seemed tender, even after the bruises were gone. I developed little rituals, patterns, for going to bed and for washing my hair. They provided some structure for my anxiety but didn't really take away the fear."

Emotional reactions to rape and sexual assault are primarily the feelings of fear—that is, the fear of bodily harm, death, or mutilation—and other feelings such as anger, humiliation, and self-blame. Frequently, the victim experiences heightened emotional reactions and overreactions in other situations not related to the rape. Increased irritability, impatience, tearfulness, and anger can cause the victim to feel out of control and out of touch with herself. Incessant thoughts about the event and sudden memory flashes at unlikely and unexpected times add to the victim's feelings of loss of control during this initial phase.

> "The first couple of weeks at work I was so busy, I didn't have much time to think about what had happened. Nights at home were the worst part. But there was one person at work that I just couldn't be around. He is a very nice, friendly person but physically, he reminded me of the guy. Just his outgoing, friendly chatter would make me nervous and I'd feel myself withdrawing and feeling threatened and vulnerable. It's an awful way to feel about someone who is just trying to be nice."

The length of the acute phase may vary from a few days to a few weeks. Frequently, the symptoms of the acute phase carry into the long-term adjustment.[15,31,36]

Long-term Process: Reorganization

Reorganization refers to the process of adjustment and adaptation during the months following the rape or sexual assault. Of the 81 victims followed up at 4 years after the rape, Burgess and Holstrom found that 74% of the women felt recovered from the assault.[7] Half of these women felt recovered within months following the attack, and the other half said that it took years before they recovered from the rape. Some of the women (26%) did not yet feel recovered 4 years after the rape. Comparison of 35 rape victims to nonabused, matched control subjects found the victims to be significantly more depressed, more generally anxious, and more fearful than control subjects, irrespective of the number of years that had passed since

the rape. The researchers concluded that sexually assaulted women have definite long-term psychological problems.[36]

The period of months or years in which reorganization occurs involves regaining equilibrium in physical, psychological, social, and sexual lifestyles. The period of reorganization closely resembles the grief process described by Lindemann.[26]

The intermediate process of regaining equilibrium has been described as an interim period in which the victim appears to have adjusted and returns to the normal routines of life, school, or work.[28] This interim period is followed by a period of resolution in which feelings toward the self and the rapist, feelings about sexuality, and feelings of loss are gradually assimilated.

Issues that are important to the rape victim during the reorganization process include the following:

1. Regaining a feeling of physical well-being and safety
2. Working through fears and phobias
3. Coming to terms with losses, such as loss of self-esteem and loss of trust
4. Assimilating the event into one's sense of self

Unresolved Sexual Trauma

Unresolved sexual trauma occurs when the person experiencing the sexual assault does not deal with the feelings or reactions to the experience. Years after the event, the woman has neither assimilated nor adapted to the sexual assault. Typically, unresolved sexual trauma occurs more often in women who have little or no intervention to support them during the acute phase of rape trauma or who experience subsequent victimization. Women who, at the time of the attack, face chronic life stressors, lack social support, suffer a negative self-esteem, or have undergone prior victimization are also more likely to experience unresolved sexual trauma.[3,7,15,31,36] Another risk factor in unresolved sexual trauma is the woman's place in the life cycle; young females and those for whom the sexual assault was their first sexual experience may have delayed recovery from rape trauma. The nurse or other mental health professional may suspect unresolved sexual trauma when the following conditions are present:

1. The individual develops persistent phobic symptoms, such as fear of being alone or going out
2. The individual experiences retreat from sexual themes, lowered self-esteem, and guilt feelings
3. A relatively minor event triggers the symptoms of the rape trauma

4. The anniversary date of the sexual assault brings on symptoms of the rape trauma
5. The individual totally avoids contact with members of the opposite sex
6. Relationships with family and friends shift in negative ways—toward withdrawal, unusual anger, or silence; negativity may represent displacement of feelings toward the assailant

A type of unresolved sexual trauma is seen in a silent reaction to rape, wherein the rape victim has never discussed the sexual assault with anyone.

Recovery from Rape Trauma

A community intervention program can help the victim of sexual assault recover from rape trauma. This program is a coordinated effort to bring together all the bureaucratic systems—medical, legal, police, and judicial—and the support systems of the victim and family toward the common goal of helping her resolve the crisis and reorganize her life. Public education and community awareness are other essential components of a comprehensive community intervention program.

Aims of community intervention include the following:

1. The police are knowledgeable and concerned about the crime and effective in apprehending the assailant.
2. Medical care is administered caringly and produces good evidence-collection.
3. The District Attorney's office works closely with the police, medical, and forensic science departments to insure apprehension and conviction of the assailant.
4. The public is educated and assured of the effectiveness of responses from the various systems involved with the victim of rape or sexual assault.

When these aims have been met, victims of sexual assault are more willing to report the assault and have a greater opportunity to work successfully through the events surrounding the attack. It is important that the victim experience careful, caring interactions with each of the systems she encounters after the assault.

Trained counselors available through victim support programs can also assist the individual and her family and friends by providing crisis counseling during the immediate trauma and through the periods of resolution and reorganization. When a crisis center or victim support program is not available, hospital and emergency room nurses can utilize crisis intervention techniques to offer supportive counsel-

ing to the woman experiencing rape trauma syndrome.

Application of the Nursing Process to Victims of Rape and Sexual Assault

Assessment

Nursing assessment of a victim of rape or sexual assault begins with the nurse's initial encounter with the woman. This may take place in an emergency room, a hospital, physician's office, or a counseling center.[2,8,34]

Assessment of the woman's physical status is necessary to determine the extent of external and internal injuries and to begin planning appropriate medical interventions. It is important that the victim's appearance and the condition of her body not be altered, because the physical evidence of the rape or sexual assault is essential in the apprehension and prosecution of the assailant. First aid may be administered to the victim, but further medical attention should be conducted in conjunction with the medical team responsible for the collection of evidence in sexual assault cases.

While assessing the victim's emotional state, the nurse first attends to the primary concerns of the woman and offers information and reassurance in those areas before addressing other issues. Some women will focus on concerns for physical safety. Others will have anxiety about significant others, when, for example, a woman asks, "What will I tell my husband?" Acceptance of these concerns and the provision of supportive care can be calming to the victim and can begin the establishment of a therapeutic alliance. Emotional assessment also includes determination of the victim's perception of the event, her coping behaviors, and her situational and social supports. (See Chart 34-1, "Making Contact with the Rape Victim.")

Of particular importance in assessment is the role of self-blame. The distinction between maladaptive and adaptive uses of self-blame is extremely important. The nurse must carefully assess, on an ongoing basis, the victim's use of self-blame. *Behavioral self-blame* represents adaptive, control-oriented responses. Attribution is made to a controllable, modifiable source ("I should not have walked home so late at night. I won't do that again"). The victim can believe that similar experiences can be avoided in the future and thereby has a sense of regaining control and lessened helplessness. *Characterological self-blame* is mal-

CHART 34-1
Therapeutic Dialogue

Making Contact with the Rape Victim

Ann B., a 20-year-old college student, called the crisis line of a metropolitan hospital. She was referred to the obstetrics-gynecology clinic of the hospital and spoke with a staff nurse in the clinic.

Client: I'm calling for some information.

Nurse: Yes, I'm Miss Smith, how may I help you?

Client: I've been staying with a friend for the afternoon. We were going to watch the game on television. He went out to get some things at the grocery. The doorbell rang and a man wanted to use the phone to get his car started. He came in and then, and then, well I don't know what to do. I'm alright, he didn't hurt me but I don't know what to do. He left, I'm okay, Johnny came back and, and what should I do?

Nurse: I think you are telling me that you've been attacked. I'd like to help, could you tell me your name? Your first name is fine if that's all you want to share now.

Client: Ann.

Nurse: Ann, I am a nurse here in the clinic. When a woman has been attacked she can come here. We can help you and see that you have medical attention. A rape crisis counselor is available to stay with you while you see the doctor and talk with the police.

Client: Oh, do I have to talk to the police? I'm really all right, he didn't hurt me, I don't have any cuts or anything, but I don't know what to do. It was so dumb of me to let him come in. I don't know how I could have been so dumb!

Nurse: Ann, you weren't dumb. You did what many people would do when they wanted to be helpful. Lots of women have done the same thing. You may not have been hurt but you may need medical attention. The best thing you can do now is come in. You don't have to talk to the police if you don't want to. The crisis counselor can talk with you and explain what the police can do and then you can decide. But it would be good to see

a doctor. John can come with you and he can be with you. You don't have to come by yourself. We don't have to tell anyone about this, but you do need to see a doctor.

In this initial contact, the nurse is establishing a climate of supportiveness for Ann by providing her with information and being directive in regard to the immediate steps that she must take to meet her health care needs.

Nurse: Ann, I'm going to be here when you come in. I'll look for you and introduce you to the counselor. The doctor will want to examine you. You need to have some medicine so you won't get an infection. Would you like John to bring you?

Client: Yes, I guess so, he can bring me.

Nurse: That will be good. It will be better if you come now. Don't take a bath or shower but just come now as you are. Can I give John directions?

(The nurse then talked with John and gave him directions to the hospital and the clinic.)

Nurse: John, I know this must be upsetting for you.

John: That crazy s.o.b., I'd like to find him and string him up. I don't know how this could have happened. If I'd just stayed home....

Nurse: John, I know you are angry. Right now, though, Ann needs you to be calm. She is blaming herself for what's happened. She may think your anger is at her for doing something she thinks is stupid, letting the man in the house. Ann needs medical attention now and, while you're here, you can talk with the rape crisis counselor to decide what to do next.

Discussion

During an initial contact with a rape victim, it is essential to address the state of disequilibrium that the victim experiences after the attack by providing her with information and specific actions that she can take. These directions offer her structure and a sense of control to counteract her feelings of helplessness and of being overwhelmed. The information should be given in a warm, supportive, personal manner. This form of interaction opens an avenue through which the victim can begin to develop a trusting relationship with the nurse or other health care provider.

In this situation, the nurse assessed John's immediate reactions to the rape and his ability to support Ann during the initial phase of the crisis. After allowing John to express his anger and acknowledging his feelings, the nurse focused on providing directives to him on how he could help Ann at this time. In this way, the nurse assisted John in gaining a sense of control and purposefulness for his feelings.

Note that in this initial contact, the nurse did not probe for information about the attack. The primary goal of the interaction was to begin the process of trust-building and provide information about the specific steps that the woman needed to take. The nurse did not initiate discussion of issues that are common to rape victims, but addressed only those issues brought up by Ann; that is, her feelings of shame and guilt.

After trust has been established and the immediate need for medical attention has been met, Ann and John will be counseled individually to assess their perceptions of the event, their situational supports, and their coping mechanisms. Planning for therapeutic interventions will be based on these assessments. Ann and John will also be counseled together to facilitate their understanding and sharing their feelings. Separately and together, Ann and John will be involved in anticipatory planning for the events and feelings to come.

adaptive and associated with depression and helplessness. Attribution is made to one's character—an internal, relatively nonmodifiable source.

Behavioral self-blame can serve three needs in positive adaptation. They are the need for perceived control over one's life, the need to preserve belief in a just world, and the need to find meaning for negative life experiences. Anxiety is reduced by providing a reason for the rape through self-blame. When self-blame is helpful to the victim, and therefore used, it may be inaccurately viewed by others, who may try to dissuade the victim from the self-blame beliefs. Awareness that expression of negative affect and behavioral self-blame may be very helpful can assist the nurse in carrying out the nursing process. Further, the nurse must have realistic expectations about the length of recovery time (months and years) to be most effective.[13]

Nursing Diagnosis

When analyzing the assessment data provided by the rape victim and her significant other, the nurse may arrive at many possible nursing diagnosis formulations. Some of the accepted nursing diagnoses that are appropriate in guiding nursing intervention for the rape victim include the following:

Physical needs
    Potential for infection
    Potential for injury: trauma
    Alteration in nutrition: less than body
        requirements
    Alteration in comfort: pain, acute
    Sleep pattern disturbance
    Sexual dysfunction
Emotional needs
    Anxiety
    Rape trauma syndrome
    Spiritual distress
    Impaired social interaction
    Powerlessness
    Fear
    Disturbance in self-concept: body image; self-
        esteem; role performance; personal
        identity
    Ineffective individual coping
    Ineffective family coping: compromised;
        disabling
    Alteration in family process
    Alteration in growth and development
    Impaired verbal communication
    Knowledge deficit concerning physical and
        emotional responses and health care
        needs

Planning

Goal-setting for the victim of rape or sexual assault includes plans to aid the woman during the immediate, interim, and long-range phases of rape trauma syndrome. Immediate concerns are the promotion of the victim's physical well-being and the collection of evidence to be used in legal proceedings. Planning during the first hours after an assault should include the following.

1. Medical attention to the victim
2. Notification of significant people in the victim's life
3. Plans for the victim's leaving the medical facility
4. Plans for the victim's immediate safety
5. Plans for follow-up contact with a crisis counselor during the interim period

The interim period refers to the first few days after an assault. During this time, plans must be made to recontact the victim, refer her to a victim support center, or continue supportive counseling. Long-range plans should include the provision of support at certain times of stress for the woman, such as police investigations, court proceedings, and the anniversary of the attack.

Intervention

Building Rapport and Trust

The primary goal of nursing intervention is the establishment of a therapeutic alliance with the victim of rape or sexual assault. An important means to this goal is through nonjudgmental acceptance of the victim. It is not unusual for the woman to feel "dirty," guilty, or in other ways unacceptable. She must feel that the revulsion society expresses about sexual assault in general is not directed at her in particular. The nurse should respond to the woman's verbal and nonverbal expressions of need. Because the victim may misinterpret any questions or comments not directly related to her immediate situation as blaming or rejecting her, the nurse should delay probing questions until the therapeutic alliance is established. The woman's recent experience of objectification intensifies her self-consciousness. She is much more sensitive to the reactions of others, yet less able to interpret others' behavior rationally.

> "My memories of going to the emergency room are blurred. What stands out is how repulsive I felt when I went into the Ob-Gyn waiting room. Who else would be in an Ob-Gyn waiting room in the middle of the night but pregnant women? I had to find a small corridor to be in where no one could see me, where I couldn't upset a woman about to give birth or be confronted with the horrible travesty of sexual intercourse I had just experienced. Later, I could view the irony of the situation—at the time I just felt so exposed and repulsive."

Preparing the Woman for Medical Events

After establishing rapport with the victim of rape or sexual assault, the nurse should begin to prepare her for the events she will encounter in the emergency room and during interactions with hospital, police, and other personnel. Preparation for these events is essential, because most women will not have any prior knowledge or experience to guide them in the immediate crisis.[18] The nurse should give the woman brief, concrete explanations of what is going to happen to her and why. This information provides the victim with a needed sense of control and boundaries. Preparation for the physical examination helps the victim view the exam as essential to her well-being, rather than as further physical intrusion. Her calmness and cooperativeness also assist in the collection of evidence for the apprehension and prosecution of the rapist. In this immediate rape crisis, the nurse determines the emotional needs of the victim.

Does she want a support counselor to stay with her?
Does she want family or friends called?
Does she need assistance from the social services department of the hospital?

Encouraging Ventilation About the Assault

Once the physical needs have been addressed, the victim can use the therapeutic relationship to begin her necessary ventilation about the assault. She should be encouraged to talk about the event and about her feelings. Early and full ventilation helps the woman regain a sense of control; by experiencing acceptance in the face of the degrading details of the rape, she is assisted to regain self-worth. When the assault is reported to the police, the victim will be questioned by many individuals, all of whom will be strangers to her. Few of these individuals will have sufficient time to develop a strong therapeutic alliance with her. The initial talking-out of the experience with a nurse or other mental health professional will prepare the victim for the investigations to follow.

Exploring Physical Safety Concerns

During the immediate contact with the victim of rape or sexual assault, the nurse explores the woman's concerns for her own physical safety. Where will she go after leaving this initial contact? With whom will she leave? How can the nurse intervene to increase the woman's feeling of physical safety at this time?

> "I had to feel safe again. The first things I did were to make physical changes for safety. A locksmith changed and added new locks; a carpenter changed the windows and doors. I was lucky I could afford to do these things, because they helped. I could be alone in my house. But still, the vulnerable feeling stayed with me a long, long time. Even now, 2 years after, I sometimes feel edgy at night and get up to check the locks several times at night. It helps to have a 'safe room.' The police recommend this—have one room, preferably your bedroom with a phone in it. Add deadbolt locks to any door leading

into the room. Any suspicious sound or activity, you can lock yourself in the room and call the police."

Anticipatory Guidance for Significant Others

It is likely that the rape victim will express concern for her family and friends. The nurse offers anticipatory guidance to significant others by talking with them and guiding them in their responses to the victim. Helping family and friends explore their feelings, particularly feelings of anger, can free them from the intensity of these feelings and enable them to be more sensitive to, and supportive of, the victim. It is not uncommon for significant others to engage in a "conspiracy of silence," because they believe "the less said, the better." This silent approach only intensifies the victim's feelings of guilt, shame, and unworthiness of love.

Making Follow-Up Plans

The victim and nurse must agree on an intermediate follow-up plan. The nurse may refer the victim to a counseling center or decide to continue working with the victim through telephone counseling. It is important for the nurse to note several phone numbers at which the woman may be reached. Frequently, the woman does not return home, particularly if the assault occurred in her home, but chooses to stay with family or friends for several days. The victim should not be called at work, unless she agrees to this in advance.

Preparing the Woman for the Interim Phase

The victim of rape or sexual assault should be instructed about the medical follow-up she will need during the interim phase. Although the woman may appear calm and in control at this time, do not assume that she will be able to recall any verbal information given to her. Always give her written instructions for medication and doctors' appointments and reinforce these with verbal instructions. The written information can be reassuring to the woman at the moment and in the future.

> "I know they told me why I had a shot of penicillin. I know I knew it but when I called my doctor for a follow-up appointment, they scheduled me for blood work. I asked what for. It was as though my mind couldn't deal with the possibility of VD and had rejected that information completely when I was in the emergency room. It made me nervous about what else I had forgotten . . . was I taking the antipregnancy medication the right way, so it would work?"

Promoting Reorganization

It is important that the victim feel she can recontact the nurse in the days following the assault to ask questions, talk, and share feelings. The nurse can assist the woman by giving her specific, written instructions about how to reach her and when are the best times to call.

During the period of reorganization, the nurse intervenes by counseling on the telephone or through face-to-face contact or by monitoring the woman's coping and adaptive behaviors. Anticipatory guidance is extremely helpful to the victim during the weeks and months following the attack.

If apprehension of the rapist occurs, the woman should be provided information about the court process. At times, it may be helpful for her to rehearse giving testimony to prepare her for the painful retelling in front of strangers. She may also benefit from exploring how she will feel relating the events in front of strangers. Often, the apprehension of the assailant and the court proceedings occur after the woman has begun reorganizing her life. She may have moved past the acute phase of rape trauma syndrome and may have begun to adapt and live her life once again. The prospect of the trial will renew her feelings of vulnerability and fear. This stress-point in her life can be navigated with the support of a nurse counselor. The woman needs to be prepared for the potential outcome of the trial, needs to explore her feelings about it, and needs to consider how she will cope with the actuality. Not every case is prosecuted. Not every rapist is convicted.

> "I think I was the craziest during the trial. I kept telling myself it was nothing compared to the real thing but I was even more consumed with thoughts about it all than I had been in the first weeks after the rape. I guess my denial system was not as strong then as it had been right after the rape. It never occurred to me that there might not be a resolution, one way or the other. I had thought about the possibility of the guy getting off, I had thought about how I would feel when I saw him again. But it never occurred to me that there could be a hung jury! No resolution, and the thought of doing it all again was almost more than I thought I could cope with. I was so ready to have it done and over with, finally. Not to have that finality was crushing."

Feelings and Attitudes of the Nurse

Just as society has stereotypical views about rape and sexual assault, so does each individual. The nurse must face her own fears about rape, her anger, and her feelings of helplessness. Understanding and acknowledging these feelings allows the nurse to attend to the victim's feelings. There may be times and circumstances, however, for which the nurse has not prepared. Some events may be so gruesome that the nurse finds them intolerable at the time. A supportive network is as valuable for the nurse as it is for the victim. It is essential that the nurse have someone with whom she can share her feelings about the events she

Nursing Care Plan 34-1

The Client Who Is a Victim of Rape or Sexual Assault

Nursing Diagnosis	Client Behavior Outcome	Intervention
Potential for injury	Physical health care needs will be assessed and met	Provide physical care to treat injuries (lacerations, bruises), prevent pregnancy, and treat infection Insure accurate evidence collection to promote apprehension and conviction of the assailant
Potential for infection		Give clear, concise explanations to the victim about procedures and their rationale Give specific, written directions regarding follow-up medical appointments and medication administration
Rape trauma syndrome	Trust will be established	Approach the client in a consistent and nonthreatening manner Do not introduce probing questions about the details of the attack until after trust has been established Communicate nonjudgmental acceptance through nonverbal means (tone of voice, facial expression, touch)
Anxiety	Anxiety will be decreased	Provide opportunities for the victim to talk freely about the event, the feelings aroused, and the meaning of the event to her
Potential for ineffective individual coping	Effective coping skills will be exhibited	Encourage the victim's family and friends to ventilate their feelings and help them identify ways to demonstrate understanding and acceptance of her Identify with the client ways to restore feeling of physical safety Develop a plan for ongoing opportunities to talk about the event and subsequent feelings as they evolve over time Provide anticipatory guidance for police investigations, medical questioning, and court proceedings

encounters. It is also beneficial for nurses and other health care professionals to take active roles around the theme of sexual assault. Organize a rape prevention seminar for colleagues or friends. Contact police to evaluate your home for physical safety. Taking active steps to insure your own safety can be reassuring and can counteract feelings of helplessness and fears of victimization.[1,9,14,22,38]

Evaluation

Few women are prepared for rape or sexual assault. The feelings that result from this experience are overwhelming in kind and intensity. Although recovery from rape trauma may follow a generalized pattern of behaviors, each woman brings to the experience a unique array of personal coping skills, personality characteristics, past history with stress, and social networks. The nurse must evaluate each encounter with the victim to monitor the progress of the woman's coping and the effectiveness of the interventions provided. Through this evaluative process, the nurse may determine that another mode of therapy would be more beneficial to the woman. For some women, the assault will precipitate a major breakdown in coping skills, or adequate coping skills will not be available. Individual therapy with a clinical nurse specialist, psychologist, psychiatrist, or social worker may be the referral of choice.[35]

Summary

This chapter has discussed the theoretical perspectives of sexual assault, the findings of recent research about rape and its victims, and the possible therapeutic interventions of nurses and other mental health care providers who work with the victims of sexual assault. Some of the major points included in this chapter are as follows:

1. Theoretical perspectives of rape and sexual assault include historical references, legal definitions, psychological reactions, and sociological views as means of examining types of assaults and characteristics of assailants.
2. Rape trauma syndrome is the process of adaptation experienced by the victim of rape as she strives to overcome her feelings of vulnerability, fear, and helplessness, and as she tries to regain her sense of equilibrium. It can be viewed as a post-traumatic stress disorder.
3. Unresolved sexual trauma and silent reaction to rape delay or inhibit a woman's recovery from the rape crisis.
4. Community intervention programs encompass

the medical, legal, police, and judicial institutions with which the victim of rape or sexual assault must interact.

5. Nursing assessment of the victim of rape or sexual assault focuses on the woman's physical and emotional state, concerns for physical safety, anxiety about significant others, perception of the event, coping skills, and the availability of people supportive to her.
6. Planning for the victim who has just been assaulted includes medical attention and the provision of physical safety for her; intermediate and long-range planning consists of continued contact with the victim, supportive counseling, and helping her reorganize her life.
7. The aim of nursing intervention for the victim of rape or sexual assault is to develop a therapeutic alliance that will help her begin to ventilate her feelings and explore what life changes she wishes to make.
8. Preparation for medical events, police investigations, and court proceedings helps demystify these procedures for the woman.
9. Anticipatory guidance is necessary for the family and friends of the rape victim to help them explore their own feelings and identify ways to become more supportive of her.
10. Follow-up plans for medical appointments and supportive counseling help the victim reintegrate and reorganize her life.
11. To enhance their therapeutic potential, nurses must recognize and face their own fears and stereotypical views of rape and sexual assault.

References

1. Alexander CS: The Responsible Victim: Nurses' Perceptions of Victims of Rape. J Health Soc Behav 21 (March): 22–23, 1980
2. Antognoli-Toland P: Comprehensive Program for Examination of Sexual Assault Victims by Nurses: A Hospital-based Project in Texas. J Emergency Nursing 11 (May–June): 132–135, 1985
3. Braen GR, Martin CA, Warfield MC, Engelberg J: Rape and the Rape Trauma Syndrome. South Med J 78 (October): 1230–1235, 1985
4. Brownmiller S: Against Our Will. New York, Simon and Schuster, 1975
5. Burgess AW: Rape Trauma Syndrome: A Nursing Diagnosis. Occupational Health Nursing 33 (August): 405–406, 1985
6. Burgess AW, Holmstrom LL: Rape Trauma Syndrome and Post Traumatic Stress Response. In Burgess AW (ed): Rape and Sexual Assault: A Re-

search Handbook, pp 46–60. New York, Garland, 1985

7. Burgess AW, Holmstrom LL: Recovery from Rape and Prior Life Stress. Res Nurs Health 1:165–174, 1978

8. Burgess AW, Holmstrom LL: The Rape Victim in the Emergency Ward. Am J Nurs 73 (October): 1740–1745, 1973

9. Burgess AW, Holmstrom LL: Accountability: A Right of the Rape Victim. J Psychiatric Nursing 13 (May): 11–16, 1975

10. Burgess AW, Holmstrom LL: Rape: Crisis and Recovery. Bowie, MD, Robert J Brady, 1979

11. Burt MR: Cultural Myths and Supports for Rape. J Pers Soc Psychol 38 (February): 217–230, 1980

12. Calhoun L, Selby J, Warring L: Social Perception of the Victim's Casual Role in Rape: An Exploratory Examination of Four Facors. Human Relations 29:517–526, 1976

13. Damrosch SP: Nursing Students' Assessments of Behaviorally Self-Blaming Rape Victims. Nurs Res 34 (July–August): 221–224, 1985

14. Damrosch SP: How Perceived Carelessness and Time of Attack Affect Nursing Students' Attributions About Rape Victims. Psychol Rep 56 (April): 531–536, 1985

15. Ellis E: A Review of Empirical Rape Research: Victim Reactions and Response to Treatment. Clinical Psychology Review 3, 473–490, 1983

16. Feild HS: Attitudes toward Rape: A Comparative Analysis of Police, Rapists, Crisis Counselors, and Citizens. J Pers Soc Psychol 36: 156–179, 1978

17. Feldman-Summers S: Conceptual and Empirical Issues Associated with Rape. In Walker MJ, Bradsky SL (eds): Sexual Assault: The Victim and the Rapist. Lexington, MA, DC Heath, 1976

18. Flynn L: Interview: Women and Rape, Medical Aspects of Human Sexuality 8 (May): 183–197, 1974

19. Frazier P, Borgida E: Rape Trauma Syndrome Evidence in Court. Am Psychologist 40 (September): 984–993, 1985

20. Greer JG, Stuart IR (eds): The Sexual Aggressor: Current Perspectives on Treatment. New York, Van Nostrand Reinhold, 1983

21. Groth AN, Burgess AW, Holmstrom LL: Rape: Power, Anger, and Sexuality. Am J Psychiatry 134, 1239–1243, 1977

22. Holmstrom LL, Burgess AW: The Victim of Rape: Institution Reactions. New York, John Wiley & Sons, 1978

23. Irving J: The World According to Garp. New York, EP Dutton, 1978

24. Irving J: Hotel New Hampshire. New York, EP Dutton, 1981

25. Kanin EJ: Date Rapists: Differential Sexual Socialization and Relative Deprivation. Arch Sex Behav 14 (June): 219–231, 1985

26. Lindemann E: Symptomatology and Management of Acute Grief. Am J Orthopsychiatry 45: 813–824, 1944

27. McCarthy BW: A Cognitive–Behavioral Approach to Understanding and Treating Sexual Trauma. J Sex Marital Ther 12 (Winter): 322–329, 1986

28. MacDonald J: Rape: Offenders and Their Victims. Springfield, IL, Charles C Thomas, 1971

29. Masters WH: Sexual Dysfunction as an Aftermath of Sexual Assault of Men by Women. J Sex Marital Ther 12 (Spring): 35–45, 1986

30. Moore HA, Zusman J, Root GC: Noninstitutional Treatment for Sex Offenders in Florida. Am J Psychiatry 142 (Aug): 964–967, 1985

31. Popiel DA, Susskind EC: The Impact of Rape: Social Support as a Moderator of Stress. Am J Community Psychol 13 (December): 645–676, 1985

32. Resick PA, Jackson TL: Attitudes toward Rape Among Mental Health Professionals. Am J Community Psychology 9:481–490, 1981

33. Riesenberg D: Motivations Studied and Treatments Devised in Attempt to Change Rapists' Behavior. JAMA 257 (February): 899–900, 1987

34. Riesenberg D: Treating a Societal Malignancy—Rape. JAMA 257 (February): 726–727, 1987

35. Rose DS: Worse Than Death: Psychodynamics of Rape Victims and the Need for Psychotherapy. Am J Psychiatry 143 (July): 817–824, 1986

36. Santiago JM, McCall-Perez F, Gorcey M, Beigel A: Long-Term Psychological Effects of Rape in 35 Rape Victims. Am J Psychiatry 142 (November): 1338–1340, 1985

37. Walker MJ, Brodsky SL (eds): Sexual Assault: The Victim and the Rapist. Lexington, MA, DC Health, 1976

38. Wilcox BL: Social Support, Life Stress, and Psychological Adjustment: A Test of the Buffering Hypothesis. Am J Community Psychol 9: 371–387, 1981

39. Wyer RS, Bodenhausen G, Gorman TF: Cognitive Mediators of Reactions to Rape. J Pers Soc Psychol 48 (February): 324–338, 1985

35 Violence Within the Family

Cheryl Lindamood Anderson

Peter, Peter pumpkin eater
Had a wife and couldn't keep her.
He put her in a pumpkin shell
And there she lived very well.

There was an old woman who lived in a shoe.
She had so many children she didn't know what to do.
She gave them some broth without any bread.
She whipped them all soundly and put them to bed.

There was an old woman in Surry,
Who was morn, noon and night in a hurry,
Called her husband a fool,
Drove the children to school,
The worrying old woman of Surry.

The Real Mother Goose,
1916

Chapter Preview

Physical, emotional, or verbal abuse can appear in any human relationship. Outbreaks of violence in the family are usually quickly denied and concealed in order to maintain the ideal image of the family as nurturing, protecting, and guiding its members. The fact that violence occurs in the parent-child relationship, however, has been recognized and researched for more than two decades. More recently, studies of violent child-parent and male-female partner relationships have emerged; however, society still does not understand a great deal about violent families.

Violence among family members is a complex issue. It is intertwined with many factors, such as alcohol, poverty, stress, and an ongoing cycle of violence. These factors are not necessarily the causes of violence within the family but may have varying degrees of influence upon the development of family violence.

The overview of violence in the family will be specifically directed at the abused woman, the abused elder, and the abused child. This chapter will describe sexual and emotional abuse but will concentrate on physical abuse of children, women, and elder victims. It is important to remember, however, that violence may exist in other family relationships as well, either as isolated occurrences or concomitantly. The incidence, the traditional and current theoretical applications, and the dynamics of family violence will be discussed. A major emphasis is the nursing process—assessment, nursing diagnosis, planning, intervention, and evaluation—as it is applied to the abused individual and family.

Learning Objectives

On completion of the chapter, you should be able to accomplish the following:

1. define the six types of child abuse
2. discuss the difficulty in documenting abuse
3. identify some predictors of potential child abuse
4. identify some predictors of parents who are at high risk to abuse their children
5. contrast the characteristics of the battering mate and the battered spouse
6. contrast the characteristics of the adult batterer and the battered elder
7. describe the strengths, limitations, and usefulness of the legal system in dealing with child, spouse, and elder abuse
8. apply the nursing process to the care of the abused individual and the abusing family
     assess the verbal and nonverbal behaviors of the abused individual and the abusing family member(s)
     list the problems, potential problems, and nursing diagnoses of all family members involved in the abusive situation
     plan nursing goals and actions designed to alleviate the identified problems of the abused or abusing client
     formulate a nursing care plan for the abused or abusing client and his family
     evaluate the effectiveness of the nursing action
9. discuss the relevance and application of past and current theories to the problem of family violence
10. recognize and discuss your own feelings, experiences, and behaviors that may affect your therapeutic effectiveness when working with abused and abusing clients

Child Abuse

Types of Abuse

Child abuse is difficult to define precisely; as a result, various definitions have emerged. Parents Anonymous recognizes the following six types of child abuse:

1. Physical abuse—acts of commission, such as burning or beating a child
2. Physical neglect—acts of omission or inadequate parenting abilities, such as improper feeding or clothing
3. Emotional abuse—attitudes directed toward the child that may be harmful to his emotional development
4. Emotional neglect—the lack of parent-child interaction
5. Sexual abuse—involvement of the child with a parent or adult family member in sex play or actual intercourse
6. Verbal abuse—assaults on the child that are verbally degrading, such as constant ridicule[47]

Documenting any type of abuse, except obvious physical abuse, is difficult; therefore, health care providers must be aware of specific clues that indicate potential or suspected child abuse. While some clues commonly occur in many families, the nurse must recognize that all violent families are not alike. They differ in their specific situations, in the circumstances surrounding the abuse, and even in the degree or nature of abuse directed at the child.

Physical Abuse

The Model Child Protective Services Act defines an "abused or neglected child" as a child (*i.e.,* a person under the age of 18 years) whose physical or mental health or welfare is harmed or threatened with harm by acts of omission on the part of the responsible caregiver.[30] Physical abuse may be those injuries resulting from excessive corporal punishment. Table 35-1 gives physical and behavioral indicators of four types of child abuse and neglect.

Sexual Abuse

Sexual abuse is defined as contact or interaction between a child and an adult in which the child is being used as an object of gratification for the adult's sexual needs or desires.[78] The sexual abuse of the child can include pornographic photos, rape, molestation, child prostitution, and incest; however, other sexual experiences such as exhibitionism, fondling, "french" kissing, ejaculation, masturbation, oral sex, and anal sex may be more common. Rape and actual intercourse may represent only 10.5% of reported cases of sexual abuse in children.[18] Sexual abuse may interfere with the child's normal, healthy development by producing a situation with which the child is unable to cope physically, emotionally, or intellectually. Often, a sexually abused child suffers feelings of anxiety, shame, or guilt.

Incidence of Sexual Abuse. The actual incidence of sexual abuse is unknown because no precise national statistics exist; however, it has been estimated that its incidence may be higher than the incidence of physical abuse.[79] The National Center on Child Abuse and Neglect estimates a current annual incidence of 60,000 to 100,000 cases, generally not including the number of children who are victims of child prostitution or pornography.[74] As many as 80% of sexual abuse victims are abused by people known to them.

Characteristics of Sexually Abusing Adults and Their Victims. Two general characteristics may describe those who sexually abuse their children—lack of impulse control, sometimes as a result of transient stress or as a characteristic of the abuser, and a confusion of roles, wherein the child is regarded not as a child but as the object of the adult's needs. These characteristics of the parent-surrogate may be seen in all types of child abuse.[79] Other characteristics of the

father (usually, but not always, the offender), who may be passive, introverted, sociopathic, alcoholic, socially isolated, or inadequate are described in the literature.

Victims of sexual abuse are frequently characterized as being the oldest daughter of a family, approximately 8 years old when the incestuous relationship begins, and involved in the relationship for an average of 5½ years. Behavioral responses of these children toward the abuser and the abusive incident can be described as passive. The children expect other adults to "see" what is happening and protect them. When this may not happen, the child's level of trust diminishes.[18] Later, if the victim enters therapy, she is generally 20 to 25 years old, married, of either blue-collar or white-collar occupational status, having either completed college or lacking a high school diploma, and presenting to the therapist with marital problems.[79]

In a few cases, the offender may be the mother; however, the father-daughter incest relationship is more common. When the mother is not the offender in an incestuous relationship, she almost always knows of the situation, either consciously or unconsciously, and thereby condones it by her lack of action. The mother may be frightened to intervene because of the father's violent nature or may welcome the situation, as the daughter now fills a role in the family previously filled by the mother. In examining the dynamics of the family as a unit the following three characteristics have been observed:

1. Distant, inaccessible parents
2. Parental stimulation of a sexual climate in the home
3. Family secrets, such as extramarital affairs[62]

Emotional Abuse

Emotional abuse and neglect and verbal abuse may be considered together as emotional maltreatment, due to the similar predictors and consequences of their occurrences. The emotionally maltreated child may or may not be also physically or sexually abused, but physically abused children are always emotionally maltreated. For a parent-child relationship to be emotionally abusive, there must be an action or series of actions or omissions by the parent(s) that can be shown to have caused emotional injury or harm to the child.[40] The causation and extent of injury due to emotional abuse can be assessed only by a qualified professional. It is unfortunate that often the true extent of injuries inflicted by emotional abuse cannot be seen until later in life; even then, the observable and

Table 35-1.   Physical and Behavioral Indicators of Child Abuse and Neglect

TYPE OF CHILD ABUSE AND NEGLECT	PHYSICAL INDICATORS	BEHAVIORAL INDICATORS

Physical Abuse	Unexplained bruises and welts:
	  On face, lips, mouth
	  On torso, back, buttocks, thighs
	  In various stages of healing
	  Clustered, forming regular patterns
	  Reflecting shape of article used to inflict (electric cord, belt buckle)
	  On several different surface areas
	  Regularly appear after absence, weekend, or vacation
		Wary of adult contacts
		Apprehensive when other children cry
		Behavioral extremes:
		  Aggressiveness
		  Withdrawal

	Unexplained burns:
	  Cigar, cigarette burns, especially on soles, palms, back, or buttocks
	  Immersion burns (sock-like, glove-like, doughnut-shaped on buttocks or genitalia)
	  Patterned like electric burner, iron, etc.
	  Rope burns on arms, legs, neck, or torso
		Frightened of parents
		Afraid to go home
		Reports injury by parents

	Unexplained fractures:
	  To skull, nose, facial structure
	  In various stages of healing
	  Multiple or spiral fractures	

	Unexplained lacerations or abrasions:
	  To mouth, lips, gums, eyes
	  To external genitalia	

Physical Neglect	Consistent hunger, poor hygiene, inappropriate dress Consistent lack of supervision, especially in dangerous activities for long periods of time Unattended physical problems or medical needs Abandonment	Begging, stealing food Extended stays at school (early arrival and late departure) Constant fatigue, listlessness, or falling asleep in class Alcohol or drug abuse Delinquency (*e.g.*, thefts) States there is no caretaker
Sexual Abuse	Difficulty in walking or sitting Torn, stained, or bloody underclothing Pain or itching in genital area Bruises or bleeding in external genitalia, vaginal, or anal areas Venereal disease, especially in preteens Pregnancy	Unwilling to change for gym or participate in physical education class Withdrawal, fantasy, or infantile behavior Bizarre, sophisticated, or unusual sexual behavior or knowledge Poor peer relationships Delinquent or runaway behavior Reports sexual assault by caretaker

Emotional Maltreatment	Speech disorders
	Lags in physical development
	Failure to thrive
		Habit disorders (sucking, biting, rocking, etc.)
		Conduct disorders (antisocial, destructive, etc.)
		Neurotic traits (sleep disorders, inhibition of play)
		Psychoneurotic reactions (hysteria, obsession, compulsion, phobias, hypochondria)
		Behavior extremes:
		  Compliant, passive
		  Aggressive, demanding
		Overly adaptive behavior:
		  Inappropriately adult
		  Inappropriately infant
		Developmental lags (mental, emotional)
		Attempted suicide

(Reproduced from Heindl C, Krall C, Salus M, Broadhurst D: The Nurse's Role in the Prevention and Treatment of Child Abuse and Neglect. Washington, DC, HEW publication #(OHDS) 79-30202, 1979) perhaps disordered behaviors of the adult may not be connected to the emotional abuse he received as a child.

An emotionally maltreated child and an emotionally disturbed one may display similar behavior, but their parents' actions may help to differentiate the cause of the problem. Parents of an emotionally disturbed child generally recognize that there is a problem and seek help, whereas the parents of an emotionally maltreated child may blame the child for the problem and refuse offers of help. The parents of the emotionally maltreated child may at times appear unconcerned about the welfare of their child.[30]

Spouse Abuse

The most common legal definition of domestic violence refers to acts of criminal conduct that include the following elements:

1. An intimate relationship between assailant and victim who in most cases are, or were, married
2. An act of physical violence
3. A private setting[75]

In any marriage, marital conflict is a possibility. Its occurrence is due to a difference between partners in individual needs and capacities to adapt. Wife battering may be regarded as a failure of adaptation, which means a failure to acquire the necessary social lessons, whether on account of an incapacity to learn, the lack of teaching, or a temporary or permanent destruction of lessons from internal or external influences.[61]

There is increased evidence and recognition that wife battering is often associated with such problems as alcoholism and drug abuse, unemployment and underemployment, and child or parent abuse. It has been estimated that as many as 90% of women batterers were victims of abuse as children.[75] Furthermore, it has been estimated that one in three battered women batter their children as well.[59] Because of the strong association between wife and child abuse, this chapter will discuss the incidence, theories, and dynamics of abuse and the nursing process in relation to both child and wife abuse victims. The terms wife abuse and spouse abuse are found most often in this chapter, but abuse occurs between live-in lovers and common-law couples as well; hence, the term battered women is also used.

Additionally, spouse abuse may refer to the battered husband. Husband abuse is not uncommon, although it is easily dismissed or ignored by many. It is likely that more than one million husbands are abused by their wives annually.[63] The problem is largely ignored because of men's embarrassment in reporting the abusive incident(s). A strong young "macho" male saying, "The little lady did it" is considered by many to be a joke. The battered man may fit the "macho" stereotype but be very cautious of his use of power, or he may be ill, feeble, old, passive, dependent on the woman, and self-blaming. These men stay in violent marriages for many of the same reasons battered women do, including emotional dependence, economic dependence, or custody of children.

Elder Abuse

Attention has recently turned to another violent relationship, that of the adult elder parent. Demographic changes in society, such as the increase in the number of elderly individuals, explain some of the increased awareness of elder abuse. As elderly people increase, more adult children will be caring for them, owing to the shortage in home care and long-term facilities. The frustration and stress encountered in caring for some elderly, along with the possible financial stress, medical problems, and potential marital strain of keeping an elder parent in the home, are some of the factors leading to elderly abuse.

Elder abuse takes many forms; not always does it involve physical abuse. The following four definitions of abuse are considered:

1. Physical abuse—willful and direct infliction of pain and injury
2. Neglect—lack of attention, abandonment, or confinement of the elderly by family members or society
3. Psychosocial abuse—withholding decision-making power and affection from the elderly or socially isolating them
4. Exploitation—dishonest or inappropriate use of the elder's money, property, or other resources[54]

Methods of defining and categorizing abuse of the elderly rely almost solely on those cases that come to professional attention. This makes it extremely difficult to determine the extent of the problem. It is believed that elder abuse is seriously underreported.[57]

Incidence and Significance of the Problem

Statistics on the number of children, women, and elders abused each year within the family vary widely.

The First National Family Violence survey estimated in 1975 that 1.5 million children between 3 and 17 years of age and living with two parents were abused. A replication of that study in 1985 showed a 47% decline in abuse, indicating that 705,000 fewer children were the victims of violence in 1985.[26] This optimistic report was not fully credited in the scientific community; however, it may illustrate the efforts of society to deal with the major problem of child abuse. Nevertheless, each year 2,000 children die in circumstances suggestive of abuse or neglect.[76]

Estimates of the number of women who are abused each year range from 1 million to 28 million.[32,39,43] One study reported that nearly 1,300 women were killed by their spouses in a 1-year period.[66] The same study showed that the frequency and intensity of the violence varies; 28% of the study subjects reported at least one violent incident in their marriages, and 5.3% experienced violence that was considered a beating. The most frequent violent incident reported was pushing or shoving the spouse, followed by slapping and, less frequently, beating.[66] Female batterers tend to throw things, kick, bite, hit with objects, and threaten their victims with knives or guns. Male batterers punch, grab, shove, slap, beat, and use guns or knives.

Statistics place the range of elder abuse between 500,000 and 1.5 million cases annually.[57] Because reporting is sparse, various studies offer other estimates of elder abuse. Additional information and research are needed to provide a more comprehensive knowledge base concerning the incidence, nature, and prevalence of elder abuse.

The actual incidence of child and wife abuse also is only estimated, because of the problems in documenting and reporting. Abuse in the home may be underreported because those engaged in violent incidents are conditioned to regard as "normal" the part that violence plays in the family system. The ongoing cycle of violence from generation to generation may make abuse an expected part of life.

The victim's or the abuser's shame or guilt may also contribute to the failure to report the abuse. Such violent acts as being hit with objects, beaten, or attacked with a knife are often too painful to report. Many incidents of wife abuse are not reported because of fear of retaliation or lack of opportunities to change the abusing situation. Many battered women, elders, and battering parents describe the abuse as an accident.

Unfortunately, health care providers may also discourage the reporting of abuse by their actions or comments. Although most parents believe that some physical punishment should be given to their children as a means of discipline, society is very judgmental about parents who resort to more severe punishments. A parent may know he is exceedingly harsh with his child's discipline and seek help, only to face ridicule and debasement from the health care professional. A battered woman may drop the charges when reporting abuse for fear of retaliation or because of feelings toward the abuser. This action may also lead to ridicule by the health professional.

Every state now has a mandatory law for reporting child abuse, with the underlying intention that one who does not report suspected child abuse is committing a misdemeanor. In addition, no state requires that the reporter of abuse have actual proof of abuse or neglect before reporting. The law may specify that a person must report "suspected" incidents or include the phrase "reason to believe" in the report.[12] The report of "suspected" child abuse states that a child *may* be abused, not that his parents are abusers. Responsibility for the abusive actions should be determined by a qualified professional. Laws regarding the report of elder or wife/woman abuse are less clear and consistent. (See Chart 35-1.)

Theories of Violence and Aggression as They Relate to Family Violence

Impulse and Maladaptation

Various disciplines have participated in developing theories that explain violence in general or a particular aspect of family violence. Freud discussed the "death wish" in some of his later writings. In *The Ego and the Id*, he postulated the dichotomy of life instincts (*eros*) and death instincts (*thanatos*).[21] The death instinct, Freud believed, is directed against the organism itself and is therefore a destructive drive that may be turned against the self or others. According to Freud's theory, aggression is not a reaction to stimuli but a constantly flowing impulse rooted in the constitution of the human organism.

Freud's work provided a framework for Lorenz's study of aggression.[45] Lorenz believed that aggression was an inherited instinct in man and animal that had to be released. He also believed that the unlearned biologic drive of aggression evolved because of its adaptive value to the species. Aggression was therefore seen not necessarily as a destructive force but, in man's case, as a distorted maladaptive behavior. Both Freud's and Lorenz's work, however, could be criticized for the ambiguity of their concepts and the lack

CHART 35-1
Legal Issues in Family Violence

Child Abuse

Less than 20 years ago, only 11 states had laws requiring the reporting of child abuse. Many times, professionals hesitated in reporting abuse because of not knowing what to report or to whom to report it to. The question of protection rights for the professional who did report "scared off" physician or nursing personnel who wished to report suspected child abuse.[36]

Today, however, there is a mandatory reporting law for child abuse in all states. Failure to report is a misdemeanor. Reports can be made to the Child Welfare Service, a county attorney, or a law officer. Problems still exist in reporting cases of abuse because all states have different reporting statutes in regard to the following areas:

1. Types of instances that must be reported
2. Persons who must report
3. Time limits for reporting
4. Manner of reporting (written, oral, or both)
5. Agencies to which reports must be made
6. Degree of immunity conferred on reporters[80]

The major purposes of mandatory reporting laws are to protect the victim of abuse from repeated attacks, to provide social services to families, and to improve the methods of identificaton and investigation of suspected abuse cases. Investigation into the reported child abuse is the second step of involvement in the situation and is a direct consequence of a filed report. An investigation has three purposes, as follows:

1. To determine if abuse or neglect is occurring
2. To determine if the child is at risk within the home
3. To determine if that risk is serious enough to warrant intervention guaranteeing the child's safety[80]

Battered Women

Legal protection for the battered woman is less well developed. Many times, the legal system encourages the wife to return home rather than to file a legal complaint against the batterer.

Different states have various civil remedies for battered women, such as protection orders, restraining orders, or vacate orders that generally include time limits. Other civil remedies can be issued only if the wife is filing for, or has been granted, a divorce. Shelter services are minimal to nonexistent in some states. Special police training to handle domestic abuse is also rare. Some police will still not issue a warrant for arrest unless the actual violent acts are observed by legal authorities. Spousal abuse is considered a misdemeanor in some states and a felony in a few states; most states continue to view spousal abuse as a private matter to be worked out by the couple.[73]

Elder Abuse

When it comes to protecting elderly individuals and determining nurses' legal responsibilities, each state has its own legislation. There is no federal policy.

Seventeen states report laws specifically covering abused elders (over 60 years of age); 21 states cover protection of the elderly and disabled adults (over 18 years of age) together; and 4 states have "voluntary reporting" laws for elder abuse. In every case the nurse must report, and in all but three states the nurse is protected from civil or criminal liability connected to the report. Each state designates who to report to. The time between reporting and investigating the abuse, however, differs from state to state. In most states, the definition of abuse covers physical abuse, neglect, and exploitation of the elderly; however, many specifics are identified by each state's law.[68]

Although some progress has been made concerning the legal issues in family violence, much more is necessary. Children, women, and the elderly still are not safe from abuse within their own families; society appears at times to condone the violence. This "private matter" of family violence must be turned into a public matter. Only increased awareness of its presence and consequences will lead to changes in our legal system.

of differentiation between violence and types of aggression.[37] Neither Freud's or Lorenz's work may be useful for the basis of family violence.

Social Learning Theory

A more useful and recent approach to the study of aggression is the social learning theory. This theory is directed at the question of whether aggression is, or could be, socially learned. Bandura and his associates conducted numerous experiments with children to determine if, once the child saw an aggressive act, he would later incorporate it into his repertoire of behaviors under similar circumstances. In these studies, children were found to imitate the aggressive behavior they had observed, even when it was unrelated to the solution of the problem.[6] Conceivably these aggressive children could become aggressive adults, thus creating the cycle of violence.

Psychobiologic Theory

An association between poor mother-infant interaction and potential child abuse is the basis for Restak's psychobiologic theory of the origin of violence.[55] This theory proposes that the infant deprived of motion and physical closeness fails to develop adequate brain pathways that mediate pleasure. Expression of pleasure, therefore, cannot be transmitted through the appropriate parts of the brain because there are fewer possible connections. As the infant is deprived of movement and touch stimuli, fewer impulses are relayed to the immature cerebellum (the coordinator of movement), causing it to develop abnormally. Consequently, fewer connections are made between the pleasure centers of the brain and the cerebellum; later, the individual may have difficulty experiencing pleasure. In this absence of pleasure, the propensity for a dysfunctional state of violence predominates, creating the potential for a cycle of violence.

Environmental Theory

An environmental theory of aggression has emerged from the discipline of sociology.[60] According to this theory, the violent behavior of man or animal is caused by acute social disorganization, which is the result of a lack of meaningful values or the inability of society to impose its values on its members. Children brought up in the inner cities are believed more likely to be socialized into a world of every kind of violence—poverty, malnutrition, lack of jobs, poor education, sickness, and racial discrimination. These children learn aggressive behaviors in order to survive.[60] Therefore, these aggressive children could grow up as potentially aggressive adults.

Systems Theory

Established theories considered useful in other areas are now being applied to the study of family violence. The general systems theory approach, for example, has been applied to family functioning and relationships and, more recently, to family violence.[65] The major assumption underlying this theory is that violence between members of a family is the product of a system rather than a chance aberration or the product of inadequate socialization or disturbed personalities.

Symbolic Interactionism

One interesting approach using an established theory of violence is Athens's application of symbolic interactionism to violent crimes.[4] This theory proposes that people commit violent crimes only after they have formed violent interpretations of the situations that confront them. In addition, some persons are thought to have violent, and others nonviolent, self-images. Those who commit violent acts are seen as having violent self-images and a violent "other" to support the violent action. Furthermore, these violent persons cause people who have a nonviolent self-image and a nonviolent "other" to commit violent criminal acts.[4] Athens's work could be useful in examining battering couples' behavior.

Additional theoretical applications, such as the conceptual framework of the cycle of violence, the theory of learned helplessness and the battered woman, and the theories of exchange and conflict can offer worthwhile contributions to the study of family violence.[14,64,69]

Theoretical Frameworks of Child Abuse

Several theories are specific to the phenomenon of child abuse. Research more than a decade ago examined the mental stability or instability of the parent and supported a premise that parents who abuse their children are usually mentally ill. The psychiatric model evolved as one of the first potential theoretical frameworks of child abuse (and spouse abuse). Although this theory is still held by some mental health caregivers, other research has led the way to new discoveries and potential theoretical frameworks of child abuse.

Research has demonstrated that the factors of stress and environmental violence also influence the occurrence of child abuse. Through the environmental-stress model of child abuse, sociologists began to approach the understanding of child abuse in relation to the high level of violence in the United States and the stress level of the family.

The best-known theory of child abuse may be that promulgated by Helfer and Kempe. In its most simplistic fashion, this theory suggests the possibility of abuse any time a "child," a "parent," and stress are present within a family.

Years of continued research on child abuse have illustrated, however, that all three of these theories are limited in scope and characterize, perhaps, only a small number of abusive families.[15] Not all abused children have mentally incompetent or psychotic parents and not all stressful families abuse their children. The inability of these theories to describe all abusive families and the knowledge that several factors appear to occur together to elicit abuse have led to the development of the human ecological model of child maltreatment.

The development of the human ecological theory of child abuse comes from the separate ideas and work of Garbarino and Belsky, which draws heavily on Bronfenbrenner's model of the ecology of human development.[9,13,23] The basic premise of the theory is that a relationship exists between humans and their environment. This premise allows for a much clearer understanding of child abuse that considers its multiple causes, such as individual personality and environmental stressors. Separate work by Garbarino and Belsky has led to a theoretical framework consisting of four levels of analysis that subsume almost all explanations of child abuse to date. These levels are as follows:

1. Ontogenic development, which considers the history of abuse in abusing parents and parental expectations of children
2. The microsystem, which considers infant/child characteristics and marital stress or conflicts
3. The exosystem, which considers the world of work and the neighborhood
4. The macrosystem, which considers the attitude of society about violence in general

The ecological theory of child maltreatment is extremely useful to explain child abuse. This theory considers multiple etiologies including parental characteristics, stress, history of abuse of the abusing parents, characteristics of the neighborhood, infant/child characteristics, and the general attitude of society about violence. Anderson is continuing to develop the ecological model of child maltreatment.[1,2]

Considering additional theoretical frameworks for child abuse, Millor has developed a theoretical framework based on three existing models that provides the nurse with an approach to examining and comparing the influences of children's temperaments in shaping parental responses in abusive, neglectful, and normative families.[48] Continued research and the

development of conceptual and theoretical frameworks will expand the knowledge of family dynamics that contribute to family violence.

Characteristics of Abusing Family Members

Abusing Parents

Although the potential or actuality of abuse may not be outwardly obvious, certain common characteristics of abusers have been identified. Earlier research in the area of child abuse characterized abusing parents by particular personality deficits and distinguished the battering as controlled or uncontrolled. The psychotic personality, the inadequate personality, the passive-aggressive personality and the sadistic personality were included in the classification of uncontrolled battering. Controlled battering was classified into two additional categories—the displacement of aggression, and the cold, compulsive disciplinarian.[10]

The psychotic abuser sees the abused child as playing some idiosyncratic role in his fantasies.[10] This type of abuser received much attention in the literature years ago; recent research, however, has discovered that the psychotic abuser is not very common.[16]

The abuser with an inadequate personality is irresponsible, immature, and impulsive. He or she has a very low threshold for frustration. As parents, these abusers are often separated or relate to one another superficially. Characterizing this family may be a disorderly home, eviction, alcoholism, and the inability to maintain an established line of work. These families are noted for their neglect of children as well as injury to them; the needs of the dependent child conflict strongly with the needs of the immature, impulsive parent.[10]

In families where the abuser is considered passive-aggressive, one child is usually abused. The child is seen as a source of competition or as a symbol of the battering parent's failure to meet necessary role expectations. The child may be illegitimate or a stepchild of the abuser. The main personality feature of the passive-aggressive abuser is dependency. These abusing parents are generally unresponsive and unemotional regarding the abuse, are defensive about their feelings, are generally depressed, and will never admit guilt.[10]

Sadistic abusers have long-established patterns of behavior without feelings of guilt, lack of emotional involvement with the act of abuse, no signs of anxiety, and possible masochistic tendencies. Similar to the psychotic abuser, the sadistic abuser is not common.[16]

One example of controlled battering is abuse associated with the displacement of aggression. The abuser who displaces aggression is often the mother who is experiencing marital conflict. This parent finds she cannot express her aggression to its primary object (her spouse); instead, she displaces the aggression onto the defenseless child. After committing the abusive act, the mother generally feels guilty and regrets her actions; however, she may never understand why she acts as she does.[10]

The cold, compulsive disciplinarian is generally characterized by his compulsiveness. This parent asserts his right to punish his own children as he sees fit; he believes this is the privilege of a parent.[10]

Behavioral indicators of abusing parents may include some of the following traits:

1. Lack of concern about the child
2. Attempt to conceal the child's injury or protect the identity of the abuser
3. Routine use of harsh, unreasonable, and age-inappropriate punishment to a child
4. High demands from his own parents
5. Inability to provide emotionally for himself as an adult
6. Expectations that his children will fill his emotional void
7. View of the child as a small adult capable of meeting his needs[30]

Fulfillment of the parenting role is different in abusive and nonabusive parents. Abusers are more likely to report stress-related symptoms, such as health problems or depression, that are linked to the parenting role. Abusers display reciprocal patterns of behavior to both children and spouse that are more aversive and less prosocial than nonabusers.[71]

Abusive mothers may be more hyperresponsive to their children's acts. Bauer and Twentyman reported that their sample of abusive mothers consistently ascribed more malevolent intentionality to their children than the nonabusive mothers. In stage I of a recently developed four-stage cognitive-behavioral model of abuse, the abusive parent sets unrealistic expectations for the child. In stage II, the child disconfirms the expectations. In stage III, the parents assumes the child's action to be caused by intentional motivations, such as spite. In stage IV, the abusive parent reacts excessively, often severely harming the child.[8] (For additional indicators of abusive parents, see the section on Assessment in this chapter.)

Abusing Spouses

Some of the characteristics of abusing parents also describe abusing spouses (within the psychiatric model). The abusing couple's association, for example, has been described as a sadistic–masochistic relationship. The woman who elected to stay in an abusive situation was considered a masochist, whereas the male batterer was considered the sadist. It may be necessary, though, to reconsider the situation before adopting this view of abusing couples. Due to inadequate finances, lack of job skills, and fear of abuser retaliation, many women see no alternatives to leaving an abusive situation.[61]

Some batterers are characterized as enjoying participating in sports and hunting, having had past military service, generally employed with high incomes but having little job satisfaction, having more education than their wives, having more children than the traditional families, and having a degree of marital happiness.[22] These men believe that arguing between spouses is common. It is uncertain whether high or low income or high or low educational level has any influence on the incidence of spouse abuse.[16,25,78] Batterers are not believed to be psychotic, but are unsure of themselves, lacking both necessary self-control and a realistic view of marriage.[16] They feel powerless and inadequate.

Elder Abusers

Research on the elderly victim of abuse indicates an abuser profile of the caregiver useful to health professional in the assessment of possible elder abuse. It includes the following elements:

1. Middle-aged or older
2. Daughter or son of the victim
3. Experiencing stress, such as financial problems, medical problems, marital conflict, substance abuse, or unemployment
4. Increasing demands of caretaking role depleting family resources
5. Resents role reversal with parent
6. Low self-esteem
7. Impaired impulse control
8. May have been abused child[54]

Additionally, the caregiver may exhibit the following behaviors during their contacts with the elder victim:

1. Act excessively concerned or unconcerned
2. Treat elder like a child or nonperson

3. Show minimal eye contact or verbal contact with the elder[54]

As the health care professional interacts with the caregiver, other presenting behaviors may be noticed, such as refusal to permit hospitalization of the elder, failure to visit the elder if admitted to a hospital, blame of the elder for the injury, or refusal to allow the elder to be interviewed alone.[54]

The dependency of the elderly victim on the caregiver (sometimes elderly also) seems to be a strong indicator for abuse due to the stress that such a burden of care presents; however, health care providers may also need to consider that some elderly support the dependent abuser and stay in an abusive situation because they perceive that their children still need them.[53]

Effect on Victim and Family

Effect on the Child

The most obvious and life-threatening consequence of abuse is the physical damage to the victim. The most common physical findings of child abuse are internal and head injuries, spiral fractures, and elbow and knee injuries due to pulling or jerking the child by his extremities.[76] Physically abused children may show evidence of neurologic impairment, including spasticity, paraplegia, or blindness. A high incidence of mental and language retardation is also found in children who are abused.[20] Vaginal tears and bruises are observed on the child who has been sexually abused.

Abuse within the home affects the child either immediately or later. The abused child may be characterized by any of the following behaviors:

1. Appears wary of physical contact with adults
2. Seems frightened of his parents
3. Stares in a vacant or frozen manner
4. Seeks affection from everyone
5. Manipulates adults to get attention
6. May not cry when approached by an examiner or react in a frightened manner during painful procedures[30]

As battered children grow older, male children often become aggressive, fight with their siblings or peers, and throw temper tantrums when they are frustrated. Girls may develop more psychosomatic complaints and become withdrawn, clinging, passive, and anxious.[81] Some investigators have found correlations between a history of abuse as a child and juvenile delinquency, fire-setting,[29] and even murder in later life.[20,28] Simply witnessing abuse in the home influences the child's later adult behavior; male children who witness abuse show more abusive behavior as husbands than boys who do not.[56,72] Female children raised in an environment of "approved" violence may be more likely to marry violence-prone men.[25] Women who are frequently struck by their parents as children may tolerate more blows from their husbands.[11]

Children who are not directly abused themselves but are caught in the middle of parental marital discord may also demonstrate behavior problems, such as anxiety disorders, truancy, or aggression. The learning of a cycle of violence may also be demonstrated later in parent abuse by adult offspring.

Effect on the Woman

The physical effect of abuse on the woman is generally recognized through injuries of the head, neck, or shoulders, with "black eyes" being the most common lesion. Other injuries may result from being pushed against walls or down stairs.

Characteristic behaviors of battered wives include appearing frightened, distant, or jumpy; being unable to look the helping professional in the eyes; or assuming a stiff, rigid posture.[44] Other characteristics of the abused wife may include emotional and financial dependence, rigid adherence to patriarchal sex roles, low self-esteem, and emotional insecurity.[11] In addition, these women become victims through socially learned behavior as the abuse is continually repeated.[70]

Sometimes the battered woman retreats to alcoholism or has a mental breakdown. The crime of shoplifting is frequently perpetrated by the abused wife to escape a bad situation. More severe outcomes, such as suicide of the abused woman or eventual homicide of the abusive spouse, are also possible.[39,61]

Battered women's reactions to abuse vary greatly; some women seek shelter and temporary or permanent severance of the spousal relationship, others appear to do nothing. Although women may initially call the legal authorities, the introduction of the legal system into what is considered by many to be a "private matter" does not necessarily work in favor of the abused woman (see Case Study 35-1). Unless the abuse is witnessed by the police, no arrest of the abuser may be made, despite the presence of the woman's bruises or other injuries. Once the police leave the home, the man may retaliate with another beating because the wife called the police. Many law-

Case Study 35-1

Maria, a Battered Wife

Maria and James lived together for several years in a common-law relationship. They rented a small but adequate apartment in the poorer section of Los Angeles. Although the first few years together had been good, lately James had begun to drink more heavily and to hit Maria. One night, Maria was hurt badly by his physical abuse and required a 3-day stay in the hospital. Maria realized then that her situation was not going to improve and made plans to file charges against James and move from their apartment.

Pursuing the issue to court was hampered by several legal obstacles, but Maria persisted. In court, the judge asked James to leave Maria alone and James promised that he would comply.

Three months later, Maria had found a new apartment and a job; however, James discovered where Maria lived, barged in on her and hit her, which led to another hospitalization for Maria. Again in court, the judge asked James to leave Maria alone, and, once again, James promised that he would.

Several months later, James returned. Maria tried to fight, but in the struggle, Maria's eye was "put out" with a broom handle. After her hospitalization Maria again returned to court and heard the same exchange between the judge and James. She was terrified and moved to another location, but James found her again and beat her severely. After that hospitalization, Maria told the court she had done everything possible to prevent James from finding her and described her multiple hospitalizations. Still, the judge only asked James to stay away from Maria. When Maria returned to her apartment that night, she took out the small gun she had bought for protection. Unable to use it on another human being, she shot herself. She died before reaching the hospital.[39]

Questions for Discussion

1. What are some of the common characteristics of abusive families illustrated by this violent family?
2. Discuss the legal ramifications and failures involved in this case history. What should have been done?
3. When Maria was in contact with health care professionals, what could have been done to prevent future abuse?
4. Outline a nursing assessment of Maria and James and parallel interventions for them.

Source: Langley, R., and Levy, R. *Wife Beating: The Silent Crisis.* New York: Simon and Schuster, 1977, pp. 71–84.

---

yers feel that there may not be a feasible legal solution to family violence.[75]

In some cases, a restraining order may be considered for the protection of the wife. Often, however, the restraining order is ignored by the batterer and not encouraged by the judge. Some lawyers advise women to hide. Pressing assault charges may also prove ineffective and may anger the batterer. The imprisonment of the batterer or the levying of a fine may have economic repercussions on the abused woman as well as her husband.

Many women who report the abuse and file a complaint against the batterer drop the complaint shortly thereafter. Women may change their minds and drop the charges because of fear of retaliation from the batterer or a court system that often appears to discourage filing complaints against the batterer. Many women who leave their homes at the time of acute abuse return home later, again and again.

Usually a number of separations are necessary before the woman can leave a battering environment. Some battered women may be separated from the abusive partner as many as 20 times before leaving the abusive situation permanently.[42] The process of seeking help appears to proceed in a wavelike fashion rather than a direct route. Several contacts with several helpers are more likely than a single consultation to result in the violence ending.[43]

Why do women return to a battering situation? Some of the reasons are obvious and some less so—lack of job skills,[42] fear of losing custody of the children on the grounds of abandonment, social isolation, and cultural or religious constraints.[7] The abused woman fears that there is no place to go, that she may be followed and beaten for her actions, that her children may be harmed if they try to protect her from the abuser, and that the future, without her husband, would be worse than the present situation. In general, fear may be the most understandable, and yet most commonly disregarded, reason for the battered wife's return to the abusing situation.[46] Abused women who return home generally do so on the promise that the husband will reform.[24] Often, the wife loves the batterer and does not wish to file for divorce or leave the husband; in fact, some abused women believe that their marital relationship is better than most.[46] Finally, many people believe that it is the wife's sole responsibility to keep a marriage intact; therefore, the violent situation continues.[11]

The health care professional's attitude also affects the woman who is abused. The fact that many women alternate frequently between battering homes and emergency facilities appears to anger many professionals and calls into question the effectiveness of previous interventions. Many battered women are believed to be evasive, uninterested in working out their problems, irresponsible for caring for themselves, and generally "troublesome."[38] These beliefs prevent many professionals from addressing the battering side of the case; therefore, assessments and interventions specific to the direct problem are never made or given.

Effect on the Elderly

According to the four definitions of elder abuse discussed previously, physical consequences of abuse on the elderly may be noted as unexplained alopecia, bruises, abrasions, fractures, falls, welts, hematomas, grip marks, or bleeding. Signs of neglect of the elderly may be dehydration, malnutrition, poor skin, unkempt appearance, muscle contractures, oversedation, or lack of needed hearing aid or glasses. Indicators of psychosocial abuse may be low self-esteem, invalid guilt, passive or withdrawn behaviors, or hopelessness. Exploitation of the elderly may be noted in the hospital or the community by such indicators as paternalism by health care professionals, lack of understanding or unnecessary custodialism, victimization by "con artists," and illegal use of the elder's money or property by the family or others.[54]

The effect of abuse on the elderly victim usually creates much embarrassment, which prevents many elderly people from reporting the abuse to anyone. In other situations, the elder accepts the abuse as deserved because, as a caregiver, he or she abused the now abusive adult when the adult was a child. Elders also fear retaliation by the abuser if the violence is reported and lack alternatives.

Sadly enough, society's response to elder abuse has been long in coming. The broken body of a small child always stirs the emotions, but the broken body of an elder may not. The elderly and the infirm are not treated with respect; they are warehoused in boarding homes where they are stored like furniture rather than being regarded as humans.[17] No wonder the idea of abuse against the elderly has only recently been recognized.

Effects of Violence on Family Members

Some of the most common effects of family violence on adult family members include the following:

1. Depression
2. Difficulty obtaining, maintaining, and adjusting to employment
3. Emotional abuse and deprivation
4. Breakup of the family unit
5. Recurrence of violent behavior with a new partner
6. Expansion of violence into the community[7]

Some of the major effects of family violence on children, however, are different from those on adults and include the following:

1. Death by homicide or suicide
2. Emotional injuries, such as lowered self-esteem
3. Depression
4. Runaway episodes
5. Alcohol and drug experimentation
6. Early marriage with continuation of violence[7]

Application of the Nursing Process to Family Violence

Assessment of the Battering Family

Assessing and Diagnosing the Battered Child
Whether in a prenatal clinic, a postpartum unit, an intensive care nursery, or an emergency room, the nurse is in a unique position to detect potential or actual abuse within families. The nurse's response to this challenge could save a life.

Prenatal Predictors. Assessing potential abuse of a child is guided by the nurse's knowledge of specific behavior predictors. Some prenatal predictors may be helpful in identifying expectant parents who may later abuse their child:

1. Parental overconcern about the infant's sex
2. Parental overconcern about the infant's performance
3. Denial of the pregnancy
4. Severe maternal depression
5. Lack of support for the expectant mother from the family
6. An earlier wish to terminate the pregnancy that was not carried out[30]

Perinatal Predictors.   During the perinatal period, potential child abuse may be signaled by several events surrounding the birth of the child. The mother who has a difficult delivery or lacks an understanding of infant care, or the parents who are unprepared for the infant at home should be more carefully assessed regarding their parenting capabilities.[30]

Other possible indicators of future child abuse can be determined through assessment of parent-child interaction at birth. For example, a new mother who is not adapting readily to her newborn may see her infant as ugly or unattractive, may allow the infant's head to dangle without support, may hold the infant away from her body, may avoid eye contact with her infant or stare fixedly into his eyes, or may fail to coo and "talk" with her infant.[50]

Postnatal Predictors.   Sometimes parental behaviors during the postnatal period signal potential child abuse or neglect. When parents are disappointed over the sex of their child or respond either negatively or not at all to their infant, their behavior should be interpreted and monitored for parenting problems and possible child abuse. The nurse who is involved in the care of the family must be alert to the situation and work toward strengthening the parent-infant bond and finding methods of substituting socially acceptable behavior for violent episodes as needed. Other postnatal predictors of potential abuse include situations in which parents resist or are repulsed at changing diapers, the parents are unreliable concerning regular medical care, and the father is jealous of the time the mother and infant spend together and of their mutual affection.[30]

Vulnerable Infants.   Certain infants have been identified as susceptible or vulnerable to later child abuse. These include the following:

1. Low birth-weight infants
2. Infants of unwanted pregnancies
3. Infants of drug-using or alcohol-using parents
4. Infants of a multiple birth
5. Infants with birth defects

6. Children who take on characteristics of a disliked parent or traits the parent dislikes in himself
7. Premature infants who experience little maternal-infant contact[35,66,77]

Screening Families for Possible Child Abuse.
An Index for Suspicion has been developed to screen families for child abuse. Four types of family structures or behavioral patterns known to foster maltreatment of some children are classified as the following radar alerts:

Radar alert 1: Parents are authoritarian, highly structured, and inflexible in disciplining techniques; attempts at family–staff interaction are either suppressed or rechanneled into superficial conversation
Radar alert 2: Drug or alcohol use of parent(s)
Radar alert 3: Psychiatric disturbances of documentable psychosis, neurosis, or mental deficiency of parent(s)
Radar alert 4: Emotional immaturity of parent(s) and loose or ill-defined family structure[52]

Many indicators have been suggested in the literature as descriptive of potentially abusing families. A classification of indicators results in nine categories of items. Each is worthy of nursing assessment. These nine categories of items are as follows:

1. Generational abuse (history of abuse/attitude of violence)
2. Prenatal characteristics
3. Intrapartal characteristics (labor and delivery history)
4. Postpartal characteristics
5. Infant/child characteristics
6. Parental characteristics (drug or alcohol history)
7. Family characteristics (unemployment)
8. Stress and life crisis
9. Social isolation

Current research by the author has led to the development of a tool based on these most significant indicators for identifying potential parenting problems and subsequent child abuse[1,2] (Chart 35-2). Additional efforts aimed at more effective identification of mothers who are at risk for problems in parenting have been made by others.

Any of these predictors alone or in combination with others may not result in abuse; however, they are signals to health professionals of needed interventions for optimal parenting and healthy families.

CHART 35-2
Assessing Parenting Behaviors and Subsequent Child Abuse

Parenting Profile Assessment[1]

Assessment of Client (through mother)	Yes	No	Unsure
Moderate to Severe Discipline as a Child (5)	___	___	___
Past or Present Spousal Abuse (3)	___	___	___
Perception of Stress (4.5)	___	___	___
Moderate to Severe Life Change Unit Score (4.5)[2]	___	___	___
High-school Education or Less (3)	___	___	___
Rare Involvements out of Home (1.25)	___	___	___
Little or No Prenatal Care (2.5)	___	___	___
Does Not feel Good About Herself (3.5)	___	___	___
Feels Like Running Away (3)	___	___	___
Age at First Birth Under 20 (2)	___	___	___

Assessment of Family (through mother)	Yes	No	Unsure
Unlisted or No Phone (1)	___	___	___
Difficulty Communicating with Family Members (3.5)	___	___	___
History of Unemployment over a 2-Month Period (of usual provider) (2)	___	___	___
Currently Under- or Unemployed (usual provider) (2)	___	___	___
Family Involvements with Police (2)	___	___	___
Less Than $20,000 a Year Income (2.5)	___	___	___

Assessment of Discipline Methods (through mother)[3]	Yes	No	Unsure
Curses at Child(ren) When Disciplining (3.5)	___	___	___
Child(ren) Show(s) Evidence of Punishment after Disciplining (Cuts, bruises, missed school) (3)	___	___	___
Perceives Discipline of Child(ren) as Harsh (3)	___	___	___
Calls Child(ren) Names When Disciplining (3.5)	___	___	___

Scoring of Risk Assessment

Scores for each variable are located in parentheses beside the variable. The scores match the scoring value on the original data collection instrument.

For each "yes" answer, add in the appropriate score. Unsure statements are not scored. More than 3 "unsures" compromises the validity of the risk assessment score.

After totaling the score, review the assessment for the *presence of all five following variables:*

Income under $20,000 a year
High-school education or less
Family involvements with police
Perceives discipline of child(ren) as harsh
Moderate or severe life change unit score

Alert for Abuse

Possible parenting problems and risk for child abuse: over 21 points or the presence of all five variables (these families require a follow-up home visit).

Minimal parenting problems and low risk for child abuse: 21 points and under and absence of one to five variables (follow-up for families is optional).

Uncertain risk: no additional children at home for immediate assessment of discipline methods by mother or three or more "unsures" checked (follow-up required for additional information).

Check Appropriate Box

Possible Parenting Problems
Risk for Child Abuse _____

Minimal Parenting Problems
Low Risk for Child Abuse _____

Uncertain Risk _____

Follow-up
Scheduled for _____

---

[1] Timing of a repeat home assessment is indicated by the at-risk status of the mother. A reassessment of variables may be required to determine additional areas of risk and necessary interventions.

[2] Tool to assess life change unit score must accompany this tool.

[3] If assessment made in hospital between mother and first newborn, observations of this area will need to be deferred until home follow-up.

(Copyright 1986, Anderson C. Reprinted with permission from *Pediatric Nursing.*)

Investigating Child Abuse. Once a report of suspected abuse or neglect is made, an investigation of the family commences. The first item in a complete social assessment of the family is the determination of whether or not the abused child is safe in his present surroundings. Assessing the level of danger to the abused child is accomplished by examining the following issues:

1. Are there weapons available to the abuser?
2. Have weapons been used, or may a weapon possibly be used, in the present abusive situation?
3. Is there use of alcohol or a history of abuse of alcohol?
4. Is there talk of murder or suicide?

Following the assessment of the danger to the child, the remainder of the social assessment, including both the strengths and weaknesses of the family, is completed.

Evaluating the Child's Health. During the assessment process, the nurse assists with the medical evaluation of the child, including the proper referrals for physical examination, x-rays, and laboratory studies. Medical personnel are also called upon to cooperate with a representative of the child protective services and to share medical information that will contribute to a thorough social assessment and subsequent interventions.

The nurse is responsible for obtaining specific health data, such as the parental explanation of the child's injury, whether the explanation correlates with the type of injury, and the child's history of previous trauma or health problems. It is important, for example, to further investigate the status of the child who is "accident prone" or who has frequent health problems.

Physical assessment of the child should focus particularly on the condition of the skin—does the child have bruises, scars, or lacerations? Preventive health practices are determined by questioning whether the child's immunizations are current and whether the child is examined by a physician on a regular basis. Abusing parents may list the names of several physicians for the child, because they have sought medical care from a variety of doctors for the various injuries the child has suffered. The child's nutritional status is assessed through his dietary history and the age-appropriateness and adequacy of his diet.

The Child's Psychosocial Status. Information about the child's social history, family supports, composition of the household, and economic status is gathered by the nurse and other medical and child protective personnel. The nurse asks about the child's typical daily activities, the parent's description of the child, the child's school performance, extracurricular activities, and developmental level of functioning. Specifically, during this phase of the assessment process, the nurse notes whether the parents describe positive or negative aspects of the child's character and whether the parents see the child as doing well in school and at home.

The nurse must pay particular attention to the quality of the parent-child interaction. In addition, the nurse evaluates the degree of parental cooperation with, or resistance to, medical treatment, the degree of parental concern about the situation, and the adequacy of the parents' coping abilities. Do the parents see a need for change in their home situation? Are they aware of their own involvement in the abuse or neglect? Do the parents wish to keep the family intact and work together to solve their problems? Descriptive assessments of the affectional ties within the family and the available supports for the parents are essential pieces of information for health care workers.[30] Are there, for example, any other adults or older children at home who can help assume some family responsibilities?

A child brought into the emergency room as a suspected victim of abuse should be admitted to the hospital. Hospital admission allows time for thorough evaluation and protects the child from an immediate abusive situation. Generally, the parents permit this admission of their child and may feel relieved that the child is removed from the home; however, if the parents do not wish to leave the child at the hospital and health care workers require additional time to complete the evaluation of the suspected abuse, the hospital can request a court order to retain the child for a specific length of time.

Diagnosis of Abuse. The nurse and other health care providers should consider several factors when formulating a diagnosis of child abuse. Do the parents present a contradictory history? Is the cause of injury projected onto another person? Did the parents appear to wait an unduly long period of time before seeking attention for the child's injury? Is there poor maternal or paternal attachment? Is a history provided that does not adequately explain the injury? Are the parents reluctant to share information with medical personnel? Have the parents "shopped around" from one hospital to another? Are the parents difficult to locate after the child's admission to the hospital?[31]

Certain factors to consider in diagnosing abuse specifically concern the child at risk. Does the child have an unexplained injury? Does the child show evidence of poor care, malnutrition, repeated injuries, fractures, or skin injuries? Does the child appear to take care of the parent?[31]

Legally, it is mandatory that professionals, and even neighbors or friends, who suspect the occurrence of child abuse must report their suspicions to the appropriate authorities. In the hospital or medical setting, if the responsible health care provider fails to report suspicions of child abuse, it is the nurse's responsibility to do so within the proper direction and authority of the hospital.

Assessing and Diagnosing the Battered Wife

An identification of child abuse may be tied to the abuse of a spouse (man or woman) as well. Some mothers, abused by their mates, abuse their children, or a husband abuses both wife and children. An alert nurse may identify abused women in almost any health care facility, such as an outpatient clinic, emergency room, prenatal clinic, or even at home through a visit by a public health nurse. Several guidelines are helpful in making a positive identification of spouse abuse.

Identifying the Battered Woman.

The acutely battered woman in the emergency room is likely to come to the hospital without her partner, state that she has no private physician, and present with the complaint of an "altercation" or a "fall." These characteristics, along with a high incidence of skull and facial contusions, assist the nurse in identifying a victim of battering. The nurse may also note a delay between injury and seeking medical treatment, hesitancy in providing information regarding the injury, or minimization of the injury.[28] Sometimes, battered women may enter the emergency room with a battered child, or present with drug overdose or alcohol intoxication, which contributes to the difficulty in formulating an accurate assessment of the underlying problem.[16] A history of repeated injuries, particularly around the head, neck, or breasts, or a type of injury that is not adequately explained, should alert the nurse's suspicions and encourage her to investigate the woman's situation more closely.[81]

In screening high-risk women for potential or current abuse, knowledge of family background and interaction patterns are helpful. Consider the history of abuse in the spouses' family of origin, spousal abuse in previous marriages or relationships, child abuse of either spouse or children of the couple, and history of alcohol or drug abuse.[42] Additional signs to assess when interviewing the woman are clues to unequal power positions in family, helplessness, possessiveness of mate, depression, and low self-esteem.

Between the acute battering incidents, the woman may visit her family doctor and complain of insomnia, abdominal pain, headaches, or "nervousness." The woman's anxiety, accompanied by its physical manifestations, is frequently precipitated by her knowledge that the battering is cyclical and that the next episode is approaching. Unfortunately, many clinicians fail to investigate the reasons for these complaints and prescribe sedatives and tranquilizers for the woman.[81]

Diagnosis of Abuse.

The history of the battered woman is likely to reveal serious bleeding injuries, broken bones of the vertebrae, pelvis, jaw, or extremities, and burns from scalding water, cigarettes, or hot appliances.[59] Like the abused child, the battered woman may show signs of both old and new wounds.[44] If there is sufficient suspicion to warrant the collection of a complete history for signs of possible abuse, it must be approached with sensitivity to the woman's embarrassment, hesitancy, or evasiveness. The nurse or other health care professional should be alert to the usual excuses that her "accident" occurred as a result of walking into a door or having a tooth pulled.[44]

The battered victim may offer subtle clues about her situation; therefore, the health care professional should remain alert to their appearance. The abused woman may hint or state directly that she wishes to speak privately with the health care provider. Any woman evidencing the trauma of having been battered should be suspected and assessed as an abused woman, unless there is evidence to the contrary.[44]

Other behaviors characterizing the battered woman appear to fit the pervasive pattern of a self-defeating behavior disorder. The person may avoid pleasurable experiences, be drawn to situations where there is suffering, or prevent others from helping her.[19] Because of this observation, psychiatrists and feminists have battled the possibility of including the self-defeating personality disorder in the DSM-III-R, "a diagnostic bible of mental illnesses."[19] A decade of research has shown that all eight criteria describing the self-defeating personality appear in female victims of violence.[19] Feminists fear that labeling the battered woman as self-defeating would strip her of custody of her children by labeling her mentally ill—all and all, a step backward in recognizing and intervening in the social problem of battered women.

Assessing and Diagnosing the Battered Elder

Several clues may suggest abuse or neglect of the elderly client to health care professionals. Many of these clues are applicable to the assessment of any possible victim of violence. They include the following:

1. Client brought to health care facility by other than caregiver
2. Frequent repeat visits to health care facility for various injuries
3. Suspicious history of "doctor hopping"
4. Delay between time of injury and seeking help
5. Inconsistency between explanation of injury and clinical findings[57]
6. Any of the previously mentioned behaviors by victim or caregiver
7. Any of the previously mentioned signs of injury or abuse

Particular high-risk situations may be more prone to violent incidents, placing the elderly at greater risk for abuse. These situations include the following:

1. Care needs exceed or soon will exceed caretaker's abilities
2. Caregiver is experiencing frustration in giving care
3. Caregiver is demonstrating signs of stress
4. Living situation includes substance abuse of caregiver
5. Family has a history of abuse[57]

When any of these clues present to the health care professional, definite plans must be made to speak with the family regarding abuse. In many cases the caregiver is elderly as well, and the "abuse" may be far from deliberate. These families need understanding and help regarding alternatives for care and other necessary resources. The characteristics of the elderly victim or caregiver in isolation do not necessarily lead to maltreatment of the elderly, but in association with a crisis they can.[33]

Nursing Diagnosis

With increasing awareness of family violence and its implication to the field of nursing, the potential for violence was introduced in the taxonomy of nursing diagnoses in 1980. Most leading researchers in the field of family violence agree that more attention should be focused on the prevention of violence within families than on curing the existing dysfunctional family. Several predictors have been identified that may influence a family to become violent. These predictors can readily be observed in many of the clinical areas that employ health care professionals;

for example, neonatal intensive care units, postpartum units, and emergency departments.

Specific indicators for potential family violence can be classified as occurring in the prenatal period, intrapartal period, postpartum period, or as characteristics of the infant/child, parent(s), family structure, or community. Additional indicators of the potential for abuse include stress and history of abuse. Each of these predictors may serve as an etiology for various nursing diagnoses regarding the potential for violence.

The following examples of nursing diagnoses may guide the care administered by health care professionals in and out of the hospital setting:

Nursing Diagnosis: Potential for family violence (specifically, child abuse) related to

Predictors: Lack of family support and medical care during pregnancy; increased length of labor and use of general anesthesia during delivery; increased length of separation between mother, father, and infant immediately following delivery; identification of unliked traits in the child that are seen in one or both parents

Nursing Diagnosis: Potential for family violence (specifically, child or spousal abuse) related to

Predictors: Increased daily use of alcohol and drugs; inability to communicate effectively among all family members; lack of social involvements with family and friends; increase in perceived or actual stress currently or continuing for long periods of time; history of child abuse to one or both parents

Nursing Diagnosis: Potential for elder abuse related to

Predictor: Adult caregivers' history of abuse as a child by elderly; increased caregiver stress due to increased dependency of elder

The use of nursing diagnoses will enable nurses to better understand, assess, and intervene with the violent or potentially violent family.

Planning

Planning the treatment of abusing and abused individuals must be approached by health care professionals who are aware of their own feelings concerning battering incidents and who display a nonjudgmental attitude toward the family. Prior knowledge of, and experience with, abusing families will help the nurse create an accepting atmosphere. A judgmental remark uttered irresponsibly will only intensify the family members' shame and guilt. Acceptance and willingness to work openly with the family, on the other hand, will promote the attainment of long-term goals to prevent further abuse.

One of the major goals in working with violent families is the promotion of trust between the health care professional and the abused victim and the abusing family member. This goal may or may not be reached, depending, in part, on the kinds of experiences the family has already had with health care professionals. Trust is encouraged and accomplished only with time.

Discussion and planning with the violent family should be conducted in a private, quiet place that is a nonthreatening environment for the family. The nurse should encourage the family to verbalize some of their goals. The active participation of the family in the planning process reminds them that the role of the health care provider is not to make the family's decisions or tell them what to do. The family should be asked what changes they want to occur within the family and how they see these changes taking place. Comprehensive planning always incorporates the family's own goals.

Available alternatives for the family are provided by the health care professional. For example, this is an important part of planning treatment with the battered wife, because she may not view her immediate departure from the family as a viable alternative. When a battered woman chooses to remain with her abusing mate, plans must be made to maintain her safety within the home. Sometimes, a woman will delay her decision to leave the battering environment until a later date, when she is financially prepared or has developed greater confidence in her abilities. It should be noted that counseling of a battered woman or elder may best be done without the family at first. Victims of abuse may not provide information to health care professionals in the presence of an abusive family member.

Information about another alternative, seeking a shelter, is provided to the battered woman. Within the safety of a shelter, the wife may learn how to become more independent through the development of skills that will prepare her financially if she decides to leave the family unit. Child care alternatives are also discussed with the woman. Health care personnel may also help the woman locate a new place to stay. Some shelters have emergency funds to help the battered victims with essential, immediate expenses.

Because of the increased demand for shelters and their scarceness in some communities, most shelters impose a time limit on the woman's stay; therefore, the woman must make some decisions about her future. It is unfortunate that there are relatively few intermediate shelters where a woman can stay as she continues to work out her plans for the future. An intermediate (stage two) shelter allows the woman to continue to develop her job skills and care for her children within a protected environment.

A heightened awareness of the battering phenomenon by society will lead to greater community involvement and the development of more shelters for the acute and intermediate stages of abuse. This awareness will also promote the activities of support groups, such as Parents Anonymous for abusive mothers or support groups for abused elders. Rather than being turned away to rely on their own coping abilities and often to deteriorate into a deeper cycle of violence leading to death, disability, and future generations of violence, abused and abusing individuals will be helped by health care providers to make the necessary changes in their lives.

Intervening With the Violent Family

Dealing With Your Own Anger

Effective intervention can be achieved only after the nurse or other health care provider has established trust and rapport with the abusing family; however, during the nurse's involvement with the family, she is exposed to information about the abuse that is often painful to acknowledge and accept. Admittedly, the nurse may feel a certain amount of anger or disgust when intervening with an abusing family. Working with helpless infants and children who have been beaten, for example, stirs up a wide spectrum of feelings in any person who is concerned with the health and well-being of others. It is, therefore, necessary that the nurse be actively involved in a supportive group with which she can ventilate and work through her feelings. Before any effective intervention with the violent family, the nurse must face the anger within.[67]

Intervening With the Abused Child

Nursing interventions for the abused child begin with the required medical and surgical care; however, it is important that in the midst of the child's physical treatment, his emotional needs are not forgotten. To initiate a trusting relationship with the abused child, the nurse should explain all tests and procedures to him, in terms he can understand, and in advance of their occurrence. The nurse should talk, sing, and play with the child to establish rapport with him. She is aware that her touch may not be welcome to the child and ascertains first that the child will permit her touch before approaching.

Planning the Child's Care. After the immediate danger to the child's life has passed, the nurse begins to formulate goals relating to the child's future safety and psychosocial development. These major goals include improvement of the child's self-esteem, development of more positive interpersonal relationships between the child and family, helping the child to communicate feelings either verbally or through play, and helping the child channel aggression constructively.

Therapeutic play opportunities will allow the child to vent aggression and communicate pent-up feelings.[40] Consistency in limit-setting with the child will help promote a sense of security and predictability.[67] Acceptance of the child, recognizing and commenting on abilities, and providing activities in which the child excels will help build a more positive self-esteem. If the parents are unable to change their behaviors, the only safe place for the child may be a foster home or a temporary shelter. Consistency and follow-up of care are essential in treating the abused child and family.

Intervening with the abused child, once the danger period is over, requires comprehensive planning and working toward the accomplishment of a series of long-term goals. Repairing the physical and emotional damage of the child takes time, as does the unlearning of a cycle of violence.

Intervening With the Abusive Parents

Accepting the Parents. Intervening with abusing parents immediately after an abusive incident may severely test the nurse's ability to remain nonjudgmental and accepting of her clients. If the parents have been made to feel they can honestly relate their feelings to a trusting, nonjudgmental professional, they will generally provide some information during the admission interview. The nurse must allow the parents to ventilate their feelings. If the nurse or other professional is not able to allow this, another health care professional should be found who is capable of working with the family.

Keeping the Parents Involved With Their Child. When counseling or interviewing the parents, it is best to retreat from any busy area to a quieter, more relaxed setting. The initial interview should be fairly brief. Be honest with the parents and keep them informed of what is happening to their child. Let them know if a report for abuse is filed and what will result from this action.[67] The nurse must, at the same time, communicate her faith in the parents' abilities. Do not begin an interview by pointing out the inadequacies of their parenting skills (after all, they

have surely heard this before); just sit, chat, and observe.[49] Full visitation rights of parents to the hospitalized child should be allowed and encouraged, except in extreme cases as determined by the court.[67] Be available to the parents.

Safeguarding the Abused Child. The safety of the child who is returned home after an abusive incident is a major concern of the health care professional. Working on the unmet needs of the parents—their frustrations, stresses, and poor self-images—can help provide a safer environment for the child. Paying attention to the parent, at some time, without focusing on the child helps to raise the parent's poor self-concept.[67]

Using Community Resources. Health care providers who work with abusive families must know of the resources and services available to help abusing parents. Referrals to community resources, such as parenting classes, foster grandparent programs, day care centers, family guidance centers, Planned Parenthood, individual therapy, or group therapy may benefit battering parents. A special application of self-help therapy to the problem of abusive parents is Parents Anonymous (PA).

Emphasis in PA is on teaching the parent to identify needs that are not being met, to establish a support system within the group, to increase interpersonal skills, and to take action toward meeting needs for affiliation, nurturance, and self-esteem.[34] Many changes in abusive mothers have been reported, especially after 18 months or more of continuous involvement in the group. Mothers state that they have become more assertive and self-confident and better able to handle stress. They demonstrate better parenting skills, appear less impulsive, and take more responsibility for their own behaviors.[34] (See Chart 35-3, "An Open Letter from a Member of Parents Anonymous.")

The court may require some parents to undergo psychiatric consultations or therapy before it will allow the abused child to be returned to the home. Such referrals can help the battering parents to communicate their feelings and frustrations more appropriately, develop a more positive self-concept, arrange time for themselves, learn appropriate developmental expectations for their child, and recognize that their problem is not unique.

Approaching the Entire Family. Nursing intervention must be directed at the entire family, not at one particular individual. In fact, the true abuser of the child within the family would not necessarily have

CHART 35-3
An Open Letter from a Member of Parents Anonymous

Dear Friends,
I feel to get my point across, I must reach out and touch each of you with some of my innermost feelings. I'll call myself Sally, although Parents Anonymous (PA), the author, and editor have respected the philosophy of PA, which allows me to remain unknown. It has taken me 28 years of searching to find out who I am and like her! I am a Parents Anonymous parent.

When I heard Parents Anonymous deals with child abuse, I couldn't believe *I* abused my children! I've never left a cut or bruise on my kids; they have no scars—or do they?

In society today, we see child abuse mentioned in the paper when Jane Doe burns her child in hot bath water, or Fred Smith beats his girlfriend's child to death, or Mary Jones, 16 years old and only a child herself, leaves her baby in the care of a stranger, who then disappears with the child. Abuse and neglect can muster feelings like, "Hang 'em from the nearest tree," or "What kind of awful person would do such a thing?" It's true, these things happen every day, everywhere in the world. My questions to you are these: What brings a person to the point of hurting someone they love? Since when is whipping with belts, paddles, hairbrushes, and shoes a "normal" form of discipline? When is leaving children alone 2 to 6 hours a day to avoid babysitting costs, calling them derogatory names, or forcing a child to eat every bit of food an adult puts on his plate "normal" child-rearing?

Not only physical and sexual abuse turn our children into abusive adults. Abuse is a cycle and is passed on, in one form or another, from generation to generation. Child abuse "hunters" can only intensify the problem by putting parents in jail, removing children from their homes, and so on.

Parents Anonymous is a self-help support group, which simply means the group supports you in your efforts to become better parents. Parents Anonymous is a support system with no guarantee that if you attend six meetings, your abusive traits will go away. What PA does is emotionally support you as you cope with the tasks of being a parent while struggling to live in a tough world.

When I attended my first meeting of Parents Anonymous, I thought that no one could ever understand what I was feeling. I heard some of the problems of members of the chapter and realized that not only did we have a lot in common, I left feeling like things weren't nearly as bad for me as they were for others!

Not everyone can attend group meetings such as MADD, AA, or PA. This should be understood and parents should not be pressured into a group atmosphere. The key word is support and this support can be sought from clergy, therapists, counselors, good friends, or close relatives. It is important to know that somebody cares. Any of us becomes very defensive when confronted with our own family's problems. Being nonjudgmental of the parents and what they've done is an important part of beginning a trusting relationship with the parents. If a child has never "driven you crazy," it will be very hard for you to understand what a parent goes through before and after an abusive episode.

Child abuse has no economic class—as a matter of fact, it can't be pinpointed to any race, creed, or color. There are, however, many common denominators such as stress, employment, and finances, but one significant factor is the generational cycle. If you were abused as a child, chances are you will have a tendency to abuse your children. We were raised hearing "tapes". "Don't do as I do, do as I say," "A good spanking never hurt you." As parents, we "replay" those tapes. By seeking help and learning to admit to ourselves that we can never be "perfect" parents, we start to grow as better people and better parents.

I have three children. They are now 10, 6, and 2 years old. My problems are not larger or smaller than when I joined PA (my children were 5 and 2 then). They are just *different* ones now. I've come to grips with the fact that my problems will never go away; they will just keep changing. What I have learned is a new way of coping with them so the stress in my life doesn't affect my children as much. Learning this takes each person his or her own time, and some people never learn it at all. I have learned this with support and guidance from PA chapters.

Parents Anonymous builds self-esteem. If you've heard all your life that you're worthless, you begin to feel that way about yourself. If you don't like yourself, even a little, then nothing much else makes you happy. Parents Anonymous helps you find the "good guy" and the "ugly green monster" in yourself. To recognize and separate these, to learn what triggers your anger, and why your kids "push buttons" are all a part

(Continues on p. 692)

of PA. Through a chapter meeting we can take one, or several, problems to the group each week and get many ideas on what to do the next time it occurs. Options! Support! Hope!

Many parents come with the same frustrations and just knowing "I am not alone" helps. It takes time and patience to work through years of feeling the anger, hurt, despair, and frustration that has led to abuse problems. Parents Anonymous helps work through those times to break the cycle of child abuse in the family.

I started out as a parent in PA with great needs, and in the chapter in Springfield, Illinois, I discovered the self-worth and strength to get through some really tough times. Now I want to help special families learn to deal with their tough times. With every meeting, training session, seminar, or workshop, I learn more about the ifs and whys of family violence. I have so many caring friends at Parents Anonymous that these groups have become families in themselves. Now, I am a chapter sponsor with great

hopes of helping families the way mine was, and still is, by being involved in PA.

My advice to you as nurses who may come in contact with family violence is to remain open. It takes a great deal for a parent to arrive at the point of abuse. Be willing to listen without judgment while remaining honest about your feelings and open to growth. I also warn you to be sufficiently aware of your own feelings, so that you might "pass," if the case or situation warrants it.

I've talked about hope, support, encouragement, openness, honesty, caring, trust, and love. I've told you from my heart how I feel about Parents Anonymous.

I wish each of you success in your nursing education and career and, most of all, in your parenting experiences, which are, however stressful, the most rewarding of all.

Sincerely,

Sally

to be identified for effecive interventions to be implemented with the abusive family.

When intervening with the family, the nurse must maintain the confidentiality of the family, establish realistic goals within a time frame, formulate short-term objectives that are measurable and observable, define specific plans for each involved agency in order to prevent duplication of services, and promote consistency of care through the involvement of as few people as possible.[30]

Intervening With the Abused Spouse

In the immediate phase of intervention, the battered woman's injuries must be treated medically or surgically as required. If her injuries are not severe enough to warrant hospitalization, the health professional must consider letting the woman go home.[59] Thorough assessment and accurate record-keeping in cases of suspected abuse are extremely important.

Interviewing the Abused Woman. If an interview is possible after the battering incident, it is best to interview the woman alone. Never demand a private interview with the woman against the couple's wishes, however, or the battering husband may retaliate later against the wife. In preparing for the interview with the abused wife, be ready for what you may hear. Be

prepared to listen attentively, or the woman may feel a second sense of rejection.[44] Encourage the woman to share her story. Explore with her what she has done about her situation and what she would like to have done; do not, however, tell her what to do.[44]

The battered woman may indicate that she expects the abuse as part of being a wife. Wife-battering continues to be accepted and expected in many cultures.[32] The battered woman may state or demonstrate that she wishes to stay with her husband. Professionals who express shock or dismay over this reaction only reinforce the battered wife's feelings of shame and guilt.[32] The health care provider must remember that the battered woman's self-respect is at an extremely low level and that she sees no alternatives to her situation. If the nurse or health care provider believes that the injury is due to battering and not an accident, it is best to ask the victim directly.[32]

Not all battered women are easy to interview. Immediately after an abusive incident, some battered women appear to "just give up." Unfortunately, some health care professionals label these women as unresponsive and disinterested in themselves, hence cutting off the lines of communication and necessary interventions. Other women may be difficult to interact with due to drugs, alcohol, combative behaviors, or other "crazy" and inappropriate actions.[38] In these cases the battering may be ignored if only the medical priorities are addressed and the woman is quickly sent from the health care facility. Before assessing for actual abuse on planning interventions, the health professional must examine his or her own feelings about wife abuse.

Identification of the Battered Wife. When a battered woman is identified, the nurse must create a situation in which the woman can be comfortable, supported, and free to discuss her feelings confidentially. The nurse must know and provide the available referrals for the battered wife, such as women's shelters and legal aid agencies.

The nurse may recommend marital counseling for the couple if both partners see the abusing problem as one needing intervention; however, more often, the woman seeks counseling or group therapy alone and then later drops out. Battered women have a high drop-out rate from psychotherapy for the following reasons:

1. Fear of the partner's retaliation
2. Stigma of being in therapy and being a battered wife
3. Therapy is seen as another promise of help that will ultimately fail
4. Some women are seriously locked in their abusive situations and do not wish to scrutinize their problem further
5. The offer of help is premature through poor timing[58]

Battered spouses appear to pass through an abuse cycle which may influence the battered woman's use of referrals. One stage, the *tension build-up stage,* is characterized by increased verbal abuse and minor physical abuse, decreased meaningful communication, and increased levels of anxiety or anxious depression. The battered woman may seek help because of complaints of psychosomatic problems such as headaches and insomnia; she may appear, at this time, more amenable to using resources.

The following stage, the *acute episode,* begins the acute phase. Tension exceeds the couple's ability to cope. Battering may be initiated by either the man or woman, and precipitated by an acute impersonal argument or increased stress from outside the home. During this stage, the battered woman may present in the emergency room in need of first aid. Denial and humiliation may make the diagnosis of abuse difficult, but once it is made, the woman may be amenable to assistance.

The last stage, *reconciliation,* is entered when the couple temporarily resolves the state of increased tension. The reconciliation stage is generally shorter than the previous stage and the battering couple can re-enter it again and again. As the couple reconciles more and more frequently, this stage becomes shorter. Resources or referrals are generally not considered or accepted at this time.

Treating the Batterer. Working with the man who batters can also be a very challenging role for the health professional. As with abusive parents, health professionals must be nonjudgmental and open, but not condoning, of the situation. Nearly 150 men's programs have emerged in the past 5 years. These programs are aimed at improving control of impulses and anger and also at offsetting the imposing social and institutional supports that predispose men to commit violence against women.[27] Agencies that do exist suggest group sessions; however, it is difficult to get men to attend group sessions because they are many times intimidated by other men when asked to share feelings and emotions. Other interventions for male batterers are to keep a diary or "anger journal," to record physical signs of anger, and to learn to take "time outs."[51] If the batterer can become involved in a therapy or self-help group and get in touch with his feelings and emotions regarding the abuse, the violence can be stopped.

The Battered Pregnant Woman. Nurses and physicians in obstetrical areas are in a unique position to detect battered women, because the injuries of many battered women first occur during pregnancy. Trauma to the abdomen, for example, may be the cause of antepartal hemorrhage or premature labor.[59] Violence during pregnancy may, in effect, be the husband's attempt to terminate the pregnancy and therefore eliminate the stress of an additional child in the family.[59] Battered women have three times the number of abortions and two times the number of miscarriages as nonbattered women.[82] The pregnant woman who leaves her husband enters a very complex prenatal period. The progress of the mother and the fetus must be safeguarded through close prenatal supervision.[59] The battered pregnant woman may need to visit the health professional more frequently and may need to be seen without appointments during the more disorganized periods of her life.[59] Intrapartally, caregivers must be made aware of the abusive situation and must focus their care on raising the battered woman's self-esteem and providing understanding and support.

The Postnatal Period. After the battered woman gives birth, pediatric caregivers need to offer additional support. If the abused woman elects to return home with the newborn, the nurse must be com-

CHART   35-4
Adolescent Abuse: A Less-Recognized Form of Abuse

Adolescent abuse appears to include family dynamics somewhat different from abuse involving younger children and families. Much of the stress related to an occurrence of adolescent abuse may result from the parent's experience of stress at the same time the adolescent is facing the stresses of identity, independence, and autonomy. Parents of adolescents appear to be facing their own developmental crisis—that of midlife—when the children are teens. The increased strain from the two concurrent developmental crises can place the adolescent at risk for maltreatment.

It has been suggested that there are three distinguishing patterns of adolescent maltreatment. They are as follows:

1.   Parents are disorganized and overwhelmed with life and see their teen as disrespectful and unresponsive
2.   More violent means of control are searched for as the adolescent becomes stronger and bigger
3.   Families are described as child-oriented; therefore, the abuse begins when the child tries to separate from the family

Individual personalities and inherited traits, developmental stages of the individuals involved, reactions to these developmental stages, and so-cial, cultural, and situational factors structure and limit the ways in which a person may respond to stress, *e.g.*, by becoming abusive.

Adolescent maltreatment is not a commonly recognized form of abuse because a bigger, stronger adolescent victim of abuse evokes less sympathy than a smaller child victim. It is assumed the teen can take care of himself or leave the situation—as many do, becoming teen runaways.

Some differences have been noted between maltreated teens and maltreated younger children. In the case of adolescent maltreatment, the perpetrator is often male and the victim is female, the opposite to abuse of younger children. Adolescent abuse is often self-reported rather than reported by other individuals. Many adolescents who are abused come from families with histories of alcohol or drug abuse by parents and of spousal abuse, rather than childhood abuse to the teen. Education and income levels may be higher in the family of adolescent abuse than in families abusing the younger child. Because the adolescent is a victim of abuse from a family with different dynamics and, as a teen, requires different services for different needs, the adolescent victim cannot be overlooked.

(Adapted from Doueck H, Ishisaka A, Sweany S, Gilchrist L: Adolescent Maltreatment. J Interpersonal Violence. 2(June): 139–154, 1987)

mitted to including the husband in the plan of care. With the crisis of parenthood, caregivers may need to prepare for future abuse of the wife.[41] Health care providers may have no alternatives except to prepare the wife for possible abuse with plans for her own safety and that of the child. Before the new mother returns to her home, the nurse encourages her to know the location of the nearest shelter, to obtain extra keys to the car, to keep a few necessities packed and hidden away until needed, and to keep handy the name of someone to call for support and assistance. The first arrival of an infant or small child into the home is one of the most common events precipitating the occurrence of wife abuse.[70]

Unplanned or unwanted pregnancies have also been identified as significant precipitating factors in wife abuse. Birth control information and Planned Parenthood agencies are helpful resources for the battered woman to help her select an appropriate method of child spacing.[59]

Intervening With the Battered Elder
When addressing the elder victim use last names rather than first. This offers respect, which is appreciated by the client. Find a quiet and comfortable place to talk with the family. Be friendly and helpful. Families are often confused or alarmed by the events taking place. Be a good listener and pick up subtle clues to the possibility of abuse. Be considerate of the feelings of the elderly victim; abuse is embarrassing to discuss with strangers.[17]

When the client is comfortable with the technique, assess for the signs and symptoms previously discussed as signals to abuse and neglect. Knowledge of the facts, however, is not enough. Know the community resources that may be helpful to the battered victim and caregiver. These resources can help the elderly lead active and fulfilling lives. Specific resources for the elderly could include legal aid, medical assistance, visiting nursing, nutrition services, physical and occupational therapy, adult day care, counseling and educational services, and shelters. Informal support systems and self-help groups are important to the elderly victim and caretaker.

Community Education

What can nurses do in our society to help battered victims and families? Participation in public workshops and forums on family violence will help to raise the community's consciousness and prompt the establishment of task forces on battered women, support groups for elders, and additional shelters. Nurses frequently answer "hot lines" for battered women and organize self-help support groups. Community education can help by making the victim aware of nearby shelters, emergency funds, and community mental health centers. The experience, knowledge, and research of nurses can also be utilized by authorities to help train police who answer domestic calls. At present, 20% of deaths of police officers occur while they are trying to break up family fights.[73]

Evaluation

The effectiveness of treatment for abusing and abused individuals depends strongly on society and its awareness of battering within the family. The community's involvement with the problem of abuse will influence how readily it provides needed shelters and education about the violent family. Changes in the legal system and special task forces in the police departments that deal with the family will determine the effectiveness of treatment for the family who exhibits violence.

The nurse's evaluation of the therapeutic interventions must first address the issue of the client's safety—is the individual who has been a victim of abuse safe from the likelihood of future abuse? The family's participation in the planning and implementation of treatment will increase the acceptance, and therefore the value, of the treatment.

An effective network or support group is needed to help rehabilitate abused and abuser family members. Follow-up with violent families must be continued until the learned pattern of violent behavior is extinguished. The evaluation process should be a continuous one. As more health care professionals become knowledgeable about the situation, progress will be made by the individual, his family, and society.

Summary

This chapter has summarized some of the literature of the past two decades in the area of child, elder, and woman abuse. Sibling abuse was not discussed; however, this omission does not imply that sibling abuse is a problem of lesser importance or magnitude.

The information presented about child, elder, and woman abuse has included the following major points:

1. The six specific types of abuse recognized by Parents Anonymous are physical abuse, physical neglect, emotional abuse, emotional neglect, sexual abuse, and verbal abuse.
2. Physical abuse is more empirically observable than emotional abuse and therefore predominates in the available literature on family violence; however, physical abuse may be the least frequently occurring form of abuse within the family.
3. Emotional maltreatment and sexual abuse are probably more common than major physical trauma to children.
4. The incidence, significance and impact of all forms of family violence are tremendous.
5. Family violence can be directed at any family member, including husband or fetus, sibling or child, wife or elder.
6. There exist several decades of multidisciplinary work on the development of theories and the application of these theories to the issue of violence in general and family violence in particular.
7. Although early research on the causes of family abuse emphasized the personality deficits of abusers, more recent studies have focused on financial stress, drug dependency, marital discord, and other factors.
8. The nurse must recognize the characteristics of abusing families and the effect of abuse on the entire family, rather than limit attention to the individual victim.
9. Nursing assessment of the battered child includes the identification of the predictors of abuse and vulnerable infants, physical and psychosocial information about the child, and specific data about the injury.
10. Assessment of the battered woman often reveals a history of repeated injuries, psychosomatic complaints, and drug and alcohol abuse.
11. Awareness of elder abuse has been slim due

Nursing Care Plan 35-1

The Battered Child (Victim of Physical Abuse)

Nursing Diagnosis	Outcome	Intervention
Disturbance in self-concept; self-esteem	To develop improved sense of self-esteem	Communicate acceptance through verbal and nonverbal means; create situations wherein the child can excel; reward the child's good work or efforts
	To interrupt the cycle of guilt and feelings that the abuse towards him is deserved	Interview the older child privately and confidentially regarding the abusive situation; discuss why parents abuse children and what can be done to help the family; reassure the child that he is not to blame for being abused
Fear	To establish rapport	Intervene in the abusing situation as a caring, supportive adult; provide appropriate discipline

The Battered Child (Victim of Sexual Abuse)

Nursing Diagnosis	Outcome	Intervention
Fear Anxiety Powerlessness Hopelessness	To help the child understand what has happened	Assure the child that he is not to blame; interview the child alone (if verbal); encourage the child to recount the experience either verbally or through pictures or drawings, role-playing, or therapeutic play; record particular words of the child and clarify with parents for proper interpretation, if the meaning is questionable
	To help the child deal with fear and guilt	
	To help the parents control emotionalism and work through guilt	Help parents show continued love and support to the child

The Battered Wife and/or Battered Elder

Nursing Diagnosis	Outcome	Intervention
Fear Hopelessness Ineffective individual coping	To establish rapport	Approach client in a nonjudgmental manner; interview client privately and confidentially regarding the abuse
	To decrease shame and guilt	Be available as a listener and source of support; provide information about community resources and services, such as nearby woman's shelters and legal aid; assist client in planning for the development of job skills, care for children, and so on
	To help woman leave situation (if desired)	Involve the client in assertiveness training workshops and consciousness-raising groups as appropriate; provide an opportunity for the woman to vent feelings and relate the complete story of the abuse; provide an opportunity for client to dis-

The Battered Wife and/or Battered Elder		
Nursing Diagnosis	Outcome	Intervention
		cuss what she has done about the problem and what she would like to do; encourage client to set her own priorities
Disturbance in self-concept: self-esteem	To promote increased self-esteem	Assist the client in identifying her own strengths; provide positive reinforcement for reaching out, even if she is unsure about future; help her reach an awareness that she is not alone

to the limited respect that society gives to the elderly.

12. It is difficult for the health care professional to document abuse within families.

13. The goals and principles of intervening with the abused victim and family focus on an accepting, objective, and nonjudgmental approach to the family.

14. Health care providers must be familiar with the available community resources and their usefulness to the client and family.

15. Because child abuse, wife abuse, and elder abuse often occur together in a family, the nurse or other health care professional may need to intervene on behalf of more than one family member.

16. The nurse must become aware of, and face, her own feelings about working with the violent family.

17. Nurses need to become involved in the area of social change through consciousness-raising, community education, and the legal process.

References

1. Anderson C: Assessing Parenting Potential: Alerting Nursing Professionals of Risk for Child Abuse. Ped Nurs. pp. 323–329 Sept-Oct, 1987

2. Anderson C: A Preliminary Profile of Abusive and Non-Abusive Mothers. Unpublished Ph.D. dissertation, Texas Woman's University, 1985

3. Appleton W: The Battered Woman Syndrome. Ann Emer Med 9 (Feb): 84–92, 1980

4. Athens L: Violent Crime: A Symbolic Interactionist Study. Symbolic Interaction 2 (Spring): 56–69, 1978

5. Avison W, Turner J, Noh S: Screening for Problem Parenting: Preliminary Evidence on a Promising Instrument. Child Abuse Neg 10: 157–170, 1986

6. Bandura A: Aggression: A Social Learning Analysis. Englewood Cliffs, NJ, Prentice-Hall, 1973

7. Barnett E, Pittman C, Ragan C, Salus M: Family Violence: Intervention Strategies. US Department of Health and Human Services, Washington, DC, 1980

8. Bauer W, Twentyman C: Abusing, Neglectful and Comparison Mothers' Responses to Child-Related and Non–Child-Related Stressors. J Consult Clin Psychol 53: 335–343, 1985

9. Belsky J: Child Maltreatment: An Ecological Integration. Am Psychol 35 (Apr): 320–333, 1980

10. Boisvert M: The Battered Child Syndrome. Social Casework 53 (October): 475–481, 1972

11. Bowerman K: Family Violence: Children Within the Cycle. Austin, TX, Texas Commission on the Status of Women, Office of the Governor, 1978

12. Broadhurst D: The Educator's Role in the Prevention and Treatment of Child Abuse and Neglect. Washington, DC, HEW publication #(OHDS) 79-30172, 1979

13. Bronfenbrenner U: The Ecology of Human Development. Cambridge, Harvard University Press, 1977

14. Burr W, Hill R, Nye F, Reiss I (eds): Contemporary Theories About the Family, Vol 2. New York, Free Press, 1979

15. Campbell J, Humpreys J: Nursing Care of Victims of Family Violence. Reston, VA, Reston Publishing Company, 1984

16. Dunea G: The Joy of Wife Beating. Br Med J 2 (August): 565–566, 1977

17. Fitch J: Stopping Elderly Abuse. TEMS (April): 50–53, 1986

18. Flynn E: Preventing and Diagnosing Sexual Abuse in Children. Nurse Pract 12 (February): 47–54, 1987

19. Franklin D: The Politics of Masochism. Psychology Today (January): 53–57, 1987

20. Freeman M: Violence in the Home. London, Saxon House, 1979

21. Freud S: The Ego and the Id. Riviere J (trans), Strachey J (ed). New York, WW Norton, 1962

22. Frieze I: Factors Correlated with Men Who See

Spousal Violence as More Common. Handout at Annual Research Conference of the Association for Women in Psychology, Dallas, 1979

23. Garbarino J: The Human Ecology of Child Maltreatment: A Conceptual Model for Research. J Marriage Family 39: 721–732, 1977

24. Gaylord J: Wife Battering: A Preliminary Survey of 100 Cases. Br Med J 1 (Jan): 194–197, 1975

25. Gelles R: The Violent Home, Beverly Hills, Sage Publications, 1972

26. Gelles R, Strauss U: Is Violence Towards Children Increasing? Journal of Interpersonal Violence 2 (June): 212–223, 1987

27. Goadolf E: Men Who Batter: An Integrated Approach for Stopping Wife Abuse. Holmes Beach, FL, Learning Publications, 1985

28. Gorline L, Ray M: Examining and Caring for the Child Who Has Been Sexually Assaulted. MCN 4 (March/April): 110–114, 1979

29. Gruber A, Heck E, Mintzner E: Children Who Set Fires. Am J Orthopsychiatry 51 (July): 484–487, 1981

30. Heindl C, Krall C, Salus M, Broadhurst D: The Nurse's Role in the Prevention and Treatment of Child Abuse and Neglect. Washington, DC, HEW publication #(OHDS) 79-30202, 1979

31. Helfer R, Kempe CH: Helping the Battered Child and His Family. Philadelphia, JB Lippincott, 1972

32. Hendrix MJ, LaGodna G, Bohen C: The Battered Wife. Am J Nurs 78 (April): 650–653, 1978

33. Hirst S: The Abused Elderly. J Psychosoc Nurs Ment Health Care 24 (Oct): 37–45, 1986

34. Hunka C, O'Toole A, O'Toole R: Self-help Therapy in Parents Anonymous. J Psychosoc Nurs Ment Health Care 23, 24–31, 1985

35. Hunter R, Kilstrom N, Kraybill E, Loda F: Antecedents of Child Abuse and Neglect in Premature Infants: A Prospective Study in a Newborn Intensive Care Unit. Pediatrics 61 (April): 629–635, 1978

36. Jacobziner J: Rescuing the Battered Child. Am J Nurs 64 (January): 92–95, 1964

37. Johnson R: Aggression in Man and Animals. Philadelphia, WB Saunders, 1972

38. Kurz D: Emergency Department Responses to Battered Women: Resistance to Medicalization. Social Problems 34, 69–81, 1987

39. Langley R, Levy R: Wife Beating: The Silent Crisis. New York, Simon and Schuster, 1977

40. Lauer J, Lourie I, Salus M, Broadhurst D: The Role of the Mental Health Professional in the Prevention and Treatment of Child Abuse and Neglect. Washington, DC, Health, Education & Welfare publication #(OHDS) 79-30194, 1979

41. Lemasters E: Parenthood as Crises. Marriage and Family Living 19 (November): 352–356, 1957

42. Lichtenstein V: The Battered Woman: Guideline for Effective Intervention. Issues in Mental Health Nursing 3 (July-September): 237–251, 1981

43. Limandri B: The Therapeutic Relationship with Abused Women. J Psychosocial Nursing 25 (Feb): 9–16, 1987

44. Loraine K: Battered Women: The Ways You Can Help. RN 44 (Oct): 22–29, 1981

45. Lorenz K: On Aggression. New York, Harcourt, Brace, 1966

46. Martin D: Battered Wives. San Francisco, New Glide Publications, 1976

47. McKeel N: Child Abuse Can Be Prevented. Am J Nurs 78 (Sept): 1478–1483, 1978

48. Millor G: Theoretical Framework for Nursing Research in Child Abuse and Child Neglect. Nurs Res 30 (Mar-Apr): 78–83, 1981

49. Mitchell B: Working with Abusive Parents, A Caseworker's View. Am J Nurs 73 (Mar): 480–484, 1973

50. Morris M: Maternal Claiming-Identification Processes: Their Meaning for Mother-Infant Mental Health. Parent–Child Relationship: The Role of the Nurse. Paper presented at Continuing Education Workshop, Rutgers University, Newark, NJ, 1968

51. Nikstaitis G: Treatment for Men Who Batter. J Psychosoc Nurs Ment Health Care 27, 33–36, 1985

52. Olsen R: Index of Suspicion: Screening for Child Abusers. Am J Nurs 76 (January): 108–110, 1976

53. Pillemer K: The Dangers of Dependency: New Findings on Domestic Violence Against the Elderly. Social Problems 33 (December): 146–158, 1985

54. Podnieks E: Elder Abuse: It's Time We Did Something About It. Canadian Nurse (December): 36–39, 1985

55. Restak R: The Brain: The Last Frontier. New York, Doubleday, 1979

56. Rosenbaum A, O'Leary K: Children: The Unintended Victims of Violence. Am J Orthopsychiatry 51 (October): 692–699, 1981

57. Ross M, Ross PL, Ross-Carson M: Elderly Abuse. The Canadian Nurse (February): 37–39, 1985

58. Rousaville B, Lifton N, Bieber M: The Natural History of a Psychotherapy Group for Battered Women. Psychiatry 42 (February): 73–78, 1979

59. Sammons L: Battered and Pregnant. MCN 6 (July/August): 246–251, 1981

60. Scott J. In Endleman S (ed): Violence in the Streets. Chicago, Quadrangle Books, 1968

61. Scott PD: Battered Wives. Br J Psychiatry 125 (November): 433–441, 1974

62. Smith H, Isreal E: Sibling Incest: A Study of the Dynamics of 25 Cases. Child Abuse Negl 11: 101–108, 1987

63. Steinmetz S: The Battered Husband Syndrome. Victimology: An International Journal 2 (March): 499–509, 1977–1978

64. Steimetz S: The Cycle of Violence: Assertive, Aggressive, and Abusive Family Interaction. New York, Praegle Publication, 1977

65. Straus M: A General Systems Theory Approach to a Theory of Violence Between Family Members. Social Science Information 12 (June): 105–125, 1973

66. Straus M: Wife Beating: How Common and Why? Victimology: An International Journal 2: 443–457, 1977–1978

67. Tagg P: Nursing Intervention for the Abused Child and His Family. Pediatric Nursing (September–October): 36–39, 1976

68. Thosaben M, Anderson L: Reporting Elder Abuse. Am J Nursing 85 (April): 371–374, 1985

69. Walker L: Battered Women and Learned Helplessness. Victimology: An International Journal 2, 525–534, 1977–1978

70. Walker L: The Battered Woman. New York, Harper Colophon Books, 1979

71. Wolfe D: Child-Abusive Parents: An Empirical Review and Analysis. Psychol Bull 97: 462–482, 1985

72. Wolfe D, Jaffe P, Wilson S, Zak L: Children of Battered Women: The Relationship of Child Behavior to Family Violence and Maternal Stress. J Consult Clin Psychol 53, 657–665, 1985

73. Battered Women: Issues of Public Policy. A Consultation Sponsored by the United States Commission on Civil Rights, Washington, DC, 1978

74. Child Sexual Abuse: Incest, Assault, and Sexual Exploitation. Washington, DC, HEW publication #(OHDS) 79-30166, 1978

75. Domestic Violence. A resource paper distributed by the National Indian Child Abuse and Neglect Resource Center. Tulsa, OK, 1980

76. Handout on child abuse at the Texas Nurses Association Conference on Family Violence. Dallas, 1978

77. Maternal Attachment and Mothering Disorders. A Round table discussion sponsored by Johnson and Johnson. Edited by Klaus MH, Kennell JH, 1974

78. National Analysis of Official Child Neglect and Abuse Reporting. Washington, DC, DHHS publication #(OHDS) 80-30271, 1980

79. Sexual Abuse of Children: Selected Readings. Washington, DC, DHHS publication #(OHDS) 78-30161, 1980

80. The Police Perspective in Child Abuse and Neglect. Gaithersburg, MD, International Association of Chiefs of Police, 1977

81. The Battered Woman. Emer Med 11 (April): 25–29, 1979

82. Anon: Trouble and Strife. Nursing Times (Aug): 32–33, 1986

36   Crises of Perinatal Loss and Depression

Patricia Murphey Lucas
Katherine Pritchett

Those who living fill the smallest space,
In death have often left the greatest void.

W.S. Landor,
Geri

700

Chapter Preview

Pregnancy and birth are considered to be a situational and/or maturational crisis.[3,4] The loss of a baby through miscarriage, stillbirth, or neonatal death is an additional crisis—a tragic and devastating experience for the parents and their families. Many times, health care providers are not prepared to offer the necessary psychological support when a perinatal loss occurs.

The emotional disorder of depression in the postnatal period is another unique entity resulting in crisis for the childbearing woman and her family. The symptomatology and management of this disorder are similar to those of depression occurring at any other time in life. Therefore, only information relating to the incidence and etiological theories of postpartum depression will be presented here. (See Chap. 23 for a complete discussion of the mood disorder of depression.) The focus of this chapter is the crisis of perinatal loss; its goal is to enable the nurse to assist the client and family through the process of mourning.

Learning Objectives

On completion of this chapter, you should be able to accomplish the following:

1. discuss depression as an emotional disturbance in the postpartum period
2. identify types of perinatal loss
3. discuss crisis theory as it relates to pregnancy
4. describe the grief process that occurs with perinatal loss
5. apply the nursing process to a client and her family who are experiencing a perinatal loss
    identify assessment data applicable to perinatal loss
    formulate appropriate nursing diagnoses and goals for the client and family with a perinatal loss
    implement nursing actions to facilitate the mourning process for the client and family with a perinatal loss
    evaluate the effectiveness of nursing actions for the client and family experiencing the death of an infant
6. discuss the effect of a perinatal loss on health care providers
7. describe the elements of a perinatal loss program
8. formulate a comprehensive nursing care plan

CHART 36-1
Terminology

Grief—the subjective experience and behaviors that occur after the psychological recognition of a loss

Mourning—the process a person must go through to resolve stages of grief and adapt to loss

Pathological grief and mourning—intensification of normal grief reaction; the person becomes overwhelmed, the mourning process does not progress, and the person resorts to maladaptive behavior

Perinatal—the time before, during, or shortly after the process of giving birth

Stillborn—an infant born dead

Miscarriage—an abortion that occurs naturally

Neonatal death—an infant who dies within the first 28 days of life

Postpartum (puerperium)—the time after birth

Postnatal—the time after birth

---

for the client and her family experiencing a perinatal loss

Depression in the Postnatal Period

Incidence and Etiological Theories

Some authors view depression in the postnatal period as indistinguishable from depression occurring at any other time in life.[26] However, studies also support the idea that this depression has enough unique symptoms to be considered a distinct entity.[6,7,10] In the DSM-III-R, however, a psychotic depression in the postpartum period is now included in the classification of the major psychotic disorders. The particular psychotic disorder diagnosed is determined by the specific symptoms and behaviors that the client presents.[1] Current research indicates that the risk of admission to a psychiatric hospital is greater during the first year after delivery than at any other time in a woman's life.[10]

Within the childbearing period, the mental health problems most commonly seen include maternity blues, postpartum depression, and postpartum psychosis. *Postpartum or maternity blues*, a self-limiting, mild transient alteration in mood, occurs in 30% to 80% of new mothers. Symptoms usually occur between the 3rd and 10th day after delivery and last approximately 24 to 48 hours. These symptoms include episodes of crying, fatigue, insomnia, irritability, and difficulty in concentrating.[5] The presence of maternity blues is found to be positively associated with a history of premenstrual tension and hormonal instability. Postpartum blues is often considered a normal variant rather than a clinical syndrome.[6,7]

Postpartum depression, on the other hand, occurs in approximately 20% of new mothers. Symptoms may appear early (within the first 3 months after delivery) or up to 1 year following the birth of the infant. These symptoms are comparable to those of depression at other times in life.[26] The etiology of depression during the postpartum period is not established. However, several possible influencing factors are being studied. An example of biologic factors is the changing levels of neurotransmitters and hormones during the postpartum period. Examples of psychological factors include a preexisting negative attitude toward childrearing and occurrence of recent stressful life events. Social factors may include a lack of support from the husband and the poor quality of the marriage relationship. Cases of depression during the postpartum period often recur, and symptoms may persist for 1 or more years. Studies indicate a positive correlation between a mother's depression and adverse outcomes for her child. These outcomes may include low birth weight, behavior problems, somatic complaints, and poor growth patterns.[26]

Postpartum psychosis is clinical similar to a nonpostpartum depressive psychosis. This condition is rare; the occurrence rate is only 1 or 2 mothers per 1,000 deliveries. Symptoms usually occur within 3 to 4 weeks after birth. These symptoms include delusions, hallucinations, and grossly disorganized behaviors. Women who develop a psychosis during the puerperal period appear to have more confusion and manic symptoms, whereas nonpuerperal women have more schizophrenic symptoms.[10,12] Etiology of psychotic depression in the postpartum period may be associated with changing hormonal levels, psychological and physical stressors as related to motherhood, and inadequate support systems.[5]

Perinatal Loss

Incidence

The loss of a baby—whether by miscarriage, stillbirth, or in the neonatal period—may be the "greatest tragedy parents feel they have ever experienced."[22]

Studies in the past 10 years indicate that a perinatal death can result in a grief and mourning response as severe as the death of a spouse or other adult family member. The national perinatal death rate is 14.7 per 1,000 live births.[25] Klaus and Kennel concluded from their review of long-term studies that "the mother suffers a tragic outcome in one-third of perinatal deaths."[13] Parents who experience a perinatal death go through an observable grief and mourning response.[8,11,22]

Etiological Theories

Pregnancy is viewed as an emotional crisis because of the major changes that occur in both physical and psychological equilibrium. The crisis of pregnancy is normally resolved in the birth of the child. A pregnancy that results in a perinatal loss creates an additional crisis. A bereaved mother must resolve the crisis of perinatal loss in addition to the crisis of pregnancy.

Perinatal death is a narcissistic loss for the mother. Such a loss can be described as losing part of oneself, which can be more difficult to mourn than the loss of a separate person. The mother identifies with the growing fetus throughout the pregnancy. Thus the mother perceives perinatal death as a threat to her own developing maternal self-worth.

During the pregnancy, a woman fantasizes about her "child-to-be"—his personality traits and particular characteristics. The loss of the infant means the end of both a real life and a fantasy. The fantasies of the "child-to-be" make the loss of the real child even greater. "What has been lost is not a child one did not know as much as fantasies of one who will never be."[16]

In order to appreciate the depth of the perinatal grief response, one must understand the concepts of attachment and detachment during the mourning process. Klaus and Kennell describe the attachment process as a series of steps that parents go through during pregnancy and birth. These steps include the following: planning, confirming, and accepting the pregnancy; feeling fetal movement and accepting the fetus as an individual; giving birth; hearing, seeing, touching, holding, and caring for the infant. It is significant that many of the steps occur before the birth of the infant. Since bonding has already begun, parents can at birth experience an acute grief reaction. The concept of detachment is also an important part of the mourning process. This phase of the process involves "letting go."[2,13]

The expression of grief and the process of mourning following the death of an infant are similar to the normal grief stages identified by Elisabeth Kübler-Ross. These five stages are as follows:

1. Denial and isolation
2. Anger
3. Bargaining
4. Depression
5. Acceptance[14]

Searching and yearning and disorientation have been added as specific to stages of perinatal grieving.[15]

Lindemann, in his work on acute grief, has also described phases of mourning. These phases are as follows:

1. Shock and disbelief
2. Developing awareness and acute mourning
3. Resolution and acceptance[17]

Physical and emotional symptoms of grief as identified by Lindemann are listed in Table 36-1.[17, 23]

Application of the Nursing Process to the Client with a Perinatal Loss

Assessment

After a perinatal loss, grief expressions typically follow the stages of grief and mourning that have been identified by Lindemann and Kübler-Ross. During the period of disbelief and denial, parents have difficulty concentrating and making decisions. Mood swings and emotional turmoil may also be observed. Somatic manifestations often noted include dizziness, pallor, perspiration, palpitations, and aching arms.[14, 17]

As the reality of the perinatal death is felt, behaviors of the next phase begin to appear. Anger and guilt predominate among the feelings of confusion, anxiety, and sadness. Authors have referred to this phase as a period of yearning and searching. In the following phase of disorientation, which occurs several months after the loss, disorganization, despair, and depression can be noted. Feelings of loneliness and emptiness intensify and there is a preoccupation with the deceased infant.[15] Within the acceptance or resolution phase, the preoccupation with the loss of the baby begins to subside. Reorganization of life begins to take place.

Lindemann believed that the normal acute grief response would be resolved within 4 to 6 weeks. Current belief is that the normal acute grief response may take up to 12 weeks, with resolution of grief extending over 1 to 2 years.

Pathological grief may manifest itself in several possible ways. There may be an absence of grief or a delay in reaction to loss in the first 2 weeks. A prolonged or a distorted grief reaction may also signal pathological bereavement. Other possible indicators may be anxiety symptoms, unrealistic idealization of the fetus, and a desire to have a replacement child.

Risk factors have been identified that increase the incidence of pathological grieving. These factors are as follows:

1. A reported crisis during the pregnancy, *e.g.*, death of a loved one, marital conflict
2. Perceived or experienced lack of emotional support from husband and/or family
3. Seeing but not holding the baby
4. Conception of another pregnancy within 5 to 6 months of the perinatal death
5. A surviving twin
6. Previous history of emotional disorders, *e.g.*, depressive reaction
7. Intense ambivalent feelings about pregnancy
8. Strong cultural view of the mothering role[11, 15]

Table 36-1.   Symptoms of Grief

I. PHYSICAL	II. EMOTIONAL
A. Loss of appetite	A. Guilt
B. Sleep problems—insomnia, vivid dreams or nightmares	B. Depression
C. Tightness in throat or chest—called by some "heartache"	C. Empty, lonely feeling
D. Choking sensation	D. Irritability, hostility, or anger directed toward those one is close to or those trying to help
E. Shortness of breath	E. Increased emotional distance from others
F. Sighing	F. Inability to return to usual pattern of conduct
G. Fatigue—lack of strength, exhaustion	G. Loss of femininity
H. Aching arms—some mothers say their arms "hurt" from their not being able to hold the baby	H. Sense of futility

(From Sahu S: Coping with Perinatal Death. J Reproductive Med 26, 3 [March]: 130, 1981)

The nurse also needs to be aware of individual differences in the process of grieving among mother, father, siblings, and other family members. Fathers follow the same grief response as do mothers; however, a man may feel a need to be strong for the sake of his wife and not add to her grief. Fathers may feel angry and cheated at the loss of the "proud father" role. The difference between the mother's progress through the stages of grief and the father's may be related to the mother's prenatal emotional attachment to the baby. This difference in the process of grieving has been termed "incongruent grieving."[20] Confusion and resentment may result if partners equate the length of time spent grieving to the intensity of the loss.

Siblings, especially young children, who may have perceived the pregnancy as a rival may experience guilt feelings over the death of a new baby. It is not uncommon for young children to wish for a new baby to go away. Thus they may feel responsible for the death of the new baby. The young child's distorted concepts of illness and death may cause him to have fears related to the possible death of his parents.[23]

Grandparents may also feel the intensity of grief and mourning of the perinatal loss. They grieve for the grandchild they will never have and for the depth of suffering their own child is experiencing.

Nursing Diagnosis

In caring for the woman and family suffering a perinatal loss, the nurse analyzes assessment data gathered to determine actual and potential problems and formulate appropriate nursing diagnoses. Examples of nursing diagnoses for the bereaved mother and family include the following:

Grieving, anticipatory/dysfunctional related to fetal or neonatal death or birth of a newborn with a defect or disorder as evidenced by crying, depression, withdrawn behavior, disrupted sleep and/or eating patterns, other somatic complaints

Anxiety or Self-concept, disturbance in: self-esteem related to lack of understanding of the grieving process as evidenced by feelings of guilt, inadequacy, and inferiority

Spiritual distress related to perinatal loss and grieving process as evidenced by expressed anger at God, questioning of established religious beliefs and/or values, failure to seek spiritual assistance from clergy or attend usual religious activities

Social isolation related to death of infant as evidenced by failure to interact with others, continued loss of interest in outside activities, increased signs of pathological grieving

Knowledge deficit: discharge teaching related to perinatal loss as evidenced by expressions of guilt and misconceptions over the cause of infant's death, anxiety concerning future pregnancies[9]

Planning

Perinatal loss represents a crisis to the individual and to the family. The goals of crisis intervention that enable a person to regain emotional equilibrium should be utilized (see Chap. 33, "Crisis Theory and Intervention"). Inherent in goal-setting for a woman and her family experiencing perinatal loss is the promotion and protection of individual self-esteem and self-worth throughout all phases of the mourning process. In goal-planning with bereaved parents, it is important to keep in mind that their preoccupation with thoughts of the lost child may interfere with their participation and understanding. An example of a planning guide for parents who are experiencing perinatal loss is found in Table 36-2. This guide includes both short- and long-term goals to help parents and family members through the mourning process.

Intervention

It is essential that the caregiver understand that the initiation of intervention strategies must begin whenever awareness of a loss occurs for the childbearing woman and family. Interventions should be designed to help the client and her family cope with the immediate significance of loss, to facilitate the process of detachment, and to help make this experience an opportunity for growth. The following strategies should be incorporated in your plan of care for the client and family experiencing loss.

Facilitating Understanding of the Mourning Process

Perinatal loss presents a special challenge in mourning. Differences exist according to the loss at varying gestational ages of the infant. For example, with a first trimester miscarriage, the pregnant woman perceives the fetus as part of herself and thus mourns self-loss rather than loss of a separate being. The loss of the parent role must also be considered. In a stillbirth or early neonatal death, there is often a lack of anticipatory grieving. The suddenness of the loss precludes preparation for grieving. With the birth of a preterm infant or a baby with a congenital defect, parents must mourn the loss of their expected perfect child.[19] The grieving couple must mourn not only the child that

Table 36-2.   **Objectives of Perinatal Grief Crisis Intervention**

PRIOR TO DISCHARGE	4–6 WEEKS POSTPARTUM	4–6 MONTHS POSTPARTUM	1-YEAR ANNIVERSARY
1. Provide basic human comfort and support	1. Share preliminary autopsy report	1. Share final autopsy results	1. Facilitate expression of sadness at anniversary date
2. Help make loss real	2. Assess patient's progress	2. Reassess emotional progress	2. Refer for psychotherapeutic support if pathologic reaction evident
3. Encourage expression of emotion	3. Facilitate emotional release	3. Reassess social support	3. Provide support if subsequent pregnancy planned or undertaken
4. Encourage open communication among family members	4. Describe incongruent grieving	4. Explore possible problems in marital or sexual relationship	
5. Prepare for encounters in community	5. Assess couple's progress	5. Schedule anniversary visit	
6. Assess response in preparation for future meetings	6. Discuss local support groups		
7. Record information	7. Assess social support		
8. Schedule 4–6 week appointment	8. Discuss plans for subsequent pregnancies		
	9. Schedule 4–6 month appointment		

(From Lake M et al: The Role of a Grief Support Team Following Stillbirth. Am J Obstet Gynecol 146, 8 (August 15): 879, 1983)

they have lost, but also the child that will never be. Interventions should not only assess the couple's progress through the mourning process, but should also facilitate their understanding of this process. Information on grief response should include normal behaviors, common somatic discomforts, realistic expectations, and time parameters for grieving. It is important for the nurse to realize that even after perinatal death has been mourned and there is a return to normal living patterns, the mother or couple may continue to grieve on birthdates and other dates that signify "hoped for" expectations of the lost child. If incongruent grieving occurs, the nurse needs to encourage open communication between family members.

Encouraging Reality of Loss
Important to the grieving couple is the encouragement and support by the health care team of the parent's decision to see, touch or hold the infant after death. This private time when the couple can say goodbye to their infant helps make their loss real. Assisting the parents to plan funeral arrangements is another way of allowing the baby's existence and death to become real. Concrete reminders of the baby's birth and death can be provided by the be-

reavement team. Examples of articles confirming the reality of death include photographs, identification bracelets, footprints, and documentation of the baby's weight and length. Parents should also be encouraged to name their baby. If the infant has an anomaly, the nurse should prepare the parents for what they will see. If the parents do not view the baby because of the anomaly, their fantasized picture of the child may be more frightening than is actually true. Miscarriages present a unique difficulty for the parents in that there can be no keepsakes of the baby. This lack of tangible keepsakes can create an "unreal" event for the grieving parents.[2, 15, 22]

Communicating with Sensitivity
The nurse's role is of primary importance in creating a therapeutic environment in which the grieving family feels comfortable in expressing loss. Through verbal and nonverbal communications, the nurse can help bereaved parents integrate the loss into their lives. Statements that acknowledge the loss may convey to the parents the nurse's concern and empathy and may assist parents in their grief expression. An example of such statements is "I am so sorry about your baby. It must be so difficult for you to be here alone." The bereaved parent may have difficulty com-

Nursing Care Plan 36-1

The Client and Her Family Who Experience Perinatal Loss

Nursing Diagnosis	Client Outcomes	Interventions
Grieving, anticipatory/dysfunctional	Client/family communicates awareness of stages of grief process, expresses emotion appropriately, demonstrates progress in process of mourning	Assess for normal and pathological grief reactions Assess understanding of stages of grief and mourning Supplement information as applicable Create therapeutic environment for expression of emotion Acknowledge depth of loss through appropriate therapeutic intervention Encourage open communication of family members Promote reinforcement of reality—encourage parents to see, touch, hold infant; provide pictures of infant, footprints, blanket, identification bracelet for memory packet to give to parents or place on file for parents at later time Refer for appropriate psychotherapy as applicable to occurrence of pathological symptomatology
Self-concept disturbance in: self-esteem	Client/couple expresses and demonstrates feelings of self-worth, recognizes feelings of guilt, anger	Encourage verbalizations of feelings of anger and guilt Provide nursing care with warm, nonjudgmental approach
Knowledge deficit: discharge teaching relating to perinatal loss	Client/family demonstrates valuing of need for continuing follow-up care and participation in self-help group, verbalizes realistic information related to perinatal loss	Provide client/family with appropriate literature, *e.g.,* guides for parents experiencing perinatal loss Allow discussion to clarify perceptions of events surrounding death of infant Provide information concerning availability of self-help groups Employ anticipatory guidance techniques in preparing couples for encounters in community Provide information relating to planning of subsequent pregnancies Set up time parameter for future contact visits

CHART   36-2
Losing a Baby
Renee Gaston Hoke

Few events in my life have affected my attitudes and emotions as profoundly as the loss of a baby—babies in our case, since my husband Greg and I lost twins at birth almost 10 years ago. I remember those first few days in the hospital vividly even today, and I remember clearly the care I received from the hospital staff.

My pregnancy had been normal in every way, so our loss was first and foremost a complete surprise. For several days, my primary emotions were disbelief and a great, dark emptiness. It would be weeks and months before I wrestled with deeper spiritual needs and emotions connected with our loss. For those first few days, I felt only numb ... and very, very empty.

The first hours were a fog of physical pain and exhaustion. I was moved to the last room on the maternity hallway, but I could clearly hear crying babies being carried to their waiting mothers. Since this was my first pregnancy, I could only guess what it must be like for those mothers to nurse their new babies.

These were normal, happy sounds. I could hear them very clearly because my own room was so quiet. When Greg was not visiting, I turned off the television and stared silently out the window into the winter sky. There were no calls or visits from my friends and relatives yet—most of our friends had not yet heard the news and our immediate relatives were making plane reservations to attend the funeral. Two or three days later Greg and I were surrounded by more love and nurturing than we could have dreamed possible. But those first few days were silent.

Who became the only living, breathing humans in my world during those empty days? The nurses—making their rounds, taking my temperature, delivering meals or medication. I remember that most of them entered and left my room uttering only the few words necessary to do their jobs. They performed their tasks in seconds, almost as if they were being timed for efficiency. I felt contagious. Soon the door would close and I would hear them move down the hall to the next room, where they would chat comfortably with the next patient.

I understand now how they must have felt in my presence. I was the abnormality—the woman *without* a baby. If they stopped to chat with me, would I burst into tears? Would I blame them for my loss? Would I ask them to explain how something so terrible could happen?

Far from it! I was not in search of answers yet. In fact, I wasn't even sure of the questions. What I needed most was a friendly voice to talk with me about the weather or a new recipe, to distract me from my loss and remind me that normal, ordinary life continues no matter what.

A nurse can be a wonderful, comforting distraction for a grieving patient. As she or he bustles around your room, taking your pulse or straightening your bed, you are transported back to your childhood and the tender loving care that mom or grandmother lavished on you. How special you feel to have someone near whose only thought is for your well-being! How nice to feel the touch of a hand or hear a kind word!

I do remember one nurse who knew just what I needed in the midst of my ordeal. She cared for me in recovery, when my pain was still more physical than emotional. As she fluffed my pillow and brushed back my hair, I thanked her.

"You're welcome," she answered softly, and then she paused. "This just isn't fair, is it?"

That was all I needed. A voice, a human being who cared. The burning spiritual and philosophical questions could wait until another day. For now, what I wanted was ordinary sights and sounds to remind me that life goes on ... regardless. For a while, thanks to those kind words, the emptiness was more bearable.

municating because of the intensity of her grief. The nurse must not push the client to communicate, but should allow her to communicate when ready. This is an appropriate time for the nurse to listen to parents, to touch, and simply to be with them. The nurse should not try to hide her feelings to protect parents.

It is okay if the nurse cries. Parents will long remember sincere expressions of empathy.

Nurses should be careful to avoid stereotypical statements such as "I know how you must be feeling, you're young, you can have other babies," "It must be God's will, it must be for the best," "You were just

C H A R T 36-3
Perinatal Loss Support Program

Joan N. Yanda, M.S.N., R.N.
Clinical Nurse Specialist
Maternal Child Nursing
Methodist Medical Center
Dallas, Texas

At Methodist Medical Center in Dallas, we have a multidisciplinary Perinatal Loss Support Program for parents and families who lose infants through ectopic pregnancy, miscarriage, stillbirth, and neonatal deaths.

Upon the death, the nursing supervisor, social worker, and chaplain are notified. The nurse caring for the infant initiates a Perinatal Loss Checklist to coordinate all supportive efforts. The chaplain visits to facilitate the grieving process; the chaplain also explains the funeral arrangements and autopsy. The nurse takes pictures of the infant, providing a background that makes a treasured picture. She offers the pictures to the parents and encourages them to see and hold their infant. The mother must give permission for grandparents or other family to see or hold the infant. A memory packet is provided. It contains a lock of hair, footprints, bracelet, crib card, and birth certificate. If the parents refuse either the photograph or the packet, it is filed and kept indefinitely; the parents often change their minds. The mother is recovered in a private area to allow her to display her feelings. After recovery, the mother is transferred to a floor where there are no babies—only other woman patients. A grief symbol on a door card is placed on her door to alert staff and ancillary help that a grieving family is in this room. Depending on the type of loss, appropriate grief literature is given to the family as well as booklets to grandparents and siblings. The social worker provides information on parent support groups. The parents are leaving the hospital with broken hearts and empty arms, but not without support. The social worker writes or calls each family after discharge to see how they are doing, that is, whether they are sleeping, eating, and have someone to talk to.

In addition, we train interested staff to be Perinatal Loss Counselors and to serve as resources for other staff members who are not as comfortable with death. Six sessions of 1½ hours each are planned to discuss personal feelings about death; how women, men, and children deal with death; common feelings following a miscarriage, a stillbirth, and a neonatal loss; what to say when counseling parents; ethnic differences in grief expression; funeralization process; autopsy; picture-taking; and support following discharge. The counselors are given articles to read and come prepared to discuss the information in class. Upon "graduation" they receive a certificate and a pin made to resemble the grief symbol.

barely pregnant, it is fortunate you really didn't get to know this baby." These statements negate the mother's feelings and interfere with the process of attachment and detachment needed for normal grief resolution. (See Chap. 4, "Communication," for therapeutic techniques.)

Providing for Human Comfort and Support

Parents experiencing perinatal loss often feel isolated or undesirable because the staff are hesitant to become involved in physical and emotional care. Nurturing is important to feelings of self-worth and esteem. In providing for the client's physical care, the nurse should carry out activities with gentleness and concern. In implementing care, the nurse acknowledges the client's cultural and religious values.

Planning for the Future

Bereaved parents must be aware that friends and even family members may respond in well-meaning but nontherapeutic ways. Anticipatory guidance from the bereavement team may allow the client to respond to these difficult situations more effectively. Written information concerning available resources (*e.g.*, support groups and helpful literature) should be provided, as parents initially may be unable to hear due to their intense grief and preoccupation with the baby. Follow-up counseling to answer parents' unanswered questions—about the baby's medical condition, or the events surrounding the death—is important. Follow-up contact can also be a time for discussing the possibilities of future pregnancies. Parents are usually advised to wait 6 or more months before having another pregnancy in order to avoid the replacement child syndrome; the new baby should not be thought of as a replacement for the infant who died. Follow-up visits can also be a time to assess for any signs of pathological grief. If symptoms are present, appropriate referral for psychotherapy should be made. An example of one hospital's approach to perinatal loss intervention is included in Chart 36-3, "Perinatal Loss Support Program."

Evaluation

Evaluating the effectiveness of interventions relating to perinatal loss requires an ongoing assessment throughout each of the stages of the mourning process. Specific observations should be made to determine if projected client outcomes have been achieved. Evaluation of the resolution of perinatal loss is dependent on the strength of follow-up interventions, as in a perinatal loss program. Because the significance of perinatal loss has only been recognized over the past 10 years, the long-range effect of interventions on psychological aspects for the woman and her family experiencing perinatal loss have yet to be established. Further studies are needed to validate the significance of such interventions as are included within present perinatal loss programs. Further clinical research is also needed to distinguish early symptomatology of pathological grief responses.

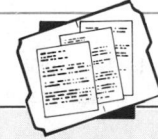

Case Study 36-1

Planning Care for the Client Who Has Experienced A Perinatal Loss (Stillbirth)
Joan N. Yanda, M.S.N., R.N.

Bob and Sue have been married 6 years. They met in high school and still live in the same town where they grew up. Bob is a policeman and Sue is a receptionist. They have a 4-year-old son, Kevin. Sue, is 38-weeks gestation.

She calls her physician because she has not felt her baby move in 24 hours. Sue and Bob arrive in Labor and Delivery for a sonogram. There are no fetal heart tones. There is no fetal heartbeat visible on the sonogram. The doctor tells Bob and Sue that their baby has died. Bob is confused and asks if something can be done—a Cesarean—something! The doctor explains that nothing can be done.

Labor is induced. During labor, Bob and Sue are quiet, but show no tears. After 8 hours of labor, Sue delivers an 8 pound, 2 ounce girl with blond hair. The delivery room is very quiet. Bob looks away as the infant is born. The nurse weighs the infant and wraps her in warm blankets. She asks if they would like to see the infant. They say no. In a private recovery room, Sue and Bob sob uncontrollably in each other's arms. The nurse takes pictures of the infant. She asks the parents if they would like to see the picture and tells them that their daughter looks as if she is sleeping. They agree to see the picture and then ask to see the baby. Through tears, the mother sees that the little girl has her family's nose and her husband's chin. The nurse asks what name they had chosen for her—it was "Jennifer." The chaplain visits and answers questions about funeral options. The father holds his daughter. The parents unwrap the infant, counting fingers and toes. The nurse leaves them alone between vital signs and lochia checks. The father requests pictures of the three of them, saying, "It is the only chance we will get." This picture is taken and added to the memory packet, which contains a lock of hair, footprints, birth certificate, bracelet, and crib card. The packet is given to the parents. After recovery, the mother is transferred to a gynecology floor, where she stays overnight. The nursing staff makes time to allow the mother and father to verbalize their feelings about their daughter Jennifer. The parents are given a book about grieving for support after discharge. The social worker provides information and the phone number of a parent support group. Sue is discharged to home the next day.

Questions for Discussion

1. Discuss the different types of crises involved in this obstetrical situation.
2. Identify the symptoms and behaviors of the grieving process that can be observed in the bereaved couple.
3. Discuss behaviors that may indicate potential problems occurring in the mourning process.
4. List those nursing interventions that facilitated the concept of attachment and detachment.

Nurse's Feelings and Attitudes

Involvement in the physical and emotional care of a family experiencing perinatal loss causes a grief response in the nurse similar to that experienced by the bereaved parents. Emotional sequela of staff need the same consideration as those of the client. Dealing with grief and loss is exhausting work for health professionals. To avoid emotional burnout, strategies such as group sessions to receive information and emotional support are necessary for team members. The strength of perinatal loss strategies, as implemented in a perinatal loss program, is contingent on the emotional well-being of the staff and their commitment to the value of the program.

Summary

This chapter has explored the topic of perinatal loss and its effect on the client and her family. Information about depression as a psychological disturbance occurring in the postnatal period has also been presented. The major points of this chapter are as follows:

1. Perinatal loss can create a situational crisis in addition to the existing maturational crisis of pregnancy.
2. There exists a difference of opinion as to whether depression during the postnatal period is a distinct entity.
3. The DSM-III-R includes depression in the postpartal period with classifications of other major psychotic disorders.
4. The client and family with a perinatal loss must progress through the normal grief and mourning stages.
5. The assessment of a client and her family experiencing the death of a baby may include normal symptoms and behaviors of grief and indicators of potential pathological bereavement.
6. Specific short- and long-term goals are formulated for the client and family in order to facilitate the accomplishment of each stage of the mourning process.
7. Intervention strategies are designed to promote the concept of attachment and detachment in the resolution of the mourning process.
8. Evaluation of the specific perinatal grief crisis interventions determines whether projected client outcomes have been achieved.
9. Because of the difficulty of working with par-

ents who have experienced a perinatal death, the nurse must have adequate and available support and encouragement.

References

1. American Psychiatric Association: Diagnostic and Statistical Manual of Mental Disorders, 3rd ed., rev. Washington DC, American Psychiatric Association, 1987
2. Beckey RD et al: Development of a Perinatal Grief Checklist. JOGNN, (May–June): 194–199, 1985
3. Benedek T: Toward the Biology of the Depressive Constellation. J Am Psychoanalytic Association 4: 389–427, 1956
4. Benedek T: Parenthood as a Developmental Phase. J Am Psychoanal Assoc 7:389–417, 1959
5. Bobak IM, Jensen MD: Essentials of Maternity Nursing. The Nurse and the Childbearing Family, 2d ed. Washington, DC, CV Mosby, 1987
6. Casiano ME, Hawkins DR: Major Mental Illness and Childbearing: A Role for the Consultation-Liaison Psychiatrist in Obstetrics. Psychiatr Clin North Am 10 (March): 35–51, 1987
7. Chang SS, Renshaw DC: Psychosis and Pregnancy. Compr Ther 12 (10): 36–41, 1986
8. Condon JT: Management of Established Pathological Grief Reaction After Stillbirth. Am J Psychiatry 143 (August): 987–992, 1986
9. Doenges, ME, et al: Maternal/Newborn Care Plans: Guidelines for Client Care. Philadelphia, FA Davis, 1988
10. Gjerdingen DK et al: Postpartum Mental and Physical Problems—How Common Are They? Postgrad Med 80 (December): 133–143, 1986
11. Hall RCW, Beresford TP: Grief Following Spontaneous Abortion. Psychiatr Clin North Am 10 (September): 405–419, 1987
12. Herzog A, Detre T: Psychotic Reactions Associated With Childbirth. Dis Nerv Syst 37 (4): 229–235, 1976
13. Klaus M, Kennell J: Maternal-Infant Bonding. St. Louis, CV Mosby, 1982
14. Kübler-Ross E: On Death and Dying. New York, Macmillan, 1970
15. Lake M et al: The Role of a Grief Support Team Following Stillbirth. Am J Obstet Gynecol 146 (August): 877–881, 1983
16. Leon IG: Psychodynamics of Perinatal Loss. Psychiatry 49 (November): 312–324, 1986
17. Lindemann E: Symptomatology and Management of Acute Grief. Am J Psychiatry 101 (September): 141–148, 1944
18. Nichol MT et al: Maternal Grieving Response After Perinatal Death. Med J Aust 144 (March): 287–289, 1986
19. Pederson DR et al: Maternal Emotional Responses

to Preterm Birth. Am J Orthopsychiatry 57 (January): 15–21, 1987

20. Peppers LG, Krapp RJ: Motherhood and Mourning. New York, Praeger, 1980
21. Raphael B: Grieving Over the Loss of a Baby. Med J Aust 144 (March): 281–282, 1986
22. Rappaport C: Helping Parents When Their Newborn Infants Die: Social Work Implications. Soc Work Health Care 6 (Spring): 57–67, 1981
23. Sahu S: Coping with Perinatal Death. J Reprod Med 26 (March): 129–132, 1981
24. Schweibert P, Kirk P: When Hello Means Goodbye (A Guide For Parents Whose Child Dies Before Birth, At Birth, or Shortly After Birth). Portland, University of Oregon Health Sciences Center, Department of Obstetrics and Gynecology, 1985
25. Vital Statistics of the United States 1985. Mortality. Vol II, Part A. Washington, DC, DHH Services, 1985
26. Zuckerman BS, Beardslee WR: Maternal Depression: A Concern for Pediatricians. Pediatrics 79 (January): 110–117, 1987

37 Suicide

Patricia Flatley Brennan
Bruce Payne Mericle

I am now the most miserable man living. If what I feel were equally distributed to the whole human family, there would not be one cheerful face on earth. I must die to be better, it appears to me.

Abraham Lincoln

Chapter Preview

Every 11 seconds, someone attempts to end his life.[24] One of every 10 of these individuals succeeds on the first attempt; another one of those 10 persons will try again and succeed.[21] What is this desperation called suicide? Suicide has been described as follows:

"a response to an invitation, originating from others, that [one] stop living"[13]
"a behavior that seeks and finds the solution to an existential problem by making an attempt on the life of the subject"[3]
the failure of all defense mechanisms

As an isolated act, suicide appears to be an individual's last message to the world. From another viewpoint, suicide is but one of a range of behaviors that directly or indirectly result in the ending of a life.[9] Drug abuse, alcoholism, noncompliance with medical protocols, and excessive risk-taking may all lead to the death of the participant; however, not all persons who engage in such behavior can be called "suicidal." The purpose of this chapter is to help the reader understand the nature of suicidal behavior and to assess and care for persons at risk for suicide.

Throughout this chapter, the reader is introduced to methods for interpreting the various meanings of suicidal behavior. The etiology of suicidal behavior and the development of suicide in an interpersonal context are examined. The steps of the nursing process—assessment of the client's needs, analysis of the data, planning, identification, implementation of appropriate nursing strategies, and evaluation of the effectiveness of the interventions—are applied to individuals manifesting suicidal behavior.

Learning Objectives

On completion of the chapter, you should be able to accomplish the following:

1. define suicide as a type of self-destructive behavior
2. discuss factors related to the incidence of suicide and the populations affected
3. discuss the biologic, sociologic, and psychological theories of the development and dynamics of suicide
4. apply the nursing process to the care of clients exhibiting suicidal behavior
   use communication techniques to assess the meaning of, clues to, and degree of risk of the individual's wish to die
   formulate short-term and long-term goals for the suicidal client
   describe the ethical and legal responsibilities of the nurse caring for a suicidal client
   identify nursing interventions to provide safety, explore stressors, and promote effective coping for the suicidal client
   evaluate the effectiveness of nursing interventions
5. recognize and discuss your own feelings and behaviors that affect the suicidal client, his family, or his survivors

Incidence of Suicide and Populations Affected

Studies of the records of suicide prevention centers and regional mortality offices paint a picture of the degree and nature of suicidal behavior in the population.[12, 27] Although women make significantly more suicide attempts than men, men are more likely to kill themselves. Women tend to use less lethal methods of suicide than men.

Suicide behavior appears in all age groups (see Chart 37-1, "Adolescent Suicide"). Children kill themselves as deliberately and as desperately as the elderly. The likelihood of successful suicide, however, increases with age. Most persons who make attempts to end their lives have experienced a stressful situation prior to the suicide attempt. The most common stressors preceding the suicidal behavior include divorce, rape, death of a significant other, and loss of a significant part of one's life, such as a job.[17, 18, 30]

Social patterns emerge as one examines the demographic information about suicide. The suicide rate among many American Indian tribes is twice that of the national average. Suicide among blacks, especially adolescents and young adults, is increasing. Marriage, once thought to protect an individual from suicide, no longer offers that protection. Increasing economic status has also been associated with an increase in suicide rate.

The demographics of suicide reflect neither the individual's true motivation for taking his own life nor an accurate picture of the suicidal individual in the community. The statistics of suicide are frequently inaccurate, due to the social stigma of suicide, and this leads to inaccurate reporting of the number of actual suicides.[27] Furthermore, statistical assessments merely describe suicide as a social trend, not as the crisis of an individual and his significant others.

CHART 37-1
Adolescent Suicide

Gregg E. Newschwander, Ph.D., R.N.
Assistant Professor
Coordinator, Adolescent and Young Adult Nursing
Marquette University College of Nursing
Milwaukee, Wisconsin

There was just nothing left, nobody there. I felt like I was all alone.

Sandy, age 15

I just wanted the feelings to go away. They were there all the time. No matter what I did, I still felt like a waste. I guess it boiled down to it was better to feel nothing at all than to feel nothing but bad.

Jim, age 17

Suicide is the third leading cause of death among adolescents, exceeded only by accidents and homicide. It is the second most common cause of death among college students.[1] Reported adolescent suicides, however, may not accurately reflect true incidence.

When a young person commits suicide, the family physician may report it as an accidental death to spare the "reputation" of the family. In addition, many suicides are difficult to distinguish from accidental deaths. Deaths resulting from automobile accidents, for example (especially single-vehicle crashes), are often attributed to loss of vehicle control or driving while under the influence of alcohol or drugs; therefore, these deaths are listed as accidents, not suicides.

In the adolescent population, the ratio of suicide attempts to completions may be as high as 100 to 1. As more than 5,000 young people commit suicide each year,[1] one could predict nearly half a million attempts—roughly one every minute of every day.

In the past 25 years, suicide rates among adolescents have increased nearly 250%.[3] One recent study of high school students indicated that 10.5% of all the students surveyed had made a suicide attempt and 65% of all students reported some degree of suicidal thoughts or action.[2]

Not only are the numbers growing, but so, it seems, is the determination on the part of adolescents. Girls have always outnumbered boys in attempts and boys outnumbered girls in completions. However, recent trends see the girls closing the gap on completions. While girls have traditionally used less violent means, they now seem more likely to use guns than ever before.[1,2]

For some, it is difficult to understand why an adolescent, a member of a group that is generally considered to be full of life, with unlimited future potential, would want to take his or her own life. After all, some adults contend that adolescents today have many luxuries that young people 25 or 50 years ago did not. The impression is that growing up today is somehow easier.

The adolescents quoted above would be quick to disagree. They are living in a complicated age. The technology responsible for the luxuries known by young people today is the same technology responsible for the fear they live with daily. The very success that enables parents to give their children more than they had growing up has taken the parents out of the home—and has perhaps decreased parents' abilities to give their children the time and attention they need. The upward mobility that takes families to higher socioeconomic planes simultaneously takes adolescents away from schools, friends, and cherished routines.

Adolescents confront insecurity on every level. They no longer feel "safe" among family, friends, and community, or even as a member of the human race. The ties that bind have loosened greatly, and the quest for social cohesion has become an increasingly difficult one.

Some adolescents verbally threaten suicide, others do not. Although impulsive suicidal behavior is seen in adolescence perhaps more frequently than in any other developmental group, most adolescents who are contemplating suicide give some clues reflecting their intentions.

These clues can generally be found in the following three main areas:

Personal habits
Changes in appetite
Changes in sleep patterns
Dramatic changes in personal appearance
Unexplained personality changes
Frequent somatic complaints
Increased use of alcohol and drugs
Increase in risk-taking or self-destructive
    behaviors
Continuous self-deprecation

School behavior
Increased truancy
Decline in academic performance
Boredom, apathy
Disrupting class
Aggression or hostility toward teacher or other authority figure
Family and social relationships
Decreased interaction with peers
Change in friends
Heightened or lack of interest in romantic relationships
Getting his or her life in order
"Willing" objects or possessions to friends
Running away

Although it should be understood that the appearance of one or more of these behaviors does not necessarily indicate a potential for suicide, efforts should be made to explore what is troubling this adolescent. It is tragic that parents, friends, and relatives are usually shocked when they learn of an adolescent's suicide attempt—not because no warning signals were given, but because the clues were not recognized and dealt with.

When an adolescent threatens suicide or gives clues that an attempt might be forthcoming, the young person must be taken seriously. He or she should not be dismissed as an attention-getter or challenged in any way, but should be dealt with immediately and openly. The adolescent should be made to understand that he or she needn't carry out the threat in order to be believed.

Intervention with the suicidal adolescent centers on open, caring communication. The adolescent needs someone to listen to—**and hear**—what he has to say. The simple fact that there is someone who really cares about him may be enough to discourage a suicide attempt. Through the development of this supportive, caring relationship, the adolescent will be helped to find other ways to cope with the problems he faces.

As a relationship with the young person is being established, his family must also be included in counseling. The family is a major source of support for the adolescent—a support which he may believe has been lost. The suicide threat or attempt has a great effect on family members. As a unit, the family may experience anger and dismay at the deliberate attempt, guilt at having failed the adolescent, and possibly resentment for having been "socially embarrassed."

Nurses, especially school nurses, can and must play an active role in suicide prevention. They are in a position to plan programs focusing on awareness, prevention, and risk assessment. If students perceive them as safe, knowledgable sources, nurses can form therapeutic relationships with students that could be instrumental in preventing the attempt. When a suicide does occur, nurses can help students work through their bereavement or deal with their depression; this may be a key to preventing the occurrence of "cluster" suicides.

It is a sad commentary that suicide is a leading cause of death in what is generally considered a "healthy population." Nurses, physicians, teachers, and parents must become more aware of the warning signs of adolescent suicide and must begin to act on this—with understanding and foresight.

1. National Institutes of Mental Health. Useful Information on Suicide. Rockville, MD, Department of Health and Human Services, Alcohol, Drug Abuse & Mental Health Administration, 1986
2. Smith K, Crawford S: Suicide Behavior among "Normal" High School Students. Suicide Life Threat Behav 16, 313–25, 1986
3. Valente SM, Saunders JM: High School Suicide Prevention Programs. Ped Nurs 13, 2 (March/April): 108–112, 1987

Etiologic Theories

Views differ concerning the variables that result in a suicide. Although no one theory or set of ideas fully explains suicidal behavior, some theories offer partial explanation. Emphasis is placed on biologic, sociologic, and psychological influences.

Biologic Factors

The search for explanations for the cause(s) of self-harmful behaviors has yet to identify, definitively, a biologic theory of suicide. Several research studies link depression, physiological changes, and suicidal behavior to alterations in the number of serotonin 2 receptors in the brain. For example, a recent study demonstrated a significant increase in the number of serotonin 2 receptors in the frontal cortices of people who committed suicide by violent means.[14]

Nurses need to become familiar with the biologically focused research and its implications for nursing practice. As noted by Simmons-Alling,[25] there is an increasing tendency to explain depression and suicide through psychobiology. These new models will require that psychiatric nursing practice include consideration of psychobiological premises.

Much more research is needed before we fully understand the relatonships of biologic alterations to suicide behavior; nonetheless, it is an area that promises to provide some answers in the future.

Sociologic Viewpoint

Durkheim, the father of modern suicidology, based his observations of suicidal behavior on the social statistics available in Europe in the late 19th century.[6] He studied suicide as a social phenomenon and drew explanations for suicidal behavior from social trends, such as reactions to social order, or the lack of social order.

Durkheim postulated that all suicidal behavior falls into one of three categories—anomic, egoistic, and altruistic. Both anomic and egoistic forms of suicide represent an individual's isolation from society. *Anomic* suicide stems from the normlessness of society, which leaves the individual without a sense of social order. A lack of meaning or purpose in life leads to *egoistic* suicide. *Altruistic* suicide occurs when the individual gives up his life for some greater good. The overdose of a solitary poet, in response to his despair at the modern world, is an example of anomic suicide. Egoistic suicide is exemplified in the behavior of those who lost fortunes and jobs during the depression. Soldiers on a "suicide mission" approach death as an altruistic suicide.

Psychological Influences

Psychoanalytic View

Early psychological theories of suicide proposed that suicide was the result of the individual's drive or desire for death. Freud defined two drives basic to all people—*thanatos,* the drive toward death, and *eros,* the drive toward life. Suicidal behavior resulted when the "death drive" of the individual took precedence over the "life drive." This shift in the driving forces of an individual, Freud believed, occurred in response to the real or imagined loss of a loved one. The image of the loved one, with all its concomitant feelings, was internalized. The individual who felt abandoned by the lost love experienced anger, and this anger, lacking an outlet, was turned toward the self. The ultimate act of self-destruction resulted as the depressive response to a loss.

"Partial Suicide"

Menninger viewed suicide as more than the depressive response to a loss.[14] He hypothesized a tripartite source of suicide in everyone—the wish to kill, the wish to be killed, and the wish to die. The core of the suicide act, he postulated, was anger and despair. Menninger viewed suicide not merely as a single act, but also as a group of behaviors he termed "partial suicide," such as polysurgeries, substance abuse, and self-mutilation. When the individual lacked one of the three components of suicide, a "partial suicide" occurred.

Interpersonal View

Later psychological theorists, although not completely rejecting Freud's and Menninger's ideas, viewed suicide as the result of an *interpersonal* as well as an intrapsychic crisis. The individual in crisis becomes distraught about his interpersonal relationships, experiences ambivalence about continuing to live, and chooses suicide as a means for resolving the ambivalence concerning his relationships.[23]

Dynamics of Suicide

A person contemplating suicide generally perceives himself as isolated, hopeless, and helpless. He may also experience feelings of worthlessness and anger. The isolation may be evident in actual physical distance from others or as a psychological barrier between the individual and other people. The suicidal person is unable to initiate or respond to social interactions. Through the act of suicide, the individual communicates his final message to others.

As a result of discussions with suicidal clients and examination of suicide notes, theorists have gleaned an understanding of the emotional components of suicide. The emotional state of the suicidal person is characterized by depression, anger, and feelings of hopelessness and helplessness. The suicidal person experiences a desire to kill himself or to be dead and a simultaneous wish to be saved or rescued. Talking about suicide or making a suicidal gesture carries in it a message to others. The meaning of the message is unique.

Baechler proposes four main themes.[3] *Escapist suicides* occur as a desire to remove oneself from an intolerable situation. In *aggressive suicide,* the individual uses the self-induced death as a means of causing suffering or revenge to another. An *oblative suicide* stems from the desire to transform the self to a more pleasurable reality. In *ludic suicide,* death is the unintended result of taking excessive chances with one's life.

The etiology of suicide and the meaning of suicidal behavior serve to heighten the nurse's awareness of the dynamics of suicide. Suicidal behavior occurs in individuals with many psychiatric diagnoses, such as depression, schizophrenia, anxiety disorders, and adjustment reactions. The nurse uses the understanding of the dynamics of suicidal behavior as a basis for providing care to the suicidal client and his family.

Application of the Nursing Process to Suicide

Assessment of the Suicidal Client

Accurate assessment is the key to the care of the suicidal client. Through observation and careful listening, the nurse examines the client's behavior and verbalizations for clues of suicidal intent. In the assessment process, the nurse explores the client's request for help, the presence and nature of a suicide plan, the client's mental state, the availability of support systems, and the client's lifestyle. Nursing knowledge and judgment guide the nurse to evaluate suicide risk amid a complex set of behaviors and thoughts.

Clues to Suicide

Most people who try to kill themselves give a clue of their intention to others.[24] Some people leave suicide notes; others give cryptic verbal messages to friends or family. Clues to suicide are found in behavior and may be classified as direct or indirect and verbal or nonverbal. Table 37-1 offers some examples of these clues to suicide.

A person may display one clue or any combination of clues to communicate suicide intention. Individuals who give direct clues to suicide have not been found to be more likely to make suicidal attempts than those who give indirect clues or no clues at all.

Behavioral Changes.

Clues to suicide are frequently subtle and difficult to interpret. Change in expected patterns of behavior is, perhaps, the most important indicator of suicide risk. The turmoil of a person considering the option of suicide is evident in his behavior; he is likely to exhibit anxiety, insomnia, poor concentration, anorexia, and somaticism. Expressions of anger and despair are also common behavioral indicators of the person's distress.

A sudden calmness in the distraught client may indicate that he has made a decision to die. Depressed people frequently think about suicide but lack the energy to act on their thoughts until the vegetative symptoms of fatigue, anorexia, and psychomotor retardation lift. The apparent improvement in the depressed client's behavior lulls those around him into assuming that the risk of suicide has passed, when, in fact, the client has decided to kill himself.

People close to the suicidal individual are in the best position to monitor changes in his behavior. The nurse on the inpatient unit or a member of the client's family may be the first to notice changes in behavior that may indicate a risk of suicide. The nurse should also be aware that certain factors, such as being older than 50, overwhelming stressors in one's life, and alcohol abuse increase the risk of suicide.

Risk Periods.

Certain times of the year have been identified as "peak periods" for suicide. Suicides increase in the spring. Some believe that suicides increase around holiday periods.[19] For some individuals, the decision to die is linked to disappointment or a sense of isolation during the holiday seasons, which are considered to be a time for family togetherness. For others, the holiday rituals decrease their loneliness and despair and lead to a diminishing of the will to die.

In inpatient psychiatric settings, certain times are risk periods for increased incidence of suicide, especially between 10:30 A.M. and 6:30 P.M., around "change of shift" time, and between Friday morning and Monday evening.[29] These times are usually pe-

Table 37-1.	**Clues to Suicide**	
	VERBAL	**NONVERBAL**
Direct	"I can't stand it—I'm going to kill myself." "I could die without pain by taking all my pills."	Actions such as taking pills, cutting wrists, making a noose Writing suicide notes
Indirect	"My family would be better off without me." "Pray for me." "I won't be here when you get back."	Risk-taking lifestyles Giving away personal possessions Purchasing a cemetery plot Sudden onset of sense of peacefulness

riods of decreased observation by, and interaction with, staff members.

Goals of Assessment

Clues and acts of self-harmful behavior do not always indicate that the individual wishes to die. These behaviors must be viewed as the individual's attempt to communicate a dramatic message.[10] In order to understand and respond to the message being communicated, the nurse observes and identifies the client's behavior and explores the meaning of the behavior with the client. The goals of assessment are as follows:

1. To establish the probability that the individual will act to harm himself
2. To determine the meaning of the self-harm
3. To initiate a therapeutic relationship with the client

Data are obtained through direct interview of the client and through discussions with family members and significant others. The nurse's own values and attitudes influence the interpretation of these data.

Interviewing

Assessment of the client at risk for suicide is an interpersonal process. During the initial interaction, the nurse uses the skills of the dyadic, or one-to-one, relationship to establish an atmosphere of warmth, concern, and interest. Calling the client by name demonstrates an attitude of respect and caring. Verbally acknowledging the client's perception of the situation and his own fears and desperation helps to convey the nurse's willingness to understand his situation. Touch may be used judiciously to establish a bond of reassurance and support. To carry out a complete assessment, the nurse asks clear, direct questions and responds to both the feeling and the content expressed by the client. It is best to avoid euphemisms such as "ending it all" and "doing yourself in" in the interview. The essence of an effective and accurate assessment of the suicidal client lies in clear, specific communication.

Gathering Information from Family

Assessment of suicidal risk also includes discussions with the family members or friends of the client. This is particularly important if the client is comatose following the ingestion of pills or self-induced trauma. Data gathered from significant others aid the nurse in identifying the precipitants to the client's suicidal act and his patterns of behavior. Health care workers who have aided the client (emergency room nurses, ambulance drivers) may also provide valuable information. Questions directed to the family or friends must be phrased in a manner that protects the client's rights to confidentiality. Contact with the family or significant others permits the nurse to offer support to those experiencing the crisis with the suicidal individual while gathering data about the crisis.

Clients who are hospitalized in general medical–surgical units, as well as in psychiatric units, may discuss suicidal thoughts or wishes before making an attempt on their lives. The assessment process of a suicidal client in an inpatient psychiatric unit does not differ markedly from that of a suicidal client in any other setting. Questions addressing past or present suicidal ideation provide additional data about the client's prior coping strategies as well as previously undetected suicide risks.

Values and Attitudes of the Nurse

Because suicide assessment is a dyadic process, the nurse's own values, moral beliefs, and attitudes toward self-destructive behavior have great influence on responses to the client. Before working with clients at risk for suicide, the nurse examines her own feelings about suicide and people who choose to terminate their own lives. The following questions address some of the issues that the nurse must consider:

Is suicide ever justifiable?
Are people who attempt suicide with nonlethal
methods merely trying to get attention?
Are all suicides preventable?

Answering these questions and discussing the responses with peers will help the nurse identify personal feelings and reactions to the suicidal person. This self-awareness will help the nurse respond to the client with greater objectivity and empathy.

Although suicide is no longer a criminal act, most societies and cultural groups consider suicide an immoral act. Religious groups generally believe that suicide is a sin and promulgate rules against suicidal behavior. At times of social crisis, such as war, proscriptions against suicide may give way to the value of giving one's life for a greater good. The social sanctions against suicide help to dissuade potential victims from carrying out suicidal acts. At the same time, these social sanctions contribute to the stigma attached to suicidal persons and their families.

Content of the Assessment

In the assessment of the client at risk for suicide, the nurse must explore the following six areas: how the client entered the health care system; the client's intent; presence of a suicide plan; current mental status; available support systems; and predominant lifestyle. The nurse may explore these topics in any order deemed appropriate.

Entry into the Health Care System. Assessment of the client at risk for suicide includes an examination of how the person initially sought help. Did the person call a suicide hotline? Did he call his physician? Did he call a friend who brought him into the hospital? The greater the individual's volition in seeking help, the greater the chance that early intervention will prevent a death by suicide.

The Client's Intent. Determining the meaning of the self-destructive thoughts or acts for the individual is an ongoing process. Initially, the nurse uses questions and active listening to identify the nature of the immediate crisis and the effect the person desires from the act of self-harm. The nurse listens for clues to the client's intent in his words—does he seek relief from stress? Escape from an intolerable situation? Revenge against a loved one? Death? By examining the desired goal, the nurse gains a framework within which she can assess and intervene to provide safety and to meet the need expressed by the client.

Because clients at high risk of killing themselves display severe anxiety and poor concentration, the exploration of the meaning of suicide is limited initially to overt, conscious motives. In-depth exploration of the factors leading to the suicide attempt is delayed until after the crisis has passed and the person is no longer at risk of acting on his suicidal impulses.

All people think about suicide; however, to certain individuals, suicidal ideation is not an intellectual tour through the options of life and death, but an actual plan to end one's life. In the assessment process, the nurse distinguishes between clients who use self-destructive behavior to end their lives and those who use self-destructive behavior to reach some other goal. Through a systematic suicide assessment, the nurse examines the content of the client's suicide ideation for the how, where, when, and what of self-destruction.

Suicide Plan. The nurse assessing a suicidal individual asks him directly if he has a plan for ending his life. Suicidal plans include a description of the method (shooting, hanging, overdose, self-immolation), location (at home, in the client's room), agent (gun, type of pills), and time (on discharge, when the client's wife is at work) of the proposed suicide. The more specific the plan verbalized by the client, the greater is the risk of suicide.

In addition, certain plans are more lethal—that is, likely to result in death—than others. Suicide by shooting or hanging carries a greater potential of success than suicide by cutting one's wrist. For example, compare the plan of the young man who stated he would hang himself with a bed sheet in his room as soon as the staff member left, with that of a middle-aged woman who threatened to "take a few pills and end it all." Suicide plans are evaluated based on the specificity of the plan and the lethalness of the method. (See Table 37-2.)

Mental State. After determining whether or not a client has a plan for ending his life, the nurse evaluates his mental state, which includes anxiety level, mood, and thought organization. Clients with a moderate-to-severe level of anxiety are at the greatest risk of deliberately acting on the suicide thoughts. In a panic state of anxiety, the person may make impulsive, haphazard attempts at suicide; low levels of anxiety rarely cause the person to act dramatically to alter his life situation. Immediately prior to a suicide gesture, the anxiety level of the client may drop. Generally, the mood of the suicidal person is depressed and hopeless. Suicide risk is increased when disorganized thinking and impaired judgment leave the individual vulnerable to an accidental suicide.[2]

Support Systems. The nurse explores with the client the interpersonal support systems that are available to him. Although the presence of family members or friends usually lowers the risk of suicide, problems in the relationships with significant others may have precipitated the suicidal gesture.[1] The nurse must realistically assess the supports available to the client, because his sense of isolation or estrangement may make him incapable of using the available support systems.

Lifestyle. Examination of the client's usual and current lifestyle is important also. What type of coping mechanisms does the client use—defense-oriented or task-oriented? Has there been a change in the client's interest in food, sex, sleep, or interpersonal relationships? A marked decrease in the appetites of life usually precedes suicidal behavior; an increase in these appetites can also be a warning sign. Another factor to consider is the stability of the client's lifestyle. Is the suicide ideation the result of a sudden, catastrophic crisis, or has the person been slowly dying for years? A history of a stable lifestyle, including job and social functioning, reduces the risk of suicide.

Determination of the Risk for Suicide

Once the nurse completes the initial assessment of suicide potential, she must interpret the data in order to make a determination of the suicidal risk. The extent of suicidal risk is not absolute; rather, the nurse uses clinical judgment skills to infer understanding out of the available clinical data. It is better to assume

Table 37-2.   **Assessing the Degree of Suicidal Risk**

BEHAVIOR OR SYMPTOM	INTENSITY OF RISK		
	Low	*Moderate*	*High*
Anxiety	Mild	Moderate	High, or panic state
Depression	Mild	Moderate	Severe
Isolation/withdrawal	Some feelings of isolation, no withdrawal	Some feelings of helplessness, hopelessness, and withdrawal	Hopeless, helpless, withdrawn, and self-deprecating
Daily functioning	Fairly good in most activities	Moderately good in some activities	Not good in any activities
Resources	Several	Some	Few or none
Coping strategies/ devices being utilized	Generally constructive	Some that are constructive	Predominantly destructive
Significant others	Several who are available	Few or only one available	Only one or none available
Psychiatric help in past	None, or positive attitude toward	Yes, and moderately satisfied with	Negative view of help received
Lifestyle	Stable	Moderately stable	Unstable
Alcohol/drug use	Infrequently to excess	Frequently to excess	Continual abuse
Previous suicide attempts	None, or of low lethality	One or more, of moderate lethality	Multiple attempts, of high lethality
Disorientation/ disorganization	None	Some	Marked
Hostility	Little or none	Some	Marked
Suicide plan	Vague, fleeting thoughts but no plan	Frequent thoughts, occasional ideas about a plan	Frequent or constant thought with a specific plan

(From Hatton CL, McBride S: Suicide: Assessment and Intervention. Norwalk, CT, Appleton-Century-Crofts, 1984)

a greater risk of suicide than a lesser risk until staff have a better understanding of the client and his potential to commit suicide.[5] Table 37-2, "Assessing the Degree of Suicidal Risk," provides some guidance for determining a client's risk for suicide.

Careful, accurate documentation of the six factors—suicide clues, means by which the client sought help, suicidal plan, mental state, support systems, and lifestyle—provides for continuity of care and meets the nurse's legal responsibilities. Documentation includes notations in the client's chart and the written nursing care plan.

Nursing Diagnosis

The formulation of nursing diagnosis is an essential component of the nursing process. The client's potential for self-harm, level of coping skills, degree of hopelessness, and use of support systems can be described in the nursing diagnosis. In turn, the diagnosis guides or prescribes nursing intervention.

Some examples of nursing diagnoses for the suicidal client include the following:

Hopelessness related to rejection by husband

Ineffective individual coping related to impulsivity, characterized by multiple suicide attempts
Potential for injury related to high risk of suicide

Planning

Planning involves bringing together the nurse's skill and judgment with the client's participation to formulate an appropriate approach to treatment. The nurse assesses the degree of suicide risk, validates this assessment with the client and other team members, and discusses with the client the type of nursing care most appropriate to meet his needs.

The nurse designs, with the client, the measures needed to protect him while supporting the maximum degree of autonomy that he is capable of. Nurses sometimes limit their response to the suicidal client to the provision of safety measures because of the overwhelming fear that the client may actually die while under the nurse's care.

At the same time, repeated contacts with chronically suicidal clients lead to feelings of frustration and anger in the nurse. The sense of futility that nurses experience while caring for the person with repeated nonlethal suicide attempts may lead them to underestimate the client's need for safety.

Treatment Settings

When planning care, the nurse considers both the immediate environment of the client in treatment and the usual living situation of the client. In the inpatient setting, the nurse uses the resources of nursing and non-nursing team members collaboratively to formulate and implement the treatment plan. The plan must be developed within the policy and procedural guidelines of the institution. Community care of the suicidal client demands that the nurse and client together discuss supports to which the client has access, such as family members or crisis hotlines. Planning within the community setting requires that the nurse recognize the limits of her ability to protect the client and be knowledgeable in the appropriate referral to community resources.

Short-Term Goals

Nursing care plans for the client with suicidal thoughts or behaviors are directed toward providing safety and interpersonal support to the client. Short-term goals include the following:

1. Client will not act on the suicidal plan
2. Client will talk with the nurse about suicidal thoughts
3. Client will take steps to resolve relationships and lifestyles that increase the suicide risk

Long-Term Goals

Long-term goals focus on helping the client to resolve the issues that precipitated the suicide crisis and to develop less destructive coping mechanisms. Long-term goals include the following:

1. Client will be free of suicidal ideation
2. Client will use task-oriented reactions to stress
3. Client will take steps to resolve relationships and lifestyles that increase the suicide risk.

Intervention

Nursing Intervention for the Suicidal Client

The nurse encounters the suicidal client in the community hospital, in emergency rooms, on psychiatric units, and through telephone calls to crisis intervention hotlines. Although the settings in which nursing care is provided vary, nursing actions center on the following three areas of concern:

1. Reducing the risk of suicide
2. Exploring, with the client, the lifestyles or stressors that precipitated the suicide crisis

3. Assisting the client in developing new ways of coping

All three actions are important, but the emphasis placed on each varies depending on the client situation. The interventions described below may be used by nurses in any setting but are grouped by where they most commonly appear.

Intervening in the Community

Understanding the Meaning of the Crisis. To respond effectively to the client, the nurse must understand the meaning of the suicide crisis to the client and to those around him. By exploring precipitating stressors and by responding to the client's words and feelings, the nurse helps the client identify the meaning of the suicide crisis. The nature of the crisis is that it is time-limited, and the client is most likely to be receptive to assistance during the crisis period.[1]

The nurse asks the client what type of assistance he needs. Questions such as "What can I do for you?" and "What would be helpful to you?" indicate the nurse's interest and decrease the client's sense of despair and hopelessness. The use of the problem-solving process helps the client to establish a plan of assistance, such as arranging for further treatment. The client should be encouraged to contact the crisis service whenever needed. The initial contact with the suicidal client is not terminated until he can state a specific plan of action for preventing self-destructive behavior in the future. In other words, he must identify effective coping skills.

Mobilizing Coping Skills. The nurse works with the suicidal client in the community to mobilize his existing coping strategies. To achieve this goal, the nurse explores with the client his perception of the situation at the time of the contact, encourages the client to report feelings and needs, and asks him to define actions he views as necessary. In a calm, direct manner the nurse emphasizes the client's desire to continue living as evidenced by his request for help. While acknowledging the client's desire for both death and life, the nurse makes clear her willingness to help the client respond to his desire to live. When the client is unable to mobilize effective coping strategies, hospitalization is warranted.

The Need for Hospitalization. A client at high risk for suicide in the community should be encouraged to enter a psychiatric inpatient unit of a hospital or treatment facility. The nurse may enlist the assistance of family members or friends to convince the client of the need for hospitalization. If the client refuses hospitalization, the nurse continues to talk with the client to identify a person with whom he can remain until the crisis has passed. The nurse must never indicate to the client that she, or anyone else, can magically protect him from his impulses. Once the client is hospitalized, several interventions are likely to be used.

Intervening in the Hospital or Treatment Center

Provide Environmental Support. The suicidal client in the hospital may already have made one suicide attempt but remains at risk to make another, or he may have entered the hospital as a means to resist acting on his suicidal impulse. In addition to the interpersonal support used in the community setting, the nurse uses the safe environment of the hospital to provide environmental support to the client.

Clients at high risk for suicide are placed on a closed unit or in some type of protected environment. Closed units provide for safety by restricting access to potentially hazardous objects such as scissors, glass bottles, light bulbs, and knives. Care is taken to preserve the client's sense of dignity; personal or clothing objects such as belts and shoe laces are removed from him only when absolutely necessary. The nurse administering medication to the highly suicidal client must insure that all medications are consumed. It is necessary to remember that the client may sequester medications for use in a suicide attempt.

The highly impulsive client may require closer observation even while in a protected environment. Nursing personnel may need to remain in close proximity of the client or even keep him in direct view. Nurses should not hesitate to employ environmental supports, such as a quiet room, to provide safety for the client. Explain the purpose of the support to the client in brief, direct sentences. Inform the client that you are concerned for his safety and will help him control his impulses to harm himself.

Verbalize Concern and Offer Help. While providing environmental support to the client, the nurse uses interpersonal techniques to decrease his sense of isolation. Verbal contact with the client every 1 to 2 hours reinforces the nurse's interest and concern. Realistic reassurances can be offered to him, such as informing him that the suicidal crisis will pass, and that the staff will work with him to help him resist the suicidal urge.

Conversation with the client should address his healthy, functional parts. This focus may include activities of daily living, such as his self-care, eating, and dressing. It is wise to avoid extensive discussion and exploration of the reasons for the suicidal behavior until the client's risk of suicide has decreased.

The severe isolation of the high-risk suicide client can be combatted by regular, frequent contact with consistent personnel. Nurses and other psychiatric staff must approach the client; he will not actively seek out the staff. The number of staff working with the client should be limited to the lowest necessary number. The nurse should inform the client when she will be available to him, how often she will make contact, and how to notify the nurse if he desires contact.

Establish a "No Suicide" Contract. The nurse establishes a "no suicide contract" with the client at moderate to low risk of suicide.[28] In this contract, the client repeats to the nurse a statement that he will not accidentally or on purpose kill himself. The "no suicide" contract specifies the length of time for which the contract is valid; it is renewed before it expires.

If a client is unable to make the "no suicide" contract, his ambivalence is evident in his attempt to alter the wording of the contract. For example, the client might say, "I will *try* not to kill myself" or "I *might* be able to keep the agreement." Insistence on the exact words of the contract promotes honesty and reinforces to the client that it is his responsibility, not the nurse's, to control the suicide impulse. If a client is unable to make a "no suicide" contract, environmental supports, such as a closed psychiatric treatment unit, may be offered. Praise should be offered for the client's ability to make and maintain the contract.

Promote Decision-Making and Autonomy. Suicidal clients are frequently preoccupied with their suicidal thoughts. Simple decisions required to carry out activities of daily living can be overwhelming and perplexing. The nurse helps the client make decisions, such as what to wear or when to bathe, thereby helping him to maintain a level of self-esteem and autonomy. Aiding the client in decision-making decreases his isolation by providing contact with a helping professional; it also maintains a sense of dignity through self-direction.

Explore Client Strengths. The suicide crisis should be viewed as a dramatic, but ineffective, means of communication. The client is trying to send others an important message. An immediate need of the client is to identify the stressors contributing to the suicide risk. Talking with the client about the stressors provides him with reassurance that his anger, despair,

Nursing Care Plan 37-1

The Suicidal Client: Moderate Risk

Nursing Diagnosis	Outcome	Intervention
Ineffective individual coping, characterized by moderate risk of suicide, related to hopelessness	Client will not act on suicide impulse	Suicide assessment each shift and as needed Document level of risk and appropriate plan on client's chart Establish a no-suicide contract with the client; renew the contract each shift and as needed Establish a support plan with client (*e.g.*, have client check in with and speak to nurse every half-hour) The primary nurse is to explore client's feelings and motives regarding suicide once a day If suicide risk increases, implement a high-risk plan and inform involved psychiatric–mental health staff
	Client will maintain activities of daily living and social interaction	Assist client with decision-making by pointing out options and supporting his decision Make a written activity schedule with client for a 2-to-4-hour period Focus the client's discussion on events and activities of the day; explore the client's satisfactions and disappointments Encourage the client to attend unit activities and meals (accomplished through verbal discussion and encouragement or by accompanying the client to the activity)

and frustration are being heard. The nurse helps the client break the problem into small pieces of solvable units, see the options available to him, and make his choices. Take care to focus on the healthy, functional parts of the client—focus not only on the suicide risk of the client, but on his realistic strengths and abilities.

Clients who make or threaten suicide gestures have poorly developed coping patterns. Nursing interventions are directed toward strengthening existing coping skills or toward developing new coping strategies. This process begins by helping the client understand and accept the implications of his suicide attempt. Discussing possible substitutions of coping mechanisms for the suicide helps the client identify other ways of dealing with the stresses in his life. The nurse identifies and reinforces those effective methods of coping that the client already possesses and of which he may be unaware due to his distorted image of himself.

Protect the Client Who Is Thought-Disordered. Clients who have thought disorders have trouble organizing their thoughts and may be at risk for making impulsive, self-destructive gestures. Schizophrenic clients may use self-harmful behaviors as a means of reality-testing or in response to auditory, command hallucinations.[2,22] Assessment of the potential for suicide in such clients should include whether the client is hallucinating and the nature of the hallucinations. If the potential exists that the person may impulsively attempt suicide, the risk may be diminished by providing a safe environment and by presenting reality for the client.

Prevention and Postvention

Prevention of suicide is the primary goal of treatment. The interventions previously described are intended to prevent suicide of persons already in health care systems. Suicide prevention centers provide access into the health care system for persons considering suicide but not yet being treated.

Suicide Prevention Services. The pioneering work of the Los Angeles Suicide Prevention Center illustrated the effectiveness of crisis intervention services in helping potentially suicidal people postpone the decision to kill themselves.[21] Since the late 1950s, volunteer groups and professional clinics have established crisis services to deal with the suicidal person. These services provide anonymous telephone hotlines and limited face-to-face counseling to persons at risk of suicide. Workers in a crisis intervention service use communication skills and crisis theory to help the individuals postpone the decision to kill themselves and to obtain needed therapy.

Community members other than those providing formal crisis intervention services encounter and work with suicidal individuals. Clergy, public health nurses, and occupational health nurses all provide support and counseling to the suicidal individual. In England, The Samaritans have offered support and counsel to the suicidal person since the early 1900s.[23] This group of lay volunteers was founded by a clergyman who discovered that suicidal persons benefit from the availability of a compassionate listener.

Despite the availability of effective psychiatric and nursing care, some persons can and do kill themselves. The suicide act is an interpersonal act and touches all those significant to the client. Nursing intervention does not end with a completed suicide act; the nurse continues to work with the survivors in resolving their reactions to the suicide.

Survivors of Suicide. The term *survivor-victim* is used to describe the dual role of the survivors of suicide.[23] Those left behind in a suicide act experience anger, frustration, guilt, and ambivalence in addition to the grief associated with a death.[6] Family members describe a sense of shame and embarrassment following a suicide, accompanied by an estrangement from well-meaning relatives who do not know how to respond to the loss through suicide.

Resynthesis of Survivor-Victims. Using Resnick's model of resynthesis, the nurse guides the survivor-victims through the stages of resuscitation, rehabilitation, and renewal.[20] In the *resuscitation* stage, the first 24 hours following notification of the suicide, the nurse offers assistance with the shock of the death. Emphasis is placed on the funeral and burial as well as helping the survivor-victims to acknowledge the death of the person who committed suicide. During *rehabilitation,* the nurse uses group or individual intervention to allow the survivor-victims to mourn the death as well as to express their unique reactions to the suicide. The *renewal* phase, characterized by acceptance, is a time for helping the survivor-victims integrate the suicide experience into their lives.

Psychological Autopsy. When a client suicides, the nursing and other psychiatric–mental health staff also experience feelings of anger and guilt.[15] Frequently, a suicide elicits a sense of failure among nursing personnel. In a *psychological autopsy,* staff gather to review the client's behaviors and actual death act.[23] The psychological autopsy does not attach blame; rather, it is a process to examine what clues, if any, were missed and to learn from the evaluation of a particular situation. Following the suicide of a client by overdose, the staff of one inpatient unit met on three occasions to discuss the death and their reactions to it. Staff members verbalized feelings of frustration at their lack of power to keep the client from killing himself as well as anger at the client for "doing it to them." Examination of clues revealed that the client, a chronically depressed young man, had not established a therapeutic alliance with any of the staff on the unit. No changes in eating or sleeping patterns were observed during his hospitalization. Based on the final evaluation of this client and his behavior in the treatment facility, the staff modified the existing assessment protocol on their unit to include a verbatim report of an interaction with every potentially suicidal client during every shift.

Evaluation

Evaluation of the care of the suicidal individual includes examining the assessment, planning, and intervention phases of the nursing process.

The first goal in the care of the suicidal client is identification; that is, did the nurse correctly identify all clients at risk for suicide? Expertise in suicide assessment comes not only from following a systematic process, but also from actually performing suicide risk assessments and receiving verification from colleagues. Evaluation of the assessment process should reveal that the nurse accurately assessed the suicide risk of all persons in her care.

Evaluation of the planning and implementation of care provided for persons at risk of suicide is an ongoing process. The information gathered in the daily evaluation of nursing care plans forms the basis of the assessment of the client's suicide risk.

CHART 37-2

Therapeutic Dialogue

Assessing Suicidal Risk

Nurse: (during admission interview) Mike, I'd like to know more about why you came to the hospital.

Client: Well, after I lost my job, I just stayed around the house. The kids, you know (looking at the floor), after they go to school, I'm pretty much alone. And my wife, well, it's awful, but she's gotta work. We really need the money.

Nurse: Uh, huh. (trying to reestablish eye contact with client) You're alone most of the day, and your wife and children are busy with work and school. Sounds like you've felt lonely and a bit worthless.

Client: You don't know what it's like! (meeting nurse's eye contact) There's just no other choice. They're all caught up in their own things. They don't need me, I'm just a burden. (mournful facial expression)

Nurse: Mike, you're telling me that you feel like a "burden" and that you have no other choice. What is the choice?

Client: Well, I thought it would be better for them, and anyway, what's left for me? I'm not a man any more.

Nurse: You seem quite desperate. I wonder if you've thought of killing yourself?

Client: Uh, no, uh, well, there's the insurance but she wouldn't hear of it. She's the one that called the doctor. I just don't know. (twisting wedding ring on his finger)

Nurse: (slowly and softly) Sometimes, when a person's life seems worthless and hopeless, he sees suicide as a reasonable choice.

Client: Yeah—I know. (hesitates) I had those pills from my wife's operation and the kids were at school. I would've been alone, and I could've slept.

Nurse: Let me make sure I understand you— you've been thinking about killing yourself and had a plan. Is that right?

Client: Well, yeah, but she came home for her purse and saw the pills out and started yelling. I wasn't really sure—I still don't know. Then she made me come here.

Nurse: How are you feeling now that you're here?

Client: I guess it's okay. She really is right.

Nurse: Do you still have thoughts of killing yourself?

Client: I don't know. Sometimes. I don't know.

Nurse: I'm sure the past few weeks have been rough for you. For now, I want to work with you to keep you from killing yourself, and to help you figure out what you want to do to make things different.

Discussion

The client in this interview displays a moderate risk of suicide. He experiences suicidal thoughts, has a specific plan of moderate lethality but low accessibility to the means or method. The client demonstrates a depressed affect with feelings of hopelessness and worthlessness. His risk of suicide is also judged as a moderate risk based upon the significant factors of job loss, role change, and loss of status. The client expresses ambivalence about dying and appears to have a supportive family structure. The fact that the client agreed to be hospitalized for psychiatric treatment suggests that he has some degree of motivation.

The nurse uses therapeutic communication techniques to establish rapport with the client and to gather assessment data. She responds to both the feelings and the content expressed by the client. The nurse directly inquires about the client's suicidal thoughts and involves him in establishing a treatment plan that will promote autonomy and provide support.

Evaluation is an inherent factor in the assessment process. The nurse examines the goal statements for appropriateness. Through evaluation based on the goals of therapy, the nurse determines whether intervention strategies should continue to promote safety, begin exploration of the precipitants to the suicide, or focus on the development of new coping strategies. Evaluation helps the psychiatric–mental health staff to identify which actions were effective in the care of the client.

Nurses participate in the evaluation of care individually when reviewing their own treatment plans and the attainment of goals. Care of the suicidal client may also be evaluated during team conferences and peer review sessions, or through "change of shift" reports and psychological autopsies.

Ethical and Legal Responsibilities

When planning care for a suicidal individual, the nurse has both legal and ethical responsibilities to the client and to the caregiving agency. The situation in which the client is encountered influences the legal responsibilities of nurses in community settings. In a personal or private relationship, the nurse's responsibilities to the suicidal individual are primarily ethical, whereas in a caregiving agency, such as a clinical facility, the nurse also has a legal responsibility to fulfill.

Nurses are legally bound to follow agency policies and procedures regarding suicide precautions, and a nurse may be found negligent for omitting or not following necessary precautionary procedures. The importance of documentation in verifying the observation of suicide precautions cannot be over-emphasized.

The law and administrative orders in most states define the legal basis of nursing care. Based on the interpretation of these laws, the nurse is responsible for making professional nursing assessments and analysis and for implementing the appropriate nursing actions in the care of the suicidal client.

Summary

All forms of self-destructive behaviors are potentially life-threatening. This chapter has focused on the assessment, planning, intervention, and evaluation of the person at risk for suicide. Some of the major points of this chapter include the following:

1. Suicide occurs as a response to life situations in an intrapersonal or interpersonal context.
2. Although some evidence suggests a biochemical basis for suicidal behavior, the most commonly held etiologic theories define suicide as the result of an interpersonal or intrapsychic crisis.
3. The suicidal person experiences feelings of ambivalence, anger, isolation, and desperation.
4. The suicide act has many meanings and serves to communicate a dramatic message to others.
5. The nurse uses the nursing process to determine the degree of suicide risk of an individual and to discover the message expressed through the suicidal behavior.
6. In assessment, the nurse examines six factors: the presence of clues to suicide, the means by

which the person sought help, the suicidal plan, the person's mental state, his support systems, and his lifestyle.

7. Nursing care is planned in conjunction with the suicidal individual and other resource personnel, including psychiatric staff and the client's significant others.
8. Nursing interventions, based on the degree of suicidal risk of the client, focus on providing safety and establishing a therapeutic alliance.
9. One goal of nursing care is to help the client express his unique message.
10. The nurse uses dyadic skills to help the client learn less destructive means to cope with stressors.
11. Nursing intervention continues after a completed suicide through postvention activities with the survivor-victims of the suicide.
12. Evaluation of nursing care is based on two questions: Were the clues identified early enough to permit intervention? Was the intervention appropriate and effective?
13. Nurses and other psychiatric–mental health care providers need opportunities to express their feelings of anger and frustration at the behaviors of suicidal clients and to work through these feelings to achieve objectivity and empathy.

References

1. Aguilera D, Messick J: Crisis Intervention, 5th ed. St Louis, CV Mosby, 1986
2. Anderson N: Suicide in Schizophrenia. Perspect Psychiatr Care 11, 106–112, 1973
3. Baechler J: Suicides. New York, Basic Books, 1979
4. Burgess AW, Baldwin B: Crisis Intervention Theory and Practice. Englewood Cliffs, NJ, Prentice Hall, 1981
5. Campbell L: Depression: Acute Care in the Hospital. Am J Nurs 1986, 288–291
6. Durkheim E: Suicide (trans). Glencoe, IL, Free Press, 1951
7. Hatton C, Valente SM: Bereavement Group for Parents who Suffered a Suicidal Loss of a Child. Suicide Life Threat Behav 11 (Fall): 114–150, 1981
8. Farberow N: Suicide. Morristown, NJ, General Learning Corporation, 1974
9. Farberow N (ed): The Many Faces of Suicide. New York, McGraw-Hill, 1980
10. Farberow N, Schneidman E (eds): The Cry for Help. New York, McGraw-Hill, 1961
11. Hankoff L: Physiochemical Correlates. In Hankoff L, Einsidler B (eds): Suicide Theory and Clinical Aspects. Littleton, MA, PSG Publishing, 1979

12. Holinger PC: Violent Deaths as a Leading Cause of Mortality: An Epidemiologic Study of Suicide, Homicide, and Accidents. Am J Psychiatry 137 (April): 472–476, 1980

13. Jourard S: Suicide: An Invitation to Die. Am J Nurs 70: 269, 1970

14. Mann JJ et al: Increased Serotonin 2 and B-adrenergic Receptor Binding in the Frontal Cortices of Suicide Victims. Arch Gen Psychiatry 43 (October): 954–959, 1986

15. Marshall K: When a Patient Commits Suicide. Suicide Life Threat Behav 10 (Spring): 23–40, 1980

16. Menninger K: Man Against Himself. New York, Harcourt, Brace and World, 1938

17. Miller M: The Geography of Suicide. Psychol Rep 47, Part 1 (December): 699–702, 1980

18. Miller M: Suicide After Sixty: The Final Alternative. New York, Springer-Verlag, 1979

19. Phillips D, Lio J: The Frequency of Suicides Around Major Public Holidays: Some Surprising Findings. Suicide Life Threat Behav 10 (Spring): 41–50, 1980

20. Resnick HP: A Clinical Approach to the Survivors in a Death by Suicide. In Cain A (ed): Survivors of Suicide. Springfield, IL, Charles C Thomas, 1972

21. Resnick HP, Rubin H: Emergency Psychiatric Care (NIMH). Bowie, MD, Charles Press Publishers, 1975

22. Robins E: Psychosis and Suicide. Biol Psychiatry 21, 7, (June): 665–672, 1986

23. Schneidman E: An Overview: Personality, Motivation, and Behavior. In Hankoff L, Einsidler B (eds): Suicide Theory and Clinical Aspects. Littleton, MA, PSG Publishing, 1979

24. Schneidman E, Farberow N (eds): Clues to Suicide. New York, McGraw-Hill, 1957

25. Simmons-Alling S: New Approaches to Managing Affective Disorders. Arch Psychiatr Nurs 1, 4 (August): 219–224, 1987

26. Snyder S: Biological Aspects of Mental Disorders. New York, Oxford University Press, 1980

27. The Reliability of Suicide Statistics: A Bomb Burst. Suicide Life Threat Behav 10 (Summer): 267–269, 1980

28. Twiname BG: No Suicide Contract for Nurses. J Psychiatr Nurs Ment Health Serv 19 (July): 11–12, 1981

29. Vollen K, Watson C: Suicide in Relation to Time of Day and Day of Week. Am J Nurs 75 (Mar): 263, 1975

30. Wilson M: Suicidal Behavior: Toward an Explanation of the Differences in Female and Male Rates. Suicide Life Threat Behav 11 (Fall): 131–139, 1981

PART 8

Community Care from Crisis to Long-Term Intervention

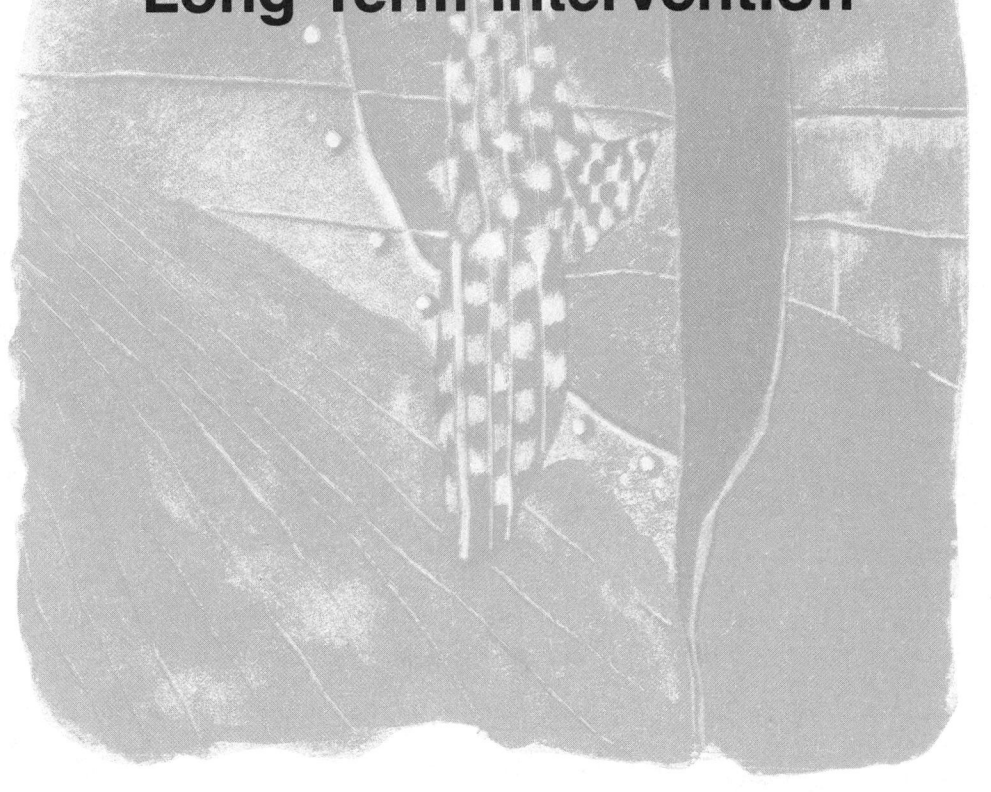

38

Community Mental Health

Marilyn Jaffe-Ruiz

A good part of the struggles of mankind center around the single task of finding an expedient accommodation—one, that is, that will bring happiness—between this claim of the individual and the cultural claims of the group; and one of the problems that touches the fate of humanity is whether such an accommodation can be reached by means of some particular form of civilization or whether the conflict is irreconcilable.

Sigmund Freud,
Civilization and Its Discontents

Chapter Preview

"Community mental health" is an idea, a philosophy, an enactment that came to fruition in 1963 with the late President John F. Kennedy's "Bold New Approach."[25] Before that time, interest in the care of mentally ill people in the community waxed and waned, depending upon the political, social, and economic climate of the times. Through the 1960s and early 1970s, the community mental health movement enjoyed momentum and prosperity, but had again waned in the late 1970s and early 1980s. By the latter part of the 1980s, concern for the homeless and the homeless mentally ill prompted renewed interest. Although enthusiasm and political support for community mental health have diminished, many important principles of care can be applied to an evolving form of psychiatric–mental health treatment in which nurses can, and do, play an important role.

This chapter will present a brief history of community mental health—its current determinants and parameters—and provide a look at the existing trends as well as a forecast for the future. The role of the nurse in community-focused mental health care delivery is essential for providing comprehensive mental health services.

Learning Objectives

Upon completion of this chapter, you should be able to accomplish the following:

1. define community mental health
2. describe the philosophy upon which community mental health is based
3. identify five essential services of the community mental health care delivery system
4. differentiate among primary, secondary, and tertiary prevention in community mental health nursing
5. analyze various factors that influence trends in community mental health
6. describe the role of the nurse in community mental health

Defining Community Mental Health

Community mental health is best defined both philosophically and operationally. The phrase *community mental health* describes a change in focus of psychiatric–mental health care from the individual to the individual in interaction with his environment. It also describes a place where comprehensive care is delivered; that is, outside of hospitals, in the least restrictive setting, and, it is hoped, at home or as close as possible to where the client lives. Community mental health is "all activities undertaken in the community in the name of mental health."[9]

Additionally, community mental health focuses on an assessment of the community—its populations, stressors, and strengths. Mental health problems are seen not only as residing within an individual whom it would be advantageous to treat in a noninstitutional setting, but as residing within specified groups as well. To accomplish treatment for these groups, the Community Mental Health Centers Act of 1963 identified five components of service, which have become almost synonymous with community mental health. These five components of community mental health care are as follows:

1. Inpatient services
2. Outpatient services
3. Partial hospitalization
4. Emergency services
5. Consultation and education

Primary, Secondary, and Tertiary Prevention

The treatment focus incorporates public health precepts of prevention of occurrence (or primary prevention), early case finding and prompt intervention (or secondary prevention), rehabilitation (or tertiary prevention), and mechanisms for continuity of care.

On a community level, prevention is geared to individuals and to larger specialized populations. For example, early childhood–parent education programs, infant stimulation programs, and early socialization play groups attempt to effect *primary prevention* of mental disorders. Although these programs would be valuable for most families, they are considered especially preventive in those families where there are more apparent risk factors (*e.g.*, in families with pregnant teenagers, homeless families).

Secondary prevention is provided by crisis intervention services, including hot lines, walk-in services, brief psychotherapy, and hospitalization when necessary. Consumer education groups and self-help groups also play a role in providing support to individuals and families during periods of increased stress or exacerbation of symptoms of mental disorders. Psychoactive medications are also therapeutic measures of secondary prevention.

Rehabilitation, or *tertiary prevention*, and continuity of care need to be available to all socioeconomic groups in the way of family supports, home services, residential placements, and halfway houses. Liaison workers, reliable friends, family members, or sponsors need to be helped to negotiate complex systems of care and to advocate for the client. Short-term and long-term hospitalization may be necessary for certain clients and should be available as a part of the mental health service delivery system.

Changes in the focus of mental health care during recent years also brought about a belief that the patient (frequently now called the client) should be an active participant in his care and should be a co-partner in his treatment planning. The mental health worker does not have to be a doctor or a trained professional, but could be an indigenous worker who would be knowledgeable and responsive to the community members and who could also, therefore, gain employment.[9] The ambiguity in the definition of mental health worker is similar to the ambiguity in the definition of client. There is a need to differentiate the individual who responds to stress with recognizable mental illness, the one who responds with a milder stress state, and the one who is chronically ill.

Philosophical Bases of Community Mental Health

Today, there is an important new philosophical premise of community mental health: a shift from the belief that all mental illness is intrapsychic and amenable to psychoanalytic treatment to a belief that whole populations may need psychiatric treatment. The interaction of man and his environment, rather than his early psychological struggles, is viewed as the cause of emotional disorders. Societal stressors are seen as contributing to, if not causing, a person's ills.

Another premise of community mental health is the belief that mental health services should be available to all who need them regardless of personal characteristics, such as age, ability to pay, or place of residence. Individual freedom, long-term relationships in small groups, and community organization are valued activities and qualities that have been incorporated into the community mental health movement.[38] There has been a change from the biologic or medical model to a biopsychosocial model, encompassing services from all of the health and social science disciplines.

Service delivery to clients has been modified to include the elimination of long-term custodial care and the exploration of new avenues for treatment in free-standing community mental health centers, in treatment units of general hospitals, and, more recently, literally in the streets, where teams of mental health workers deliver treatment to the homeless in need.[18] Nurses and other mental health professionals have become increasingly involved in the assessment and treatment of social ills. Mental health workers have undertaken involvement in tenant advocacy, legal issues, and school problems, as well as traditional psychological issues.

Community mental health has tried to be all things to all people, perhaps to its detriment. Now, however, is the time for mental health professionals to determine how they can best provide comprehensive services to those in need.

History and Influences on Community Mental Health

The community mental health movement has been hailed as a revolution in psychiatry, with the shift of care from individuals in institutions to populations in the community. This change in the focus of care, or movement, may be viewed as having the same magnitude of impact as that of Phillippe Pinel removing the chains from mental patients and Sigmund Freud introducting psychodynamic concepts.[32]

Advances in psychopharmacology have played a large, but often unstated, role in community-based mental health treatment. With the advent of major tranquilizers in the early 1950s, individuals could be treated in less restrictive environments and were psychologically amenable to other treatment modalities, such as the verbal therapies of individual, group, and family therapy.

Although the Community Mental Health Centers Act of 1963 was the first piece of federal legislation aimed at large-scale funding for the building and staffing of treatment centers for the mentally ill, important events preceded this major one.[8] It is interesting to note that, before 1963, responsibility for care and treatment of the mentally ill fell to state and local governments; currently, there is a trend to return this responsibility to state and local governments. (Chart 38-1, "Historical Review of Community Mental Health," presents a brief review of these events.)

The historical overview tells a story of increasing federal responsibility for funding of mental health services through the 1970s. Mandated by the 1963 Community Mental Health Centers Act, the focus of mental health care shifted from the individual in institutions to communities organized into catchment areas of populations between 75,000 and 200,000.[8] Community mental health centers were built and staffed to provide comprehensive and continuous care with an emphasis on prevention. Minorities, children, and the elderly were identified as particular groups whose needs were incorporated into the legislation of the 1970s. Direct service gave way to indirect services that provided consultation and education to schools, religious organizations, courts, non-

CHART 38-1
Historical Review of Community Mental Health

1930s	Two Federal Narcotics Hospitals were established.
1946	Congress passed the National Mental Health Centers Act. The National Institute of Mental Health was created.
1955	Mental Health Study Act—Congress establishes the Joint Commission on Mental Illness and Mental Health.
1960	Report of the Joint Commission on Mental Illness and Mental Health, *Action for Mental Health,* was published.
1963	Report from the President on Mental Illness and Mental Retardation to Congress—stimulated Community Mental Health Centers Act. Congress passed Community Mental Health Centers Act to provide federal funding for building and staffing of Community Mental Health Centers.
1973	Joint Commission on Mental Health of Children established.
1975	Congress extends Community Mental Health Centers Act.[30]
1978	Report to the President from the President's Commission on Mental Health.[31]

(From Beigel A, Levinson A: The Community Mental Health Center: Strategies and Programs. New York, Basic Books, 1972)

psychiatric health professionals, and others in the community.

Community Mental Health and the Nursing Process

The community mental health nurse has the opportunity to work with the individual and the social system in which he lives. Stressors that impinge upon people in the human–environment interaction are often social in nature. At the same time, the human–environment interaction provides the health professional with an opportunity to supply interactions to improve a persons' coping ability.

Historically, nurses have played a key role in providing mental health services in the community by combining public health and psychiatric nursing knowledge. One study identified 22 roles nurses play in community mental health; the most frequently identified roles included therapist, co-therapist, collaborator on the interdisciplinary team, consultant, liaison, case finder, and crisis intervention worker.[32] Nurses have also begun to do research on the factors that would influence positive integration of individuals into the community.

Assessment and Nursing Diagnosis

The community mental health nurse assesses the individual and his community resources, living arrangements (including housing and significant others), job status, economic status, cultural background, and religious affiliation. Stress in any one or more of these areas may interact with a vulnerable individual to produce psychiatric–mental health problems.

The nurse's assessment of the client in the community takes in the following factors. Generally, *economic conditions* contribute to the rate of mental hospital admissions. There is a relationship between a depressed economy and increased social stress resulting in an increased number of psychiatric hospitalizations.[11] For that reason, the nurse asks the following questions: What is the current economic, social, and political climate? How is it likely to affect the client system? What additional services might need to be provided during times of financial need?

Sociocultural status often affects economic conditions of a particular client. Many minority groups in this country are disproportionately represented among the underemployed and unemployed members of our society. Additionally, many people use health care providers who are indigenous to their cultural group. In some communities, "medicine men," herbalists, and spiritualists may be front-line primary care providers. The nurse needs to be sensitive to how the health care system is viewed by the client and vice versa. Often, because of economic, cultural, or language barriers, obtaining health care has been a frustrating or discouraging experience for the client.

Transportation to a health-care agency is often a problem. How accessible is the agency to the client? Are outreach services provided? Are alternative means of transportation available? Is reimbursement provided? Transportation is of particular concern for the elderly.[20]

It is commonly agreed that, when a client has a strong *support system,* he will be better able to solve his problems effectively. Who are the important persons to the client? What are their relative states of health or illness? How involved are they able to be or willing to be? What role or roles does the client serve for them?

Many people who are mentally disturbed, especially if they are chronically ill, live in isolation. What service groups are available? Religious groups? Self-help groups?

Some clients are representatives of *populations with special needs* and communities have organized services around such people. Examples of special populations are the elderly, the young, substance abusers, and the developmentally disabled. Does this client or his family fit into any of those or other categories of individuals with special needs? If so, what resources are available for referral in his community?

The type of *living facilities* available certainly reflects how a person cares for himself. In what type of dwelling does the client live? Is it safe? Is there adequate plumbing, heating, refrigeration, and so forth? Can this person live without supervision? Are there halfway houses, group homes, or adult homes available, if necessary? How receptive is the community to the mentally ill individual?[23, 30] Services for the homeless mentally ill must include finding homes and the proper supports to assist the client in the community.

The community mental health nurse assesses both the client's needs and the services available to him. For example, if the nurse thinks a client could manage at home if he could attend a day treatment program, but there is not any day treatment program available, acute care hospitalization may be necessary.

The nurse analyzes the data gathered about the client and his life situation and determines the level of his needs. This analysis leads the nurse to identify nursing diagnoses that, in turn, prompt plans and nursing interventions.

Planning

The nurse and other members of the treatment team estimate carefully the client's needs and the community resources before beginning the planning process. Planning takes into consideration the goals the mental health care providers, the client, his family, and his significant others want to achieve. Realistic, attainable, short-term goals are imperative to reduce frustration and facilitate successful treatment outcomes.

Intervention

Community mental health intervention is planned along the public health model of primary, secondary, and tertiary prevention. The nurse may be a primary care provider by working with clients—individuals, families, or groups—to identify their needs and facilitate treatment through collaboration and referral.

Primary Preventon

Primary prevention aims at preventing illness or disorder before it occurs. To accomplish this goal, the nurse must anticipate the needs of special populations and provide counseling and other needed services; for example, to those undergoing a developmental or situational crisis. Brief, short-term, supportive services to families undergoing bereavement or experiencing other losses fall under the rubric of primary prevention. Nurses provide these services in public health as well as mental health settings by identifying and strengthening coping abilities; for instance, the nurse might foster an individual's use of intellectualization in order to mobilize his energies to find resources during a family crisis. Another nursing intervention is the development of appropriate community mental health services, such as the implementation of senior citizens' hot-lunch and drop-in programs to reduce the isolation of the elderly and meet their nutritional needs. Children of homeless families need a tremendous amount of intervention to prevent psychological, physical, social, and cultural disturbances.

Goals of primary prevention are tailored to the individual, to the entire community, or both. For example, a husband who lost a wife at a recognized disaster (*e.g.,* the collapse of a midwestern hotel) may engage in bereavement therapy. At the same time, the surrounding community may use crisis intervention groups to deal with the effect of the disaster on their lives.

Another example is that of a middle-aged male who is depressed after losing a job due to a particular industry's slowdown. The man may require individual therapy to intervene in the depression, while his family may need help adjusting to the modification of roles resulting from this loss. On a community scale, food subsidies, housing programs, and stimulation of employment may be needed to promote mental health (see Case Study 38-1, "Intervening in a Family's Crisis").

Secondary Prevention

Secondary prevention reduces prevalence through early case-finding and prompt intervention. Rapid, available, and accessible treatment and referrals to appropriate services are essential. Short-term hospitalization, intensive outpatient treatment, medication, and partial hospitalization are some of the approaches through which secondary prevention is accomplished. Nurses frequently provide this care in emergency rooms to the suicidal client, in inpatient units, and in

Case Study 38-1

Intervening in a Family's Crisis

Mr. Alan is a 45-year-old engineer in the aircraft industry. He lives with his 42-year-old wife and two daughters, Mary, age 14, and Jane, age 18.

The aircraft plant in their community has recently been shut down because of a slowdown of growth in that industry. Mr. Alan has lost his $35,000-a-year position, as have most of his neighbors.

Mrs. Alan is a homemaker. She has not worked outside the home since her older daughter was born. Prior to that time, she worked as an executive secretary. Periodically during their marriage, Mrs. Alan suffered from periods of depression, specifically after the loss of her parents and when the family moved from an urban to a more suburban environment. Each episode of depression was treated by brief psychotherapy and antidepressant medication.

This year, Jane has begun college in a neighboring state and Mary is a freshman in high school. Mary has had increasing difficulty academically. She has been truant from school and her grades have fallen from her usual As to barely passing marks. In the classroom, she seems lethargic and demonstrates a poor attention span. Because of these problems, the home-room teacher referred Mary to the school nurse.

The school nurse took a complete health history and performed a physical assessment of Mary. In the course of the interview, Mary told the nurse that she is upset and worried about her parents. She said that they have been fighting constantly since her father lost his job 1 month ago and she's worried that her mother will get "sick" again. Mary also told the nurse that she has been frightened and unable to sleep.

During their conversation, the nurse observed that Mary's speech was slurred and her reaction time slowed. The nurse asked Mary if she was using any drugs. Mary stated that since she has been unable to sleep, she has been smoking marijuana and sometimes takes "downs" a friend gave her.

The nurse realized that in order to help Mary, she would have to meet with the whole family. She told Mary that she was going to call her parents in to meet with them and Mary's teacher together.

The next day, the meeting took place. Mr. and Mrs. Alan were very concerned about the teacher's report of Mary's behavior. They, too, were upset about their home situation and were therefore not paying as much attention as usual to Mary, although they noticed and were worried about the changes in her behavior. Mrs. Alan admitted to feeling depressed and worried that she might not be able to function in a job outside her home. Mr. Alan expressed that he felt numbed by his job loss. Their financial problems are further compounded by the expenses of Jane's tuition and room and board. Also, because Mr. Alan's job is terminated, so are his health insurance benefits.

The school nurse helped the family recognize their need for help and suggested that she refer them to the community mental health center. The family seemed relieved by the suggestion and cautiously accepted the referral.

The Alan family (including Jane) visited the community mental health center 2 days later. The community mental health center nurse gathered the initial intake and assessment information. She identified the family to be in crisis precipitated by Mr. Alan's recent job loss. This loss of job has meant a loss of family income, alteration in roles with resultant marital discord, and drug abuse by the younger daughter. The older daughter, Jane, felt guilty about being away, worried, and angry about the possibility of being made to return home from college.

After the assessment and during the planning of strategies for intervention, the nurse realized that, even though the Alan family is unique, these same issues were confronting many other families in the area. The family as a whole, as well as each individual member, needed assistance.

The nurse analyzed her data and shared with the Alan family her assessment, validating their concerns and desires. She elicited their thoughts and ideas about the interventions, which she then presented to the Mental Health Center's treatment team.

Her suggestions are incorporated into Nursing Care Plan 38-1.

psychiatric and other health care clinics. The nurse intervenes by fostering a therapeutic relationship, by restructuring the environment, by bringing in services, by providing respite or halfway-house care, and by using psychopharmacological agents to strengthen the client's coping mechanisms. For the homeless, liveable and safe shelter is an imperative treatment intervention.

Tertiary Prevention

Tertiary prevention aims to reduce long-term disability through a program of rehabilitation, after care, and resocialization. Its aim is also to prevent the exacerbation of acute symptoms or a worsening of symptoms. The nurse assesses individuals' stress levels and coping behaviors and encourages them to develop new patterns of adaptive behavior and to adopt new coping skills. One goal of a client, for example, may be to learn to talk out his problems rather than attacking someone.

Deinstitutionalization of large numbers of psychiatric clients during the late 1960s and 1970s made the tertiary prevention level of care the focus of much attention by communities, politicians, and health care workers. Many communities with insufficient resources were not equipped to absorb large numbers of psychiatric clients into their neighborhoods. Additionally, the stigma attached to psychiatric illness and the possible occurrence of deviant social behavior resulting from mental disturbance make this type of disorder not acceptable to the vast majority of people. Much work remains to be done in the areas of public attitude, education, and support of communities to cope effectively with the care of people with psychiatric illness who are in the community.

The overall goal of community mental health nursing is to provide the optimum level of mental health for a community and its members. It is not sufficient to treat the individual's ills without treating the larger societal issues. It is counterproductive for a person who has been deinstitutionalized to come to a mental health clinic and receive medication, supportive psychotherapy, supplemental security income, and food stamps if he has inadequate or no housing and no meaningful work.

Nurses in community mental health assist clients, through the nursing process, by identifying needs, problems, strengths, and resources, by making referrals, by offering therapeutic support, and by encouraging the use of an effective problem-solving process. In addition, the nurse needs to work actively as an advocate toward promoting legislation for innovative approaches to preventing and caring for the mentally disturbed in our communities.

Evaluation

Legislative pressures are moving the mental health system from process to outcome evaluations. Funding, policy-setting, and clinical issues are dependent on the clarity of outcome studies. To say a client is or is not better, or that a community has mental health services adequate for its population is difficult in the absence of clear-cut criteria.[35] Identified areas for study include the following:

1. Program quality that conforms to standards
2. Values of specific treatment
3. Safety and efficacy, rather than usual and customary practice
4. Administrative structure
5. Program designs
6. Target populations of clients
7. Outcome indices, such as reduction of symptoms and vocational and social rehabilitation[35]

Unfortunately, even if ideal conditions are set up for research, little research in the social sciences shows direct cause-and-effect findings. Instead, results are likely to be descriptive and inconclusive. The ambiguities of the social systems model, though frustrating, offer the mental health practitioner an opportunity for diverse and creative practice. A shift from a single-causality to a multicausality mode of explanation of emotional disorder, which includes biologic, psychological, sociologic, and spiritual stressors, is essential for providing holistic care.

Trends Affecting Community Mental Health Care Delivery

The hopes, enthusiasm, and plentiful federal funding that characterized 1963 have diminished in the 1980s. Inflation, the state of the economy, unemployment, homelessness, high crime rates, and a conservative political climate all serve to diminish the prospects of community mental health making a significant impact in reducing the ills of the individual in this country. Nevertheless, these times may spawn some new ideals for effective community-based mental health services in which nurses may play an important therapeutic role. Much research is needed to demonstrate beneficial outcomes with cost-effective service. Preventive treatment, identification of potential at-risk populations, and diverse treatment modalities using a variety of practitioners need to be examined.

Some gains of the community mental health movement include a reduction of population and an unlocking of doors of state mental hospitals, both lit-

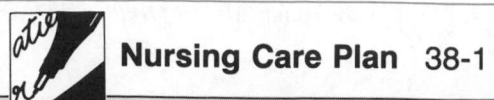

Alan Family Care Plan

	Outcomes	Intervention	Evaluation
Mr. Alan	Will grieve his loss of position and establish new employment	Participate in support group with others who have lost their jobs; vocational counseling with job placement	Mr. Alan successfully finds new employment
Mrs. Alan	Will evidence no signs of further depression	Individual, brief psychotherapy; possible medication; opportunity for job placement; support group for women re-entering job market	Mrs. Alan mourns the loss of status and is able to be flexible in assuming a new role without incapacitating depression
Mary	Will find alternative ways, besides drugs, of coping with her feelings and family events	Drug-abuse therapy program; group for adolescents	Mary is able to stop abusing drugs and is able to form positive identifications in an adolescent group
Jane	Will find alternate payment options at school; will learn to cope effectively with family crisis	Explore school work/study program or part-time job to help defray college living expenses; apply for scholarship aid; telephone availability to clinic staff with referral to college health service	Jane is able to stay at college and participate in decision-making regarding family's and her own future
Whole family	Will resolve family role and functions	Financial assistance; health-insurance provisions; food subsidy program; family therapy	Family members are able to be more flexible in roles while satisfying their individual and family needs
Community	Will assist specialized groups to maintain optimal health	Education about effects of job loss and its consequences; drug consultation and education to the schools; community action involving legislators, business people, clergy, and health professionals to prevent further community problems	Legislative programs are established to prevent social, economic, and psychological breakdown in the community

Questions for Discussion

1. Which of the five essential components of community mental health did the nurses use to intervene with the Alan family?
2. What other alternatives, based on the principles of community mental health, might the school nurse have suggested if a community mental health center was not available in the community?
3. Which of the interventions planned for the Alan family are examples of primary prevention? Which are examples of secondary prevention?
4. What are the various biopsychological stressors that contributed to the Alan family's problems?
5. How is the role of the community mental health nurse similar to, and different from, other nursing roles?
6. How do you compare the principles and philosophy of community mental health with other treatment approaches?

erally and figuratively, to operationalize the notion of treatment in the least restrictive setting; a decreased emphasis on expensive analytic therapies as a major form of psychiatric treatment; and a de-emphasis on psychiatrists as the only legitimate care providers in order to enable other professionals (*e.g.,* registered nurses, social workers, psychologists, and paraprofessionals) to play a more active role in care. Mental health care providers have broadened the scope of services available to a wider range of the population.

The plight of the homeless mentally ill has prompted a reexamination of the issues surrounding "asylum"—for those who have the need and the right to treatment yet may not be in a position to seek it voluntarily. Forced intervention raises the complementary question regarding the right of the individual to refuse treatment.

Community mental health must provide for comprehensive and continuous care, available and accessible to all members of the population. It must involve the orderly uninterrupted movement of clients among the diverse elements of the service delivery system. Strong linkages and communication networks need to be established without a duplication of efforts or negation of important components.[4]

There remains a need to develop, in a systematic way, primary prevention ranging from prenatal care to care for the elderly. Secondary prevention, acute care, and early case-finding should be available through community hospitals. Those persons with emotional disorders require services to alleviate stressors and to strengthen coping skills; these services (or tertiary care) include financial, housing, food, recreational, and social services in a homelike setting with backup services as needed.

Greater emphasis and appreciation should be given to self-help groups, transitional facilities, and respite facilities. Families of the mentally ill are better equipped to provide supportive care on a continual basis if they, too, have support services as well as a chance for separation from the disturbed family member.

It is clear that the need for mental health services will not diminish; if anything, it will increase in the future. Fifteen percent of the American population suffers from some emotional disorder, and of these 32 million people nearly 7 million do not receive any care.[34] At the same time, unfortunately, funding for mental health services is disappearing. With the shift of funding from the federal level to the state level, mental health services, including research and aid to the handicapped, are being reduced. The "Bold New Approach" of the 1960s must be evaluated and redesigned to preserve the humanistic intent of community mental health as we move toward the 21st century.

Summary

This chapter has traced the development of the community mental health movement in the United States and the current challenges facing our communities. Other points of the chapter include the following:

1. Community mental health services are designed to provide comprehensive, continuous care to populations of people who need them.
2. The aims of community mental health are the prevention of illness or disorder (primary prevention), limitation of disability (secondary prevention), and rehabilitation (tertiary care).
3. Mental health workers, professional and paraprofessional, are used in addition to psychiatrists to provide mental health care to individuals, families, and communities.
4. The shift in funding from the federal to state level has reduced mental health services and endangered the viability of community mental health.
5. The community mental health nurse applies the nursing process—assessment, nursing diagnosis, planning, intervention, and evaluation—to provide comprehensive services to clients.

References

1. Aiken L: Unmet Needs of the Chronically Mentally Ill: Will Nursing Respond? Image 19:3 (Fall): 121–125, 1987
2. Albee G: Psychiatry's Human Resources: Twenty Years Later. Hosp Community Psychiatry 30:11 (November): 783–786, 1979
3. Albee G: The Fourth Mental Health Revolution. J Prevention 1, 67–70, 1980
4. Bachrach L: Community of Care for Chronic Mental Patients: A Conceptual Analysis. Am J Psychiatr 138:11 (November): 1449–1451, 1981
5. Barton W, Sanborn C: An Assessment of the Community Mental Health Movement. Lexington, DC Heath, 1975
6. Bellak A, Mueser K: A Comprehensive Treatment Program for Schizophrenia and Chronic Mental Illness. Community Ment Health J 22, 3 (Fall): 186, 1986
7. Bellak L: A Concise Handbook of Community Psychiatry and Community Health. New York, Grune & Stratton, 1974
8. Biegel A, Levinson A: The Community Mental Health Center: Strategies and Programs. New York, Basic Books, 1972
9. Bloom B: Community Mental Health: A General Introduction. Monterey, Brooks/Cole, 1977

10. Bloom B: The Logic and Urgency of Primary Prevention. Hosp Community Psychiatry 32:12 (December): 839–843, 1981

11. Brenner MH: Mental Illness and The Economy. Hosp Community Psychiatry 26:7 (July): 451, 1975

12. Butler R: Psychiatry and the Elderly: An Overview. Am J Psychiatr 132:9 (September): 893–900, 1975

13. Caton C: The New Chronic Patient and the System of Community Care. Hosp Community Psychiatry 32:7 (July): 475–478, 1981

14. Chu F, Trotter S: The Madness Establishment. New York, Grossman, 1974

15. Cohen G: Mental Health Services and the Elderly: Needs and Options. Am J Psychiatr 133:1 (January): 65–68, 1976

16. Estroff S: Making It Crazy. Berkeley, University of California Press, 1981

17. Fagin C: Psychiatric Nursing at the Crossroads: Quo Vadis. Perspect Psychiatr Care XIX(3, 4): 79–106, 1981

18. Flaskerud J: The Effects of Culture-Compatible Intervention on the Utilization of Mental Health Services by Minority Clients. Community Ment Health J 22:2 (Summer): 127–140, 1986

19. Freud S: Civilization and Its Discontents. New York, WW Norton, 1961

20. Hagebak J, Hagebak B: Serving the Mental Health Needs of the Elderly: The Case for Removing Barriers. Community Ment Health J 16(4): 263–275, 1980

21. Hollingshead August de Belmont, Redlich F: Social Class and Mental Illness. New York, John Wiley & Sons, 1958

22. Howard L, Baker F: Ideology and Role Function of the Nurse in Community Mental Health. Nurs Res 20, 5 (September/October): 450–454, 1971

23. Johnson P, Beditz J: Community Support Systems: Scaling Community Acceptance. Community Ment Health J 17:2 (Summer): 153–160, 1981

24. Joint Commission on Mental Illness and Mental Health: Action for Mental Health. New York, Basic Books, 1961

25. Kennedy JF: Message from the President of the United States Relative to Mental Illness and Mental Retardation. House of Representatives, Document No. 58, 88th Congress, 1st Session. Reprinted in Bloom B: Community Mental Health: A General Introduction. Monterey, Brooks/Cole, 1977

26. Lamb HR, Zusman J: A New Look at Primary Prevention. Hosp Community Psychiatry 32:12 (December): 843–848, 1981

27. Lancaster J: Prospects for Mental Health in the 80's. Responding to Stress: Community Mental Health in the 80's, pp 1–9. New York, National League for Nursing, 1981

28. Laster R: Community Mental Health. J Psychiatr Nurs Ment Health Serv 15:3 (March): 19–22, 1977

29. Leiberman EJ (ed): Mental Health: the Public Health Challenge. Washington DC, American Public Health Association, 1975

30. Ozarin L: Community Alternatives to Institutional Care. Am J Psychiatr 133:1 (January): 69–72, 1976

31. President's Commission on Mental Health: Report to the President from the President's Commission on Mental Health, Vols 1 and 2. Washington DC, Government Printing Office, 1978

32. Ramshorn MT: Mental Health Services. In Haber J et al (eds): Comprehensive Psychiatric Nursing, pp 10–17. New York, McGraw-Hill, 1978

33. Report of the Task Force on Community Mental Health Programs. Am J Psychiatr 139:5 (May): 705–708, 1982

34. Reiger DA, Goldberg ID, Taube CA: The De Facto U.S. Mental Health Services System. Arch Gen Psychiatry 35 (June): 685–693, 1978

35. Schulberg H: Outcome Evaluations for the Mental Health Field. Comm Ment Health J 17:2 (Summer): 132–142, 1981

36. Weissman CM, Klerman GL: Epidemiology of Mental Disorders: Emerging Trends in the U.S. Arch Gen Psychiatry 35 (June): 705–712, 1978

37. Yolles S: The Future of Community Psychiatry. In Barton W, Sanbonn C (eds): An Assessment of the Community Mental Health Movement. Lexington, DC Heath, 1975

38. Zusman J: The Philosophic Basis for a Community and Social Psychiatry. In Barton W, Sanbonn C (eds): An Assessment of the Community Mental Health Movement. Lexington, DC Heath, 1975

39 · Psychosocial Home Care

Nina A. Klebanoff

Heidegger sees that home means more than a house and the merely casual possession of domestic things. Hestia makes a house a home by endowing it with soul. It is her gift to reveal how my dwelling serves as an outward expression of my inward self and how the image of the inmost center of a dwelling, its hearth, serves as the most adequate, the most inevitable, image of the essence of self.

Martin Heidegger
Remembrance of the Poet

Chapter Preview

Deinstitutionalization of psychiatric inpatients has not solved the problem of providing the best care for people with long-term or enduring mental illness. Home health care nursing, specifically psychosocial home health care nursing practice, is a service that strives to meet the challenge of providing accessible and equitable care to persons in need.

Home health care is an aspect of home care. Home health care nursing provides skilled nursing care, usually on an intermittent—that is, visiting—basis, where people usually live. Psychosocial home care nursing practice is a focused component of home health care. "Psychosocial" is used in this chapter to indicate an approach that is complementary to but distinct from the medical, or disease, model of mental health and mental illness. "Psycho," from the Greek *psyche* signifies the human mental, behavioral, and emotional structure—mind, soul, consciousness, or spirit. "Social" signifies the individual client, his family, the community in which they reside, and their relationship to, and interaction with, humanity or society in general. For reasons that will be discussed below, many clients in the community must receive health care services in their homes, or prefer to do so.

This chapter will further define home health care and psychosocial home health care nursing practice. This discussion will include an overview of the historical, philosophical, and theoretical foundations of psychosocial home health care nursing. The role of the nurse in the provision of psychosocial home health care will be covered. Selected issues, as well as trends, will be explored.

Learning Objectives

Upon completion of this chapter, you should be able to accomplish the following:

1. define home health care nursing and identify the need for psychosocial home health care nursing
2. describe the historical, philosophical, and theoretical foundations upon which psychosocial home health care nursing practice is based
3. identify the essential components of psychosocial home health care nursing practice
4. discuss the appropriate candidates for referral to psychosocial home health care nursing service
5. differentiate among the role aspects and functions of the psychosocial home health care nurse
6. discuss the attitudes and feelings of the psychosocial home health care nurse
7. apply the nursing process to the care of a client and family in their home
8. analyze various factors that influence trends in psychosocial home health care
9. explore the relationships among psychosocial home health care nursing, community or public health, and community mental health

Defining Psychosocial Home Care

Home care is one part of a comprehensive health and mental health care system. It aims to provide an array of health-related services to individuals and families in their places of residence. These residences include residential care facilities, group homes, and the private homes of clients or their family members. Home health care is an aspect of community health nursing,[92] *not* an alternative to institutional care. The delivery of home health care services is one of the most rapidly growing and changing fields in health care today, even though it is one of the oldest forms of ambulatory health care in existence.

Serving Client and Family Needs

Because nurses are the major service providers of home care, they can coordinate and manage home health care effectively. Other suitable service components for home care, singly or in a multitude of combinations and sequences, include—but are not limited to—the following:

Medical services
Social work services
Psychological services
Physical therapy
Occupational therapy
Vocational therapy
Speech therapy
Recreational therapy
Respiratory therapy
Dental services
Pharmacy services
Intravenous and parenteral therapy
Enterostomal/wound therapy
Nutritional services
Homemaker/home health assistant/companion
   services
Transportation services
Laboratory services
Use of durable and disposable medical supplies and
   equipment

CHART 39-1
Sources of Payment for Home Health Care Services

Psychosocial home care services may be paid for in the following five ways:

1. Medicare, the program of the federal government, will pay for psychosocial home care services if the client has a primary psychiatric diagnosis; has been evaluated by a psychiatrist (and reevaluated every 60 days by one); and is homebound. "Homebound" status, in general, means that a client is unable to leave home either due to illness or injury (*e.g.*, physical reasons such as unsteady gait, shortness of breath after 10 feet, or a fracture) or because psychiatric illness, to some degree, makes it unsafe to leave home unsupervised, or because of a refusal to leave the place of residence.

2. Medicaid, a federally and state-funded program, is a state-administered program of reimbursement for home care services, among other functions. Each state has its own criteria for eligibility and reimbursement for psychosocial home care services.

3. Many third-party payors (private health insurance companies) follow the guidelines set forth by Medicare. Others, however, adhere to their own rules and regulations which may or may not cover psychosocial home care nursing services. With the presence, increase, and benefit of home care services, some health insurance companies are paying for home care services on a case-by-case basis.

4. Some individuals pay directly for psychosocial home care services, mainly because they do not meet the criteria for Medicare, Medicaid, or private health insurance coverage or do not have private health insurance. Yet they desire this type of service and are willing to pay for it. Some agencies or providers charge a flat rate, while others have a sliding fee scale (based on the client's ability to pay). People also may choose to pay directly for psychosocial home care services in order to continue desired services in the home beyond the period authorized by an insurance company or the government programs.

5. Some agencies and individuals have in their budgets funds to pay for home care on a charity basis for individuals in need of psychosocial home care services but for whom no funding sources exist.

Two recent articles discuss the proper planning, delivery, and documentation of home care nursing services that will help to assure that home care visits are reimbursed.[24,71]

The individual needs of the client and his family determine which services are to be arranged and coordinated in the home. In home care, the word "family" is used to mean anyone in the client's life who is able and willing to take some responsibility for helping the identified home care client.

Providing Home Health Care

Various organizational arrangements, which are discussed in greater depth in textbooks of community health nursing, administer home care services. In general, home health care services are provided in the following six ways:

1. Official or public agencies operated by state or local governments
2. Private and voluntary nonprofit agencies operated by boards of directors
3. Combinations of official and voluntary nonprofit agencies operated by both sources or a new board
4. Hospital-based agencies administered by the hospital's board of directors
5. Proprietary (for profit) agencies administered by the owner
6. Individual or group partnerships of nurses or other health professionals providing home care services on a private or charitable basis

See Chart 39-1 for the ways in which these types of service are reimbursed. Chart 39-2 identifies the various sources of home health care referral sources.

Every home care situation has greater or lesser psychosocial aspects. Home care services are customized for each client, depending on his needs or problems as well as the needs of the home health care provider and the reimburser. Because of the psychosocial and wellness orientation of community health nursing, a psychiatric nurse working in this setting is

C H A R T   39-2
Referral Sources for the Psychosocial Home Health Care Nurse

Hospital Discharge Planners
Nurses
Physicians
Social Workers
Clients
Former Clients
Family Members
Landlords, Neighbors
Health Departments
Police and Fire Departments
Community Agencies
Interdisciplinary Staffings

more aptly titled a psychosocial than a psychiatric nurse.

Goals of Psychosocial Home Health Care

The two goals of home health care are to gain, regain, maintain, or restore the client's optimum state of health and independence, and to minimize and rehabilitate the effects of illness and disability either before or after institutionalization.

Specific goals of psychosocial home care nursing are to prevent hospitalization and to provide the least restrictive alternative for treatment. For example, a client might be able to go to his own home following discharge from a psychiatric hospitalization, rather than to a nursing home or the home of a family member, because of the availability of psychosocial home care services.

Psychosocial home care nursing can help relieve or resolve psychological and social problems facing clients and their families when the clients return home; an example is care following a hospitalization for depression. Medicare outlays for home health care increased 21.1% between 1984 and 1985, and more than 1.6 million Medicare recipients received home health care services during that period.[64] It is likely that the need and demand for psychosocial home care nursing services will continue to increase because of the following factors:

Most people prefer to remain in their homes and to be as independent as possible
Psychiatric inpatients have been deinstitutionalized to an increasing degree
Home care cases are increasingly complex

Consumers increasingly expect holistic care, which includes the psychological, social, spiritual, and environmental or ecological realms, in addition to the physical factors of health care
Home care in general is cost-effective[51]

The Psychosocial Clinical Nurse Specialist

Fig. 39-1, "Role Aspects of the Psychosocial Clinical Nurse Specialist in Home Care," outlines the components of the three roles of psychosocial nurses in home care. A Psychosocial Clinical Nurse Specialist (PCNS) is defined as follows:

> The Psychosocial Clinical Nurse Specialist is a master's-prepared nurse with psychiatric and mental health assessment and intervention skills who is eligible for, or has already received, the American Nurses' Association certification as a specialist in adult psychiatric and mental health nursing.[51]

It is generally agreed that, as minimal preparation, a nurse should possess a baccalaureate degree in nursing to function as a generalist nurse in community health or home health care. A specialist is prepared to provide advanced practitioner skills as a clinician, administrator, teacher, or researcher. It is recommended that psychosocial home care services be provided by a master's-prepared and certified nurse. The American Nurses' Association Standards pertaining to home health care nursing practice differentiate the roles and functions of the generalist and the specialist nurse, as well as their educational requirements.[7] By definition, the specialist is also able to operate as a generalist. The nature of the administration of home health care services, client needs, provider needs and preferences, the home care setting, and home care problems will determine who provides psychosocial home care nursing services and how. This chapter will cover only the home care of adults. There are also, however, specialized home care services for infants and children.

Historical, Philosophical, and Theoretical Foundations

A conceptual model of home health care takes into account cultural, historical, professional, economic, political, philosophical, social, pharmacological, technological, and ecological factors. The exploration of all of those aspects is either covered elsewhere in this text or beyond its scope. However, this section explores three elements critical to understanding psychosocial home care nursing. They are its historical

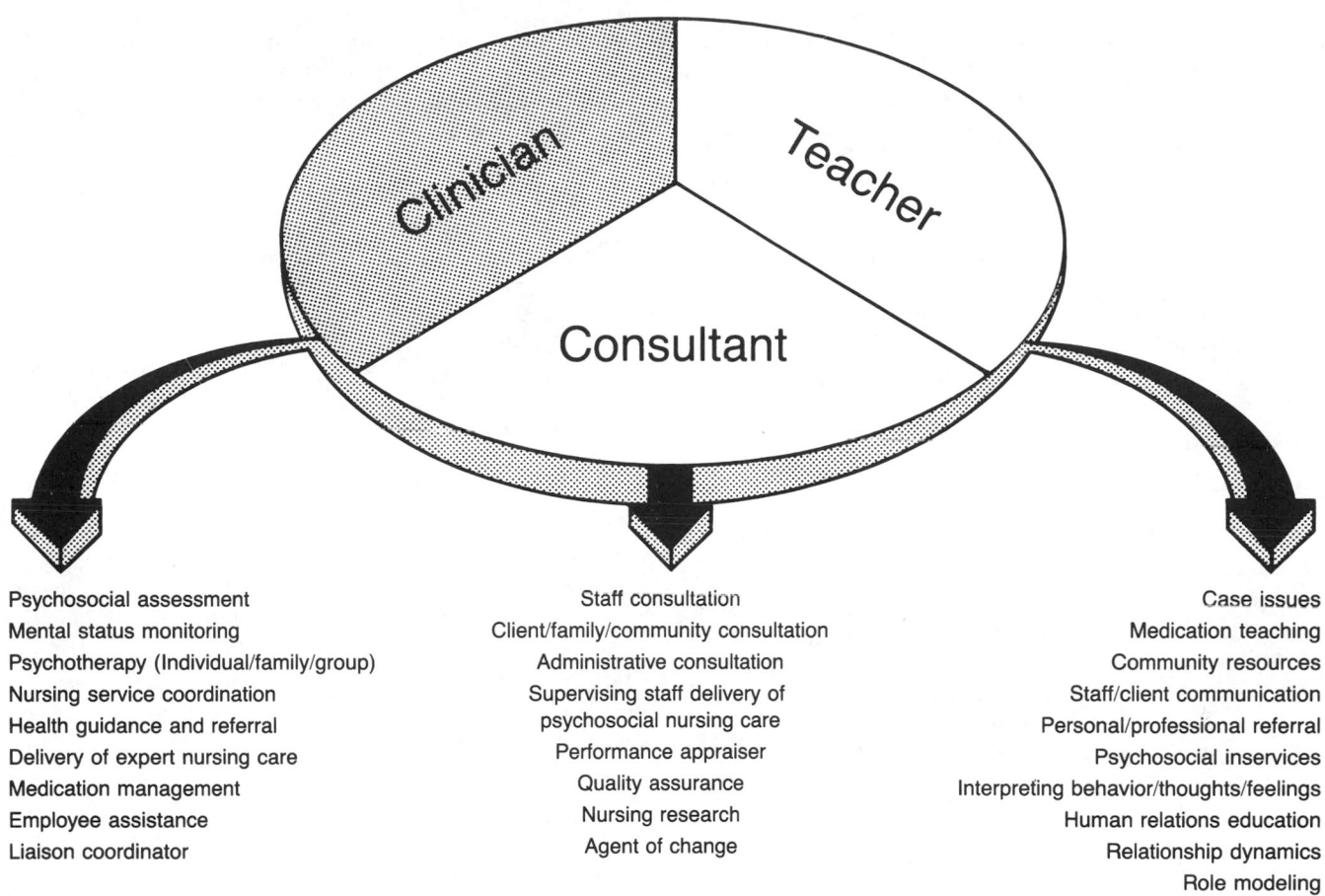

Clinician	Consultant	Teacher
Psychosocial assessment	Staff consultation	Case issues
Mental status monitoring	Client/family/community consultation	Medication teaching
Psychotherapy (Individual/family/group)	Administrative consultation	Community resources
Nursing service coordination	Supervising staff delivery of	Staff/client communication
Health guidance and referral	psychosocial nursing care	Personal/professional referral
Delivery of expert nursing care	Performance appraiser	Psychosocial inservices
Medication management	Quality assurance	Interpreting behavior/thoughts/feelings
Employee assistance	Nursing research	Human relations education
Liaison coordinator	Agent of change	Relationship dynamics
		Role modeling

Figure 39-1. *Role aspects of the psychosocial clinical nurse specialist in home care.*

Reprinted with permission from Home Healthcare Nurse, Vol. 4, No. 6, 1986. (Hospital Publications, Inc.) Klebanoff NA, Casler CB: The Psychosocial Clinical Nurse Specialist: An Untapped Resource for Home Care. Home Healthcare Nurse 4:37, 1986.

underpinnings, its philosophical foundations, and the theoretical bases that are particular to it. Stanhope's and Lancaster's text on community health nursing provides a comprehensive treatment of the history of public health nursing and general home health care.[92]

The 1983 report of the Joint Commission of Mental Illness and Health sped the process of supporting mental clients in society through the deinstitutionalization of mental inpatients and a focus on community care instead of hospital-based care.[47] Home care had been delivered in the United States as early as the 1950s.[100] These approaches were patterned after one that was delivered in Amsterdam, Holland.[79] In the late 1960s and early 1970s, during the height of the community mental health movement, efforts were directed toward providing home care for the mentally ill, especially the elderly mentally ill.[100] Since the late 1970s, the literature has contained accounts of psychiatric or psychosocial home care nursing in the United States and other countries. References can be found at the end of this chapter.

In addition to the philosophical bases of community mental health and community health/public health nursing, which psychosocial home care nursing shares and overlaps, there are philosophical assumptions that are particular to home care nursing in general and to psychosocial home care nursing in particular.

Principles of Psychosocial Home Care

In general, most home care agencies subscribe to a common set of basic principles and share a common philosophy.[94] These beliefs are as follows:

As long as it is medically, socially, and economically possible, adults want to remain in their own homes and communities and should be permitted to do so

Clients who need long-term care often present many overlapping challenges and problems

The whole individual must be considered

Services must be coordinated and integrated

Cost-effective care requires direct payment at the level of program delivery

Quality long-term care is affordable

Additionally, the following premises guide the clinical approach of the psychosocial home care nurse and a psychosocial specialty team:

Client care is maximized when integrated into a comprehensive care plan that takes into account the client and family and their environment, self-concept, functioning level, coping mechanisms, stressors, and sociocultural perspective

An individual's or a family's reaction to an alteration in mental health status, mental disability, or mental illness is often influenced by whether the condition is permanent, temporary, degenerative, or unknown

Care of a client is based on the idea of therapeutic use of self, the setting and attaining of goals for health status enhancement, and the development of the client's ability to develop his own resources within a realistic level of functioning

Eclectic Approach

The biopsychosocial model interacts with theories from adaptation, behaviorism, systems, cognitive therapy, community mental health, communications, crisis intervention, family therapy, developmental perspectives, self-care, interpersonal, social learning, and nursing models, as well as from other theoretical models discussed elsewhere in this textbook, to provide fertile ground for an individual approach to psychosocial home care. Usually, the psychosocial home care nurse will employ a blended or eclectic approach to meet the needs of home care clients.

Application of the Nursing Process to Psychosocial Home Care Nursing

The psychosocial home care nurse has the unique privilege of working with the client and the family on their own turf, as psychosocial home care nursing services are delivered in the place of residence. But the nurse must remember that the home is part of a larger community and social system, and that the provision of home care services involves many different disciplines and services. It is very important to note also that cultural influences will play a large part in the planning and delivery of psychosocial home care nursing services. Some cultural differences that are pertinent to home care are identified in Chart 39-3, "Cultural Factors Influencing Psychosocial Home Care Nursing Practice."

C H A R T 39-3
Cultural Factors Influencing Psychosocial Home Health Care Nursing Practice

The following cultural factors should be assessed in each psychosocial home health care situation:

1. Family structure
2. Race and ethnic origin
3. Countries lived in
4. Dietary habits and nutritional variables
5. Religious and spiritual practices
6. Ways of communicating, use of language
7. Use and appreciation of art, music, drama, etc. in the home
8. Dress and clothing habits
9. Health and mental health behavior, beliefs, patterns
10. Illness and mental illness behavior, beliefs, patterns
11. Healing beliefs and practices
12. Influence of external beliefs
13. Perceptions of health care providers
14. Other family beliefs, values, customs, rituals, and behaviors about health and mental health, illness and mental illness, disease, health and mental health care providers, and health and mental health care systems
15. Available cultural and ethnic institutions
16. Risk factors, vulnerabilities, or resistances

Community health nursing textbooks invariably contain helpful family assessment guides that include cultural and ethnic variables to be considered.

Chapter 6 in this book, "Sociocultural Aspects of Care," gives specific information about various cultural groups.

CHART 39-4
ANA Standards of Home Health Nursing Practice

Standard I. Organization of Home Health Services

All home health services are planned, organized, and directed by a master's-prepared professional nurse with experience in community health and administration.

Standard II. Theory

The nurse applies theoretical concepts as a basis for decisions in practice.

Standard III. Data Collection

The nurse continuously collects and records data that are comprehensive, accurate, and systematic.

Standard IV. Diagnosis

The nurse uses health assessment data to determine nursing diagnoses.

Standard V. Planning

The nurse develops care plans that establish goals. The care plan is based on nursing diagnoses and incorporates therapeutic, preventive, and rehabilitative nursing actions.

Standard VI. Intervention

The nurse, guided by the care plan, intervenes to provide comfort, to restore, improve, and promote health, to prevent complications and sequelae of illness, and to effect rehabilitation.

Standard VII. Evaluation

The nurse continually evaluates the client's and family's responses to interventions in order to determine progress toward goal attainment and to revise the data base, nursing diagnoses, and plan of care.

Standard VIII. Continuity of Care

The nurse is responsible for the client's appropriate and uninterrupted care along the health care continuum, and therefore uses discharge planning, case management, and coordination of community resources.

Standard IX. Interdisciplinary Collaboration

The nurse initiates and maintains a liaison relationship with all appropriate health care providers to assure that all efforts effectively complement one another.

Standard X. Professional Development

The nurse assumes responsibility for professional development and contributes to the professional growth of others.

Standard XI. Research

The nurse participates in research activities that contribute to the profession's continuing development of knowledge of home health care.

Standard XII. Ethics

The nurse uses the code for nurses established by the American Nurses' Association as a guide for ethical decision-making in practice.

Psychosociocultural Assessment

Indications for Care

Critical indicators of the need for psychosocial home care include the following:[51]

Mental health status changes
Health status changes
Changes in material welfare
Changes in the home environment
Family changes
Changes in social support network
Changes in psychosocial functioning
Changes in motivation
Need for health/medication teaching
Need for anticipatory guidance

Psychiatric crisis or emergency
Changes in leisure or diversionary time interest/
   activity

Standards of Care

The psychosocial home care nurse assesses the individual and the family, as well as available personal and community resources. This is in keeping with the Standards of Home Health Nursing Practice (see Chart 39-4). These standards have been developed by the American Nurses' Association (ANA) Task Force to Develop Standards of Nursing Practice for Home Health Care, under the direction of the Executive Committee of the Council of Community Health Nurses.[17] See also the ANA Standards of Community

C H A R T   39-5
National Associations and Organizations Concerned with Home Health Care

American Hospital Association
Division of Ambulatory and Home Care
  Services
840 North Lake Shore Drive
Chicago, IL 60611
(312) 280-6000

American Association for Continuing Care
1101 Connecticut Avenue, N.W.
Washington, DC 20036
(202) 857-1194

American Federation of Home Health Agencies
1320 Fenwick Lane, Suite 500
Silver Spring, MD 20910
(301) 588-1454

American Nurses' Association
2420 Pershing Road
Kansas City, MO 64108
(816) 233-2428

Council of Community Health Services
National League for Nursing
10 Columbus Circle
New York, NY 10019
(212) 582-1022

Home Health Services and Staffing Association
2101 L Street, N.W.
Washington, DC 20037
(202) 547-7424

National Association of Home Care
205 C Street, N.E.
Washington, DC 20002
(202) 547-7424

National Homecaring Council
67 Irving Place
New York, NY 10003
(212) 674-4990

Health Nursing Practice and the ANA Standards of Psychiatric and Mental Health Nursing Practice.[5,6]

The legal necessity of documenting all nursing activities in the home supports the use of the nursing process as guided by the Standards of Home Health Nursing Practice. Additionally, most states have enacted legislation that details the rights of populations receiving care at home, especially the elderly. National associations (see Chart 39-5, "National Associations and Organizations Concerned with Home Care") have printed materials outlining the rights of people receiving care in their homes.

In accordance with Standard III, Data Collection, the nurse continuously collects and records data that are comprehensive, accurate, and systematic. Information that is asssessed prior to discharge from a health care facility, during the initial home care visit, and during all subsequent visits will guide the formulation of a nursing diagnosis, the planning of interventions based on sound scientific and theoretical foundations (Standard II, Theory), and the evaluation of nursing care. Data collection for assessment purposes includes the following in conjunction with Standard III:

1. Physical, emotional, intellectual, psychological, social, cultural, religious, spiritual, community, and environmental history; support systems; lifestyle factors; and stressors

2. Client's and family's growth and development, dynamics, perceptions, vulnerabilities, risk factors, and current and past coping strengths or mechanisms

3. Sleep, rest, and activity patterns; appetite and nutritional–metabolic patterns; elimination patterns; other patterns and habits affecting health, knowledge, and motivation

4. Self- and role-relationship enactments and patterns, including sexuality–reproductive patterns

5. Mental and emotional status, including thought processes, perceptual patterns, and cognitive functioning

6. Understanding of and receptivity to home care, expectations of the psychosocial home care program

Objective and subjective data are collected, in a standardized, succinct, and systematic manner, regarding the psychosocial indicators for home care, resources, and parameters for assessment. Many sources are available from which to collect these data.

CHART 39-6
Client/Family and Environment Checklist

This checklist is a guide to be modified as needed depending upon the client and circumstances.

Family:
Members in the Home:
    Name(s):
    Age:
    Sex:
    Ethnicity:
    Family position (*e.g.,* mother):
    Status (*e.g.,* single):
Extended Family Members:
    Name(s):
    Place of residence:
    Frequency and length of contact:
Educational Level Attained:

Vocational Interests:

Hobbies and Other Interests:

Occupation and Job Satisfaction:

Financial Resources:
    Sources:
    Total income:
    Adequacy of income to meet needs:
Religious/Spiritual Practices:
    Preferences:
    Involvement:
    Importance:
    Rituals:
Recreational Interests:
    Around home:
    Outside home:
    With whom:

Residence:
    Type of housing:
    Number of rooms:
    Condition in general:
    Furnishings:
    Privacy:
    Sleeping arrangements:
    Adequacy of bathroom facilities:
    Adequacy of food preparation (*e.g.,* cooking, cleanliness, refrigeration)
    Adequacy of:
        Water supply/source:
        Waste/garbage disposal:
        Lighting:
        Heating/cooling ventilation:
        Laundry facilities:
        Telephone:
Safety provisions:
    Smoke alarms:
    Crime prevention:
    Emergency telephone numbers:
Safety hazards:
    Noise level:
    Crowding:
    Storage of medicines/cleaners/ poisons:
    Tools out:
    Unsafe toys:
    Loose rugs/clutter:
    Swimming pools:
    Fire dangers:
    Air Pollution:
    Traffic flow:
Condition of yard:
    In general:
    Pets:
    Automobiles:

(Adapted from Stanhope M, and Lancaster J, Community Health Nursing: Process and Practice for Promoting Health. St. Louis: CV Mosby Co., 1984)

Methods of Data-Gathering

A client and his family member(s) or other significant people (*e.g.,* neighbors or a rabbi) are the primary sources for assessment data through history-taking, interviewing, physical assessment, mental status examination, and reporting that various diagnostic and psychological tests were performed. The nurse will need objective, independent verification of information gathered in the home. The home environment itself provides valuable assessment information.

(Chart 39-6 "Client/Family and Environment Checklist" provides a guide for assessing a residence.)

Various flow sheets and forms of nursing progress notes are available for use in data collection in home health care and psychosocial home health care nursing. Usually, the agency offering the home health care services provides these forms for the nurse's use.

As data are collected and organized, nursing diagnoses relative to the mutually identified problems

C H A R T   39-7
Summary of Client/Family Health Assessment

Demographic profile:

Environment—strengths and problems regarding home, neighborhood, and community:

Structure, process, functions–strengths and limitations, existing and/or potential problems:

Coping profile:
    Conflict management—strengths and limitations:
    Life changes—strengths and limitations regarding coping with changes:
    Support Systems—strengths and limitations:
    Life satisfaction profile:

Health behavior profile:
    Health history—existing and/or potential problems:
    Health status—existing and/or potential problems:
    Activities of daily living—strengths and limitations/problems:
    Risk profile—for family unit and family members:
    Health beliefs—profile of values, attitudes, and beliefs regarding health and illness:
    Self-care—strengths and limitations:
    Health care resources—adequacy, availability, accessibility, attractiveness, use, general practices:
    Community health nursing services—attitudes and expectations:

Stanhope M and Lancaster J: Community Health Nursing: Process and Practice for Promoting Health, p. 891. St. Louis: CV Mosby Co, 1984

---

are formulated. The nurse includes the client and his family in the nursing process, for they are integral to the planning, implementation, and evaluation of home care services. Also, during the assessment phase, once the necessity for and acceptance of home care have been established, the nurse determines the resources, equipment, and disciplines that will be needed in the home and initiates referrals for them.

Nursing Diagnosis

The data-collection during the psychosociocultural assessment—subjective verbal data, objective non-verbal data, symptoms, signs, etiology, risk factors, and critical indicators—ends the assessment phase of the nursing process and begins the decision-making process: formulating a nursing diagnosis.

Standard IV, Diagnosis, of the Standards for Home Health Nursing Practice addresses this phase. Prioritizing the nursing diagnosis(es) starts with identifying actual health problems or needs requiring immediate attention. The nurse also notes potential problems that can be altogether prevented or can be dealt with quickly if they become actual problems. (See Chart 39-8, "Nursing Diagnoses and Actual or Potential Client/Family Health Problems or Needs." While many of these client conditions, health problems, or needs may be encountered in any number of other settings, they are the ones most likely to be en-

countered in the home health care setting.) Because of the added complexity of home care, it is likely that clients will have more than one nursing diagnosis.

Planning

Goal-Setting

Nursing diagnoses give the psychosocial home health care nurse needed information which can be used to formulate short- and long-term goals with the client and the family. Some examples of short-term goals in psychosocial home care are the following:

The client/family will participate in the home physical therapy program three times for at least 10 minutes in each 24-hour period

The client will not attempt to harm himself in any way until the psychosocial home care nurse returns within 24 hours

The client/family will identify in writing at least five factors that lead to anxious feelings within 48 hours of the client's admission to home care services

Short-term goals are usually immediate, realistic steps that are to be taken in order for long-term goals to be met. The time perspective in home care is longer than that of an acute care psychiatric hospital. For example, at the onset of home care services, the nurse may visit daily, which would facilitate setting 24-hour goals,

CHART   39-8
Nursing Diagnoses and Actual or Potential Client/Family Health Problems or Needs

Anger
Anxiety: mild, moderate, severe, panic
Body image, alteration in
Chemical dependency: alcohol, drugs, prescriptives
Cognition, impairment in
Comfort/pain, alteration in
Communication process, impairment in
Coping mechanisms, impairment in individual/family
Denial
Depression: mild, moderate severe
Developmental level, delay in
Environmental conditions, altered
Family dysfunction, impairment in dynamics, structure, support systems
Fears
Grieving: anticipatory, normal bereavement, maladaptive
Health management, impairment/emotional response to illness/disease
Hospice care

Independence/dependence, altered/delayed
Knowledge, impairment in
Medication: reactions, interactions, responses
Nutrition, impairment in
Parenting, impairment in
Perception, impairment in
Psychosomatic/psychophysiological/psycho-biological states
Rape/incest trauma
Role patterns, alteration in
Self-concept, impairment in
Self-esteem, impairment in
Sensory perception, impairment in
Sexuality, impairment in
Sleep/rest/activity patterns, alteration in
Socialization, impairment in
Spiritual integrity, alteration in
Stress reaction
Therapeutic regimen, response to
Translocation syndrome
Values/beliefs conflict
Violence, actual or potential

(From Gordon M: Nursing Diagnosis—Process and Application. New York, McGraw-Hill, 1982. In Klebanoff NA, Casler CB: The Psychosocial Clinical Nurse Specialist: An Untapped Resource for Home Care. Home Healthcare Nurse, 4, 38, 1986. Adapted with permission of Hospital Publications, Inc.)

whereas if home visits are made weekly, biweekly, or monthly, the client/family and the nurse will couch their goal statements in longer time frames. Because home care services are currently provided on an episodic, intermittent basis, very long-term or enduring goals will usually not be met for months or years after discharge from psychosocial home care services. A few examples of long-term goals appropriate for the psychosocial home care setting are as follows:

The client will perform relaxation exercises for at least 15 minutes daily for the next 6 months
The client/family will attend monthly Alliance for Mental Illness support group meetings
The client will reestablish and maintain sexual activity at the level specified prior to the onset of depression

Client/Family Outcomes
Some general outcomes are expected in psychosocial home care nursing. Two such outcomes are the maximization of the client's level of independence through health promotion, maintenance, and restora-

tion, and the prevention of complications in the home (and the concomitant lessening of the effects of psychiatric illness and disability) through health teaching, education about psychoactive medication, and the sharing of information about community resources. Anticipating a psychiatric crisis and creating plans to avert or minimize it can often prevent a visit to an emergency room or a hospitalization. Psychosocial home care nursing can also facilitate the transition to home after hospitalization (or vice versa, often lessening the amount of time spent in the hospital). This adds to the overall continuity of care for the psychosocial or psychiatric–mental health client and his family members. The provision of home-based care may delay admission to a nursing home or other long-term care facility.

Other long-term outcomes that can result from psychosocial home care services are the ability of the client to maintain ties with the family network and community and his ability to maintain a greater sense of control by helping to determine his own health, mental health, or mental illness care needs. Home and community assessment contributes to effective, efficient, and appropriate discharge planning. Psychosocial home care nursing contributes invaluable insight to the client, the family, and other team members; this insight influences the overall plan of care, support, and follow-up.

The nursing care plan written for use in psychosocial home care nursing practice outlines the specific actions that will be taken by the nurse, the client, and the family unit to achieve the mutually agreed-upon goals and outcomes to the identified needs or problems.

Intervention

The psychosocial home care client's specific goals and outcomes lead to individual interventions in the home. Interpersonal, intellectual, and technical skills are used during this phase of the nursing process, which is addressed by Standard V, Intervention.[7] Direct interventions that are used in the home by the psychosocial home care nurse include the following:

Comprehensive in-home assessment
Crisis intervention
Medication administration, monitoring, and teaching about responses, indications, actions, and interactions
Individual, couple, family, and group counseling and psychotherapy
Health guidance and referral
Client advocacy
Case management activities
Mental, emotional, physical, and spiritual observation, interpretation, and evaluation
Health care team coordination
Liaison activities
Reporting to physician about client response to home environment, medication responses, medical follow-up, new signs and symptoms relative to the client's status
Supervision of team members (*e.g.*, home health assistant)
Role-modeling/social skills education
Teaching about
    Diet/special diet
    Disease/illness
    Management of illness
    Stress reduction
    Risk factors
    Safety measures/accident prevention
    Management of activities of daily living
    Emergency measures
    Positive coping behaviors
    Administration of treatments, medications
    Rehabilitative exercises, when indicated
    Community resources to help attain state of

optimal functioning, client well-being, and psychosocial rehabilitation

The process of making verbal or written contracts with clients, a behavioral approach that is used in other health care settings, can easily be adapted to the psychosocial home care setting.

Much of what is taught to clients in the home is not documented because it is thought of as advice or common knowledge. But most of what nurses share with and teach to clients and their families is based on sound theory, knowledge, and experience gained through a professional nursing education and career. Learning outcomes help guide teaching, which can be documented. In home care, anything that is done to assist the client in reaching his highest level of wellness, to improve functioning, or to manage illness in a safe and healthy way, is teaching.

The nurse who works in the home care setting also intervenes in indirect ways. Indirect home care includes the nurse's actions that affect the home care situation but do not involve personal contact with the client or family.

Telephone or one-to-one consultation with another home care team member or member of a hospital or emergency room staff is an instance of indirect care. The psychosocial home care nurse may be called upon to provide an in-service for the home care agency staff or a community group, another example of indirect care. Participation in agency orientations, team conferences, discharge planning meetings, and recertification sessions are other examples of the indirect functions and interventions of the psychosocial home care nurse. Most indirect functions in the home care arena, including client and legislative or political advocacy, improve the continuity and coordination of services for the best use of resources and services toward the end of providing optimal client care and recovery.

Thus, psychosocial nursing interventions take place prior to the initial home visit, during home visits, and after home visits have been made. The client and family are the ones who are to follow through with the plans for recovery and improvement in the home and are, therefore, active participants in home care. The nurse intervenes to help the client return to an optimal level of health and functioning. The client, the family, and the psychosocial nurse continually evaluate the status of the client throughout the course of psychosocial home care.

Evaluation

Standard VII, Evaluation, reads as follows: "The nurse continually evaluates the client's and family's responses to interventions in order to determine

C H A R T   39-9
Crisis Home Care Visits

A major challenge in community mental health and psychosocial home health and illness care is providing emergency or crisis services in a timely and humane way. Developing and implementing a crisis-oriented psychosocial home care service is one way to meet this need. Often clients are in crisis at home and are unable or unwilling to be transported to a mental health center or psychiatric emergency room.

Crisis team approaches are described in the psychosocial/psychiatric nursing and medical literature.[15–17,34,36,38,52,54,102] The crisis-oriented team is made up of a psychiatrist, psychosocial or psychiatric nurse(s), and sometimes a combination of other mental health professionals, such as a mental health worker, social worker, or psychologist. Two members usually are able to manage the in-home crisis, if one is a pre-scribing physician (should the need for medications be present). Some programs recommend that a psychosocial home crisis team go into the home during the crisis; others are concerned with the provision of alternative family home sites. This involves removing the client in crisis from his setting and temporarily placing him in the home of a community family instead of admitting him to a psychiatric hospital. Difficult issues include finding and training suitable families, the availability of providers, transportation, telephone screening, other physical problems of the clients, and safety. Psychosocial crisis-oriented home care services can provide an effective and cost-efficient way to manage people in crisis in the community, either in their own homes or the homes of alternative families.

progress toward goal attainment and to revise the data base, nursing diagnoses, and plan of care."[7]

Plans for discharge from home care services are made early in the span of home care, ideally during the initial visit. This helps the client reach measurable, customized goals. The nurse and the client/family determine whether the goals for home care have been met. In home care, the needs and status of clients often change. This necessitates a dynamic and continual revision of, and addition to, the data base, nursing care plan, and interventions. Chart audits, reviews by regulatory agencies, peer reviews, and the various home health agency certification processes also provide ways to evaluate the quality and effectiveness of home care services.

All of those involved in the home care case—client, family, nurse, other home health care team members, physician, and others—evaluate the client's progress toward and attainment of goals. As the client and family become increasingly able to care for the client, the nurse and other home health team members decrease the intensity and frequency of their visits. Discharge from home care services includes the making of provisions for aftercare, if indicated, and other types of case management and coordination of community resources (see Standard VIII, Continuity of Care).

Other Considerations

As in any health care setting, safety factors are of utmost importance. Safety hazards to be noted and fixed or improved during the provision of psychosocial home care nursing include the following:

Structural integrity
Heating, cooling, ventilation
Stairways and ramps
Storage of dangerous objects and fluids
Storage of medications
Mats and throw rugs
Gas and electrical appliances
Number of people per square footage
Cooking and bathing facilities
Nature of neighborhood
Sanitation

Problems with safety measures often occur because of an additional stressor found in psychosocial home care situations—the issue of financial constraints. As listed in Chart 39-1, there are five sources of payment for home health care services.

Two related practices in home nursing care overlap psychosocial home health care. They are hospice care and care of the person living with AIDS (acquired immune deficiency syndrome). Many excellent texts and articles cover the realm of hospice care, which is also discussed in Chapter 44 of this book. Many psychosocial issues enter into nursing care of a person with AIDS related complex (ARC), person with AIDS (PWA), or a person living with AIDS.

Although a person with AIDS may be hospitalized repeatedly, most persons living with AIDS are taken care of in their residences. We now know that the virus thought to be responsible for the manifestation of AIDS, human immunodeficiency virus (HIV), attacks the central nervous system, leading to many neurological and psychological problems. A full and broad range of symptoms is associated with a diagnosis of AIDS or ARC. Anxiety and depression are the most common psychological responses to these diagnoses. Most people with AIDS are likely to experience some neurological involvement, often in the form of encephalopathy, which initially resembles depression. Not all persons with AIDS will develop neurological involvement; in those who do, such involvement may occur at any point in the course of the illness. *AIDS dementia* begins with forgetfulness and diminished concentration. These are followed by psychomotor retardation, decreased alertness, apathy, withdrawal, lessened interest in work and usual activities, and loss of libido. Some persons living with AIDS later develop utter confusion, disorientation, hallucinations, seizures, mutism, profound dementia, and finally coma leading to death.[65] Menenberg discusses the accompanying behavioral patterns and psychological changes, as well as the measures that can be taken to cope with and adjust to living with AIDS.[60]

A full range of services and caregivers is required to care for a person with AIDS in the home. Local lesbian and gay organizations, volunteer agencies, and church groups furnish "buddy" programs and a cadre of other people who can greatly enhance the professional and family care delivered to the person living with AIDS at home. Because most care given to persons with AIDS takes place in the home, articles and books on the subject written by nurses and other health and mental health care professionals are available; their number is expected to increase.

Nurses' Attitudes and Feelings

Although one study found that psychiatric nurses were more likely to be well received in the homes of clients and families than other mental health professionals and workers (*e.g.*, psychiatrists, psychiatric social workers, mental health therapists, psychology interns, and chemical dependency counselors), psychosocial nurses still have a range of feelings and attitudes related to providing home health care services.[87] Certain characteristics or traits are helpful for the performance of this nursing role and function. According to Burgess, these are as follows:

Being a self-starter
Possessing good physical assessment skills
Having superb clinical judgment
Having the ability to communicate effectively with clients, family members, other health team members, and others in the community
Practicing efficient organizational skills
Using well-honed time management techniques
Having the ability to prioritize one's work
Being able to function independently, with minimal supervision
Having a good and growing working knowledge of community, state, and national resources and referral sources[19]

Additionally, it is helpful if the psychosocial home care nurse is comfortable in a variety of settings with a diversity of home and family arrangements. This ensures that responses to vast differences are accepted and do not compromise or prevent the nurse's acknowledgement of the intrinsic dignity, worth, and value of clients and their significant others. Finally, a nurse working in this arena must be able to explain health care benefits to clients and their families and to feel comfortable discussing financial arrangements with responsible parties. Discussing financial arrangements, and in some instances collecting fees, can lead to anxious feelings in a nurse who is not accustomed to these matters.

Unfortunately, however, home health care nurses are isolated from one another, from other health care professionals, from their supervisors, and from a shared work setting. For these reasons, the home health care nurse is susceptible to frustration, resentment, sadness, and fear. Additionally, home health care nursing requires an unusually large amount of paperwork and necessary documentation that must be completed within stringent time spans; this adds to the potential for "burnout."

Two other main features of home care can be viewed as disadvantages. The first is the considerable overlapping of professional and personal boundaries in this realm, which can lead to a myriad of feelings on the part of the psychosocial home care nurse. The second is the fact that the psychosocial home care nurse may not have as much privacy and control over the environment in the home as is found in an institutional setting. Many families who receive home care have multiple problems, and the psychosocial home care nurse may experience a sense of helplessness, sadness, or anger in attempting to provide comprehensive care in a limited time with less-than-ideal resources.

On the other hand, home health care nurses enjoy a high level of responsibility, autonomy, decision-making, direct access to clients and families, the satisfaction of working collaboratively with other interdisciplinary health team members, the opportunity to work as a client advocate, primarily weekday hours, and some measure of control over their schedules, which allows them to complete work at home. The psychosocial home care nurse is able to observe and work with people on their own "turf," where clients are perhaps more likely to share information with the nurse; and the psychosocial nurse can "see" the obvious and subtle details that influence a client's optimal functioning. Another advantage of home care is that it is often more economical and cost-effective than institutional care. This appeals to the many psychosocial nurses who want to "work with" clients and their families, as opposed to "doing to" them. Last, in keeping with the notion of giving care in the least restrictive setting possible, home is often the first choice if the appropriate supports are in place.

An awareness and processing of your own emotional and physical feelings is of utmost importance if you decide to practice in the psychosocial home health care nursing arena. Psychosocial home health care nurses need support. Meetings with interdisciplinary team members provide a time for all to share their thoughts and feelings and to gain support from each other—also to share successes and the rewards of this kind of work. Conferences with peers or supervisors can also serve this purpose. To continue to meet the challenge of this aspect of our complex health care system, the psychosocial nurse must rest and rejuvenate often. It is also important for the nurse to reflect upon the positive aspects of providing psychosocial home health care; this requires some regular recreation and distance from the career.

Trends Affecting the Provision of Psychosocial Home Health Care Nursing

The future of psychosocial home health care nursing practice in the United States will be affected by the incidence of mental illness, by demographics, and by legislative and political trends. The same factors that diminish the prospects of community mental health impinge upon psychosocial home health nursing practice. Although psychosocial home health care nursing has yet to be proven cost-effective, general home health care services have been demonstrated to be cost-effective. Studies must document the benefits and effects of psychosocial home health care nursing. Currently, studies are being conducted to determine whether psychosocial home health care nursing reduces recidivism among clients.[56] Research is also concerned with collecting data about the average length of service and the interventions and nursing diagnoses that are used in providing psychosocial home health care nursing.

Approximately 2 to 5 million people with long-term or enduring mental illness live in the United

CHART   39-10
The First Home Visit

A psychosocial nurse often experiences a moderate level of anxiety and anticipation during the first home visit. Subsequent visits to the same home are much more comfortable, but each time the nurse visits a home, some excitement and anxiety are bound to arise. Usually, these feelings lessen with experience. The nurse's level of anxiety can be diminished or heightened by the amount or type of information the nurse receives prior to, or in arranging for, the first home care visit. Burgess discusses obtaining pre–initial visit data as a way to decrease the nurse's anxiety and gives case examples, as well as useful information about preparing for initial visits, obtaining entrance into the home, and personal safety.[19]

States, and most of them live in their communities. Long-term services, though not of a custodial nature, are needed to support this population in the home. However, most home care services are reimbursed on a short-term or intermittent basis. Legislation to authorize long-term home care services has been proposed but remains to be enacted. Bills permitting directly reimbursable community nursing services, including home health care, are also in various stages of the federal legislative process.

Respite care for family members of clients who live at home is needed to prevent hospitalization, institutionalization, caretaker burnout, client abuse, and overload. This is an important need that the psychosocial home health care nurse can advocate in the community and in the legislative process.

The impending implementation of diagnostic related groups (DRGs) in both the psychiatric institutional setting and the home health care realm will pose many challenges to the administration and delivery of psychosocial home health care nursing services.

Our elderly population is growing at a dramatic rate. Alzheimer's disease affects 5 to 10% of the population over 65 years of age and increases proportionally in the over-85 group. Maintaining a person affected by an organic brain disorder in the home, or facilitating his transfer to a temporary or permanent facility, is often a function of the psychosocial home health care nurse. In the future, this nursing role will become more and more common. Women and elderly people from minority groups are especially susceptible to mental health and mental illness problems

(Text continues on p. 759)

Case Studies/Nursing Care Plans 39-1

Psychosocial Home Care Case Studies

Two client populations are appropriate for referral for psychosocial home care nursing services. They are as follows:

1. Clients and families who demonstrate actual or potential nursing diagnoses and client/family conditions suitable for psychosocial home care. This includes psychoactive medication management for clients who are newly diagnosed with, or have exacerbations of, psychiatric (medical) disorders
2. Clients with new or exacerbated nursing or medical diagnoses (not of a psychosocial, psychiatric, or mental illness/health nature) complicated by the presence of factors described in item 1 above

The most common specific population groups to be served include the elderly, people with problems in living, people with psychosocial responses to their health conditions (especially after accidents or with long-term physical problems such as COPD and cancers), and people with long-term or enduring mental illness. An example from each of the two main client populations and selected aspects of their psychosocial nursing care plans follow.

Ms. B.

Ms. B. is a 76-year-old black female with no previous history of psychosocial or psychiatric difficulties. However, a neighbor reported to her nephew that she had seen Ms. B. frequently talking out loud to herself and crawling under her house, staying in the crawlspace for up to 2

hours, shortly after Ms. B's spouse suffered a massive and fatal heart attack in their home of 52 years. The nephew called a nurse friend and was referred to a home health care agency. The admitting nurse and the nephew agreed to meet at Ms. B's home after he had obtained permission from his aunt to do so.

The admitting nurse referred Ms. B to the psychosocial nurse after the initial assessment detected that the client had altered thoughts (probably delusions and possibly hallucinations) and was not sleeping or eating. Ms. B. refused to leave her home, but the psychosocial nurse learned that the client had a great deal of respect for the physician who had treated her husband for diabetes mellitus and cardiovascular problems. Together the nephew, the psychosocial nurse, and the physician were able to assist Ms. B. in resolving this crisis in her life through reality-testing, family and social support, and regulation of her sleeping and eating patterns.

For 2 weeks, until a sister from a neighboring state was able to come and stay with Ms. B, a home health assistant provided personal care, prepared meals, and changed linens. The nurse visited three times a week for 2 weeks and maintained telephone contact with the nephew, who agreed to spend nights at his aunt's home. Thereafter, the nurse visited twice a week for 3 weeks in order to teach the sister how to care for and monitor Ms. B. Prior to discharge from home care services, the nurse visited Ms. B. once a week for 1 week and then two more times every other week. The nephew paid for those visits that were not covered by Medicare.

Nursing Care Plan: Ms. B.

Nursing Diagnosis	Client Outcome	Intervention
Grieving, maladaptive or dysfunctional with alterations in thought processes, sleep patterns, and impairment in nutrition	Ms. B. will identify verbally and symbolically the loss (death) of spouse during each home care visit Ms. B. will verbalize her feelings regarding the death of spouse during each home care visit Ms. B. will discuss her response to assistance from her nephew, sister, nurse and physician Ms. B. will verbalize an under-	Encourage Ms. B. to express her feelings about the loss of spouse in whatever way she is most comfortable (*e.g.*, talking, crying, drawing, reminiscing) Spend at least 15 minutes during each home visit allowing Ms. B. to express her feelings Assess and monitor thought processes via observation, interaction, and reports from significant others

Nursing Diagnosis	Client Outcome	Intervention
	standing of the grief process	Assess for potential for harm to self, others
	Ms. B. will seek out additional support systems (*e.g.,* church, social clubs, neighbors)	Assess for evaluation of psychoactive medication treatment
	Ms. B. will experience the grieving process with other members of her family and on her own	Explore the meaning of Ms. B's retreat into the crawl space under the house for clues to help her resolve her grief
	Ms. B. will begin to resolve any unresolved thoughts and feelings about her marriage and spouse	Assist Ms. B. in making realistic plans and goals for the present and the future
	Ms. B. will begin to make plans for the future	Instruct family members to promote as much independence and self-care as possible on the part of Ms. B.
	Ms. B. will identify the factors that hinder her sleep	Encourage Ms. B. to make use of available support systems
	Ms. B. will sleep 7 hours a night (the number of hours she was sleeping 1 year ago)	Educate Ms. B. and her family members about existing support groups in the community
	Ms. B. will lose no more weight	Refer Ms. B. to an appropriate mental health professional for follow-up care when she is able to leave her home
	Ms. B. will consume a minimum of 1000 calories per day for the first 2 weeks of home health care services	Provide opportunities for Ms. B. to talk about the factors that keep her from eating
	Ms. B. will consume 2000 calories per day by the time she is discharged from home care service	Observe and record Ms. B's caloric and fluid intake
	Ms. B. will verbalize an understanding of the emotional and psychological factors that interfere with her eating	Monitor bowel and bladder patterns
		Assess knowledge base about nutrition
		Encourage high-protein, highcaloric snacks between meals
		Weigh and record weight every other day at same time of day
		Instruct about sleep aids and hindrances
		Promote regular, daily activity/ rest patterns
		Promote regular, daily diversional activities
		Monitor and instruct about regulation of sleep patterns
		Educate about relaxation methods and techniques
		Assist in the creation or re-creation of a bedtime ritual

(Continues on p. 758)

Mr. J.

Mr. J. is a 34-year-old white male who has a history of bipolar disorder, which has been treated in the past with lithium carbonate and intermittent hospitalizations. Hospitalizations have occurred roughly every 2 years since Mr. J. was first diagnosed as having "manic-depressive illness" in his early 20s. Recently his spouse filed for divorce and he became suicidal. They have no children and have been married for 7 years.

Mr. J. was hospitalized following an automobile accident in which he sustained multiple internal injuries and a broken left leg. He had stopped taking the lithium before his accident; during the hospitalization he was given phenothiazines. Shortly before his discharge, he was again started on lithium carbonate. His spouse moved out of their condominium while he was in the hospital, but she agreed to assist with his care at home until he was able to be more independent. A hospital-based social worker made the referral to a home care agency that had a psychosocial clinical nurse specialist on staff.

After the initial visit, the nurse made a referral for a physical therapist to provide services in the home. The nurse visited three times the first week following discharge from the hospital to monitor his potential for harm to himself, his response and adherence to the lithium therapy, the status of his broken leg, supportive psychotherapy, referral to community resources, and instruction to and support of his spouse regarding all aspects of his care in the home.

As Mr. J. became more independent, nursing visits were decreased to twice a week for 2 weeks, followed by once a week for 2 weeks for a total of nine visits. Physical therapy was provided for help with activities of daily living, gait training, safe transfers, electrical stimulation, and strengthening. His serum lithium levels were monitored weekly for the first 4 weeks of home care nursing services and again at the end of the span of care. During the course of psychosocial home care nursing, Mr. J's spouse began to attend support group meetings held by the local chapter of the Depressive and Manic Depressive Association.

Nursing Care Plan: Mr. J.

Nursing Diagnosis	Client Outcome	Intervention
Violence, potential for harm to self	Will discuss feelings that precipitated the suicidal feelings, for at least 15 minutes during the first four home visits and as needed thereafter Will call the 24-hour suicide and crisis telephone hotline as needed Will seek ongoing follow-up with a mental health professional Will formulate and act on ways to reduce personal, relationship, and environmental stress	In the home and on the telephone, approach and interact with Mr. J. and spouse in a nonjudgmental, caring, warm manner Listen carefully to what client verbalizes and demonstrate understanding of his views Continually assess risk for harm to self or others Assess home environment for dangerous objects and weapons and have them removed from the home, at least temporarily Suggest to the physician limiting the amount of medication prescribed at any one time Contract a no-suicide agreement verbally and in written form Instruct spouse and other home health team members to notify the psychosocial nurse and/or physician of indications of suicidal ideation and/or intent Make appropriate referrals to mental health professionals in the community

Nursing Diagnosis	Client Outcome	Intervention
		Provide short-term individual psychotherapy
		Provide short-term couples therapy with Mr. J. and spouse
		Provide Mr. J. and spouse with telephone numbers and other information about community resources and information (*e.g.*, 24-hour telephone hotlines, support groups, community organizations, crisis centers, clinical nurse specialists, psychologists, social workers, psychiatrists, clergy)
		Assist Mr. J. in mobilizing his coping skills and resolving or reducing personal, relationship, and environmental stress
		Formulate an emergency or crisis plan; hospitalize if necessary

and will increasingly need attention in terms of psychosocial home health care. Improving coping methods and strengthening family care bonds will help to meet this burgeoning demand.

The American Nurses' Association identifies societal and political forces that influence and shape the delivery of home health care nursing services.[7] The societal forces include the following:

1. The rate of living older Americans is increasing disproportionately to the total population
2. Traditionally, women have provided health care for youth and aging parents; more than half of all adult women now must work or choose to work outside the home and are therefore not available to care for family members
3. The traditional support system of the extended family has been almost eliminated by the increasing mobility of society and the ever-increasing rate of single-parent family units and female heads of households

Governmental responses to societal demands, changes, and spending trends have changed health care financing patterns. Political forces identified by the ANA that influence the provision of home health care services include the following:

1. Increased private third-party payment and government-financed health care programs, beginning in the 1960s, have promoted an increase in the demand for and use of health care services
2. Shorter hospital stays with earlier discharges of more acutely ill clients from institutions have called attention to the need for home health care services; these shorter hospital stays have been prompted by prospective, diagnosis-related, and managed health care plans[7]

Summary

This chapter has discussed home health care in general and psychosocial home health care nursing practice in particular. Some of the major points of the chapter include the following:

1. Home health care nursing and psychosocial home health care nursing are aspects of community health nursing and the community health movement.
2. Psychosocial home health care nursing is *not* an alternative to institutional care; the reverse is the case.

3. The goals of psychosocial home health care are to assist the client/family to gain, regain, maintain, or restore the optimum state of health and independence; to minimize and rehabilitate the effects of illness and disability either before or after institutionalization; and to prevent institutionalization altogether when possible.

4. The nursing process is used by the psychosocial home health care nurse to provide comprehensive services to clients in their places of residence.

5. Various social, legislative, and political forces make it likely that the need and demand for psychosocial home health care services will continue to increase.

References

1. Abrogast RC, Scratton JM, Krick JP: The Family as Patient: Preliminary Experience with a Recorded Assessment Schema. J Fam Prac 7: 1151, 1978

2. Ahmed M: The Process of Establishing a Collaborative Program Between a Mental Health Center and a Public Health Nursing Division: A Case Study. Am J Nursing 64 (9): 880–885, 1974

3. American Association of Retired Persons: A Handbook About Care in the Home. Long Beach, CA, American Association of Retired Persons, 1982

4. American Medical Association: Physician Guide to Home Health Care. Monroe, WI, American Medical Association, 1979.

5. American Nurses' Association: Standards of Community Health Nursing Practice. Kansas City, MO, American Nurses' Association, 1973

6. American Nurses' Association: Standards of Psychiatric and Mental Health Nursing Practice. Kansas City, MO, American Nurses' Association, 1982

7. American Nurses' Association: Standards of Home Health Nursing Practice, Kansas City, MO, American Nurses' Association, 1986

8. American Nurses' Association. ANA Addresses Physician Reimbursement. Capitol Update 4, 1, 5, 1986

9. American Psychiatric Association. Diagnostic and Statistical Manual of Mental Disorders, 3d ed, rev. Washington, DC, American Psychiatric Association, 1987

10. Baer ED: A Philosophical Argument Supporting Primary Care Nursing. In Mezey MD, McGivern DD (eds): Nurses, Nurse Practitioners: The Evaluation of Primary Care, pp 15–28. Boston, Little, Brown, 1986

11. Beck CF, Rawlins RP, Williams SR (eds): Mental Health–Psychiatric Nursing: A Holistic Life-Cycle Approach. St. Louis, CV Mosby, 1984

12. Bennet JA: Nurses Talk About the Challenge of AIDS. Am J Nursing (September) 9: 1148–1155, 1987

13. Betts VT, Gale MN, Gibson JM: Ethical and Legal Issues. In Critchley DL, Maurin JT (eds): The Clinical Specialist in Psychiatric Mental Health Nursing: Theory, Research and Practice, pp 453–473. New York, John Wiley & Sons, 1985

14. Briscoe M: Identification of Emotional Problems in Postpartum Women by Health Visitors. Br Med J (Clin Res) 10, 292 (May): 1245–1247, 1986

15. Britton JG, Mattson-Melcher DM: The Crisis Home: Sheltering Patients in Emotional Crisis. J Psychosocial Nursing Ment Health Serv 23:12 (December): 18–23, 1985

16. Brook B: Community Families: An Alternative to Psychiatric Hospital Intensive Care. Hosp Comm Psychiatry 3, 195–197, 1976

17. Brook B: Community Families: A Seven-Year Perspective. J Comm Psychology 8, 147–151, 1980

18. Burgess AW: Psychiatric Nursing in the Hospital and the Community, 3d ed. Englewood Cliffs, NJ, 1981

19. Burgess W, Ragland EC: Community Health Nursing Philosophy, Process, Practice. Norwalk, CT, Appleton-Century-Crofts, 1983

20. Callender M, LaVor J: Home Health Care: Development, Problems, and Potential. Washington, DC, Office of the Assistant Secretary for Planning and Evaluation, Social Services and Human Development, HEW, 1975

21. Chenoweth B, Spencer B: Dementia: The Experience of Family Caregivers. Gerontologist 26 (3): 260–266, 1986

22. Critchley DL, Maurin JT: Psychiatric Mental Health Nursing Perspectives. In Critchley DL, Maurin JT (eds): The Clinical Specialist in Psychiatric Mental Health Nursing: Theory, Research and Practice, pp 514–521. New York, John Wiley & Sons, 1985

23. Cunningham B: Nursing Assessment of Depression in the Aged Adult. Home Health Care Nurse 2 (4): 9–16, 1984

24. Daubert E: Strategic Planning in Home Care. Am J Nursing 9 (September): 1161–1163, 1987

25. DiCicco-Bloom B, Space S, Zahourek R: The Homebound Alcoholic. Am J Nursing 86 (2): 167–169, 1986

26. Edison C: Family Assessment Guidelines. In Hymovich D, Barnard MU (eds): Family Health Care, 2nd ed, p 1. New York, McGraw-Hill, 1979

27. Fagin C: Family Centered Nursing in Community Psychiatry. Philadelphia, FA Davis, 1970

28. Fenton FR, Tessier L, Siruening EL, Smith FA, Benoit C: Home and Hospital Psychiatric Treatment. Pittsburgh, University of Pittsburgh Press, 1982

29. Fitting M, Rabins P, Lucal MJ, Eastham J: Caregivers for Dementia Patients: A Comparison of Husbands and Wives. Gerontologist 26:3 (June): 248–252, 1986

30. Flitterman M, Fulmer B: The Alzheimer Caregiver: Prisoner of Love. Calif Nurse 82:6 (July–August): 3, 1986

31. George LK, Gwyther LP: Caregiver Well-being: A

Multidimensional Examination of Family Caregivers of Demented Adults. Gerontologist 26:3 (June): 253–259, 1986

32. Gilleard CJ: Family Attitudes to Caring for the Elderly Mentally Infirm at Home. Fam Pract 3:1 (March): 31–36, 1986

33. Godchaux SM: The Challenge of Chronicity. In Critchley DL, Maurin JT (eds): The Clinical Specialist in Psychiatric Mental Health Nursing: Theory, Research and Practice, pp 406–425. New York, John Wiley & Sons, 1985

34. Greenblatt M, Chien CP: Depression in the Elderly: Use of External Support Systems. In Breslau LD, Haug MR (eds): Depression and Aging Causes, Care, and Consequences, pp 193–207. New York, Springer Publishing Co, 1983

35. Hall AD, Baud WR, Elliston EB: Comparing Staff Attitudes and Patient Satisfactions in a Home Health Agency. Home Health Rev 4:1 (June): 4–11, 1982

36. Halloran T, Huggins M: A Five-year Directional Statement and Plan for Mental Health Services for the Adult Chronically and Seriously Ill. Hennepin County, MN, Mental Health Division, Department of Community Services, 1980

37. Harris M, Solomon K: A Study of Client Acceptance of Various Professionals in Psychiatric Home Visits. Hosp Comm Psychiatry 28 (9): 661, 1977

38. Hatch C, Schut L: Description of a Crisis-oriented Psychiatric Home Visiting Service. J Psychiatric Nursing 18 (4): 31–35, 1980

39. Health Care Financing Administration: Conditions of Participation for Home Health Agencies, subpart I, section 405.1229, evaluation. Washington, DC, DHHS, 1982

40. Health Care Financing Administration: Conditions of Participation, subpart I, reg 8, section 405.1201. Washington, DC, DHHS, 1982

41. Health Care Financing Administration: Health Care Financing Review, Vol II, No 2, Washington, DC, HCFA office of Research, Demonstration, and Statistics

42. Hildebrandt DE, Davis JM: Home Visits: A Method of Reducing the Pre-Intake Dropout Rate. J Psychiatr Nurs Ment Health Serv 13:5 (September–October): 43–44, 1975

43. Hirschfeld M: Homecare versus Institutionalization: Family Caregiving and Senile Brain Disease. Int J Nursing Studies 20 (1): 23–32, 1983

44. Home Health Care Team—Randomized Trial of a New Team Approach to Home Care. National Center for Health Services Research, Grant #HS03030, 1982

45. Home Health Services: Commerce Clearinghouse Medicare and Medicaid Guide, paragraph 1401. Washington, DC, DHHS, 1982

46. Jenkins J, Spencer F: Mental Health Nursing: Home Benefits. Nursing Times 82 (3): 15–21, 1986

47. Joint Commission on Mental Health and Mental Illness: Action for Mental Health: Final Report. New York, Basic Books, 1961. In Breslau LD, Haug MR

(eds): Depression and Aging Causes, Care, and Consequences, p 201. New York, Springer Publishing Co, 1983

48. Julavits WF: Psychiatric Home Care: An Evolving Legal Standard. Psychiatric Clinics of North America 8 (3): 577–586, 1985

49. Kerfoot K, Crowell CM: Maintaining Patients with Chronic Mental Health Conditions in the Community: A Joint Project of a College of Nursing and a Mental Health Center. J Nurs Ed 23: 269–271, 1984

50. Kivimake K: Psychiatric Home Nursing in Pohjois-Karjalassa. Saraahhoitaja (Finland) 50 (8): 18–21, 1974

51. Klebanoff N, Casler C: The Psychosocial Clinical Nurse Specialist: An Untapped Resource for Home Care. Home Healthcare Nurse 4 (6): 36–40, 1986

52. Krauss JB, Slavinsky AT: The Chronically Ill Psychiatric Patient and the Community. Boston, Blackwell Scientific Publications, 1982

53. Laben JK, McLean CP: Legal Issues and Guidelines for Nurses Who Care for the Mentally Ill. Thorofare, NJ, Slack, 1984

54. Leaman K: A Hospital Alternative for Patients in Crisis. Hosp Comm Psychiatry 38:11 (November): 1221–1223, 1987

55. Leavitt MB: Families at Risk. Boston, Little, Brown, 1982

56. Lesseig DZ: Home Care for Psych Problems. Am J Nurs 87:10 (October): 1317A–1320H, 1987

57. Levert D, Quellette P: Psychiatric Home Care. Canadian Infirmary 19 (10): 18–19, 1977

58. Marvan-Hyam J: Occupational Stress of the Home Health Nurse. Home Healthcare Nurse 4 (3): 18–21, 1986

59. Mayers M: Home Visit—Ritual or Therapy. Nurs Outlook 21 (5): 328, 1973

60. Menenberg SR: Somatopsychology and AIDS Victims. J Psychosocial Nursing and Mental Health Services 25:5 (May): 18–22, 1987

61. Medicare Regulations for the Home Health Agency. Washington, DC, DHHS, 1978

62. Munjas BA: Care of the Chronically Mentally Ill: A Continuing Challenge to Nursing. Iss Ment Health Nurs 8: 203–212, 1986

63. Naegle MA: Primary Care Concepts in the Psychiatric Nursing Role. In Mezey MD, McGivern DD (eds): Nurses, Nurse Practitioners: The Evolution of Primary Care, pp 218–235. Boston, Little, Brown, 1986

64. National Association for Home Care: 1986 Health Care Fact Sheet. Washington, DC, National Association for Home Care. 1986. In Omdahl DJ: Preventing Home Care Denials. Am J Nurs 8 (August): 1031–1033, 1987

65. National Institute of Mental Health. Coping with AIDS: Psychological and Social Considerations in Helping People with HTLV-III Infection. Rockville, MD, DHHS, 1986

66. National League for Nursing: Utilization Review—Guidelines for Home Health Agencies. New York, NLN, 1971

67. National League for Nursing: Criteria and Standards Manual for National League for Nursing/American Public Health Association Accreditation of Home Health Agencies and Community Nursing Services. New York, NLN, 1980

68. National League for Nursing: Cost and Charge for Home Care of Sick Service—1981. New York, NLN, 1981

69. Nielsen E, Nielsen N: Psychiatric Home Nurses' Cooperative Relationships and Work Environment: Psychiatric Home Nursing Creates Teamwork. Sygeplejersken 76 (42): 22–24, 1976

70. O'Brien AM, Oerlemans-Bunn M, Blanchfield JC: Nursing the AIDS Patient at Home. AIDS Patient Care 1 (1): (June): 21–24, 1987

71. Omdahl DJ: Preventing Home Care Denials. Am J Nurs 8 (August): 1031–1033, 1987

72. Orr J: Supporting the Family: Trouble and Strife. Nurs Times 82:32 (August 6–12): 32–33, 1986

73. Pai S, Nagarajaiah: Treatment of Schizophrenic Patients in Their Homes Through a Visiting Nurse—Some Issues in the Nurse's Training. Int J Nurs Stud 19:167–172, 1982

74. Pai S: Home Care for Chronic Mental Illness in Bangalore: An Experiment in the Prevention of Repeated Hospitalization. Brit J Psychiatry 147 (August): 175–179, 1985

75. Palermo E: Mental Health Consultation in a Home Care Agency. J Psychiatr Nurs 16 (9): 21–23, 1978

76. Paykel E, Mangen S, Griffith J, Burns T: Community Psychiatric Nursing for Neurotic Patients: A Controlled Trial. Br J Psychiatry 140:573–581, 1982

77. Phillips L, Rempusheski V: Caring for the Frail Elderly at Home: Toward a Theoretical Explanation of the Dynamics of Poor Quality Family Caregiving. ANS 8 (4): 62–84, 1986

78. Pownall M: Health Visiting: A Family Affair. Nurs Times 80 (43): 58–61, 1985

79. Querida A: The Shaping of Community Mental Health Care. In Breslau, LD, Haug MR (eds): Depression and Aging Causes, Care, and Consequences, p 201. New York, Springer Publishing Co, 1983

80. Richmond and Hopkins Family Coping Index (Appendix A). In Freeman RB, Heinrich J (eds): Community Health Nursing Practice, 2d ed, pp 555–565. Philadelphia, WB Saunders, 1981

81. Schipske G: Documenting Care for the Patient at Home. The Coordinator 3, 4, 19–21, 1984

82. Schulberg HC, Killilea M: The Modern Practice of Community Mental Health. San Francisco, Jossey-Bass, 1982

83. Sharpe D: Community Nursing—Psychiatry in the Home. Nursing Mirror 150, 2, 34–36, 1980

84. Silliman RA, Fletcher RH, Earp JL, Wagner EH: Families of Elderly Stroke Patients: Effects of Home Care. J Am Geriatr Soc 34:9 (September): 643–648, 1986

85. Slavinsky AT: Psychiatric Nursing in the Year 2000: From a Nonsystem of Care to a Caring System. Image 15(1): 17–20, 1984

86. Smith AM: Alternatives in AIDS Homecare. AIDS Patient Care 1:1 (June): 28–32, 1987

87. Solomon K, Harris MR: A Study of Client Acceptance of Various Professionals in Psychiatric Home Visits. Hosp Comm Psychiatry 28:9 (September) 661–665, 1977

88. Soreff SM: Indications for Home Treatment. Psychiatr Clin North Am 8(3): 563–575, 1985

89. Soreff SM: New Directions and Added Dimensions in Home Psychiatric Treatment. Am J Psychiatry 140: 1213–1216, 1983

90. Spradley BW: Community Health Nursing: Concepts and Practice, 2d ed. Boston, Little, Brown, 1985

91. Staggs K, Egli H: Home Health Team—An Overview of the Core Elements in the Home Care Team. The Coordinator 3(4): 14–16, 1984

92. Stanhope M, Lancaster J: Community Health Nursing: Process and Practice for Promoting Health. St. Louis, CV Mosby, 1984

93. Stanton L, Heymans G: A Pilot Study to Evaluate Visiting Nurses' Services to Chronic Psychiatric Patients. Hosp Community Psychiatry 28 (2): 97–101, 1977

94. Steffl BM, Eide I: Long-Term Care: Discharge Planning, Home Care, and Alternatives. In Steffl BM (ed): Handbook of Gerontological Nursing, pp 498–512. New York, Van Nostrand Reinhold, 1984

95. Stomboni J: The Home Visit: Taking Responsibility for the Mental Patient in His Home by the Community Psychiatric Nurse. Soins Psychiatric (France) 31: 19–23, 1983

96. Todd J: Community Nurse: CPN—A Life Line Keeping Psychiatric Patients at Home. Nursing Mirror 147(15): 46–48, 1978

97. Utah Nurses' Association. Reimbursement Battle. J Psychosoc Nurs Ment Health Serv 23 (7): 5, 1985

98. Warhola C: Planning for Home Health Services: A Resource Handbook. Washington, DC, Public Health Service, DHHS, 1980

99. Wasson W, Ripeckyj A, Lazarus LW, Kupferer S, Barry S, Force F: Home Evaluation of Psychiatrically Impaired Elderly: Process and Outcome. Gerontologist 24:238–242, 1984

100. Weiner LW, Becker A, Friedman TT: Home Treatment: Spearhead of Community Psychiatry, pp 201, 202. Pittsburgh, University of Pittsburgh Press, 1967. In Breslau LD, Haug MR (eds): Depression and Aging Causes, Care, and Consequences. New York, Springer Publishing Co, 1983

101. Weinstein S: Specialty Teams in Home Care. Am J Nurs 84, 3: 342–345, 1984

102. West DA, Litwok E, Oberlander K, Martin DA: Emergency Psychiatric Home Visiting: Report of Four Years' Experience. J Clin Psychiatry 41, 4, 113–118, 1980

103. Subjective Burden of Husbands and Wives as Caregivers: A Longitudinal Study. Gerontologist 26:3 (June): 260–266, 1986

40   Community Support and Rehabilitation

Mary Huggins

The clanging was back in her head but she refused to believe that she had come all that way, endured all she had, to die on the wrong side of the river.

Toni Morrison
Beloved

Chapter Preview

The general definition of a community support system is a "network of caring and responsible people committed to assisting a vulnerable population to meet their needs and develop their potentials without being unnecessarily isolated or excluded from the community."[14] This general definition encompasses a basic philosophy of care meant to address humanely the needs of adults with severe and persistent mental illnesses that seriously limit their ability to function in the primary areas of daily living. Prior to the Community Support Program (CSP), a federal initiative, these individuals had been labeled "deinstitutionalized." In the 1970s, a General Accounting Office Report publicly recognized that the social policies surrounding deinstitutionalization were not effectively addressing the basic needs of persons with severe and persistent mental illness.

In an attempt to address these issues, the National Institute of Mental Health (NIMH) established a Community Service System Branch to promote community support systems in all areas of the country. This movement, which has just celebrated its first decade, has made an amazing impact on the delivery system of broad-ranged services and support needed for this special population to live in the least restrictive environment. The movement also recognizes the need for quality of life. Over this decade much has been learned—much is left undone. This chapter presents a historical and philosophical context for the development of community support systems, explores the effects of the community support movement on delivery systems, and projects trends that will affect the continued delivery of community-based care.

Learning Objectives

Upon completion of the chapter, you should be able to accomplish the following:

1. define community support system
2. describe the philosophical context of the community support initiative
3. identify the ten essential components of a community support system
4. explain the relationship of case management, or service coordination, to the effectiveness of a community support system
5. compare at least five models for the delivery of community support systems
6. describe the impact of community support systems on consumers and their families
7. identify the trends that affect social policy regarding the care of persons with severe and persistent mental illnesses
8. describe the role of the nurse in a community support system

Definition of Community Support System

Like community mental health (see chapter 38), a community support system must be defined both philosophically and operationally. The changing focus and locale described in the definition of community mental health is built upon and refined in the definition of community support systems. Not only does an effective community support system require all the components of community mental health, it also requires elements found in systems theory, *i.e.*, the whole is only as effective as its parts. Thus, a community support system can be seen as a systems model for the delivery of community-based care for a specific population that formerly required admission to hospitals for significant portions of their lifetime. This system includes a range of life supports—health, mental health, and rehabilitation services, as well as the social networks, housing arrangements, and educational and employment opportunities. Additionally, the community support system is a program that delivers these specific services and can be exemplified by several program models. Conceptually, a community support system operates on the systems level by the linkage of a network of agencies dedicated to the provision of services to support seriously and persistently mentally ill persons in the least restrictive alternative; on the program level, community support systems operate through various program models. (See Chart 40-1 on the components of a community support system.)

The network is coordinated by a single agency—many times called the core service agency—responsible for the organization and coordination of the system, as well as for negotiation among the various agencies forming the network of services. This core service agency articulates the philosophical and operational basis for the network and allows for active participation of all persons with an investment in the system—consumer, family member, government official, and provider. The community support system is not a single model but embraces and incorporates many models in order to provide comprehensive service arrangements to meet the diverse needs of the population. To achieve the comprehensiveness needed to address the needs of persons with severe

CHART 40-1
Components of a Community Support System

Ten essential components define a Community Support System. They are as follows:

1. **Identification of and outreach to the population at risk**

   This includes informing the population of the available services and assuring access to the needed services, such as transporting the client to the service or the service to the client.

2. **Assistance in the application for entitlements**

   This includes assistance in obtaining food, shelter, clothing, general medical and dental care, and personal safety.

3. **Provision of adequate mental health care**

   This includes prescribed medications and medication monitoring, diagnostic evaluations, periodic reviews, and community-based treatment services.

4. **Provision of 24-hour crisis services**

   This includes ready assistance on a 24-hour basis for individuals and families in crisis and treatment options that allow the clients to remain functioning members of the community.

5. **Provision of a variety of psychosocial and vocational services that offer different possibilities for treatment environments and expectations**

   These choices should focus on the improvement or maintenance of the individual's normally functioning social roles.

6. **Provision of a range of rehabilitative and supportive housing options**

   These options should offer the support needed by the client, but should also encourage him to accept increasing responsibility for his own life.

7. **Provision of backup support, assistance, education, and consultation to families, friends, landlords, employers, and community agencies**

   This involvement will provide the support necessary for individuals to remain in the community and will minimize the associated problems.

8. **Recognition and involvement of concerned community members and the client's natural support system in the development of community support systems**

   These groups might include consumer and family self-help groups, churches, community organizations, industry, and commerce.

9. **Presence of grievance procedures in the community support program**

   This will provide for the protection of client rights.

10. **Provision of case management (a single person or team responsible for helping the client make informed choices and assure timely access to needed services)**

    This coordinates all services to meet the client's needs and goals.

and persistent mental illness, a community support system maintains flexibility, allowing for the incorporation of the positive elements of several generic models, such as the medical, rehabilitation, and social support models. (For more information regarding severe and persistent mental illness, see Chap. 24 on schizophrenia.)

The ten essential components defining a community support system are as follows:

1. Identification and assertive outreach to the population at risk, including client outreach, to inform the individual of the available services and to assure access to needed services. This may include arranging for needed transportation, transporting the individual to the service, or the delivery of the service in vivo.

2. Assistance in the application for entitlements, such as income, medical, housing, and other benefits critical to meeting basic human needs. This includes assistance in obtaining food, clothing, shelter, and general medical and dental care, as well as assistance in assuring that personal safety has been taken into account.

3. The provision of adequate mental health care, including diagnostic evaluations, prescribed medications, periodic reviews, and monitoring

of psychotropic medications, as well as community-based psychiatric, psychological, and/or counseling and treatment services.

4. The provision of 24-hour quick-response assistance to enable both the family and the consumer to cope more effectively with crises while maintaining the consumer's status as a functioning community member. This element requires crisis options to be available on a 24-hour basis, to be provided by trained professionals, and to be available at a variety of sites, including at-home and on-the-job when necessary.

5. Psychosocial and vocational services provided through a variety of options ranging from high to low expectations and environments. These options should be provided for an indefinite duration and should assist clients to evaluate their strengths and weaknesses, including training in daily living and community living skills; development of social skills, interests, and leisure activities; and assistance in finding and making use of appropriate employment and vocational services. These options focus primarily on the improvement or maintenance of the client's ability to function in normal social roles.

6. The provision of a range of rehabilitative and supportive housing options that offer the necessary degree of support while providing incentives and encouragement for the client to accept increasing responsibility for his own life.

7. The provision of backup support, assistance, consultation and education to families, friends, landlords, employers, community agencies, and the like. This is essential to maximize the benefits of individuals living in the community and minimize problems associated with their presence.

8. Recognition and involvement of concerned community members as well as the endorsement of the natural support system, including client and family self-help groups, churches, community organizations, commerce, and industry, in the development and implementation of community support systems on the systems level. In individual community plans, these elements are also basic to the success of community support systems.

9. All program components must have grievance procedures to provide for the protection of client rights.

10. Case management is the "glue" that holds the system together at the client level; it means that a single person or team is responsible for helping the client make informed choices and ensuring timely access to needed assistance. Case management provides opportunities and encouragement for self-help and coordinates all services to meet the client's goals.

Overriding all of these components, the community support system is based upon the respect for the dignity and the individual needs of each person and upon empowerment rather than dependency. The overall goal of a community support system is to enable persons with severe and persistent mental illness to remain in the community and to function at optimal levels of independence. Because the individuals who constitute this population are diverse and have unique concerns, abilities, motivations, and problems, and because that population comprises a variety of subgroups, the guiding principles of the community support system are as follows:

Client self-determination
Individualization of services
Normalization of services and service settings
Service provision in the least restrictive appropriate settings
Maximization of mutual assistance and self-help[8]

The Community Support Program has effectively focused attention on persons with severe and persistent mental illness at all levels of government. Effective community support programs "have positive sanction for their activities and service function from the highest level of local and state administration."[8] This includes visibility and continuing support from all levels of government—city, county, and state—in order to effect services at the systems level, *e.g.*, police, housing authorities, and local planning boards. This attention has publicized the conditions under which this vulnerable population must exist and has identified the needs of these individuals as a priority.

Background Information

When the Community Mental Health Centers (CMHC) Act began the establishment of community mental health centers throughout the nation, a series of pharmacological breakthroughs led to the development of several new drugs. This combination "promised" a new era in the treatment of long-term mental illness and led to the policy of *deinstitutionalization*. By 1974, residents in public mental institutions had declined from 559,000 in 1955 to 216,000.[15] Community placement, however, occurred without the needed supports to maintain basic living in the community. Community mental health centers and other programs were ill-equipped and not organized or prepared to assume responsibility for the needed support services. Thus deinstitutionalization resulted in a depopulation of public mental institutions without the concomitant establishment of needed supports and/or adequate funding for community alternatives.

Deinstitutionalization, however, is not the sole cause of the system's problems. Long periods of neglect and shunning of the needs of these individuals are at least equally responsible. Since the establishment of asylums, mentally ill persons and their needs have been ignored or, at best, met with minimal regard. As the era of depopulation progressed, former patients of the state hospitals began the *revolving door syndrome*. With the lack of community alternatives and the tightening of admissions to the state hospital, recidivism was imminent. As numbers grew, attention turned to the living conditions under which "deinstitutionalized" individuals must live. "Some critics noted that the conditions in communities were as bad as those in institutions—the mentally disabled were isolated, neglected, untreated and, in some cases, abused."[13]

Along with this population and as a direct result of the policy of deinstitutionalization, a number of younger mentally ill individuals began to be extruded from their home communities. In past years, this younger population would have been institutionalized. But with the closing of public hospitals and the tightening of admissions criteria, beds were unavailable. Therefore, added to the increasing number of "deinstitutionalized" individuals were young, mentally ill persons who had never been institutionalized. In recent years, homeless mentally ill persons joined this population. In this environment, the Community Support Program was conceived. Several studies, including a report from the General Accounting Office as well as newspaper, magazine, and television accounts, focused on the "failure" of deinstitutionalization. Attention was brought to bear on the lack of a range of services to promote growth and autonomy and to support individuals in the community. As a result, in 1974 NIMH formed an ad hoc committee that culminated in a task force recommendation to establish community alternatives encompassing ten essential components needed for mentally ill persons to live in the community. With unexpended federal funds from Hospital Improvement Program grants, the Community Support Program initiative was launched on a shoestring in 1977. Since that time, all 50 states, the District of Columbia, and two United States territories have been involved in the Community Support Program initiative.

Philosophical Basis of Community Support Systems

Community support systems encompass a philosophy that is based upon a set of values that act on three levels. These levels are the client, the service agency, and the service network. The values are centered on the individual; therefore, the client is central to the community support system. As such, the client maintains involvement in decisions that affect the needed services. The central theme of community support systems is empowerment, which recognizes the following three principles:

1. All people are valuable and should be afforded dignity, respect, and the opportunity to take full advantage of their human, legal, and social rights
2. Every human being is capable of growth, development, and learning
3. Services should be provided in a normative and socially valued way

Principles of Psychiatric Rehabilitation

These values can be embodied in a variety of settings. However, certain principles have been identified as basic to most psychiatric rehabilitation settings.[1] They are as follows:

1. The primary focus is on the improvement of the capabilities and the competence of the person with psychiatric problems, even the most disabled. The alleviation of symptoms is secondary.
2. Insight is not a primary goal; rather, this model focuses on the ability to function.
3. The model is eclectic and utilizes a variety of therapeutic constructs.
4. Improvement of vocational outcomes is a central focus.
5. Emphasis on positive expectations and hope is essential to the process.
6. A deliberate increase in dependency, as in sheltered settings, may be a first step in the process.
7. Active participation and involvement of clients in rehabilitation, in the operation of programs, and in the delivery of services to other clients are sought in order to provide rehabilitation *with*, rather than *to*, the client.
8. Client skill development and environmental resource development are fundamental interventions in the rehabilitation process.

Thus, the comprehensive network of services recognizes and emphasizes continuity of care, which, in many cases, is provided with an indefinite time frame.

Access

An effective community support system embraces a comprehensive spectrum of services for persons with serious and persistent mental illness and their relatives. These services are not related to the specific content of a particular program model, but "are rather part of the program's philosophy, operating style, and leadership."[8] Although several models of community support systems have been identified, access to a community support system is primarily through five major models or their derivatives.[13] These models may be developed singly or in combination. Each of these program models must contain the ten components of an effective community support system either within the program or by means of linkages to the provider system. Although all of the program models have similarities, they differ in their comprehensiveness and in the degree to which services are provided for or brokered. Additionally, these program models are based on individually tailored program plans with realistic goals based on an assessment of the individual client's strengths and weaknesses.

Program Models

The services in these program models are delivered for the most part in real-life community settings, that is, *in vivo*, to promote the transfer of learning through modeling and immediate reinforcement. These in vivo sites include, but are not limited to, home, school, and work. Each program model is described below. (This description is not intended to be complete; for further information, see material specific to each model.)

Psychosocial Rehabilitation Model

The psychosocial rehabilitation model evolved from Fountain House, which was begun by a group of clients in New York City in 1948. This model is generally organized as a clubhouse with members (clients) who are full participants in the operation of the program. Services are usually divided into the following four major areas:

Social/recreational
Vocational
Residential
Educational

Members are provided the opportunity to participate in a wide variety of activities relating to the management of the program, such as meal preparation, publication of a newsletter, and janitorial services, as well as decision-making regarding program operation.

Evaluation indicates that this model is effective in the reduction of hospitalizations and in improved community functioning, particularly in the areas of vocation and independent living for long-term members.[2]

Fairweather Lodge Model

The Fairweather Lodge model generally comprises two basic components; one is hospital-based, the other community-based. This program model, which began in 1960, uses the hospital as a training center for a group of patients who subsequently moves to the community to operate a small business. Group norms and peer support form the foundation of this model. All members of the lodge participate fully both in the lodge and the work place, utilizing appropriate work roles and habits. Evaluation indicates a reduction in recidivism and an increase in community employment activities.[6]

Training in Community Living Model

The training in community living model is a model of assertive involvement in community treatment of the long-term mentally ill person. This model (also known as the program of assertive community treatment, or PACT) was begun in the 1970s in Madison, Wisconsin. It involves the in vivo teaching of basic coping skills in the client's environment. It is an extremely directive approach, taking treatment to the client through role-modeling and support as well as treating the client as a responsible citizen. The hospital is utilized only in extreme cases. This model emphasizes the importance of clinical management, including appropriate medications and medication monitoring. It teaches the client about his symptoms, the relationship of the symptoms to stress, and how to control the symptoms.

Research indicates that this model is effective in helping clients maintain stability in the community. Stability is exhibited by a doubling of work productivity, decreased symptomatology, decreased hospitalization, decreased unemployment, and increased satisfaction with life.[16]

Consumer Run Alternative Model

The consumer run alternative is a model that endorses the planning, administering, delivery, and evaluation of services for consumers by consumers. Philosophically, this is a self-help model. Its core is voluntary participation, consumer control, and empowerment. Several such alternatives have been developed. Social, recreational, and educational services frequently are added to the usual drop-in center, which may also include community and public education and advocacy at both the individual and public policy levels. Other consumer alternatives have been started in the areas of residential, crisis, and vocational services.

Little formal evaluation of the consumer run alternative is available; however, Michigan and Ohio have provided some avenues for future research. The Michigan Department of Mental Health has collected data that indicate a highly successful experience overall. This evaluation is based on a high attendance rate and on high levels of reported satisfaction. Additional research has been recommended to assess the negative effects on consumers who staff these alternatives.[10] The State of Ohio has established an office in the State Department of Mental Health that is specific for consumer issues. Additionally, Ohio has made an evaluator available to assist consumer run programs in the development of a sound and consumer-acceptable evaluation. It is hoped that these efforts will be the impetus for future evaluation efforts of this model.

Community Worker Model

The community worker model relies on ordinary citizens to provide a range of community support services. These services are generally provided on a part-time basis and may be either paid or volunteer work. They include friendship, emotional support, teaching of community living skills, and assistance in accessing appropriate services. The community worker complements professional mental health services by modeling appropriate behaviors and by monitoring the client's level of functioning. Two primary variations of this model exist.

The community supportive care variation (also called the Rhinelander model) pays lay citizens to function as community support workers. This variation originated in rural Wisconsin and emphasizes the one-to-one relationship.

The Compeer variation utilizes volunteers to provide caring, supportive relationships. It originated in Rochester, New York, as an adjunct to therapy and to fill the gap left by a lack of supportive natural support systems.

Evaluation of these variations suggests a reduction in rehospitalization rates and days, as well as positive changes in the client's ability to socialize and cope in the community.[3,5]

As indicated above, several community rehabilitation program models have been established. These five models are only the most common ones.

Public Policy and Trends

The community support system program is a system change initiative. A number of public policy issues needing attention have been discussed or are identified by the development of an effective community support system. However, certain areas of concern have become obstacles at worst, or challenges at best, to the delivery of community-based care for persons with serious and persistent mental illness.

Chronic Mental Illness and Its Effects

A growing body of knowledge identifies mental illness as a disease of the brain (see Chap. 24 on schizophrenia for more information). Therefore, serious and persistent mental illness must be recognized as a chronic condition, much like multiple sclerosis, chronic heart disease, and other chronic, debilitating diseases. This recognition would counter the myth that there is a "quick cure" for all mental illness. It would also diminish the belief that people with serious and persistent mental illness can live without supportive treatment such as medication and availability of varying degrees of treatment intensity and length as the need arises. Additionally, gross confusion between the disease and the symptoms occurs, perpetuating the myth that serious mental illness precludes the individual from opportunities for rehabilitation. According to Pepper, "In failing to specify the differences between chronic mental disorder and long-term social disability, we perpetuate the myth that they are synonymous. In fact, the social disability is separate and its development is neither inevitable or incurable. Such confusion victimizes patients with a chronic disorder by denying them the opportunity for rehabilitation of their social disability."[11]

Resources

Conflicting federal, state, and local mandates preclude the targeting of resources (funds and staff) to the community. This can be best documented simply by looking at the dramatic shift of funding responsibility over the past 25 years or so.

In the late 1960s, the majority of costs for this population rested with state governments (primarily in state hospitals). More recently, responsibility for the provision of community-based care has rested at the local government level, with federal payments and reimbursements to support the individual. However, responsibility for overall planning and policy-making remains at the state level. The role of Medicaid (MA) and Supplemental Security Income (SSI) is central to the realities of this scenario. Although these funding bases were not intended to support the mentally ill, they are in fact at the core of community-based funding. Medicaid is the major source of health care funding for poor people and thus for most seriously and persistently mentally ill persons. However, Medicaid levels of support for non-institutional (that is, hospital and nursing home) care are extremely limiting. Thus persons with serious and persistent mental illness are in some cases admitted inappropriately to nursing homes and in other cases must go without appropriate health care. In some states, commitment laws have been promulgated in an attempt to stem inappropriate admissions to state hospitals. Families of mentally ill persons are becoming active in attempts to loosen these laws. This activity is due both to the difficulty in admitting their loved ones and to their sense that hospitalization is necessary because the community lacks alternatives that can appropriately address the needs of the loved one.

Reliance on SSI as the sole source of financial support for seriously and persistently mentally ill individuals allows little opportunity for choices. Many of these individuals live in unlicensed facilities with little or no follow-up care. The average monthly stipend is such that little is left after paying the "rent." Opportunities are limited or nonexistent due to the lack of funds for recreation, clothing, and transportation. Additionally, these limited stipends can only buy a level of housing that is most generally found in the poorer areas of the inner city; thus the "social service ghetto" is established.

Further, regulations prevent recipients from making more than a limited amount of money while receiving these "benefits." Therefore, an individual who gets a job risks losing his "health insurance" if more than the allotted amount is earned. This situation is further complicated by the mental illness, which, in many cases, is exacerbated by stress. An individual who is re-hospitalized or is unable to work on a long-term basis loses both benefits and medical insurance as well as the potential for broader health benefits. Thus the poverty spiral continues.

Regulations and Legislation

Regulation and legislation must emphasize the establishment of community support systems, including case management and interagency cooperation, in all local areas. Data have underscored the effectiveness of case management and community supports in the increased quality of life for individuals in these programs. However, Medicaid and other sources of fund-

ing and licensing requirements set up for larger institutions historically have not recognized adequately these community-based options. Recent trends point toward allowing payment for services such as day treatment, case management, and psychosocial programs, and to increasing the coverage for other outpatient services under Medicaid. Also, in many areas, private insurers are including mental health coverage. This latter benefit may, however, be somewhat overshadowed by the federal catastrophic health insurance regulations, which are not as favorable to mental health care as had been hoped.

Other mainstream funding sources have begun to recognize their responsibility in funding opportunities for this population (*e.g.,* HUD and RSA). Mainstream resources at the local and state level are equally important in the development of effective community-based alternatives.

Stigma

Ignorance on the part of the general public regarding mental illness is perpetuated by the media, leading to varying responses. Sometimes this ignorance is exhibited as frustration over the mentally ill person's inability to be cured. Sometimes it is exhibited as fear of the mentally ill person's perceived "differentness." Whatever the basis, many times the outcome is stigma and discrimination. Stigma may take place at the job location, so that mentally ill persons are not hired or are hired only for entry-level, low-expectation positions. Stigma may occur in housing alternatives, resulting in the refusal to rent to persons with mental illness or the development of restrictive zoning regulations regulating where these persons can live. Stigma may take place on the street, when passersby avert their eyes so not to be "engaged" in a conversation. Although it is clearly discriminatory to refuse jobs and housing based upon an individual's diagnosis, fear regarding personal safety and community welfare has allowed these practices to continue. Further, the frustration of seeing an individual with "an obvious illness" not being cared for has escalated the stigma and the lack of community acceptance of these individuals.

Consumer Movements

At the forefront of the antistigma campaigns are the recently endorsed consumer and family movements. These groups demand to be involved in the development of treatment alternatives. They provide advocacy and knowledge regarding the disease—including realistic expectations—to other consumers, family members, and the general public. In many parts of the country, consumers and families are involved in antistigma media watches as well as public education and advocacy.

Consumers and family members also are becoming increasingly involved at the decision-making levels of government, thus helping shape the policies and practices of the future. In many states, legislation requires consumer and family member participation at the decision-making level; one example is the newly promulgated Minnesota Comprehensive Mental Health Systems Act.

Reinstitutionalization

Due to the fundamental lack of public policy to date, serious problems are surfacing associated with reinstitutionalization of individuals into hospitals and jails. As responsibility for seriously and persistently mentally ill persons remains in limbo, local government has become increasingly overwhelmed by the large numbers of homeless or inadequately housed mentally ill persons in our large cities. As governments attempt to deal with this increased number of obviously needy people, a trend toward reinstitutionalization is beginning to take shape. New York City, for example, instituted a program for involuntary hospitalization of seriously mentally ill persons living on the street. The current national interest in reinstitutionalization "seems to have come about as a result of discrepancies between the public's knowledge of mental disorders and its understanding of current public policies dealing with treatment of severely disturbed/mentally ill persons, as well as a gross discrepancy between stated public policy and actual practice in most American communities."[11]

Reforms

It is imperative that certain social reforms be assessed to ascertain their effectiveness as proposed public policy. Although total agreement on needed reforms has not been reached, the following reforms are being viewed with some unanimity:

1. The development of a comprehensive policy for seriously and persistently mentally ill persons in the least restrictive alternative. This policy should range from prevention to hospitalization (noting that in *some* instances hospitalization is the least restrictive alternative) and should include accommodations for acute episodes within the framework of the service continuum. This policy should recognize the need for supportive housing as well as other community support services such as recreation, jobs, and medical/dental/mental health services.[4,11,12]

2. Government policy and funding must be directed toward the development of a comprehensive, unified network of community support services in each community. According to Pepper, "state governments, being the repositories of constitutional responsibility for the mentally ill, [must] take the initiative in developing policies" addressing the following areas: entitlement of citizens to intensive interventions funded by private insurance when it is available and by public funding when it is not; comprehensive, integrated outpatient alternatives and community support services when needed; and integrated services for persons with dual disabilities.[11]

3. Active initiatives are needed from the federal government in the development of federal policy regarding financial resources and regulations so that quality community-based alternatives can become a reality.[11]

4. Antistigma efforts should focus on the population at large in promoting an understanding of mental illness that incorporates new knowledge based upon recent research that identifies the illness as a chronic disease.

Although many other needs in the area of public policy are evident, initiatives begun by the federal Community Support Program must continue so that trends resulting in untoward outcomes—such as large-scale reinstitutionalization in hospitals and jails—are halted or reversed. The federal Community Support Program has been identified as the logical "unifying agency for these efforts"; its role in working with existing resources in the development of community alternatives has been acknowledged.[12]

The Nurse's Role

As in community mental health, the nurse is in a unique position of assessing both individual and community needs for community support programs. Further, nursing equips the professional with the ability to focus on a particular situation while retaining a holistic approach. Such an approach blends the physical, mental, and social needs of an individual with community environmental norms.

Nurses are unique in their ability to bridge the gap between the hospital and the community, between the psychiatrist and the community caregiver, and between the public and other health care providers. Nursing education includes an emphasis on teamwork and sharing of responsibility with other individual caregivers that is rarely if ever found in other professional training. Nurses understand the needs and responsibilities of 24-hour programming. When included on community teams, nurses enhance the teams' understanding of treatment alternatives, medications and side effects, and the importance of client education and client teaching to reduce stress in the individual and thus alleviate episodes.[7] Nurses understand the importance of physical movement to decrease muscle atrophy and the other long-term effects of not utilizing a full range-of-motion, a problem frequently associated with the long-term ingestion of psychotropic medications.

The combination of inpatient, public health, and psychiatric nursing knowledge based upon good physical assessment skills is imperative in community-based programs. Understanding the role of stress in the consumer's system affords the nurse the ability to provide the integrative link among community resources, housing, vocation, social relationships, and psychiatric episodes. Of primary importance is the separation of the disease from the social disability.[11] Extensive nursing knowledge and education place nurses in a position not only to educate the consumer regarding the client's disability, side effects, and the effect of stress on the mental disorder, but also to educate other professionals and the community in areas such as medication effects, side effects, and interventions to diminish harmful effects.

Nurses have traditionally worked with natural support systems in developing client care plans. In many parts of the country, nurses have initiated contact with tribal healers, curanderas, midwives, or other healers in the implementation of the care plan. It is therefore a logical extension of the nursing role to integrate natural support persons into the treatment plan for seriously and persistently mentally ill persons.

The nurse's role in community support services is primary. Nurses are responsible for building upon the assessments and analyses described in the community mental health chapter, for integrating these outcomes into input for public policy, and for becoming change agents in the community. Thus, the nursing process is applied at all levels of the community support system in the provision of comprehensive services to individuals with serious and persistent mental illness living in the community.

Summary

Research over the past decade indicates that community support services are critical to quality-of-life residence in the community for individuals with serious and persistent mental illnesses. This chapter has highlighted the following points:

1. The National Institute of Mental Health has documented that local sites all over the nation are organizing Community Support Systems and that states are mobilizing financial and legislative resources dedicated to the seriously and persistently mentally ill.[9]

2. The research surrounding Community Support Programs has demonstrated that, when clients participate in Community Support Programs, inpatient hospitalization is reduced by 50%; approximately two-thirds of clients show improvement or no deterioration over a 1-year period; and there has been an increase in the number of clients in Community Support Programs, from 4,200 in 1980 to 350,000 in 1984.[9]

3. Nurses have a leadership role in the development of a comprehensive community support service system that is committed to the holistic approach of intervening on both the client and the system level.

4. As we face the challenge of choosing between an easy answer (reinstitutionalization) and the development of long-term social policy reforms to stimulate and support individuals in community alternatives, nursing must not only accept the challenge but must remain in the forefront of these developments.

References

1. Anthony W, Cohen M, Cohen B: Psychiatric Rehabilitation. In Talbot J (ed): The Chronic Mental Patient: Five Years Later. New York, Grune & Stratton, 1984

2. Bond G, Dincin J, Setze P, Witheridge T: The Effectiveness of Psychiatric Rehabilitation: A Summary of Research at Thresholds. Psychosoc Rehab J 7 (4) (April): 1984

3. Cannady D: Chronics and Cleaning Ladies. Psychosoc Rehab J 5, 1 (January): 1982

4. Carling PJ, Ridgway P: A Psychiatric Rehabilitation Approach to Housing. In Anthony W, Farka M (eds): Psychiatric Rehabilitation: Program and Practices. Baltimore, Johns Hopkins University Press, in press

5. Compeer Program: Annual Report 1984–1985. Rochester, NY, Compeer

6. Fairweather G: The Prototype Lodge Society: Instituting Group Process Principles, New Directions for Mental Health Services—The Fairweather Lodge: A

Twenty-Five Year Retrospective. San Francisco, Jossey-Bass, 1980

7. Huggins M: A Model Case Management System in a Local CSS: Community Support Network News Vol 4, No 4. Boston University Center For Psychiatric Rehabilitation, December, 1985

8. Liberman R, Kuehnel T, Phipps C, Cardin V: Resource Book For Psychiatric Rehabilitation: Elements of Services for the Mentally Ill. Camarillo, CA, Center for Rehabilitation Research and Training in Mental Illness, UCLA School of Medicine, 1984

9. Manderscheid RW: CSP Research Accomplishments: Community Support Network News Vol 4, No 2. Boston University Center For Psychiatric Rehabilitation, October, 1987

10. Mowbray C, Chamberlain P, Jenning M: Final Report: Consumer Run Alternative Services: Demonstration and Evaluation Projects 1982–1984. Lansing, MI, Research and Evaluation Division, Michigan Department of Mental Health, 1984

11. Pepper B: A Public Policy for the Long-Term Mentally Ill: A Positive Alternative to Reinstitutionaliza-tion. Am J Orthopsychiatry 57, 3 (July): 452–457, 1987

12. Searight HR, Handal PJ: Psychiatric Deinstitutionalization: The Possibilities and the Reality. Psychiatr Q 58 (3): (Fall): 153–166, 1986–1987

13. Stroul B: Models of Community Support Services: Approaches to Helping Persons with Long-Term Mental Illness. National Institute of Mental Health, Community Support Program, 1986

14. Turner J: Comprehensive Community Support Systems for Severely Mentally Disabled Adults: Definitions, Components and Guiding Principles, rev. National Institute of Mental Health, 1977

15. U.S. Department of Health and Human Services: Toward a National Plan for the Chronically Mentally Ill: Report to the Secretary by the Department of Health and Human Services Steering Committee on the Chronically Mentally Ill. Washington, DC, DHHS, 1980

16. Weisbrod BA, Test MA, Stein LI: Alternatives to Mental Hospital Treatment II: Economic Benefit-Cost Analysis. Archives General Psychiatry 37 (April): 400–408, 1980

PART 9

Mental Health Intervention with the Medical Patient

41

Trauma, Surgery, and Critical Care

Cynthia Ann Pastorino

Surgical Ward

They are and suffer; that is all they do;
A bandage hides the places where each is living,
His knowledge of the world restricted to
The treatment that the instruments are giving.

And lie apart like epochs from each other
—Truth in their sense is how much they can bear;
It is not talk like ours, but groans they smother—
And are as remote as plants; we stand elsewhere.

For who when healthy can become a foot?
Even a scratch we can't recall when cured,
But are boist'rous in a moment and believe

In the common world of the uninjured, and cannot
Imagine isolation. Only happiness is shared,
And anger, and the idea of love.

WH Auden,
Collected Poems

Chapter Preview

Trauma, surgery, or an acute illness requiring a hospital stay is a stressful event. Both the individual patient and the involved family face the stresses of the illness heaped upon preexisting personal and interpersonal life stressors. The individual's usual problem-solving abilities, energy and resources, and available supports influence his ability to cope with the stress of a major physiological onslaught. The injured or seriously ill person often experiences the psychological themes of denial, threatened body image, and emotional lability. Nurses generate interventions that assist the individual and his family by preserving and nurturing adaptive responses.

Learning Objectives

On completion of the chapter, you should be able to accomplish the following:

1. describe the personal, environmental, and injury-related stressors confronting the person experiencing trauma, surgery, or critical illness
2. describe a problem-solving method of coping with the stressor of illness or injury
3. apply the nursing process to the care of persons experiencing trauma or critical illness
    describe the behaviors of patients at the various phases of their injury—impact, resistance, and resolution
    formulate nursing diagnoses for the injured or acutely ill patient
    identify goals and interventions that help the individual and family cope with specific trauma reactions
    evaluate the effectiveness of nursing interventions
4. discuss the major concerns of family members of severely injured or critically ill patients during hospitalization
5. describe the effect of working with trauma and seriously ill patients and their families on the nurse
6. identify coping measures that assist the nurse who cares for victims of trauma and critical illness

Effect of Trauma and Surgery

Severely traumatized patients and those undergoing major surgeries account for millions of hospital days per year in the United States. The cost of trauma—financially, physically, and emotionally—to the injured and their families is staggering. Aside from the physical effects of the trauma or surgery, the individual suffers emotional or psychological consequences, which comprise a stress response.

Stress is a part of everyday life. People respond to stress in a total or holistic manner as they try to reestablish or maintain a steady state, or equilibrium. This stress-response cycle is characterized by the following factors:

1. The stressful event or stressors
2. The interpretation or perception of the meaning of the event
3. Conditioning factors or characteristics of the individual, such as his past experiences and goals
4. The individual's available coping mechanisms[38]

Stressors Confronting the Seriously Ill Patient

The seriously ill patient experiences stress due to a combination of preexisting life stressors, stressors inherent to hospitalization, and injury- or illness-related stressors. Stress may have a negative connotation, such as death of a loved one, or a positive connotation, such as an increase in salary. Both of these examples suggest a change of some sort, and any change interrupts the individual's equilibrium, thereby creating stress. Not all changes result in maladaptation, however; stress may induce a person to grow and develop more effective responses to his environment.

Stressful Life Events

Certain life events that occur normally in the course of a lifetime may add to the stress of the seriously ill patient. Death of a spouse, divorce, or financial problems are highly stressful events due to the amount of change that occurs at those times.[18] These stressful life events drain the resources of the individual. When they are closely spaced, they increase the likelihood of illness. It is not unusual, for example, for the surgical patient to give a history of recent major life stress. Inadvertently, the nurse may focus on the present event, the patient's illness or injury, and ignore or dismiss the importance of the previous stressful events in his life. Nevertheless, those previous events may have precipitated the current illness, and they definitely affect the healing capabilities of the individual.

Stressors Due to Hospitalization

Hospital-related stressors compound the injured or ill patient's preexisting life stresses. These stressors include unfamiliarity of the surroundings, loss of independence, separation from loved ones, and financial problems. It has been found that people reporting high levels of life stress also report high levels of hospital-related stress.[41] In addition, these people who experience higher-than-normal levels of stress require a longer period of convalescence before returning to their previous or usual activities.[45] Often, the patient may be unaware of the amount of stress with which he is coping. In this situation, nurses may help the patient develop insight into his life and recognize and manage his stress.

Illness-Related Stressors

If stressful life events and hospitalization have not overwhelmed the patient, consider the stressors confronting the critically ill patient; that is, the *illness-related stressors*. These stressors include physical, chemical, biologic, and physiological assaults.[39] Physical stressors include changes in environmental temperature and disturbances in the patient's natural body rhythms of rest and activity. The constant activity of the critical care areas of the hospital, such as the noise and lights throughout the day and night, cause the patient to lose those indicators of night and day. While environmental effects confuse the patient, drugs may add to his disorientation by disturbing normal body functions. Pain and other physiological factors contribute to the problem.

ICU Syndrome. Illness-related stressors also contribute to a phenomenon, most often seen in the intensive care unit (ICU), called "ICU psychosis," "ICU syndrome," or "ICU-itis." The onset of this syndrome is heralded by a change in orientation (person, place, or time), usually preceded by major physiological assault (trauma or surgery) and accompanied by sleep deprivation.[15] Patients at risk for the development of this syndrome tend to be over 50 years of age, to have a personal history of inflexible modes of coping under stress, and to have been in the intensive care unit for more than 3 days.[30] The onset of this syndrome usually occurs 3 to 7 days after the surgery or trauma.

With improved surgical techniques, diligent postoperative monitoring, and increased sensitivity of staff to psychological needs of patients, the incidence of this syndrome has decreased dramatically over the years. If the ICU syndrome is left untreated, or unrecognized, however, the change in cognition develops into full-blown psychosis with the patient experiencing visual hallucinations, paranoid ideation, and strange bodily sensations.[14] Nursing interventions to prevent the development of this syndrome will be discussed later in this chapter.

Stressors related to life events, hospitalization, and illness or injury elicit both a physiological and psychological stress response. Ineffective coping per-petuates the stress syndrome and results in maladaption, at the least, and illness or death, at the extreme. How these stressors are perceived governs the effectiveness of the patient's response.

Perception and Problem-Solving

Understanding how stressors are perceived and how problems are defined and solved is crucial in assisting patients through surgery, trauma, or any other crisis event. Adults who have been responsible and functioning in society have learned how to meet their needs and how to make sense out of their environments. These same adults, however, when hospitalized, are lost in a strange place. The patient's predicament may be likened to driving in a foreign city in search of a specific place. The ill or injured patient is ignorant of the hospital's rules and customs and is dependent upon caregivers who are unfamiliar to him, yet he attempts to understand and react appropriately to the strange environment.

Perception of an event is a highly individualized phenomenon based on values, instincts, personality, past experience, problem-solving ability, and many other factors.[11] These factors contribute to the individual's ability to define the problem, generate possible solutions, and choose the solution that is most likely to be effective.[19]

When a patient's resources (*e.g.*, his attention span or verbal abilities) are compromised, satisfactory resolution of the stressful situation or problem is hampered. For example, when a patient is treated with analgesics, his problem-solving ability is likely to be affected.

Several obstacles may hinder the individual's effective resolution of a problem. They include the following:

1. The problem may tax the individual beyond his capacity to respond
2. The problem may be insoluble
3. The solutions to the problems are contradictory.[19]

When stress is overwhelming, the patient cannot mobilize sufficient energy to overcome it. An example of this effect of overwhelming stress is the compromised ability of a person to cope with several successive family deaths. An insoluble problem, for instance, may be extensive multisystem organ failure. Contradictory solutions to problems pose an ever-present quandary in patient care; for example, how to provide comfort to a patient with extensive orthopedic injuries who also has head trauma. Nevertheless, solutions must be found, because the stress will perpetuate itself if the problem remains unresolved.

Conditioning Factors

The intensity and duration of the stress response depend not only on perception and problem-solving, but also on other characteristics of the individual. These characteristics, or conditioning factors, include genetic predispositions, nutritional status, types and variety of coping mechanisms, available situational supports, cultural inheritance, health history, and developmental level.[1]

Adults and children differ in their perception of their injuries and the meaning of hospitalization. Children's perception of hospitalization is largely dependent on their age and stage of development. Preschool children are convinced that some great misbehavior caused their injury. Their limited understanding of any procedure causes them to resist any treatment. Schoolage children may feel singled out, and they too express feelings of guilt and self-blame. Adolescents vary in their responses to trauma and treatment depending on their level of maturity, but tend to feel isolated and alone.[43]

An individual with a deficit in these factors is at risk for more adverse effects of trauma, surgery, or critical illness. For example, a diabetic patient undergoing major surgery is more likely to experience complications and a prolonged recovery period than a nondiabetic patient. Likewise, an injured person who uses only acting-out behavior as a coping method and who hasn't any friends has limited resources at a time when he needs maximum resources.

The Critically Ill Person and the Nursing Process

Assessment

Nursing care of patients who have suffered trauma or serious illness or who have major surgery relies on a data base of information concerning previous life experiences, responses to stressful life events, and other factors. The particular response of the patient to trauma or surgery depends on several factors. They include the following:

1. The extent and type of injury
2. The meaning that the injury has for the individual
3. Other situational factors[27]

The overall goal of nursing care of these patients is to return them to the highest possible level of functioning, with healing of both physical and psychological wounds. This healing requires a gradual shift from life-or-death considerations to self-actualization considerations. At the time of injury, the person's energy expenditure is at the level of compensation, or constantly trying to "catch up" with physiological and psychological needs. As these needs become satisfied, the injured person can direct his energies toward coping with the environment and, finally, toward growth.[33] Nursing care focuses on conserving the patient's energy to enable growth to occur. Patient response to injury or critical illness is studied through the phases of impact, resistance, and resolution.[38]

Impact

At the time of serious illness or injury, the individual is placed in an unfamiliar environment and is expected to adapt, although his bodily energies are focused at the life–death level. Some of the behavioral manifestations of the phase of impact include denial, threatened body image, loss of control, and altered cognitive abilities.

Denial. Denial is perhaps the most frequent initial response to injury or serious illness. Patients may deny the extent of their injuries, the consequences of the injuries, or that they are injured at all. It is not uncommon for a person with a fractured leg to attempt to walk on it, despite the severe pain. Patients who are spinal-cord injured may rationalize the paralysis as temporary and may imagine movement. Even in the face of obvious clues (monitors and so on) and frank conversation to the contrary, patients may verbalize being "okay."

Denial is used to minimize the degree of threat of the injury and to "buy time" needed for the patient to call on his resources.[26] Denial allows the patient to focus energies on physiological healing while preserving other energies for later needs. Denial may be maladaptive when it is so encompassing that it threatens the patient's health, or when great amounts of energy are required to maintain the denial. Often, denial and awareness coexist and usually progress to some kind of reality-testing.[44] Although a patient may use denial when talking to others, this does not necessarily imply that he is deceiving himself.

Threatened Body Image. Threatened body image is another frequent response to trauma, serious surgery, and illness. The whole, functioning body that the patient once knew and loved is now changed. The patient may feel betrayed by his body. In the critical care unit, as well as in general units of the hospital, the person is connected to intravenous infusions, catheters, monitors, traction, and respirators, all of which provide basic functions that were once taken for granted.

Body image, which develops from early childhood, is largely associated with freedom of movement and autonomy.[21] Our culture greatly esteems the ability to function independently. An important criterion of independence is movement, yet movement is greatly restricted in the critically ill. In injured patients, not only is the mental picture of oneself altered, but the means of assessing the amount of damage done is also denied.

Behavioral manifestations of threatened body image vary and change over time. The patient often verbalizes a feeling of change in body function or structure; he may have a pet name for the body part involved; he may refuse to look at the affected part; or he may be depressed, anxious, or guilty.[12, 16]

Loss of Control. While the patient is seriously ill and basically dependent, he experiences loss of control and helplessness. The more serious his illness and the further removed he is from his family, the greater are his feelings of helplessness. If the patient attempts to solve problems originating in the hospitalization or illness, and the desired outcomes are not attained, his feelings of helplessness will increase and he may give up trying.[35] For example, a patient may cooperate with painful breathing exercises to prevent pulmonary complications of bedrest, but develops pneumonia anyway; he then sees no relationship between his actions and the outcome, which magnifies his feelings of being out of control and powerless.[34]

Behavioral manifestations of loss of control may include verbalization of powerlessness, such as, "I don't see why I should try, it won't work anyway," worthlessness, such as, "I don't know why you bother with me," and passivity. The patient may be unable to recognize any area of his life over which he may exert some measure of control.

Altered Cognitive Abilities. During the impact phase, the patient may experience a change in cognitive abilities and sensory overload. *Sensory overload* is a phenomenon wherein the individual, having lost the ability to distinguish, weigh, and interpret environmental cues, attempts to attend to all stimuli. Ordinarily, people are aware of a few stimuli at any one time, and all others are ignored. The ill person, however, feels the hardness of the strange bed, the roughness of the sheets, the pinching of the tape, the burning of the intravenous solution, the pain of the incision, the lightness of the room, the noise of the monitor, the conversations of the staff, and so on. The ICU syndrome is detected by a change in cognitive ability in persons stressed by major assault, sleep deprivation, and limited coping strategies.

It is not uncommon for critically ill persons to have fantasies of being dead (not dying) or of being held prisoner.[25] These feelings are very confusing and frightening for the patient. It is not difficult, though, to understand why a patient might experience these feelings, because he is restrained, looking through the bars of the bed's siderails, and may be unable to speak because of a new tracheostomy.

Resistance

The next phase, resistance or stabilization, is characterized by increasing attempts by the individual to come to terms with the injury, illness, or surgery. The individual's energy stores are depleted and he is unable to focus his energy in any direction. The emotional responses of this phase include anger and hostility, guilt, vulnerability, and grief.

Anger and Hostility. The patient's anger and hostility may be directed at himself, family members, staff, or those who have been spared injury.[22] Whereas once the patient was passive, he now becomes hostile and difficult to please. If the injury is permanent, the patient may be reluctant to express any anger for fear of alienating future care providers.[45] Often, the patient succeeds in turning away loved ones who may be bewildered by these outbursts.[16]

Guilt. The patient's emotional outbursts may trigger feelings of guilt at having been angry, at having been injured, or at any wrongdoings.[22] The patient may feel guilt or shame for his behavior early in the hospital stay. Nurses may hear the patient talk about what he "should have" or "wished he would have" done, as he expresses responsibility for the injury, illness, or surgery. The conclusions reached by the patient may be far-fetched; for example, when the automobile-accident victim states he "should have taken the bus" when he never before rode the bus.

Vulnerability. The feeling of vulnerability implies that the individual is not coping well; it is characterized by a distressed mood and by feelings of being flawed, breakable, or exposed to harm. The patient may express lack of confidence in significant others and caregivers.[44] He scrutinizes each staff member for clues as to whether or not he or she can be trusted. Although clinically he may be improving, the patient sees little future for himself. He may feel abandoned, in part because of the less frequent visits by health care workers and families during the patient's improvement. These feelings of vulnerability seem to increase and decrease depending on the patient's energy.

Grief. During the resistance phase, the patient has time to think about the injury and begins to tally his losses. The patient grieves for all that has been changed or lost, and the losses are many. These losses, which may be potential, actual, or irreversible, include the following:

1. Changes in body parts or functioning; that is, self-care activities, agility, consciousness, mental acuity, and others
2. Changes in rest or comfort
3. Changes in self-concept; that is, self-esteem, body image, personal identity, and role performance
4. Changes in significant other; that is, availability of support group and emotional and financial security
5. Changes in availability of inanimate objects, such as personal belongings
6. Control over the environment
7. Existential changes, such as choice, hope, freedom, and individuality
8. Changes in life dreams and goals
9. Changes in certainty or predictability.[12]

The realization of the extent of the losses may come as a surprise to the patient, especially if he has previously used denial. If the injury, illness, or surgery has resulted in a permanent handicap or disfigurement, the patient has a constant reminder of the loss and, therefore, the potential for constant grieving.[45] The feeling of grief may flood the patient at unpredictable times, and this unpredictability further increases his feelings of distress. The increased awareness of the effect of the trauma or surgery signals the beginning of the third stage of the response syndrome: resolution.

Resolution

During the resolution phase of the response to critical illness or trauma, the patient comes to terms with the assault. Coping is defined as the satisfactory resolution of distress. Through these stages of stress, patients try a variety of coping measures until equilibrium is attained. This equilibrium may not be achieved for months after the injury or serious illness, or may not be achieved at all. Exhaustion results from failure to cope with the injury or illness, and is characterized by depleted energy stress, continued distress, and impaired psychophysiological functioning.[38] Exhaustion is precipitated by errors in problem-solving, altered perception, and deficits in biologic functioning.

Not all people recover psychologically from trauma, just as all do not recover physically. Individuals may be left with fears and uncertainties, especially when confronting situations similar to those surrounding the accident or illness. If the individual was injured in an automobile accident, it is not unusual for that person to be afraid to drive again or even to approach the geographical area where the accident occurred. At times the fear may be disabling, or it may evidence itself in reluctance to go on driving vacations.[23]

Coping generates energy for growth. The goal of the resolution phase is the establishment of quality of life to the patient's ability and satisfaction. By this time in the course of the injury or illness, the patient has defined more clearly the problems, has generated some options for himself, and is attempting to reconstruct his life. The patient has plans for reentry into a social life and his energies are now directed toward growth. Major themes of the patient during the resolution phase include framing memories of the accident or illness, divided time, and existential and spiritual concerns.

Framing Memories of the Accident or Illness. In an attempt to pull together the events surrounding the injury or illness, the patient will begin to frame memories of the accident or illness.[10] He may also express embarrassment about some of his past behavior, or fear of the trauma happening again. The patient attempts to place the accident or surgery in perspective, and in his past. This is accomplished through telling and retelling his story. Some people may even keep a scrapbook of souvenirs from their hospital stay.

Divided Time. With the trauma or surgery safely in the past, the injury is used as a marker with which to divide time.[35] The patient places events "before the accident" (or illness or surgery) or "after the accident," as though the event were a convenient way to remember other unrelated events. A daughter's wedding is now remembered as occurring "before my accident," or Uncle Joe died "after my accident."

Existential and Spiritual Concerns. Along with framing memories and using the assault to divide the past, individuals may also experience increased attention to existential and spiritual concerns.[40] Some patients view the accident or surgery as a lesson. The patient may realize unfulfilled hopes and dreams and set new goals. These goals often revolve around promises to give to charity or attend church services more often. The trauma may have provided an opportunity for the patient to grow.

Effect on the Critically Ill Patient's Family
The individual patient is not alone in experiencing the stress of trauma or major illness; the family, as

a unit, also encounters stressors. These family stressors include interpersonal problems, debt, unemployment, problems with child care, and illness of other family members. The family also experiences hospital-related stressors, such as loss of social contact with the injured member, role changes, changes in eating and sleeping habits, and relocation to a strange environment. These stressors often affect the health of family members and may cause exacerbations of their preexisting health problems.

Assessing Family Members. The nurse assesses the family's strengths and weaknesses by examining the following factors:

1. Adaptation, or use of resources in a crisis
2. Partnership, or shared decision-making
3. Growth, or the self-fulfillment achieved by family members through mutual support
4. Affection
5. Resolve, or the commitment to each other[37]

How the family perceives this illness and its effect on family life will determine the amount of threat that is experienced. If the family perceives the patient's illness or injury as affecting all family roles, life dreams, and relationships, then the family is at risk for emotional problems. The basic needs of the family are to hope, to know, and to be close.

Family Responses. Typical responses of the family with a critically ill member are high anxiety levels, denial, anger and rage, and, finally, resolution.[5]

Manifestations of high anxiety levels are observed in the family members' tense facial expressions and posture.[5] "Is he alive?" is their main concern. The family members often huddle together, supporting each other and attempting to make sense out of what has happened. The nurse functions as the main source of information about the hospital and about their injured or ill family member. The nurse is the family's lifeline to the injured member; the family attempts to interpret every piece of information it receives.

Denial serves the same purpose for the family as it does for the individual—it maintains hope. At times, one family member is designated the "strong one" and denial helps that member maintain the posture of strength.[8] Family members using denial say, "He looks okay," when the patient has multiple monitors, IVs, and massive dressings. They see the patient as they want to see him—alive and basically well.

The family's anger and rage may be focused at the patient, the hospital, society, or other family members. Not infrequently, a family member will react to some trivial irritant, such as the tone of someone's voice, with an explosion of anger. In reality, the family unit has been severely disrupted by the patient's injury or critical illness. Families need reassurance that their anger is understandable and needs to be expressed.

It is hoped that the family resolves the crisis adaptively. They make plans to resocialize the injured or ill family member into the fold. The members once again laugh with each other and begin to act as a family unit. (See Chart 41-1, "Therapeutic Dialogue: Recognizing and Responding to the Anxiety of Family Members.")

Nursing Diagnosis

From the assessment data, the nurse formulates nursing diagnoses that will guide the planning and implementing of nursing care for the patient. Some of the nursing diagnoses which may be appropriate for these patients include the following:

Sensory-perceptual alteration related to cerebral hypoxia, other physical disorders resulting from trauma, illness, or surgery, evidenced by disorientation, disordered thought sequencing, inappropriate responses, visual and auditory distortions

Disturbance in self-concept: body image related to effects of physical trauma or illness, evidenced by verbalization of negative feelings about body, fear of rejection or reaction by others, change in social involvement

Impaired verbal communication related to facial or neck trauma, tracheostomy, disorientation, fear, evidenced by fact that he does not or cannot speak

Dysfunctional grieving related to absence of anticipatory grieving, thwarted grieving response to a loss, bereavement overload, evidenced by difficulty in expressing loss, labile affect, developmental regression, denial of loss

Anxiety related to situational crisis, threat of death, threat of self-concept, trauma of injury or illness, unmet needs, evidenced by restlessness, visual perceptions of traumatic event, fear of dying, feelings of unreality

Planning

Goal-Setting

Planning nursing care for patients experiencing trauma or critical illness poses serious problems for the care provider. Much attention is focused on the patients' technical and physical needs; obviously, the priority is the patient's life. Nevertheless, just as pro-

CHART 41-1
Therapeutic Dialogue

Recognizing and Responding to the Anxiety of Family Members

Nineteen-year-old M. C. was involved in a major automobile accident. He underwent extensive surgery for abdominal and multiple orthopedic injuries. His condition is stable at this time.

Father: How's he doing?

Nurse: He spoke to me awhile ago and said he was okay, but was having pain in his leg.

Mother: Did you give him a shot? He doesn't like needles.

Nurse: He had a shot about 1 hour ago, so . . . .

Mother: Well, the other nurse said he can have it anytime!

Nurse: No, not really . . . .

Father: Well, I wish you'd all get your stories straight!!

Nurse: We seem to be getting off on the wrong foot here. I know you must be scared and worried half to death about M. I would be, too, about my child. And the intensive care unit is pretty confusing—especially with all the different doctors and nurses and machines.

Father: Everyone says something different.

Nurse: Sometimes that's true; sometimes we don't hear everything because we're so worried.

Mother: Well, that's true . . . .

Nurse: I think there's a way we can get together. We have what we call a care plan where we write down the most important aspects of M's care. I think you can help us by letting us know about M. so we can help him better. Some things we may not be able to do while he's here in intensive care, but when he goes back to the orthopedic unit, the nurses there will know just how to care for him.

Discussion

Being in the intensive care unit is an anxiety-producing experience for both the patient and the family. Although the patient's parents verbalized their need for information, their anxiety and fear hindered their understanding.

There are times when the communication process goes badly, as when the nurse and parents began to discuss the patient's injections for pain. The nurse recognized the parent's emotional need, redirected the conversation (although it would have been easy to become angry or defensive), and proceeded with a more constructive interchange. The family also hinted at other avenues that need to be explored; for instance, other incidents that led the family to hear conflicting stories, and the need for reassurance that their son's pain management is of great concern to the nursing staff.

---

tocols for physical care must be planned, so must nurses recognize and plan care to meet the patient's psychosocial needs. General goals to promote the mental health of patients and families include the following:

1. Maintaining previously adequate coping styles and encouraging flexibility of coping
2. Preventing untoward side effects, such as distrust, despair, and ICU syndrome
3. Maintaining the patients' support system

Incorporating Psychosocial Concerns into Care

Although these goals may seem obvious in the context of this chapter, the "real-world" situation is often problematic. When the focus of care is crisis-oriented and the priority is the preservation of life, psychological issues assume less importance. It is, therefore, imperative that nurses and other caregivers incorporate psychological support into the patient's care, beginning with his entrance into the hospital.

Social workers, chaplains, and clinical nurse specialists often serve as liaisons between hospital staff and the patient and family and help facilitate the development of trust and understanding. These health care professionals usually have flexibility in the geographic areas in which they work and may be able to link the intensive care unit with the general hospital units for the patient and family. The concept of continuity of care is vital in the care of seriously ill patients. When staffing problems prohibit continuing

CHART 41-2
Nursing Diagnosis of the Critically Ill

Diagnosis	Supporting Data
Sleep pattern disturbance	Critically ill and surgical patients are frequently awakened throughout the day for assessment of physiological parameters and necessary activities. Patients may verbalize feeling tired, or may be restless, confused, apathetic, and unable to perform customary activities, such as bathing, turning, or feeding self.
Impaired verbal communication	Patients may be unable to communicate because of facial or neck trauma, tracheostomy, fatigue, disorientation, or fear. Speech may require more energy than is available for the patient, resulting in halting speech or shortened phrases. This results in frustration for staff and patient and reliance on nonverbal communication, which, by its nature, may be incomplete or misinterpreted.
Impaired thought process	Patients demonstrate a decrease in attention span, memory deficits, and a change in problem-solving ability related to excessive sensory stimulation when acutely ill.
Disturbance in body image	The patient's body image is challenged by illness or trauma, resulting in feeling unfamiliar with self and capabilities. The patient can become preoccupied with the involved body parts, feel negative about the body, and fear rejection by others because of perceived changes in his body.
Impaired home maintenance management	The patient/family express difficulty in being able to care for patient because they are unfamiliar with care regimens or lack the resources (personal, financial) to provide assistance, or because the regimens are too complex, difficult, or disruptive to family's lifestyle.
Dysfunctional grieving	The grieving process is normal after injury/trauma, especially when that injury has lasting effects. The inability to resolve the feeling of grief may result in a lack of physical progress and exhaustion of the patient and family. Patients may verbalize distress, guilt, anger, and, in general, may experience disruption of the usual patterns of living, eating, sleeping, and work.

care by the same nurse, a written plan of care becomes increasingly essential. If nurses use standardized care plans or guides, interventions directed at emotional/psychosocial issues should be listed along with other items.

Nurses should be rewarded for attending to patients' and families' emotional needs. Often, the outcome of the psychological intervention is not realized until long after the patient has left the intensive care unit. Skill in addressing and alleviating the patient's and family's emotional problems should be incorporated into the nursing career ladder along with technical skills. Critical care nurses also need to be allowed and encouraged to visit former patients as they recover on the general hospital units. This visiting allows the nurse to evaluate the effectiveness of her psychosocial interventions and reinforces their importance. Visiting with the critical care nurse also provides the patient with the opportunity to fill in blank areas of his memory and put the experience into perspective.

Intervention

Nursing interventions for critically ill patients and families involve three main areas for consideration—structuring the environment, sharing information, and providing emotional support.

Structuring the Environment

Monitoring Environmental Stimuli. Structuring or controlling the environment involves monitoring the amount and intensity of environmental stimuli reaching the patient. Stimuli easily amenable to restructuring include lowering the noise level of the unit, providing a light and dark cycle to promote sleep, condensing nursing activities so that the patient is minimally interrupted, and providing privacy for the patient. Calendars and clocks will help patients stay aware of the passage of time.

The pros and cons of restricted visiting hours in critical care areas continue to be debated. Proponents of limited visiting (for example, for 10 minutes of every 2 hours) believe that the patient is better able to rest without interruptions and that care is facilitated. Opponents of severely restricted hours believe that the nearness of loved ones promotes a more normal atmosphere and that patients are less likely to become disoriented and families less likely to become angry and suspicious.[14]

Providing Safety and Comfort. From the family's perspective, waiting rooms need to be geographically close to the patient and should have nearby bathrooms and comfortable chairs.[28] Although these may seem like minor points, they become very important to the family who waits for hours and days.

The patient and family need to feel safe in their new environment. The family may bring objects from home, such as pillows, pajamas, or pictures of loved ones, which will increase their feelings of being safe. These objects also make a statement about the patient as a person and reaffirm his personhood to himself and others.

Sharing Information

Because the way in which individuals and families cope with stress is based on the processing of information or stimuli, it is essential that caregivers share information with them. Nurses recognize the importance of sharing information with the patient and family. Nurses may not realize that, in addition to the data they share, they are conveying a sense that the loved one is being cared for by competent professionals. Nurses may assume that it is obvious that the ICU and its resources are top-rate, but the family has no such knowledge, and needs to be reassured that their family member is well cared for.[31] This sharing of information helps the individual define the problem, generate options, and think of consequences to those options. The sharing process also provides patients with feedback on their progress toward the achievement of their goals.

Preparing the Patient and Family. Information sharing begins at admission with a discussion of the hospital admitting procedure. Where to wait while the patient is undergoing surgery and how various members of the health care team function are examples of the information needed by family members to help them cope with hospitalization.[36]

Information shared with family members during the initial hours of treatment usually involves the patient's general condition, such as vital signs and comfort level, and an interpretation of that information. If the patient is scheduled for surgery, he and his family should be given information about the surgery and what to expect pre- and postoperatively. Although patients vary in their abilities to recall the information given preoperatively, they have a need to know.[32]

Sensory Preparation for Medical Events. The use of sensory information, coupled with relaxation measures, is a potent nursing intervention for helping patients cope with treatments and hospitalization.[20] Sharing information about how the treatment will look, taste, feel, sound, or smell prepares the patient for those sensations so that they are not alarming. For example, when a patient is going to ambulate after surgery, knowing that the incisional area usually feels tight to most postoperative patients helps him to interpret the sensation as "normal."

Facilitating the Patient's Move Out of Intensive Care.

When the patient is to be moved from the intensive care unit to another unit of the hospital, he may both welcome and dread the move. Although the move usually signifies an improvement in the patient's condition, it also means a loss of the now-familiar critical care area and relationships with the critical care nursing staff. Patients and their families become dependent on the staff and the physical environment of the ICU and express feelings of trust and security. At transfer to a general unit, they may feel ambivalent and anxious. Now they must learn a new staff and routine. It's not uncommon for them to feel that the new caregivers are less watchful and do not appreciate how ill the patient was and what the family has been through.[24] To ease the transfer, patients need to know, upon admission, that their stay in the intensive care unit is temporary, that the general medical or surgical unit is different from the intensive care unit, and that the plan of care formulated with the patient in intensive care will be continued, with modifications, on the other hospital unit.[24]

Probably the most effective nursing intervention is a combination of information-giving and caring.[29] Although sharing information assists the patient and family in problem-solving, caring and providing emotional support are also essential for patient healing.

Providing Emotional Support

The nurse's provision of emotional support helps the patient resolve the multiple responses to his injury or illness. The caring attitude softens any "bad news" or difficulties that the patient encounters. Patient goals include the following:

1. Maintenance of hope
2. Establishment of feelings of control
3. Grieving for losses
4. Reentry into the social world

Maintaining Hope.

The ability of a patient to maintain a feeling of hope is related to his level of trust; both help the individual face adverse times. It has been said that both trust and hope are strong enough to withstand truth.[44] These thoughts are useful to consider when the nurse is caring for a person or family who deny the seriousness or consequences of the illness.

Because the patient's denial is protective at this time, the nurse supports his response. On the other hand, the nurse realizes that inaccurate information undermines the patient's trust and shatters hope. If the nurse has established, through listening and sharing, a warm and caring relationship with the patient and family, this warmth will cushion the realities of their situation.

The patient's and family's need to be physically close to each other signifies hope in a tangible way.[8] Very often, patients remark, "I guess they're still there—they haven't given up on me yet." Tailoring visiting hours and supporting families when they spend the night with the injured patients are only two ways to foster hope. If there is no hope for survival, there can still be hope for peaceful death.

Maintaining Control.

The nurse helps the patient establish and maintain feelings of control by continually involving him and his family in decision-making and by informing them of areas in which they can be in control. Simple nursing measures, such as placing the call light and telephone within reach and in the patient's control, will alleviate some feelings of powerlessness. A call light that slips off the bed is terrifying to a patient. Minimal use of restraints, while ensuring patient safety, will also ensure feelings of control. If the patient is able to maintain a record of his breathing and leg exercises, intake and output, or turning, he will have a feeling of accomplishment and may be diverted from the stress of the injury through this activity.[6]

Mourning the Losses.

The patient's grief for losses incurred through his illness or injury may become evident as anger, hostility, or sad feelings. The explosive anger of the resistance phase is, in part, related to the patient's losses. Continuing anger of the patient may drive away family and hospital staff. The patient needs to know that his anger is understandable, but that the energy consumed by his anger might better be channeled into rehabilitation or constructive activities.

Vulnerability is, in a sense, precipitated by the patient's ineffective coping and diffusion of energy. The feeling of being open to hurt is distressing because the patient and family increase their surveillance and lose sight of the objectives of care. Nurses need to protect the individual from unwise energy expenditure and to reinstill the feeling of hope by acknowledging and praising any small increment of progress or lack of regression.

If the patient's losses entail a significant change in lifestyle—according to the patient's, not the staff's, perception—he will need to learn new ways of managing his resources of energy and supports. Perhaps, if the patient is a college professor, teaching a class of 100 students might be beyond his capabilities, but he might be able to manage a class of 25 students.

Probably the most important intervention to help patients deal with loss is to encourage them to ventilate their feelings and grief. Patients whose illness or injury leaves them very much unlike their former selves face a constant reminder of their loss; their families are also constantly reminded of the loss. The patient and family's mourning is not a once-and-forever thing.[45] Although patients may adapt to illness or handicap, most probably continue to wish for lost functions and abilities.

Reentering the Social World. Planning for discharge from the hospital or rehabilitation setting presents a new set of challenges for the patient and family. Nurses have always stated that discharge planning begins at admission but now, with new reinbursement policies, that saying is a reality. It is not unusual for families to express anger at the discharge planner and staff for discussing the subject or to feel anxious or not ready to leave. This discharge anxiety can be related to the following factors:

1. The family has not emotionally recovered from the event
2. The illness may have caused role changes—temporary or permanent–that the family members are grappling with
3. Care that was the staff's responsibility will now be the family's, and this care has become complex and highly technical
4. The patient and family must now refocus from the past, *i.e.,* the injury or illness, to the future, *i.e.,* active problem-solving
5. The financial effect of the illness is now being realized[3]

When the patient has progressed to leaving the hospital or rehabilitation center, he needs to rehearse for social situations. Most patients carefully decide whom they will see or visit while convalescing, and when they will allow visitors. For patients who have a lasting handicap or change in appearance, this rehearsal for reentry into society is vital.

If a disfiguring surgery, such as a mastectomy, is planned, the nurse and patient have the luxury of time to explore the significance of the body part to the patient and the meaning of the surgery, and to plan for the postoperative course. Unfortunately, this period of time to deal with the upcoming event is not possible when an individual undergoes trauma. The victim of trauma may not be aware of the extent of his injuries and the consequences of the trauma for some time after the accident. As he becomes aware of the extent and ramifications of his injury, he may retreat from social contacts. Patients and families benefit from visits from recovered patients and members of self-help groups, such as Reach to Recovery for mastectomized women. In these groups, patients can help and be helped by sharing common problems and concerns. These groups provide patients with hope, guidance, and an opportunity for catharsis.[35]

Evaluation

The ultimate effect of nursing interventions may be difficult to determine because much of the patient's healing continues after he is discharged from the health care setting. The establishment of a lifestyle satisfactory to the patient may or may not be possible. Realistic expectations for the patient probably exist somewhere between being locked into his anatomy, or limited by it, and the feeling that anything is possible.[45]

If good coping means good solutions for old problems, adequate solutions for new problems, and resourceful solutions for unexpected problems, then effective nursing measures elicit these adaptive responses.[44] Nursing intervention has been effective when the patient trusts, hopes, feels in control, and is ready to take on the world (or his portion of it). It is necessary to make early recognition of, assessment of, and intervention with patients and families who lack resources, are overwhelmed with stressors, or react in a rigid manner. These patients and families may need more intensive counseling continuing beyond hospitalization.

Effects on the Nurse

Working with people who are anxious, depressed, physically ill, or stressed by normal life events can be both exhilarating and draining to the nurse. When profession-related stressors are coupled with job-related stressors, such as rotating shifts, the result is devastating because of the energy drain on nurses. No area of nursing is immune from this energy drain, nor does this drain affect nurses in critical care areas more than on general medical or surgical units.[9]

Nurses need to provide the same supportive actions for themselves and each other that they provide for patients. The physiological indicators of professional stress syndrome include changes in eating habits, insomnia, lethargy, muscle tension, rashes, and gastrointestinal symptoms. Psychologically, the nurse feels disoriented, fragmented, frustrated, and indecisive. The nurse may exhibit angry, suspicious, or all-knowing behavior and may begin taking excessive risks.[9]

To prevent professional stress syndrome, nurses are encouraged to do the following things:

CHART 41-3
Moral and Ethical Dilemma

Patsy Keyser, M.S.N., R.N.
Director of Nursing
Nursing Resources/Oncology/Psychiatry
Methodist Medical Center
Dallas, Texas

The practice of nursing has experienced significant and thought-provoking changes in recent years. There have been astonishing advances in health care science and technology. This technological revolution highlights the likelihood that nurses' actions and potential actions may conflict with nursing's "human values" and with its notion of ethical appropriateness. Nurses today occupy a pivotal position in the ever-changing health care field. Of all health care providers, nurses are most directly involved in the day-to-day care of the patient; nurses mediate among patient, doctor, and health care institution.

Because of this critical and pivotal position, nurses experience conflicting loyalties, responsibilities, and expectations, often in situations where the lives of patients are the primary concern. Nurses face ethical conflicts and decisions for which their education has only partially prepared them and for which they receive little or no support from the institutions that employ them. Examples of moral or ethical dilemmas confronting nurses include the issues of allocation of scarce resources and of whether or not to resuscitate a patient—the issue, in fact, of life itself versus quality of life.

In these dilemmas, nurses continually ask, "Am I accountable to the patient, institution, physician, or myself?" Although nursing's code of professional ethics places emphasis on the nurse–patient relationship—that is, the nurse's obligation to the patient—this emphasis is difficult to maintain in practice. Nursing practice takes place within a complex interaction of social and political values. Because of the particular mix of obligations impinging upon them, nurses know that even when they practice responsibly, it is still possible to suffer recriminations or job loss. The dual position of professional and employee occupied by nurses makes it a struggle for them to preserve the autonomy needed for ethical decisions. These nursing problems are particularly important due to the nature of interpersonal relationships and patient contacts, for it is within the nurse-patient relationship that human interactions of practice are structured. Moral values that promote human dignity and welfare are incorporated into these relationships.

At a time when nursing education is more technical, the need for compassionate caring is increasing. As technology increases health care's impersonal approach, the need for an ethical dimension based in human concern increases in importance. This ethical dimension of care cannot be merely a question of competing rights and rules. Ethical issues are embedded in the very nature of social life, with its competing obligations, power, and resources. We cannot answer ethical questions from a set of principles without considering the values, behaviors, and kinds of power that condition our acting on these principles. Nursing in all settings must be actively concerned with making assessments of moral issues and gaining the autonomy necessary to make ethical decisions.

1. Become aware of the stresses in their lives
2. Establish peer group support
3. If possible, change work activities or settings
4. Pursue recreational interests
5. Set realistic goals
6. Attend conferences and seminars away from the hospital interruptions
7. Take and give credit for a job well done[7]

"Burnout" perpetuates more "burnout"; inadequate staffing perpetuates itself through a high level of nurse turnover. When they have fewer negative feelings with which to deal, nurses will have more energy for patient care and personal growth.

Summary

This chapter examines the stresses of, and responses to, major trauma, surgery, and critical illness. Some of the emphases of the chapter are as follows:

1. The assessment of the patient's response to

(Text continues on p. 792)

Case Study 41-1

Recovering from the Loss of a Limb

D. R. is a 70-year-old man who underwent an above-the-knee amputation secondary to arterial occlusion. Immediately after recovering from the anesthetic in the intensive care unit, he became confused and combative. Within 24 hours of surgery, he was alert and oriented to person, time, and place. He was returned to the general surgical unit where his vital signs and general medical status stabilized. Because of the extent of other concurrent medical conditions, however, D. R. was expected to have a prolonged hospital stay.

The loss of his leg rekindled feelings of other losses D. R. had experienced in his life—especially the loss of his beloved wife 5 years previously. He repeatedly recounted stories of their life together and of their three children. His feelings of grief affected how he felt about life in the hospital. He grieved over his loss of control over the environment, the meal selections, his daily schedule, visiting hours, and his lack of contact with friends. During this time, the loss of his leg with resultant loss of mobility, though temporary, seemed to him an insurmountable obstacle. He wished he had died.

D. R.'s personal turmoil influenced his perceptions of the caregivers. He was distrustful of them; he felt that they didn't know what they were doing and that they withheld information from him. He maintained close ties with one nurse, but even when this nurse talked with him, he continually increased the volume on the television. He later referred to these days as "those dark times."

His adjustment to his new body took many weeks. At first, he did not look at his stump or touch the dressings. Gradually, he began to supervise the dressing changes, but was not interested in more active participation for some time.

The turning point in his adaptation, or coming to terms with his surgery, began about 10 days postoperatively. Within one day, he felt relatively painfree, was given a peanut butter sandwich (his favorite food) for lunch, received out-of-town visitors, and began to work with a new physical therapist. In therapy, he saw others "in worse shape than I'm in," and those who were "just as bad as me, but getting somewhere."

The therapy sessions provided a means for him to measure his progress and encouraged his maximum effort. He throve on the challenge.

Then D. R. began to redefine what had happened to him. Perhaps, he said, he "could still golf after all." He began dressing his stump and became very assertive about his care. The time arrived for his discharge to a rehabilitation hospital.

The rehabilitation hospital was definitely not home but, because it encouraged self-care, D. R. could be responsible for himself. Although he complained about the "rules," he realized the benefits. He spoke of the "dark times" at the acute care hospital and began to place that experience in perspective. He recognized his capabilities and accepted help for what he was unable to do. He finally consented to allow his grandchildren to see him, because, he asserted, "I'm still the same old grandpa—even with only one leg."

D. R. was discharged from the rehabilitation hospital 8 weeks after his amputation. At that time, he had a prosthesis and was able to take care of himself very well. If he were granted one wish, he would still wish to have two legs, but he had gained a respect for "what I can do if I set my mind to it." His son, with whom he had never had a deep relationship, became his most fervent supporter. He began to establish new relationships with a few people in his neighborhood.

Discussion

D. R's recovery from an amputation of his leg reflects the course of hospitalization and resolution of grief of many trauma patients. The loss of his limb was compounded by the loss of his wife 5 years before the surgery. He suffered the effects of hospitalization and experienced loss of control over daily events. The nurses strove to reestablish his sense of control over the situation and provided information, emotional support, and even peanut butter sandwiches. The combined efforts of the nurses, other members of the medical team, D. R., and his family helped reduce his feelings of isolation and challenged and encouraged him to continue.

Nursing Care Plan 41-1

Responses to Trauma

Nursing Diagnosis	Client Outcome	Intervention
Sensory-perceptual alteration	Client will experience reduced sensory input	Decrease sensory stimulation—turn down lights, provide privacy, decrease number of people who come in contact with the patient Interpret meaning of sensory input to patient—explain how procedures will look, feel, taste, smell, sound; explain meaning of alarms
Hopelessness	Client will demonstrate a more hopeful attitude	Establish a relationship with patient through a calm, caring demeanor Encourage verbalization of feelings Reinstill feelings of hope, by acknowledgement of small increments of progress, or lack of regression Protect the patient's energy stores by providing rest, adequate nutrition, and pacing activities according to his capabilities Focus on small, easily tackled problems
Anxiety	Client will reestablish feelings of control	Identify aspects of care in patient's direct control—for instance, arrange room according to patient's desire, place call light and phone within reach, serve patient's food preferences *Together* plan the day, incorporating the patient's wishes Ask the family to bring into hospital patient's personal items from home
Dysfunctional grieving	Client and family will resolve their grieving	Establish trust and hope through an honest, caring relationship Acknowledge that the losses occurred Help the patient and family verbalize the meaning of losses Help generate options—what have the patient and family gained from this experience?
Disturbance in self-concept: body image	Client will experience a reopening of his social world	Plan a gradual widening of his social circle—initially, only family and very close friends permitted to visit, then other acquaintances Walk with the patient in the hall or to the hospital lobby Arrange for a visit by a self-help group of recovered patients for sharing and support

trauma, surgery, or critical illness depends on his usual coping methods, problem-solving ability, and conditioning factors, such as available supports, previous health status, developmental level, and cultural background.

2. The response to trauma or serious illness varies from individual to individual, but generally follows a course of shock or impact, through resistance to, it is hoped, resolution.

3. Some of the emotional responses of patients to injury or critical illness include denial, body image disturbances, feelings of loss of control, vulnerability, angry outbursts, and grief.

4. Family members of the critically ill patient also experience overwhelming anxiety, denial, anger, and rage.

5. Psychosocial interventions should be incorporated in the plan of care for the critically ill patient and his family, beginning with the patient's entrance into the hospital.

6. The focus of nursing intervention is the promotion of hope, control, trust, appropriate grieving, and reentry into the social world through sharing information, structuring the environment, and supporting the individual and family.

7. To provide optimal care to the injured or seriously ill, the nurse also needs to care for herself and accept peer support and recognition.

References

1. Antonovsky A: Health, Stress, and Coping. San Francisco, Jossey-Bass Publishers, 1979
2. Auden WH: Selected Poetry of W. H. Auden. New York, Modern Library, 1958
3. Blazyk S, Canavan M: Managing the Discharge Crisis Following Catastrophic Illness or Injury. Soc Work Health Care 11 (Summer): 19–32, 1986
4. Eisendrath S: ICU Syndrome Revisited. Critical Care Update! 9 (May): 31–35, 1982
5. Epperson M: Families in Sudden Crisis. Soc Work Health Care 2 (Spring): 265–273, 1977
6. Gal R, Lazarus R: The Role of Activity in Anticipating and Confronting Stressful Situations. J Human Stress 1(4):4–19, 1975
7. Gardner E, Hall R: The Professional Stress Syndrome. Psychosomatics 22 (August): 672–680, 1981
8. Geary M: Supporting Family Coping. Supervisor Nurse 10 (March): 52–59, 1979
9. Gentry WD, Parkes K: Psychologic Stress in Intensive Care Unit and Non-Intensive Care Unit Nursing. Heart Lung 11 (January–February): 43–47, 1982
10. Giacquinta B: Helping Families Face the Crisis of Cancer. Am J Nurs 77 (October): 1585–1588, 1977
11. Goosen G, Bush H: Adaptation: A Feedback Process. Advances In Nursing Science 1 (July): 51–66, 1979
12. Gordon M: Manual of Nursing Diagnosis. New York, McGraw-Hill, 1982
13. Gunta K: The Assessment of Losses Related to the Immobility of Orthopedic Patients. Master's Paper, Marquette University, Milwaukee, Wisconsin, 1981
14. Heater B: Nursing Responsibilities in Changing Visiting Restrictions in the Intensive Care Unit. Heart Lung 14 (March): 181–186, 1985
15. Helton MC, Gordon SH, Lunnery SL: The Correlation Between Sleep Deprivation and the Intensive Care Unit Syndrome. Heart Lung 9 (May–June): 464–468, 1980
16. Henkler F: Body-Image Conflict Following Trauma and Surgery. Psychosomatics 20 (December): 812–820, 1979
17. Hohmann G: Psychological Aspects of Treatment and Rehabilitation of the Spinal Cord Injured Person. Clin Orthop 112 (October): 81–87, 1975
18. Holmels TH, Rohe RH: The Social Readjustment Rating Scale. J Psychosom Res 11:213–218, 1967
19. Howard A, Scott R: A Proposed Framework for the Analysis of Stress in the Human Organism. Behav Sci 10:141–160, 1965
20. Johnson J, Fuller SS, Endress MP, Rice V: Alluring Patients' Responses to Surgery: An Extension and Replication. Res Nurs Health 1 (May–June): 111–121, 1978
21. Kolb L: Modern Clinical Psychiatry. Philadelphia, WB Saunders, 1977
22. Krupnick J, Horowitz M: Stress Response Syndromes. Arch Gen Psychiatry 38 (April): 428–435, 1981
23. Kuch K, Swinson RP, Kirby M: Post-traumatic Stress Disorder After Car Accidents. Can J Psychiatry 30 (October): 426–427, 1985
24. Lawson CA, Werner R, Nugent SK: Parental Stress During and After Pediatric ICU Hospitalization. Indiana Med 78 (May): 372–375, 1985
25. Lenehan GP: Emotional Impact of Trauma. Nurs Clin North Am 21 (December): 729–740, 1986
26. Lazarus R: Positive Denial: The Case for Not Facing Reality. Psychology Today 13 (November), 44–60, 1979
27. Mattsson E: Psychological Aspects of Severe Physical Injury and Its Treatment. J Trauma 15 (March): 217–234, 1975
28. Molter N: Needs of Relatives of Critically Ill Patients. Heart Lung 8 (March–April): 332–338, 1979
29. Mumford E, Schlesinger H, Glass G: The Effects of Psychological Intervention on Recovery from Surgery And Heart Attacks. Am J Public Health 72 (February): 141–151, 1982
30. Nadelson S: The Psychiatrist in the Surgical Intensive Care Unit. Arch Surg 111 (February): 113–117, 1976
31. Norris LO, Grove Sk: Investigation of Selected Psychosocial Needs of Family Members of Critically Ill

Adult Patients. Heart Lung 15 (March): 194–199, 1986

32. Reading A: Psychological Preparation for Surgery. J Psychosom Res 25:57–62, 1981

33. Ryden MB: Energy: A Crucial Consideration In The Nursing Process. Nursing Forum 16:71–82, 1977

34. Seligman M: Helplessness. San Francisco, WH Freeman, 1975

35. Scarlon-Schilpp A, Levesque J: Helping The Patient Cope with the Sequelae of Trauma. J Trauma 21 (February): 135–139, 1981

36. Selva MC: Effects of Orientation Information on Spouses' Anxieties and Attitudes toward Hospitalization and Surgery. Res Nurs Health 2, 127–136, 1979

37. Smilkstein G: The Family Apgar. J Fam Pract 6 (June): 1231–1239, 1978

38. Smith M, Selye H: Reducing the Negative Effects of Stress. Am J Nurs 79 (November): 1954–1957, 1979

39. Stephenson C: Stress in the Critically Ill Patient. Am J Nurs 77 (November): 1806–1811, 1977

40. Tomlinson W: Psychiatric Complications following Severe Trauma. J Occup Med 16 (July): 451–454, 1974

41. Vollicer B: Hospital Stress and Patient Reports of Pain and Physical Status. J Human Stress 4 (June): 28–37, 1978

42. Vollicer B, Burns M: Pre-existing Correlates of Hospital Stress. Nurs Res 26 (November–December): 408–415, 1977

43. Waechter EH: Dying Children, Patterns of Coping. Issues Comp Ped Nurs 8, 1–6, 51–68, 1985

44. Weisman A: Coping with Cancer. New York, McGraw-Hill, 1979

45. Zola CK: Denial of Emotional Needs to People with Handicaps. Arch Phys Med Rehabil 63 (February): 63–67, 1982

42

The Child at Risk: Illness, Disability, and Hospitalization

Sally Francis

Whenever I approach a child his presence inspires two feelings in me. Affection for what he is now, and respect for what he may one day become.

Louis Pasteur

There is virtue in the search for some form of precise intervention, but there remains the discomforting awareness that the future environmental demands that all children must face, whatever their degree of vulnerability to psychopathology, are so great that a broader program of intervention seems necessary. Skill and competence develop, as Bruner has observed, by small daily accretions of experience from infancy throughout childhood. Such skills lead to new mastery, and this, in turn, encourages the development of other skills that generate a deep competence that may be the necessary inoculant that stays the ravaging effects of disorder.

Norman Garmezy,
in Anthony EJ,
Koupernik C (eds):
The Child in His Family:
Children at Psychiatric Risk,
1974

794

Chapter Preview

This chapter focuses on a child's illness, disability, and hospitalization, events in a child's life which place him and his family at risk for psychosocial disturbance and disruption to ongoing development. Because a child is an integral part of a family, the adaptation required in response to the stresses of illness will be influenced by, and required of, the family as well as the child. The interaction between nurse, parent, and child is foremost in the delivery of nursing care to the child. The nursing process—assessment, nursing diagnosis, planning, intervention, and evaluation—supports the child's and family's positive adaptation to these crisis events.

Communication and self-understanding are essential to the nurse's personal coping with the illness of a child and to the nurse's professional role of assisting the child and family at risk. Additionally, the nurse's role as an advocate for the child and family within the health care environment is discussed.

Learning Objectives

On completion of the chapter, you should be able to accomplish the following:

1. Discuss the overlay of illness, disability, and hospitalization on the developmental needs of children
2. Describe the influences of hospitalization, parent–child attachment, and communication on the child's and family's positive adaptation
3. Apply the nursing process to the care of ill, disabled, or hospitalized children

    Assess the child's developmental level, environmental influences on the child (including the child's family), and idiosyncratic attributes of the child

    Discuss the concepts of trust, understanding, and mastery, on which the nurse bases nursing plans and interventions

    Formulate nursing diagnoses for children at risk due to illness, disability, or hospitalization

    Evaluate the psychosocial care of physically ill, disabled, or hospitalized children and their families

4. Describe the nurse's role of advocacy for children in health care and for their families
5. Discuss the nurse's use of personal coping measures and collegial support in the provision of psychosocial care to children at risk due to illness, disability, or hospitalization

Development and the Overlay of Illness, Disability, and Hospitalization

All individuals arrive at adulthood having developed from the dependency of an infant who must rely on the external world for survival. Successful passage through the phases of development leads to a sense of the self as both separate from the external environment and capable of using the external world to provide for one's own survival. The individual becomes self-reliant, as well as interdependent with others in the environment. This is accomplished through the years of childhood as the individual acquires skills and resolves developmental crises.[30]

The crises of illness, disability, and hospitalization are frequently added to the normal, although monumental, developmental vicissitudes. These events may place the individual at risk not only for physical survival, but also for successfully managing the developmental tasks that lead to satisfying, productive adulthood.

The events of illness, disability, and hospitalization place the child at risk, but they also provide opportunities for the child and family to acquire skills for coping with, mastering, and adapting to stress.[19,52] The stresses on the child are also stresses experienced by the family.[55,69,106]

A developing child is an integral part of a family unit; the stresses of illness, disability, and hospitalization are disruptions for the family as well as for the child; for example, the family's daily routines are altered by trips to the health care setting. The parents' relationship is altered by sleeping arrangements and family responsibilities divided between home and hospital. Siblings experience disruptions as they become secondary to the ill child and are cared for by neighbors or relatives.[53,55,60,65] Hospital bills, medication costs, and time off work result in unusual financial strains on the family. As one child takes on the patient role, other family members shift in their roles and functions within the family.[64] These disruptions in the family's daily living, routines, and roles require adaptation by all members of the family.

Adaptation becomes more complex when the illness represents a chronic condition or disability. The family unit must make ongoing adjustments with each phase of the child's illness.[96] Consider the family in which a child is diagnosed with leukemia. At the time of diagnosis of the disease, there is an acute phase of stress and disequilibrium. The family begins adjusting with the onset of remission of the child's illness. As the remission extends over time, the family adapts; however, disruption occurs again when the child relapses, necessitating adjustment that may be followed by another period of the disease's remission. Stress, disequilibrium, adjustment, and adaptation may take place several times as the disease process and treatments continue.[55, 110]

When the chronic illness or disability extends over months and years, the child and family must make new adjustments and adaptations with each developmental phase through which the child passes.[45, 47, 50, 63] For example, the child with congenital abnormalities must cope with disruptions in daily living resulting from staged surgical corrections, while the evolving processes of body image, sexual identification, self-esteem, and mastery take on different emphases with each stage of psychosexual development. This overlay of illness on developmental behaviors is also seen when the usual storm and stress of adolescence is compounded in the child with diabetes who uses noncompliance with treatment as a vehicle for expressing typical adolescent rebellion.[23]

The parents' feelings of grief and guilt for what the child is, or could have been, further complicate the family's adaptation. The family may mourn the loss of the fantasized child. The family's feelings about the disability and perceptions of the stresses influence its adjustment to the stressors.[96] The support available to the family and the understanding and acceptance of their feelings also influence adaptation.

Adaptation is the end state of adjusting to the changes brought about by the illness, disability, and hospitalization. How the child and family perceive the stress influences their manner of coping. The nurse affects the perceptions, understandings, and responses to stress of the child and family and, subsequently, their adaptation. By providing support and assistance in the mastery of stress, the nurse mediates the adaptive responses of the family. To facilitate this help for the family, the nurse must understand the effects of hospitalization, parent–child attachment, and communication as factors influencing the child at risk.

Hospitalization

Whether as a mental health consultant or as a pediatric clinician, the nurse often becomes involved with a child and family on admission into the hospital. Admissions generally take one of the following three forms:

1. Emergency admissions for which there is little time for advance preparation
2. Planned admissions for elective events, such as diagnostic work-ups and surgery
3. Episodic admissions; that is, one of multiple hospitalizations for a chronic condition

Entry into the health care system is a time of stress for the child and family. The amount of stress experienced by the child and family and the opportunities for mediation of the stress vary with the type of admission. The nurse has a greater opportunity to initiate planned interventions with a child's planned or episodic admissions than with emergency admissions.

Admission to the hospital carries the potential for psychological upset, which will have a disruptive effect on the child's development (see Chart 42-1, "The Psychosocial Needs of Children in Hospitals"). This disruption, in fact, occurs in about 25% of all pediatric hospitalizations. Children with multiple admissions during the first 4 years of life are the most vulnerable to the effects of psychological upset; however, another 25% of children admitted to the hospital appear to benefit psychologically from hospitalization. The remaining 50% of children admitted into hospitals are neither unusually negatively affected nor benefited psychologically, by hospitalization.[24, 89, 90, 118, 120]

The statistics just mentioned affirm an imperative of pediatric health care—to examine a child's experiences in hospitalization. The goal of this examination is to minimize the potential negative psychological effects and to maximize the opportunities for psychological benefit from hospitalization. Benefits can occur when the child and family view hospitalization as a stressful event that can result in positive adaptation, an event which can lead to growth in self-confidence, self-esteem, and mastery. As hospitalization supports the physical well-being of the child, it can support—and can, in fact, enhance—the child's emotional well-being.

Hospitalization at the time of initial diagnosis of a chronic illness or disability begins the process of adjustment for the family. Whether diagnosis is made at the time of the child's birth or later, the family experiences initial feelings of shock and disbelief. Disruption occurs and adjustment begins. The Rochester Child Health Group conducted extensive studies of families with children with chronic conditions and families of well children and proposed that early identification of families at risk for successful adaptation is an essential intervention to assist the child with a chronic condition.[97] One scale, devised to detect families at risk, rates components of psychosocial family functioning to identify the risk factors for the family with a chronically ill child.[61]

Recent research on protective factors, in addition to risk factors, has focused on *resilience*—the individual response to risk.[101] Three broad sets of variables have been identified as protective factors for children. They are personality features, as in self-esteem; family cohesion and absence of discord; and

C H A R T   42-1
The Psychosocial Needs of Children in Hospitals

A Historical Perspective

Reports of hospital conditions during the first part of the 20th century described stringent aseptic conditions, enforced to counteract the threat of untreatable cross-infections. In these hospitals, children were isolated from one another, contact with staff was restricted, and parents were permitted very limited visiting.

The studies of maternal-child separations in the 1940s by Rene Spitz and Anna Freud brought the term *maternal deprivation* into focus. James Robertson, a colleague of Anna Freud, applied the study of mother–child separations to hospitalized children. His findings, published in 1958, documented adverse effects of hospitalization on children and brought about reforms in pediatric care in English hospitals.

In the United States, interest in the emotional care of hospitalized children developed throughout the 1950s. Impetus came from the first major United States study to document the psychological effects of hospitalization on children. Conducted by Dane Prugh in Boston, the study found that adverse psychological disturbance resulting from a child's hospitalization could be mediated by unlimited parental visiting, provision of play and preparation programs for children, and support of staff and parents.

Research and clinical concern continued in the 1960s and led to the formation of a multidisciplinary organization focused on the psychosocial needs of children in health care—the Association for the Care of Children in Hospitals.

(In 1980, the name of this organization was changed to the Association for the Care of Children's Health to reflect changing patterns of health care, such as the expanded role of outpatient care in chronic illness.)

The thrust of research from the mid-1960s through the 1970s focused on the use of preparation to decrease children's anxiety in health care. Clinical settings also developed or expanded therapeutic play programs as means of providing emotional support to children. The development of the clinical nurse specialist role and primary nursing in pediatrics further strengthened the provision of care based on the developmental needs of children. Research studies by Douglas, reported in 1975, and a supporting study by Quinton and Rutter documented the prolonged trauma experienced by some children as a result of hospitalization and identified children at psychiatric risk.

Unfortunately, the research findings of the past 3 decades have not found uniform expression in the organization and delivery of health care to hospitalized children in the 1980s. Concern for the psychosocial needs of children and families expressed in the provision of play and preparation programs, rooming-in, primary nursing, and clinical nurse specialists has yet to become common to all pediatric settings. However, a growing awareness of the need for family-centered care in the late 1980s and 1990s may bridge the gaps in pediatric health care.

the availability of external support systems that encourage and reinforce a child's coping efforts.[42] The identification of families at risk turns attention to the child who is hospitalized and to efforts to support protective factors.

Parent–Child Attachment

Research evidence clearly indicates the necessity for the presence of the child's primary emotional support figure during the hospitalization.[12,94,111] The anxiety aroused in the child by unfamiliar surroundings and people and by painful events is secondary to the anxiety aroused by separation from his primary object relation. Although this is evident for young children, it is also applicable to older children for whom re-

gression is a normal response to the physical and emotional demands of illness and hospitalization.[27,41] Providing emotional support to the child must begin with efforts to continue the support provided by the child's primary attachment. Except in unusual instances, this primary attachment is to the parents, particularly the mother.

On admission of the child into health care, the nurse plays an important role in the continuance of the parent–child attachment. The nurse explains to the parents the need for *rooming-in;* that is, allowing the parents unlimited stay in the child's room. The nurse refers the parents to the social work department to acquire financial assistance, or to other services, such as child care, that will make the parents' rooming-in possible.

After assuring continuation of the parent–child attachment, the nurse next directs her efforts toward decreasing the parents' anxiety.[14,31,35,47,50,70,76] Young children mirror the anxiety of their parents. Interventions to reduce the parents' distress result in the reduction of a child's anxiety.[80,108,128]

The nursing process is based on the child's needs and the parents' ability to meet the health care and emotional needs of their child. This is not always as easy as it appears. The nurse continually examines her personal feelings toward the parents. For example, it may be easier to provide comfort and support to a 2-year-old child who has ingested cleaning fluid than to be supportive of the negligent parents; however, the parents' perceptions of health care, formulated during this initial hospitalization, will influence the family's positive adaptation to future multiple admissions, surgical procedures, and clinic visits. The acceptance and support offered to the parents by the nurse help them clarify their own feelings of guilt. This may lead to greater receptiveness to the nurse's instructions for home care and to role-modeling and education promoting more effective parenting, limit-setting, and discipline for their child.

The nurse who does not acknowledge her own feelings of blame toward the parents may unconsciously exclude them from participation in the child's physical and emotional care. As the parents become increasingly uncomfortable in the climate provided by the nurse, they may withdraw from the nurse's efforts at instruction and, perhaps, withdraw from their child. By ignoring or discounting feelings evoked by the parents, the nurse unwittingly sabotages her own efforts to implement the nursing process and to promote the child's adaptation.

Communication

The nurse conveys attitudes and feelings that influence the behavior of the recipients of care. Communication is a key element in caring for children at risk from illness, disability, and hospitalization.[2,67] Verbal communications convey warmth, acceptance, empathy, and caring; however, the communication of these attitudes through nonverbal means is more important.

The nurse has many functions and duties to perform in pediatrics. These activities include the administration of drugs, therapies, treatments, and other tasks relating to machines and equipment. How the nurse performs these functions communicates a level of caring that influences the child's and family's coping. For instance, the necessary physical restraint of a child during a lumbar puncture can convey caring and support of the child's efforts, however limited,

for self-control, or can indicate punitive retaliation against the child's actions, which are judged as willfully immature and hostile. The difference is observed in the nurse's physical handling of the child, tone of voice, and facial expressions. Through these communications, the nurse can convey a supportive, humanistic concern for the child as a person or can convey a mechanical, task-oriented outlook, in which the child is perceived as an object to be controlled. The former attitude is health-inducing, because it promotes the child's coping with stress; the latter attitude, in its dehumanization of the child, adds to the child's psychological stress and places him at further risk.

Successful communication with a child and family is built on an understanding of their problems, needs, and strengths obtained from the nursing assessment, and on the recognition and acceptance of personal feelings and attitudes.

Application of the Nursing Process to the Child at Risk Due to Illness, Disability, and Hospitalization

Each child and family are different from all others. Each course of hospitalization of a child differs from others. There are many physical diagnoses and concomitant treatments. The degree of physical disability and psychological distress resulting from illness varies from child to child.

The complexity of facts and possibilities and the feelings they arouse may overwhelm us; however, by keeping the goal—minimizing psychosocial distress in pediatric nursing—in focus, the nurse maintains and acts on the commitment to children at risk from illness, disability, and hospitalization. The nurse assists the child's and family's positive adaptation by performing tasks within the perspective of providing emotional support. The nursing process provides a framework within which information is organized and nursing intervention is planned.

Assessment of the Child

The nurse has an opportunity to assist the child and family in defining the stressors as opportunities for growth, rather than as events that are overwhelming, beyond personal control, and leading to disorganization and disturbance.[62,129] How the nurse best supports the child's positive adaptation is addressed through the nursing process, beginning with the first step, assessment.

The goal of assessment is to gather and organize

information in such a way that it assists the nurse in caring for the child at risk in health care. The assessment incorporates information about the child, the family, and the resources available in the health care setting (see Chart 42-2, "Assessment Outline").

Developmental Level

The assessment of the child begins with an understanding of the child's developmental level. What psychosocial issues is the child dealing with?[30] How does the child process events and information? What fears, general and specific to health care, are typical of children at a particular age?[4,9,11,32,78] (Chart 42-3 lists common fears and anxieties of children in health care.) Chronological age, combined with an understanding of theories of psychosexual, ego, and cognitive development, provides guidelines for nursing assessment.[39,40,46,79,83]

Environmental Influences

Environmental influences affecting the child's response to the stresses of illness, disability, and hospitalization are assessed by gathering information about the child's specific illness or disability, his previous life experiences, and his family.[35,74,109]

Nature of the Illness or Disability. Research has not substantiated a causal relationship between a specific illness or disability and a psychological disorder in a child. Nevertheless, knowledge about specific diagnoses does provide the nurse with information about the typical kind of hospitalization that is required, treatments that are prescribed, and medical

---

CHART 42-2
Assessment Outline

> **I.** Assessment of the child
>   **A.** Developmental level
>   **B.** Environmental influences
>   **1.** Specific illness or disability
>   **2.** Child's previous life experiences
>   **3.** Child's family
>   **C.** Idiosyncratic (personal) attributes
> **II.** Assessment of the health care setting
>   **A.** Resources in the physical environment
>   **B.** Departmental and program resources
>   **C.** Resources in the affective environment

---

events that the child will encounter. Furthermore, the nurse's knowledge of the illness or disability gives her indications about the pain and physical discomfort, about the type and number of intrusive procedures that the child will experience, and about the changes in the child's appearance—outward physical signs of the disease or disability and required treatments—to which the child and family must adjust.[86,105,110]

The nature of the child's illness or disability gives the nurse information about the acuteness or chronicity involved, information about the probable number of hospital admissions required, and some indication of prognosis for life expectancy. This and other information related to a specific illness or disability has implications for the nurse in planning and carrying out interventions to support the child's adaptation.[35]

Previous Life Experiences. The child's response to the stress of illness and hospitalization at a given point in time is influenced by prior experiences, particularly those perceived as stressful. For some young children, hospitalization may be the first stressful experience encountered by the child and family. The repertoire of responses and skills available to the child will therefore be limited because there has been little prior need for, or practice with, responding to stress.

Other children may have had many opportunities to develop coping skills in response to stress. The child whose family moved a great distance 2 months prior to the child's hospitalization, or whose mother began full-time work after giving birth to the family's second child, will certainly have had practice with coping. Despite their suggested callousing effects, these recent changes in the child's life may intensify the child's vulnerability and feeling of insecurity.

Previous stressful life experiences may influence the child's perception of the immediate stress. What, for example, is the possible meaning of hospitalization to a 10-year-old girl whose maternal aunt died in a hospital, 3 months earlier, with cancer? Knowing about the child's previous life experiences that are perceived as stressful by the child and family assists the nurse in understanding the child's responses to the immediate stress and affects her plans and interventions.

The Child's Family. The greatest environmental influence in the life of a child is the child's family. The family constellation, the ability to organize daily activities, the socioeconomic level, the cultural–ethnic makeup, and the previous life experiences of the family have implications for the delivery

CHART 42-3
Common Fears and Anxieties of Children in Health Care

Developmental Phase	Fears, Anxieties
Infancy	Separation anxiety
Toddlers	Separation anxiety
	Fear of the unknown
	Fear of strangers
Preschool Ages	Separation anxiety
	Anxiety about body intrusions, intense need for body intactness
	Anxieties aroused by egocentric thought, fantasies, magical thinking
	Fear of punishment aroused by guilt, as child feels he is the cause of the illness or disability
	Fear of body mutilation
School-age	Fear of body injury
	Fear of pain
	Fear of loss of respect, love, and emerging self-esteem
	Anxiety related to guilt continues
	Fear of anesthesia
Adolescence	Fear of loss of identity and control
	Anxiety about body image and changes in physical appearance
	Fear of loss of status in peer group
	Anxiety related to long-term implications of illness or disability

of nursing care to the child.[1, 16, 54, 99, 109] Several of these factors relate to the child's vulnerability to psychological disturbance resulting from hospitalization. For example, children from chaotic, disorganized families experiencing chronic family stresses—referred to as families with high psychosocial disadvantage—have the greatest risk for psychiatric disturbance resulting from hospitalization.[24, 90]

Assessment of the family's cultural–ethnic orientation has obvious implications for the delivery of nursing care.[10, 56] What language does the family speak? What language can they read? Can they understand the language that the nurse speaks? Perhaps less obvious are the cultural implications for behavioral responses to health care. For example, in families with strong hispanic orientations, it is more difficult for a mother to remain with her child in the hospital and to make decisions if she is not accompanied by her husband.[68]

The religious orientation of families and strong ties with a particular religion influence a family's perceptions and coping with stresses of illness. For exam-

ple, the refusal of blood transfusions by members of Jehovah's Witnesses may complicate medical care and increase the anxiety of staff, which, in turn, compounds the stress of the family.

The previous life experiences of the family will alert the nurse to changes to which the family may still be adjusting and which may have depleted their resources for dealing with the stress of the child's illness. Of particular concern is information about loss and grief. Is the family mourning the illness or death of a significant person at the time of the child's hospitalization? How emotionally available are the parents and family members to the child as the child experiences the stresses of illness, disability, and hospitalization?

The mother of an 18-month-old child was observed sleeping throughout the remainder of the day of the child's admission to the hospital and the following day. The mother seldom roused when the child cried or fretted. In talking with the mother, the nurse explored possible reasons for the extended sleep.

Suspecting a depressive reaction, the nurse

questioned the mother about recent events in the family's life. Although there had not been other illness in the family, the mother's aunt, a close emotional support to her, had died immediately in a car accident 2 days previously. This information not only assisted the nurse's assessment and plans for care of the child, it also facilitated the nurse's interaction with, and personal reactions to, the family. The information enabled the nurse to extend empathy and acceptance to the mother, rather than to judge her a "bad" mother because she was unresponsive to her child.

Idiosyncratic (Personal) Attributes of the Child

Assessment of the developmental level of the child and the environmental influences on the child must be augmented with an understanding of the child as an individual. What is the temperament and personality of the child?[20,116] Does the child typically move toward new experiences or is he shy? What is the child's pain tolerance?[26,105] What coping mechanisms does he use to defend against stress?[80,127] What words does the child use to refer to body parts and functions? Does he have a transitional object that provides comfort, such as a blanket or doll? What are the child's preferences—dietary, play activities, nap and bedtime routines? By what name does he prefer to be called? What was he like prior to the illness; that is, his premorbid personality? Answers to these questions will be unique to each child. Gathering and analyzing information about the child specific to his personality and temperament increases the nurse's understanding of the child and the child's responses to the stressors in illness, disability, and hospitalization.[57] It also allows the nurse to implement nursing actions in ways that minimize the strangeness of the health care setting and convey to the child and family the nurse's deep commitment to the child as a person, not an object, in health care.

The nurse analyzes the assessment data to determine the health problems of child and family and to formulate nursing diagnoses. Analysis also helps the nurse understand and clarify personal feelings toward a child and family. Understanding that a child's physical expression of anger is a typical response of 2-year-olds, that a child's refusal to find comfort in the nurse's arms is usual when he is initially reacting to separation anxiety, and that this particular child is described as "a difficult baby" by the mother helps the nurse remain supportive of the child. Through understanding based on assessment of the child, the nurse remains supportive, rather than withdrawing due to personalizing the child's rejection of her nursing efforts.

Assessment of the Health Care Setting

The Physical Environment

A final aspect of assessment that influences the implementation of the nursing process is the health care setting's ability to meet the psychosocial needs of the child and family. What resources are provided by the physical environment?[75] What departmental or program resources are available? Finally, what is the affective environment of the health care setting? The assessment of the child and family is combined with an assessment of the health care setting's ability to provide for the needs of the child; this total assessment affects the plans and interventions of the nurse.

No setting is ideal. All hospitals and health care settings have assets and limitations that affect the delivery of care to patients. One setting may be particularly supportive of the needs of young children, but meet few of the typical needs of adolescents. For example, the pediatric unit may have a large playroom but no space that affords privacy or peer interaction for the teenagers. If there are limited provisions for rooming-in, what will the nurse have to do to make the parent comfortably available to the child? If there is not a playroom on the pediatric unit, what can the nurse improvise as space for children to be actively engaged in constructive play?

Department and Program Resources

Departments within the health care setting offer resources the nurse utilizes in planning care. For example, the dietary department assists in meal planning to meet individual preferences; this will both enhance the child's nutritional intake and provide more familiar, comfortable mealtimes. The social work department provides financial referrals for families and support and counseling for parents. The child life–child development department (sometimes known as play therapy or children's activities departments) provides developmental assessments, supervised play and activities based on assessments, and support for children's understanding and mastery of the health care experience.[21] The volunteer department is available as "parent surrogates" for children whose parents must return to work. Foster grandparent programs are used in this capacity in many children's hospitals in the United States.

The Affective Environment

A final consideration is the affective environment of the health care setting. Does the formal philosophy of the health care setting and nursing department emphasize the psychosocial needs of children and families? Does the informal group attitude welcome parents or feel they are a nuisance? How much support will the nurse receive from the other staff and departments as she tries to meet the psychosocial needs of families?[7,71] The answers to these questions help the nurse plan for the time and energy she must expend as she integrates psychosocial care into the physical care of children.

Nursing Diagnosis

The nurse caring for the child who is physically ill or disabled and his family uses the assessment data to formulate nursing diagnoses that guide intervention. Appropriate diagnoses for the child may be as follows:

Alteration in growth and development related to prolonged or repeated hospitalizations, chronic illness, physical disability

Fear related to invasive and/or painful procedures, inadequate comprehension of the medical event, lack of opportunity to use medical play to work through the procedure or event, parental anxiety

Ineffective individual coping related to overwhelming stimuli of medical environment, lack of comprehension of the medical experience

Ineffective family coping: compromised, related to serious illness of child, separation of siblings during child's hospitalization, absence of parent from home while staying with hospitalized child

Deficit in diversional activity related to separation from home and usual activities, separation from siblings and peer group, restrictions of illness/disability and treatment

Planning

Development of Trust, Understanding, and Mastery

Treatment plans are drawn from the information provided in the assessment of the child and family and the health care setting. The process of planning includes setting of goals, utilization of resources, and discharge planning.

Three concepts are common to the processes involved in planning for the child at risk—trust, understanding, and mastery. If the nurse uses these concepts in planning and organizing interventions, the psychosocial needs of the child and family will be integrated into nursing care.

The nurse must ask, How can I assist in the child's and family's development of trust? How can I assist in their understanding? How can I assist in their development of mastery of the stresses they encounter in health care? What goals can I establish around these concepts? How can I plan to utilize the resources

available to assist in their trust, understanding, and mastery? What discharge plans are necessary to continue their mastery? These concepts of trust, understanding, and mastery are essential to nursing planning and interventions that support psychosocial needs.

Goal-Setting

Without goals, the nurse has limited knowledge and limited ability to direct the nursing process. Although treatment plans for physical care of pediatric diagnoses may be standardized in some settings, plans for psychosocial care cannot be standardized. The interplay between the diagnosis, the child, the family, and the health care setting necessitates individualization of treatment plans. The nurse plans the performance of required physical care in an emotionally supportive manner.

Although treatment plans should not be standardized, they should share some common goals. The primary goal should be to minimize the potential for psychosocial disturbance in the child as the state of physical health is being restored or supported. A second goal should be to maximize the opportunities for psychosocial benefit as the state of the child's physical well-being is restored or supported. A further goal common to treatment plans in pediatrics should be to help the child develop trust, understanding, and mastery of the stressful experiences in health care.

Goals specific to an individual child and family, which may lead to positive adaptation, should also be made in the planning process.[14,35,76] These goals should include the utilization of resources available in the health care setting.

> A 5-year-old child is admitted for intravenous antibiotic therapy to treat cystic fibrosis. The admission is one of many admissions the child has experienced; the hospital and treatment are familiar to the child; however, the child has great difficulty with intrusive procedures. As the nurse plans for the child's care, a specific goal for this child will be "to develop positive coping with intrusive procedures." Resources available in this particular setting that the nurse plans to utilize are primary nursing assignments and the child life–child development program.

Primary nursing facilitates the child's development of trust. The formation of a therapeutic alliance with the primary nurse assists the child in perceiving intrusive procedures as necessary steps to feeling better, rather than as retaliation or punishment. The child life–child development program provides unhurried opportunities for the child to play out feelings and anxieties aroused by medical procedures. This play, often referred to as *medical play,* facilitates the child's mastery of aggressive, angry feelings. The presence of the child life specialist during medical play provides support and boundaries for the child's expression of feelings.

Discharge Planning

Discharge planning begins with the assessment of the child and continues throughout hospitalization. For example, instructing parents in home care is most successful when a therapeutic alliance has been formed with the family, a process which begins on admission. The child's specific illness or disability may dictate particular referrals needed. Informing the child and family about the referral, the particular agency, or the treatment provides preparation for discharge. Discharge planning also includes preparing the family for changes in the child's behavior, those that are specific to the diagnosis or expected as common reactions to hospitalization.[36,76] Discharge plans should also include follow-up contact to assess the child's adjustment and any concerns of the parents.

Finally, discharge planning should include the concept of closure; that is, the ending of an experience marked by a sense of resolution, which can include feelings expressed by the individuals toward one another. This is particularly important for a child who has experienced a lengthy hospitalization. Closure of the hospital experience gives the child permission to move on in the process of adaptation—to move back into the family and home and other relationships while retaining the esteem of the people left behind in the health care setting.

> A simple closure device is saying to the child, "John, you have done it! You have been here with people you didn't know and you had things done to you that hurt. But you did it! And you made new friends in the playroom, you painted your mom some pictures, and you took your medicine which helped you feel better. And now you get to go home. You did it! And you helped me and the doctor help your kidney. Thank you!!"

This small speech, accompanied by a congratulatory handshake, conveys a strong message of mastery to a 7-year-old, yet takes very little time from the nurse's busy routines.

Intervention

Nursing interventions to support a child at risk due to illness, disability, and hospitalization are directed to the following:

1. External or environmental factors, which influence the child and family's experience of the stressors

2. Influencing the child and family's perceptions of the stressful experience (see Chart 42-4)
3. Support for family-centered care

The concepts of trust, understanding, and mastery are applied to both internal and external factors. For example, providing rooming-in for the parent of a 4-year-old, an environmental intervention, enhances the child's ability to trust. Providing the child with preparation for surgery enhances the child's understanding and mastery by influencing the way in which he thinks and feels about the surgical procedure.[57,81,114]

Setting Priorities

Nurses establish priorities based on the assessment, goals, and plans for individual patients. Establishing priorities gives the nurse a guide and mandate for allocating the resources of time and energy. The nurse's priorities should reflect the degree of vulnerability of a child for psychosocial disturbance in illness, disability, and hospitalization. Children most vulnerable to psychiatric disturbances are those in the first 4 years of life who have had multiple hospital admissions and who are from psychosocially disadvantaged families. These children should have the greatest allocation of the nurse's time and energy that

---

CHART 42-4

Family-to-Family Support

A diagnosis such as *diabetes* may be perceived as devastating by one family. The child is viewed as a normal child no longer. The parents respond with overprotectiveness, hovering, and restricting the child's activity. When introduced to another family who has a similar-aged child with the same diagnosis, the newly diagnosed family has a model of coping on which to base their understanding of what can reasonably be expected for their child. They can see that their child, in fact, can continue usual activities just as the other child has done.

This parent-to-parent support can be utilized in many situations of different diagnoses. Careful assessment of the families should be made to assure their positive potential. Some settings utilize parent support groups, parent consultants, and training for parent models to increase their effectiveness with families of children newly diagnosed with illness or disability.

can be devoted to psychosocial care. Needless to say, these priorities must coincide with the priorities for required physical care.

Other priorities are those children, of any age, who are assessed as vulnerable to stress in illness, disability, and hospitalization. Vulnerability is seen in the following instances:

Children who have recently experienced severe stress, such as a death in the family, parents' divorce, or parental illness

Children who have experienced a recent series of stressful events

Children who are in mild to moderate psychological distress prior to the hospital admission

Children who cannot understand communication as it is usually performed in the health care setting, who communicate in another language, or who have severe hearing or visual deficits

Children who have limited life experiences and limited repertoires of behaviors with which to respond to stress

Children who have experienced recent illness or hospitalization that may or may not be related to the present condition

Children who have defects from birth, such as blindness or deafness[3, 74, 102]

Finally, the nurse considers as priorities those interventions that, for all patients, will be growth-producing.[87, 114, 121] The child's psychosocial growth is enhanced as he experiences positive adjustment to the stresses of illness, disability, and hospitalization.

Not all nursing interventions can be planned in advance; some take place in an acute, crisis manner. As the nurse gains experience working with children at risk, greater flexibility in intervening in acute, emergency situations will result. Nevertheless, the nurse must first have a firm commitment to, and understanding of, the possible and desirable interventions.

> A 6-year-old with esophageal varices began hemorrhaging. The child was alert as the 'stat' call was made; the room filled with staff and a cardiac monitor was rushed in. The child looked at the monitor, which had not yet been activated, and cried out in extreme fear, "I'm dying! I'm dead! The line is straight, the line is straight!!"
>
> Those participating in this acute emergency will certainly be sensitive to the need for simple explanations in future emergencies when the child is alert and aware of the activities.

In a global sense, and in each specific instance, the nurse must ask, How can I promote this child's development of trust, understanding, and mastery? These three concepts will be used to organize nursing interventions.

Interventions to Support and Develop Trust

Interventions to support and develop trust involve external factors, such as changes in the physical environment, in conjunction with interpersonal behaviors, such as communication. The nature and flavor of the interventions vary according to the assessment data. Development of trust with a 15-month-old focuses on the presence of the parenting figure; development of trust with a 15-year-old depends on verbal communications and their congruence with nonverbal messages.

Interventions in the physical environment include the following:

Maintenance of tie with primary emotional support figures (rooming-in)

Continuity of care in nursing assignments, particularly primary nursing

Maintenance of tie with family (sibling visiting)

Maintenance of tie with peer group, for older children and adolescents

Structuring delivery of care so that intrusive procedures are not done in the patient's bed or in the patient's room

Structuring delivery of care so that as many routines and rituals associated with activities of daily living as possible (meals, naps, bathing, bedtime, and so forth) can be continued during hospitalization

Nursing interventions to support trust, which are based on interpersonal behaviors, include the following:

Spending nonstructured, non–task-oriented time with child patient and parents

Postponing intrusive procedures, whenever possible, until the child and parents recognize the nurse as a trusted individual

Communicating openness and "trustworthiness" through nonverbal signals and congruence of verbal and nonverbal messages

Using communication skills of active listening, inviting requests, attending, showing warmth, self-disclosure, and feedback[37, 126]

Interventions to Support and Develop Understanding

Developing and supporting the child's and family's understanding directly affects their levels of stress as the nurse mediates their perceptions of the stressors. Observation of young children in health care shows that their fantasies of what will happen are often more frightening than the real events. Through preparation the child learns about the reality—what he will see, hear, feel, and be expected to do. Sensory preparation has been found to be successful in decreasing children's anxiety during health care procedures.[51] Sensory preparation is preparation that imparts information about what will be felt, seen, and heard.

The nurse reduces the child's anxiety by relating to his concrete feelings rather than explaining the medical routines. For example, an explanation of what happens during the surgery is not appropriate, because the child will not feel during this time. Explaining that a mist that feels cool and soft will be blowing in his face when he awakens after surgery is important, however. Experiencing the feeling of the mist during presurgery preparation enhances sensory preparation for the child.

Understanding, developed through preparation and patient education, has been extensively reported in research and clinical literature.[5, 25, 117] Interventions to promote understanding include the following:

Preadmission preparation[34]

Stress-point preparation, which is preparation immediately before each potentially stressful experience, such as injections, venipunctures, or going to a new location in the hospital[123]

Preparation for diagnostic procedures[25, 100, 101, 125]

Preparation for surgical procedures[112, 117, 120, 128]

Patient education to teach child and parents about in-patient and home care; for example, teaching a child newly diagnosed with diabetes to give insulin[77, 80, 128]

The nurse integrates the concept of developing understanding through preparation into all nursing tasks. This means that at each point of potential stress, the nurse will give the child some advance knowledge of what to expect, particularly what the child will feel. How the nurse presents the information depends on the child's cognitive development, what the child can expect sensorially, and a brief explanation of why.

The question of "why" is important to interventions to develop understanding, for the child as well as for parents and other family members. Children's concepts of illness and causality follow developmental trends aligned with cognitive development as described by Piaget.[4, 9, 15, 18, 26, 59] This means that young children functioning at the concrete operational level need brief, specific, unambiguous, object-related explanations of why things are being done to them.[9]

Older children who can grasp cause and effect relationships will benefit from simple analogies.[85] Adolescents who have begun abstract thinking may require more detailed information with explanations of the implications of the treatment.[28] Giving suitable explanations for health care events lets the child understand that there is a plan for his care, that he is not being subjected to disturbing events at the whim of more powerful individuals, and that there are boundaries and limits that are known and shared. The impact of regression in health care must also be considered in the child's understanding. It is not unusual for individuals to regress to a lower level of cognition during stress.[11]

A further aspect of interventions to support understanding relates to the structuring of events.[124] As much as possible, the nurse should structure routines of care to follow a course that can be made known to the child. It is desirable, wherever possible, to follow routines the child experiences at home. For school-aged children, simple charts of the daily activities and calendars to mark the days and special events will help them understand the process and reinforce the ending of the hospitalization.

By developing a child's understanding of what is to happen, when it is to happen, and why, the nurse intervenes in the child's perception of the stress. Fantasies become anchored in reality. Overwhelming fear of the unknown becomes a manageable known. Parents' perceptions take on more realistic concerns, thereby decreasing the anxiety they project to the child.

A wide array of media has been developed for pediatric preparation and patient–parent education. These media include movies, filmstrips, coloring books, and children's books. Although there is still much to be researched in the use of media for preparation of children for health care events, those materials that most closely approximate the reality and provide behavioral modeling for the child most effectively decrease children's anxiety.[117]

Interventions to Support and Develop Mastery

A final group of interventions uses the development of trust and understanding to activate the child's coping with stressors. *Mastery* is the term that describes the positive coping with stress, which encourages adaptation.

Illness, disability, and hospitalization present as life crises, events that disrupt reality as experienced by the child and family. These life events involve changes to which the child must react. Coping is the process, or series of steps and sequences, through which the child comes to terms with the changes in reality. Coping devices are the choices in ways of using resources, new structures, and integrations developed by the child to respond to the changes in the environment. Defense mechanisms are also part of the overall coping effort.[41, 62, 96]

Changes and stressors in the environment demand coping of the child. Adaptation is the result of coping, a return to equilibrium. Mastery is positive adaptation; it is the successful use of coping devices to come to terms with the environment. Mastery is the child's ability to respond to, and use, the environment constructively.[44,72,73,127]

One of the early studies of coping with psychosocial stress in illness involved patients of all ages in a medical center for polio care.[122] Effective coping was found to be patterns of behavior, thoughts, feelings, and actions, that facilitate one or more of the following functions:

1. Keeping distress within manageable limits
2. Generating encouragement and hope
3. Maintaining or restoring a sense of personal worth
4. Maintaining or restoring relations with significant others
5. Enhancing prospects for physical recovery
6. Enhancing prospects for favorable situations—interpersonal, social, economic—after maximum physical recovery has been attained

In one study of chronic illness in children, four adaptive patterns were identified, from the onset of their illnesses, in children who did not develop debilitating psychological symptoms during the course of their diseases. These adaptive patterns were as follows:

1. Intellectualization
2. Identification with medical staff
3. Denial in the service of hope
4. Idiosyncratic rituals[43]

Interventions to support these adaptive patterns from the onset of the illness or disability lead to mastery. *Intellectualization* involves the sense of organization it contributes to the ego's assimilation of anxiety (see Chart 42-5, "Supporting Children's Use of Intellectualization"). *Identification with medical staff,* when combined with intellectualization, fosters a strong desire to care for one's own body.

> Identification is seen when a child develops a trusting bond with a particular nurse. The child likes the nurse and knows from pleasurable interchanges between them that the nurse likes him. Because this nurse believes a particular treatment will be helpful to him and his body, the child, too, adopts this belief and wants to do what will help him.

Denial in the service of hope alleviates the painful external reality of sickness and allows courage and hope to assist the endurance of unreasonable suffering.

Idiosyncratic rituals are patterns of behavior developed by children to cope with, or get through,

---

CHART 42-5
Supporting Children's Use of Intellectualization

A common misconception of young children is that they have somehow caused their illness.[15,49] Telling the child many times, in different ways, that she did not cause the illness develops appropriate intellectualization, which reduces guilt and anxiety.

A 3-year-old playing with a doll picked it up, gave it a big swat on the bottom and said, "You've been bad! You have to go to the hospital!" An observing health care provider said to the child and her mother, "Lots of children think they have been bad and that's why they come to the hospital. But you know, you haven't been bad; those other kids haven't been bad. You came to the hospital so your hurt in your stomach would be helped to go away. Your mother knows you weren't bad. She brought you to the hospital so we can help you feel better and help the hurt go away." The mother then picked up the child and gave her a big hug, echoing these statements and adding, "Mommy and Daddy love you." Later, the child was playing with the doll and imitated the words and actions of the mother. This child was using intellectualization; that is, thinking about her experience in ways appropriate to her developmental level, as a coping mechanism.

Intellectualization in an older child was graphically illustrated when an 11-year-old requested that pictures be taken of him while he underwent a lumbar puncture. Previously, he had great difficulty with the procedure, was uncooperative, and could not maintain positioning. He could not mentally visualize what was being done to him. The pictures provided him with a device for seeing what was being done, thinking about what was happening, and understanding why positioning and his cooperation were important. The pictures were additionally important as concrete means to think about the experience after it was over and develop mastery. For several days after the procedure, the boy would say to adults entering his room, "Say, do you want to see what I did?" He would then display his pictures with pride at his accomplishment.

particular aspects of illness or treatments. The rituals serve to bind staff and patient together in a shared, nonpathological routine. Unless the ritual self-destructively interferes with the patient's care, the staff should not disrupt the rituals because they offer a playful, yet formalized, sequence that provides boundaries for the child's anxiety. The ritual enhances the child's feeling of belongingness and of personal distinctiveness.

> A 6-year-old having difficulty with intravenous injections begins chanting, "I think I can, I think I can, I think I can," when he sits down in the treatment room and continues this chant throughout the procedure. This chant is taken from the children's book, *The Little Engine That Could.* At the conclusion of procedures, the child and nurse exclaim together, "I knew I could!" This ritual is repeated whenever the child has intravenous infusions started. It brings shared mastery to the child and nurse, as well as recognition and praise for the child's attempts to hold his arm immobile and cooperate as a team member in his physical care.

Another example of rituals is one hospital's use of finger puppets. Laboratory technicians follow finger sticks for blood tests with the presentation of a finger puppet to be worn over the child's bandaid. If the technician forgets, children often remind the technician and ask for the puppet. The finger puppet is a pleasurable, ritualized ending to this procedure.

In considering these adaptive patterns of behavior that allow the child to manage and master the changes in the environment, one sees that the patterns relate both to the internal and external perceptions. Interventions may support mastery through mediating the child's internal environment or external, physical environment. Play is a most useful means for supporting mastery. Provision for a child's play becomes an essential intervention in the nursing process.

Play. What is play? It is not the equivalent of adult recreation. Says Erikson:

> The playing adult steps sideward into another reality; the playing child advances forward to new stages of mastery. I propose the theory that the child's play is the infantile form of the human ability to deal with experience by creating model situations and to master reality by experiment and planning.[30]

Play, he further states, is "an indispensable harbor," one that is used for "overhauling of shattered emotions after periods of rough going in the social seas." Play is a device for mastery of anxiety-producing aspects of hospitalization and illness or disability. Piaget views play as a means of assimilation. New experiences, such as the stressful events of illness, are assimilated and accommodated into the child's structure.[84] One study looked specifically at the use of play in hospitals by children 3 to 8 years of age. The youngest children first established a trusting relationship with the adult in the play setting and then moved to the manipulation of toy objects. Older children used toys rather than the adult to orient, establish familiarity, and then achieve pleasure in the mastery of function. Once familiarity was established, they moved into supportive peer play.[119]

The play environment and the child's use of play can be used in assessment and to support trust and understanding.[8, 17, 22, 29, 87, 88, 113] Play interventions support mastery by affording the child the opportunity to be actively involved in structuring, controlling, and recreating the stresses of the hospital and illness events. This is most dramatically seen in the use of *medical play,* dramatic play using props of real medical equipment in which the child plays about being a patient and a caregiver. When this play is nondirective (*i.e.,* not designed toward a specific learning objective), the process of mastery is facilitated.

Expression of Feelings. Other interventions that support mastery encourage and allow the child's expression of feelings through art, storytelling, the use of children's books, and peer-group discussions.[33, 38, 48, 82, 91, 95] Efforts to facilitate communication between parents and child in order to overcome the "conspiracy of silence" lead to shared mastery of feelings.

Stress Immunization

Many activities the nurse can carry out with the child serve as protective mechanisms or stress immunization. As with all interventions to increase the child's understanding, both cognitive and affective, preparation and play activities afford an opportunity to anticipate the stress event. The child can mentally rehearse the event, become desensitized, and practice coping strategies. This process of early preparation for a future stress event immunizes the child to the negative effects of the stress experience. Successful management becomes protective as the child's cognitive appraisal is altered from a negative to a sense of accomplishment. For example, one intervention to decrease a child's fear of needles combined reading a story about the event, drawing pictures, discussing fears and fantasies, reading a poem, and playing with medical instruments. This process of intervention was found successful in decreasing children's anxiety and fear during injections and increasing their cooperation.[32] Two additional techniques require few materials and little time and can be taught to parents. Parents can carry out the techniques with their child, thereby activating both the child's and the parents' coping skills. These techniques are thought-stopping and relaxation training. Both have been found successful with children 5 years of age and older.

Thought-stopping involves substituting reassuring information each time the child begins to think about an upcoming stress event. The child, with the parent and nurse, generates the reassuring information and memorizes short phrases that convey the meaning.[100] For example, a child with daily venipunctures used these positive statements: "It doesn't take too long; I get a prize when it is over; it will help the doctors help me." Her reassuring facts were: "My mother can stay with me; I can go to the playroom when it's over." When the child has a set of positive, reassuring statements to substitute whenever fear thoughts begin, the fear responses are gradually weakened. In addition, the child develops a resource of her own, which decreases feelings of helplessness and increases mastery.

Relaxation training teaches the child to focus attention on his body, tighten and relax different muscles, and breathe deeply. The same progression should be used each time so that the process becomes very familiar to the child. The training should take place many times in a nonstressful setting. When the child has learned the process of relaxation, the parent can coach the child in the process during a more stressful event.[87]

Positive Feedback to Child and Family.   The nurse further supports mastery through interventions that mediate the child's self-esteem.[42, 103] The Roy Adaptation Nursing Model discusses this as interventions in the self-concept mode.[92] One's self-concept is determined through interactions with others.[66] The nurse intervenes through positive feedback to the child and family about their successes, however small (see Chart 42-6, "Reinforcing the Child's Self-Esteem").

School Activities.   Providing school activities for the child who is hospitalized or homebound builds the child's self-esteem as he successfully learns new academic skills and information. Provision of school activities is an intervention in the physical environment that enhances the internal perceptions of the child.[111]

C H A R T   42-6
Reinforcing the Child's Self-Esteem

"Amy, I know it hurts you to have your injections. When you held your leg still, counted to three, squeezed your mom's hand, and said, 'Ouchie!' you helped me! Thank you!!"

It is not uncommon to observe children's anger expressed in play. Children will say to a doll, "I'm the nurse and I'm going to give you a shot. Don't you cry or I'll give you another one!" The nurse who observes such expressed anger may feel dismay to realize her careful support of the child has, seemingly, gone unrecognized by the child.

However, what is really happening is ventilation of natural anger and retaliation in an acceptable way. It is important to know that children do have anger, should be allowed to express it, and that it need not represent a personal rejection of the nurse's efforts. If one finds it difficult to accept the display of children's anger, the nurse might need to question her personal support system and look for ways to feel good about herself that are not dependent on a child's total acceptance.

In one setting where psychosocial care is a priority, the nurses try to have some pleasant physical interaction with young children after an invasive procedure. The nurse will say, "Judy, I know the needle I gave you hurt. I wish I didn't have to hurt you but that is the only way to give this medicine. Now that the hurt is over, can I give you a hug? I want to help you feel good, too." Most children eagerly and positively respond to this request. Parents also seem to appreciate this extra display of caring for their child. Occasionally, a child will refuse. If the nurse takes this refusal as a personal rejection, further distress is placed on the child. When the nurse accepts the child's refusal and says, "That's okay, Judy, some other time maybe we can do something nice together— when you want to," the nurse conveys a deep acceptance of the child as an individual, as well as a belief in the child's basic worth and hope for a better time to come for them.

Helping Families at Risk. Additional interventions that enhance mastery have been identified from research on the effects of chronic illness and disability.[97,98] Three interventions found beneficial in decreasing risk to the child's adjustment to chronic conditions and development include the following:

1. Early identification of families at risk; for example, families with low functioning are two times as likely to have a child whose adjustment to illness is poor as are other families of children with chronic conditions

2. Determining and making known to the family and health care staff who is in charge; that is, identifying the primary orchestrator of the child's care

3. Provision of an "outreach person" to meet the needs of the family on an intensive, sustained, caring, and creative basis

This outreach individual influences the child's and family's perceptions of themselves and gives support and feedback on their successes in coping with specific stressors. Through her role in a specialty clinic, the nurse may function as this person or may advocate and demonstrate the need for such a person in the child's health care.

Evaluation

The final component of the nursing process, evaluation, is actually an ongoing process that begins with the child's entry into the health care system. Evaluation serves as a "feedback loop" for the nursing process. At any point in the process, or system, evaluation is used to determine the success or correctness of other parts of the system.

Evaluation in the nursing process is based on observation and analysis. Observing a child's behavior, analyzing it, and thinking about its meaning and probable causes confirm or modify the analysis of assessment data and subsequent plans. Evaluating the child's response to interventions may lead to developing other interventions, planning the continuation of present interventions, or developing a new plan of care.

Self-Reflection

Evaluation also offers the nurse an opportunity for self-reflection. How am I doing? How do I feel? How am I coping? What stresses am I experiencing in working with this child and family? The use of self as a therapeutic tool in working with the child at risk is a primary organizing factor in the nursing process. The self as an open, accepting, and warm person actualizes the development of trust. Understanding, developed through preparation, depends on clear, appropriate communication between the nurse and child and family. Ego strength in the nurse is necessary to allow, and accept, the child's negative feelings.

At times, the nurse's defense mechanisms may aid in coping. At other times, their use may interfere with her personal coping and with assisting the child and family in positive coping. An example of this interference is the nurse's use of denial of pain when, in truth, bearing the child's pain is difficult for her. When a nurse says to a child, "There, that was just a little stick. It didn't really hurt so bad. Don't cry," she is really saying that she hates to hurt children, please don't cry, because then she will have to face the fact that she did hurt the child. The nurse is really saying, "Please help me continue my denial of this unpleasant part of my job." The nurse must continually evaluate the effectiveness of her defense or coping mechanisms and processes.

Working with ill or disabled children in a hospital or health care setting can be emotionally painful and draining. There are times of helplessness—the child's physical pain continues, the disability cannot be reversed, the progress of the disease cannot be arrested, perhaps death is an approaching reality. The projected increase of infants born with AIDS is an example of a condition that lends itself to feelings of helplessness. The limitation of medical knowledge is a reality that must be faced and dealt with by the effective nurse. Anger is a natural expression of helplessness. How and where the nurse directs anger is important to consider. Evaluating one's professional and personal effectiveness is enhanced by awareness of other defensive or coping mechanisms such as denial, repression, projection, intellectualization, and overidentification.

Need for Personal and Professional Supports

Working with children can stir up the "child" in each of us. Unresolved issues in our developmental past may be brought into preconscious awareness and may evoke unpleasant feelings. Acknowledging and accepting these feelings, understanding one's self, and developing personal support systems and professional support systems within the work setting all aid in the process of caring for children at risk.[7,71]

The Nurse's Role As an Advocate

While knowledge of the psychosocial needs of children in health care has progressed, the application of such knowledge has lagged behind.[117,118] What are the explanations for this lag? The primary reason is that health care systems are bureaucracies and change is

C H A R T 42-7
Prolonged Hospitalization and Immobilization

Special needs arise when infants, children or adolescents experience prolonged hospitalizations. At greatest risk are infants.[63] Organization of the environment to facilitate the development of trust and cognitive processes is essential.[30,83] The challenge to the nurse is to collaborate creatively with the family and other health care disciplines to "normalize" the environment, *i.e.*, to incorporate essential life experiences into the hospital setting. Included can be such activities as the development of a schedule for the baby's day, which promotes predictability and decreases disruptions and unnecessary people; the use of adaptive toys (homemade or commercial products) that enhance stimulation and organization of sensory modes; and the provision of support programs for *all* members of the family, such as respite time for the parents and sibling involvement with the infant in the hospital.

Equally challenging to the nurse's creativity is the immobilized child patient. Whether he is immobilized by treatment and equipment as in an intensive care unit, or as a result of surgical intervention as in orthopedic care, the child's experience of powerlessness can be a risk to positive coping and eventual adaptation. Again, environmental manipulation can counteract the necessary restrictions. Most important is the recognition that mobility is the child's primary way of exerting control, expressing tension and anxiety, and exploring the environment. The nurse must recognize the child's attempts to compensate for the loss of mobility and must facilitate adaptive behaviors that give the child feelings of control and mastery.[6]

A common response to immobilization in an intensive care unit is for a child to withdraw from the environment by refusing to make eye contact. Another common behavior is seen when a child in traction uses the "nurse call" button incessantly. Providing choices for the child in a realistic way is a first step in assisting the child to regain feelings of control. Providing outlets for tension and anxiety, through verbalization and adaptive activity, further assists the child in compensating for the loss of mobility. Support and structure are also provided by increasing peer contacts and continuing normal routines such as schoolwork.

Peer contact was maintained for a child who was in traction and in isolation through daily bingo games held in the playroom; the child participated by telephone. Audiotapes made by the child and sent home to siblings, who sent their own tape-recorded messages back, provided an outlet for the child's energy as well as a readily available comforting device. Daily sessions with fantasy, such as reading stories involving action, allowed the child to identify with and vicariously become an active hero, mastering challenges. Through assessment and planning, the nurse can help the child regain feelings of control to counteract the powerlessness of immobility.

---

always slow. Decisions about the allocation of funds and resources are frequently made by individuals far removed from the literature and research findings. The medical model, built on concrete observations and manipulation of observable data, is frequently resistant to the "soft" sciences. Changing routines of care to meet psychosocial needs of children acknowledges that the provision of health care can be detrimental to children's development; those caring for children are reluctant to admit that, while helping, they do inflict pain. Regardless of these and other explanations, the need to provide for the psychosocial requirements of children and families exists. As an advocate, the nurse educates about, facilitates, and models more effective care of individual children and all children in health care.

Advocacy takes place when the nurse shares with other health care providers information that helps them understand the child and family. This may be done through verbal communication, as when giving a change-of-shift report or in written communications in the nursing progress notes and Kardex. Advocacy may also take the form of volunteering to present nursing inservice education programs organized around psychosocial issues. Frequently, advocacy for individual children takes the form of sharing information that makes caring for the child easier for other staff and, consequently, for the child. For example, the nurse may share "tricks of the trade" with a lab technician who must collect blood samples from the child or with a physician who is starting an IV.

Advocacy also takes place when the nurse shares information with the parents.[76] It is not uncommon to see parents placing unrealistic demands for behavior

CHART 42-8
Family-Centered Care

Advances in medical technology, economic trends in health care and rising hospital costs, the development of home health care services, the consumer movement, and federal initiatives in health care (as well as in education) for the handicapped provided momentum in the 1980s for emphasis on family-centered care.

The U.S. Surgeon General, C. Everett Koop, directed attention to the needs of families with children who have chronic illnesses or handicapping conditions through a series of conferences incorporating parent–professional collaboration. The Division of Maternal and Child Health of the U.S. Public Health Service extended this focus through funded projects implementing family-centered approaches.

As described by the Association for the Care of Children's Health, the elements of family-centered care are as follows:[108]

1. Recognition that the family is the constant in the child's life, while service systems and personnel within the systems fluctuate
2. Facilitation of parent–professional collaboration in all levels of health care (care of the individual child, program develop- ment, implementation and evaluation, and policy formation)
3. Sharing of unbiased and complete information with parents about their child's care in appropriate, supportive ways on an ongoing basis
4. Implementation of policies and programs and provision of emotional and financial support to meet the needs of families
5. Recognition of family strengths and respect for different methods of coping
6. Understanding and incorporating developmental needs of children and their families into health care delivery systems
7. Encouragement and facilitation of parent-to-parent support
8. Design of health care delivery systems that are flexible, accessible, and responsive to families

The nurse, incorporating these elements in the organization and delivery of care, provides support to children that increases the psychosocial support to families and, therefore, decreases risk to children in health care.

---

on their child. "You're a big boy now, don't cry!" the parents might say to their child. By explaining pain and the usefulness of expressing pain for the child's emotional and physical well-being, the nurse promotes quality care of the child.

At times, advocacy is best accomplished when the nurse can help others identify, intellectually and emotionally, with the child and family. One child used a ritual of stalling and gaining control before he could participate in intrusive procedures. He seemed to need more time than other children typically requested. This need for time was interpreted by one staff member simply as stalling that served no useful purpose, other than taking up her time. Another nurse observed, "Did you ever dive off the high-dive board when you were little? I can remember climbing the ladder, getting to the top, walking out to the end of the board, and I just couldn't make myself jump. I wanted to. I would back up a little, take forward steps, and then stand again. I just couldn't do it at first. I'd take another try and finally I would be able to. I think this is what Jeff does. He's just getting himself ready for the big plunge." The first nurse, with a strong remembrance, exclaimed, "I used to do that when I was doing backward dives off the high dive. Was I ever scared!" With an analogy she could appreciate, this nurse was able to understand the child's need for "just a little more time" to get ready for frightening events.

Advocacy also occurs during staff meetings when a group of health care providers discusses ideas and reaches decisions about routines of care for child patients and their families. Speaking up on ways to provide health care that meet both the institution's needs and the psychosocial needs of children and families demonstrates for others the importance and possibility of combining and meeting both needs. How to accomplish this comes from many sources— reading journals, talking with people from other health care settings, attending educational conferences—all of which impart information about how best to care for children and families in pediatric settings.

Accepting the role of advocate comes with realizing that advocacy can minimize the potential for psychosocial disturbance and can maximize the opportunities for benefit to children by facilitating physical care. By reducing the emotional stress component of the patient's illness, the child is left with more of his metabolic resources in reserve to deal with the onslaught of disease.[13]

Summary

This chapter has discussed the child in health care from the perspective of stress/adaptation theory. Illness, disability, and hospitalization are life crises for a child and family; the impact of these events can affect the developmental progress of a child. Some of the major points of the chapter include the following:

1. Long-lasting psychological disturbance has been found in 25% of pediatric hospital admissions.

2. Children with multiple admissions to the hospital in the first 4 years of life are the most vulnerable to psychological disturbance.

3. The influences of hospitalization, parent–child attachment, and communication are factors that the nurse recognizes and analyzes when applying the nursing process.

4. Assessment of the child at risk for psychosocial disturbance in health care includes gathering information about the child's developmental level, the environmental influences on the child (such as the nature of the specific illness or disability, the child's previous life experiences, and the child's family), and personal attributes of the child.

5. Planning and interventions for the child who is ill, disabled, or hospitalized are evaluated for effectiveness in supporting the child's and family's development of trust, understanding, and mastery of the stresses involved in health care.

6. Preparation for experiences encountered in health care and the use of play are common, yet critical, psychosocial interventions.

7. Mastery allows the child to be active on his own behalf, to turn from a passive victim to a participating role.

8. Interventions to support mastery are those that allow the child active exploration of feelings, as in nondirective play and expressive arts; that enhance the child's and family's self-concept and self-esteem; and that promote family-centered care.

9. Evaluation of the effectiveness of nursing intervention is based on observation and analysis of the child's and family's behavior and self-reflection.

10. The nurse's acceptance of the advocate role, coupled with the responsibility to minimize potential psychological disturbances and to maximize growth potentials, affords the challenges and rewards of nursing children.

References

1. Abu-Saad H: Cultural Components of Pain: The Arab-American Child. Issues Comp Ped Nurs 7: 91–99, 1984

2. Anthony EJ, Koupernik C (eds): The Child in His Family: The Impact of Disease and Death. New York, John Wiley & Sons, 1973

3. Anthony EJ, Koupernik C (eds): The Child in His Family: Children at Psychiatric Risk. New York, John Wiley & Sons, 1974

4. Astin EW: Self-Reported Fears of Hospitalized and Non-Hospitalized Children Aged Ten to Twelve. Matern Child Nurs J 6 (Spring): 17–24, 1977

5. Azarnoff P, Woody PA: Preparation of Children for Hospitalization in Acute Care Hospitals in the United States. Pediatrics 68 (September): 361–368, 1981

6. Baumann DR: Coping Behavior of Children Experiencing Powerlessness from Loss of Mobility. In Miller JF (ed): Coping with Chronic Illness, pp 61–84. Philadelphia, FA Davis, 1983

7. Beardslee WR, DeMaso DR: Staff Groups in a Pediatric Hospital: Content and Coping. Am J Orthopsychiatry 52 (October): 712–718, 1982

8. Betz CL, Poster EC: Incorporating Play into the Care of the Hospitalized Child. Issues Compr Pediatr Nurs 7 (6): 343–355, 1984

9. Bibace R, Walsh ME (eds): New Directions for Child Development: Children's Conceptions of Health, Illness, and Bodily Functions, no 14. San Francisco, Jossey-Bass, 1981

10. Blitzer EC et al: Another Myth: Reduced Hospital Visiting by Inner-City Mothers. Pediatrics 71 (April): 504–509, 1983

11. Blos P: Children Think About Illness: Their Concepts and Beliefs. In Gellert E (ed): Psychosocial Aspects of Pediatric Care, pp 1–18. New York, Grune & Stratton, 1978

12. Bowlby J: Separation: Anxiety and Anger. New York, Basic Books, 1973

13. Bovard EW: The Effects of Social Stimuli on the Response to Stress. Psychol Rev 66 (September): 267–277, 1959

14. Broome M: Working with the Family of a Critically Ill Child. Journal of Critical Care 14 (July): 368–372, 1985

15. Broome ME, Hellier AP: School-Age Children's Fear of Medical Experiences. Issues Compr Pediatr Nurs 10 (Spring): 77–86, 1987

16. Burns CE: The Hospitalization Experience and Single Parent Families: A Time of Special Vulnera-

bility. Nurs Clin North Am 19 (June): 285–293, 1984

17. Burson JZ, Brannigan CN: The Use of Play in the Nutritional Support of Hospitalized Children. Issues Compr Pediatr Nurs 7, 4–5, 283–289, 1984

18. Campbell JD: Illness is a Point of View: The Development of Children's Concepts of Illness. Child Dev 46 (March): 92–100, 1975

19. Caplan G (ed): Prevention of Mental Disorders in Children. New York, Basic Books, 1961

20. Chess S, Thomas A: Temperamental Differences: A Critical Concept in Child Health Care. Pediatr Nurs 11 (May–June): 167–171, 1985

21. Committee on Hospital Care: Child Life Programs for Hospitalized Children. Pediatrics 76 (September): 467–469, 1985

22. D'Antonio IJ: Therapeutic Use of Play in Hospitals. Nurs Clin North Am 10 (June): 351–359, 1984

23. Denholm CJ: Hospitalization and the Adolescent Patient: A Review and Some Critical Questions. Children's Health Care 13 (Spring): 109–116, 1985

24. Douglas JB: Early Hospital Admissions and Later Disturbances of Behavior and Learning. Dev Med Child Neurol 17 (August): 456–480, 1975

25. Droske S, Francis S: Pediatric Diagnostic Procedures. New York, John Wiley & Sons, 1981

26. Eiser C, Patterson D: Children's Perceptions of Hospital: A Preliminary Study. Int J Nurs Stud 21, 1, 45–50, 1984

27. Eissler RS, Freud A, Kris M, Solnit AJ (eds): Physical Illness and Handicap in Childhood. New Haven, Yale University Press, 1977

28. Elkind D: Teenage Thinking: Implications for Health Care. Pediatr Nurs 10 (6): 383–385, 1984

29. Ellerton ML, Caty S, Ritchie JA: Helping Young Children Master Intrusive Procedures through Play. Children's Health Care 13 (Spring): 167–173, 1985

30. Erikson E: Childhood and Society. New York, WW Norton, 1950

31. Etzler CA: Parents' Reactions to Pediatric Critical Care Settings: A Review of the Literature. Issues Compr Pediatr Nurs 7 (6): 319–331, 1984

32. Fassler D: The Fear of Needles in Children. Am J Orthopsychiatry 53 (July): 371–377, 1985

33. Fassler J: Helping Children Cope: Managing Stress Through Books and Stories. New York, Free Press, 1978

34. Ferguson BF: Preparing Young Children for Hospitalization. Pediatrics 64 (November): 656–664, 1979

35. Ferraro AR, Longo DC: Nursing Care of the Family with a Chronically Ill, Hospitalized Child: An Alternative Approach. Image 17 (Summer): 77–81, 1985

36. Fletcher B: Psychological Upset in Posthospitalized Children: A Review of the Literature, Matern Child Nurs J 10 (Fall): 185–195, 1981

37. Fosson A, deQuan MM: Reassuring and Talking

with Hospitalized Children. Children's Health Care 13 (Summer): 37–44, 1984

38. Frank JL: A Weekly Group Meeting for Children on a Pediatric Ward: Therapeutic and Practical Functions. Int J Psychiatry Med 8, 3, 267–283, 1978

39. Freud A: Normality and Pathology in Childhood: Assessments of Development. New York, International Universities Press, 1965

40. Freud A: The Ego and Mechanisms of Defense. New York, International Universities Press, 1966

41. Freud A: The Role of Bodily Illness in the Mental Life of Children. In Eissler RS, Freud A, Kris M, Solnit A (eds): Physical Illness and Handicap in Childhood, pp 1–12. New Haven, Yale University Press, 1977

42. Garmezy N: Stress Resistant Children: The Search for Protective Factors. In Stevenson J (ed): Recent Research in Developmental Psychopathology, pp 67–85. Oxford, Pergamon Press, 1984

43. Geist RA: Onset of Chronic Illness in Children and Adolescents: Psychotherapeutic and Consultative Intervention. Am J Orthopsychiatry 49 (January): 4–23, 1979

44. Gohsman BN: The Hospitalized Child and the Need for Mastery. Issues in Comprehensive Pediatric Nursing 5 (March–April): 67–76, 1981

45. Goslin ER: Hospitalization as a Life Crisis for the Preschool Child: A Critical Review. Journal Comm Health 3 (Summer): 321–346, 1978

46. Greenspan S: The Clinical Interview of the Child. New York, McGraw-Hill, 1981

47. Hayes E, Knox JE: The Experience of Stress in Parents of Children Hospitalized with Long-Term Disabilities. J Adv Nurs 9 (July): 333–341, 1984

48. Hughes MC: Chronically Ill Children in Groups: Recurrent Issues and Adaptations. Am J Orthopsychiatry 52 (October): 704–711, 1982

49. Hunsberger M, Love B, Byrne C: A Review of Current Approaches Used to Help Children and Parents Cope with Health Care Procedures. Matern Child Nurs J 13 (Fall): 145–165, 1984

50. Jessop DJ, Stein REK: Uncertainty and Its Relation to the Psychological and Social Correlates of Chronic Illness in Children. Social Science and Medicine 20 (10): 993–999, 1985

51. Johnson JE, Kirchhoff KT, Endress M: Easing Children's Fright During Health Care Procedures. Am J Matern Child Nurs 1 (July–August): 206–210, 1976

52. Kliman G: Psychological Emergencies of Childhood. New York: Grune & Stratton, 1968

53. Knafl KA, Dixon DM: The Role of Siblings During Pediatric Hospitalization. Issues in Comprehensive Pediatric Nursing 6 (January–February): 13–22, 1983

54. Knafl KA, Dixon DM: The Participation of Fathers in Their Children's Hospitalization. Issues Compr Pediatr Nurs 7, 4–5, 269–281, 1984

55. Knox JE, Haynes VE: Hospitalization of a Chron-

ically Ill Child: A Stressful Time for Parents. Issues in Comprehensive Pediatric Nursing 6 (July–August): 217–226, 1983

56. Korbin JE, Johnston M: Steps Toward Resolving Cultural Conflict in a Pediatric Hospital. Clinical Pediatr 21 (May): 259–263, 1982

57. LaMontagne LL: Children's Locus of Control Beliefs as Predictors of Preoperative Coping Behavior. Nurs Res 33 (March–April): 76–85, 1984

58. LaMontagne LL: Three Coping Strategies Used by School-Age Children. Pediatr Nurs 10 (January–February): 25–28, 1984

59. Lambert SA: Variables That Affect the School-Age Child's Reaction to Hospitalization and Surgery: A Review of the Literature. Matern Child Nurs J 13 (Spring): 1–18, 1984

60. Lavigne JV, Ryan M: Psychologic Adjustment of Siblings of Children with Chronic Illness. Pediatrics 63 (April): 616–627, 1979

61. Lawson BA: Chronic Illness in the School-aged Child: Effects on the Total Family. MCN 2 (January–February): 49–56, 1977

62. Lazarus R, Folkman S: Stress, Appraisal, and Coping. New York, Springer Publishing, 1984

63. Liakopoulou M, Patterson A, Samaraweera S, Finnegan L: Developmental Interventions in Infancy During Lengthy Hospitalizations. J Dev Behav Pediatr 4 (September): 213–217, 1983

64. Litman TJ: The Family as a Basic Unit in Health and Medical Care: A Social-Behavioral Overview. Soc Sci Med 8 (September): 495–519, 1974

65. McKeever P: Siblings of Chronically Ill Children: A Literature Review with Implications for Research and Practice. Am J Orthopsychiatry 53 (April): 209–218, 1983

66. Mack JE: Self-esteem and Its Development: An Overview. In Mack JE, Ablon SL (eds): The Development and Sustaining of Self-esteem in Childhood, pp 10–22. New York, International Universities Press, 1983

67. Marten GW, Mauer AM: Interaction of Health-Care Professionals with Critically Ill Children and Their Parents. Clin Pediatr 21 (September): 540–544, 1982

68. Martinez RA (ed): Hispanic Culture and Health Care. St Louis, CV Mosby, 1978

69. Mattsson A: Long Term Physical Illness in Childhood: A Challenge to Psychosocial Adaptation. Pediatrics 50 (November): 801–811, 1972

70. Mischel MH: Parents' Perception of Uncertainty Concerning Their Hospitalized Child. Nurs Res 32 (November–December): 324–330, 1983

71. Moynihan RT, Outlaw E: Nursing Support Groups in a Cancer Center. J Psychosoc Oncology 2, 1, 33–48, 1984

72. Murphy L, Moriarty AE: Vulnerability, Coping and Growth, New Haven, Yale University Press, 1976

73. Murphy L et al: The Widening World of Childhood. New York, Basic Books, 1962

74. Nagera H: Children's Reactions to Hospitalization and Illness. Child Psychiatry Hum Dev 9 (Fall): 3–16, 1978

75. Olds A: Psychosocial Considerations in Humanizing the Physical Environment of Pediatric Outpatient and Hospital Settings. In Gellert E (ed): Psychosocial Aspects of Pediatric Care, pp 111–132. New York, Grune & Stratton, 1978

76. Pass MD, Pass CM: Anticipatory Guidance for Parents of Hospitalized Children. J Pediatr Nurs 2 (August): 250–258, 1987

77. Paulson JA: Patient Education. Pediatr Clin North Am 28 (August): 627–635, 1981

78. Perrin EC, Gerrity S: There's A Demon in Your Belly: Children's Understanding of Illness. Pediatrics 67 (June) 841–849, 1981

79. Perrin EC, Perrin JM: Clinicians' Assessments of Children's Understanding of Illness. Am J Dis Child 137 (September): 874–878, 1983

80. Peterson L, Shigetoma C: The Use of Coping Techniques to Minimize Anxiety in Hospitalized Children. Behavior Therapy 12, 1–14, 1981

81. Peterson L, Toler S: An Information-Seeking Disposition in Child Surgery Patients. Health Psychology 5 (Fall): 343–358, 1986

82. Petrillo M, Sanger S: Emotional Care of Hospitalized Children. Philadelphia, JB Lippincott, 1972

83. Piaget J: The Language and Thought of the Child. New York, Meridian Books, 1953

84. Piaget J: Play, Dreams and Imitation in Childhood. New York, WW Norton, 1962

85. Pidgeon V: Characteristics of Children's Thinking and Implications for Health Teaching. Matern Child Nurs J 6 (Spring): 1–8, 1977

86. Pless IB, Roghmann KJ: Chronic Illness and its Consequences: Observations Based on Three Epidemiologic Surveys. J Pediatr 79 (September): 351–359, 1971

87. Poster EC: Stress Immunization: Techniques to Help Children Cope with Hospitalization. Matern Child Nurs J 12 (Summer): 119–134, 1983

88. Poster EC, Betz CL: Allaying the Anxiety of Hospitalized Children Using Stress Immunization Techniques. Issues Compr Pediatr Nurs 6 (July–August): 277–233, 1983

89. Prugh D et al: A Study of the Emotional Reactions of Children and Families to Hospitalization and Illness. Am J Orthopsychiatry 23 (February): 70–106, 1953

90. Quinton D, Rutter M: Early Hospital Admissions and Later Disturbances of Behavior: An Attempted Replication of Douglas' Findings. Dev Med Child Neurol 18 (August): 447–459, 1976

91. Rie HE, Boverman H, Grossman BJ, Ozoa N: Immediate and Long-Term Effects of Interventions Early in Prolonged Hospitalization. Pediatrics 41 (April): 755–764, 1968

92. Riehl J, Roy Sr C: Conceptual Models for Nursing Practice, New York, Appleton-Century-Crofts, 1974

93. Ritchie JA, Caty S, Ellerton ML: Concerns of Acutely Ill, Chronically Ill and Healthy Preschool

Children. Res Nurs Health 7 (December): 265–274, 1984

94. Robertson J: Young Children in Hospitals. New York, Basic Books, 1958

95. Robertson M, Barford F: Story Making in Psychotherapy with a Chronically Ill Child. In Schaefer CE (ed): Therapeutic Use of Child's Play. New York, Jason Aronson, 1976

96. Robinson K et al: Concepts of Stress for Nursing. Issues in Mental Health Nursing 4 (July–September): 167–176, 1982

97. Roghmann K, Pless IB (eds): Child Health and the Community. New York, John Wiley & Sons, 1975

98. Rose MH: The Concepts of Coping and Vulnerability as Applied to Children with Chronic Conditions. Issues Compr Pediatr Nurs 7, 2–3, 177–186, 1984

99. Rosenberg JA: Health Care for Cambodian Children: Integrating Treatment Plans. Pediatr Nurs 12 (March–April): 118–125, 1986

100. Ross DM: Thought-stopping: A Coping Strategy for Impending Feared Events. Issues Compr Pediatr Nurs 7, 2–3, 83–89, 1984

101. Ross DM, Ross SA: Stress Reduction Procedures for the School-age Hospitalized Leukemic Child. Pediatr Nurs 10 (November–December): 393–395, 1984

102. Rutter M: Prevention of Children's Psychosocial Disorders: Myth and Substance. Pediatrics 70 (December): 883–894, 1982

103. Rutter M: Psychosocial Resilience and Protective Mechanisms. Am J Orthopsychiatry 57 (July): 316–331, 1987

104. Sabbeth BF, Leventhal JM: Marital Adjustment to Chronic Childhood Illness: A Critique of the Literature. Pediatrics 73 (June): 762–768, 1984

105. Savedra M et al: Description of the Pain Experience: A Study of School-Aged Children. Issues Compr Pediatr Nurs 5 (September–December): 373–380, 1981

106. Schulman J: Coping with Major Disease: Child, Family, Pediatrician. J Pediatr 102 (June): 988–991, 1983

107. Shelton TL, Jeppson ES, Johnson BH: Family-Centered Care for Children with Special Health Care Needs. Washington, DC, Association for the Care of Children's Health, 1986

108. Skipper JK, Leonard RC: Children, Stress and Hospitalization: A Field Experiment. J Health Soc Behav 9 (December): 275–287, 1968

109. Speer JJ, Sachs B: Selecting the Appropriate Family Assessment Tool. Pediatr Nurs 11 (September–October): 349–355, 1985

110. Spinetta JJ: Behavioral and Psychological Research in Childhood Cancer: An Overview. Cancer 50 (November suppl): 1939–1943, 1982

111. Spitz R: Hospitalism: An Inquiry into the Genesis of Psychiatric Conditions in Early Childhood. The Psychoanalytic Study of the Child 1:53–74, 1945

112. Tarnow J, Gutstein S: Children's Preparatory Behavior for Elective Surgery. J Am Acad Child Psychiatry 22 (July): 365–369, 1983

113. Terr L: Forbidden Games: Post-Traumatic Child's Play. J Am Acad Child Psychiatry 20 (Autumn): 741–760, 1981

114. Tesler M, Savedra M: Coping with Hospitalization: A Study of School-Aged Children. Pediatr Nurs 7 (March–April): 35–38, 1981

115. Tesler M et al: Coping Strategies of Children in Pain. Issues Compr Pediatr Nurs 5 (September–December): 351–359, 1981

116. Thomas A, Chess S: Temperament and Development. New York, Brunner/Mazel, 1977

117. Thompson RH: Psychosocial Research on Pediatric Hospitalization and Health Care. Springfield, IL, Charles C Thomas, 1985

118. Thompson RH: Where We Stand: Twenty Years of Research on Pediatric Hospitalization and Health Care. Children's Health Care 14 (Spring): 200–210, 1986

119. Tisza V, Hurwitz I, Angoff K: The Use of a Play Program for Hospitalized Children. J Am Acad Child Psychiatry 9 (July): 515–531, 1970

120. Vernon D et al: The Psychological Responses of Children to Hospitalization and Illness. Springfield, IL, Charles C Thomas, 1965

121. Vipperman JF, Rager P: Childhood Coping: How Nurses Can Help. Pediatric Nursing (March–April) 6: 11–18, 1980

122. Visotsky H, Hamburg D, Goss M: Coping Behaviors Under Extreme Stress. Arch Gen Psychiatry 5 (November): 423–448, 1961

123. Visintainer M, Wolfer J: Psychological Preparation for Surgical Pediatric Patients: The Effect on Children's and Parents' Stress Responses and Adjustment. Pediatrics 56 (August): 187–202, 1975

124. Volz DD: Time Structuring for Hospitalized School-Aged Children. Issues in Comprehensive Pediatric Nursing 5 (July–August): 205–210, 1981

125. Wear E, Covey J, Brush M: Facilitating Children's Adaptations to Intrusive Procedures. In Fochtman D, Foley G (eds): Nursing Care of the Child with Cancer. Boston, Little, Brown, 1982

126. Whaley LF, Wong DL: Effective Communication Strategies for Pediatric Practice. Pediatr Nurs 11 (November–December): 429–432, 1985

127. Yates A: Stress Management in Childhood. Clin Pediatr 22 (February): 131–135, 1983

128. Zastowny TR, Kirschenbaum DS, Meng AL: Coping Skills Training for Children: Effects on Distress Before, During, and After Hospitalization for Surgery. Health Psychology 5 (Summer): 231–247, 1986

129. Ziemer MM: Coping Behavior: A Response to Stress. Topics in Clinical Nursing 4 (July–September): 4–12, 1982

43 Issues in Women's Health Care

Rhea P. Williams

Your health is bound to be affected if, day after day, you say the opposite of what you feel, if you grovel before what you dislike and rejoice at what brings you nothing but misfortune . . . [Our soul] can't be forever violated with impunity.

Boris Pasternak,
Doctor Zhivago

Chapter Preview

Women are the largest group of consumers of health care. They account for about 60% of all patient visits to a doctor.[27] Women present a variety of common, yet unique, health issues. For many years, these concerns have been closeted as "female problems." Over the past two decades, however, the interest in women's health care has grown steadily and encouraged open discussion of women's health care needs.

To provide competent and sensitive care to women, the nurse must be aware of these health care issues and their meanings to women. This chapter focuses on the psychological significance of women's health care issues, problems, and needs. It examines the politics of women's health care and discusses the notions of self-concept, loss, anxiety, powerlessness, and stress as they relate to women in health care. The issues of childbearing and parenting, menopause, and the surgical interventions of hysterectomy and mastectomy are studied and the nursing process is applied to each of these issues in women's health care.

Learning Objectives

On completion of this chapter, you should be able to accomplish the following:

1. identify needs and conflicts of the female client seeking health care
2. compare and contrast the traditional and emerging roles of women
3. discuss the politics of women's health care
4. describe adaptation of the health care system to the needs of women
5. discuss the application of mental health principles to the concepts of loss, anxiety, self-concept, stress, and powerlessness
6. apply the nursing process—assessment, nursing diagnosis, planning, intervention, and evaluation—to the health care of women facing childbearing and parenting, surgical interventions (mastectomy and hysterectomy), and menopause.

Developing Roles of Women

The 1980s are both an exciting and a difficult time to be a woman. As their horizons broaden, women claim greater freedom to make choices and define their own courses of action. Despite society's changes, however, this is also a difficult era for women working for their equal place, because they are becoming increasingly susceptible to the pressures and stresses of contemporary society.

In response to changes in society, today's woman is undergoing significant life changes. She faces questions such as these:

"What are my expectations of myself?"
"Am I prepared and capable?"
"Need I change?"
"What are the consequences?"

Change invariably brings conflict. Conflict produces stress; unresolved conflict produces distress, which can lead to disruption or pathology. To ease this stress and distress, the nurse must understand the many conflicts and needs of the woman seeking health care.

Traditional Role of Women

Traditionally, from infancy, a little girl was programmed or socialized into the feminine role. The proclamation at delivery, "It's a girl," started the socialization process. Infant girls are held, cuddled, and kissed more often than male babies.[6] These behaviors directed toward baby girls may foster the emotional and dependent responses seen in the traditional female.

Girls have also been socialized into the female role in other ways. Girls were dressed in pink, a color shown to contribute to calmer and more passive behavior. Wearing a dress was part of learning to act feminine, because this article of clothing was certainly meant to discourage rough-housing, ball-playing, and other forms of active child play. Little girls were given dolls, toy brooms, dishes, and similar toys to help them enter the domestic experience. In her early play, a girl was frequently reminded to be ladylike and not to be a tomboy. She was praised for being "Mommy's helper." She was taught to have low aspirations; too much education or success, she was warned, might scare away the boys.

Female role models depicted in books and the mass media were often emotional and dependent thinkers. The important names learned in history class were, overwhelmingly, those of men. A woman, the little girl was taught, was best suited to be a wife and mother. Girls took classes in home economics and typing and were encouraged to fear math and anything mechanical. The woman's ultimate status would be dependent on her husband's, not her own, skills. Her unmarried sisters were viewed as "poor dears" or misfits.

The traditionally socialized girl was a conforming person, bound by cultural values and social expectations. In accordance with the expectation that they would devote their lives to others, women were trained to be sensitive to, and respond to, other people.[19] Women were defined by the image of their domestic responsibilities; that is, they were perceived as actual or potential wives and mothers to the exclusion of other roles. The image of the ideal wife and mother as a warm, nurturent, supportive person defined what all women were supposed to be.[3]

Emerging Role of Women

Although the socialization process held clear-cut expectations, there were always women who didn't fit this clear-cut role. Coupled with the messages that they should be feminine, women were exposed to other messages. During school and through the media, girls learn the value society places on achievement, success, competition, leadership, and productivity. Parents are proud of their daughters' achievements in school, but often deliver the double message, "Do well, but don't do too well."[19]

Throughout the last two decades, women have questioned their place in society. They have asked, "Why should I not do as well?" Women have struggled with their dissatisfaction and with what Betty Friedan, in 1963, called "the problem that has no name."[11] The women's movement brought about many alterations in the traditional woman's role.

Every woman is affected by the uncertainty of the woman's role today. Some women cling to traditional values and defend the roles of wife, mother, and homemaker as fulfilling, rewarding, and important ones. They would argue for a return to the past.

The modern woman, liberated from the confines of tradition, perceives the role of women as changing. She believes in her ability to achieve whatever she desires and become whatever she wants to become.

There are also those women caught in the middle. They have internalized the traditional role of women, but still feel a nagging dissatisfaction. They frequently ask, "Is that all there is?" The internalization of traditional values is too binding to bring about an immediate role change; therefore, this group of women experiences a "role addition." The woman who is in or approaching the middle years during the 1980s is particularly at risk for conflict. Although she has been socialized as a traditional female, she is bombarded by her own feelings, the media, and literature about the modern female. Her ambivalence and conflict about women's roles may be passed along to her daughter in the form of mixed messages, such as, "Girls can be anything...but act ladylike."

The emerging role of women has many con-

sequences for the mental health of women. Nurses must help women deal with conflict, change, and stress.

The Politics of Women's Health Care

Women make up the largest number of health care consumers in a system dominated by male physicians, a system that, over the years, has kept women in a passive role. Women are often, therefore, the recipients of care delivered from a male viewpoint at the most private and vulnerable times of their lives.

Women's acceptance of male dominance in medical care is not surprising in light of their traditional socialization. The physician represents everything one admires—intelligence, independence, omniscience, decisiveness, dominance, and power. He commands respect. He often calls the woman by her first name and may refer to her as a "good girl," but he is always called Dr. _____. Many women feel that their symptoms are treated less seriously than those of men, because most medical problems of women are approached as though they are psychosomatic in origin.[10]

The medical profession's literature is replete with examples of a sexist view of women. Eighteenth- and nineteenth-century medicine regarded women as feeble creatures who needed to invest their limited energies in their primary task of reproduction. Overdevelopment of the brain, it was felt, might atrophy the uterus.[18]

In a textbook of obstetrics and gynecology published as recently as 1971, women are seen as self-sacrificing, dependent beings whose mental health and life fulfillment are derived from the achievements of their loved ones, primarily their husbands and children. The book also explains that a woman's visit to a physician often places her in a "parent–child" situation. The woman is depicted as placing her trust and faith in the knowledgeable physician in much the same way that she trusted her parents when she was a child.[35]

Even the popular modern authority on child care, Dr. Benjamin Spock, expresses the view that women are innately passive. He believes that women derive more pleasure from life when they are non-competitive.[29] One can only speculate how these attitudes influence the advice given to so many women.

There are also those who believe that visiting a doctor is a feminine way of coping with stress and ailments of any nature. If the doctor in attendance has been successfully socialized into the medical profession, the woman patient is likely to meet a physician who views her as a dependent, emotional person to be looked after.

Medicine's traditional beliefs and teaching have contributed to the inferior status of women. Because physicians are highly esteemed by society, their beliefs about women help to perpetuate those views.[18]

The subordination of women is also reflected in the sexual structure of the organization of medicine; in a field where women comprise the majority of health care workers, the power control of the medical hierarchy is solidly in the hands of the male physician.[10] In light of such confining medical and social stigma, nurses have a responsibility to plan and implement strategies to assist women to become more independent and powerful in matters of their own health care.

Adaptation of the Health Care System

The Women's Health Movement

The traditional system of providing health care to women is now being questioned. Prompted by the women's movement, the women's health movement has played a major role in the adaptations of the health care system. The women's health movement originally focused on the issues of birth control, abortion, and maternity care, but has expanded to include all aspects of preventive health, including nutrition and exercise, respiratory health problems, occupational health, and aging. The literature of the women's health movement combines shared experiences, health information, and political comment.[12]

Nursing's Adaptation to Women's Health Needs

In addition to society, nursing is also involved in a period of transition as it attempts to adapt its practice to the needs of women. Leonide Martin's message is important for all nurses working with women.

> The nurse is in a particularly favorable position to bring about many of the changes women desire in their health care. As an occupational group consisting mainly of women, nurses have a built-in propensity to understand and respond empathetically to women's concerns. Men in nursing also have an advantage in responding sensitively to women's health needs through their close association with many women and the socialization process of the profession. Professional norms and values internalized through nursing education emphasize the patient as an individual and promote practice which considers the person's unique needs, relation to the family and community, psychological and social factors as well as physical, and concentrate much of nursing care on the meaning and impact of illness rather than the illness itself. Nursing also emphasizes education about health and maintenance of well being as a major function of the profession.[19]

Applying Mental Health Principles to Women's Health Needs

By reviewing women's past and present roles and expectations, persistent themes of change, role addition, and conflict surface. These stressors (change, conflict, and so forth) produce physiological and psychological stress. For example, when one's self-concept is threatened, the individual becomes distressed; to restore and maintain a state of eustress, or optimal stress level, the individual's self-concept must adapt.

Self-Concept

The *self-concept* is the composite of an individual's beliefs and feelings about himself at a given time. This self-concept is formed from perceptions of others' reactions to the individual, and directs his behavior. There are two components of self-concept—the physical self and the personal self.[7]

The *physical self* or *body image* is the person's appraisal of his physical being; that is, his image of himself physically. The physical self includes one's physical attributes, appearance, physical performance, sexuality, and level of wellness.

The *personal self* involves the person's expectation of himself—his dreams, his standards, his evaluation of himself, and his need to maintain a consistent or stable self-image that says, "I can and should be; therefore, I am and will be tomorrow." When an individual's self-concept is high, his self-esteem, or his perception of his worth, is also high.

How a woman sees herself and feels about herself is an important issue for nurses to assess because it influences her health care needs. The traditionally socialized woman has learned continually to seek the approval of others; for this woman, what others think of her is critical in the development of her self-concept.

Development of Self-Concept

The development of the self-concept may be discussed as parallel to the developmental stages described by Erikson.[9] At each stage of development, the individual passes through a growth period wherein new coping mechanisms are learned and used to promote adaptation to the environment. During each of these periods, the individual takes on a new view of himself, thereby adapting his self-concept.

These life periods have been called "crisis points" in a person's life. Resolution of each crisis encountered builds on the resolution of the previous crises and, in turn, contributes to how the person will meet the next crisis.

For the female, particularly, these crisis points may have been resolved with ambivalence. The 3-year-old to 5-year-old, faced with the task of initiative versus guilt, strives to determine what kind of person she will be. She asks, "What can I be?" This time of subtle but distinct differences between male and female is reflected in the toys given to children and the play that is encouraged or discouraged. When a girl senses more excitement in boys' play and prefers to play like a boy, she may develop a subconscious feeling of guilt. Her initiative may falter when she is reprimanded, and her self-concept suffers.

The next stage of development, industry versus inferiority, is a critical one for girls. Schools send messages about what girls can achieve; for example, it is not unusual to hear that "girls can't do math." If a feeling of inferiority or inadequacy develops at this stage, the girl's self-concept is impaired, and her future adult functioning may be affected.

During the period of intimacy versus isolation, all individuals strive to develop an important, intimate relationship. Often, however, this relationship allows a woman to experience her self-worth only through another, a situation leading to isolation.

When a woman has achieved only through the accomplishments of others, she may face another crisis during the stage of generativity versus stagnation. The need to be needed can lead to emptiness and depression when the children are gone.

At the final stage of development, ego integrity versus despair, the woman must determine whether her younger and present selves are good enough. When this task is accomplished successfully, the woman's self-concept is secure and filled with affirmative reflection; if she develops despair, she views her life with much regret.

Loss

The experience of a loss to the physical or personal self often leads women to seek assistance from health care agencies. *Loss* is defined as a state of being deprived of, or being without, something one has had.[23] For example, a woman who has experienced unsuccessful resolutions of various developmental crises is deprived of a secure sense of self. On the other hand,

she may lose positive attitudes about the self, such as pride, esteem, attractiveness, independence, or control, as well as more obvious losses, such as loss of body parts and loved ones.

An individual who suffers a loss goes through a well-defined grief response. A frequent consequence of this response is depression. A greater number of women experience depression than men, and this depression is often related to the loss of a love object.[27]

Anxiety

Anxiety is a response to a threat to the personal self—particularly the self that yearns to maintain a consistent and stable self-image. Tradition has always been a core of the culture, and therefore, when the feminine tradition is threatened, both women and men may become uncertain of their places and roles. An individual's perception of threat, however, varies according to many factors, which include sociocultural background, education, financial resources, support system, self-esteem, and previous experience with change. The stressors that cause the anxiety response and the response itself are highly individualized.

A woman's attempt to adapt to threatening stressors may be either successful or unsuccessful. She may face up to the stressor ("fight") or withdraw from the situation by physically or mentally removing herself ("flight"). Often, the woman who deals directly with the threat may appear to be a healthy, self-actualizing person, or she may present with various psychophysiological diseases, such as insomnia, hyperactivity, ulcer disease, or hypertension. The woman who withdraws from stressors, on the other hand, is often depressed and dependent.

Stress

Contemporary society bombards women with numerous stressors. These stressors may interfere with the fulfillment of individual needs. Women's responses to these stressors make stress an inevitable force in their lives. Because prolonged stress is unbearable to the equilibrium, the individual must adapt to these forces and maintain eustress and a feeling of well-being.

The differences in response to stress, on the basis of sex, are shown in Table 43-1. As you examine this chart you could speculate that hormonal changes in response to stress in women seem to play a part in their increased incidence of anxiety and depression.

Powerlessness

Roy describes *powerlessness* as "the perception on the part of the individual of a lack of personal or internal control over events within a given situation."[26] Each woman perceives herself as what she would like to be

Table 43-1. **Sex Differences: Male and Female Responses to Stress**

	WOMEN	MEN
Stress	↓ Epinephrine	↑ Epinephrine
	↑ Behavioral inhibition	↓ Behavioral inhibition
Normal conditions	↑ Circulating estrogens	↑ Circulating androgens
	↑ Circulating high-density lipoprotein	↓ Circulating high-density lipoprotein
Exercise	↓ Physical working capacity	↑ Physical working capacity
	↓ Lung capacity	↑ Hemoglobin capacity
	↓ Blood volume	↑ Energy expenditure (aerobic)

(With permission from Martinson I, Anderson S: Male and Female Response to Stress. In Kjervik D, Martinson I [eds]: Women in Stress: A Nursing Perspective, p 91. New York, Appleton-Century-Crofts, 1979)

and what she expects herself to be. This includes some sense of power or control over her being. When the individual does not fulfill her expectancy and self-ideal, an important part of the self-concept, she is likely to feel powerless.[26]

Childbearing and Parenting

Childbearing is a significant event in the life of a woman; parenting is a significant role addition. Both childbearing and parenting lead to important consequences regarding a woman's self-concept. Positive adaptation to these events enhances a woman's level of wellness.

Childbearing and parenting were once seen as natural and expected norms of adult female functioning. In 1970, nine out of ten married women between the ages of 40 and 44 had at least one child; this implies that practically every fertile couple claimed parenthood.[3] Today, however, these presumed expectations of women are being questioned. The emerging roles of women and dependable methods of birth control allow women to explore choices and make conscious decisions about whether, and when, to bear children and parent. Even in our so-called modern society, however, these decisions are seldom reached easily. Both internal and external pressures affect a woman's decision to mother. Indeed, pregnancy is a biologic process invested with great social meaning and surrounded by values, customs, and law in all human societies.[30]

The present period is a time of social transition, when values are changing—a time when old and new norms coexist. It is so much a part of feminine identity to bear children that, for both traditional and nontraditional women, the decisions of whether to mother and when to mother are frequently met with significant conflict.[3]

Crisis Events

Both childbearing and parenting are crisis events. Pregnancy is a major turning point or crisis in the life of a woman, especially the primigravida, calling for far-reaching psychological adaptations.[2]

The crisis of parenthood occurs when old patterns of coping are inadequate to deal with these sharp or decisive life changes. Some of the problems resulting from these changes include the following:

1. Adjusting to being "tied down" or restricted to the home
2. Getting accustomed to being awake at all hours
3. Inability to keep up with the housekeeping and decline in housekeeping standards
4. Tiredness and exhaustion
5. Feelings of neglecting the spouse[8, 17]

The elements of fantasy and romance, which are so prominent in our culture, contribute to the crises of pregnancy and parenting.

In one study of the perceptions of motherhood, it was found that prospective mothers do imagine what it will be like to have a baby and be a mother. Some of these views are unrealistic, with elements of imagination, idealization, and romance. Many prospective mothers imagine the storybook baby who smiles and coos much of the time. Prospective mothers seldom think about a crying baby and the daily work involved in caring for a newborn. New parents are seldom prepared for the effect of parenting on their individual lives and their life as a couple.[34]

Whether the periods of childbearing and parenting develop into crises or not, most women must make adjustments and adaptations. Through the nursing process, the nurse helps the woman adapt to the roles of childbearing and parenting in a changing society.

The Nursing Process

Assessment

To determine the woman's perceptions and present level of adaptation to pregnancy and parenting, the nurse completes an assessment of both biologic and psychosocial components. Using an accepted theoretical reference for biologic assessment, the nurse determines the client's biologic state of adaptation and subsequent energy for psychosocial adaptations.

One aspect of the psychosocial component of assessment is the consideration of cultural influences. Examples of some cultural differences are identified in Chart 43-1.

The following assessment tool for pregnancy and parenting is based on the Roy adaptation model of nursing.

Psychosocial Assessment

I. Assessment of self-concept
   A. How do you feel about being pregnant?
   B. How do you feel about the changes in your body since you became pregnant (example: abdomen, breast, weight gain, skin, and so on)?
   C. What do you think people think of you now that you are pregnant?
      1. Husband
      2. Family
      3. Friends
      4. Coworkers
   D. Many women find that they act or feel different when they are pregnant
      1. Have you noticed any difference in your moods or temperament?
      2. How do you react to this?
   E. Contraception
      1. Was this a planned pregnancy?
      2. Did you use a contraceptive before you became pregnant?
      3. Have you thought of using a contraceptive after the baby is born?
      4. Do you need any information about birth control?
   F. How do you feel about becoming a mother?
   G. Do you think the new baby will change your present functioning as a person?
II. Assessment of role mastery
   A. Educational background
   B. Job
      1. Are you working outside the home?
      2. Do you plan to return to work outside the home after the baby is born?
      3. If yes, how do you think this will affect your job and your mothering?
   C. If this is a first pregnancy,
      1. What do you like most about being a wife?
      2. Do you think this will change when the baby comes?
      3. What are you looking forward to most about being a mother?
      4. What are you looking forward to least about being a mother?
      5. Have you ever taken care of a baby before?

6. Do you feel confident about baby care?
7. Have you attended any baby care classes?
8. Do you think newborn babies sleep very much?
9. How do you think you might feel about having to get up in the middle of the night with the baby?
10. Have you thought about the baby crying? What do you think you will do when the baby cries?
   D. If second (or third, fourth, and so on) baby,
      1. Did you find that your role as a wife changed after your first child?
      2. What do you enjoy most about being a mother?
      3. What do you enjoy least about being a mother?
      4. Do you think the new baby will change your present functioning as a mother?
III. Assessment of interdependency or interrelationships
   A. 1. Have family and friends given you special attention since you have been pregnant?
      2. How do you feel about it?
   B. Has your relationship with your husband changed since pregnancy (or motherhood)?
   C. Has your relationship with friends and coworkers changed since pregnancy (or motherhood)?
   D. Do you plan to have any help when you return home with the baby?
   E. What will you expect whoever helps you to do?
   F. In what ways do you expect your husband to help?
   G. Are there any particular cultural practices or customs around childbearing or childrearing in your family that you will follow?
   H. In what way can we help?

Nursing Diagnosis

Identifying Adaptation Problems. The assessment data are analyzed to determine actual and potential problems. These problems must be validated with the woman. In many instances, what may be considered a problem for many women (or for the nurse) may not be a problem for another woman. Some common nursing diagnoses that might be anticipated by the nurse include the following:

Disturbances in self-concept related to: body image changes associated with pregnancy and delivery

Anxiety related to: ambivalence about combining parenting and career responsibilities; guilt about plans to return to work outside the home after birth of baby

Knowledge deficit related to: biologic changes dur-

CHART 43-1
Cultural Beliefs and Practices: Childbearing and Parenting

Most of these cultural beliefs and customs reflect the traditional culture and are not universally practiced by all members of the cultural group. Variables such as degree of acculturation, educational and income levels, and amount of contact with older generations influence the extent to which these customs are practiced.

Cultural Group	Pregnancy	Childbirth	Parenting
		Labor	**Newborn**
Mexican-American[15]	1. Pregnancy desired soon after marriage 2. Expectant mother influenced strongly by mother or mother-in-law 3. Cool air in motion considered dangerous during pregnancy 4. Unsatisfied food cravings thought to mark the baby 5. Some pica observed in the eating of ashes or dirt (not a common practice) 6. Milk avoided because it causes large babies and, thus, difficult deliveries 7. Many predictions about the sex of the baby 8. Unacceptable and frightening to have pelvic examination by male doctor 9. Use of herbs to treat common complaints of pregnancy 10. Drinking chamomile tea thought to assure effective labor and uncomplicated separation of the placenta, starting during the 8th month of pregnancy	1. Use of "partera" or midwife preferred because they do not rush the delivery 2. After the delivery of the baby, the mother's legs brought together to prevent air from entering the uterus **Postpartum** 1. Diet restricted after delivery, for first 2 days only boiled milk and toasted tortillas permitted, then followed by pieces of chicken or chicken soup for next 2 to 3 days; no fruits or vegetables, which are considered too "acid" or "cold;" pork and chili thought to harm breast milk, therefore avoided for 40 days 2. Bed rest for 3 days after delivery 3. Mother's head and feet protected from cold air—bathing permitted after 14 days 4. Mother often cared for by her own mother 5. Forty-day restriction on sexual intercourse	1. Breast feeding begun after the 3d day; colostrum may be considered "filthy" 2. Olive oil or castor oil given to stimulate the passage of meconium 3. Male infant not circumcised 4. Female infant's ears pierced 5. Belly band used to prevent umbilical hernia 6. Religious medal worn by mother during pregnancy; placed around infant's neck 7. Infant protected from the "evil eye" 8. Various remedies used to treat mal ojo and fallen fontanel
		Labor	
Asian[5]	1. Pregnancy considered time when mother "has happiness in her body"	1. Mother attended during labor by other women 2. Father does not	1. Concept of the family is important and valued 2. Father is head of

(Continues on p. 824)

Cultural Group	Pregnancy	Childbirth	Parenting
		Labor	**Newborn**
	2. Pregnancy seen as natural process 3. Strong preference for female physician 4. Belief in theory of hot and cold 5. May omit soy sauce in diet to prevent dark-skinned baby 6. Prefer soup made with ginseng root as general strength tonic 7. Milk is usually excluded from diet because it causes stomach distress	actively participate during labor **Postpartum** 1. Must protect self from yin (cold forces) for 30 days Ambulation limited Shower prohibited Chinese mother avoids fruits and vegetables 2. Diet Some patients are vegetarians Korean mother is served seaweed soup with rice Chinese diet high in hot foods (*e.g.,* chicken soup made with pig knuckles)	the household; wife plays a subordinate role 3. Birth of a boy is a particularly joyful event
		Labor	**Newborn**
Black American[4]	1. Acceptance of pregnancy depends on economic status Middle-income family usually shows acceptance of pregnancy Pregnancy of lower-income family may be accepted or rejected depending on circumstances 2. Pregnancy thought to be state of "wellness," which is often the reason for delay in seeking prenatal care, especially by lower-income blacks who seek medical care only when "sick" 3. Old wives tales Having your picture taken during pregnancy will cause stillbirth Birthmarks are the result of emotional frights or the un-	1. Use of "Granny midwife" 2. Stoic behavior exhibited to avoid calling attention to selves 3. Mother may arrive at hospital in far-advanced labor 4. Often, cries to the Lord; for example, "Lord have mercy." 5. Emotional support often provided by other women, especially own mother **Postpartum** 1. Vaginal bleeding seen as sign of sickness; tub baths and shampooing of hair prohibited 2. Sassafras tea thought to have healing power 3. Liver thought to cause heavier vaginal bleeding because of	1. Feeding very important: "Good" baby thought to eat well "Good" mother thought to have baby who eats well Early introduction of solid foods May breast or bottle feed; breast-feeding may be considered embarrassing 2. Parents fearful of spoiling baby 3. Commonly call baby by nicknames 4. May use excessive clothing to keep baby warm 5. Belly band used to prevent umbilical hernia

Cultural Group	Pregnancy	Childbirth	Parenting
		Labor	**Newborn**
	satisfied food cravings during pregnancy Reaching up will cause the cord to strangle the baby 4. Craving of certain foods Nutritionally acceptable foods include chicken, greens Unacceptable foods or pica include clay, starch, dirt	its high "blood" content 4. Pregnancy may be viewed by black men as a sign of their virility 5. Self-treatment for various discomforts of pregnancy Constipation treated with epsom salts, castor oil Nausea, vomiting and headache treated with herb teas Heartburn treated with vinegar, baking soda	6. Abundant use of oil on baby's scalp and skin 7. Strong feeling of family, community, and religion

The discussion of cultural practices is not intended to stereotype clients. It is important, rather, that the nurse become familiar with the woman client as an individual and validate the cultural beliefs that are meaningful to her.

Equipped with this knowledge, the nurse supports and nurtures those beliefs that promote physical or emotional adaptation; however, if certain beliefs that might be harmful are identified, the nurse should carefully explore those beliefs with the client and use them in the reeducation and modification process.

ing pregnancy and the puerperium, infant care

Parenting, alterations in related to impaired maternal–infant attachment (bonding), breast feeding difficulties

Grieving related to actual or perceived loss such as change in lifestyle following pregnancy and childbirth; unexpected cesarean section delivery

Planning

After validation of problems, the nurse and woman client formulate realistic objectives for the adaptation process. The woman's participation in goal formulation allows her to accept the goals as part of herself. The nurse remembers that goals are the client's behavioral outcomes. By providing the woman with optimal control over these outcomes, the nurse helps to enhance the woman's self-concept and self-esteem. In some instances, however, the nurse may have to provide more input into the goal-setting for those women experiencing high levels of anxiety or crisis.

Goal Statements. A general objective for the care of a client experiencing pregnancy or parenthood follows:

The woman will make a positive adaptive response (state specific behavioral outcome) to pregnancy or parenting, while achieving and maintaining a secure self-concept (state measurable behavior[s] to detect secure self-concept).

An example of a specific objective for the nursing care of this client might be the following:

The woman will state realistic perceptions of infant behaviors and show confidence (through her statements and actions) in dealing with the infant's behavior by the end of the fourth trimester.

After validating the actual or potential problems and determining the objectives, the nurse is ready to intervene.

Intervention

Personalizing Care. The nurse examines both the apparent cause of the client problem and the corresponding influencing factors, or variables, that make the problem unique and personal to the client. Pregnancy and parenting, for example, may be viewed as two of life's most personal experiences. As the nurse and client examine and deal with each influencing factor, either to change or to support it, the nurse intervenes to provide truly personalized nursing care. For example, sensitivity to the woman's sociocultural and spiritual practices helps to individualize care and make it more acceptable to her.

Supporting the Significant Other. The nurse also supports the woman client's significant other during intervention. This requires initially determining the father's perceptions of the pregnancy and parenting. In addition, his feelings about the traditional and emerging roles of women and his own role as father will be important information for the nurse to use in planning care.

Promoting Optimal Control. The nurse intervenes in a way that promotes the woman's feelings of being in control. One nursing approach used to attain this goal is an attitude of collaboration of care; that is, doing things with, not to, the client. The use of therapeutic communication will enable her to explore her feelings and to identify her problems and their best solutions. Encourage the woman to ask questions about things that are important to her. If she does not understand something, she should ask for an explanation.

Choosing the Setting and Timing. The setting in which the nurse intervenes may influence whether the woman client experiences adaptation or maladaptation. Some interventions are presented most effectively in a group setting, whereas others are most effective on a one-to-one level.

The timing of interventions is also a critical factor in planning nursing care. The identified psychological tasks of pregnancy indicate that a woman faces certain tasks during each of the three trimesters of pregnancy.[30] These tasks suggest that the woman's interest in, and need for, information will vary according to each trimester of pregnancy.

Offering Information. The provision of learning opportunities for the woman client usually revolves around the biologic facts of pregnancy and the puerperium, and preparation for childbirth and child care activities. This information should include some of the known realities of parenting, such as a realistic picture of the wide range of normal infant behavior and of the mother's role. The nurse should also offer information about resources that can assist the woman

during the pregnancy and parenting experience; for example, child care resources and various support groups for the family. An increase in knowledge increases the client's security and self-confidence and therefore strengthen's her self-concept. Praise reinforces the client's increased knowledge and self-esteem.

Communicating Therapeutically. Therapeutic communication allows the woman to explore her feelings about pregnancy and parenting. By encouraging open communication with significant others, the nurse helps her examine the effects of pregnancy and parenting on relationships. Although, today, greater numbers of men are participating in child care activities, the nurse cannot assume that all fathers will wish to do so; each family's plans for parenting should be discussed and clarified. The woman is also encouraged to explore her own career plans and to find solutions for herself.

Evaluation

The evaluation process leads the nurse to review the objectives or goals of intervention and reassess the client's behaviors. How closely, the nurse asks, do the outcome behaviors resemble those stated in the objectives? How well has the woman client adapted to childbearing and parenting in today's society? Does her adaptation represent, for her, a high level of wellness?

This organized problem-solving process, the nursing process, and identified intervention strategies offer the nurse guidelines for assisting women to cope with the tasks and challenges of childbearing and parenting (see Nursing Care Plan 43-1).

Surgical Alterations: Hysterectomy and Mastectomy

Each year, thousands of women in the United States enter hospitals to undergo surgical procedures that strike at the internal and external symbols of feminine identity. The United States Bureau of the Census reports that in 1984, 664 hysterectomies per 1,000 procedures for inpatients discharged from short-stay hospitals were performed.[31] It is estimated that 123,000 new cases of breast cancer were reported in the U.S. during 1986. "About one out of 11 women will develop breast cancer at some time during her life." Most of these cancers are treated by various forms of mastectomy.[1]

Hysterectomy and mastectomy mean far more to these women than simply the physical recovery after a surgical procedure. These operations can have

Nursing Care Plan 43-1

Adaptation to Parenting

Assessment and Nursing Diagnosis	Planning (Objectives/Goals)	Intervention

Parenting, alterations in, related to: impaired parental–infant attachment

Behaviors
1. Holds infant tensely, at arm's distance
2. Refers to infant as "it"
3. Says "He's so little"
4. Asks "Why does he cry so much?" and "Nurse, will you change his diaper?" (makes a face when nurse changes diaper)
5. Watches television most of time while infant is in room, including during feeding
6. Asks that infant be returned to nursery right after feeding

Influencing Factors
1. 19-year-old mother
2. No previous experience with infants
3. Hoped for a female infant
4. Maternal physiological discomfort

Short term
The mother will begin to show signs of maternal infant bonding by the end of the shift, as evidenced by calling the infant by name and holding the infant closely

Long-term
The mother will continue to show signs of increased bonding with infant before discharge, by participating in infant care and using affectionate terms when referring to infant

Intervene to provide physiological comfort and meet mother's dependency needs

Initiate conversation with mother

Use therapeutic communication techniques to assess mother's feelings about the infant; for example, "Beth, tell me how you are feeling now that your baby boy is here," or, "Sometimes mothers feel disappointed when the baby is not the sex they had hoped for"

Accept mother's feelings without judgment

Call the infant by name

Provide brief, frequent opportunities for the mother to be with the infant, suggest times when favorite shows are not on television

Make positive statements about the infant

Demonstrate to mother how to hold infant; explain that baby can see her best when held close

Explain crying behavior of infants and suggest specific techniques for comforting infant

Praise mother for any positive maternal–infant interactions; for example, "you look so good together; he looks so comfortable in your arms"

Assess the mother's readiness for learning infant care and begin teaching specific infant care activities

(Continues on p. 828)

Adaptation to Parenting

Assessment and Nursing Diagnosis	Planning (Objectives/Goals)	Intervention
		Provide the mother with opportunities for return demonstration of baby care
		Praise her efforts to care for baby
		Gradually increase length of time mother spends with the baby
		Encourage the mother to ask questions about infant behavior, needs, and care, and about her own needs

far-reaching, and sometimes devastating, effects on a woman's self-concept. Although health care practitioners may anticipate many common responses such as grief, anxiety, fear, depression, anger, and powerlessness, the ultimate effect of the surgery is unique for each woman. Her experience of the grief process depends on the reason for the surgery and her perception of femininity, lifestyle, support system, sociocultural orientation, stress responses, and personality factors.

Hysterectomy and mastectomy need not produce pathological responses. A knowledgeable, understanding nurse can help the woman client deal with these stressors and grow as a result of the experience.

Common Responses to Surgical Alterations

From childhood on, women have been informed about their "private parts." They anticipate the growth of their breasts and await the external sign, menstruation, which signifies that the uterus within functions. Loss of either of these organs, uterus or breast, causes the woman to experience loss and grief.

Loss and Grief

The grief process results from the losses to both the physical self and the personal self. Besides the loss of the body part, the uterus or breast, the woman also faces the perceived or actual loss of good health, especially if cancer is diagnosed. When a woman's breast is removed, she may fear that others will discover she has had a mastectomy and she may have concerns about her physical attractiveness. Undergoing a hysterectomy may cause the woman to worry that she will experience acceleration of the aging process, weight gain, or decreased sexual interest. Her personal self may question whether her dreams for longevity will be realized. She may examine her life plans and ask, "Can I now really expect this for myself?"

Anxiety and Fear

Anxiety and fear follow both the woman's realization of the need for the surgery and her realization, afterward, that the surgery has taken place. The impact of an altered state of wellness may cause the woman to turn inward. She must use a great deal of mental energy to deal with the unknown—energy that is drawn from every aspect of her life.

Anger and Powerlessness

Anger is another part of the grief response. If the woman believes that she has somehow done, or not done, something to cause her illness, she may direct her anger at herself, often leading to depression. Often, she directs her anger at medical personnel if she believes she has not been told the truth about her condition. For example, she may wonder whether the hysterectomy was absolutely necessary. If the woman is unclear about a one-step biopsy and mastectomy procedure, she may awaken from surgery feeling deceived by the surgeon. Anger and powerlessness, or frustration at the lack of control of her body, must be acknowledged and dealt with.[32]

Depression

Depression is also a stage of the grief reaction and may be a pronounced response to surgical alterations. The meaning of these surgeries to the woman and the perceived loss of femininity are often causes of her depression following mastectomy and hysterectomy.

Factors in the Response to Surgical Alterations

Reason for the Surgery

The indications for hysterectomy are surrounded by controversy. Some women and physicians share the opinion that, if a woman has completed her family or desires no more children, a hysterectomy relieves her of a useless, bleeding organ that may become cancerous. On the other hand, some believe that American surgeons are performing too many hysterectomies.[25]

When a woman is ambivalent about the need for an operation, she loses a certain degree of trust in the physician and experiences increased anxiety. If a woman begins to question the necessity of the operation after she has undergone the surgery, she may express anger toward herself and others. Women seem to be more accepting of a total hysterectomy (removal of the uterus) than a total hysterectomy and bilateral salpingo-oophorectomy (removal of the uterus, ovaries, and fallopian tubes).

Before undergoing a hysterectomy, a woman may have lived with the symptoms and the thought of surgery for a period of time. Anticipatory grieving and the mobilization of resources often occur during the presurgical period. If nurses, physicians, and significant others use this time to prepare the woman physically and psychologically, she is more likely to experience successful postoperative adaptation.

A mastectomy is generally performed when a life-threatening disease, breast cancer, is detected. With more treatment options now available to women with breast cancer, the necessity of a mastectomy may be debated. Once the woman and her physician decide on the need for this surgery, however, she is forced to face the reality of having a life-threatening illness. Usually, little time elapses between suspicion of breast cancer and determination of need for the operation. The crisis nature of this situation provides a woman with little time to deal with her acute feelings of grief, anxiety, powerlessness, and depression, or to mobilize her strengths. Immediate intervention by family, friends, nurses, and other health care professionals is crucial to help the woman cope effectively with the disease and the treatment that will follow.

Perception of Femininity

Our culture emphasizes women's breasts as a sign of femininity. As a girl grows into womanhood, the development of her breasts give her and "the world" external evidence of her femaleness. The functioning of the internal female organs comprises another value in the process of becoming a woman. Menstruation is the first visible sign of the functioning uterus and corroborates its existence.[25] The breast and the uterus, then, are likely to symbolize a woman's femininity and to form an essential component of her body image. Her reaction to losing either breast or uterus will depend, to a great extent, on the value she places on these organs as symbols of being a worthwhile woman. For example, it has been found that women who have considerable emotional investment in their breasts are more likely to suffer severe depression after mastectomy.[28]

Studies have also demonstrated that some women view the uterus as a badge of femininity and, after hysterectomy, perceive themselves as less attractive and fear rejection by their spouses or other men. In addition to reproduction, they attribute to the uterus the functions of excretion, regulation of body processes, expression of sexuality, and maintenance of health, vitality, youth, and attractiveness.[14] The woman who values her body as a measure of self-worth and social acceptance may have more difficulty incorporating the loss of a breast or uterus into an acceptable altered body image than the woman who places greater value on intellectual qualities.[14]

Lifestyle

Lifestyle variations influence the woman's acceptance of surgical alterations. For example, the woman whose body image and role in life are dependent on her external appearance, such as a model or dancer, may be more severely threatened by potential or actual breast loss than a woman whose career is not based on physical attributes.[32] Likewise, for the woman who has not completed her family, the prospect of a hysterectomy comes as a severe blow. The threat of cancer and its potentially debilitating physical effects alter a woman's lifestyle and role performance. It is usually difficult for an independent woman to alter roles and accept help from others.

Support System

An individual's self-concept is partially dependent on the response of others; what others think of us is important in affirming our self-esteem. As she alters her perception of herself in the face of these surgeries, the woman also tries to determine what others now think of her.

The reaction of others following her surgery is a critical determinant of her emotional adaptation to the event. For example, it has been found that, following hysterectomy, a woman is more apt to be depressed if her significant male is distant or detached, shows little concern for her feelings, or believes that she is less attractive than before her surgery.[25] Similarly, when a woman undergoes a mastectomy, her feelings about the loss of her breast are deeply affected by the reaction of her significant male. Most women interpret a negative response from a significant male as physical rejection and interpret avoidance as pity.

In addition to coping with the loss of the specific organ, the significant others must cope with their feelings about the presence of cancer, if that diagnosis has been made. Family members and friends suffer many of the same anxieties, fears, and grief responses as the woman client; their feelings and reactions affect her adaptation.

Sociocultural Orientation

We live in a cancer-fearing society. The American Cancer Society reports that most people associate cancer with death and pain.[32] Women with breast cancer who wish to enter or re-enter the job market may face discrimination through company policies. Although such discrimination policies are illegal, the American Cancer Society of California has reported discrimination against cancer patients in all aspects of employment.

Because the American culture places such a high value on breasts, many women believe that the size and shape of their breasts define their acceptability as women.[32] Recent social trends, however, may help ameliorate society's traditional emphasis on the breast as woman's most valuable attribute.

Various cultural groups hold particular views about the uterus and its functions in maintaining health, youth, and attractiveness. Following a hysterectomy, therefore, a woman of one of these cultural groups might perceive herself as unattractive, unhealthy, and aging.

Response to Stress

An individual's reactions to the crises of life are unique responses influenced by her own personality, philosophy of life, and characteristic coping behavior. Emotionally charged surgical procedures, such as hysterectomy and mastectomy, challenge one's ability to cope and maintain ego integrity. The nurse is able to support and facilitate psychosocial adaptation to these surgical alterations through the systematic approach of the nursing process.

The Nursing Process

Assessment

The woman undergoing surgical alterations experiences both physical and emotional trauma and fatigue, which impede healing of the body and mind. Care provided to both body and mind begins with the physical and psychosocial nursing assessment. As the woman client begins to feel better physically, she also

begins to improve psychologically. Freedom from pain, infection, and complications greatly eases emotional distress. It is often through the preoperative and postoperative physical care that the nurse begins to build a trusting relationship with the client. The development of a trusting relationship is essential before psychosocial assessment and intervention can be accomplished.

The psychosocial assessment example that follows is based on the Roy adaptation framework. Suggested questions and observations regarding the assessment of self-concept, role, and interrelationships are included. The nurse varies or alters the questions according to the client's response and the nurse's comfort level. Some of these issues are best approached preoperatively, others postoperatively; some in a formal manner, others informally. Exploring these areas helps the nurse obtain information needed to plan nursing interventions, which, eventually, promote the client's positive adaptation (see Chart 43-2).

The nurse should inform the client that obtaining this information will help to anticipate some of her needs and insure optimal care. When possible and appropriate, the nurse also involves the client's sexual partner in the assessment process to identify concerns and feelings about the proposed surgery and the degree of support available to the woman.

Psychosocial Assessment.

I. Assessment of self-concept (and body image)
   A. How would you describe yourself?
      1. Your appearance?
      2. Your outlook on life?
   B. How would you describe your general state of health?
   C. What is your understanding of why this operation is necessary?
   D. Can you recall your reaction when you first learned that this operation was necessary?
   E. Can you describe what will happen during the operation?
   F. Do you anticipate any changes?
      1. In your body's functioning?
      2. In your body's appearance because of the operation?
   G. How do you feel about these anticipated changes?
   H. How would you describe a feminine woman?
   I. How would you describe your usual response to a stressful situation?
   J. Do religious practices have meaning for you?
   K. How has your present illness affected your religious beliefs and practices?
   L. What questions do you have about the surgery or anything related to the surgery (preoperatively)?

C H A R T   43-2

Excerpts from an Interview with a Postoperative Mastectomy Client

I. Assessment of self-concept:
  A. How would you describe yourself?
    1. Your appearance?
       "Not very good. Awful, I look awful."
    2. Your outlook on life?
       "Cheerful, with a coverup."
  B. What is your understanding of why this operation was necessary?
     "To keep me alive, and keep the cancer from spreading."
  C. Can you recall your reaction when you first learned that this operation was necessary?
     "I thought, 'This couldn't be real.' I was angry and hysterical."
  D. Do you anticipate any changes?
    1. In your body's functioning?
       "Yes. I wonder if I will be able to do everything I did before."
    2. Your body's appearance?
       "Oh yes. How will I look in my clothes? Will everyone notice the difference?"
  E. How do you feel about these anticipated changes?
     "Bewildered and confused."
  F. How would you describe your usual reaction to a stressful situation?
     "I always try to keep my cool."
  G. Do religious practices have meanings for you?
     "Yes. It's what will carry me through this experience. It's made me stronger."
  H. How are you feeling about your surgery now?
     "I am grateful to be alive. Sometimes I wonder, 'Did they get it all, and are they lying to me?'"
II. Assessment of role
  A. Educational background?
     "B.S."
  B. Do you work outside the home?
     "No."
  C. With whom do you live?
     "My husband and two children; they are teenagers."
  D. Will you describe your activities at home?
     "General housework, care of the family, and gardening."
  E. What kind of activities do you do for fun?
     "Swimming, sailing."
III. Assessment of interrelationships
  A. Has your present illness affected your relationship with your husband, family, friends, or coworkers?
     "No. But I now appreciate them more."
  B. Do you anticipate any changes in your relationships with your husband?
     "Yes, some. I wonder how he will look at me. I don't feel sexy."
  C. Do you anticipate needing help with your usual routines when you return home?
     "No, I will be able to manage fine myself."

Discussion

It is important to remember that the assessment data do not need to be gathered at one time. Some client responses require immediate intervention; others lead to further questioning and analysis. The client may need to express her feelings about one issue before moving on to the next.

This assessment interview shows some typical, yet unique, responses from a client who has undergone mastectomy. The nurse analyzes the data and notes the client's reference to her "coverup" and her concerns about survival, body image, and role performance. Beginning interventions include encouraging further expression of feelings and giving concrete and direct information. This might also be an appropriate time to involve her with a Reach to Recovery volunteer.

The nurse also notes the client's concern about her relationship with her husband and deems that an area of high priority for intervention.

The client's responses indicate that she is independent and feels she will need no help with usual activities upon her return home. It is expected that the recovery period will extend beyond the hospital stay. The nurse is responsible for exploring the client's perceptions of the recovery period and offering concrete suggestions about activities to the client and her family.

M. How are you feeling about your surgery now (postoperatively)?

Observations:

A. Words used to describe herself
B. Ease or uneasiness as she speaks
C. Age
D. Personal appearance
E. Nonverbal behaviors and affect
F. Willingness to look at operative site
G. Use of religious articles

II. Assessment of role mastery
A. What is your educational background?
B. Do you work outside the home?
C. Will you describe the type of activities necessary for your job?
D. With whom do you live?
E. Will you describe your responsibilities at home?
F. What kinds of activities do you engage in for fun?

III. Assessment of interrelationships
A. Describe how you view your relationship to
   1. Men
   2. Women
B. Has your present illness affected your relationship with anyone in your life?
   1. Husband or significant other?
   2. Family?
   3. Friends?
   4. Coworkers?
C. How did your family and friends react when they first learned about your surgery?
D. Do you anticipate any changes in your relationships after the surgery?
   1. With husband?
   2. With family?
   3. With friends?
   4. With coworkers?
E. Do you anticipate needing help with usual routines when you return home?
F. Whom do you expect to help you?
G. How do you feel about needing this help?

Observations:

A. Visitors? How often? Who?
B. Family involvement
C. Response to others in the hospital environment (*e.g.,* doctors, nurses, roommate)
D. Willingness to accept help or do for self

Identifying Nursing Diagnoses. After analysis of the assessment data, the nurse identifies nursing diagnoses and validates them with the woman client.

Some psychosocial adaptation problems experienced by women undergoing hysterectomy and mastectomy include the following:

Self-concept, disturbances in, related to perceived or actual body image problems
Knowledge deficit related to anatomic and physiological changes after surgery

Anxiety related to: actual or perceived threat to self-concept; loss of valued body part; actual or perceived threat to biological integrity
Fear related to: loss of body part; diagnosis of cancer and future implications
Grieving related to: loss of body part; surgery; future childbearing ability
Potential altered sexual patterns related to personal significance of loss of body part and implications of loss on lifestyle
Potential social isolation related to fear of response of others

Planning

The plan for her health care must be acceptable to the woman client. Participation in the decision-making process fosters the development of her self-esteem. A broad or general goal for the client undergoing hysterectomy or mastectomy follows:

The client will perceive herself as a worthwhile individual who understands what is happening to her and will possess a realistic outlook and the ability to problem-solve in the future.

The nurse also formulates specific, measurable objectives for each actual or potential problem of the client.

The client will make positive statements about her appearance before discharge from the hospital.
The client will correctly describe the function of the uterus and the effects of its removal on her body.

Intervention

Before intervening with women clients undergoing hysterectomy or mastectomy, the nurse must look at her own feelings about the loss of female organs, cancer, and these surgical alterations. Confronting and dealing with her own responses will prepare the nurse to promote the client's adaptation to these losses. The nurse must face the question, "Am I strong enough to hear what the client has to say?" Although the general guidelines that were discussed in the section Childbearing and Parenting are also appropriate here, some specific interventions for the woman with surgical alterations follow.

Communicating Therapeutically. The use of therapeutic communication allows the woman freedom to express her feelings about these surgical procedures. This expression of her feelings will be encouraged by the nonjudgmental statements and open-ended questions of a warm, caring health care provider. The nurse also encourages the woman to discuss her feelings and concerns with her loved ones. If the woman is unable to express her feelings verbally, she may be encouraged to express them through the medium of writing. Informing the woman of your availability when she is ready to talk will help her realize that you are genuinely interested in her well-being.

The nurse empathizes with the woman client and accepts her feelings as real and worthy of attention (see Chart 43-3). For example, the nurse conveys, through words and attitude, "I can understand how you could feel that way...."

Providing Physical Care. Providing for the woman's physical well-being and comfort is the basis for competent nursing care. Freedom from incisional pain, abdominal distention, and fatigue will allow the client to rest, mobilize her resources, and, eventually, deal with the physical and emotional implications of her surgery. The nurse also assists the client to maintain her personal appearance, which, in turn, enhances her self-esteem.

Fostering Independence. In the early stages of her recovery, the woman is permitted, and even encouraged, to satisfy her dependency needs. This period of dependent behavior allows her time to mobilize her strengths. The nurse then begins to foster the client's independence as soon as, and to whatever degree, she is able to do for herself. Praising her independent behavior reinforces its occurrence.

There are times, however, when the woman's regression and dependency should be supported. Certain predictable, stressful times require the presence of a caring health professional. During the woman's first look at her mastectomy scar, for example, she needs privacy and the nurse's presence, acceptance, and, perhaps, touch.

Discharge Teaching. Several areas of concern should be addressed with the woman client undergoing surgical alterations prior to her discharge from the hospital. This should include information about the drugs she will be taking, the available community resources, and the perceived effects of surgery on sexual activity.[49] After mastectomy, the woman will need information about the fitting of a prosthesis.

Two examples of valuable community resources are as follows:

1. The American Cancer Society's Reach for Recovery. Through this program, women who have undergone mastectomy help other breast cancer patients during their initial recovery period; the woman client's physician must make the referral.
2. Encore (Encouragement, Normalcy, Counseling, Opportunity Reaching out Energies re-

---

C H A R T   43-3
Therapeutic Dialogue

Exploring the Feelings of a Woman After Mastectomy

Two days ago, Mrs. C. B. underwent a mastectomy of the right breast. The nurse who has been caring for her since her admission to the hospital now enters the client's room and finds her crying.

Nurse: (with hands on Mrs. B.'s shoulder, waits quietly for a few minutes)

Client: (still crying, but more softly, looks at the nurse)

Nurse: (softly, conveying care, and maintaining eye contact) Mrs. B., you seem upset. Is there anything you would like to talk about?

Client: My whole life has changed.

Nurse: Your whole life has changed?

Client: Well, yes, just look at me... (pauses and looks down at her chest) I don't even feel like a woman anymore.

Nurse: You feel that, without your breast, you are not a woman?

Client: I... I don't know, it's hard to say. (a period of silence) I feel so confused.

Nurse: Will you tell me a little more about what being a woman means to you?

Discussion

The client postmastectomy frequently has a need to cry. Crying will help her release pent-up emotions and should be accepted by others. Standing near her, making physical contact, and using periods of silence help the woman feel accepted and cared for. By acknowledging and encouraging the expression of her feelings, the nurse explores with the client what being a woman means to her.

---

vived). This program of the YWCA focuses on exercises performed on land and in water that aid women in rebuilding their physical and emotional strengths after mastectomy.

A summary of other programs available in various cities may be found in The Breast Cancer Digest.[32]

Evaluation

If objectives are realistic and interventions are appropriate for each identified client problem, the nurse will assess positive signs of emotional adaptations to hysterectomy and mastectomy. Often, the adaptive process is just beginning at the time of the woman's discharge from the hospital; the continued support of family, friends, and community resources is necessary. During the evaluation process, the nurse may identify adaptation problem areas of the client in which the nurse is unable to intervene. Such problems should be referred to another health care professional with the necessary expertise.

Menopause

The menopause is that period in a woman's life that marks the permanent cessation of menstrual activity. It can be diagnosed retrospectively, after one year has elapsed.[24] Menopause is not a disease, however, but a normal physiological process.

The terms *menopause, female climacteric,* and *change of life* have been used interchangeably not only to describe the biologic occurrence, but also to indicate that the menopausal woman is middle-aged and quickly approaching old age.[13] Because of the myths surrounding menopause, many women anticipate this time in their lives with dread and respond to it as if in physical and emotional pain (see Chart 43-4, "Myths and Misconceptions About Menopause"). The continuous message in American society, that these are years of declining usefulness and value, proves stressful to women. It is important, then, for nurses and other health care providers to understand the impact of this physiological process and its associated stressors for the woman client and to promote psychological adaptation and well-being.

Significant Life Changes

"Change of life" is an accurate description of the middle years because of the many major changes taking place in the life of the middle-aged adult.[13] The significant life changes that expose a woman to stress at this time include the following:

1. Children reaching maturity and leaving home
2. Possible alteration in marital (or other significant) relationship
3. Returning to the work force (and possible unpreparedness for, or reassessment of, one's place in the work force)
4. Significant physical changes

The menopause occurs at a time in a woman's life—at the average age of 49 years in the United States—

CHART 43-4

Myths and Misconceptions About Menopause

1. Menopause brings on depression and mental illness.
2. Menopause is a deficiency disease.
3. The hot flashes associated with menopause occur at any time and they are unbearable.
4. A menopausal woman will become old, fat, and wrinkled overnight.
5. The menopausal woman loses interest in sex and becomes sexless.
6. Menopausal women drive their husbands to other, younger women.
7. The menopausal woman is always tired.
8. Menopause is the end of womanhood, because womanhood is equated with fertility.
9. Menopause is *the* change of life.

---

when the traditional role assigned to her by society, that of mothering, is essentially complete. A woman's crisis during menopause, therefore, is often one of lost identity. With no clearly defined and socially accepted role for the later years, the middle-aged woman sees menopause as a symbol of profound loss.[19] She may increasingly question her self-worth as she seeks to redefine herself, an inevitable characteristic of the developmental task of the middle years. During this stage of generativity versus stagnation, a woman's need to be needed can lead to emptiness and depression when the children are gone.

As their children mature and leave home, the woman and her husband must adapt to being a couple again. Their communication may have centered on the children for so long that they now find it difficult to express needs as individuals. The perimenopausal woman may even discover she has no supportive person to help her. Often, couples face the prospect of divorce during these years because they have, sometimes unknowingly, drifted apart.

The perimenopausal woman often faces the dilemma of how to use her excess time. In the past, women frequently turned to volunteerism. Faced with the reality of today's economy, however, many women are forced to enter the work force; for some of these women, it may be the first time in their lives to hold a job outside the home. In the 1980s, unfortunately, many of these women are ill-prepared to enter the work force. They often hold low-paying and boring jobs, another contributor to low self-esteem. As a result of societal changes, future generations of menopausal women may be less affected by this potential stressor.

Physical Changes

Changes in body functioning occur during the middle years. The most obvious change, cessation of menstruation, results as the ovaries finally stop functioning. Other physical effects may include vasomotor instability, atrophic vaginitis, osteoporosis, coronary atherosclerosis, and skin and muscle changes. If a woman has been dependent on a youthful body for affirmation of her femininity, she may find it difficult to accept the changes associated with menopause.

Perception of the Menopause

When the woman perceives the menopause as a loss, such as the loss of the mothering role or the loss of purpose, youth, femininity, and self-esteem, she will experience a grief response.

Some of the more frequently observed responses to the menopause include emotional lability, anxiety, feelings of tension and nervousness, insomnia with resultant fatigue, vague bodily aches, and depression. Individual reactions to the menopause, however, are highly variable. Some women respond to the climacteric with no notable behavioral changes, whereas others respond to it with all the typically described behaviors. A woman's response seems to depend greatly on her feelings about herself and her womanhood. If youth, motherhood, and femininity have been the major sources of her self-esteem, she may have a more severe, and, perhaps, destructive, reaction to the menopause than a woman with a number of interests and fulfilling activities outside her home.[13]

On the other hand, many women do not view the end of fertility as a tragedy. Moving into the middle years can be a special time for a woman.[19] Such women are questioning sexual stereotypes and the concomitant confining social roles.

The Nursing Process

The nurse's role in helping the perimenopausal woman meet her needs is to approach her as a unique individual reacting to physical and environmental stressors. The nurse or other health care provider strives to minimize the effect of these stressors and maximize the client's adaptation and growth.

Assessment

A thorough assessment of biopsychosocial factors is important to determine to what extent the client's present distress results from the impact of the menopausal experience. Biologic assessment includes a complete menstrual history and consideration of the presenting physical symptoms. To obtain the psychosocial assessment, it is again suggested that you use the Roy adaptation framework to help you organize data about the woman's self-concept, role, and interrelationships, which are affected during the perimenopausal years. The following serves as a guide to this important information:

I. Assessment of self-concept
   A. How would you describe yourself?
     1. Your appearance?
     2. Your outlook on life?
   B. Have you noted any changes in your body during the past years? (If not, do you anticipate any changes?)
   C. How do you feel about these changes?
   D. How would you describe your general state of health?
   E. Describe what comes to mind when you hear or think of the term "menopause."
   F. During this time of their lives, women sometimes report feeling "different." Have you noticed any differences?
     1. In your mood or temperament?
     2. In your energy level?
   G. How do you feel about these differences?
   H. How have you reacted in the past to changes occurring in your life?
   I. How would you like to describe yourself?
     1. In the next few years?
     2. Ten years from now?

II. Assessment of role mastery
   A. Educational background
   B. Marital status and number of children
   C. Do you presently have children living at home?
   D. Did you work outside the home while your children were growing up?
   E. Can you describe how you felt when your last child left home?
   F. Are you presently working outside the home?
   G. What do you like most about your job?
   H. What do you like least about your job?
   I. What other interests do you have outside the home and your job?
   J. How important are these interests to you?

III. Assessment of interdependency or interrelationships
   A. Marital status and years of marriage
   B. Who is the most important person to you?
   C. For whom are you responsible?
   D. (If married) Have you noted any changes in your marital relationship?
     1. During the last year?
     2. Since your children left home?
   E. How would you describe your present relationship with your children?

F. How do you feel about this relationship (or these relationships)?

G. To whom would you turn if you needed help?

H. Have you spoken to your husband (or significant other) regarding the changes occurring in your body?

Depending on the woman and her concerns, other assessment data may be necessary to complete the picture within this framework.

Nursing Diagnosis

Identifying Adaptation Problems. Analysis and validation of the assessment data often reveal the following psychosocial nursing diagnoses for the menopausal client:

Alteration in self-concept
Grieving related to perceived loss of body function
Anxiety related to: actual or perceived threat to self-concept; actual or perceived threat to biological integrity
Knowledge deficit related to expected physical changes during menopause

Planning

Together, the nurse and the woman client formulate a realistic plan to promote adaptation during the menopause and thereby enhance the client's self-esteem. The woman's desired view of herself in the future guides long-range planning. Specific behavioral objectives are determined jointly to address each identified problem. An example of a specific objective is that the menopausal client will state that she views herself and her physical appearance in a positive manner.

Intervention

Women in the menopausal years during this transitional time in American society are often dependent on others for their feelings of worth. The nurse incorporates these significant others into the plan of care.

Communicating Therapeutically. The nurse realizes that it is important that the client expresses how she feels about this time of her life and how the perceived changes are affecting her. The woman needs to examine the multiple influences in her life and discover which factors are creating stress. For effective and therapeutic communication, the nurse must encourage open expression of the woman's feelings within a nonjudgmental atmosphere.

Health Teaching. The nurse draws from her knowledge of the physiological bases of menopause to clarify the myths and misconceptions that surround it.

The individual who understands what is going on within her body is better able to cope with it. The nurse explains health maintenance through proper nutrition, rest, exercise, and various treatment modalities, such as the use of estrogen therapy. "Not knowing what to expect is still seen as the worst thing about menopause and is seen as the rationale for nursing interventions."[22] The study conducted by Millette also recommends educating men about menopause as husbands are ranked as the first source from whom women seek support in times of stress.[22]

Anticipatory Guidance. The client is guided in using problem-solving techniques to identify her strengths and resources. The nurse supports, praises, and thereby reinforces the woman's positive attempts to determine solutions to her own problems. Encouraging the menopausal client to share her experiences with other women may help to demystify the event.

Evaluation

The nurse evaluates the responses of the woman client by reviewing the behavioral outcomes. Is there evidence that her self-esteem has increased? Does the woman now express more positive feelings about herself and her abilities? Is she able to view the menopause as another natural occurrence in her life during which her own inner strength and support system will guide her to new horizons?

Summary

This chapter emphasizes the significance of applying mental health principles while providing nursing care to women's health needs. The issues of childbearing and parenting, surgical alterations of hysterectomy and mastectomy, and the menopause provide examples of how these principles can be utilized. Other issues in women's health care, such as infertility, menstrual problems (*e.g.,* premenstrual syndrome), abuse and battering, and rape, are equally important. Through application of mental health principles while using the nursing process, the nurse ensures a holistic approach to the health care of women. This chapter has included the following points:

1. Today's female seeking health care faces conflicts related to the traditional and emerging roles of women in our society.

2. Women's traditional place within the health care system has been a subordinate one, but that is presently being questioned.

3. Many of women's health problems are related

to how the individual perceives her physical and personal selves.

4. The nurse frequently deals with the recurring themes of loss, anxiety, stress, and powerlessness in the health care of women.

5. Application of the nursing process to the specific issues of childbearing and parenting, the surgical alterations of hysterectomy and mastectomy, and the menopause includes consideration of the psychosocial significance of these events.

6. Psychosocial assessment of the woman client in the health care setting is based on the Roy adaptation framework, addressing the client's self-concept, role, and interrelationships.

7. General interventions to promote adaptation to these common health alterations include therapeutic communication, mutual goal-setting, health care teaching, and anticipatory guidance.

8. By designing nursing care to meet the needs of the whole person, nurses can have a significant effect on the woman client experiencing childbearing and parenting, surgical alterations, or menopause, as well as other issues in women's health care.

References

1. American Cancer Society: Facts and Figures. New York, American Cancer Society, 1986

2. Bibring B et al: A Study of the Psychological Process in Pregnancy and the Earliest Mother–Child Relationships. Psychoanalytic Study of the Child 14:25–26, 1959

3. Bradwick JM: In Transition. New York, Holt, Reinhart, 1979

4. Carrington BW: The AfroAmerican. In Clark AL (ed): Culture, Childbearing, Health Professionals, pp 35–51. Philadelphia, FA Davis, 1978

5. Chung HJ: Understanding the Oriental Maternity Patient. Nurs Clin North Am 12 (March): 67–75, 1977

6. deChateau P: The Influence of Early Contact on Maternal and Infant Behavior in Primiparae. Birth and the Family Journal 3 (Winter): 149–155, 1976–1977

7. Driever MJ: Theory of Self-Concept. In Roy SC (ed): Introduction to Nursing: An Adaptation Model, pp 169–179. Englewood Cliffs, Prentice-Hall, 1976

8. Dyer ED: Parenthood as Crisis: A Restudy. In Parad H (ed): Crisis Intervention, Selected Readings, pp 312–323. New York, Family Service Association of America, 1965

9. Erikson E: Childhood and Society, 2d ed. New York, WW Norton, 1963

10. Fee E: Women and Health Care: A Comparison of Theories. In Dreifus C (ed): Seizing Our Bodies, pp 279–297. New York, Vintage Books, 1977

11. Friedan B: The Feminine Mystique. New York, WW Norton, 1963

12. Fruchler RG et al: The Women's Health Movement, Where Are We Now? In Dreifus C (ed): Seizing Our Bodies, pp 271–278. New York, Vintage Books, 1977

13. Galloway K: The Change of Life. Am J Nurs 75 (June): 1006–1011, 1975

14. Hogan R: Human Sexuality: A Nursing Perspective. New York, Appleton-Century-Crofts, 1980

15. Kay MA: The Mexican American. In Clark AL (ed): Culture, Childbearing, Health Professionals, pp 88–108. Philadelphia, FA Davis, 1978

16. Lake A: Our Own Years, What Women Over 35 Should Know About Themselves. New York, Random House, 1979

17. LeMasters EE: Parenthood as Crisis. In Parad H (ed): Crisis Intervention, Selected Readings, pp 312–323. New York, Family Service Association of America, 1965

18. Levinson R: Sexism in Medicine. Am J Nurs 76 (March): 426–431, 1976

19. Martin LL: Health Care of Women. Philadelphia, JB Lippincott, 1978

20. Martinson IM, Anderson S: Male and Female Response to Stress. In Kjervik DK, Martinson I (eds): Women in Stress: A Nursing Perspective, pp 89–95. New York, Appleton-Century-Crofts, 1979

21. Maslow AH: Motivation and Personality. New York, Harper & Row, 1954

22. Millette BM: Menopause: A Survey of Attitudes and Knowledge. Issues in Health Care of Women 3: 263–276, 1981

23. Peretz D: Development, Object-Relationships, and Loss. In Schoenberg B et al (eds): Loss and Grief: Psychological Management in Medical Practice, pp 3–19. New York, Columbia University Press, 1970

24. Perlmutter JF: A Gynecological Approach to Menopause. In Notman MT, Nadelson C (eds): The Woman Patient: Medical and Psychological Interfaces, pp 323–335, Vol 1. New York, Plenum Press, 1978

25. Roeske NA: Hysterectomy and Other Gynecological Surgeries: A Psychological View. In Notman MT, Nadelson C (eds): The Woman Patient: Medical and Psychological Interfaces, Vol 1, pp 217–231. New York, Plenum Press, 1978

26. Roy Sr C: Problems in Self Ideal and Expectancy: Powerlessness. In Calliota R: Introduction to Nursing: An Adaptation Model, pp 224–231. Englewood Cliffs, NJ, Prentice-Hall, 1976

27. Scaff M: The More Sorrowful Sex. Psychology Today 12 (April): 44–52, 89–90, 1979

28. Schoenberg B, Carr AC: Loss of External Organs: Limb Amputation, Mastectomy, and Disfiguration. In Schoenberg B et al (eds): Loss and Grief: Psychological Management in Medical Practice, pp 119–131. New York, Columbia University Press, 1970

29. Spock B: Decent and Indecent. New York, Fawcett World, 1971

30. Tanner LM: Developmental Tasks of Pregnancy. In Bergersen BS et al (eds): Current Concepts in Clinical Nursing, Vol 2, pp 292–297. St. Louis, CV Mosby, 1969

31. US Bureau of Census. Statistical Abstract of the US: 1987 (107th edition). Procedures for Inpatient Discharges from Short-Stay Hospitals 1975–1984, p 98. Washington, DC, 1986

32. US Department of Health and Human Services: The Breast Cancer Digest. Bethesda, MD, National Cancer Institute, May, 1984

33. Weideger P: Menstruation and Menopause: The Physiology and Psychology, The Myth and the Reality. New York, Alfred A Knopf, 1976

34. Williams R: The Perceptions of Motherhood as Viewed by Primigravidas. M. N. Thesis, University of California at Los Angeles, 1972

35. Willson JR, Beecham CT, Carrington ER: Obstetrics and Gynecology, 4th ed. St Louis, CV Mosby, 1971

44 Death and Dying

Patricia N. Mahon

You hurry on—
but for one brief moment
saw the anguished night of darkness,
heard the echoes of fear and terror,
felt both human strength and weakness.

You hurry on—
but for one brief moment
knew that you made all the difference.
And—for one brief moment prayed.

P. Mahon

Chapter Preview

Death is an inevitable event that every living organism faces as the end of life and living. Death, said Jung, is probably the only irreversible and unequivocal process we experience that is directed toward a goal, a state of complete rest.

This chapter discusses the theoretical, philosophical, religious, and "American" viewpoints on death and dying. The stages of dying are described in relation to the dying client, his significant others, and the professionals involved in his care. The chapter also examines mourning and societal rites. Nursing care of the dying client and his family—both physical and psychological care—is explored.

Learning Objectives

On completion of the chapter, you should be able to accomplish the following:

1. Discuss theoretical, philosophical, religious, and "American" perspectives of death and dying
2. Discuss the meaning of death to the client, his family and friends, and the health care professionals caring for him
3. Compare the behavior of clients, significant others, and health care providers during various levels of awareness of dying
4. Provide examples of clients' and family members' behavior during each stage of dying
5. Discuss the implications of certain special circumstances of death, such as sudden death and death of a child
6. Describe physical and psychological nursing care of the dying individual and his family

Perspectives on Death and Dying

Theoretical Viewpoints

The meaning of death has troubled man from the beginning of time; its meaning and relationship to life have been the philosopher's enigmas. From the time of the ancient Greeks, death's mysterious relationship with life has been examined. The major religions of the world deal intimately with death and view it as a commencement or transformation to another type of existence. At one end of the continuum, death may be perceived as the ultimate threat of nonexistence; at the other end, as a blessed relief for those in agony.

Psychologists and sociologists have theorized about death and have made it a topic of study. Freud believed that the ego of man was incapable of understanding the possibility of his own future nonexistence. He proposed that people experience, simultaneously, anxiety over death and a death instinct.[9] In strong disagreement with Freud, Carl Jung presented the idea that the most important and positive aspect of individuation, or unique development of self, is recognition and acceptance of one's mortality and fulfillment of the tasks to prepare for death.[17] The integration of death into the process of living may be viewed existentially as an essential aspect of development and a way to diminish the individual's vulnerability to a neurotic denial process.[28]

Systematic investigations into the generally tabooed topic of death began after the appearance of Feifel's book *The Meaning of Death* in 1959.[7] In the 5 years following the book's publication, its effect was reflected in the scientific community in the appearance of a greater amount of social, psychological, and medical literature on death, dying, and grief than had appeared in the previous century. In 1973, the Center for Death Education and Research at the University of Minnesota published a bibliography of more than 2600 references on the topic of death and related issues.[12]

One author examined the individual denial reactions to death and categorized them according to the following degrees:

1st degree—denial of the clinical facts
2d degree—denial of the implications of the clinical facts
3d degree—denial of extinction or nonexistence[38]

An individual may reach a level of "middle knowledge" or vacillation between complete denial and acceptance. On the other hand, an individual may experience both acceptance and denial of death at the same time, which may serve as an adaptational process in the preparation for death.[8]

The American View of Death

The thought of death elicits anxiety and denial in modern man. Death has become an enemy that evokes our greatest fears. American society, with its emphasis on the "to be" and the young, has little room for the concept of "no future." Death, therefore, has the power to stir our fear and hostility and to set into motion a process of denial. Many view death as the final loss of identity, complete extinction, or the annihilation of the individual's significance.

The coping mechanisms of our culture have attempted to disguise death or pretend that its finality does not exist. An example of this pretense is the elaborate burial rite in which the body is prepared "to look natural" for the funeral at the cost of many thousands of dollars. In addition, the language or phrases we use to communicate that an individual has died reflects yet another ritual of denial. Phrases such as "he passed on" or "she's gone," utilized by lay and professional persons alike, are common attempts to avoid discussing death directly. The American funeral has been sarcastically described as "grief therapy" for those who try to "buy off" the grief process in dollars and cents.[27]

The American way of death primarily reflects the Judeo-Christian orientation of our society. There are two basic reactions to death in our contemporary world—avoidance, and preoccupation with death as a destructive force. Death delivers with it separation, from the body as well as from loved ones, and reawakens the childhood threat of abandonment.[26] Most individuals readily admit that they will die, but view their own death and the deaths of their loved ones as events that are far removed and in the distant future. The prevalent attitude in our society, says Kübler-Ross, is "It shall happen to thee and thee but not to me."[21]

In direct counteraction to these views of death is the "happy death movement," which attempts to promote a change in the American society's taboo on death.[25] The three main components of this movement are immortality, positivity, and expressivity. Immortality is associated with a belief in an afterlife, positivity is the breaking away from secularism and materialism of society, and expressivity is the open expression of feelings about dying. There will, however, always be individuals who will wish to prolong life at any cost, emotional or monetary. There will be others who will not, or cannot, express feelings about living or dying. Still others may see themselves as failures if they are unable to "grow" in this final chance for achievement and end their lives as they have viewed themselves during life.

Death is inevitable, no matter what ritual, thoughts, or actions we attempt to use to magically control or alter the reality. Both professionals and lay persons continue to experience the ambivalences of death and continue to move closer to a new understanding and realistic acceptance of what is inevitable as a stage of potential growth. We must use the strengths of the new philosophy of caring for the dying, while maintaining objectivity about its limits.[2]

Meaning of Death

Meaning of Death to the Client

Relocation of Care
Medical progress in the past few decades has proven to be a double-edged sword to the dying individual. This progress has not only altered the care and treatment of the dying, but has relocated the place of death and the interaction of the dying with loved ones. Rarely does an individual die in the privacy of home and family; rather, he is subjected to the institutional "public square" of the impersonal hospital. This transfer to the institution of what was once an intimate, personal, and private process reinforces our denial of death and breeds isolation and loneliness for the dying individual.

Fear of Abandonment
Loneliness is the experience that results from the dying person's exposure to the abandonment of others and the isolation in the institutional setting.[19] The lengthier the process of dying, the greater the feelings of abandonment and isolation that are experienced by the dying individual (see Chart 44-1, "Living with a Terminal Illness"). The dying patient manifests three basic levels of fear—fear of pain, fear of loneliness, and fear of meaninglessness.[41]

The interaction between the dying patient and his family or staff has been described as "premortem dying."[40] The individual's isolation is potentiated by the nonverbal gestures of dimming the lights and drawing the blinds, and the verbal gestures of whispering and giving stereotyped answers to the patients' questions. Despite increasing public and professional attention to the subject of death and dying, dying still remains a lonely and isolated event in which the patient often feels "dehumanized, impersonalized, and mechanized."[20]

The "Sick Role"
The process of dying also places the individual in a dependent position with many role expectations. Society has carved out a unique position for the ill individual. The expectations associated with the illness role include the rights to be dependent, to accept help from those whom the patient previously has not known, and to anticipate that he will be cared for. To possess these rights, patients must conform to the bureaucratic structure and expected behaviors of the health care system. Those who do not conform to the role expectations and bureaucratic structures cause much annoyance to health care providers and

C H A R T   44-1
Therapeutic Dialogue

Living with a Terminal Illness

Dave is a 16-year-old diagnosed with terminal bone cancer. In the last year, he has undergone two surgeries and chemotherapy. This interview took place at a recreational center where Dave spends time with his friends. Dave was expecting the interviewer and was aware of the topic of the interview.

Nurse: Hi Dave, I'm Dr. M.

Client: Yeah, hi...I've been expecting you. Let's go sit under the tree by the courts.

Nurse: You look like you're having fun.

Client: Yep, it's about time...I was letting myself die too long...until I finally got a little smarts and I said to myself, this death thing...you've been just going down, down...you've got to LIVE! You know you can make the decision to die, like my doctor said, just give up, lay there and finally die.

Nurse: Did that happen to you?

Client: Oh yeah, for a long time all I did was stay in bed in my room...didn't do a thing.

Nurse: Just stayed alone...and did you experience anger?

Client: Yep, when I was laying there I used to think over and over again, why me, why me...why did I get picked out for cancer? It seemed like I just finally said to myself, "Dave, you're just gonna have to die or live—not live just like I was—you're gonna have to really LIVE!! I just can't do everything I used to do before. So I went back to my regular school and did most of what I used to. Most my friends knew I was going to die—and it was hard—nobody would say anything at first and they didn't invite me to do all the things we all used to. But it got better— I guess they just forgot about me dying.

Nurse: That was difficult.

Client: Yep, for a while it made me more scared, but now it's okay....

Nurse: You might have to have more surgery....

Client: That's what they wanted...but after my last surgery when I finally woke up...I said to myself, "No way am I ever going to go back for any more. My mom said that I had the choice, and I don't want to go through all that pain any more for nothing. I know that they can't cure it...and that's okay. It hurts my mom, but she understands.

Discussion

One of the greatest stressors experienced by the dying is the isolation from family and friends. Sometimes this occurs when significant others avoid conversations dealing with the client's feelings about his illness and impending death. Nurses and other health care professionals can fill this need for openness and truthfulness by accepting the client's expressions. The nurse listens to, acknowledges, and refrains from making judgments about these expressions.

The individual who is living with a terminal illness faces multiple, real losses. Interpersonal or social support should not have to be one of these losses when health care providers intervene therapeutically.

may be viewed as demanding or "difficult patients," or may be subtly avoided.

By accepting the sick role, the individual patient loses control over his environment, loses the right to make decisions about basic functions such as eating and sleeping, and loses his familiar and secure social roles, such as father, mother, boss, worker, breadwinner. These losses, which are inherent in the sick role, and the change in role expectations place the individual in a vulnerable, dependent, childlike position, and may prompt him to view himself at the mercy of the professional staff. (Chart 44-2, The Living Will, illustrates one recently adopted alternative to the terminal patient's complete loss of control.)

The Stigma of Nonexistence

The dying person not only confronts new experiences and new roles, he is also saddled with a stigma; he represents what all of us fear—our own nonexistence.[15] Instead of dealing with our death fears, we tend to view the dying individual as "different," thereby protecting ourselves, in some magical way, from the horror of death. This process of stigmatization further isolates the dying individual and compounds the loneliness of the dying process.

It is almost an impossibility to be truly prepared for death, because we cannot imagine ourselves as nonexistent. Although fear of death is a part of the human experience, we find that, many times, the older individual seems to be less fearful than the young person and, consequently, is more often concerned about the deaths of his loved ones, friends, and pets. In a lengthy terminal illness, an individual may even welcome death as a release from pain. A client's religious belief or philosophical orientation may alter his acceptance of death and may individualize his dying process.

The acceptance of death as an inevitable and individual process may begin early in life for one person, whereas, for another, this realization may not be reached until he experiences the physical signs and deterioration of aging. A small group of individuals may attempt to deny death to the very ends of their lives.

Meaning of Death to Family Members and Loved Ones

The Experience of Loss

The loss of a loved one is experienced not only through death, but also through lengthy illness, divorce, and separation. The experience of each loss requires adjustment to the specific life circumstance. All losses in life, including the loss of a loved one through death, involve a part of the "self"; therefore, the experience is unique for each individual. Sur-

vivors experience difficulty in reintegrating as a family unit and as individuals. The dying process and the accompanying loss are often more difficult for the survivors than for the dying person. Every family in which a loss by sudden, unexpected, or expected death has occurred is defined as a family at risk or in crisis.[4]

Anticipatory Grief

During the hospitalization of a terminally ill family member, the other family members begin to experience intense feelings of loss. This phenomenon is termed *anticipatory grief* and occurs when the family and loved ones know for sure that the individual will die.

Anticipatory grief is a contemporary phenomenon that has been identified by professionals concerned with the mental health of the public. Identifying and nurturing anticipatory grief are vital aspects of pre- and postdeath counseling and the reconstruction and reintegration of the survivor's emotional and social life. This phenomenon aids in the grief transition and acceptance of the death of the loved one, and therefore frees the survivor's energy to function in the decision-making of everyday living. Although anticipatory grief work may function as a positive experience in the adjustment of the survivor, it presents itself as a double-edged sword to the dying individual. The dying individual must not only deal with his own loss, but must also attempt to cope with the loss of emotional support of the loved one.

Another backlash of anticipatory grief is felt when the loved one's actual death and funeral are confronted. Historically, funeral rites have functioned as ceremonies to provide emotional support to the survivors and to strengthen familial, friendship, and community bonds. When anticipatory grief has helped the survivors separate from the dying client, their expected mourning behaviors are minimized and they may be criticized for coldness or lack of love of the dead individual. Traditional funeral rites will not disappear because of anticipatory grief work, but, for a large number of individuals, they will change significantly.

Coping with the Loss

From the earliest investigations, it has been observed that under "normal" circumstances, "normal" individuals will experience "normal" grief reactions and return to a "normal" state of functioning. It has, however, been observed that if the pattern is disrupted in any way, such as when there is a lack of evidence that death has occurred (*e.g.,* war deaths) or when the primary denial reaction is not overcome, then a maladaptive reaction to the loss may occur, such as a

CHART 44-2
The Living Will

In caring for the dying, it is critically important to respect the individual's decisions and wishes. The Living Will is one attempt to communicate to family, friends, and physician that one wishes to be allowed to die when that event becomes inevitable.

Although it has little legal power except in California, the Living Will is a legal document and, therefore, must be signed in the presence of two witnesses; notarization is not necessary. It is suggested that the individual who wishes to utilize the Living Will provide copies to his physician and significant others and discuss with them his decision about terminal care. The individual must also carry a copy of the Living Will on his person to guarantee that his wishes will be known to health care providers. A copy of the Living Will follows.

TO MY FAMILY, MY PHYSICIAN, MY LAWYER, MY CLERGYMAN;

TO ANY MEDICAL FACILITY IN WHOSE CARE I HAPPEN TO BE;

TO ANY INDIVIDUAL WHO MAY BECOME RESPONSIBLE FOR

MY HEALTH, WELFARE OR AFFAIRS

Death is as much a reality as birth, growth, maturity and old age—it is the one certainty of life. If the time comes when I, _____ can no longer take part in decisions for my own future, let this statement stand as an expression of my wishes, while I am still of sound mind.

If the situation should arise in which there is no reasonable expectation of my recovery from physical or mental disability, I request that I be allowed to die and not be kept alive by artificial means or "heroic measures." I do not fear death itself as much as the indignities of deterioration, dependence, and hopeless pain. I, therefore, ask that medication be mercifully administered to me to alleviate suffering even though this may hasten the moment of death.

This request is made after careful consideration. I hope you who care for me will feel morally bound to follow its mandate. I recognize that this appears to place a heavy responsibility upon you, but it is with the intention of relieving you of such responsibility and of placing it upon myself in accordance with my strong convictions, that this statement is made.

Signed _____

Date _____

Witness _____

Witness _____

Copies of this request have been given to _____

_____

_____

_____

major pathological depression, or even psychosis in certain instances.

Family members and friends begin to cope with the loss of an individual through death before the actual death occurs and continue to deal with their loss after the death. *Coping behavior* may be defined as all of the mechanisms utilized by individuals to deal with significant threats to their psychological stability and to enable them to function in daily living.[37] Coping behaviors are responses to environmental factors that assist the individual regain control or master the situation and successfully adapt to the stressor.

The Process of Mourning

During the initial stage of mourning, *impact,* the mourning individuals have difficulty determining their own needs and lack the initiative or energy to search out the needed helping service. The second phase, or *middle stage* of mourning, may extend beyond 1 year after the death, during which the family and friends acutely feel the losses. During this second phase, the mourner experiences loneliness and a need to speak about the deceased. The third phase, *accommodation,* overlaps the first two phases, from 3 months to 2 years after the loss. Those who have experienced anticipatory grief appear to have less severe grief reactions and to enter the accommodation stage earlier.

The dying individuals and their families may move through the stages of dying identified by Kübler-Ross—denial, anger, bargaining, depression, and acceptance—although not necessarily at the same time or at the same pace. Successful mourning brings comfort when the family or friends attain a sense of peace or acceptance with the death. To grieve is to allow expression of the sorrow and other feelings but not to grasp the feelings as an excuse to avoid the gift of life that the mourners still possess.

In the process of grieving, the deep feelings of ambivalence—that is, love, anger, and guilt toward the lost loved one—are the emotions seen in a major depression. Although these emotions of the grieving person are, in varying degrees, identical to those of major depressions, they differ in origin and process. The grief process is healthy, necessary, and growth-producing; major depressions are personality structure–oriented and growth-blocking processes.

The length of the grieving reaction and the final adjustment made to a new social environment depends on the success of what is called the "grief work"; that is, freedom from the bondage to the deceased, reorientation to the environment in which the deceased is no longer present, and establishment of new relationships.[24] Some individuals resist accepting the discomfort and distress of mourning. They may choose to avoid the intense pain connected with the grief experience and the expression of the feelings associated with grieving. The avoidance or disruption of normal grieving may be the prelude to a morbid grief reaction. This morbid reaction may be reflected in both physiological and behavioral responses, ranging from psychosomatic conditions such as asthma, ulcerative colitis, and rheumatoid arthritis, to antisocial behavior and even psychosis.[24]

Certain factors must be considered when dealing with a bereaved individual because they can aid in understanding and predicting reactions and facilitating the helping relationship. These critical factors include the following:

1. The degree of significance the deceased played in the life of the survivor
2. How others react behaviorally to the death
3. The ages of the deceased and the survivor
4. The emotional and physical state of the survivor
5. Previous loss experiences
6. The presence of close friendships
7. Role changes necessitated by the death
8. The degree of the survivor's dependence upon the deceased

In addition, professionals must recognize the typical behaviors seen in a healthy response to the death of a significant other. Grief may be manifested in tears, overwhelming feelings of loss, desires to withdraw, imagined guilts over omissions, and a multitude of physical symptoms such as anorexia, headache, and dizziness. Health care professionals must accept grief-related behaviors because these behaviors help individuals reorganize and resume productive, functional living. These behavioral expressions loosen the ties to the deceased, which, in turn, frees the survivor to form new ties. It is particularly helpful for survivors to understand that the emotions they are experiencing are common phenomena and that the deep hurting does come to an end.

The grieving process does not necessarily take place only after the physical death of the loved one. During a long illness, family members and significant others may actively move through the stages of mourning and may "let the other go"; in this way, they accept the person's death before his death actually takes place. Therefore, when the death finally occurs, the survivors may express, through verbal and non-verbal behavior, a sense of relief and peaceful acceptance.

Although none of us is able to control the inevitability of death, we can control the process by which the separation from life and loved ones takes place; we can create either a life-accepting or life-rejecting stage of development.

Meaning of Death to the Health Care Professional

Outside their own natural life experiences, many health professionals are as unprepared to deal with death and dying as is the lay person. Health education focuses on health, living, and the extension of life and neglects to teach coping skills in the care of the dying and their families. Because the underlying and subconscious goal in the ministering to the sick is health, a dying individual is difficult for health care providers to handle. Symbolically, the health care professional may experience death as a frontal attack on the professional goal of health promotion and life.

In addition to the professional threat, working with the dying stirs a more personal reminder of our own death, nonexistence, and abandonment. Nurses and other health care providers may avoid the dying by busying themselves with other patients, make short and only necessary contacts with the dying individual, move the dying person out of their constant vision and hearing, or overtly avoid the dying person and his family on the hospital unit.

One study found that a number of factors affected the physician's behavior toward the dying patient, including the patient's age, the patient's response to therapy, the rank or social worth of the patient, the ability of the patient or family to pay for services, the patient's attractiveness, the appeal of the disease, and the physician's own personality; that is, his optimism, conservativism, or radicalism.[23]

Nurses seem better able to face death than their co-workers. As one nurse succinctly stated:

> We readily care for those whom we can help cure, and it feels good...knowing a patient is going to die doesn't mean we can't receive just as much reward....[36]

In an investigation involving 15,400 nurses, it was found that a significant number felt that a dying person most needed to be allowed to die in peace, which included the right to refuse treatment. Sixty percent of the nurses believed that the patient should be told as soon as possible that he is dying.[29] One nurse therapist utilized role-playing to help the nursing staff in the coronary care unit deal with death. Staff members played the roles of the dying patient, the family, and the staff to reenact and work through difficulties they experienced in patient care situations. The therapist identified two major reactions. The majority of the nursing staff was willing to deal directly with the patient and his problems with dying; others attempted to ignore the problem of death, became involved with technical tasks, and proceeded to tell the patient that he was doing well.

It is necessary for the health care professional to accept and recognize his own mortality and examine the personal meaning of death to be effective in caring for the dying. Even when these steps have been accomplished, death is still difficult to view and the feelings accompanying it are painful.

Theories of Dying

Research and theory development regarding death and dying have increased dramatically in the past 20 years. Glaser and Strauss conducted a long-term sociologic study of dying and, from this intensive investigation, they published their work describing aspects of the process of dying.[13,14]

Levels of Awareness of Dying

The dying client and his family, friends, and professional staff may experience awareness that the client is dying but each may be at different levels at any given time. The levels of awareness are as follows.

1. *Closed awareness,* or "keeping the secret." The client in this situation is not aware that he is dying but the family and professional staff are.
2. *Suspicion awareness.* The client has a suspicion that death may occur but cannot obtain sufficient information to verify it.
3. *Mutual pretense awareness,* or "let's pretend time." All individuals involved in the situation are aware of the active dying process, but a ritual of pretense is carried out by all.
4. *Open awareness.* All involved in the situation are aware of the active dying process and demonstrate their awareness in actions, communications, and the taking care of unfinished business.[13]

Expected Death Patterns

In a later publication, Glasser and Strauss discussed death expectations and professional care patterns.[14] A terminal patient, for example, cared for on a particular service (emergency room, cardiac intensive care unit, oncology unit, and so forth) is expected to die over an expected time period and in a predictable way.

Professional staff may assess when a patient will die and may, therefore, plan their work in light of their expectations. The death patterns have been divided into five categories:

1. Too sudden death
2. Vacillating pattern

3. Certain to die on time
4. Short-term reprieve
5. Lingering

When the health professional's assessment closely parallels the actual death pattern of the patient, the professional staff's work with all patients, the dying individual and other patients, is made easier and care is delivered more smoothly.[14]

Process of Dying

The time involved in the process of dying has also been subdivided into last weeks, last days, and last hours. During the last weeks, nurses need to rearrange care activities for the patient, while he ties up the loose ends and begins to take leave of life. The phenomenon of social isolation of the dying patient is more evident during these last weeks. During the last days, the family and professional staff are faced with the decision of whether to prolong the life of the individual and make decisions concerning where the final stage of his dying will occur—home, hospital, or nursing home.

During the last hours, three levels of behavior—the death watch, the death scene, and the final death—occur. The death watch is carefully handled by the caregivers to prevent an unpleasant death. Physiological control through promotion of sleep, elimination of pain, and relief from restlessness is the focus of care. It is of utmost concern to the health care providers and family and friends that the patient not die alone. The death scene is usually brief and terminates at the actual physiological death with the ritual pronouncement of death. Family members are usually most intimately involved in this final stage of dying.

Stages of Dying

What of the patient? Once diagnosed as dying—what comes about next? In 1969, Kübler-Ross presented a framework for understanding the process of dying. Her extensive case study investigations with the terminally ill, their families, and professional staff for the past 20 years and her many books and workshops on death and dying have profoundly affected how society thinks about death.

Kübler-Ross identified five possible stages of dying experienced by the patient and his loved ones.

Stage 1—denial
Stage 2—anger
Stage 3—bargaining
Stage 4—depression
Stage 5—acceptance

Denial

In the first stage of dying, the initial shock and its concomitant denial are reactions to the overwhelming threat of nonexistence. Denial is a necessary and protective mechanism that may be present for a few minutes or may be utilized for periods of months.

Anger

The initial stage is followed by felt and expressed anger. The dying person's anger is directed at self, God, and others who have a future and do not face the loss of existence.

Bargaining

The anticipation of the losses through death brings about a time of bargaining. Through this bargaining, the individual attempts to postpone or reverse the dreaded moment of death. The individual may pray for more time to complete important goals in his life, to see a new grandchild born, or take the special trips he had always planned. During this time, promises are made to alter lifestyles, go to church more often, and give to charity; the individual usually promises something in exchange for life.

Depression

When the full effect of his diagnosis is felt and the loss can no longer be delayed, the individual moves into the stage of depression. This depression is a therapeutic state and a necessary way of aiding the individual to detach from life and living and thereby accept his death.

The depression of the process of death and dying is viewed differently from the pathological depressions seen in the process of life. Pathological depressions must be treated and their cause or causes must be dealt with; in the process of dying, depression is a necessary stage of growth rather than a regression.

Acceptance

To accept death is to pass beyond the emotional turmoil inherent in its process. The word, acceptance, is an ambiguous word. The individual who "gives up" by refusing medication, treatment, or food can, in a sense, be said to have accepted death. Or has he just "refused" life? Though the physical fact of the cessation of life is the same, the emotional freedom and sense of peace that accompany acceptance may not exist with the person who "gives up."

Kübler-Ross's theory of the stages of dying is currently being questioned, because of her lack of a controlled research design. The stages she described, says one critic, have not been clearly demonstrated and no strong evidence has been presented that individuals do, in fact, move through stages in dying.[18] Nevertheless, the greatest value of Kübler-Ross's work may be an increased sensitivity to the needs of the dying person and attention to the possibility that adaptive stages may be at work in the terminal process.

Disengagement

The theory of disengagement has evolved with the growth of the field of gerontology. This theory proposes that the elderly or dying person acts voluntarily in giving up his or her roles in life, slowly loses interest in the active world, and pulls away or withdraws from significant others. The individual would not be defined as happy and may, in fact, experience emotional deprivation, but is at peace. This state is comparable to the stage of acceptance described by Kübler-Ross.

According to the disengagement theory, society and the individual mutually engage in the process of withdrawal from each other as a normal aspect of aging and the ending of life. This theory further states that an individual will deal with aging and dying similar to the way he dealt with other problems and losses in his life.[3]

Other studies have shed doubt on the idea of mutual withdrawal or the disengagement theory. One investigator, for example, found that aging individuals generally move toward activity and social contacts, and questioned whether the disengagement process is a result of environmental conditions, rather than a natural process of tying up loose ends and preparing to withdraw from life.[5]

From the work with the terminally ill, we can learn something about living—if death is a final separation, what of other separations in life, such as divorce, graduations, loss of a job, a move? If there is a parallel in the processes, then each of us in daily living is preparing ourself for the final "letting go."

Death and Special Circumstances

Sudden Death

Much work has been done with the survivors of victims of sudden or unexpected deaths. Sudden deaths are related to a greater amount of emotional turmoil and shock in the survivors than with those whose significant other was ill. The survivors of victims of sudden death have no time to engage in anticipatory grief and often have no alerting, warning time. The most disturbing and unbalancing feature of a sudden death is the element of unexpectedness.

Many times, interpersonal circumstances existing prior to the death, such as periods of emotional stress, anger, or hurt, may result in severe guilt feelings in the survivors. The immediate reactions of the survivors are usually severe and include disbelief, guilt, fear, remorse, and despair.[16,35] There is a high incidence of suicide in the surviving mate after the sudden death of the spouse.[31]

The sudden death of a significant other is viewed as a disaster, similar to a catastrophic event. This reaction is a "disaster syndrome," which includes the initial shock followed by motor retardation, flattened affect, somnolence, amnesia, guilt feelings, exhaustion, numerous bodily complaints, and feelings of worthlessness.[10,42]

The "psychological autopsies" on the parents of adolescents who committed suicide demonstrated three basic phases in the survivors' grief process. These phases include the following:

1. Resuscitation from the initial shock, which lasts up to 24 hours
2. Rehabilitation, which extends from 1 to 6 months after the death
3. Renewal, which is a healthy tapering off of the mourning, lasting 6 months or more[33]

To help families cope with sudden death, nurses may direct survivor care toward the goals of intervening in the distortion of the reality of the event, identifying consistent support systems for the family, and enhancing the coping mechanisms of the family members.[32]

Death of a Child

The death of one's child is probably the most threatening loss that a person can experience. The parent visualizes his child as he visualizes his future and the extension of the self. With the child's death, the bubble of the future is burst and nothing remains. The parents are desolate.

One of the most difficult tasks of any health professional is attempting to help the parents of a dying child. Each parent reacts in a unique manner to the imminent death of his or her child. The impending death of an only child produces more severe reactions, ranging from psychosis to total denial. Self-recrimination and self-degradation may surface in response to perceived "selfishness" in having only one child. This dynamic has the potential of affecting the stability of the marriage.

Guilt is likely to be a prominent manifestation of the parents when their child dies and they feel responsible for what led up to the death. A common feeling is that they have nothing left to live for.

In viewing family grief, attention must also be paid to the grieving siblings. It is much too easy to overlook the emotional needs of the young. The parents' natural reaction is to remember only what is good about their dying or dead child, which may lead to a difficult family situation when the dying child is raised to "sainthood" in the eyes and feelings of the parents. The surviving siblings must then attempt to match that idealized image or may begin to exhibit antisocial, or another form of disordered, behavior in a desperate call to win their parents' love again.

Nursing Care of the Dying Patient and His Family

The goals of nursing care of the dying individual are synonymous with those designed for all individuals who cannot meet their own needs. The dying person must be treated as a unique individual, not as a diagnosis or entity, within the institution's confines. The nursing care should foster the optimum quality of life for the individual at that point in time; he and his family need to be dealt with in a secure and protected atmosphere.

Physical Care

The priority of nursing care for the dying patient is meeting his physical needs. This priority must be met before the nurse can continue to intervene meaningfully on an interpersonal level to provide emotional care of the dying patient and his family. Prevention or alleviation of physical problems reassures the dying individual and his loved ones that they need not be anxious about the adequacy of his care. Physical care of the dying includes attention to the following:

1. Hair—cared-for hair has a great influence on the self-image and self-esteem of the individual
2. Mucous membranes—nose, mouth, and eyes need to be kept moist and clean; the use of oils and mouthwashes is desirable
3. Skin—skin should be clean, lotion should be applied to provide moisture, and pressure areas should be protected from skin breakdown and decubitus formation
4. Elimination—the nurse should keep the incontinent patient clean, dry, and odor-free, and should assess him for the presence of an impaction; the nurse's attitude when dealing with the incontinent patient may communicate rejection or protective care
5. Positioning—frequent positioning is needed to protect the patient from skin breakdown and to ensure that the airway is not partially or totally obstructed
6. Nutrition and hydration—small, frequent feedings of the patient's favorite foods are

likely to be accepted; ice chips or favorite soft drinks need to be constantly available to him[2]

(Extensive discussions of the physical care of the dying may be found in medical–surgical nursing texts.)

Psychological Care

Psychological care of the dying individual is not a specific, delineated set of activities or interventions, but an ongoing, individualized interpersonal process based on the personality of the individual and his specific situation and circumstances (see Chart 44-3, "Emotional Care of the Dying Patient"). The goals and needs of the patient and the philosophy of the health care professional generate the specific interventions of care. Five psychological factors that need to be incorporated into the care of the dying are as follows:

1. Information
2. Autonomy
3. Safe conduct
4. Meaningfulness
5. Appropriate death[2]

Providing Information
Patients and family members wish to be kept informed about what is happening to them. Information that is solicited but withheld is a professional's method of controlling the situation, the dying individual, and his family. Without appropriate information, the patient cannot take an active part in decisions made regarding his personal self.

The nurse's role in working with dying individuals and their loved ones is one of liaison between the patient, his family, the physician, and the hospital. The nurse also assumes the vital role of clarifier, explainer, and interpreter of symptoms, communications, hospital rules, and expectations.

Maintaining Autonomy
The ill or dying individual finds himself in a situation of extreme dependency. A balance between autonomy and dependency must be maintained as long as the patient is able to remain involved. Areas of involvement, including various aspects of self-care and decision-making, allow the individual a degree of personal power and control. An individual may be totally dependent for his physical care yet maintain autonomy through his decision-making. This is an important aspect in a health approach, rather than an illness approach, to the dying individual (see The Living Will again).

Offering personal control means allowing the individual a voice in the decisions in his care. Control over the environment—that is, where to place objects,

C H A R T   44-3
Emotional Care of the Dying Patient

Assessment and Analysis

Is the patient aware of his terminal diagnosis?

At which stage of death and dying is the individual?

Does the individual have helpful support systems (*e.g.,* family, significant other)?

Does the individual express "unfinished business" that needs to be completed?

Is a referral needed to deal with financial, emotional, or legal problems?

What are the individual's positive coping skills?

Planning

Be available, on a daily basis, to the individual.

Sit down and LISTEN. Use open statements, such as "You look sad—is there something you'd like to talk about?" "Is there something I can do for you today?" Or, the nurse may have to follow an intuitive hunch, pull up a chair next to the patient's bed, facing him, and ask, "Do you mind if I sit awhile?"

If financial, emotional, or legal problems exist, identify the area of concern and the individual's wish for assistance.

Be available to the family and significant others for information, understanding communication, and support.

Allow for as much physical and emotional independence as the individual needs and is capable of.

Intervention

Spend time daily with the individual, creating an accepting atmosphere.

LISTEN rather than talk; allow for the expression of feelings.

Allow and support the individual's own decision-making in regard to planning time of care, visitors, and so forth.

Use touch when patient indicates through verbal or nonverbal behavior (crying, relating sad stories) that it is needed.

Meet with family and significant others to answer questions, listen to feelings, provide information, and give support.

Allow as much time as the dying individual needs with family and significant others.

Make appropriate referrals, based on individual's wishes, to social worker, lawyer, minister or priest, and so forth.

Aid the individual in completing "unfinished business."

who is acceptable as a visitor, what will be eaten and when, and when treatments and medications will be administered—can lead to the assumption of control. The nurse provides the patient with the basic rights of all individuals, including that of informed consent and the alternative of saying "no" to those things that intimately affect him.

As with any behavior, extremes of the autonomy–dependency continuum may exist. Individuals who are basically dependent may react by exhibiting dictating, controlling behaviors toward health care professionals and family. A more intense look at the individual may reveal a frightened and lonely individual whose greatest fear is that of abandonment. This dynamic of behavior has probably existed throughout the individual's life with family members and significant others and will probably not change during this aspect of life.

If the client's behavior represents a major change in the way he has reacted or acted in the past, the nurse demonstrates quiet acceptance, gentle limit-setting, and trust through reliable and predictable administration of nursing care. Listening, role-modeling, and open communication with the loved ones are necessary to maintain a balance of integrity and support a continued interaction with the dying individual. The nurse facilitates family interactions and provides a place for the expression of feelings.

Assuring Safe Conduct

Safe conduct is the cautious and prudent behavior that guards another individual through peril or the unknown.[40] A promise not to abandon the dying individual comprises the corner stone of assurance of safe conduct. Social isolation is a component of the potent feeling of abandonment that may be experienced if safe conduct is not aided.

In the provision of safe conduct, the nurse meets the physiological needs that the patient cannot meet himself and supports a relationship in which the patient can express and explore feelings. The experience of safe conduct requires the reinforcement and nurturance of the patient's existing positive coping skills.

Supporting Meaningfulness

Frequently, the dying patient's world is filled with loneliness, isolation, and feelings of rejection. This triad is the source of feelings of meaninglessness in an existence that holds no purposeful actions or goal attainment activity for an individual.

Alleviation of pain, the lessening of discomfort, and positive give-and-take relationships are supportive of the dying individual during the remainder of his life. During the phases of the dying process, the presence of at least one significant other—at times, that person may be the nurse—is necessary for open sharing and expression of feelings. Dying persons, when given the opportunity and appropriate milieu, tend to be frank and direct in expressing their feelings and thoughts.

Communication with the dying individual should be composed of active listening and a minimum of idle chatter. Many times, all that is needed is a mutual silence in which the nurse is comfortable. During the active listening, the nurse carries on the ongoing assessment of the client's feelings and coping abilities. The dying individual may express concern about specific problems or unfinished business that he must complete before reaching any sense of peace or acceptance. Together with the nurse or other health care provider he can then make appropriate plans.

The exploration of feelings may be appropriate at any time in the dying process. When dealing with human beings, it is too global to assume that certain feelings are occurring because the individual is dying. Examining expressed feelings opens the way for sharing deeper or more submerged ones, thereby releasing energies that may be used in more successful coping.

When curing is not possible, the nurse can be involved in a healing–caring process. Through a healing–caring process, the dying individual is given the opportunity to maintain connectedness to the world.[6] One aspect of the healing–caring process is the nurse's role in aiding the dying individual to maintain relationships with family and significant others; such relationships may require learning new methods of interacting, even at this stage in life.

Through assessment and analysis of client and family data, the nurse makes decisions about the needs of the dying individual. These needs may vary from active communication and exploration of feelings to the acceptance of the need for withdrawal, reflection, and separation from life.

The search for meaning, which many dying individuals undertake, is an introspective process examining not only the meaning of death, but also the meaning of life. The patient may reaffirm philosophical or religious orientations of his earlier life or make major alterations in his religious or philosophical beliefs during this time. The values of his accomplishments, achievements, and relationships are examined. Relationships with family members and significant others may take on increased importance and immediacy. When all the pieces begin to fit together and some order has been put to life and death, dying can become a meaningful growth experience.

The act of leave-taking or saying goodbye may be possible when the dying patient feels a sense of order to his life and death. The nurse's role in this stage is one of support to the dying individual, family members, and significant others.

Promoting an Appropriate Death

An "appropriate death" for the client involves the following criteria:

1. Reduction of conflict
2. Reinforcement of significant relationships
3. Behavior compatible with the individual's ego ideal
4. Realization of basic instincts and wishes[40]

The appropriate death for an individual is one that reflects, and is integrated into, his lifestyle and its past meaning. The event is not alien to the client's past behavior or some magical change in behavior. It is reflective of the dignity of the individual and his personality.

Summary

This chapter has examined the philosophical, theoretical, religious, and "American" viewpoints on death. Some of the major points of the chapter are as follows:

1. Contemporary reactions to death involve avoidance and preoccupation with death as a destructive force.
2. Advances in medical practice have altered the nature and location of treatment of the dying.
3. The dying client faces the fears of abandonment, initiation into the "sick role," and stigmatization, all of which further isolate him.
4. Family and friends of the dying experience feelings of loss and anticipatory grief to prepare for the death of their loved one.
5. As a result of the grieving process, the survivors free themselves from the bonds of the deceased, reorient themselves to their environment from which the deceased is absent, and establish new relationships.
6. Working with the dying elicits both a personal and a professional threat in health care providers.
7. Kübler-Ross identified five stages of dying experienced by the patient and his family— denial, anger, bargaining, depression, and acceptance.
8. Sudden, unexpected death allows no time for the survivors to engage in anticipatory grief.
9. Competent physical nursing care of the dying patient reassures the family and significant others and adds to their emotional well-being.
10. Psychological nursing care of the dying is

CHART 44-4

Personal Reflections on Death

Felicitas Alfaro, R.N., M.Ed.
Instructor of Nursing
El Centro College
Dallas, Texas

When I stop to analyze or reflect on the major events of my life, I necessarily have to think about the significant losses that I have experienced and the tremendous impact they had on me and my development.

Six to seven hours after I was born, my mother died. When I was 2 weeks old, my oldest sister and my father brought me home to a family of two sisters and nine brothers ranging in age from 2 to 25 years. They all played a role in raising me, as did my aunts and even a friendly neighbor or two.

I grew up hearing, "That's the baby of the family—poor thing—you know her mother died when she was born." Often, I was introduced as "this is my baby sister—the one that was born when my mother died." There was no malice here, just fact; however, for many years I felt guilty. I used to think that if I'd never been born, then my mother would have never died and my brothers and sisters would have had a mother. It was not until I was in college that I was truly able to verbalize this and work it through, to realize that I had no control over my being born or over my mother's life or death.

When I was 8 years old, my oldest brother died of cancer at the age of 33. He had struggled for 7 years. The last few months of his life were the most uncomfortable. A couple of my older brothers and my oldest sister helped his wife with his care. He died at home—surrounded by those who loved him most. I remember it being a Valentine's Day because his daughters and I were comparing our Valentine's Day cards.

As an adult looking back, I am struck by the vivid memories of my brother's colostomy, his pneumonectomy scar, the whispers and the crying at home when the doctor pronounced him dead—and the Valentine's Day cards.

By the time I graduated from high school, one of my paternal aunts, who had taught me to sew and to embroider, was found to have metastatic bronchiopulmonary carcinoma. Because she had no children, she and my uncle moved in with my other aunt. My sister, cousins, and I took turns helping with her care until she died—again, very peacefully at home.

My father died a couple of months later of a massive heart attack. It was New Year's Day afternoon and we were getting ready to go to mass. I remember him walking by my room and on out to the back door where he collapsed after looking out one last time. I ran to him, sat him up and held him in my arms. He died there, but I didn't know it because I had never seen anyone actually die.

A neighbor helped me bring him into the house to his bed. I called my brother, who is a mortician, to come quickly. He arrived within minutes. He knew my daddy was dead, but he also knew that I still thought he was alive.

Daddy was pronounced "D.O.A." I could not cry just as I was not able to look at him in his coffin. After the shock wore off, all I felt was anger. I was very angry at God—I could not and did not want to understand. Then I was very depressed.

The depression was what drove me to see the doctor I had had as a child. He was hispanic and he knew my family well. He was very sensitive and gentle with me and helped me to realize that I had to get out of the "poor me's" and get on with living.

I became a volunteer in the clinics at the county hospital and it was that experience that led me to become a nurse—the one thing I had sworn I would never be.

Since then, I have lost all my aunts and uncles and several very close and dear friends, as well as a sister-in-law who died suddenly and tragically.

I have to think of all that uncalled-for guilt of a child who did not understand. I reflect on the years when anger would surface and then subside. I'm glad that it is finally resolved. I'm thankful for all the love and support from my family and friends, the love and support that I believe is a reflection of God's love and support.

It is the enduring love, the steadfast love, the patient love, the quiet love of those around us that keeps us going.

The interesting thing is that, even after many years, I still cry and I still miss them. The feelings never go away—the changes in understanding and the tears are different—but the feelings never go away. I'm sure some of you can understand what I am saying.

based on the patient's and family's goals and needs and incorporates the provision of information, autonomy, safe conduct, meaningfulness, and appropriate death.

References

1. Becker E: The Denial of Death. New York, Free Press, 1973

2. Burns N: Nursing and Cancer. Philadelphia, WB Saunders, 1982

3. Butler RN, Lewis MI: Aging and Mental Health. St Louis, CV Mosby, 1982

4. Caroff P, Dobrof R: The Helping Process and Bereaved Families. In Schaenberg B et al (eds): Bereavement: Its Psychosocial Aspects. New York, Columbia University Press, 1975

5. Carp FM: A Future for the Aged: Victoria Plaza and Its Residents. Austin, University of Texas Press, 1966

6. Castles MR, Murray RB: Dying in an Institution: Nurse/Patient Perspectives. New York, Appleton-Century-Crofts, 1979

7. Feifel H: The Meaning of Death. New York, McGraw-Hill, 1959

8. Feifel H (ed): New Meanings of Death. New York, McGraw-Hill, 1977

9. Freud S: Thoughts for the Times on War and Death, Part II: Our Attitudes toward Death, pp 289–300. Standard Edition 14 (1915). London, Hogarth, 1957

10. Friedman P, Lum L: Some Psychiatric Notes on the 'Andrea Doria' Disaster. Am J Psychiatry 114: 426–432, 1958

11. Fulcomer DM: The Adjustment Behavior of Some Recently Bereaved Spouses. Unpublished Doctoral Dissertation, Chicago, Northwestern University, 1942

12. Fulton R (ed): A Bibliography on Death, Grief, and Bereavement. Minneapolis, Center for Death Education and Research, 1973

13. Glaser BG, Strauss AL: Awareness of Dying. Chicago, Aldine Publishing, 1965

14. Glaser BG, Strauss AL: Time for Dying. Chicago, Aldine Publishing, 1968

15. Goffman E: Stigma. New Jersey, Prentice-Hall, 1963

16. Goldstein S, Heidmann EM: Sudden Death and Coronary Heart Disease. Cardiovasc Nurs 12, 11–15, 1976

17. Jung CG: Modern Man in Search of a Soul. New York, Harcourt, Brace, 1933

18. Kastenbaum R: Death, Society, and Human Experience. St Louis, CV Mosby, 1977

19. Kneisel CR: Dying Patients and Their Families: How Staff Can Give Support. Hospital Topics 45, 37–39, 1957

20. Kübler-Ross E: On Death and Dying. New York, Macmillan, 1971

21. Kübler-Ross E: On Death and Dying. JAMA 221, 174–179, 1972

22. Kübler-Ross E: Death—the Final Stage of Growth. New Jersey, Prentice-Hall, 1975

23. Lasagna L: Physicians' Behavior Toward the Dying Patient. In Brins O et al (eds): The Dying Patient. New York, Missel Sazeton, 1970

24. Lindemann E: Symptomatology and Management of Acute Grief. Am J Psychiatry 1011 (September): 141–148, 1944

25. Lofland LH: Toward a Sociology of Death and Dying. Beverly Hills, Sage, 1976

26. May WF: The Sacred Power of Death in Contemporary Experiences. In Macks A (ed): Death in American Experience. New York, Schacken, 1973

27. Mitford J: The American Way of Death. Greenwich, CT, Fawcett, 1963

28. Pattison EM: Help in the Dying Process. In Wilcox S, Sutton M (eds): Understanding Death and Dying: An Interdisciplinary Approach, 2d ed. Sherman Oaks, CA, Alfree, 1981

29. Popoff D: What Are Your Feelings About Death and Dying? Nursing 75, 5, 15–25, 39–50, 55–62, 1975

30. Ramsey P: The Indignity of 'Death with Dignity.' In Steinfels P, Veatch RM (eds): Death Inside-Out: The Hastings Center Report, Institute of Society, Ethics and Life Sciences. New York, Harper & Row, 1975

31. Rinear EE: The Nurse's Challenge When Death Is Unexpected. RN 38 (December): 50–55, 1975

32. Ryan MA: Helping the Family Cope with a Cardiac Arrest. Nursing 74, 4 (August): 80–81, 1974

33. Schneidman ES: The Death of Man. New York, Quadrangle, 1973

34. Silverman P et al (eds): Helping Each Other in Widowhood. Health Sciences 7, 1974

35. Surawicz FG: Psychological Aspects of Sudden Cardiac Death. Heart Lung 2 (November–December): 836–840, 1973

36. Ufema JK: Dare to Care for the Dying. Am J Nursing 76, 88–90, 1976

37. Visotky HM, Hamburg DA, Gross ME, Lebovitz BA: Coping Behaviors under Extreme Stress: Observations of Patients with Severe Poliomyelitis. Arch Gen Psychiatry 5, 423–448, 1961

38. Weisman A: On Dying and Denying. New York, Behavioral Publication, 1972

39. Weisman AD: The Psychiatrist and the Inexorable. In Feifel H (ed): New Meanings of Death. New York, McGraw-Hill, 1977

40. Weisman AD, Hackett TD: Predictions to Death: Death and Dying as a Psychiatric Problem. Psychosom Med 23, 232–256, 1961

41. Williams JC: Understanding the Feelings of the Dying. Nursing 76, 6, 52–56, 1976

42. Wolfenstein M: Disaster: A Psychological Study. Glencoe, DE, Free Press, 1957

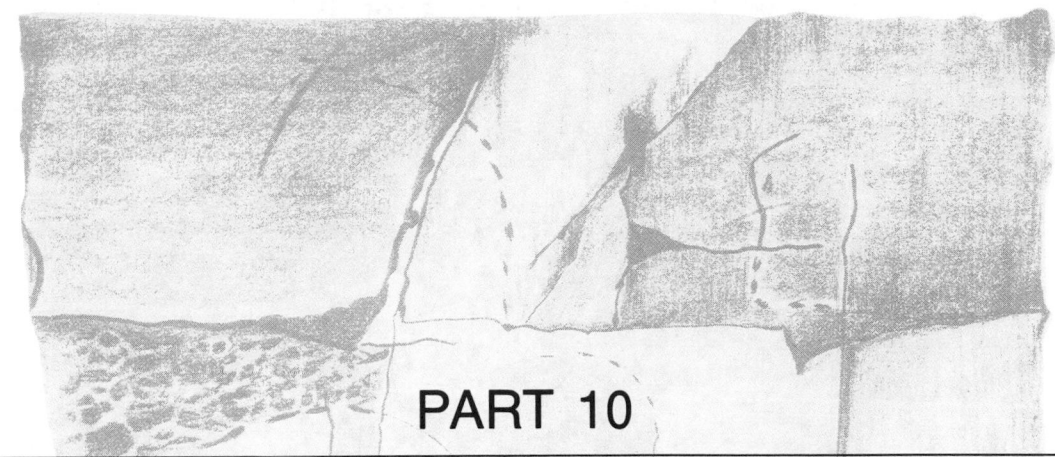

PART 10

Professional Issues in Psychiatric–Mental Health Nursing

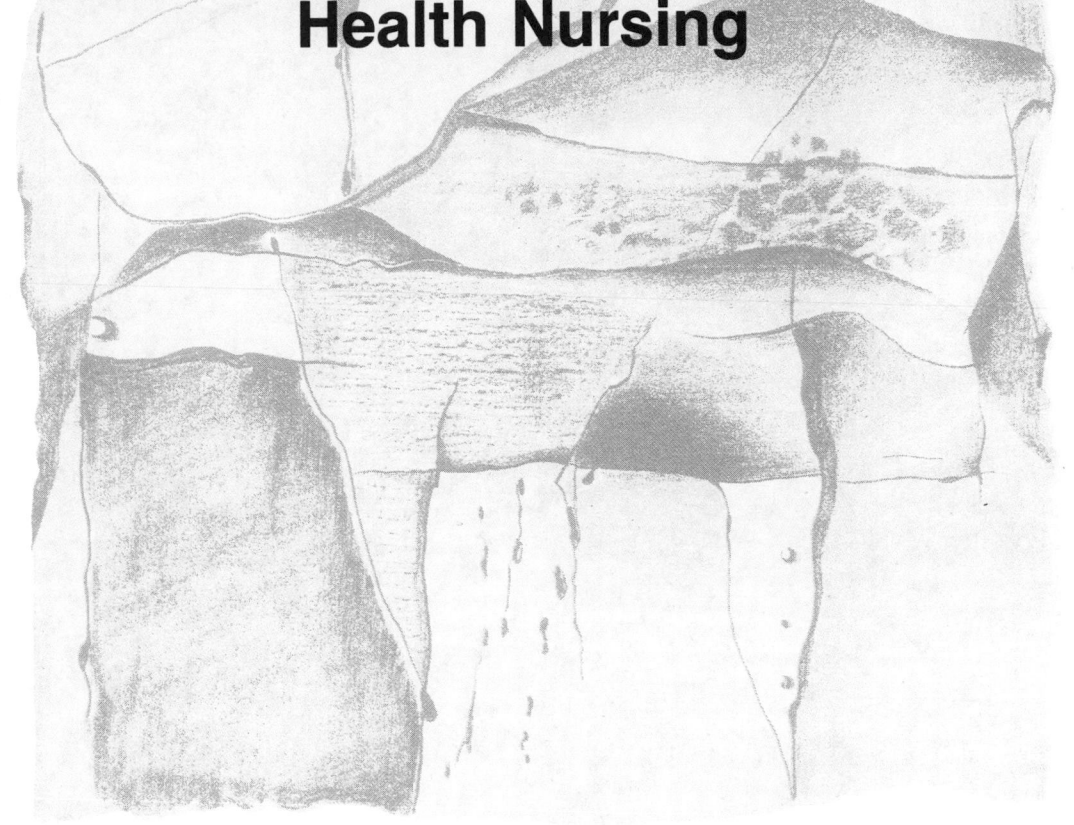

45

Legal Implications of Psychiatric– Mental Health Nursing

Virginia Trotter Betts
S. Robin Shanks

Like the five blind men, each grasping a different part of the fabled elephant and each describing a different beast, so the perceivers of the therapeutic state have seen in it diverse realities. Some have viewed it as a humanistic boon. Others have portrayed it as the first rational endeavor for the scientific control of deviant behavior. Still others have compared it to the infamous Star Chamber proceeding—the royal Tudor court that dispensed arbitrary punishments without proper regard for the safeguards that the law usually provided for the liberty of the subject.

Nicholas Kittrie,
Informed Consent:
A Guide for Health Care
Remedies, 1981

Chapter Preview

Probably no other specialty area of nursing demands as great a need for knowledge of the law and its effect upon nursing practice than does psychiatric–mental health nursing. Consumers of health care are becoming increasingly knowledgeable about legal issues, rights, and remedies, and have improved access to legal counsel through legal clinics, the American Civil Liberties Union, and other protective rights–conscious groups (see Chart 45-1, "Past and Present Legal Trends in Mental Health," for a historical perspective). Therefore, psychiatric nurses and other health care professionals must be aware that their practice must not only meet their own professional standards, but that those professional standards must also bear close adherence to legal standards as developed through case or statutory law.

Psychiatric nurses are responsible both for the services that they perform and for those that they do not perform. They are responsible for accurate assessments, careful plans, competent implementation, and purposeful evaluation. If psychiatric nurses are not aware of the national expectations for clinical practice, the impact on clinical practice of new laws arising from cases decided in the court system, and proposed and past legislation affecting mental health care, it seems unlikely that they can provide the quality of care to consumers that would safeguard clients' rights, protect the client's safety, or further the influence or power of the nurse on the interdisciplinary mental health team.

This chapter has many purposes, the first of which is to define a standard of quality psychiatric care as set by professional nurses and to demonstrate how this standard has been affected by current case law. Another important purpose of the chapter is to clarify, for the practicing mental health nurse and for the nursing student, some of the differences in important legal concepts that may seem somewhat similar to the novice. Some of these differences include the following:

1. Competency to stand trial versus competency to handle affairs
2. The tort actions of malpractice and assault and battery
3. Voluntary and involuntary civil clients and their rights
4. Criminal or civil status of clients in inpatient institutions

It is imperative that nurses learn to value, respect, and seek out knowledge about laws, legislation, and the legal processes that regulate, impede, and facilitate the practice of professional nursing. The major goal of this chapter is to prepare nurses to include legal principles in their psychiatric–mental health nursing practice, both to benefit and protect the nurse and to enhance the quality of care that the client receives.

Learning Objectives

On completion of this chapter, you should be able to accomplish the following:

1. identify and discuss some legal issues basic to accountable nursing practice
      nursing practice and malpractice
      informed consent
      confidentiality
      record-keeping
2. identify the basic rights of the mentally ill
3. differentiate between voluntary and involuntary civil commitment
4. differentiate between criminal and civil commitment
5. discuss the differences between the competency to stand trial and general legal competency
6. differentiate between the rights of voluntary and involuntary clients
7. identify nursing implications for the right to refuse treatment and other important client rights
8. plan actions for ensuring accountability for psychiatric–mental health nursing practice
      use of the ANA Standards of Practice
      integration of quality assurance into practice
      seeking of appropriate legal consultation

Legal Issues Basic to Accountable Psychiatric–Mental Health Nursing Practice

Nursing Practice and Malpractice

Nursing Practice Acts

Nursing as a profession is given effect in each state by the promulgation of the Nurse Practice Act by each state legislature. Each state Nurse Practice Act defines nursing, describes the scope of nursing, and identifies limits on the practice of nursing within that state. Although the Nurse Practice Act may differ in each state, the definition of nursing in the Tennessee Nurse Practice Act is clearly a definition not too dissimilar from many of the acts in the nation. The act

C H A R T   45-1
Past and Present Legal Trends in Mental Health

For the last few hundred years, society has dealt with its mentally disturbed members in a variety of ways. Until recently, the principal method was to segregate them from the general population.

This isolation from society is reported in K. Jones's *Lunacy, Law & Conscience:*

16th century, deranged were expelled,
   shipped off, executed;
17th century, insane were locked up
   in jails and houses of correction;
18th century, madmen were confined
   in madhouses;
19th century, lunatics were sent to asylums;
20th century, mentally ill are committed to
   hospitals[13]

Present laws regarding the treatment of the mentally ill evolved from the Common Law of England. During the 11th century, the King of England was responsible for the care of the insane if there were no kinsmen. By the beginning of the 14th century, the church and the lord of the manor were responsible for the mentally ill. Then, in the early 14th century, Edward II proclaimed the king's responsibility toward the mentally ill. The national law of guardianships extended to this class of people, and they were again made the duty of the crown. The term *parens patriae* was used by W. Blackstone to refer to the power and the responsibility of the state to care for the disabled members of society. In Blackstone's words, "The king has the general superintendance of all charities."[16]

At first, the mentally disabled who came to the New World were dealt with informally by the colonists. Families locked up their mentally ill relatives in back rooms or outhouses. Others who had nowhere to go wandered from place to place or were confined in jails with criminals, drunkards, and other social outcasts. The *parens patriae* power of the king then was officially assumed by the states.[15]

In 1752, Philadelphia Hospital was opened. Not only was it this country's first general hospital, but it also provided treatment to the mentally ill in addition to the sick and poor. During this period, Pinel's and Luke's work in France and London, referred to as moral treatment of the mentally ill, traveled across the Atlantic. Pinel's "moral treatment" implied a mental condition that was curable in an appropriate psychological and social environment.[24]

Subsequently, other hospitals opened, but by the middle of the 19th century, it was obvious that the corporate hospitals were unable to meet the needs of the mentally disabled.[24] This, in turn, caused social crusaders such as Dorothea Dix to assist with funding, building, and enlarging public mental hospitals. Despite their humanistic purposes, these hospitals actually allowed for an era of custodial treatment by the unwarranted commitment of thousands of homeless people in overcrowded hospitals with little regard for any legal protective processes.

To combat these increasingly unacceptable conditions, the patients' rights movement developed; the movement supported the concept of deinstitutionalization of the mentally ill. During the last decade, the deinstitutionalization concept and its implementation have been at the forefront of mental health care delivery. Community mental health centers have opened their doors to provide necessary psychiatric treatment to persons who do not require inpatient hospitalization. As a result of this community approach, inpatient psychiatric numbers have decreased by more than 50% since the early 1950s. Within the past 10 years, the criteria for judicial commitment have been narrowed considerably. A person can no longer be judicially committed merely because of the presence of mental illness or the need for psychiatric treatment.

Deinstitutionalization has mandated the development of more than 2000 public mental health centers to provide care for the mentally ill for whom inpatient care is not necessary, leaving hospital facilities to care for those who are not functioning safely in society due to mental illness. The integration of the mentally ill into the general population has engendered a great deal of political and social controversy and conflict. This conflict is not likely to be resolved until the stigma attached to mental illness is replaced by an increased understanding of mental health and illness by society or until the health delivery system develops community support services such as housing, employment, and accessible after-care that facilitate social integration of the formerly hospitalized mental health client population.

Many legal rights and remedies for the mentally ill are in rapid states of evolution. One of the most frequently litigated issues is the right to refuse psychotropic medication. New statutes resulting from judicial decisions will have a major impact on the care and treatment of the mentally ill in our society in the future.

immediately highlights some recognized independent nursing practices as well as some dependent areas of nursing practice (see Chart 45-2).

It is important to review the specific activities that are mandated in the Nurse Practice Act. Clearly, only "the administration of medications and treatment as is prescribed by a licensed physician or dentist" is a service that could be considered dependent for the nurse; that is, it is dependent on the acts (orders) of someone else.[27] The rest of the mandated activities are acts that the nurse can, should, and must do on her own initiative because patients need and should reasonably expect these nursing actions. Nurses are responsible and accountable for these nursing acts and are responsible for performing them in a manner that is safe for the patient.

Nursing Malpractice

It is important to define nursing malpractice. *Malpractice* is a particular kind of tort action that is brought by a consumer plaintiff against a defendant professional from whom the consumer plaintiff feels that he has received injury during the course of the professional–consumer relationship. Malpractice is professional negligence.

In order for a plaintiff consumer to receive money damages by successfully suing a professional nurse for malpractice, the consumer plaintiff must prove the following five elements of nursing negligence:

1. The nurse professional had a duty to use due care toward the plaintiff.
2. The nurse professional's performance fell below the standard of care and was therefore a breach of that duty.
3. As a result of the failure to meet the standard of care, the plaintiff consumer was injured and the nurse's action was the proximate cause of the injury.
4. The act that the nurse engaged in could foreseeably have caused an injury.
5. The plaintiff consumer must prove his injuries.

In a malpractice action against the nurse, the proof of the standard of care becomes an essential and important ingredient. Expert witness testimony is usually presented by both sides to give the jury the perspectives of experts on professional practices and standards. The appropriate expert witness for psychiatric nursing practice is another psychiatric nurse who would have knowledge about what the standard of care in the particular case should have been.

Such expert testimony is presented in the case and is submitted with all other testimony and evidence to the jury for a decision. The jury is asked by the court to apply the reasonable man test to the facts in the case at hand. The *reasonable man test,* as applied to the nurse defendant, is what the reasonably prudent nurse would have done under similar circumstances if that nurse came from the same or a similar community (see Chart 45-3, "Practice or Malpractice?"). Therefore, in order to decrease liability for malpractice, a psychiatric nurse must keep her professional practice within the bounds that her nurse peers would consider reasonable and appropriate. The law of negligence seeks a peer standard for reasonableness of action—not a quality performance standard of excellence.

In the history of malpractice litigation, nurses have been protected from direct suits by clients due to the perception that they are either dependent on the physician for orders or employees of an institution. Attorneys, using the "deep pocket theory" of recovery, tended to sue as direct defendants either the well-insured physician or the employer-hospital rather

---

CHART 45-2
TCA 63-7-103: "Professional Nursing" Defined

The practice of professional nursing means the performance for compensation of any act requiring substantial specialized judgment and skill based on knowledge and application of principles of nursing derived from biologic, physical, and social sciences including:

a. responsible supervision of a patient requiring skill and observation of symptoms and reactions and accurate recording of the facts
b. the maintenance of health or prevention of illness of others
c. supervision and teaching of others
d. administration of medications and treatments as prescribed by a licensed physician or dentist
e. application of such nursing procedures as they involve understanding of cause and effect. The foregoing shall not be deemed to include acts of medical diagnosis or the development of a medical plan of care and therapeutics for a patient.

(From Tennessee Code Annotated, §63-7-101 et seq)

CHART 45-3
Practice or Malpractice?

A 23-year-old, married graduate student, Mr. C. T., became severely depressed over a 3-week period. He was increasingly despondent, was unable to study, and discussed suicide with his family and friends on frequent occasions during the 3-week period. He finally became so immobilized that he requested voluntary admission to the psychiatric unit of the local general hospital.

The unit was a 32-bed, open-ward therapeutic community treatment center and the nursing model was primary nursing. Mr. C. T.'s primary nurse, Ms. D., met him on admission and completed a nursing history in a hurried manner. She did not include the client's wife in the history-taking process, nor did she directly inquire about suicidal thoughts, gestures, or plans despite his obvious depression.

Ms. D.'s nursing history and her participation in the interdisciplinary team conference to develop the treatment plan for the client included information about his health status, drug allergies, the stressors of graduate school, and his deteriorated eating and sleeping habits. Information from and about the client's family was omitted, as well as the client's and his wife's perceptions of the severity of the problem and their goals for hospitalization.

After 10 days on the unit, Mr. C. T. evidenced an improved mood and energy level. He approached the nurse, Ms. D., with a request for a weekend pass. Ms. D. championed his request in the team meeting noting his increased energy, his compliance and "good" behavior, and his voluntary admission status.

The team, relying on Ms. D's judgment, agreed that she could facilitate his pass. Without further assessment or activity, Ms. D. provided him with the weekend pass. The client left the unit at 2:00 P.M., went to his home, and took an overdose of medication, part of which

was provided for him for his pass and part of which he had acquired on his own prior to admission. He died before he was discovered by his wife when she returned home from work; she had not been informed that a pass was to be granted to her husband.

The wife sued the primary nurse, the hospital, and the attending physician for negligence and wrongful death.

If you were called as an expert witness to evaluate Ms. D.'s standard of care and her possible liability, both personally and jointly, what would you consider?

1. Inadequate history-taking and initial assessment, especially lack of family participation in the process
2. Limited scope of assessment
3. Poor understanding of dynamics of depression indicated in client assessment
4. Lack of understanding of the meaning of "voluntary" status
5. No planning with the family for goals for treatment or continuity of care
6. Limited evidence of use of the ANA Standards of Practice

It is doubtful that this primary nurse and her treatment team colleagues met the "reasonable man" test in the case of Mr. C. T. As his caretakers they had a duty to do so. They breached their duty and his harm was foreseeable. Their inappropriate actions toward him were legally significant factors in his death and death is a monetarily compensable injury.

Therefore, it is likely that, by proving each element of negligence, the client's wife will be able to recover money damages from the defendants. Malpractice does occur in psychiatric settings due to acts of both commission and omission.

than the nurse. Now, with the advent of consumerism, the recognition of professional nursing as an independent discipline, and the awareness that most nurses are self-insured against malpractice liability, there is an increasing trend to sue the individual nurse as a co-defendant along with the physician and the hospital.[17]

This trend has many implications for nursing practice and for the profession. As nurses are being held increasingly responsible and monetarily liable

for nursing practice and malpractice, nursing must and will take control of nursing practice issues such as staffing, educational qualifications and competencies, and role definition on the health care team.

When nurses are found liable for less-than-adequate nursing care, employers are usually found liable to the plaintiff under the legal theory of respondeat superior. *Respondeat superior* states that the acts of employees are attributable to the employer for the purpose of being responsible for damages to injured third parties.[21] Eventually, because of joint liability and increased monetary risk, hospitals will insist on, rather than resist, nursing's efforts to direct and control its practice in order to provide a higher quality of client care. Quality client care provided by nursing greatly decreases malpractice litigation and successful recovery against both professional and corporate defendants. And, of course, quality client care can only be legally proved by clear, concise, accurate, complete, and outcome-oriented documentation. The medical record is the best source of legal protection in a malpractice suit.[11]

Informed Consent—A Basic Right

All consumer clients have a right to informed consent prior to health care interventions. The performance of health care treatments or procedures without the informed consent of the client can result in legal action against the physician and the health care agency. A client will prevail in a lawsuit alleging battery, which is the unpermitted touching of another, if it can be proved that the client did not consent to the procedure.[21]

Consent is an absolute defense to battery, and informed consent is required in health care situations. A client will prevail in a malpractice or a professional negligence suit if it can be proved that informed consent was not obtained from the client. *Informed consent* can be defined as that knowing consent that is given in an interaction or series of interactions between the treating physician and the client that allows the client to fully consider information about the treatment that is being proposed (*e.g.*, the way it will be administered, its prognoses, its side effects, its risks, the possible consequences of refusing the treatment, and other treatment alternatives).[23]

In the case of *Canterbury* v. *Spence*, the Court said that the client could truly be informed only if the physician shared with him all those things that "the patient would find significant" in making a decision on whether to permit or to participate in a particular treatment regimen.[8] Elements of informed consent include the following:

1. Adequate and accurate knowledge and information
2. An individual with legal capacity to consent
3. Voluntarily given consent[14]

Special Consent Considerations in Psychiatric Settings

A major problem with consent arises with psychiatric clients because the validity of their competence to agree to a procedure is usually questioned. Many mental health clients certainly are capable of giving informed consent. They are aware of their surroundings, they understand what is being said, they are making their decisions based on what they think is best for them, and they are doing it without coercion.

Nevertheless, it is clear that some clients are not able to give informed consent. It may be doubted whether clients already determined by the court to be incompetent for the purposes of handling their civil and business affairs possess the ability to make treatment decisions. Some clients who have not been so adjudicated are so clearly impaired by their psychiatric illness that a true understanding of what is being said is not possible, and they are therefore unable to give valid consent. Because of this unreliability, major nursing considerations in the psychiatric–mental health practice area of informed consent are the constant monitoring and observing of clients for the following:

1. A state of legal capacity or competence when they are asked to give informed consent
2. Continuing understanding of the information that they have been given
3. Power and opportunities to revoke consent at any time during a particular course of treatment[23]

Substituted Consent. When it is determined that a client is unable to give informed consent, providers of health services should obtain substituted consent for the necessary treatment or procedure. *Substituted consent* is that authorization given by another person on behalf of one who is in need of a procedure or treatment. Substituted consent can come from a court-appointed guardian or, in some instances, from the client's next of kin.

If the client has not previously been adjudicated incompetent to handle his own affairs and, if the law so permits and there is no next of kin available to give substituted consent, the health care agency may initiate a court proceeding to appoint a guardian so that the procedure or treatment can be carried out.[23]

It is important for nurses, along with other health care providers, to know the statutory requirements for obtaining substituted consent. It is also necessary for the nurse functioning in the role of client advocate to know whether a client has been adjudicated incompetent and whether consent from a next of kin or a guardian is a legally acceptable substitution for the consent of the client. Assuring legally adequate informed consent prior to treatment should be an important part of the psychiatric nursing care plan.

The Nurse's Role

In the area of informed consent, the nurse acts as the client advocate, the physician's colleague, and the hospital's excellent employee by her continuing evaluation of an individual's ability to give informed consent, as well as his voluntariness to participate and continue in a particular treatment modality. It is not the nurse's responsibility to obtain informed consent because that is an activity between the client and the primary physician. It is the nurse's prerogative to pursue actively the observations as outlined above to protect the client's rights as he is engaged in treatment. Clearly defining the nurse's role in obtaining a client signature on a consent form needs to be addressed in every agency. A joint signing between the physician and client at the time of the decision is a preferred method of documenting consent; many agency policies and consent forms reflect this preference.

Confidentiality

In nursing practice, it is well acknowledged that the data generated through both interpersonal relationships and indirect sources with and about clients are confidential. It is a professional and an ethical duty to use the knowledge that is gained about clients for the enhancement of their care rather than for other purposes, such as gossip, personal gain, or mere curiosity. The confidentiality of verbal, as well as written, material must be maintained. This is especially true in the care of the mentally ill.

Despite the modernization of society, there continues to be a tremendous stigma attached to anyone who is labeled with a diagnosis of mental illness. Any breach of confidentiality of data about clients, their diagnoses, their symptoms, their behaviors, and the outcomes of treatment can certainly affect the course of the rest of their lives in terms of employment, promotions, marriage, attainment of insurance benefits, and so forth. Psychiatric nurses cannot be too careful with their records, their reports, and their plans.

Responsible Record-Keeping

According to the Bill of Rights of the American Hospital Association, each patient has a right to a written record that enhances his care.[2] The client record should state all those concerns that must be addressed in the care of the client, including those history items that affect his current status. The record should not be so in-depth as to be voyeuristic, but it should not be so limited as to narrowly construe the client's condition.

Records are legal documents that can be used in court; therefore, all nursing notes and progress records should reflect descriptive, nonjudgmental, and objective statements. Examples of significant data include here-and-now observations of the client through the use of the nurse's senses, accurate reporting of what is said and what is done for the client, and a description of the client outcomes of the care provided.[15]

Verbal communication and data-sharing are important, especially on treatment teams and units that use interdisciplinary approaches to client care. The verbal sharing should be straightforward, forthright, descriptive, and unopinionated, and should be shared only with those individuals who are involved in the care and treatment of the client. It is wise in a psychiatric institution to have an established methodology of reminding staff about their professional and legal responsibilities for confidentiality, such as an annual signing of a form that promises the maintenance of client confidentiality.

Privileged Communication

Privileged communication is provided by statute in each state. The statute delineates which categories of professionals are given the legal privilege not to be required to reveal conversations and communications with a citizen. Although statutes differ state by state, the statutes customarily provide privilege to physicians, attorneys, clergymen, and, in some states, psychologists, nurses, and other health care providers. Psychiatric nurses should be aware of statutory privileged communication and, if the nursing privilege is limited or nonexistent, they should know what typical boundaries to set in therapeutic interviews. In the absence of statutory privileges for nurses, communications between the nurse and the client may be required to be repeated in court through the subpoena process. Therefore, sharing sensitive or incriminating data should not be encouraged.

Some cases have involved the issue of the appropriate circumstance to warrant breach of the confidential relationship with a client. A leading case in this area is *Tarasoff* v. *Board of Regents of University of California*, which held that therapists may have a duty to protect a person who is threatened by a client.[25] Subsequent decisions discuss the issues of foreseeable violence and the amount of control that the therapist could reasonably use to prevent the harm.[5] In these types of cases, courts have said that the mandate on therapists to hold clients' verbalizations in confidence is cut off when those confidences include threats on the lives of third persons.

Courts have held that, although the duty of confidentiality between client and therapist is one that should be recognized, a higher duty to protect the public safety intervenes and subsumes the duty of confidentiality. There are no nursing cases *per se* on this point, but it is important to know that threats to third persons cannot be ignored or unattended, especially when there is some reasonable opportunity for the client to follow through on these threats.

Other types of situations in which a breach of confidentiality may be required by law include child abuse allegations and allegations of sexual misconduct made against a therapist.

Providing Legally Acceptable Nursing Care: Rights Issues

Basic Rights of Psychiatric Clients

An important issue in psychiatric–mental health nursing care is the recognition of the basic rights of clients. This is particularly true because the treatment of the mentally ill tends to be more coercive, less voluntary, and less open to public awareness and scrutiny than are the treatment and hospitalization of other types of clients.

When a psychiatric client enters a hospital, he loses his freedom to come and go, to schedule his day, to choose his activities, and to control his activities of daily living. If he is also adjudicated incompetent, he loses his freedom to manage his financial and legal affairs and make many important decisions.[10]

Because of the loss of these important freedoms, the courts and the advocates of psychiatric clients closely guard and value those rights that the psychiatric client retains. Some of these rights include the right to communicate with an attorney, the right to send and receive mail without censorship, the right to visitors, the right to the basic necessities of life, and the right to safety from harm while hospitalized.

Certainly, treatment issues arise that indicate a need for a limitation on visitors or for client inclusion in a behavior modification type of treatment program that requires the earning of tokens to secure certain privileges or articles; however, clients have a right to challenge such restrictions and the treatment facility may have to prove the value or necessity of such rights abridgements.[10]

Use of restraints and seclusion as treatment approaches are considered suspect because such approaches reflect a flavor of possible punishment; therefore, the when's, where's, why's, and how long's of restraints and seclusion need to be addressed by policy in every psychiatric facility. Many states have developed statutes to define the use of restraints and seclusion within psychiatric units.

Clients have limited rights to be paid for work within institutions. Forced or even voluntary labor by clients without payment violates the principles of law in our society. The amount of payment considered adequate for client labor is still not clearly defined in each state.[10]

Clients have the right not to be subjected to experimental treatments nor to be subjects in research projects without their informed consent. Because of the complexity of informed consent issues with psychiatric clients as discussed previously, institutions having programs involving research or experimental treatment approaches must have institutional review boards to evaluate such projects and programs and to approve or disapprove them based upon strict client-protection criteria. Humane research approaches that entail no undue risks to clients but that have strong expectations of client benefit and that allow clients to withdraw from the project at any time are usually viewed favorably by these human subjects committees if clients give voluntary consent to participate.[10]

Nursing Implications for Provision of Rights

Nursing has long espoused a philosophy that one of its important roles in the health care system is to act as an advocate for the client. The advocacy role is nowhere more important than in the psychiatric care system as an assessor of, and spokesman for, the protection of client rights.

Discussing rights within treatment teams, including these rights in the nursing care plan, and ensuring that methodologies for rights protection are included in facility and unit policies and procedures are nursing activities that fulfill the client advocate role. One important resource that nursing should request is ongoing legal advice and consultation in the area of client rights.

Client Status and Specific Legal Issues

When psychiatric clients are hospitalized, the type of admission is vitally important. It is important because various admission statutes reflect differing client rights as well as staff treatment responsibilities. Civil commitment admissions are as follows:

1. Voluntary admissions
2. Emergency admissions
3. Involuntary commitments (indefinite duration)

Each state has specific statutory regulations pertaining to each admission status, and these statutes control state procedures for admissions, discharges, and commitments for treatment.

Voluntary Admissions

When clients present themselves at psychiatric facilities and request hospitalization, they are considered *voluntary admission* clients. Likewise, clients who are evaluated as being of danger to themselves or to others or being so seriously mentally ill that they cannot adequately meet their own needs in the community but who are willing to submit to treatment and are competent to do so have *voluntary admission* status.

Voluntary clients have certain rights that differ from the rights of other hospitalized clients. Specifically, voluntary clients are considered competent unless otherwise adjudicated and, therefore, have the absolute right to refuse treatment, including psychotropic medications, unless they are dangerous to themselves or others, as in a violent destructive episode within the treatment unit.[22]

Voluntary clients do not have an absolute right to discharge at any time but may be required to request discharge. This time delay gives the health care team an opportunity to initiate a procedure to change the client's admission status to involuntary if the client meets the necessary statutory requirements. Many clearly mentally ill people can be voluntarily treated but cannot be required by the state to be treated in any setting if the client refuses. Therefore, numerous mentally ill people whose behavior causes family, community, and social problems do not and cannot receive psychiatric care if they are unwilling to be voluntary clients.

Involuntary Admissions

An individual is considered to have *emergency involuntary admission* status when that individual acts in such a manner as to indicate that he is both mentally ill and, due to his illness, likely to harm himself or others, and is taken into custody and detained in a psychiatric facility.[26] The exact procedure for the initial evaluation is defined by state statute, as is the possible length of detainment and attendant treatment available.

All emergency admission individuals are admitted to facilities for the purposes of diagnosis, evaluation, and emergency treatment. At the end of the statutorily limited admission period, the client must be discharged, must be changed to voluntary status, or must attend a civil hearing, which will be held to determine his need for continuing treatment on an involuntary basis.

During the time of the emergency admission, the client's right to come and go is restricted, but he must have the right to consult with an attorney in order to prepare for his hearing. He may be forced to take psychotropic medications, especially if he continues to be dangerous to himself or to others, but more invasive procedures, such as electroconvulsive therapy (ECT) or psychosurgery, are not permitted. No treatment should impair the client's ability to consult with an attorney at the time of his hearing.[26]

An individual who refuses psychiatric hospitalization or treatment but poses a danger to himself or others, who is mentally ill, and for whom less drastic treatment means are unsuitable may be adjudicated to *indefinite involuntary admission* status in a psychiatric hospital for an indefinite period for the purpose of treatment.[26] The exact legal procedure may differ in each state but the standards for commitment are similar (see Case Study 45-1).

Certainly, to deprive an individual of liberty to the extent of involuntary commitment is a serious matter, and the legal protections are strict. A major case, *Addington* v. *Texas,* decided in 1979, requires that, in a civil hearing prior to involuntary commitment, the standard of proof of "mentally ill and dangerous to self or others" must be beyond that of a "preponderance of the evidence" (the prior civil commitment standard) and must be, instead, "clear and convincing evidence" (a much higher standard).[1] This Supreme Court standard of the protection of the right to liberty must be reflected in the statutes of each state concerning commitment procedures.

It is for that classification of clients who are indefinitely involuntarily committed that many of the issues of psychiatric client rights have been pursued. Therefore, these other "evolving" rights will be discussed in a later section.

Legal Issues of Special Client Populations

Forensic Psychiatric Clients

Mental health professionals become involved with clients who are charged with criminal acts in two major instances: first, for the evaluation of a defendant's competency to stand trial and concomitant pretrial treatment if needed, and second, for the evaluation of a defendant's mental condition at the time of an alleged crime and concomitant treatment if the defendant pleads and is acquitted on an insanity defense. This specialized area of mental health care is called *forensic psychiatry.*

Competency to stand trial refers to the mental condition of an individual defendant at the time of the trial. Mental health professionals determine whether the defendant is competent by assessing the following:

1. The defendant's ability to assist his attorney with his defense

Case Study 45-1: Committable and Not Committable

A Case of Mental Distress—Not Committable

Mrs. A., a 65-year-old widow, had lived alone for 25 years. Her neighbors frequently expressed concern among themselves and to the local authorities about Mrs. A.'s unusual lifestyle and eccentric behavior. Their complaints were generally based on tales told to them by neighborhood children. The observations of the neighborhood children included reports that Mrs. A. slept during the day but stayed up all night, ate strange foods like raw meat and 10 pounds of sugar every 2 weeks, and talked to herself aloud. The only public place in which Mrs. A. was ever seen was in the church on Sunday mornings.

Finally, a neighbor called the police who picked up Mrs. A. while she was in her yard placing tree branches in strange patterns. She was then admitted as an emergency admission to the local state mental hospital. The various psychiatric team members' assessments and psychological diagnostic testing results were presented at the hearing, along with testimony from other experts and testimony from the neighbors. The descriptive nursing observations of Mrs. A.'s behavior for the 5 days prior to the hearing were a most important part of the expert evidence and testimony.

The mental health assessment indicated that Mrs. A.'s rather odd behavior was the result of her suffering from primary degenerative dementia. The court found that, even though Mrs. A. exhibited rather bizarre behaviors at times, her mental condition, as indicated by the testimony, did not generate a tendency for her to harm either herself or others. Likewise, the testimony did not indicate that her condition would prevent her from using community resources in a manner adequate for continued self-care.

Therefore, the court determined that Mrs. A. was not judicially committable to an inpatient psychiatric unit. Nevertheless, the court did find the need for follow-up care by a visiting nurse from the local mental health center to monitor Mrs. A.'s nutrition, self-care, and any further progression of her mental illness that might eventually require hospitalization.

A Case for Involuntary Civil Commitment

Jim, a 20-year-old single white man, lived at home with his parents while attending college classes at the community college. For the past 2 months, Jim's behavior had become increasingly bizarre. Finally, he did not sleep, did not eat, and did not attend class. He left his parents' house at all times of the day and night, which caused a great deal of disturbance. When his father attempted to reason with him, he became increasingly agitated and stormed out of the house.

The parents were not aware of any drug use; however, they are aware of the fact that Jim had been drinking large amounts of beer. Jim lost a lot of weight and failed to care for his personal hygiene.

Although Jim had become very agitated, he had never made any threats toward anyone nor had he exhibited any assaultive behavior. He became increasingly preoccupied with the Bible; when his parents questioned his strange behavior, he responded that he was an apostle and that he was only doing what God told him to do. About 1 month ago, Jim's parents persuaded him to visit the local mental health center, but, when the therapist suggested inpatient treatment at a psychiatric hospital, Jim stormed out of his office.

One night, with Jim standing on the patio "preaching the gospel," and disturbing the whole neighborhood, his parents, feeling completely helpless and frightened, called the local police department. The police transported Jim to the state psychiatric facility where he stayed for 5 days on an emergency admission status, after which time he attended his hearing.

During the hearing, Jim was still hyperactive to the point that he could not sit still. Based on the testimony of both the physician and the nurse regarding Jim's mental condition and behavior, the court found that Jim met the standards for civil judicial commitment on two grounds. First, his hyperactivity secondary to his mental illness was resulting in loss of appetite, loss of weight, and insomnia to the extent that his physical health was compromised. Second, his increasing agitation and preoccupation with religion, also secondary to his mental illness, was potentially an antecedent to a situation in which he could lose control and harm others. Therefore, Jim was returned to the psychiatric hospital for continued treatment on a nonvoluntary, civilly committed basis with no judicial pronouncements about his competency status.

2. The defendant's understanding of the nature and consequences of the charge against him
3. The defendant's understanding of courtroom procedures

In many states, community mental health centers have forensic teams that visit the jails and provide these evaluations for the court, and most states have a forensic inpatient unit that provides these evaluations as well.

If the defendant is evaluated as being incompetent to stand trial, treatment begins with the defendant being judicially committed to a psychiatric hospital with a forensic unit. Treatment of incompetent defendants includes, but is not limited to, medication, individual and group psychotherapy, and groups designed to educate the defendant about courtroom proceedings as well as his current legal predicament. An important point to remember is that a defendant can be exhibiting signs and symptoms of mental illness but can still be competent to stand trial.

A decision handed down by the United States Supreme Court in *Jackson* v. *Indiana* in 1972 has resulted in state statutes designed to protect the rights of persons with criminal charges who continue to be incompetent to stand trial by virtue of their mental illness.[12] These defendants can no longer be detained for an indefinite period of time without the benefit of the same type of commitment hearing to which all civilly committed clients have a right. In other words, these pretrial defendants should be returned to court as soon as they are competent to stand trial, and this should be the primary goal of pretrial treatment.

If the defendant chooses to plead an insanity defense, mental health professionals are involved in the evaluation of the defendant's mental condition at the time of an alleged crime. Four different standards or tests are used for an insanity plea to be a valid defense.

The earliest standard that achieved wide acceptance in the United States was the M'Naughten Rule, which was established in England in 1843. This is the "right–wrong test," which states, in essence, that, if at the time of his criminal act the defendant suffered from a disease of the mind that so affected his reason that he was unaware of the nature and quality of his act or that his act was wrong, then he is to be found not guilty by reason of insanity.

The second test, the Irresistible Impulse Rule, broadened M'Naughten. This test retained the language of M'Naughten but also provided that a person acting in response to an irresistible impulse also lacked criminal responsibility even though he knew the wrongfulness of his act.

The third test, the Durham Rule, provided that a person lacked criminal responsibility if his acts were the product of a mental disease or defect. This rule was not widely used.

The fourth test, which was adopted by the American Law Institute, is most widely used today. It provides that a person is not responsible for a criminal act if he was suffering from a mental illness at the time of the act, if he was unable to appreciate the wrongfulness of his act, and if he was unable to conform his conduct to the requirements of the law.

After the forensic team uses these statutory standards in their evaluation of the defendant, it is then called to court to testify based on their evaluation of the defendant's mental status at the time of the crime. The jury uses the team's expert testimony when deciding about guilt or innocence and the appropriateness of the insanity plea.

If a defendant is found not guilty by reason of insanity, the legal implication is that, because of a mental condition, the defendant could not form the deliberate intent necessary to constitute mens rea. *Mens rea* is the mental element necessary for a defendant to be convicted of a crime; it involves a notion of deliberate criminal intent and foresight of the consequences.

When an individual is found not guilty by reason of insanity, he is involuntarily admitted to a psychiatric facility for a statutorily defined evaluation period. During this time, mental health professionals evaluate the client's need for hospitalization and any other appropriate disposition. On completion of the evaluation, the court is notified of the recommendations, at which time a hearing may be scheduled to determine the court's order for release or for continuation of mandatory commitment for treatment. As soon as the client is considered not committable, he will be released into the community, possibly with some mandatory requirements for aftercare treatment.

There is a great deal of controversy involving the verdict of not guilty by reason of insanity, much of which has surrounded the John Hinckley acquittal in the assassination attempt against President Reagan. As a result of this controversy, some states have passed "a guilty but mentally ill" plea, which is meant to mandate psychiatric treatment of the mentally ill in correctional facilities when they are serving sentences. This plea has not yet passed constitutionality scrutiny; therefore, although it is popular in principle, it may not be the final answer to a difficult balancing problem between the rights of victims and the rights of mentally ill offenders.

Ideally, the mental health team responsible for providing forensic evaluations and services is composed of a psychiatrist, a clinical psychologist, a social worker, a psychiatric–mental health nurse clinical specialist, and other nursing personnel who are active in the client's evaluation and treatment.

Nurse clinical specialists can be very valuable members of the mental health team. They are specially trained to do mental status examinations as well as to function as individual and group therapists. In some states, they are qualified to be trained in competency evaluations and to testify in court as expert forensic witnesses.

Registered nurses are, likewise, valuable in the evaluation and treatment of these clients. Their nursing assessments, nursing observations, nursing interventions, knowledge of medication, and accurate documentation contribute to the formulation and implementation of a treatment plan to ensure that these clients with very special needs are given the highest quality of care possible.

Juvenile Psychiatric Clients

A special population of psychiatric clients is minors or juveniles. Until the recent past, parents or guardians have had almost an absolute privilege to admit their minor children under 18 years of age for mental health treatment. This absolute right has been eroded somewhat by state recognition of some rights of more mature children (12–18 years) to protest such treatment.[10]

In 1979, the United States Supreme Court, in *Parham* v. *J.L. et al,* gave a more definite standard for juvenile admissions to which state statutes and hospital policy should conform.[20] The Supreme Court held that juveniles can be authorized for admission by their parents, but that accompanying the admission, some "neutral fact finder" should determine whether statutory requirements for admission are satisfied. Further, an adversarial hearing for admission is not required nor does due process require that the fact finder be legally trained or a hearing officer.[20]

By ruling in this way, the Court balanced competing interests of the rights of parents and guardians to control the lives of their children with the right of children to due process prior to a limitation upon their liberty.

Psychiatric–mental health nurses need to be mindful of these procedural protections for the benefit of their juvenile clients. Limiting hospitalization to statutory requirements is an important advocacy activity for juvenile psychiatric clients.

Major Evolving Legal Rights

Right to Treatment

The idea that psychiatric clients have a legally actionable right to psychiatric treatment began to develop in the late 1960s and culminated in the early 1970s in the Circuit Court case of *Wyatt* v. *Stickney.*[28] The case provided innovative statements about the rights of civilly committed mentally ill patients in state hospitals. The Court stated that such patients do have certain treatment rights, which include the following:

1. Treatment must give some realistic opportunity to improve or be cured
2. Custodial care is insufficient to meet treatment requirements
3. A lack of funding does not excuse a state from treatment responsibilities
4. Commitment without treatment violates the due process rights of patients[28]

Perhaps the most important pronouncement in Wyatt concerns the three determinants for the adequacy of treatment, which are a humane environment, a qualified staff in adequate numbers, and individualized treatment plans.[28] This case gave the nation guidance about treatment rights; however, because it was not reviewed by the Supreme Court, it is not totally generalizable.

O'Connor v. *Donaldson* was decided by the Supreme Court and is commonly thought to be the leading case for the right to treatment.[19] However, O'Connor instead states that no state can confine a nondangerous mentally ill individual in a state hospital who is capable of surviving safely in the community by himself or with the help of willing responsible family or friends.[19] There is still no clear national standard on the right to treatment of the involuntarily civilly committed or on the right of the state to commit involuntarily the mentally ill for the purpose of treatment. Newer cases will decide these issues.

Treatment in the Least Restrictive Environment

Over time, through dicta and decisions, courts have given guidance to the mental health system on many matters, including standards about the settings in which treatment should occur. As early as 1969, in *Covington* v. *Harris,* the courts held that an individual who is to be treated involuntarily should receive such treatment in a setting that is least restrictive to his liberty but that will still meet his treatment needs.[9]

Least restrictive environments can be community resources instead of hospitalization, open wards instead of locked wards, or outpatient care instead of inpatient care.[10] The importance of this client right to nursing is that nurses need constantly to assess the client's condition and status so that more or less restrictive treatment alternatives can be applied based upon the client's evolving needs.

Right to Refuse Treatment

As discussed previously, the doctrine of informed consent implies that clients have a right to choose or refuse medical and health treatment. Certainly, health care providers, through interpersonal relationships and client education, may try to convince clients about the need for certain treatments, but only in rare or life-threatening instances do courts intervene in the negative treatment decisions of clients.

Voluntary Clients. Following this principle of judicial noninterference, voluntary clients who have not been adjudicated incompetent have an absolute right to refuse treatment and to choose between treatment alternatives. They cannot be forced to take medications, be research subjects, or be involved in invasive treatments, such as ECT or psychosurgery. Only in rare cases of severe behavioral acting-out that threatens self or others can voluntary clients be forced to take psychotropic medications.

Involuntary Clients. The rights of involuntarily committed clients to refuse treatment are less clearly defined than are the rights of voluntary clients. *Rennie* v. *Klein* and *Rogers* v. *Okin* are the leading cases to give guidance on this unsettled issue.[22] The Courts have been prone to state that involuntary clients cannot refuse tried and true treatments that promote recovery, such as psychotropic medication; however, there must be protections applied for more risky procedures with more extreme side effects or consequences, such as ECT, insulin shock, or psychosurgery. In *Mills* v. *Rogers* (on appeal of *Rogers* v. *Okin*), the Supreme Court seemed to favor a standard that there would be no absolute right of involuntary patients to refuse treatment but that treatment decisions would be left to the judgment of professionals who would consider patient rights in their treatment decisions.[18]

Clearly, it is important for the psychiatric nurse to know that there is much continuing controversy and litigation about the rights of involuntary clients to refuse treatment; therefore, being current on the most recent case law about this issue is a must. Unit and facility policies need to remain current and should clearly reflect that, as the treatment becomes more invasive, as it has increased risk, or as it demonstrates questionable results, the more likely it is that the client's right to refuse must be honored.

Right to Aftercare

Care in the community following psychiatric hospitalization is greatly needed to prevent readmissions and to ensure the rehabilitation of former inpatients. There is no absolute legal right at this time to after-care programs unless such a right is provided by state statutes. It is not inconceivable that case laws may evolve to mandate aftercare services as a right of the mental health client.

In conjunction with other members of the interdisciplinary team, it is a nursing responsibility to plan for aftercare treatment. As knowledgeable and responsible citizens, nurses voice their concern at all levels of the political system to see that psychiatric clients have access to adequate aftercare services such as outpatient counseling, medication follow-up, vocational placement, and sheltered living environments.

Strategies for Assuring Quality and Accountability in Nursing Practice

American Nurses' Association's Standards of Practice

The nursing profession—through its professional organization, the American Nurses' Association (ANA)—has developed clinical standards of practice for both generic and specialty areas of practice. The generic standards apply to all professional nursing practice and serve as guidelines or norms for practice. A review of the generic standards indicates that nurses must use the nursing process in therapeutic relationships with clients. In other words, nurses will assess, diagnose, document, report, plan, implement, and evaluate client care with the client, the family, and the client's significant others.[4] The focus of nursing practice is on the client's attainment or restoration of physical and mental health. Practitioners of nursing are uniquely able to view the client holistically and to engage in a process *with* the client that has, as its aim, care and growth. The use of ANA Standards of Practice as a baseline for performance evaluation will assure such practice.

Quality Assurance Programming

Another major strategy for the assuring of quality and accountability in nursing is the involvement of nursing in quality assurance programs. In the 1970s, the American Nurses' Association developed a national program emphasizing that nurses would implement the standards of nursing practice through development of, and participation in, systematic quality assurance endeavors.[3]

The American Nurses' Association developed a conceptual model for quality assurance that is represented in Fig. 45-1.[3] The use of the model as the conceptual basis for quality assurance facilitates nurses' and other health care practitioners' understanding of

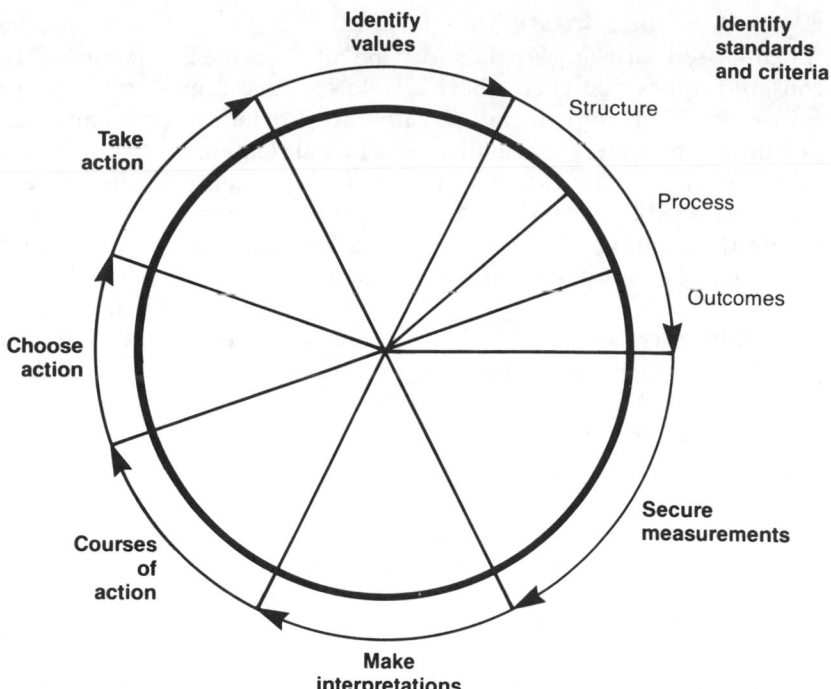

Figure 45-1. *Quality assurance model.*

quality assurance and demonstrates that quality care is assured to consumers and is not merely an exercise used for accreditation or reimbursement verification.

There are numerous nursing activities that fit into the ANA quality assurance model—client care audit, peer review, client classification and acuity rating, the nursing clinical ladder, medical care evaluation, and nursing care planning, to name a few. Psychiatric audit is a procedure through which client care in psychiatric settings can be measured for its effectiveness in providing care to population categories in psychiatric settings. The ANA Model for Quality Assurance can be used in a psychiatric audit as a way of conceptualizing the audit activity as a dynamic process. The process includes values classification, criteria development, client care measurements, identification of care successes and failures, development of alternative care approaches, and the introduction of change into the psychiatric setting.[3] The dynamic audit process is never complete until a complete re-audit is accomplished to evaluate the effectiveness of change.

Audit criteria should be written to include the measurement of the health team's awareness of the legal rights and remedies available to clients. Criteria that address the client's legal needs are very important, especially in the psychiatric setting. It is most important that nurses voluntarily and enthusiastically join in quality assurance programs for the purpose of systematically evaluating client care in an effort to improve care for all consumers.

Seeking Legal Consultation

A further strategy that needs to be employed by health professionals on the psychiatric unit is knowing how and when to obtain appropriate legal consultation on an ongoing basis. First, it would be important as a baseline to have an attorney who is aware of the issues in mental health law assess the institution's policies and procedures and provide that review for the staff in a problem-solving, rather than policing, manner.

Second, some arrangements should be made to have such an attorney offer continuing education programs on a regular basis in order to review with the staff updates on court decisions and recent legislation that would affect care in the psychiatric unit. Also, having legal consultation readily available on a case (client) consultation basis when the staff is endeavoring to ensure legal accountability is extremely valuable. Most institutions should provide this kind of legal consultation, if requested, not only for the benefit of their clients but also to protect the institution from potential liability.

Summary

The legal impact on the practice of psychiatric–mental health nursing is both immense and subtle. The psychiatric nurse who evaluates her practice in an attempt to improve the nursing profession and the

Nursing Care Plan 45-1

Legal Nursing Care

Goal	Plan	Outcome Evaluation
To prevent nursing negligence	Provide at minimum "reasonable man" standard of care in assessment, planning, implementation, and evaluation of nursing practice Know elements of negligence and problem-solve to prevent occurrences Give safe care in both independent and dependent areas of nursing practice	Malpractice suits are at a minimum and client feedback reflects satisfaction with nursing care Staff inservice periodically reviews legal malpractice problems and strategies Care shows nursing initiation of assessment, planning, implementation, and evaluation of health care and judicious implementation of the physician's treatment and drug orders
To ensure client rights to informed consent	Know the elements of informed consent Observe the client for behaviors that would indicate consent was valid—knowledge, competence, capacity Record and report any discrepancies in consent or behavior, revocation of consent, and so on to the client's physician	Staff inservice periodically reviews issues of informed consent for psychiatric clients Nurse acts as client advocate in informed consent and has interdependent role of assessment of consent, competence, and consent revocation with physician Client record reflects specific nursing assessment of current behaviors and appropriate nursing action is taken if consent is questioned or invalidated
To protect the client's right to confidentiality of health data	Records/charts are protected and data are not shared without client authorization The record is the legal document and should be chronological, comprehensive, and complete to facilitate care No verbal communication about the client should be shared except between treatment team members Nurses rarely have statutory privileged communication with clients but both confidentiality/privilege may be breached if the client threatens harm to third persons	The unit has policy/procedure for staff confidentiality and that procedure is reviewed by all staff yearly The client record reflects nursing process and descriptive charting Policy/procedures reflect nurse's duty to protect third persons in cases of prior threats and identify the procedural steps to provide the protection

(Continues on p. 872)

Legal Nursing Care

Goal	Plan	Outcome Evaluation
To protect client rights	Client rights should be made known to all staff Ensure that ward policy/procedure does not violate client rights Periodically review rights, issues of violations, and mechanisms that provide rights accountability Specifically review/reevaluate changes in voluntary/nonvoluntary status and civil/criminal commitment proceedings and treatment consequences	Inservice programs on client rights are held periodically Legal consultant periodically reviews unit policy/procedure manual to guard against rights violations and to advise staff as to protective mechanisms for full rights provisions Staff inservice periodically covers statutory/case law on admission status, procedures, and treatment Quality assurance materials reflect items that measure the status of client's rights
To protect evolving client rights	The nurse must know, and policies must reflect, the following factors: Voluntary clients are seeking treatment and nondangerous involuntary clients cannot be confined without receiving treatment Treatments need to be and occur in methods and settings that are least restrictive to the client's liberty Voluntary clients who are nondangerous may refuse all treatments, including medications, ECT, and psychosurgery Nonvoluntary clients who are nondangerous have limited rights to refuse medication and have greater rights to refuse more invasive procedures such as ECT and psychosurgery Competence to consent and procedures for substituted consent are always at issue with involuntarily committed clients	The legal consultant reviews and advises on new legislation and case law implications for mental health care Psychiatric treatment reflects differing modalities and choices for the consumer Medicine and nursing are concerned about the client's right to refuse treatment and this is reflected in policies, client records, and orders Policies and procedures clearly reflect differing rights in voluntary and nonvoluntary clients and between medication and more invasive procedures Consent procedures are clearly defined, known, and utilized by all involved staff
To provide legally sound and professionally accountable nursing care	Secure legal consultation for new decision-update, review of policy/procedures, and case consultation when needed	A yearly staff legal inservice for case update is held A legal consultant is retained and is available to staff on an "on call" basis; ANA Quality Assurance Model is used by

---

Legal Nursing Care

Goal	Plan	Outcome Evaluation
		the unit in a quality assurance program
		There is an ongoing audit on each diagnostic category of frequent client population
		Each client care plan and audit tool includes one or more elements of legal knowledge and specific need in the area of psychiatric–mental health care

---

health of her clients does so not from legal demands but from professional standards. Nevertheless, nursing practice must meet certain legal standards and must adjust its course as new legal standards evolve. It is the capable and challenged nurse who includes legal knowledge in client care and it is to her that many clients will turn for information, advocacy, and protective justice.

Some of the major points of this chapter include the following:

1. Nurses have both independent and dependent areas of nursing practice and are liable for maintenance of a responsible standard of care to clients in both of these areas of practice.

2. A failure to meet the standard of care that results in an injury to a client/consumer makes the nurse liable for nursing negligence or malpractice.

3. Nurses have a duty to participate in the issues of informed consent, which are basic rights of clients; failure to obtain informed consent from a client prior to a procedure can result in a civil action against the physician and the health care agency on the theories of assault and battery or malpractice.

4. Clients also have a right to rely on the appropriateness and confidentiality of their medical records and data.

5. Confidentiality is an ethical, professional, and legal responsibility and is, in many instances, mandated by statute.

6. Privileged communication is determined by statute for certain professional groups and their clients.

7. Some cases indicate that confidentiality must be breached when the public safety is in jeopardy, as when clients threaten to harm third persons.

8. To provide legally acceptable nursing care in psychiatric–mental health settings, nurses must be informed about a variety of issues, including recognized client rights, and they must take responsibility with other health team members to see that client rights are protected.

9. Client rights may differ due to the civil or criminal nature of commitment proceedings; the voluntariness of a civil commitment; the purpose of the criminal commitment; and the age of the client.

10. It is most important that psychiatric–mental health caregivers identify client status and client rights and secure adequate consultation as client rights evolve.

11. Three strategies for enhancing the quality of psychiatric–mental health nursing care, and thereby assuring quality care and accountability by nursing to consumers, are as follows:

    Nurses must practice by using the ANA Standards of Practice as their normative base

    Nurses must develop, and participate in, quality assurance programming, including psychiatric audits

    Nurses must request and secure ongoing continuing education and consultation with an attorney who is knowledgeable in mental health law

References

1. *Addington v. Texas,* 99 Supreme Court Reporter 1813, 441 United States Reporter 418, 1979
2. American Hospital Association: A Patient's Bill of Rights. Chicago, American Hospital Association, 1974
3. American Nurses' Association: Quality Assurance Workbook. Kansas City, MO, American Nurses' Association, 1976
4. American Nurses' Association: Standards of Practice. Kansas City, MO, American Nurses' Association
5. Beck JC: The Psychotherapist's Duty to Protect Third Parties from Harm. Mental and Physical Disability Law Reporter 2, 2 (Mar–Apr) 1987
6. Brakel SJ, Parry J, Weiner BA: Mentally Disabled and the Law, 3d ed. Chicago, American Bar Foundation, 1985
7. Calloway SD: Nursing and the Law, 2d ed. Eau Claire, WI, Professional Education Systems, 1986
8. *Canterbury v. Spence,* 464 Federal Second Reporter 772, 1972
9. *Covington v. Harris,* 419 Federal Second Reporter 617, 1969
10. Ennis B, Emery R: The Rights of Mental Patients. New York, Avon Books, 1978
11. Feutz SA: Preventive Legal Maintenance. J Nursing Administration 17, 1 (Jan): 8–10, 1987
12. *Jackson v. Indiana,* 406 United States Reporter 715, 1972
13. Jones K: Lunacy, Law, and Conscience. London, Routledge and Kegan Paul, 1955
14. *Kaimowitz v. Michigan Department of Mental Hygiene,* 2 Prison Law Reporter 433.
15. Kerr AH: Nurses Notes, That's Where the Goodies Are. Nursing 75 (Feb): 34–41, 1975
16. Kittrie N: The Right to be Different. Baltimore, Johns Hopkins Press, 1974
17. Menzes WC: The Negligent Nurse: Rx for the Medical Malpractice Victim. 12 (104) Tulsa Law Review 104, 1976
18. *Rogers v. Okin,* 478 Federal Supplement Reporter 1342 (D. Mass. 1979); aff'd in part, rev'd in part, *Rogers v. Okin,* 634 Federal Second Reporter 650 (First Circuit 1980); vacated and remanded; sub nomine *Mills v. Rogers,* 457 US 291 (1982); on remand, *Rogers v. Okin,* 738 Federal Second Report 1 (First Circuit 1984)
19. *O'Conner v. Donaldson,* 422 United States Reporter 563, 1975
20. *Parham, Commissioner, Department of Human Resources of Georgia et al v. J.L. et al,* 442 United States Reporter 584, 1979
21. Prosser W: Law of Torts. St. Paul, MN, West Publishing, 1971
22. *Rennie v. Klein,* 653 Federal Second Reporter 836, 1981
23. Rosoff AJ: Informed Consent: A Guide for Health Care Remedies. Rockville, MD, Aspen Systems Corporation, 1981
24. Sharill NL: Patients' Rights vs. Patients' Needs: The Right of the Mentally Ill to Refuse Treatment in Colorado. 58 Denver Law Reporter 567, 1981
25. *Tarasoff v. Board of Regents of University of California,* 592 Pacific Second Reporter 553, 1974
26. Tennessee Code Annotated, Section 33-6-103.
27. Tennessee Code Annotated, Section 63-7-101 et seq.
28. *Wyatt v. Stickney,* 325 Federal Supplement Reporter 781, 1971

46

Research in Psychiatric–Mental Health Nursing

Mary Anne Sweeney
James McColgan, Jr.

RULE 1. We are to admit no more causes of natural things than such as are both true and sufficient to explain their appearances.
Isaac Newton,
Rules of Reasoning
in Philosophy

Chapter Preview

This chapter presents an overview of the research process in nursing. Special emphasis has been placed on two key areas that integrate research skills with a well-rounded nursing practice base. The first area is the utilization of published research reports. Nurses need to utilize the professional literature—to learn the outcomes of studies that have already been completed. In addition, they need to develop abilities to critique research reports and to incorporate important elements of the research process into routine nursing practice. The second area of emphasis is the involvement of nurses in the steps of the research process. Because learning is enhanced by participation, practical suggestions have been included with the beginning researcher in mind.

Learning Objectives

After completion of this chapter, you should be able to accomplish the following:

1. define nursing research and recognize broad distinctions among the main types of research
2. discuss the varied ways that the research process can be incorporated into the role of the nurse
3. locate published nursing research reports and other sources of research-related information
4. read, evaluate, and utilize information from research studies
5. develop a strategy for active participation in nursing research-related activities

Understanding Nursing Research

Definition and Purpose of Research

One way of gathering and processing information related to nursing is through the use of the research process. Unfortunately, the mention of the word "research" may trigger an immediate, unfavorable response in many professionals. But although you may not have realized it, you have been doing "research" for quite some time.

If we put the research process into its proper perspective, we can deal with it more effectively. Research is one way to gather and process information, and it is used routinely by all types of professional groups. Research is the use of a series of formalized steps to gather objective information; the research process is a series of steps that can be followed by nurses, psychologists, biologists, or any professionals interested in obtaining data or information. *Nursing research* has "application to the study of all nursing problems with the goal of expanding the theoretical basis of nursing through the discovery of new knowledge."[6]

The Research Process

The steps of the research process provide a structured and consistent approach to information-gathering. Flexibility is available at each step of the research process; this enables a study to be specifically tailored to each new and individual situation. Because the major objective of conducting a research study is to add new knowledge to what is already known about nursing, some of the reasons for the formality and safeguards of the process become clear. It is critical to ensure that the information gained in the study be as accurate as possible. The information should also be useful, and, above all, it should be unbiased by the investigator's particular point of view. Many safeguards have been devised to help researchers collect "good" or "clean" information and to help them sort out its true meaning.

Scientific Method Applied to Nursing

The scientific method is a set of steps to be followed in approaching any question. Broadly defined, these steps are: identification of the question; collection of relevant facts concerning the question; analysis of these facts; development of an approach to investigate the question; investigation and collection of data; analysis of findings; and, interpretation and application of the investigation's results. These same steps are used in the application of the nursing process. When faced with the question of how best to care for a patient, the nurse in developing a nursing care plan applies these same steps. See Table 46-1 for a comparison of the steps of the scientific method with those of the nursing process.

The scientific method has been found to be the most effective way of determining relationships between variables, thereby enabling the scientist to understand, predict, and, to a degree, control their behavior.[3] The scientific process can be applied by practitioners of any professional discipline to obtain objective information.

The nursing role is presently expanding to include the use of scientific research methods at many different levels of expertise. Nursing students, faculty members, and clinical nursing practitioners in all types of different nursing settings are becoming increasingly involved in nursing research throughout

Table 46-1.   **Comparison of the Scientific Method
with the Nursing Process**

SCIENTIFIC METHOD	NURSING PROCESS
Collection of relevant facts	Assessment
Analysis of facts	Nursing Diagnosis
Development of approach to investigate	Planning
Investigation and collection of data	Implementation
Analysis of findings	Evaluation
Interpretation and application of findings	Revision

the course of their normal work routine (see Chart 46-1, "Examples of Research Studies Conducted by Nurses in Psychiatric Nursing and Mental Health Topics").

Nurses, in general, are fortunate that their work entails a variety of interesting experiences and situations. The selection of research topics can be as varied as the types of professional work that nurses perform. It usually takes only a brief period of perusing research journals to discover a study that is both interesting and useful to the reader. For instance, two faculty members at Wayne State University in Detroit, Michigan, were interested in looking at factors that influenced the success of registered nurse students when they returned to school to earn a baccalaureate degree. They examined a specific set of characteristics and found, among other things, that the type of the student's initial nursing program discriminated significantly between students who completed the baccalaureate degree and those who did not.[5]

The best introduction to the realm of research is to read about it. You are encouraged to find examples in the literature of studies that cover issues or questions that are important to you. The selected references listed in Chart 46-2 will help you locate the material you need. Your objective should be to locate,

CHART 46-1

Examples of Research Studies Conducted by Nurses in Psychiatric Nursing and Mental Health Topics

Client Expectation and Perception of the Nurse's Role in Relationship to Client Satisfaction

A Comparative Study of Widows' and Widowers' Perceived Social Support During the First Year of Bereavement

The Effects of Cognitive-Behavioral Nursing Intervention for Depressed Patients and Their Families

Factors Affecting Staff Nurses' Use of Limit-Setting with Disruptive Patients

Nurses' Attitudes Toward the Suicidal Patient

Nursing Interventions with Long-Term Patients in Regard to their Physical Appearance: An Evaluation Study

The Nurse's Therapeutic Use of Touch as Related to Withdrawn Patients

Observable Signs of Anxiety or Distress During Psychiatric Interviews Conducted by Nurses

Patient and Situational Factors That Affect Nursing Students' Like or Dislike of Caring for Patients

A Study of Alcoholic Patients' Perception of the Role of the Nurse

A Study of the Confidence Level of Nurses in Caring for Patients with Depression

A Study of Psychiatric Patients' Knowledge about Their Prescribed Medications

C H A R T 46-2
Selected References for Locating Research-Related Nursing Information

Books

Abdellah F, Levine E: Better Patient Care Through Nursing Research, 3d ed. New York, Macmillan, 1986

Brooking J (ed.): Psychiatric Nursing Research. New York, John Wiley & Sons, 1986

Burns N, Grove S: The Practice of Nursing Research: Conduct, Critique and Utilization. Philadelphia, WB Saunders, 1987

Castles M: Primer of Nursing Research. Philadelphia, WB Saunders, 1987

Diers D: Research in Nursing Practice. Philadelphia, JB Lippincott, 1979

Downs F: A Sourcebook of Nursing Research, 3d ed. Philadelphia, FA Davis, 1984

Hardyck C, Petrinovich L: Understanding Research in the Social Sciences: A Practical Guide to Understanding Social and Behavioral Research. Philadelphia, WB Saunders, 1975

Holm K, Llewellyn J: Nursing Research for Nursing Practice. Philadelphia, WB Saunders, 1986

Kerlinger F: Foundations of Behavioral Research, 3d ed. New York, Holt, Rinehart & Winston, 1986

Lieske A (ed.): Clinical Nursing Research: A Guide to Undertaking and Using Research in Nursing Practice. Rockville, MD, Aspen Systems Corporation, 1986

Mayo C, LaFrance M: Evaluating Research in Social Psychology: A Guide for the Consumer. Monterey, CA, Brooks/Cole Publishing, 1977

Meltzoff J, Kornreich M: Research in Psychotherapy. Chicago, Aldine Publishing, 1970

Polit D, Hungler B: Nursing Research, 2d ed. Philadelphia, JB Lippincott, 1983

Seaman C, Verhonick P: Research Methods for Undergraduate Students in Nursing, 2d ed. New York, Appleton-Century-Crofts, 1982

Sweeney MA, Olivieri P: Introduction to Nursing Research. Philadelphia, JB Lippincott, 1981

Journals

Advances in Nursing Science
    Aspen Publishing Inc., 7201 McKinney Circle, Frederick, MD 21701

Archives of Psychiatric Nursing
    Grune & Stratton Inc., P.O. Box 6209, Duluth, MN 55806

International Journal of Nursing Studies
    Pergamon Journals, Maxwell House, Fairview Park, Elmsford, NY 10523

Journal of Psychosocial Nursing and Mental Health Services
    Slack Inc., 6900 Grove Road, Thorofare, NJ 08086

Journal of Nursing Education
    Slack Inc., 6900 Grove Road, Thorofare, NJ 08086

Nursing Research
    555 West 57th St., New York, NY 10019

Research in Nursing and Health
    John Wiley & Sons, Publisher, 605 Third Ave., New York, NY 10158

Scholarly Inquiry for Nursing Practice
    Springer Publishing Co., 536 Broadway, New York, NY 10012

Western Journal of Nursing Research
    Sage Publications Inc., 2111 West Hillcrest Drive, Newbury Park, CA 91320

Indexes

Index Medicus and its annual cumulation, Cumulated Index Medicus, 1960 + (National Library of Medicine)

Nursing and Allied Health Literature Index and its annual cumulation, Cumulative Index to Nursing and Allied Health Index 1956 + (Glendale, CA, Adventist Medical Center Library)

Nursing Studies Index 1900–1959 by Virginia Henderson, 4 Volumes (JB Lippincott, 1972)

Abstracts

Abstracts of Reports by Studies in Nursing in each issue of Nursing Research 1960–1978

Excerpta Medica, 1947 +

Nursing Research Abstracts (England), 1979 +

Psychological Abstracts, 1927 +

---

read, and assess the results of the research project, and then if applicable use the new knowledge in your nursing activities.

There are a number of ways to implement the research process according to the objectives of the individual conducting the study. Table 46-2 summarizes the main points in six of the most frequently encountered types of research. The most prevalent type of research in the nursing literature is the survey, and it an take many forms, such as descriptive and explanatory studies. The report should clearly state, usually in the introductory section, the type of re-

Table 46-2. **Characteristics of Various Research Approaches**

	PHILOSOPHICAL	HISTORICAL	CASE STUDY	METHODOLOGICAL	SURVEY	EXPERIMENTAL
Time frame	Present, past	Past	Present, past	Present	Present	Present, future
Research objectives	Trace development and/or present status of abstract ideas	Discover exciting facts and combine to draw conclusions	In-depth analysis of subject; usually includes historical aspects	Develop instruments to measure variables; test statistical procedures for appropriateness	Discover new facts about subjects; make conclusions and interpretations	Prediction of events; discover cause-and-effect relationships under controlled conditions
Data collection Source	Documents	Personal and public documents and	Combination of data from subjects, documents and ... acts	Subjects utilized for pretesting, reliability, and validation of instruments	Subjects	Subjects
		...ative with ...ional numerical data; ...nclude ...ts or ...cts		Numerical with accompanying narrative statements	Narrative that usually includes numerical data	Narrative with great emphasis on numerical results

Handwritten note overlaying page:
Unit Test #1   (3-26)
ch. 1-7, 17

Unit Test #2   (4-2)
ch. 8-14, 16 & 24

Unit Test #3   (4-16)
ch 21-22, 25 + 26

Unit Test #4   (4-20)
ch. 31-33, 37 44 & 46

... few ... with ...

... research ... methodology, results, and discussion. Each area contains essential information for comprehension of the research project and its possible applications to nursing practice.

Introduction

The introduction of the research report describes the problem that was investigated and related background information. The problem statement is usually placed in the first paragraph of the report. Usually, a declarative statement describes the overall purpose of the study. For example, the author might state that "the purpose of this study is to investigate the relationship between blood pressure and varied levels of psychological stress."

An interrogative statement of the research problem may be used to question the nature of the relationship between the variables or factors being studied. An example of this type of problem statement is, "What is the relationship between blood pressure and different levels of psychological stress?" A simple definition of what the study is about is particularly important at this point. The focus of the study will be one or more variables. Variables may be defined as characteristics or traits. In the example given above, the variables in the problem statement are "blood pressure" and "psychological stress." The variables being investigated are identified and defined in general terms in the introduction, but are definitively refined in the methodology section of the study.

The introduction of the study should lead the reader to understand not only what is currently investigated, but why it is an important topic for scrutiny. The background of the problem is presented by a review of related literature. The scope of the literature review should be fairly exhaustive and should demonstrate a comprehensive grasp of the topic. This literature review should include key studies that have been conducted about the problem, the findings of previous investigations, and the identification of questions concerning the problem that have yet to be answered. Although the review of the literature is not intended to provide an expert level of knowledge concerning the problem area, it should give you an appreciation for where the problem under investigation "fits" into the realm of nursing theory and practice.

Methodology

The methodology portion of the research report describes the mechanics by which the investigation was conducted. It includes an explanation of the population and sample, instrument, data collection methods, and data analysis procedures. The detailed information in this portion of the study is needed to provide a clear understanding of the procedures used so they can be evaluated or replicated by other researchers.

Population and Sample. The study population will be described in this portion of the research report. The population is the entire group of subjects possessing the qualities desired by the researcher. For example, returning to our sample problem statement, the researcher may wish to investigate the relationship between blood pressure and psychological stress in American males more than 40 years of age who live in urban settings. In this example the population would include all males over 40 years of age living in American cities. The sample is a subset of the population. The sample is the group of people who were actually selected from the population to participate in the research project. Therefore, the sample of the population described above could be males more than 40 years of age living in Boston, New York, Dallas, or San Francisco—in fact, in any American city.

The research report should describe, in as much detail as possible, both the population and the criteria used to select the sample from this group. This description should include how many individuals were selected, how they were chosen, and the procedures used to obtain consent from the individuals for participation in the study.

Research Instrument. The description of the research instrument includes discussion of its format, reliability, and validity. The instrument might be a questionnaire, an interview schedule, or machinery (*e.g.*, a sphygmomanometer). In the first two types of instruments, the number, type, and some examples of the items should be included in the research report. Because of the variety of instruments available to researchers, knowledge of the particular instrument's format is important to understanding this aspect of data collection.

Reliability of an instrument refers to its consistency. Its ability to collect the same kind of data in repeated administrations, and in a variety of situations, is important. One of the more common ways of determining reliability is termed *test–retest reliability*. To establish this type of reliability, the researcher ad-

ministers the instrument, and then, after a period of time (from 2 weeks to several months), administers the same instrument to the same sample group again. If the instrument has a high degree of test–retest reliability, it will yield similar results on both occasions. The reader of the research report needs to know if the instrument is one that produces consistent results before believing its findings.

Validity is the ability of the instrument to measure the variables under investigation. There are various types of validity: face, content, construct, and criterion-related. *Face validity* is the degree to which the research instrument appears or looks related to what is being studied. The determination that a research instrument has face validity need not be made by someone who is familiar with the area under investigation. The focus of face validity is the appearance of the instrument to measure what the researcher intends to measure. *Content validity* refers to the degree to which items contained in the instrument collect representative information related to the variable being measured. The process of establishing a research instrument's content validity, like its face validity, is based on judgment. To establish content validity, the researcher asks subject matter experts from the area under investigation to assess the degree to which items in the instrument will measure the variable(s) under study. Content validity is the degree of agreement between experts that, in their judgment, the instrument will measure or collect the desired data.[8]

Construct validity is more difficult to establish. Constructs are concepts that are not directly observable, such as human reasoning, intelligence, or stress. In one means to establish construct validity, the researcher compare their results with an alternative means of measuring the variable. For example, the instrument is administered to a group that is also observed by judges for the concept. The amount of agreement between the data collected by the instrument and the observations of the judges is the level of construct validity. Another means to establish construct validity is to administer the instrument to a group known to possess the construct that the researcher wishes to measure. In our sample research problem, we might use a questionnaire to measure anxiety, because constructs are intangible and anxiety is a manifestation of the construct stress. To establish construct validity we would administer our questionnaire to a group that we know demonstrates characteristics of anxiety. Such a group might be patients with a clinical diagnosis of neurosis who display high levels of anxiety. This would be our "known group." A research instrument that has construct validity will collect data corresponding to the characteristics of the known group. If our questionnaire has construct validity, we would expect that the responses of the known group would indicate that they have high levels of stress.

Criterion-related validity is used to predict future performance. This validity is established by *post facto* identification of characteristics related to successful performance of a task. These characteristics are formulated into an instrument that should then identify individuals who will successfully perform the tasks desired. When establishing the criterion-related validity of an instrument, the researcher focuses not on the collection of data itself but rather on how well the data collected predict future events or outcomes. Instruments with criterion-related validity are often used in business and industry to identify potential employees who are able to behave in desired manners or perform desired tasks. The varied types of validity are important in assessing the value of the instrument used to obtain information from subjects.

Reliability and validity are important to your understanding of the values of a research instrument. When reading a research report, you need to know the reliability and validity of the instrument before accepting the data it collected. A research instrument that has reliability will collect similar, consistent results with each application to a particular study group. When an instrument has validity, it collects the data which the researcher is seeking. Both reliability and validity of the instrument are essential to your understanding of the research report and identifying a proper place for the study's results in your nursing practice.

Data Collection.   After describing the instrument, the research report should describe the data-collection methodology. This description concerns how the study group was selected and how the information was actually collected. In this portion of the report, the reader should find sufficient details to replicate the research project.

The description of how the study group was selected should explain its source and the criteria used to select or exclude individuals from it. Continuing with our sample research problem, we might state that our study group will be selected from male pedestrians at the intersection of Tremont and Park Streets in downtown Boston who answer "yes" to the questions "Are you more than 40 years of age?" and "Do you live in Boston?" To select our study group we would stand at the designated intersection and address these questions to males passing by. If they answer "yes" to both questions, they will be included in the study group; if they answer "no" to either one, they will not be included.

The description of the data collection method may be general or complex, depending on the instru-

ment format employed. The methodology of using mechanical instruments or paper and pencil measures with established reliability and validity may be described in general terms if the instrument's specific administration procedures have been followed by the researcher. More complex descriptions of the methodology are required when researchers adapt an instrument or its administration procedure to meet their particular needs. In the former case, the reader may be referred to the original instrument; in the latter, the researcher should report the methodology in sufficient detail to enable the reader to replicate it. In the case of our sample research problem, the description of our data collection method should include how the questionnaire was completed by the study participant and how his blood pressure was measured.

Data Analysis.   The final area in the methodology is the data analysis plan. The data analysis plan describes processing of the raw data and the procedures, usually statistical, that will be employed to tabulate the data. Processing may range from hand-scoring items on a test or questionnaire to coding data for computer analysis.

The statistical procedures used by researchers are classified as descriptive or inferential. *Descriptive statistics* are used to summarize the characteristics of the data collected. The most commonly used descriptive statistics are frequencies and mean (or average) scores. The descriptive statistics that might be included in a research report about our sample study are: highest, lowest, and average stress levels measured by our questionnaire; highest, lowest, and average systolic and diastolic blood pressures measured with our study group; and the age of the oldest and youngest participants as well as the average age of the study group.

Inferential statistics are used to test hypotheses and develop conclusions about the population from the results of the study group. Unlike most descriptive statistics, inferential statistics require the application of complex mathematical formulas. For this reason, a computer is often employed for this type of data analysis. There are many types of inferential statistical tests designed to analyze specific types of data. Each reports a numerical value for its specific statistic that is compared to a table of values for that test. If the numerical value of the statistics falls at or above the table's designated value for the level of significance desired (usually 0.05), the existence of a relationship between the variables is supported. The level of significance is important to the reader because it describes the extent to which the researcher is willing to be wrong about his conclusions. The standard level of significance used in research is 0.05. This means that the researcher wants to be correct 95% of the time when stating that there is a relationship between variables, and wrong only 5% of the time. The researcher should name the statistical test that will be used and specify the acceptable level of significance when describing the data analysis plan.

Results

The implementation of the data analysis plan is reported in the results section of the report. This discussion should focus first on the overall characteristics of the data by using descriptive statistics. The discussion itself should highlight important characteristics rather than reporting each item singly. Most of the data may be presented in tabular form; there are usually several tables in this section. Tables are an efficient means to present data to the reader. In using a tabular format, though, the researcher must focus on the clarity of the table itself. A table which is confusing or complicated to the reader makes the data it contains worthless. An important point to remember is that not every piece of data collected should be discussed individually, but the highlights of the data should be discussed thoroughly.

The analysis and interpretation of the data should follow a logical sequence. Often, research reports will analyze and interpret data following the sequence established by the order of the hypothesis or research questions. The researcher's goal is to present a clear picture of the study results. The analysis of the data should report both the obtained statistical values and the level of significance. The researcher should also state whether or not a hypothesis was supported or, in the case of research questions, a relationship was implied.

Keep in mind that research in which hypotheses or relationships are not supported also has value. The lack of significant findings in a research project has important implications, too. From this discussion of results, you should learn not only what the researchers found out from the subjects, but also how they interpret these results. The interpretation section will discuss the meaning of the findings.

Discussion

The final area of a research report that contains important information for the reader is the discussion. In the discussion, the researcher describes the conclusions drawn from the study and suggests implications of this information in regard to nursing practice. The discussion should review, in broad terms, the various aspects of the study. It should review the hypothesis or research questions, the sample, research instrument, and the major results. Often, the researcher will compare the results with other similar studies. The conclusions must be specific and must clearly be based upon the results of the study. The researcher must always keep this in mind. The results of the study direct and, at the same time, limit the conclusions which the researcher may make. The conclusions proposed by the researcher describe what has been learned from the research project. It is a summary of what was and was not found, what was answered and what remains unanswered.

In discussing the implications of the findings, the researcher suggests practical uses for the information learned. All research learning has practical applications. As an example, returning to our sample research problem, our conclusion might be that there is a direct relationship between levels of stress reported by our sample group and the measured systolic and diastolic blood pressures. The implication of our research results might then be that our study population may reduce its systolic and diastolic blood pressures by reducing its level of stress. Implications also include predictions of the impact that the results may have on the theory or practice of nursing. Again, in reference to our sample research problem, we might suggest the need for primary preventive nursing interventions. The report usually concludes with suggestions concerning the future directions of research in this area. Often the research will suggest a larger study group or different population. Sometimes, based upon the study's results, the researcher may suggest a different approach for a new investigation.

The discussion portion of a research report is considered by many readers to be its substance, but the discussion must be considered within its overall context. The conclusions and implications of a research project must be viewed in relation to specific information about such factors as the size of the study group, the soundness of the instrument, and the data analysis plan. Weakness in any of these areas reduces the value and applicability of the research conclusions and implications. The form in Chart 46-3 may help you extract, summarize, and evaluate information from research studies.

Protection of Subjects' Rights

The ethics surrounding the conduct of research projects must be considered. The nurse conducting a research project has the dual role of researcher and nurse. As a researcher, the nurse must implement the project's methodology and collect the desired data. As a nurse, the researcher continues to have the nursing responsibility of promoting the health needs of the person. The issues with which the nurse researcher should be concerned include the individual's right not to participate, informed consent, and confidentiality.

C H A R T   46-3
Research Reading Guidelines

Use the following guide to extract and summarize in your own words research studies that you read.

1. Reference identification (in bibliography format)
2. Introduction
   A. Research problem
   B. Purpose of study
   C. Summary of relevant points in the literature review
3. Methodology
   A. Variables
   B. Instrument(s)
   C. Sample
   D. Data collection plan or design
   E. Data analysis plan
4. Results
   A. Summary of main results
   B. Interesting additional findings
5. Discussion
   A. Conclusions
   B. Implications
6. Evaluation
   A. Your comprehension level of the report (easy, difficult, complicated)
   B. Overall value of the study (very worthwhile, average, questionable)

Right to Refuse to Participate

An individual has the right to refuse to participate in any research project for any reason. This is a right possessed solely by the individual. No other individual or institution may deny or override this right. Furthermore, an individual may not be coerced into agreeing to participate in a research project. Nurses should be aware of the client's involvement in a research project and the circumstances surrounding this involvement, even when they are not directly involved in the research themselves.

Right to Informed Consent

Informed consent is the term used to explain that the individual has the right to be fully informed about what participation in the research project involves, how it might affect him, the time commitment required, and any possible risks that may be involved. To obtain informed consent, the nurse researcher must explain these aspects of the study to the individual in nontechnical language. Although the researchers must be careful not to affect or bias the information that will be forthcoming from the client, they should answer all questions about the study as fully and honestly as possible. Obtaining informed consent from potential research subjects can be time-consuming for the researcher, but it will pay dividends by increasing the level of each subject's participation.

Right to Confidentiality

Confidentiality and anonymity are often considered synonymous by researchers; however, they are not. Confidentiality involves the right of the individual to privacy concerning the data that he provides to the researcher. Researchers may provide confidentiality to a research group participant's data by various methods, such as replacing the name on each instrument with a code number.

Anonymity involves the individual's right of privacy as a participant in the research group. The most common manner in which well-meaning researchers violate a subject's anonymity is by specifically identifying the source of the study group in their research report. For example, a researcher who identifies the study group as "the senior class of nursing students at Plain State College" has not provided anonymity to the research subjects. Although the research report must contain specific information concerning the criteria for selection of the study group and its characteristics, the specific source of the study group need not be revealed.

The nurse researcher must be cognizant of the rights of subjects involved in research projects. As a professional, the nurse must balance both the requirements of these rights and the research process itself. Above all, as a nurse, the researcher must be supportive and protective of subjects' rights.

Participating in Nursing Research

Developing Necessary Skills

Three broad steps help to develop the skills that are necessary to participate in nursing research. The amount of participation increases from step to step, and they should be approached in the order in which they appear.

Step 1. Read All the Studies You Can

The steps you have just learned to apply in utilizing published research studies will help you develop greater understanding of the process and increase your depth of knowledge. The confidence you display in identifying varied steps of the research process will increase markedly as you read and critique examples in the professional literature. Use the journals listed in Chart 46-2 as a starting point for locating nursing-related research articles.

Step 2. Practice Individual Steps of the Research Process

You do not have to undertake a complete study to gain experience in research-related activities. Start with one step of the research process that involves a skill you could develop to do your job better. Perhaps the skill involves summarizing and analyzing data. Look over the data analysis section of the research studies you have been critiquing. Then take some of your patient-related data and try to summarize it just as the authors did in one of the published reports. In other words, construct a table that presents the key points, and then make several summary statements about the information in your table.

Perhaps you need to present a summary of the current literature regarding a procedure at a team conference. Study the introductory sections of published research studies to see how various articles are summarized, condensed, and combined. Note how the authors give credit to the original sources and how they present reports with conflicting results.

Step 3. Replicate a Published Study

The best way to acquire an understanding of the research process is to become actively involved in it. A good way to begin is to use a previously conducted study as an example. Use it as a step-by-step pattern, just as a tailor would when making a garment. Follow it and update it as needed. For instance, check the literature to see if any related articles have been published since the date of this study. Use the same instrument, if possible, or a close facsimile. Your tables will already be laid out, but the data will be new. You'll learn a lot about the practical steps of conducting a project while having your own set of back-up instructions.

Nurses who are just starting out in research often think that they must "reinvent the wheel." Replication of previously conducted studies is a necessary step in the process of building sound theoretical knowledge. Replications of studies are also appearing more frequently in the nursing literature.

Tips on Conducting Small Research Projects

The following ten steps will help you get started on your way to becoming a professional who utilizes research in a meaningful way in any area of nursing practice.

1. Define a topic that you want to find out more about. Your interest level will help spur you on to explore the topic further. Note two things—the types of articles you tend to read when you look through professional journals, and the aspects of nursing that you puzzle over or think about a lot. The first step is to summarize your idea or interest in a few words, such as "communicating with confused patients" or "exploring nurses' reactions to dying patients." The idea doesn't need to be crystal clear, just a start in a direction that is interesting to you.

2. Find several studies that have been published on this general topic or ones that are closely related to it. Remember in your search that you may find a related study that has been done by researchers in another discipline, such as psychologists or social workers. Use these studies as a basis for your "research folder." Summarize the main points of the study or make a copy that you can put in your folder for later reference. Find several articles about the topic that may not be formal "research" studies and add them to your folder, too. The more you know about a particular

topic, the better. Note the articles your authors mention most often in their bibliographies and gather those works as well.

3. Pick out one aspect of one of the studies in your folder and draw up a plan to reconstruct this in a limited fashion. Use a study or parts of several studies as a pattern to follow. For instance, suppose one study on communicating with confused patients contrasts two different types of nursing intervention. Use the two approaches as part of your nursing care and observe the results. Keep some notes in your folder about your findings. Talk with other nurses to find out their views and experiences on the subject. With your previous reading and thinking about the topic, you will quickly be able to spot and explore new ideas. Add all this to your growing folder.

4. Talk to colleagues about your interest and the material you've gathered. See if you can find someone who would like to work with you on this type of study. It is often more stimulating to work with one other researcher or even a small group. That way, you can share the work and have built-in audiences for discussing varied aspects of the project. If you want to pursue it by yourself, try to locate someone with some research experience with whom you can consult and discuss ideas.

5. Write out a simple study plan. Define what you intend to study and outline the steps you plan to take to complete your project. Keep it simple and straightforward. You can do another project later if you wish to investigate more than one aspect of the topic.

6. Polish your proposal outline with advice from some expert source—a basic textbook or someone who has previously conducted a research project. Don't be afraid to investigate your resources; many health care institutions are providing help for employees who want to carry out small-scale studies. Try to project the time it will take you to complete the tasks on this polished version of the outline. Then multiply every number by 2 in order to give yourself leeway. Check your project calendar periodically to help keep track if you're on schedule. You'll need a tentative budget, too, but you can keep the costs of important work to a minimum, as other researchers have demonstrated.[2]

7. Identify the steps you need to follow in gaining permission to conduct your study. Usually, you will need to submit a written request to a review committee. Use your outline as a basis for the proposal to this group.

8. Watch for advertisements of workshops, continuing education classes, or university courses in research-related topics. You may even find some needed consultation or a research partner there.

9. Keep a record of all your study activities in case you want to write about the study at a later time.

10. Offer to give a small inservice program on your topic. You can communicate your procedures and findings—and, it is hoped, stimulate more interest and discussion about the project.

Summary

This chapter has explained the research process as an effective way to gather and process information and has examined some of the components of nursing research. Major points of the chapter include the following:

1. The research process can be applied by any professionals interested in obtaining data or information.

2. The safeguards of the steps of the research process provide structure and consistency to information-gathering.

3. Research reports contain four areas:
   The introduction, describing the problem investigated and related background information
   The methodology, describing the population and sample, research instrument(s), and procedures for data-collection and analysis
   The results of the report, describing the analysis and interpretation of the data
   The discussion, describing the conclusions drawn from the study and the implications of the findings in relation to nursing practice

4. The individual subject possesses the right to refuse to participate in the research, the right to informed consent, and the right to confidentiality.

5. The expanding role of nurses today includes participation in nursing research and the application of research results to nursing practice.

References

1. Downs FS: A Source Book of Nursing Research, 3d ed. Philadelphia, FA Davis, 1984
2. Holstrom L, Burgess A: Low-Cost Research: A Project on a Shoestring. Nurs Res 31 (March–April): 123–125, 1982
3. Munhall P: Nursing Philosophy and Nursing Research: In Apposition or Opposition? Nurs Res 31 (May–June): 176–177, 1982
4. Polit DF, Hungler BP: Nursing Research: Principles and Methods, 2d ed. Philadelphia, JB Lippincott, 1983
5. Raderman R, Allen D: Registered Nurse Students in a Baccalaureate Program: Factors Associated with Completion. Nurs Res 23 (January–February): 71–73, 1974
6. Sweeney MA, Olivieri P: An Introduction to Nursing Research: Research, Measurement, and Computers in Nursing. Philadelphia, JB Lippincott, 1981
7. Treece EW, Treece JW: Elements of Research in Nursing, 4th ed. St Louis, CV Mosby, 1986
8. Waltz CF, Bausell RB: Nursing Research: Design, Statistics, and Computer Analysis. Philadelphia, FA Davis, 1981

47

Trends in Psychiatric–Mental Health Care

Patricia Flatley Brennan
Maureen P. McCausland

The only way to maintain any semblance of equilibrium during the super-industrial revolution will be to meet invention with invention—to design new personal and social change-regulators. Thus we need neither blind acceptance nor blind resistance, but an array of creative strategies for shaping, deflecting, accelerating or decelerating change selectively. The individual needs new principles for pacing and planning his life along with a dramatically new kind of education. He may also need specific new technological aids to increase his adaptivity. The society, meanwhile, needs new institutions and organizational forms, new buffers and balance wheels.

Alvin Toffler,
Future Shock,
1970

Chapter Preview

Although institutional care of the mentally ill has existed since the Middle Ages, psychiatric nursing as a legitimate clinical focus is only 100 years old.[8] Throughout the 500 years of psychiatry, practitioners of the mental healing arts faced many challenges, in response to which the psychiatric and mental health nursing specialty changed and grew. Current obstacles faced by psychiatric–mental health nurses stem from changes in social awareness and population demographics, economics and legislation, technology, and the health care system itself. These obstacles demand responses from practitioners in the form of newer, more sophisticated, less costly, and more effective modes of treatment. The responses to these challenges by psychiatric–mental health nurses take the form of changes in providers, changes in practice settings, changes in the nature of care, and changes in the foci of care.

Some challenges in the past, caused by new forms of treatment such as electroconvulsive therapy or sodium amytal interviews, required nursing skills to promote safe and effective patient response to treatment. Other challenges, such as the need for psychiatric nursing support throughout the general hospital, were met through the inception of a new breed of practitioners, the clinical liaison nurse. Still other challenges were met by the community itself. The community, having grown tired of the lack of responsiveness from professional providers, encouraged the development of support groups. These self-help groups place new demands on psychiatric and mental health nurses, not for direct service, but for consultation, education and referral.

Learning Objectives

On completion of the chapter, you should be able to accomplish the following:

1. explain the influence that changes in the following have on psychiatric and mental health nursing
    population demographics and social
        awareness
    economics and legislation
    technology
    the health care system
2. assess the response of psychiatric–mental health nursing to the challenge posed by change
3. describe the foundation documents supporting the new order of psychiatric and mental health nursing
4. define the roles of psychiatric–mental health nursing
5. identify foci for psychiatric–mental health nursing research
6. trace the trends in inpatient and community psychiatric nursing practice
7. prepare responses to current and future challenges within target groups

The Challenges

Since 1950, significant events and attitude shifts have affected the nature and function of psychiatric and mental health nursing. Despite a close alliance, the field of psychiatric nursing and the field of mental health nursing are not identical. The specialty of mental health nursing resulted from the merger of community-based psychiatric nursing and psychiatric emphases in community health nursing.[14] For the purpose of this section of the chapter, however, the two fields will be discussed together, and events that affected only one field will be identified as such.

Social Awareness and Population Demographics

Changes in society's attitudes toward certain groups often accompany, or are followed by, changes in the demographic parameters of those groups. The 1960s were a time of great social change and of tremendous growth in the awareness of the social rights of many groups. The rights and needs of various groups were highlighted through civil action, enactment of laws protecting the rights of certain groups, and an increased awareness of the complexity of society. The affected groups include the elderly, women, families, and minority groups. The phenomena of change within these groups cannot be viewed in isolation of the whole of society; rather, we must examine change from the standpoint of both intragroup and intergroup influences.

The Elderly

The over-65 age group comprises an ever-growing proportion of society. Numbering greater than 25 million in 1982, the elderly will account for over 50 million by the year 2030.[13] One person of nine in America is over 65. This group presents new challenges to all economic and social support systems.

Scientific research and social activism challenge many commonly held assumptions about the elderly. Myths of inevitable senility, lack of sexuality, and lowered productivity among all aged persons are being dispelled. Limited economic resources, a need for specialized, not more, health services, and changes in social support systems certainly bring a new configuration to the lifestyle of the aging person. Living arrangements vary, but fewer than 5% of all persons over 65 reside in nursing homes.[26] The number of elderly persons living independently is also increasing. The economic status of the elderly spans a wide range, with the median income well below $10,000.[26] Although the remaining life span of a person at age 65 has increased steadily, women continue to outnumber men in the over-65 age group.

The mental health concerns of the aging population pose several unique challenges. Previously healthy adults may develop the need for mental health care arising from loss, the physiological changes associated with aging, or the developmental demands of aging. Chronically mentally ill persons, hospitalized during the 1950s, now reside among the geriatric population. Therefore, two related but separate specialty fields have emerged in the care of the elderly—psychogeriatrics and geropsychiatry. *Psychogeriatrics* refers to special psychiatric care for clients in the over-65 age group; *geropsychiatry* is the care of the aging psychiatric client.[22] This distinction is not artificial, because each group of elderly persons requires special understanding and demands the application of a different body of knowledge. In addition, nonclinical services, such as Eldercare and the Meals-on-Wheels programs, have emerged and indirectly meet the mental health needs of the elderly population.

The Gray Panthers movement of the 1960s addressed social prejudice and discrimination affecting the elderly. Of the several "isms" that social activists brought to the attention of the public, the Gray Panthers advocated liberation from the ill effects of agism. *Agism* is a social stereotype that prevents the elderly from achieving the fullness of living. Maggie Kuhn, herself an aging person, led the fight for full recognition of the abilities, talents, and liveliness of the older person. This process led to the enactment of laws protecting the older person from discrimination in the work place, in residences, and in health care.

The Family

Through the past 25 years, we have learned that there are many definitions of the word "family." Society at large has become more accepting of alternative family styles, although the traditional nuclear family is still desired and even revered. Alternative family styles have become increasingly common, and these families make their claim on the service and skills of mental health professionals. The 1980 census found an increasing number of single heads-of-households and families headed by a single parent. In many cases, that parent was a single woman—single by divorce, separation, widowhood, or choice. Unmarried couples living together and other group-living situations forced redefinition of what actually composes the family.

Awareness of the importance of the family in psychological development was enriched by the growth and acceptance of the family therapy movement. Family concepts were also incorporated into the treatment approaches to the individual and the group. Changes in family composition forced treatment providers to consider the special needs of the aging parent caring for a disabled child or the anguish experienced at the end of a long-term, live-in relationship.

The growth in family theory led to a reconsideration of the origins and etiology of psychopathology. Intrapsychic dynamics were not abandoned; rather, the care of the mentally ill was expanded to encompass exploration and experience of the individual's family relationships. Family assessments became an essential component of each contact with a health care provider. The changing family not only demanded a new type of treatment, but also forced a revision of the traditional modes of treatment.

The Feminist Movement

Women constitute the majority of psychiatric clients as well as of society.[11] The activism of the 1960s brought an awareness of the roles and rights of women. Many books and journals appeared that promulgated the new order of women. Women were viewed with a new understanding, as persons first, then as members of social groups and families, and finally as workers.

The special issue of women and psychotherapy deserves consideration. The women's movement has demanded new definitions of the concepts of mental health and mental illness.[10] Feminist psychology challenges traditional concepts of human development and the very nature of psychotherapy. Viewed from a feminist perspective, many of the "problems" experienced in living result from an oppressive, male-dominated society that rewards males and sanctions females.

The women's movement's cry for androgyny and equality led to the introduction of nonsexist language, a reduction in the sexual biases found in advertising, education, and entertainment, and a greater acceptance of the values of both "maleness" and "femaleness." Although the feminist movement has been accused of contributing to the demise of traditional values and of the nuclear family, it has also been credited with helping the society as a whole achieve a higher level of mental health. The failure of the ratification of the Equal Rights Amendment, however, threatens the permanence of the gains initiated by 20th-century feminists.

Minority Groups

America, supposedly the great melting pot, took a look at itself over the last few decades and discovered that very little melting had actually occurred. Many racial, sexual, and cultural groups make up this complex social group. Blacks, native Americans, orientals, and hispanics, for example, represent major cultural subgroups. The recent influx of refugees from Third World countries expands the diversity of cultural minorities in need of health care services. Each group has its own characteristic focus and special features. More important, however, different cultures define mental illness in their own terms.

The activism of the 1960s and the "me-ism" of the 1970s engendered an awareness of the danger and damage of social prejudices, as well as of the pride and power of membership in a minority. The melting envisioned by our forefathers gave way to a peculiar sense of nationalism, in which minority groups demanded civil rights and social acceptance without giving up the uniqueness of the subculture. Prejudice and exploitation continue to exist. The effect of minority awareness can be measured by legislation prohibiting discrimination and by the economic gains of some members of minority groups. Social prejudice and inequity cannot be legislated away.

Biases and stereotypes influence the practitioner's assessment and treatment of culturally different clients. Attempts have been made to devise bias-free psychological tests in order to evaluate clients' psychological status more accurately. Some argue that effective mental health treatment can only be designed and delivered by providers with cultural backgrounds similar to the client. Others believe that clinical education and supervision can ameliorate the effects of culturally biased assumptions in the treatment dyad.

Psychiatric mental health nurses have provided leadership in developing services that anticipate and respond to our country's changing demographics. Programs that target the new care needs of elders include day treatment and respite care for Alzheimer's patients. Community mental health nurses have developed alternative counseling centers that are feminist in orientation and philosophy. Nurses have been actively involved in family work for many years in the areas of direct treatment, research, and theory development.[18]

Economics and Legislation

The care of the mentally ill has long been tied to political, economic, and legislative issues. The community mental health movement of the 1960s flourished as federal commitment to the needs of the mentally ill was translated into large amounts of funding for construction of community mental health centers as alternatives to state hospitals for the mentally ill; direct services; education of mental health professionals; and research into the cause and treatment of mental illness.

Deinstitutionalization of the mentally ill became the predominant public policy in most states. The effect of this policy on the chronically mentally ill has been negative in many aspects. The quality of care envisioned by the architects of the community mental health movement has not been provided.[9] Many patients exist without proper continuity of services in a cycle of hospitalization, deinstitutionalization, homelessness, and rehospitalization.

In response to the failure of government programs, families and clients are uniting to bring about changes. The Alliance for the Mentally Ill is a fast-growing association of families of the chronically mentally ill. The members of this new organization are committed to reducing the stigma associated with mental illness. Their lobbying efforts increased federal funding for research into the biological and genetic factors associated with mental illness.

Legislative initiatives of importance to mental health clients and psychiatric mental health nurses include the schizophrenia initiative of 1987 at the National Institutes of Mental Health and the founding of the National Center for Nursing Research at the National Institutes of Health.

The Changing Reimbursement Environment

Beginning in the late 1970s, private insurers and federally related insurance agencies such as Civilian Health and Medical Program of the Uniformed Services (CHAMPUS), entered the funding arena. Reimbursement for mental health services is a mandated benefit in many states, a requirement for any private insurance carrier in those states.

The turbulent economic environment of the 1980s now threatens the economic viability of the mental health care system as it presently stands. Direct federal support of mental health services, education, and research is rapidly diminishing. Mental health care services are particularly vulnerable to changes in funding because the hoped-for private sector support may be hampered by the lingering social stigma of mental illness.

The United States spends more per capita on health care than any other country in the world.[15] In 1986, this amounted to $458 billion dollars and 10.9% of the gross national product. Concerns about the cost of health care led to changes in reimbursement for health care services. Under prospective reimbursement, hospitals receive payment based upon a predetermined standard cost per case. Although psychiatric services are currently exempt from prospective payment through Medicare, efforts to decrease the cost of health care have resulted in pressures on psychiatric and mental health services.

Some states are seeking to decrease the amount of mandated services for psychiatric clients. Other states have resisted including benefits for alcohol and substance abuse as a part of comprehensive care benefits. The average length of stay for psychiatric clients has decreased as a result of cost containment efforts. Psychiatric–mental health nurses are in key positions to provide discharge planning, community-based aftercare services, and support services to clients and their families.

Block Grants

A discussion of the economics of mental health care is not complete without an understanding of the block grant process. Traditionally, funding for community mental health center services was initiated at the federal level, with direct funding of local community mental health centers and some supplemental funding coming from the states. The Reagan administration's fiscal plan, presented in 1981 and implemented in fiscal year 1983, is based on the premise of shifting the responsibility for funding from the federal level to the state level. This change in attitude means that the state governments are now charged with the responsibility of administrating mental health services. Money from the federal government will be awarded to the states, under a system of block grants, in a lump sum to be dispensed in the manner decided upon by the state.[27]

A *block grant* is a federal allocation given to a state's government for a special purpose, such as mental health services. Each state will receive one block grant to fund all mental health and drug and alcohol abuse treatment services. The amount of money received by the state is a proportion of the monies received for similar services during prior fiscal periods. Each state then determines for itself exactly how it will use the money. The actual dollar amount of the block grant is expected to be less than the earlier allocations. It is not the administration's intention to replace or reduce state expenditures under the block grant program; rather, block grants will supplement state funds for mental health services.[24]

Other factors resulting from changes in the economy impinge on the mental health system. The number of jobs available for vocational rehabilitation has decreased, preventing optimal habilitation of many mentally ill persons. The "social drift" hypothesis questioned whether the mentally ill congregated in the lower socioeconomic classes by chance or whether persons in the lower social classes were more vulnerable to mental illness.[8] Resolution of this debate will not solve the mental health problems of the poor, who are both statistically more in need of mental health care services and least able to pay for such services. The economically disadvantaged are currently the focus of a glut of poorly designed services, many of which overlap the others, and none of which truly accomplishes what was originally envisioned by the service designer.

Mental health services today are more costly to provide than they were 25 years ago. The much needed economic parity for nurses has, in part, contributed to the rise in the costs of mental health services. The salaries of other mental health professionals have risen along with nursing salaries, prompting the phenomenon of "substitutibility" among the mental health professional groups.[22] With salaries rising and the measurable differences between professional groups declining, is it any wonder that mental health center administrators seek the most cost-effective staff member regardless of clinical discipline?

Legal Protection of Clients' Rights

The past 20 years have seen a growth in the clients' rights legislation. These laws led to the most significant restructuring of the legal environment of mental health care since the M'Naughten ruling.[29] Clients' rights legislation attempts to protect the client from undue restriction of personal safety or freedom. One of the negative effects of the client's rights legislation has been to preclude the involuntary treatment of persons who are in need of psychiatric care but who are not displaying behavior dangerous to themselves or others.

Technology

Technological developments of the past 25 years have created a world heretofore only imagined. Computers are commonplace, supplementing and, at times, substituting for human processes of decision-making, verbal communication, and discrimination. Advances in electronics now make possible the instant replay of a football game or a family therapy session. Television enables in-home education, entertainment, and public awareness of events as they happen. No part of daily living remains unaffected by technology.

These advances produce a mixed blessing of better, cheaper, faster living along with information overload, hazardous by-products of energy materials, and complex stressors. The television, which brings the excitement of a sports competition in to the home, also brings the terror of a bombing raid. Computer technology provides rapid access to massive amounts of data about individuals but also threatens the individual's right to privacy. The speed with which information is processed precludes the more gradual integration of knowledge into one's repertoire of skills and strategies. Modern persons are asked to develop stress responses to stressors newly created in the name of technological advancement.

Technology and Mental Health Care

Computer technology has affected the very nature of psychiatric care in addition to influencing the methods of delivering, charging for, and evaluating care. Computer programs simulate the interaction between the therapist and the client.[30] Recordings of client progress, pharmacotherapy protocols, and psychological evaluation can be recorded and stored in a computer data base. Computers assist mental health practitioners to reach clinical decisions regarding diagnosis and treatment.

Computer systems that conduct psychological tests and immediately score the results offer great assistance to community-based practitioners. Standard psychological tests, such as the Minnesota Multiphasic Personality Inventory or the Beck Depression Inventory, are stored in the memory bank along with the appropriate normative information. To undergo testing, the individual client sits at a computer terminal. The screen displays one question at a time to which the client is asked to respond. At the conclusion of the test the individual responses are recorded and analyzed. The therapist practitioner has immediate access to very sophisticated information to aid in diagnosis and evaluation.

The electronic media play a large role in the development of feelings and attitudes among the general public. The public perception of the complex of psychiatric players, including the nurse, the client, and the mental health system, is molded in part by the images conveyed through movies and television.[21] Television can also serve the public's need for mental health education. Special interest programs alert viewers to the signs of stress or to effective parenting strategies. In rural areas, mental health professionals can receive their continuing education through television. Television technology has invaded the therapy session with the use of videotaped sessions. Closed-circuit systems permit the taping and immediate review of clinical therapy sessions. Videotape techniques have become standard, not only in the training of neophyte therapists, but also as a means to enhance a group's or family's progress in self-awareness.

Developments in basic science research permit sophisticated laboratory screening for such disorders as depression or schizophrenia. In the dexametha-sone suppression test, for example, cortisol levels are evaluated 16 hours after the administration of oral dexamethasone. Elevated serum cortisol indicates that the expected response to dexamethasone did not occur, a phenomenon consistent with depression.[19] Laboratory screening for mental illness aids in the accurate diagnosis and prompt treatment of individuals with those disorders.

The Health Care System

Although it is difficult to isolate the health care system from its many component parts and interacting related systems, it is necessary to try to do so in order to understand trends and issues in psychiatric–mental health nursing.

General Medical Care

Advances in life support systems and in surgical techniques have saved the lives of persons who would have died less than 5 years ago. This process of aiding in survival from catastrophic illness and injuries has made options for life support and choices of health services more complex than ever. The economic factors of life support systems, coupled with the moral and legal ambiguity surrounding life support, add additional stress to the family members and significant others of the patient. Life support issues also cause stress among health care providers, as evidenced by the recent upsurge in the literature on the topic of burnout in the human service professions.

During the past 20 years, the medical environment has witnessed a growth in the understanding of the mind–body interaction. Psychophysiologists have taught that the presence of physical or emotional stress results in stress responses from both his body and his mind. There is, at present, a new (or renewed) awareness of the psychological needs of the hospitalized patient and a search for the physiological roots of mental distress. Traditional therapies, which relied only on the mind or the body as the site of intervention, have been challenged. Although the response to this challenge has not been a complete cessation of purely somatic therapies, many more therapies are currently being scrutinized.

Mental Health Care

Rising frustration with traditional health care providers led some groups of individuals to form self-help groups. Individuals sharing common problems or life situations banded together for the purpose of exchanging support, coping hints, and encouragement. At times, the outrage at the common enemy, traditional healers, provided an external impetus for cohesiveness among these groups. Self-help groups of the 1980s are not antiprofessional care providers; rather, they call on professional providers in a collaborative, consultative manner. Some self-help groups have received recognition from professional health care providers and are now viewed as reasonable adjuncts or alternatives to traditional professional care.

Community Mental Health. The community mental health care system is the fastest growing subgroup of the health care system. Three major factors influenced the inception and establishment of the community mental health system. First, the discovery of chlorpromazine and the antipsychotic medications during the 1950s enabled previously dependent clients to live outside of the hospital. Second, the 70% reduction in state hospital beds since 1955 placed a demand on communities to provide shelter and services for chronically disturbed clients.[28] Third, the commitment of the federal government to the care of the mentally ill during the Kennedy and Johnson administrations provided funding for the development and staffing of community mental health centers. The legacy of the community mental health movement of the past 25 years is an awareness of the tremendous mental health needs of communities and the lack of an organized, effective method for meeting the needs.

The community mental health center movement also brought about an awareness of the factors within the community that influence the development and treatment of mental illness. The original design of 1500 mental health centers scattered throughout the country was never realized; nonetheless, the consciousness-raising caused by this movement will have impact for years. The private-profit and not-for-profit sectors responded to the need for community-based treatment facilities with the development of isolated treatment centers located within the community. The network of treatment and research centers envisioned by community mental health planners never materialized, however, in part, because of the lack of clear-cut evaluation standards and processes.[23]

Community-based psychiatric treatment has not replaced inpatient care of the mentally ill. Now the majority of all admissions to public mental hospitals are readmissions. The evidence suggests that the rate of readmissions is far higher than would be expected if alternative forms of care were actually available.[1]

Gaps in Understanding. This section discussing the challenges to psychiatric–mental health nursing care would not be complete without an examination of the trends that did *not* occur. No new forms of somatic therapy have been evaluated and proven effective for such pervasive disorders as anxiety and depression; instead, a resurgence of older, somatic therapies is occurring. Science has given us greater understanding of what happens neurochemically in the presence of illness, yet we still do not know why one person develops schizophrenia and another develops an ulcer. Research tells us that dyadic relationships make people better, yet we know little how the dyad works. It is left to the future practitioners of psychiatric–mental health nursing not only to react to the demands of society, but to act to ensure the mental health of society.

The Responses

Psychiatric and mental health nurses are called upon to meet many challenges arising from population changes, an unstable economy, patients' rights legislation, developments in technology, and changes in the way health care is delivered. The process of meeting challenges can occur actively (that is, in a planned, well-designed manner based on an assessment of the needs of society and of available resources) or reactively (that is, in reaction to the challenges presented from health care consumers, colleagues, and employers). An active response to change demands vigilance and creativity; a reactive response to a challenge requires rapid mobilization of resources and adaptability. Psychiatric–mental health nursing's responses to challenges can be seen by examining four areas of change—changes in care providers, changes in roles in practice settings, changes in the activity of psychiatric–mental health nurses, and changes in the focus of care. Before examining the responses to challenges, let us examine the supporting guides for change.

Guides for Change

Within established professions, the direction for change and the needs for meeting the challenges of the future arise from within the profession. As the nursing profession grows and becomes more fully established as a profession, nurses assume greater responsibility for self-direction. The development of nursing as a self-directed profession can be traced through the American Nurses' Association's publication of four documents:

1. The Statement on Psychiatric and Mental Health Nursing Practice (1967, revised 1976)
2. The Standards of Practice of Psychiatric and Mental Health Nursing Practice (1973, revised 1982)

3. The Code for Nurses with Interpretive Statements (1976)
4. Nursing: A Social Policy Statement (1980)[3,5,6,7]

These documents present to the public a definition of nursing practice in psychiatric–mental health care, a clarification of the various roles of nursing personnel, and the established standards of nursing practice. Through the use of these documents, nurses promulgate their functions, and colleagues and consumers learn what can be achieved through nursing care.

We, as psychiatric–mental health nurses, constitute one special group among the 1.5 million nurses in the United States. We share professional colleagueship with all nurses, thereby maintaining a responsibility for intraprofessional collaboration and service. We hold claim to a specialized body of knowledge within nursing practice and yet acknowledge that psychiatric–mental health nursing concepts permeate the whole of nursing practice. Psychiatric–mental health nurses also share a professional peership with other disciplines within the mental health complex, including social workers, psychologists, physicians, and adjunctive therapists. Although our practice is derived from many of the applied human sciences, our mandate for practice rests within the nursing profession. Therefore, we develop and draw from the documents of professional nursing to guide our practice and our response to the challenges.

Definition of Psychiatric–Mental Health Nursing

The Statement on Psychiatric and Mental Health Nursing Practice defines psychiatric nursing as follows:

> . . . a specialized area of nursing practice employing theories of human behavior as its science and purposeful use of self as its art.[7]

Nursing practice in psychiatric–mental health care shares many functions with other disciplines, yet holds several unique features, notably a biopsychosocial approach to client and community and the systematic use of the nursing process. The Statement serves to interpret psychiatric nursing practice to interested others within the mental health field. In addition to an explanation of nursing, critical variables such as subspecialization and the scope of practice are defined. Nursing roles in psychiatric and mental health care include direct care functions, such as psychotherapy, provision of the therapeutic milieu, and community action, and indirect care functions, such as education, administration, and research.

Standards of Psychiatric–Mental Health Nursing

The Standards of Psychiatric and Mental Health Nursing Practice define the minimally acceptable practices of psychiatric and mental health nurses. Subsequent to the development of the Statement on Psychiatric and Mental Health Nursing, the practice division established criteria describing psychiatric and mental health nursing practice. These criteria serve as guides denoting the nature of activities that nurses are prepared to implement competently. Standards serve both to direct professional activities and to evaluate the quality of professional care. Self-direction and professional accountability contribute to a profession's ability to meet the challenges of the present and of the future. Many agencies have incorporated the Standards of Practice into the job descriptions or evaluation criteria for practicing nurses. Nurses in private practice use the standards as guides defining the nature and scope of their practice. The standards have also been entered in legal testimony as evidence of the expected professional practice of a nurse.

Code of Ethics for Nursing

The Code of Ethics for Nursing defines ethical conduct for practicing nurses in all clinical areas, not only for psychiatric–mental health nurses. The changes and challenges that affect target populations, and therefore the nature of psychiatric and mental health nursing practice, pose dilemmas for every practicing nurse. Issues of patient confidentiality, protection of society, and patients' right to treatment confront the nurse in daily practice. The Code neither supplants individual decision-making nor provides universally applicable answers to the nurse's ethical dilemma. Rather, the Code serves as a decision-making guide concerning ethical practice.

The Social Policy Statement

A landmark document titled Nursing: A Social Policy Statement emerged in 1980, slightly more than 100 years after the first training school for nurses was organized. This document delineates the nature and scope of nursing practice and serves all nurses as "an affirmation of nursing's social responsibility."[5] Although it does not replace any of the documents noted earlier, the Social Policy Statement renews and organizes the commitment of nursing to the public society it serves. Based on the premise that a social contract forms the legal right to practice, the statement defines nursing practice issues, specialization, articulation with other disciplines, and the role of theory within the social environment of nursing.

Nursing: A Social Policy Statement has particular significance for psychiatric and mental health nurses. Several leaders within psychiatric nursing contributed to the development of this document. The very nature of psychiatric and mental health nursing practice is social, involving a dyadic encounter between nurse and client.[14] The proliferation of mental health professionals within the past 25 years demands a delineation of the borders, boundaries, and dimensions of psychiatric–mental health nursing. Nursing: A Social Policy Statement provides a professional mandate for the establishment of these delineations by validating the right of self-determination among the various nursing specialty groups. It also legitimizes many of the activities already carried out by psychiatric and mental health nurses. Graduate education, certification at the generalist and the specialist levels, and clinical research have been guided by the leadership of psychiatric and mental health nurses.

Other Guides

Other guides for nursing practice are found in legislation, in agency policy, and within the nurse–client relationship. Nurse practice acts define the legal nature of nursing practice and have undergone major revisions over the past 25 years. The revisions of the laws speak more directly to expanded nursing practice in all areas, and not specifically to psychiatric–mental health nursing practice. Under the nurse practice acts of most states, however, psychiatric–mental health nurses find legal support for independent nursing functions and independent nursing practice. Agency policy, under the aegis of state and federal laws, establishes the parameters of practice within a given institution. Within the client care dyad, the nurse finds the specific directions for individualizing practice. The psychiatric–mental health nurse then draws from the professional group, the employing agency, and the client situation to formulate practice. The nurse's internalization of theory, understanding of behavioral dynamics, and self-awareness complete the composite of guides required for professional practice and the ability to meet the challenges posed by society.

The Care Providers

Twenty-Five Years Ago

Psychiatric nurses today make up a very different configuration than those of 25 years ago. As a group, we are older than other nurses, better educated—that is, with a greater proportion of master's-prepared nurses among our ranks—and more varied in our practice settings. The psychiatric nurse of 1957 grappled with the issues of moving the chronic mentally ill person out to the community and how to manage a client with mania without the use of the medication lithium carbonate. Peplau's work on anxiety and psychiatric nursing and Maxwell Jones's therapeutic milieu were both about 5 years old. Electroconvulsive therapy was the treatment of choice for depression, and sedation was a treatment for any type of emotional disorder. Medical-surgical concepts applied in the psychiatric setting served most nurses well, and the only nurse who worked in the community was the local public health nurse. Independent practice of nurses was almost unheard of, and the effect of economics on nursing practice was negligible.

Psychiatric–Mental Health Nursing in the 80s

The 1980s are witnessing many changes in the education and practice of psychiatric and mental health nurses. The growth of the profession provided the necessary intraprofessional support needed to meet the challenges of changing populations, unstable economics, technological advancements, the demands of a changing health care environment, and nurses' own health problems (see Chart 47-1, "Autobiography of a Recovering Alcoholic Nurse"). The psychiatric–mental health nursing response can be seen in the changes in the education, practice roles, and practice settings of psychiatric nurses.

Basic Education. The integrated curriculum stands as education's response to the challenge of abandoning the mind–body dichotomy of medical care. Although many definitions of the integrated curriculum exist, the concept essentially refers to the unification of nursing concepts that transcend isolated clinical areas. In an integrated curriculum, for example, students do not take a separate course in the nursing care of patients with selected medical problems. Interpersonal nursing concepts form the core of nursing practice, the nurse–client relationship. Accordingly, concepts traditionally reserved for the psychiatric nursing course, such as anxiety, stress management, and depression, are addressed throughout the nursing curriculum. The integrated curriculum has recently come under attack by nursing practice and educational leaders.[16, 20] Although the integrated curriculum enhanced the psychosocial skills of all nurses, the cost may have caused a decline in the number of nurses capable of, and interested in, entering psychiatric nursing care.

Advanced Education. The federal government has fostered the development of psychiatric–mental health nursing at the bachelor's and master's levels of nursing education. The federal government's support of community mental health centers, following the deinstitutionalization process, demanded

CHART 47-1

Autobiography of a Recovering Alcoholic Nurse

Doris Leffler, R.N.C., C.A.C.
Senior Nurse
Coordinator, Alcoholism Recovery Program
Friends Hospital
Philadelphia, Pennsylvania

I was born in New York City and raised as an only child, although I have a brother who is 15 years older. My environment, although stimulating, was generally hectic and often chaotic. I was shy, self-conscious and insecure. My father was a quiet, outwardly easy-going man and rarely demonstrative in his feelings; my mother, on the other hand, was outgoing, assertive, and often capricious.

I attended private school and was an average student. Upon graduation, I was accepted, on a probationary basis due to my grades, into a 3-year diploma nursing program at a New York city hospital. Because this was what I had wanted most in my life, I worked exceptionally hard; within the 6-month probationary period, I received my cap.

Going to class and working on the hospital ward was a very hectic, demanding, and anxiety-provoking schedule. When it became difficult to sleep, Seconals (secobarbitol) became my friend. During my third year of nursing school, I became acquainted with amphetamines while doing my psychiatric affiliation at a state hospital. I also found another friend in alcohol. Alcohol give me a warm, comfortable feeling, filled the void of emptiness, conquered all my fears and insecurities, and allowed me to function.

My life seemed perfect to colleagues and friends. I had a husband and three healthy children. No one at home or elsewhere knew I was frightened, lonely, and empty, drinking every evening, taking tranquilizers throughout the day and sleeping pills at night.

In 1972, I was employed as a psychiatric nurse in a 500-bed general hospital located in a mid-sized northeastern suburb. It was there that I met Helen H., another psychiatric nurse. I was very much in awe of Helen when we first met; she was vibrant, articulate, and one of the best nurses I had known. More than anyone else, she taught me the techniques of nursing. Though she was 20 years my senior, Helen and I became good friends.

Helen and I were working buddies and drinking buddies, joking about who drank more and which one of us had a problem with alcohol. And yet I had a fear of Helen; when she drank she became hostile and nasty. Even with our joking, I knew Helen drank too much and I knew she was sick, perhaps alcoholic. If this were true of her, I speculated, was it also true of me? In January 1975, Helen committed suicide, alone in her car with a drink in her hand.

The hospital opened an alcoholism recovery unit shortly afterward and the coordinator of the program, Helen P., a registered nurse and a recovering alcoholic, not only became my friend but also was instrumental in educating me about the disease of alcoholism.

HP, as I later referred to her, frequently visited the psychiatric unit seeking patients, as this was the unit that most commonly admitted alcoholics and drug users. HP spent much of her time talking with me, querying me about my patients and myself. She knew how to ask questions and how to share of herself, never accusing or belittling, but rather comparing feelings with compassion and dignity. I knew she understood me, and over the months, I began to trust her more and more and to face some of my fears. If HP was afflicted with the disease of alcoholism then I, too, must be an alcoholic.

Denial is the foremost symptom of the disease of alcoholism and nurses have massive denial. They are taught how to be caretakers, how to heal others but not themselves. More aware of the disease and its symptoms, I made a conscious decision to look at myself.

As a recovering alcoholic for several years, I have experienced considerable behavioral changes. I have learned to deal with life on life's terms, I have learned that feelings do not have to consume me, that it's all right to be imperfect, and, in fact, that to be human is to be imperfect. I have learned to share my feelings—to follow the principles of life we use in dealing with our patients.

While attending support groups—the only way I have found to maintain continued sobriety—I realized that recovering nurses did not share their professional problems. In June 1982, a small group of recovering nurses in Philadelphia formed a nurses' support group. This group was a safe haven to verbalize feelings of inadequacies, fears, and concerns about working with addictive drugs while continuing to practice safely. The number of active members grew steadily. Some relapsed, but the group, without being judgmental, continued supporting them with treatment.

This group, the Philadelphia Recovering Nurses Association (PRNA), is very active and involved in the community. By sharing our experience, strength, hope, and love with each other, by living one day at a time without an addictive substance, the recovering members now give lectures and seminars at hospitals and schools of nursing and help with employee assistance programs. The knowledge, education, and experience they bring to these facilities helps develop better relations in the professional field among management, employee, and student.

Through the support of PRNA, nurses were encouraged to share their addiction problems with their supervisors and peers. Although they were able to maintain abstinence from alcohol and drugs for a while, many still had difficulty at work. I believed if their supervisors were educated about the disease of addiction, nurses would have a better chance of recovering and maintaining their jobs. Hospital administrators became interested and willing to learn more about the disease.

A protocol was instituted in a few major hospitals. A nurse found to be diverting drugs or manifesting signs of drug use, such as personality changes, social changes, mental status changes, and a general job shrinkage, is confronted by two people; one, if possible, is a recovering person. The nurse is asked to surrender his or her license to the hospital and/or to an appropriate consultant to the state or therapist. If the nurse is willing to do this, a consultation is set up with a recovering nurse capable of recommending treatment. To the frightened, impaired nurse, willing to do almost anything, treatment is usually a welcome encounter. A medical leave is granted and the nurse's job is held open. If possible, the nurse meets with the hospital and nurse representatives prior to discharge from a rehabilitation center. In that meeting, a back-to-work contract, outlining the commitments of both the nurse and hospital, is agreed upon. As a result of support groups and the education of hospital personnel, recovering nurses are returning to their profession.

Statistics indicate that 15% to 20% of nurses practicing today have a substance abuse problem; many are in a program of recovery. They have learned not to idealize their profession, but to accept nursing as it is. By learning to care for themselves, they can deliver quality patient care, sharing, if warranted, their experience of this devastating disease. It has also been found that recovery lessens "burnout" and absenteeism, making it cost-saving to the hospital. The recovering nurse, dealing with her disease, returns to the profession strengthened and capable of performing an excellent job.

For nursing to be truly a caring profession, nurses must learn to care for their own in the struggle with the devastating disease of addiction. Increased awareness of addiction in the health professions and renewed education about substance abuse in general are positive trends. We are finally beginning to recognize this illness as being treatable—and if we treat ourselves, we can more effectively treat others.

---

practitioners who were skilled in the care of the mentally ill in the community. Grants available through the Nurse Training Acts of the 1960s and 1970s and through the National Institute of Mental Health (NIMH) funded master's level nursing education. As late as 1980, NIMH traineeships provided tuition and stipend subsidy for Master of Science in Nursing candidates, in significantly greater amounts than were available to other nursing specialties. Current federal cutbacks, however, portend the end of such funding. Funding for graduate study is in short supply, but programs addressing special needs of the elderly or the chronically mentally ill are most likely to be successful in obtaining funds.

Graduate education flourished under the period of federal funding from 1964 to 1980. In response to the need for clinical practitioners, consultants, researchers, and educators, special programs developed. Programs addressed such roles as clinical nurse administrator (University of Pennsylvania), psychiatric liaison nurse (Yale University), clinical nurse practitioner (Rutgers University), and clinical nurse specialist (University of Wisconsin). Although the need for such programs remains strong, recent reductions in the federal funding available for student subsidy and program development threaten both the viability of existing programs and the inception of any new programs.

Advanced preparation for the psychiatric–mental health nurse begins with the master's degree. Post-master's training options include special institutes, continuing education, and doctoral study. Special institutes focus on the development of a particular set of skills and therapeutic technique, such as family therapy. Continuing education emphasizes incidental knowledge or skill acquisition. Through doctoral study, nurses prepare for future roles as expert practitioners, clinical researchers, administrators, or nurse scientists.

Changes in Roles in the Practice Setting.
The most obvious evidence of psychiatric–mental health nursing's response to social challenges can be seen in the practice setting. Although psychiatric nurses constitute less than 5% of the entire active nursing workforce, their practice efforts permeate every type of health care setting possible.[3] Within each of these settings, nurses fulfill many roles, including staff nurse, clinical nurse specialist, liaison, consultant, administrator, and psychotherapist.

Staff Nurse.　Inpatient psychiatric nursing presently receives renewed interest. During the heyday of the community mental health movement, some suggested that the need for inpatient care was on the decline, a fact that most psychiatric staff nurses would quickly dispute. The nature of inpatient psychiatric care has changed over the past 25 years, with a greater focus on the nurses' role in the development of the milieu, the application of the nursing process to aid clients in maintaining activities of daily living, and in the provision of leadership for formal and informal client therapeutic groups. The number of colleagues of the staff nurse has increased, especially the number of nonphysician, mental health professionals.[28]

The role of the staff nurse in psychiatric inpatient facilities is multidimensional. Primary nursing and the decrease in numbers of ancillary staff have provided new opportunities for nurses. Peplau stated that psychiatric nurses did not need to bring the patient to the therapy or the therapy to the patient because *nurses are the therapy.*[25] Nurses are the therapy in the psychiatric inpatient milieu, group therapy, and family work.

Psychiatric nurses are also involved in formulating and testing nursing diagnoses in conjunction with the North American Nursing Diagnosis Association (NANDA).

Clinical Nurse Specialist.　The advent of the clinical nurse specialist in psychiatric–mental health nursing redefined many nursing roles in both the community and inpatient settings. The activities of the clinical nurse specialist vary from educational to therapeutic to consultative in nature, and are many times defined by the agency and the nurse's personality and role interests.

Clinical nurse specialists are potentially more valuable than ever in the current cost containment environment. Their expert skills can facilitate shorter lengths of stay and sophisticated interventions with patients. The clinical nurse specialist role is theoretically sound, but little research has been conducted to measure its cost effectiveness.

Psychiatric Liaison Nurse.　The liaison nurse serves patients in a general hospital setting with select psychosocial needs. Skills of consultation, nursing process, and brief psychotherapy are essential to a full actualization of the role of the psychiatric liaison nurse.[27] The client of the liaison nurse may be a patient, a family member, or a staff member. Initially, the liaison nurse faced many battles to secure her place on the hospital staff; presently, most large hospitals have a psychiatric liaison nurse, or at least a person fulfilling part of the duties of the liaison nurse. The unit-based psychiatric–mental health clinical nurse specialist may assume liaison responsibilities outside the psychiatric unit. The term *liaison* specifically refers to the mental health treatment, consultation, and educational functions in a nonpsychiatric environment.

Nurse as Psychotherapist.　The growth of master's and doctorally prepared psychiatric–mental health nurses has produced many nurse psychotherapists. Some nurse psychotherapists practice independently; others practice in group practices or in community mental health centers. Increases in the number of nurse psychotherapists forced recognition of two problems never before faced by psychiatric–mental health nurses—reimbursement for services and certification for practice. During the 1970s, some private and one government agency began reimbursing nurses directly for mental health services provided independently of a physician. This achievement meant that consumers now had a viable alternative to physician-directed mental health care. Desire for reimbursement required that nurses could certify their competency for independent practice. Not only did insurance companies demand such verification, but health care consumers also began inquiring about the credentials of the providers.

Establishing and verifying the credentials of professionals is a process managed internally by the profession. The American Nurses' Association certifies two levels of psychiatric–mental health nurses— the generalist, prepared at the bachelor's level, and the specialist, prepared at the master's level. This credential signifies to the profession, to colleagues in other professions, and to consumers that the holder demonstrated the standards and competency to practice at the identified level.

Nurses in independent practice use a variety of psychotherapeutic models—psychoanalytic, Christian healing, systems, and the like (see Chart 47-2, "The Integration of Spirituality with Psychotherapy"). No theory of psychiatric–mental health nursing exists

CHART 47-2

The Integration of Spirituality with Psychotherapy

Margaret T. Crepeau, R.N., Ph.D.
Marquette University College of Nursing
Milwaukee, Wisconsin

Among the new trends in psychiatric nursing, from primal scream to computers, it is a gift to be able to include the integration of a faith in God, or spirituality, and psychotherapy. The results are so rich, so rewarding, that it is a joy to share them, and to distinguish the elements in Christian psychotherapy from processes and strategies in traditional therapies.

On the surface, Christian psychotherapy doesn't appear very different from any other form of competent verbal therapy. But at its heart is the belief that the God who forgives, heals, and frees His broken people is an active participant in every therapy session. The differences are perhaps in content or interpretation of issues, and usually in taking the last few minutes of a session to anoint and pray with the client. These unique foci in content are as follows:

1. Emphasis on forgiveness of self and others as a key to healing
2. Getting in touch with, and letting go of, painful memories by seeing these episodes with the compassionate eyes of Christ
3. A gentle, but responsible, acknowledgement of one's own sins and how these affect a hurting life
4. Being open to the reality of grace through healing prayer

The emphasis on forgiveness in integrating spirituality with psychotherapy is a crucial one. In traditional psychotherapy, the endpoint of treatment has often been simply to get in touch with one's anger, resentment, and bitterness toward those who have been hurtful and express those feelings in an "appropriate way." Until one has really gone back and forgiven the people who have been responsible for hurts, however, it seems the anger, resentment, and bitterness do not go away.

Beginning with MacNutt's classic book, *Healing*, therapists who are working with clients toward deep inner healing recognize the power and intense freedom that accompany forgiveness.[2] Forgiveness, above all, needs to begin with self. Many can find it in their hearts to forgive others, but they somehow cling to the idea that they, themselves, are not forgivable. These destructive patterns of self-hatred, which are written out of the scripts of perfectionism, legalism, moralism, unhealthy guilt, and projecting to God a punishing image, are gently and brilliantly dealt with in Brennan Manning's *A Stranger to Self-Hatred*.[3] All healing is centered on forgiveness of self and others.

The Linns' Healing of Memories portrays the process through which clients allow the Lord to reveal those conscious and hidden memories through which He desires to heal the brokenhearted.[1] The idea is made real that out of painful experiences have also come gifts and strengths that otherwise would not have been developed. The techniques of imaging and visualizing are used, but with the added picture of Christ in each scene. The examples can be dramatic, as in the case of a young woman who had had many unhappy affairs and was locked in a vicious cycle of self-hatred and depression. A long-repressed memory surfaced of her coming into the house at the age of 16, after a date and some very innocent kissing, and her father thundering at her from the second-floor stairway, "You're a whore!" The blatant falseness of this was superseded by a lethal blow to her spirit in which she believed she was unclean and unable to love. As she went back in time and understood the dynamics that had contributed to her father saying such a thing, and forgave him and herself, she quickly made progress toward valuing herself and rediscovering a joy and purity in herself that truly changed her life. The healing of memories is often a radical turning point in the lives of people who have too long believed that nothing or no one could help them.

The acknowledgement of one's own sins and the consequences of sin in life is seemingly difficult in an age and a society that denies, for the most part, the existence of sin. (This is suggested eloquently in Menninger's *Whatever Became of Sin?*[4]) What is often forgotten or distorted is that Freud himself believed men are basically responsible for the choices they make and, therefore, for the way in which they attempt to alleviate their inner loneliness and pain. In practice, it is astounding that, once clients are freed from unhealthy guilt, there is a real willingness and relief to accept responsibility for patterns of pride, rebellion, arrogance, unforgiveness, impurity, and other subtle, and not so subtle, sins that have kept them for years in prisons of blaming others, clinging to hurt

(Continues on p. 900)

and sickness, and, in general, choosing to be a "poor me" victim.

A recent example of this blaming pattern is of a young woman who came to therapy with complaints of scrupulosity because of past involvement with the occult. She held a self-righteous contempt for her husband because of his violence toward her and their son in the early years of the marriage. As the husband joined her in the sessions, it became clear that her only method of communicating with her husband was through constant criticism, castrating judgments, and derogatory statements. Once she could stop seeing her husband only as the "bad" one, and begin to see an element of her own verbal violence in interactions, they were together able to ask each other's forgiveness and explore tenderness and support of one another that they hadn't dreamed was possible.

The healing prayer that accompanies each session is as varied as the myriad stories that accompany each person into therapy. Usually, it is a gentle lifting of all the elements of that session into the heart of God for transformation into light, freedom, and forgiveness. Barbara Shlemon's *Healing the Hidden Self* is a beautiful example of a type of prayer through all the developmental stages from conception to adulthood.[6] Leanne Payne's *The Broken Image* describes a very deep type of prayer used with persons with problems with sexual identity.[5] As the Spirit moves each therapist, so develops the prayer. It is acknowledged that some people prefer to be in therapy for many months without the dimension of prayer because they do not feel ready for it.

In whatever way the integration of spirituality and psychotherapy develops, it remains true today, as in ancient times, that the body, mind, and spirit are one, and the Lord God of all creation is healing His people in new and extraordinary ways. Nurses, along with other health professionals who are committed to bringing their gifts of faith to their healing ministries, have long been conscious of the unique broad knowledge base that nursing has as its foundation. Nurses in many areas are also aware that only lip service has been given, in many instances, to the concept of "total patient care." What has been missing is the hunger of the spirit to be fed and healed. Christian psychotherapy is one such avenue for psychiatric–mental health nurses to feed the hungry, give sight to the blind, and heal the broken.

References

1. Linn M, Linn D: Healing of Memories. New York, Paulist Press, 1974
2. MacNutt F: Healing. Notre Dame, IN, Ave Maria Press, 1974
3. Manning B: A Stranger to Self-Hatred. Denville, NJ, Dimension Books, 1982
4. Menninger K: Whatever Became of Sin? New York, Hawthorne Books, 1975
5. Payne L: The Broken Image. Westchester, IL, Cornerstone Books, 1981
6. Shlemon B: Healing the Hidden Self. Notre Dame, IN, Ave Maria Press, 1982

now; this lack of current theory stands as a challenge to the independent nurse practitioners of the future.[16]

Nurse Leader. Within facilities devoted to psychiatric care, nurses hold management positions. Rarely, however, are psychiatric–mental health nurses found in nursing leadership positions in general hospitals. Although mental health nurses in clinics may hold positions of leadership in nursing departments, very few nurses serve as clinic administrators.

The leadership roles of the psychiatric–mental health nurse are not limited to either inpatient or community settings. Psychiatric–mental health nurses hold such leadership positions as academic deans, directors of state nurses' associations, and in one case, director of a center for nursing research. Psychiatric–mental health nurses also possess and encourage a professional alliance that crosses disciplinary boundaries, and they frequently hold influential positions within interdisciplinary groups.

Activities

Issues Influencing Activities

The practice of psychiatric–mental health nursing draws heavily from developments in related fields. Growth in family theory helped broaden the understanding of family dynamics in the care of the mentally disturbed. Selected trends now indicate a need for psychiatric–mental health nurses to integrate more fully the care of the chronically mentally ill person. Economic instability and fiscal restrictions decrease the likelihood of job training and remotivation activity for clients. Fewer persons will be eligible for insurance coverage, while, at the same time, the economy threatens to increase the incidence and prevalence of stress-related illnesses. The rise in community-based treatment and the shortened hospital stay point to the need for a greater focus on daily living skills. Traditional psychotherapy has yet to either prove its effectiveness or reduce its cost in the care of the mentally ill. The future focus of psychiatric–mental health nursing care must be directed to finding more cost-effective ways of delivering services that will enable persons with emotional disorders to maintain daily independent lives that are satisfying and fulfilling.

Legal Issues. Client's rights legislation of the 1970s brought into focus a crying need—that of the client's right to choose and freedom to select care providers, treatment options, and other medical services. Throughout the country, new statutes were enacted guaranteeing basic rights to the mentally ill. No longer could treatment and restrictive confinement be induced at the request of the family.

The client's rights legislation has had two major consequences. Clients are entitled by law to comprehensive assessment and treatment in a timely fashion. Emergency court-ordered treatment for the mentally ill came under strict guidelines. The burden of proof of a person's mental incapacity rested with those initiating a treatment request.

Client's rights legislation, however, extends far beyond emergency court-ordered treatment. Informed consent agreements now detail the outcomes of treatment, anticipated therapies, and specific criteria for the use of chemical, physical, or environmental restraints. Treatment plans, progress, and evaluation must be discussed with the client.

Advocates and Gatekeepers

The nurse serves as the client's advocate when she actively pursues treatment and services that are in the best interest of the client. This advocacy occurs in several ways. Teaching a client about treatment options enables him to make informed decisions about the treatment situation. In multidisciplinary conferences, nurses coordinate the skills of the mental health team or report to the team about the client's status. Perhaps the most essential act of advocacy occurs when the nurse helps the client enter and navigate the mental health treatment maze.

Community mental health introduced the concept of the "gatekeeper." Gatekeepers are persons who, by their positions or abilities, facilitate or control the movement of other persons in or out of the mental health system. All nurses, by the nature of their preparation in mental health concepts, can function as gatekeepers. The permeable boundaries of the mental health system are known to health professionals. Nurses can aid others in defining and entering these boundaries.

Despite the much-needed benefits brought on by the client's rights legislation, these laws can work to the disadvantage of the individual in need of care. Sometimes the person who is most in need of treatment cannot be helped because he refuses treatment

voluntarily and is not commitable under the existing legislation. The paranoid person, or the elderly recluse, may not demonstrate behavior that is potentially harmful to self or others, and would therefore not qualify for court-ordered treatment. It becomes the nurse's role, when such a person is encountered, to help the person recognize the need for treatment. In the absence of treatment, the nurse may provide assistance and guidance to family members in helping them understand and cope with the disturbed family member.

Clinical Activities

The set of activities of the psychiatric–mental health nurse within the dyadic relationship has emerged as viable and essential over the past 25 years. The nurse uses the skills of the dyadic relationship to aid individuals, groups, and families in achieving effective living. The nurse participates in the care of the client receiving somatic therapies. Education, research, and leadership activities complete the set of activities of the psychiatric–mental health nurse. These activities are defined in the Standards of Psychiatric and Mental Health Nursing.

Both the nature of the activities and the proportion of time spent in each activity is now changing. Milieu development in an inpatient setting remains a critical function. Medication administration is changing to include a greater emphasis on client participation and client education. The dyadic relationship remains the core arena for psychiatric–mental health nursing practice.

The cry has gone out for research that would validate the effectiveness and value of the dyadic relationship. Although nurses have studied the therapeutic dyad from a process framework—that is, focusing on personal growth, self-awareness, and so forth—they have not examined the range of therapeutic effectiveness of dyads. Nurses seem to place a higher value on therapy than on counseling in relation to activities of daily living. Therapy is valuable, certainly, but nurses may be missing the major contribution of psychiatric–mental health nursing—encountering a person in a corrective emotional experience.

Cost-Effective Care

Economic constraints, both in the practice setting and in education, have forced psychiatric–mental health nurses to develop a sense of cost-effectiveness about their care. Nurses are now questioning how much it costs to provide emotional support, to reduce anxiety, to teach problem-solving, and to formulate a nursing care plan. This awareness of the cost of client care is healthy; gone are the days of expansiveness in treatment inspired by the federal allocations of the 1960s and 1970s. Cost containment and cost-effectiveness of services are essential to the future availability of services. To preserve the gains brought about by the community mental health movement, we require an accountable, more cost-wise group of practitioners.

Focus of Care

The net effect of changes in social awareness and population demographics has been a redefinition of the target populations served by the mental health systems. Target populations are the selected groups that will be the recipients of mental health services. Traditional target populations include youth (through primary prevention activities), the elderly, and those having identified mental disorders. The identification of additional target populations led not only to the design of new services for the specific group, but also to an increased vigilance in case finding and to alternative forms of treatment.

Target Group: Women

Social awareness of women's issues brought to light the myriad of subgroups of women who need special services. Victims of sexual assault, battered women, and women in transition are some of the newly defined target groups. Mental health services are provided in community-based shelters in consultation with police and through special groups in the workplace. Inpatient therapies for depressed women, for example, now include action-oriented foci, such as assertiveness training and preparation for return to the workplace. Recent theoretical and research advances in women's studies that identify differences in men and women's moral reasoning development and ways of knowing should be recognized by mental health professionals.[12, 17]

Target Group: The Elderly

The growing number of well and ill elderly persons demands a specialized response. Geropsychiatric service units in the hospital and in the community offer care for the complex needs of the aged mentally ill. Psychogeriatric services address the psychiatric needs of the elderly in the areas of loss, organic dysfunctions, and other health problems and concerns. Care of the older person requires collaboration of nurses with many other health care professionals.

Target Group: Criminals

Of the four major resolutions approved during the International Congress of Nurses (ICN) in 1981, two dealt specifically with mental health nursing issues.[2] In response to the worldwide increase of substance abuse, crime, suicide, and other stress-related disorders, ICN publicly acknowledged a commitment to the instruction and practice of preventive mental health care. The second resolution defined the nurse's role in the care of criminals. The decline in the availability and access to the mental health system will spill over into a greater demand for services from the criminal justice system—not because the mentally disturbed are potential criminals, but because individuals who need mental health care and cannot get it become desperate. Referrals from the criminal justice system will be more difficult to meet, thereby further taxing the health care providers already serving this population.

Target Group: The Mentally Retarded

Federal cutbacks and court rulings adjudicating the least restrictive treatment setting for the disabled will create a demand for community-based nursing services for disabled persons. Nursing is ill-prepared for this demand at present. Most psychiatric and mental health nursing curricula do not address the issue of mental retardation. The courts and funding regulations stipulate the necessity of providing nursing care in community-based treatment settings, but nursing will need to move quickly to meet this demand in the care of the mentally retarded.

Target Group: Youth

Although the birth rate is declining, the number of persons under age 24 is higher than ever. Mental health activities directed toward youth have usually focused on the primary and secondary levels of prevention. Economics currently threaten both the viability of most primary prevention activities and secondary activities that involve screening for emotional disorders. Subgroups among adolescents that require specialized services include suicidal adolescents, psychotic adolescents, and adolescents with behavioral disorders. Funding will be most available for prevention activities within existing structures, such as through the schools.

Target Group: The Chronically Mentally Disturbed

The proportion of chronically mentally ill, as defined by the number of readmissions for hospitalization or the duration of treatment, is increasing at an accelerated rate.[23]

The chronically mentally disturbed pose special challenges for the psychiatric–mental health nurse because of the complexity of their needs and the difficulty of providing services. In the face of economic cutbacks, many former conceptions of the right to treatment and the potentially curable disorders must be modified. The chronically mentally ill populations of most large cities are the poorest, the most in need of service. Services need to be directed to both the disturbed person and his social support group. Because many of the chronically mentally ill lack supportive networks, attention must be paid to developing supports through nontraditional methods.

Summary

This chapter has explored some of the significant challenges to the mental health care of society. These challenges demand the delivery of a greater amount and a greater variety of mental health services under a shrinking funding source. The major foci of the chapter include the following points:

1. Nursing's response to the challenges to mental health care has been to provide a variety of practitioners who are capable of serving clients in an inpatient or community setting.
2. Another significant nursing response to this challenge is to integrate psychiatric–mental health nursing concepts into the generic preparation of all nurses.
3. Psychiatric–mental health nurses assume leadership and practice roles in all types of health care delivery systems.
4. Presently, the most significant threat to the psychiatric–mental health nursing practice is one shared by all mental health practitioners—economic destruction.
5. Despite economic disasters and the high cost of service, mental health professionals must not lose their awareness of the pain and suffering caused by mental disorders, and they must use the available political, social, and professional avenues to alleviate that suffering.[23]
6. The demand for skill in mental health consultation will increase.
7. The need for psychiatric nurses who specialize in the care of the chronically mentally disturbed and mentally disturbed youths will continue to out-distance the number of nurses prepared in these areas.
8. Psychiatric–mental health nurses will develop new funding sources to maintain and promote the graduate educational programs necessary to carry out nursing research.

References

1. Aiken L: Unmet Needs of the Chronically Mentally Ill: Will Nursing Respond? Image 19, 3, 121–125, 1987
2. American Journal of Nursing: ICN 81. Am J Nurs 81 (September): 1664–71, 1981
3. American Nurses' Association: Code for Nurses with Interpretive Statements. Kansas City, MO, American Nurses' Association, 1976
4. American Nurses' Association: Facts About Nursing 80–81. New York, American Journal of Nursing Company, 1981
5. American Nurses' Association Commission on Nursing Practice: Nursing: A Social Policy Statement. Kansas City, MO, American Nurses' Association, 1980
6. American Nurses' Association Division of Psychiatric and Mental Health Nursing: Standards of Psychiatric and Mental Health Nursing Practice. Kansas City, MO, American Nurses' Association, 1982
7. American Nurses' Association Division of Psychiatric and Mental Health Nursing: Statement on Psychiatric and Mental Health Nursing Practice. Kansas City, MO, American Nurses' Association, 1976
8. Bloom B: Community Mental Health. Monterey, CA, Brooks/Cole Publishing, 1977
9. Borus J: Deinstitutionalization of the Chronically Mentally Ill. N Engl J Med 305, 339–342, 1981
10. Brodsky A, Hare-Mustin R: Women and Psychotherapy: An Assessment of Research and Practice. New York, Guilford Press, 1980
11. Carmen E, Russo N, Miller J: Inequity and Women's Mental Health: An Overview. Am J Psychiatry 138 (October): 1319–30, 1981
12. Clinchy B, Belenky M, Goldberger N, Tarula J: Women's Ways of Knowing. New York, Basic Books, 1986
13. Cohen G: The Older Person, The Older Patient, and the Mental Health System. Hosp Community Psychiatry 33 (February): 101–103, 1982
14. Curtin L: Privacy-Belonging to Oneself. Perspect Psychiatr Care 19 (March–April): 112–115, 1981
15. Division of National Cost Estimates, Office of the Actuary, Health Care Financing Administration: National Health Care Expenditures. Health Care Financing Review 8 (4): 1–36, 1987
16. Fagin C: Psychiatric Nursing at the Crossroads: Quo Vadis? Perspect Psychiatr Care 19 (March–April): 99–106, 1981
17. Gilligan C: In a Different Voice: Psychological Theory and Woman's Development. Cambridge, MA, Harvard University Press, 1982
18. Gillis C: The Family as a Unit of Analysis: Strategies for the Nurse Researcher. Adv Nurs Sci 5 (3): 50–59, 1983
19. Harris E: The Dexamethasone Suppression Test. Am J Nurs 82 (May): 784–785, 1982
20. Hipps O: The Integrated Curriculum: The Emperor is Naked. Am J Nurs 81 (May): 976–980, 1981
21. Kalisch P, Kalisch B: Image of Psychiatric Nurses in

Motion Pictures. Perspect Psychiatr Care 19 (March–April): 116–129, 1981

22. Lewis R: A Review and Preview of the State of the Art. Paper presented at Perspectives in Psychiatric Care '82, Washington, DC, 1982

23. Mechanic D: Mental Health and Social Policy, 2d ed. Englewood Cliffs, NJ, Prentice-Hall, 1980

24. Mental Health Reports 5: 21 (October 21): 1981

25. Peplau H: Interpersonal Relations in Nursing. New York, Putnam's, 1952

26. Redick R, Taube C: Demography and Mental Health Care of the Aged. In Birrin J, Sloan RB (eds): Handbook of Mental Health and Aging. Englewood Cliffs, Prentice-Hall, 1980

27. Robinson L: Liaison Nursing. Philadelphia, FA Davis, 1974

28. Sharfstein S: Medicaid Cutbacks and Block Grants: Crisis or Opportunity for Community Mental Health? Am J Psychiatry 139 (April): 466–470, 1982

29. Slovenko R: Law and Psychiatry. In Kaplan H, Freedman A, Sadock B (eds): Comprehensive Textbook of Psychiatry III. Baltimore, Williams & Wilkins, 1980

30. Spitzer R, Endicott J: Computer Applications in Psychiatry. In Arieti S (ed): American Handbook of Psychiatry. New York, Basic Books, 1974

48 Career Profiles in Psychiatric–Mental Health Nursing

Karen Dunne-Maxim, R.N., M.S.

Co-coordinator, Suicide Prevention
Project
University of Medicine and Dentistry
of New Jersey
Piscataway, New Jersey

In 1972, my brilliant, successful, youngest brother killed himself at age 16. We in the family failed to recognize his symptoms of depression. These symptoms were treatable, but at that time little was known about depression in childhood and adolescence and thus his death was not prevented. One year later I entered Rutgers—The Graduate School of Advanced Psychiatric Nursing—but it was not until 7 years later that I realized that the coincidence of those two events was not accidental.

Since my graduation from the Psychiatric Nursing Program, 11 years ago, I have had different responsibilities as a staff member of the UMDNJ-Community Mental Health Center. Initially I worked as an outpatient therapist, providing family, group, and individual therapy to clients from a wide variety of cultural and socioeconomic backgrounds. At the Community Mental Health Center we worked as a team, and case conferences were a multiprofessional discussion. A significant portion of my work was with inner-city multiproblem families. Several colleagues and I developed an intensive treatment model for these families titled MIFT—Multi-Impact Family Therapy.

Concerned that many of the families we were seeing were headed by mothers who had become pregnant as teenagers and were now seeing their daughters pregnant as teenagers, I became interested in adolescent pregnancy prevention.

With the support and vision of Gary Lamson, Vice President for Mental Health Services, UMDNJ-CMHC at Piscataway, I then began my career in prevention services and coordinated the Middlesex County Network on Adolescent Pregnancy.

In 1982 I became in touch with the fact that the subtle, yet clear, pressure to keep my brother's suicide death a secret was affecting my work as a therapist. With the help of Monica McGoldrick, my supervisor, I began a task force on survivors of suicide. This task force was joined by my brother, Edward Dunne, who is a psychologist. Together with other professionals who were also survivors of suicide, we began to bring the topic of survivorship "out of the closet." Our book, edited by John L. McIntosh, *Suicide and Its Aftermath,* is a direct result of our meetings with professionals and our work with families surviving suicide.

Again, it's not merely by chance that a significant portion of my current responsibilities involves youth suicide prevention. We have a suicide prevention project that provides consultation to school systems on areas of prevention and postvention. This past year I was project director for the New Jersey Central Region Youth Suicide Prevention Project.

I think the field of psychiatric nursing will continue to grow with exciting opportunities for the practitioner. So many of my former classmates are employed in interesting, challenging, and diverse positions. To a nurse entering the career I have two recommendations. First, keep involved with mental health professionals from other disciplines; the cross-fertilization is extremely nourishing. Second, find a mentor like Shirley Smoyak, Dean of the Rutgers Graduate School of Advanced Psychiatric Nursing. Her mandate to us was "Everything is possible," and it is!

Judith Ann Greene, B.S.N., M.S.N, PH.D., R.N.

Nursing Coordinator
Westcott Center for Alcohol and Drug
*   Abuse and Psychiatric Treatment*
Hamilton Medical Center
Dalton, Georgia

As a nursing coordinator, I work as a clinical specialist, including clinical, administrative, and research functions. I have the opportunity and privilege to engage in every aspect of clinical nursing—individual, group, family, and psychiatric liaison nursing. I also enjoy working with a very caring and professional team of mental health professionals who are an interestingly diverse yet like-minded group of individuals as far as clinical values and skills go. Finding them as co-workers has been a true gift. In many ways, I know that I would be here or some other similar place doing this work even if I did not have financial reasons for doing so. It is a true privilege to have the opportunity to serve the folks who come here for help. I only hope and pray every day that I will always be deserving of the trust and confidence they place in me and my co-workers.

This is hard work. Don't do it unless or until you learn to caregive rather than caretake. The difference is simple. When you caregive, you give without diminishing the person who is your client. In many ways, the client becomes more, not less, a person because of your nursing care. The opposite is true when you caretake. There are too many caretakers. If you understand the distinction I've made here, then there's probably a lot of hope for you as a psychiatric nurse provided that you are willing to submit to a rigorous academic program in psychiatric–mental health nursing. Without such preparation, you cannot function safely. Also, the lack of educational background really weakens a nurse's ability to contribute effectively as a mental health team member.

This is good work. I am thankful that I can do it and I am very, very thankful to my family and friends who are wonderful caregivers. Without the love and care they give me, the work would be unnecessarily difficult.

Nina A. Klebanoff, M.S.N., R.N., C.S.

Psychosocial Specialist
Independent, nonaffiliated private
practice
Dallas, Texas

Although I did not decide to enter nursing until I was halfway through an undergraduate degree in philosophy, there is evidence that I was interested in the field of psychology as early as age 8. As I continued to have more of an idea of my life and wanted to learn more about the interrelationships among feelings, thoughts, and actions, I followed a different path than the preconceived one. Once I entered a diploma program in nursing, after completing my undergraduate degree, it was only a matter of time before I was able to live what I had dreamed of doing. Many people advised me to work in an ICU or on a med–surg floor before seeking employment in a psychiatric hospital. That was helpful counsel, but I did not use it. I wanted to pursue a career in psych nursing and had already received good, solid experience in those other areas while in school. More education and experience were necessary to achieve my goals.

Currently, my independent practice as a psychosocial clinical nurse specialist is made of the following activities: psychosocial home health care nursing; office-based psychotherapy (individual, couple, family, and group); consultation with home health care agencies and individuals; providing in-services; report-writing; safer sex education; and professional activities in various organizations.

Working backwards, let me review my professional endeavors here. For two years prior to starting my own practice I worked for a proprietary health maintenance organization (HMO) as a nurse psychotherapist, case manager, and coordinator of a 5-week computer-facilitated, self-learning course. In addition to those functions, I also performed teaching, liaison, and consultation activities with the non–mental health group of providers within the HMO.

During my internship for psych clinical specialization while in graduate school, everyone else in my class sought hospital-based sites. It was important to me to be in a community mental health arena. I arranged to spend my time with a psych clinical specialist who was at a voluntary, non-profit home health care agency. I then worked there before and after graduation as a psych clinical nurse specialist and generalist nurse for 2 years before going on to the HMO.

My first place of employment, after finishing the diploma program while working on a B.S.N., was at a private, nonprofit psychiatric hospital and community mental health center. There I worked as a staff nurse on open and closed adult/adolescent units.

I was always curious about what happened to people when they went home after being in the hospital or what had taken place in between a series of hospitalizations. Because of that curiosity, and the desire to have a more independent nursing practice, I pursued more education and experience in psych nursing and community mental health.

But that does not let you know why I went into nursing in the first place. Working in an x-ray lab and then as a nursing assistant in a large metropolitan county hospital, I discovered that *nurses* talk and spend time with people and their families, that what nurses and nursing did had life-affirming relevance to human needs and purposes, and that as a nurse I would have a fuller appreciation and grasp of the totality of situations as well as the parts of the whole in this context and the world that we live in. Because of where I grew up (New Mexico) and other influences, I believe, as Florence Nightingale did, that healing comes from within and without (nature, the environment). Our role as nurses is to facilitate that healing, in the broadest sense of the term.

The future of psych–mental health nursing has to do, in my opinion, with healing: ourselves, our clients, the profession of nursing, and the world we dwell in. The future is now. Not only can psych–mental health nursing seek to dissolve the duality of the mind and body, it can work to eliminate the splitting of health and mental health. Nursing is a living, process world-view. Because psych nursing explores dynamics and results of ones such hope, powerlessness, rape and other forms of violence, addictions, and self-care psych–mental health nurses and nursing can facilitate a sway toward what are called feminist values—valuing and practicing life-affirming connections, esteem, interdependence, and worth in ways that are not focused on death and destruction. Toward that means and end, I suggest that a nurse interested in the field of psych–mental health nursing follow that inclination or inner voice. There is a myriad of settings and opportunities or subspecialties in which to enact and expand this role. It is essential that you work in a hospital or acute care facility at the outset to understand how systems and institutions can, and fail to, function. For example, concerns about third-party payment and the like are nonissues.

My plans include completing a Ph.D. in nursing, being more intimately involved in clinical and theoretical nursing research, and developing my nursing practice. For me this is a rewarding, fascinating, progressive, and fun profession!

Kay Peterson, M.S., R.N.

Psychiatric Clincial Nurse Specialist
Homeless Health Care Team
City of Dallas, Health and Human
*   Services*
Dallas, Texas

When I began my career in psychiatric nursing, I had no idea that I would be implementing theory into practice under bridges, in alleys, bus stations, and parks, and in the cavernous skeletons of vacant buildings. Yet the pervasive issue of homelessness for the mentally ill has created a focus for nursing, and a challenge for me, that inspires creativity in practice, adaptability in the most "grassroots" of clinical situations, and a redefining of the concept of outreach.

In reaching out to the homeless mentally ill, a level of readiness is mandated in order to adapt from moment to moment, client to client. Any moment may bring the need for tending to secondary infections caused by infestation or poorly fitted shoes, counseling a woman who has been recently assaulted, handling the crisis of the Vietnam vet who is trying to cope with the sounds of choppers over the city, or helping the hallucinating client gain control amid the relentless stimuli of the street. Reaching out may involve attempting to provide some potential for encouragement to those families searching for "lost" relatives, or perhaps redefining the perception of hope to the empty faces of those who have become economically and socially distanced from what we have come to call the mainstream.

In developing and implementing the role of the psychiatric clinical nurse specialist with the homeless mentally ill population, I have found that alliance-building is of utmost importance. There is a natural paranoia on the street that is more of a survival skill than a pathological phenomenon. Establishing rapport may take months, so patience and a nonjudgmental, unhurried approach are most helpful prerequisites; in fact, they are matters of necessity.

Other components of my role include serving as a team member on a Homeless Health Care Team, providing follow-up medication teaching after our psychiatry clinics that are set up in the shelters, and being a consultant for shelter staffs and a variety of community agencies. Managing medications on the street can be a true challenge from a nursing perspective. The side effects of many of the psychotropic medications involve the risk of dehydration with lithium therapy, of sunburn with the phenothiazines, both common problems when dealing with exposure-related situations. Social skills many times need to be relearned by clients who have been living outside of the traditional social system, perhaps as a result of their delusions. Also, teaching a client ways to promote his or her own safety can be an important part of a care plan. As public awareness grows regarding homeless issues, I have discovered a significant need, as well as a benefit, in working with advocacy groups concerned with the mentally ill. Many times the psychiatric clinical nurse specialist "on the street" may be the only link between the client and clinical services.

For me, nursing has always been a way of responding to the world, envisioning the complexity of needs, then reacting from my own expertise. The key for me is to become a participant. I believe we, as psychiatric nurses, need to utilize our knowledge base in order to envision future needs. Provision of shelters and soup kitchens, however invaluable, is politically expedient and does not address the long-term needs of housing, job training, and lifelong supportive services for the chronically mentally ill. In light of deinstitutionalization, changes in commitment laws, and the continued lack of sufficient community support, I cannot foresee any lessening in the numbers of the homeless mentally ill. This clinical area for psychiatric nurses is, unfortunately, one which is not likely to go away.

Cynthia Booth Pharis, M.S.N., R.N., C.A.D.A.C.

Co-founder & President of Pharis Institute
Dallas, Texas

As an administrator and entrepreneur, my day-to-day activities are numerous and varied. The Pharis Institute is an organization providing academic education in addictive diseases; clinical services for individuals with addictions to drugs, alcohol, sex, food, relationships and their families; and consultation with business, industry, and hospitals to design and implement educational and clinical programs. In addition, I am involved in a nursing research project with two colleagues, examining the relationship between trauma and chemical dependency in an indigent hospital population. Our goal is to increase staff awareness of their need for more education about how to help addicts and alcoholics. In order to validate this need, we are demonstrating that a large percentage of patients are admitted because behavior related to the disease of addiction caused the hospitalization (auto accident, broken bone, liver disease, and so on). Similar studies have shown that one in three of such patients is alcoholic.

Active involvement in the professional community is an important element in organizing a successful business. Being a businesswoman has also meant learning financial planning as well as marketing and community relations techniques. Developing and writing our school catalogs and bro-

chures has been accomplished with my self-taught computer and art skills.

My interest in addictive diseases originated in my own chemical dependency and subsequent recovery. After years of daily use of alcohol and other drugs, my addiction caught up with me. My nursing career almost ended when I was terminated from two jobs in two states for drug use. My recovery began at a 28-day treatment program in Minnesota and in a nationwide 12-step support group for addicts. Today, I am aware that it is my good fortune and God's grace that I am alive and sober. Most addicts die of their disease.

At the time I entered treatment, I had just completed my Master's degree and was working in labor and delivery. Early in my recovery, it became apparent to me that little or no help was available for impaired nurses and I decided that helping other impaired nurses and other addicts was going to be a part of my life and career. I started impaired nurse programs and support groups. As I began reading new literature and research, attending seminars, and working towards my certification as an alcoholism and drug abuse counselor (CADAC), my love of the whole specialty of addiction grew. With help, addicts were now able to become productive members of society.

915

The Pharis Institute started as a dream. I and my husband and co-worker, Charles, whom I met and married in sobriety, recognized the need for a multidisciplinary curriculum addressing the essentials of addictions counseling. We opened the doors to the institute in August of 1986, with fourteen students in one class. At the time of this writing (April 1988) more than 100 students enroll in several classes each quarter.

The future is bright for nurses who wish to specialize in addictive diseases. Many positions are available for interested nurses. Some programs utilize specially trained nurses as nurse counselors. The American Nurses' Association will soon be offering a certification for addictions nurses. Those who specialize in this field are on the cutting edge of new technology and knowledge that permits addicted persons to achieve optimal wellness. Incorporation of the proven principles of Alcoholics and Narcotics Anonymous into treatment programs has fostered freedom from addiction. It is my goal in writing this to spark your interest and curiosity about addictions nursing. Practicing in this challenging and rewarding specialty provides a sense of accomplishment and competency that comes from tackling a formidable but treatable disease.

Lovetta L. Smith, D.N.SC., R.N., C.S.

Assistant Professor
University of Florida College of
Nursing
Gainesville, Florida

I am a teacher of mental health nursing. I teach in the undergraduate baccalaureate nursing program at the University of Florida, Gainesville. The College of Nursing is a part of the J. Hillis Miller Health Center which encompasses six colleges of health-related professions and Shands Hospital. The College includes an upper division (junior- and senior-level studies) and graduate and doctoral programs in nursing. The mental health portion of our undergraduate curriculum is in the senior year. Every 8 weeks, I have the opportunity of introducing 30 students to the content and process of mental health nursing. It is very exciting to be a part of someone's discovery of this vibrant practice area! I team-teach the lecture portion of the course; that is, I am responsible with two other faculty members for the presentation of a total of 25 hours of material. Lecturing is interesting, but I find the greatest pleasure in clinical teaching, the supervision of experiential learning in a hands-on clinical setting. It is in this phase that the theoretical information takes on true meaning.

What prompts one to become an educator? The reasons are varied, but here are a few from my perspective: If one cares about a particular area as I do mental health nursing, there are few things more satisfying than the sense of helping, in some small measure, to continue and perhaps refine that practice area through the efforts of those you teach. It is rewarding to see individuals grow in their understanding and their appreciation of the content. Mental health is particularly fascinating because the experiences encountered in the learning process touch and transform not only the patient, but the learner as well. With "self" as the tool, the work transcends mechanical technique and at its best becomes genuine encounter. One gains a sense of unique contribution in that others may "do" the same, but others cannot "be" the same, and thus each intervention becomes one's own.

Mental health nursing is a part of a multidisciplinary world, yet even given the team approach, this is one of the most autonomous of practice areas. Each of the core mental health disciplines (psychiatric mental health nursing, psychiatry, psychology, and psychiatric social work) contributes a unique perspective and a shared repertoire of skills; thus, colleagueship is enhanced to the greater service of patients.

Although mental health nursing shares common concerns with other mental health disciplines, it is assuredly a part of nursing practice, and the future of this specialty is connected with the future of nursing in a larger sense. I predict that undergraduate curricula will have to be creative and flexible to attract applicants from heretofore untapped wells, nontraditional students who may be older or new careerists. Classes and clinical opportunities will have to occur at times and places that working students and single heads-of-households can integrate work and learning experiences. I believe that a major shift of focus will be from inpatient settings back to community-based care; learning experiences must become broader to parallel the outpatient move.

I offer the following advice to would-be educators in mental health nursing: First, have a firm foundation in the practice of mental health nursing, and continue to practice even as you teach. Such ongoing contact keeps you abreast of the issues, concerns, and questions which feed research inquiry and theory development. It augments your credibility to students and to colleagues and it grounds you in the practicalities of the "real" world of nursing practice. Second, become formally educated in the art of teaching. The "content" that comes from your practice connection must be melded with the "process" that comes from understanding "how to teach"; having only one or the other leaves one inadequately prepared for the job at hand.

Holly Skodol Wilson, R.N., PH.D., F.A.A.N.

Professor, Department of Mental Health Community and Administrative Nursing
Affiliated Professor, Aging Health Policy Institute
Affiliated Professor, Women's Health & Healing Program
School of Nursing, University of California
San Francisco, California

When I first envisioned my psychiatric nursing future in the autumn of 1960 as a beginning student at Duke University School of Nursing, I never expected that I would become a nurse scientist and writer with an academic career. Yet, as I think back over the past 28 years, I realize that I was attracted to psychiatric nursing as a speciality because of the intellectual challenges involved in the search for knowledge about the complexities of human psychology, relationships, and culture. The work I do now as a university professor-researcher in the growing field of psychogerontology and as an author of textbooks and scholarly papers sustains my interest and imagination because the intellectual challenges continue. Good ideas can open doors for solutions to important health care and social problems. Devoting my career to the sensitive generation of good ideas for nursing care and global health is worthwhile and rewarding.

An academic career offers both flexibility of schedule and contrasts in the nature of my work. While some students may view the prospect of "being in school forever" as somewhat daunting, life in my role as Professor of Psychiatric Nursing has allowed me to travel as a guest lecturer to the People's Republic of China, Japan, the Philippines, Australia, New Zealand, Hong Kong, Canada, Mexico, Argentina, England, East Africa, and Israel. It has also allowed time for contributing to professional literature in creative ways. I am the author or co-author of 11 books, including my *American Journal of Nursing* Award-winning texts *Psychiatric Nursing* (now in its third edition), *Research in Nursing,* and *Introducing Research in Nursing,* all published by Addison-Wesley Publishers and translated into many languages throughout the world. I have also written more than 50 scholarly and scientific articles for professional journals over the years. It's a great source of satisfaction to meet a young nurse at a national or international meeting who says that my work has made an important difference in his or her career or student experience.

I think of teaching and my conference presentations and keynote addresses as additional opportunities to communicate ideas—and to do so in a style that captures the intellect and imagination of the audience. It's been said of teaching that students want to be more than merely informed, they also want to be inspired and, on occasion, entertained. I keep that premise in mind every time I speak, whether it be to an international audience of hundreds or in my own psychiatric nursing and research courses in the graduate program at UCSF.

Much of the psychiatric nursing research I have accomplished since completing my master's degree at Case Western Reserve University and my Ph.D. at U.C. Berkeley is best categorized as "qualitative, theory-generating" research. My master's thesis relied on interviews with ghetto teenagers about the meaning of rock-and-roll dancing in their lives. My doctoral dissertation involved more than a year of participant observation and informal interviewing in a nontraditional, personal growth oriented, community-based healing community for young diagnosed schizophrenics that was modeled after R. D. Laing's Kingsley Hall in England. Thanks to a Kellogg National Fellowship, I did postdoctoral research on international approaches to care for the mentally disordered elderly; this has continued as my current research interest. Qualitative research emphasizes the value of grasping social and psychological processes as they are experienced in natural settings rather than relying on measurement tools to obtain quantifiable data. Qualitative, theory-generating research offers psychiatric nursing useful strategies for advancing our knowledge of human experiences associated with mental disorders and the care that's needed. Psychiatric nurses are prepared as keen observers and interviewers who can interpret what they observe and learn from clients. Qualitative research involves these very same skills, offering the clinically oriented nurse a natural approach for incorporating research into practice.

An academic career in psychiatric nursing is well suited to a person who is a self-starter and a self-pacer, a person who finds questions of "why" we do what we do as intriguing as the doing itself, a person who can take satisfaction from long-term rather than immediate fruits of efforts, a person who likes to read and is challenged to write and speak, a person who appreciates a balance of interaction and solitude in life, a person who doesn't mind living with the awareness that projects are never finished and that one's work is integral to one's life, and a person who enjoys the world of ideas—particularly when those ideas can be devoted to social good.

Recommendations for a student who feels that the preceding paragraph is an accurate self-description include the following: read widely, actively and analytically; develop a network of colleagues to provide support, direction, and critique for your work; keep in contact with the real day-to-day clinical world, either directly or indirectly through others who are collaborators; keep learning; take chances when they're for a good cause; set your own priorities and hold onto them; try to situate yourself in the center of an exciting intellectual environment; and figure out how to transcend conventional ways of doing and thinking about things, especially when your ideas and work can enlighten and improve.

Glossary

Acrophobia   fear of heights.

Acting-in   a kind of resistance that circumvents therapy through blocking, forgetting, changing the subject; trying to elicit the therapist's approval or disapproval while trying to recall or express feelings.

Acting-out   the client substitutes some kind of action for feeling or thinking; common forms of acting out include running away, use of alcohol or drugs, sexual promiscuity, and aggressive behavior.

Adolescence   the stage of development during which the physiological changes of puberty, the emergence of the self-concept, and the integration of the biopsychosocial aspects of the individual occur.

Affect   mood or feeling tone.

Aggression   any behavior that expresses anger or its related emotions.

Agoraphobia   a marked fear of being alone or in a public place from which escape would be difficult and/or in which help would be unavailable in the event of suddenly becoming disabled.

Akathisia   a syndrome characterized by motor restlessness.

Anal period   late infancy or toddlerhood, the period from ages 2 to 3 or 4 years, during which the child is involved in the development of social, emotional, and physiological control.

Anger   a physical and emotional state in which a person experiences a sense of power to compensate for an underlying feeling of anxiety.

Anorexia nervosa   self-imposed starvation, a psychiatric disorder characterized by a voluntary refusal to eat.

Antianxiety agents   psychotropic drugs used in the treatment of overt anxiety.

Anticipatory grief   the experience of intense feelings of loss that occur when the family and friends know for certain that their loved one will die.

Antidepressant agents   psychotropic drugs used in the treatment of depression.

Antipsychotic (or neuroleptic) agents   psychotropic medication used primarily to treat psychoses, that is, severe emotional disorders.

Anxiety   the initial response to psychic threat, evidenced as feelings of discomfort, uncertainty, apprehension, dread, restlessness, and uncertainty.

Anxiety disorder   a psychiatric condition characterized by the emotion of intense terror.

Assertiveness   the employment of expressive, goal-directed, spontaneous, and self-enhancing behavior.

Assessment   the gathering, classifying, and categorizing of client information that forms the basis of nursing planning.

Autocratic leadership   the exercise of significant authority and control over group members, including the lack or rare use of input from the group and minimal group interaction and participation.

Avoidance   the management of anxiety-laden experiences through evasive behaviors.

Battery   the unpermitted touching of another.

Behavior   a wide range of overt and covert responses that include emotions and verbalizations.

Behavioral contract   an agreement between client and psychiatric–mental health caregiver for a specific behavior.

Behavioral rehearsal   role-playing, that is, the client rehearses new responses to problem situations after learning new adaptive responses portrayed through modeling.

Behavioral therapy   a form of treatment that deals with changing the individual's maladaptive behavior by a planned, objective approach, such as respondent conditioning.

Bisexuality   equal, or almost equal, preference for either sex as a sexual partner.

Blocking   the client suddenly "blanks out" and is unable to finish a thought or idea, that is, he represses painful knowledge and feelings.

Body image   a mental picture of one's body.

Bulimia   episodic, uncontrolled, rapid ingestion of large quantities of food over a short period of time, or binge eating, often accompanied by self-induced vomiting, obsessive exercise, and/or use of laxatives and diuretics.

Catharsis   the emotional re-experiencing of painful, frightening, or angry feelings that are associated with the client's symptom or behavior.

Claustrophobia   fear of closed spaces.

Coitus   sexual intercourse, or penetration of the vagina by the penis.

Collaboration   working with others, as an equal, toward a common goal.

Communication   a personal, interactive system, a series of ever-changing, ongoing transactions in the environment.

Community support system   a systems model for the delivery of community-based mental health care, which includes rehabilitation, housing, physical and mental health services, educational and employment opportunities, and social networks.

Compliance   adherence to prescribed treatment regimes.

Compulsions   ritualistic behaviors that the individual feels compelled to perform either in accord with a specific set of rules or in a routinized manner and which are designed to prevent or reduce anxiety.

Consciousness   the perceptions, thoughts, and feelings existing in a person's immediate awareness.

Coping mechanisms (also called ego defense mechanisms, mental mechanisms, and defense mechanisms) mechanisms that function to protect the ego from overwhelming anxiety and that usually operate on an unconscious level.

Countertransference   an experience in which the therapist transfers his feelings for significant others onto the client.

Crisis   a turning point, a state of disequilibrium usually lasting 4 to 6 weeks.

Crisis intervention   a thinking, direct, problem-solving form of therapy that focuses only on the client's immediate problems.

Cryptic language   abbreviated language, such as speaking aloud only every fifth or tenth word of one's thoughts.

Cunnilingus   oral-genital stimulation performed on a woman.

Deinstitutionalization   the discharge of large numbers of psychiatric clients from inpatient treatment centers to the community.

Delusion   a fixed, false belief that cannot be corrected by reasoning.

Dementia   clinical behavior manifested in the insidious development of memory and intellectual deficits, disorientation, and decreased cognitive functioning.

Democratic leadership   the encouragement of group interaction and participation in group problem-solving and decision-making; the group is marked by common goals, solicitation of opinions, ideas, and input and provision of feedback.

Denial   an unconscious coping mechanism wherein a person denies the existence of some external reality.

Depression   pathologically intense unhappiness.

Development   the orderly evolution of events moving from simple to more complex.

Differentiation   a tendency of living, open systems to increase in complexity over time.

Discrimination   a specific response occurring in a given situation.

Disengagement   a theory that proposes that the elderly or dying person acts voluntarily in giving up his roles in life, slowly loses interest in the active world, and withdraws from significant others.

Displacement   an unconscious coping mechanism through which a person transfers an emotion from its original object to a substitute object.

Disqualifying   an individual fails to attend to another's message by silence, ignoring it, or changing the subject.

Distress   damaging or unpleasant stress.

Double-bind communication   the sending of an incongruent message that includes a directive to do something and a nonverbal message to do the opposite, while the receiver of the message is not permitted to comment on it.

DSM-III-R   the American Psychiatric Association's *Diagnostic and Statistical Manual, Third Edition, Revised.*

Dyspareunia   pain with sexual intercourse.

Dystonia   involuntary, jerking, uncoordinated body movements.

Early latency   the ages from 6 to 9 years, or early school-age years, during which the child focuses on learning, the acquisition of knowledge, the development of the social role outside the protection of home and family.

ECT electroconvulsive therapy, a form of treatment for depression.

Ego the structure of the human personality that has the greatest contact with reality.

Ego-dystonic that which is unacceptable to the self.

Ego-syntonic that which is acceptable to the self.

Enculturation the process by which an individual learns the expected behavior of the culture.

Enmeshment lack of clear boundaries between the parent and child subsystems and between individual family members.

Entropy the tendency of a system to be closed to the environment.

Erectile dysfunction (also called impotence) the inability to achieve or maintain erection sufficiently to perform coitus.

Erogenous zones the areas of the body that are particularly sensitive to erotic stimulation, such as the neck, breasts, inner thighs, and genital areas.

Ethnic groups a group of people with a common origin and holding basically similar values, beliefs, and means of communication.

Evaluation the process of determining the value of something in the attainment of preset goals.

Exhibitionism an erotic desire to expose one's genital or erogenous areas to others.

Existential crisis a crisis in which the individual is faced with life, in the form of aloneness, the absurdity of existence, and the responsibilities inherent in his attained freedom, and is confronted with a reorganization of the meaning of life.

Extinction the withholding of reinforcers, thus reducing the probability of the occurrence of the response.

Fading gradual reduction of the process of facilitating or accentuating the reinforcer.

Family a primary group whose members are related by blood, marriage, adoption, or mutual consent, who interact through certain familial roles, and create and maintain a common subculture.

Family structure the organization of the family.

Family therapy a form of treatment based on the premise that the member of the family with the presenting symptoms signals the presence of pain in the whole family.

Fantasy a coping mechanism through which a person engages in nonrational mental activity and thus escapes daily pressures and responsibilities.

Fellatio oral-genital stimulation performed on a man.

Female orgasmic dysfunction an inability to achieve or difficulty achieving orgasm.

Fetishism a condition of recurrent sexual urges and sexually arousing fantasies by means of the use of nonliving objects by themselves or with a sexual partner.

Flight of ideas a stream of thought characterized by a rapid association of ideas and play upon words.

Folie à deux a delusional system shared by two persons, most commonly sisters.

Foreplay the petting and fondling activities engaged in during the excitement phase of the sexual response cycle.

Formal group a group with structure, authority, and limited interaction, such as a business meeting.

Free association a primary method of treatment in psychoanalysis, the free expression of thoughts and feelings as they come to mind.

Frotteurism a disorder of recurrent, intense sexual urges and sexually arousing fantasies regarding rubbing against or touching a nonconsenting person; the touch, not the coercion, is the sexually exciting focus.

Generalized anxiety disorder a disorder characterized by chronic anxiety that is uncomfortable to the point that it interferes with the individual's daily living.

Gender identity how one chooses to view oneself as a male or female in interaction with others.

Gender role how a person's gender identity is expressed socially, in behavior with others of the same and opposite sex.

General Adaptation Syndrome (GAS) the body's manifestations of stress that evolve in three stages: alarm reaction, stage of resistance, and stage of exhaustion.

Generalization the phenomenon by which adaptive behavior specific to one situation may occur in similar situations.

Geropsychiatry the care of the aging psychiatric client.

Group three or more persons with related goals.

Group norm the development, over time, of a pattern of interaction within a group to which certain behavioral expectations are attached.

Group therapy a form of treatment in which individuals explore their problems and styles of communication in a safe, confidential atmosphere where they can receive feedback from other group members and undergo change.

Hallucination a false sensory perception, that is, without external stimuli, or a sensory perception that does not exist in reality, such as seeing "visions" or hearing "voices."

Homosexuality a male's preference of a male as a sexual partner.

Hostility a feeling of antagonism accompanied by a wish to hurt or humiliate others.

Id   the most primitive structure of the human personality; the site of the instincts.

Identification   a coping mechanism through which a person unconsciously adopts the personality characteristics, attitudes, values, and behavior of another person.

Illusion   a misinterpretation of a real sensory experience.

Imagery   a therapeutic approach in which the client pictures significant memories and present events that, combined with relaxation and role playing, increase awareness of events and behavior.

Imitation   the conscious process of identifying with another person.

Informal group   a group of members who are not dependent on each other, such as a hobby group.

Informed consent   the knowing consent given in a interaction or series of interactions between the treating physician and the client that allows the client to consider fully information about the treatment that is being proposed.

Insight   conscious awareness of the painful, angry, or socially unacceptable thoughts or feelings that the client repressed.

Intellectualization   an unconscious coping mechanism through which a person uses his intellectual abilities such as thinking, reasoning, and analyzing to blunt or avoid emotional issues.

Interpretation   a person's insight or understanding of his feelings and behavior.

Interview   a purposeful, goal-directed interaction between two people.

Laissez-faire leadership   a style of leadership in which group members are free to operate as they choose.

Latency   the ages from 9 to 12 years, or late school-age years, during which occur the harmonization of various aspects of the self-concept, especially through clubs, sports teams, and scouts.

Latent content   that content which is not discussed, which occurs on a feeling level, and which is seldom verbalized.

Lesbianism   a female's preference of a female as a sexual partner.

Libido   an energy source associated with the physiological or instinctual drives such as hunger, thirst, and sex.

Listening   focusing on all of the behaviors expressed by a client.

Lithium carbonate   a psychotropic drug used in the treatment of bipolar disorder (formerly termed manic–depressive illness).

Malpractice   a tort action brought by a consumer plaintiff against a defendant professional from whom the consumer plaintiff feels that he has received injury during the course of the professional–consumer relationship.

Mania   a mood disturbance characterized by elation, hyperactivity, agitation, and accelerated thinking and speaking.

Manifest content   the spoken words during an interaction.

Masochism   a paraphilia in which the person's preferred sexual object is the experience of pain.

Masturbation   self-stimulation of erogenous areas to the point of orgasm.

Maturational (or developmental) crisis   a crisis precipitated by the normal stress of development, such as pregnancy, birth, or adolescence.

Melancholia   depression, at one time thought to result from an excess of "black bile" in the body.

Mental health   a state of emotional well-being in which a person functions adaptively and comfortably within his society and is satisfied with himself and his achievements.

Mental health team   the groups of mental health caregivers, including nurses, occupational and recreational therapists, social workers, psychiatric nurse clinical specialists, dance and art therapists, psychologists, psychiatrists, pastoral counselors, and paraprofessionals, who work together to design and implement a therapeutic milieu for clients.

Mental retardation   a significantly subaverage general intellectual functioning existing concurrently with deficits in adaptive behavior and manifesting itself during the developmental period.

Milieu   environment or setting; in psychiatric–mental health nursing, the therapeutic milieu is the people and all other social and physical factors in the 24-hour environment with which the client interacts.

Milieu therapy   a group therapy approach that uses the total living experience of a client to accomplish therapeutic objectives.

Modeling   imitation as a method of behavior change.

Negative reinforcer   a harmful reinforcer that the client evades or avoids, thus strengthening or facilitating adaptive behavior.

Negentropy   a tendency toward openness to the environment, both inside and outside the family.

Neologism   a new, private word with idiosyncratic meaning.

Noncompliance   the failure of the client and his family to adhere to prescribed treatment regimes, such as the failure to take prescribed psychotropic medication after discharge from the treatment facility.

Nursing diagnosis   a statement of a client's response pattern to a health disruption.

Obsessions   recurrent, persistent thoughts, ideas, images, or impulses.

Obsessive-compulsive disorder   a psychiatric condition in which the individual experiences recurrent obsessions and/or compulsions.

Objective data data or information that can be measured, observed, or validated.

Oedipal period the preschool years, from age 3 or 4 to 6 years, during which stage the child's developmental needs include dealing with sexual and aggressive impulses and coming to terms with parental and societal demands.

Oral period the first 2 years of life, or infancy, during which the personality structure of the individual is centered around the issue of impulsivity.

Panic disorder an anxiety disorder characterized by recurrent, unpredictable anxiety attacks of panic proportions.

Paraphilia the investment of an adult's sexual interest in objects, events, or particular types of people.

Pedophilia recurrent and intense sexual urges and fantasies of sexual activity with prepubescent children.

Perinatal loss the loss of a baby by miscarriage or stillbirth, or in the neonatal period.

Personality an individual's consistent and stable pattern of behavior.

Personality disorder a maladaptive personality style.

Phobia a persistent, irrational fear attached to an object or situation that objectively does not pose a significant danger.

Physical dependence (addiction) a state manifested by withdrawal symptoms when the drug is removed.

Planning the structuring of needs and problems in an orderly manner to achieve an end or a goal.

Pleasure principle the employment of pleasure-seeking behaviors that reduce tension when the physiological or instinctual drives are released.

Positive reinforcer a reward, that which strengthens a behavior.

Post-traumatic stress disorder the development of characteristic symptoms after exposure to a traumatic life experience capable of psychologically harming most people.

Preconscious that material which is not immediately accessible to a person's awareness.

Primary gain an individual's symptom or behavior is defense against and/or reduction of the emotioanl pain associated with anxiety.

Primary group a group of members with face-to-face contact and boundaries, norms, and explicit and implicit interdependent roles, such as a family.

Primary prevention therapeutic approaches such as infant stimulation and parenting education programs that aim to prevent mental illness or disorder before it occurs.

Primary process thought processes deriving from the id and characterized by an illogical, confused form and preverbal, or preoperational, content.

Problem-solving using anxiety in the service of learning adaptive behavior.

Projection an unconscious coping mechanism through which a person displaces his feelings, usually feelings perceived as negative, onto another person.

Prompting the creation of a condition that facilitates or accentuates the reinforcer.

Psychoanalysis a form of long-term therapy that uses strategies such as dream interpretation, hypnosis, and free association.

Psychodrama a form of group therapy in which clients explore problems through dramatic methods.

Psychoeducation a form of intervention aimed at the family members of individuals with psychiatric disorders that explores the families' reactions to mental illness of a member and provides families with information about, and ways to help the member with, an emotional disorder.

Psychogeriatrics the special psychiatric care for clients in the over-65 age group.

Psychological dependence (habituation) the expression of a severe craving or compulsion to take a drug in order to "feel good."

Psychopathology the difference or gap between the existing emotional developmental level of an individual and the expected emotional development level that corresponds to his chronological age.

Psychopharmacology the use of psychotropic, or psychoactive, drugs to treat various emotional disorders.

Psychosis an extreme response to stress that may be characterized by impaired reality-testing, delusions, hallucinations, and affective, psychomotor, and physical disturbances.

Psychosomatization the visceral or physiological expression of anxiety.

Psychotherapy the use of a group of techniques to modify feelings, attitudes, and behavior in people by means of understanding self and being understood by another, to achieve relatedness, and to relieve emotional pain.

Punishment that which suppresses the maladaptive pattern of behavior.

Rape a crime in which forcible penile–vaginal penetration of a female occurs without her consent and against her will.

Rape trauma syndrome the process of adaptation in which the rape victim frees herself of overwhelming fear, redefines her feelings of vulnerability and helplessness, and regains control and equilibrium.

Rationalization an unconscious coping mechanism through which a person substitutes socially acceptable reasons for the real or actual reasons motivating his behavior.

Reaction formation an unconscious coping mechanism through which a person acts in a way opposite of how he feels.

Reality principle the ability to delay pleasure in favor of more socially acceptable behavior.

Reality-testing the ability to perceive reality accurately.

Reconstructive therapy deep psychotherapy or psychoanalysis that delves into all aspects of the client's life and may take 2 to 5 years or longer.

Re-educative therapy psychotherapy that involves new ways of perceiving and behaving and exploring alternatives in a planned, systematic way, often requiring more than short-term therapy.

Regression an unconscious coping mechanism through which a person avoids anxiety by returning to an earlier, and more satisfying or comfortable time in his life.

Reinforcer anything that increases the probability of a response.

Relationship a state of being related or affinity between two individuals.

Repression a coping mechanism through which a person forces certain feelings or thoughts into his unconscious.

Resistance the client resists recalling information or recalling feelings.

Sadism a paraphilia in which the person's preferred sexual object is the act of inflicting pain on someone else.

Safe sex limiting numbers of sexual partners, the use of condoms, avoidance of oral sex or "french kissing" with an unscreened partner, and the use of a glove or finger cot when exploring anal or vaginal areas and touching the penis; the general rule is to avoid contact with blood, feces, vaginal secretions, or semen.

Scapegoating the process in which a family tends to view one of its members as "different" and the cause of its trouble.

Schizophrenia a severe disturbance of thought or association, characterized by impaired reality-testing, hallucinations, delusions, and limited socialization.

Secondary gain an individual's behavior or symptom relieves him of responsibility and provides extra attention or monetary rewards.

Secondary group a group of members who do not have relationship bonds or emotional ties, an impersonal group such as a political party.

Secondary prevention therapeutic approaches such as crisis intervention, counseling, and inpatient hospitalization that reduce prevalence of emotional disorders through early case-finding and prompt intervention.

Self-concept a composite of a person's beliefs and feelings about himself at a given time.

Sex roles culturally determined patterns associated with male and female social behavior.

Sexual identity the basic recognition of one's sex.

Sexuality the expression and experience of the self as a sexual being.

Shaping a behavioral reinforcement technique used to condition close approximations of some desired adaptive behavior.

Simple phobia a persistent, irrational fear of, and compelling desire to avoid, exposure to a circumstance or class of thing other than those specific to agoraphobia or social phobia; common examples of simple phobias include claustrophobia and acrophobia.

Situational crisis a crisis precipitated by a sudden traumatic event, such as divorce, job loss, or birth of a child with a congenital defect.

Social phobia a persistent, irrational fear of, and compelling desire to avoid, situations in which exposure to the scrutiny of others may occur.

Stress the nonspecific response of the body to any demand made upon it, according to Hans Selye.

Stressors stress-producing factors, including physical stressors such as heat, cold, and illness and psychological stressors such as failure, success, and loss.

Subculture a group of people who may be distinguishable by ethnic background, religion, social status, or other similar characteristics, and simultaneously share certain features with larger segments of society.

Subjective data data that reflect the client's feelings, perceptions, and "self talk" about his problems.

Superego the structure of the human personality that contains the values, legal and moral regulations, and social expectations that thwart the free expression of pleasure-seeking behaviors.

Supportive therapy psychotherapy that allows the client to express feelings, explore alternatives, and make decisions in a safe, caring relationship.

Suppression a coping mechanism through which a person consciously excludes certain thoughts or feelings from his mind.

Suspiciousness hypersensitivity, alertness, and hypervigilance.

Tardive dyskinesia a late symptom associated with the long-term use of high-dose phenothiazine drugs; symptoms include buccolingual movements such as "fly catcher" movements, pursing of lips, jaw movements, and involvement of limbs and trunk.

Termination the dissolution of a relationship.

Tertiary prevention therapeutic approaches such as halfway houses and residential placements that aim to reduce long-term disability from emotional disorder through a program of rehabilitation, aftercare, and resocialization.

Theory   a conceptual system consisting of interrelated propositions that describe, explain, and predict selected phenomena.

Therapeutic relationship   a relationship in which the nurse and client participate with the goal of assisting the client to meet his needs and facilitate his growth.

Time-out   a period of time during which the client is removed from any form of reinforcement.

Token reinforcement   a therapeutic approach that delays the use of direct reinforcers through the administration of tokens, which can then be redeemed for actual reinforcers.

Tolerance   a state wherein an increased amount of a drug is necessary to obtain the desired effect or there is a decrease in the desired effect with regular use of the same amount of a drug.

Transcendental self   a self that exists beyond one's individual self-image, or a self in relation to the larger universe.

Transference   a tool or technique of psychotherapy whereby the client transfers feelings and attitudes held toward significant others onto the therapist.

Transsexuality   the belief that one is psychologically of the sex opposite his or her anatomical gender.

Transvestitism   a sexual desire to dress in the clothing, or adopt the mannerisms, of the opposite sex.

Treatment alliance   the ability to work together and to be invested emotionally in the task of therapy.

Triangle   a form of cross-generational clinging, such as a coalition formed by a mother and son against the father.

Unconditioned response   the response elicited by an unconditioned stimulus, for example, salivation is an unconditioned response in a hungry dog elicited by an unconditioned stimulus, food.

Unconditioned stimulus   that which elicits an unconditioned response, for example, food is an unconditioned stimulus that elicits an unconditioned response, salivation, in a hungry dog.

Unconscious   that material which is inaccessible to a person's awareness.

Unresolved sexual trauma   a state in which a person experiencing a sexual assault does not deal with the feelings or reactions to the experience.

Vaginismus   a spastic contraction or tightening of the vagina before or during penetration for coitus.

Voyeurism   a desire to watch others in sexually vulnerable or erotic positions.

Withdrawal   the behavioral or psychological retreat from anxiety-provoking experiences.

Working through   a part of the final phase of therapy in which the client's insights are discussed and reworked over time.

DSM-III-R
Classification

Mental Retardation
317.00	Mild mental retardation
318.00	Moderate mental retardation
318.10	Severe mental retardation
318.20	Profound mental retardation
319.00	Unspecified mental retardation

Pervasive Developmental Disorders
299.00	Autistic disorder
299.80	Pervasive developmental disorder NOS

Specific Developmental Disorders
Academic skills disorders
315.10	Developmental arithmetic disorder
315.80	Developmental expressive writing disorder
315.00	Developmental reading disorder

Language and speech disorders
315.39	Developmental articulation disorder
315.31	Developmental expressive language disorder
315.31	Developmental receptive language disorder

Motor skills disorder
315.40	Developmental coordination disorder
315.90	Specific developmental disorder NOS

Other Developmental Disorders
315.90	Developmental disorder NOS

Disruptive Behavior Disorders
314.01   Attention-deficit hyperactivity disorder
Conduct disorders
312.20   Group type
312.00   Solitary aggressive type
312.90   Undifferentiated type
313.81   Oppositional defiant disorder

Anxiety Disorders of Childhood or Adolescence
309.21   Separation anxiety disorder
313.21   Avoidant disorder of childhood or adolescence
313.00   Overanxious disorder

Eating Disorders
307.10   Anorexia nervosa
307.51   Bulimia nervosa
307.52   Pica
307.53   Rumination disorder of infancy
307.50   Eating Disorder NOS

Gender Identity Disorders
302.60   Gender identity disorder of childhood
302.50   Transsexualism
302.85   Gender identity disorder of adolescence or adulthood,
                     nontranssexual type
302.85   Gender identity disorder NOS

Tic Disorders
307.23   Tourette's disorder
307.22   Chronic motor or vocal tic disorder
307.21   Transient tic disorder
307.20   Tic disorder NOS

Elimination Disorders
307.70   Functional encopresis
307.60   Functional enuresis

Speech Disorders Not Elsewhere Classified
307.00   Cluttering
307.00   Stuttering

Other Disorders of Infancy, Childhood, or Adolescence
313.23   Elective mutism
313.82   Identity disorder
313.89   Reactive attachment disorder of infancy or early childhood
307.30   Stereotypy/habit disorder
314.00   Undifferentiated attention deficit disorder

Organic Mental Disorders

Dementias arising in the senium and presenium
Primary degenerative dementia of the Alzheimer type, senile onset,

290.30	With delirium
290.20	With delusions
290.21	With depression
290.00	Uncomplicated
290.1x	Primary degenerative dementia of the Alzheimer type, presenile onset
290.4x	Multi-infarct dementia
290.00	Senile dementia NOS
290.10	Presenile dementia NOS

Psychoactive Substance-induced Organic Mental Disorders

Alcohol

303.00	Intoxication
291.40	Idiosyncratic intoxication
291.80	Uncomplicated alcohol withdrawal
291.00	Withdrawal delirium
291.30	Hallucinosis
291.10	Amnestic disorder
291.20	Dementia associated with alcoholism

Amphetamine or similarly acting sympathomimetic

302.70	Intoxication
292.00	Withdrawal
292.81	Delirium
292.11	Delusional disorder

Caffeine

305.90	Intoxication

Cannabis

305.20	Intoxication
292.11	Delusional disorder

Cocaine

305.60	Intoxication
292.00	Withdrawal
292.81	Delirium
292.11	Delusional disorder

Hallucinogen

305.30	Hallucinosis
292.11	Delusional disorder
292.84	Mood disorder
292.89	Posthallucinogen perception disorder

Inhalant

305.90	Intoxication

Nicotine

292.00	Withdrawal

Opioid

305.50	Intoxication
292.00	Withdrawal

Phencyclidine (PCP) or similarly acting arylcyclohexylamine

305.90	Intoxication
292.81	Delirium
292.11	Delusional disorder

292.84	Mood disorder
292.90	Organic mental disorder NOS
	Sedative, hypnotic, or anxiolytic
305.40	Intoxication
292.00	Uncomplicated sedative, hypnotic, or anxiolytic withdrawal
292.00	Withdrawal delirium
292.83	Amnestic disorder
	Other or unspecified psychoactive substance
305.90	Intoxication
292.00	Withdrawal
292.81	Delirium
292.82	Dementia
292.83	Amnestic disorder
292.11	Delusional disorder
292.12	Hallucinosis
292.84	Mood disorder
292.89	Anxiety disorder
292.89	Personality disorder
292.90	Organic mental disorder NOS

Organic Mental Disorders associated with Axis III physical disorders or conditions, or whose etiology is unknown.

293.00	Delirium
294.10	Dementia
294.00	Amnestic disorder
293.81	Organic delusional disorder
293.82	Organic hallucinosis
293.83	Organic mood disorder
294.80	Organic anxiety disorder
313.10	Organic personality disorder
294.80	Organic mental disorder NOS

Psychoactive Substance Use Disorders

	Alcohol
303.90	Dependence
305.00	Abuse
	Amphetamine or similarly acting sympathomimetic
304.40	Dependence
305.70	Abuse
	Cannabis
304.30	Dependence
305.20	Abuse
	Cocaine
304.20	Dependence
305.60	Abuse
	Hallucinogen
304.50	Dependence
305.30	Abuse
	Inhalant
304.60	Dependence
305.90	Abuse
	Nicotine
305.10	Dependence
	Opioid
304.00	Dependence

305.50	Abuse
	Phencyclidine (PCP) or similarly acting arylcyclohexylamine
304.50	Dependence
305.90	Abuse
	Sedative, hypnotic, or anxiolytic
304.10	Dependence
305.40	Abuse
304.90	Polysubstance dependence
304.90	Psychoactive substance dependence NOS
305.90	Psychoactive substance abuse NOS

Schizophrenia

295.2x	Catatonic
295.1x	Disorganized
295.3x	Paranoid
295.9x	Undifferentiated
295.6x	Residual

Delusional (Paranoid) Disorder

297.10	Delusional (Paranoid) disorder

Psychotic Disorders Not Elsewhere Classified

298.80	Brief reactive psychosis
295.40	Schizophreniform disorder
295.70	Schizoaffective disorder
297.30	Induced psychotic disorder
298.90	Psychotic disorder NOS

Mood Disorders

Bipolar Disorders

	Bipolar disorder
296.6x	Mixed
296.4x	Manic
296.5x	Depressed
301.13	Cyclothymia
296.70	Bipolar disorder

Depressive Disorders

	Major depression
296.2x	Single episode
296.3x	Recurrent
300.40	Dysthymia (or Depressive neurosis)
311.00	Depressive disorder NOS

Anxiety Disorders (or Anxiety and Phobic Neuroses)

	Panic disorder
300.21	With agoraphobia
300.01	Without agoraphobia
300.22	Agoraphobia without history of panic disorder
300.23	Social phobia
300.29	Simple phobia

300.30	Obsessive compulsive disorder (or Obsessive compulsive neurosis)
309.89	Post-traumatic stress disorder
300.02	Generalized anxiety disorder
300.00	Anxiety disorder NOS

Somatoform Disorders

300.70	Body dysmorphic disorder
300.11	Conversion disorder (or Hysterical neurosis, conversion type)
300.70	Hypochondriasis (or Hypochondriacal neurosis)
300.81	Somatization disorder
307.80	Somatoform pain disorder
300.70	Undifferentiated somatoform disorder
300.70	Somatoform disorder NOS

Dissociative Disorders (or Hysterical Neuroses, Dissociative Type)

300.14	Multiple personality disorder
300.13	Psychogenic fugue
300.12	Psychogenic amnesia
300.60	Depersonalization disorder (or Depersonalization neurosis)
300.15	Dissociative disorder NOS

Sexual Disorders

Paraphilias

302.40	Exhibitionism
302.81	Fetishism
302.89	Frotteurism
302.20	Pedophilia
302.83	Sexual masochism
302.84	Sexual sadism
302.30	Transvestic fetishism
302.82	Voyeurism
302.90	Paraphilia

Sexual Dysfunctions

Sexual desire disorder

| 302.71 | Hypoactive sexual desire disorder |
| 302.79 | Sexual aversion disorder |

Sexual arousal disorder

| 302.72 | Female sexual arousal disorder |
| 302.72 | Male erectile disorder |

Orgasm disorders

302.73	Inhibited female orgasm
302.74	Inhibited male orgasm
302.75	Premature ejaculation

Sexual pain disorders

302.76	Dyspareunia
306.51	Vaginismus
302.70	Sexual dysfunction

Other Sexual Disorders

| 302.90 | Sexual disorder NOS |

Sleep Disorders
Dyssomnias

Insomnia disorder

307.42	Related to another mental disorder (nonorganic)
780.50	Related to known organic factor
307.42	Primary Insomnia

Hypersomnia disorder

307.44	Related to another mental disorder (nonorganic)
780.50	Related to a known organic factor
780.54	Primary hypersomnia
307.45	Sleep–wake schedule disorder
307.40	Dyssomnia NOS

Parasomnias

307.47	Dream anxiety disorder (nightmare disorder)
307.46	Sleep terror disorder
307.46	Sleepwalking disorder
307.40	Parasomnia NOS

Factitious Disorders

Factitious disorder

301.51	With physical symptoms
300.16	With psychological symptoms
300.19	Factitious disorder NOS

Impulse Control Disorders Not Elsewhere Classified

312.34	Intermittent explosive disorder
312.32	Kleptomania
312.31	Pathological gambling
312.33	Pyromania
312.39	Trichotillomania
312.39	Impulse control disorder NOS

Adjustment Disorder

Adjustment disorder

309.24	With anxious mood
309.00	With depressed mood
309.30	With disturbance of conduct
309.40	With mixed disturbance of emotions and conduct
309.28	With mixed emotional features
309.82	With physical complaints
309.83	With withdrawal
309.23	With work (or academic) inhibition
309.90	Adjustment disorder NOS

Psychological Factors Affecting Physical Condition

316.00	Psychological factors affecting physical condition

Personality Disorders

Cluster A

301.00	Paranoid
301.20	Schizoid
301.22	Schizotypal

Cluster B

301.70	Antisocial
301.83	Borderline
301.50	Histrionic
301.81	Narcissistic

Cluster C

301.82	Avoidant
301.60	Dependent
301.40	Obsessive compulsive
301.84	Passive aggressive
301.90	Personality disorder NOS

(From *Diagnostic and Statistical Manual of Mental Disorders* 3d ed, rev. Washington, DC, American Psychiatric Association, 1987)

Index